Success in the Classroom, in Clinicals, and on the NCLEX-RN®

Classroom

- Detailed lecture notes organized by learning outcome
- Suggestions for classroom activities
- Guide to relevant additional resources
- Comprehensive PowerPoint™ presentations integrating lecture, images, animations, and videos
- Classroom Response questions
- Image Gallery
- Video and Animation Gallery
- Online course management systems complete with instructor tools and student activities available in a variety of formats

Clinical

- Suggestions for Clinical Activities and other clinical resources organized by learning outcome

Real Nursing Simulations Facilitator's Guide: Institutional Edition

- 25 simulation scenarios that span the nursing curriculum
- Consistent format includes learning objectives, case flow, instructions for set up, student debriefing questions and more
- Companion online course cartridge with student exercises, activities, videos, skill checklists, and reflective questions also available for adoption

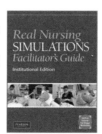

NCLEX-RN®

- Test Item Files with NCLEX®-style questions and complete rationales for correct and incorrect answers mapped to learning outcomes– *available in TestGen, Par Test, and MS Word*

D0431716

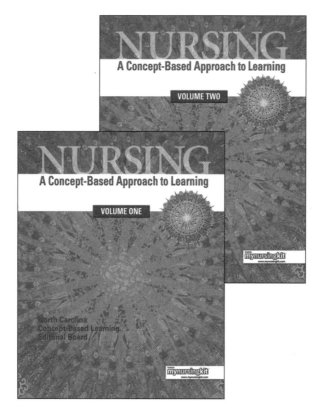

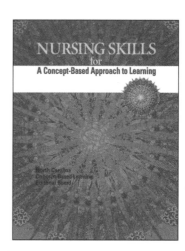

Instructor Resources

More information and instructor resources
visit www.mynursingkit.com

BRIEF CONTENTS OF VOLUME 2

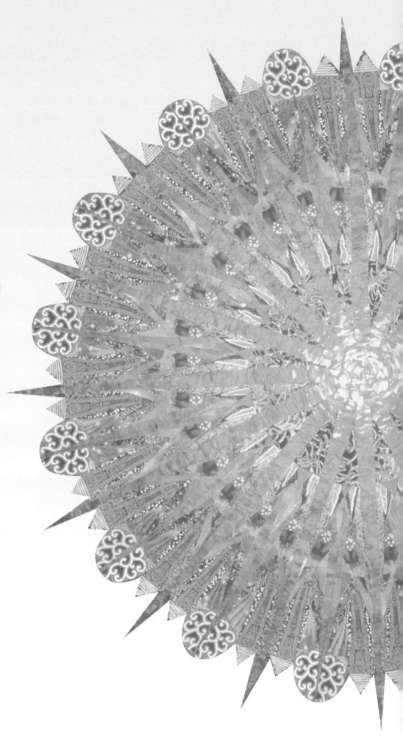

Part II: The Nursing Domain

Concept 32: Assessment
Concept 33: Caring Interventions
Concept 34: Clinical Decision Making
Concept 35: Collaboration
Concept 36: Communication
Concept 37: Managing Care
Concept 38: Professional Behaviors
Concept 39: Teaching and Learning

Part III: The Health Care Domain

Concept 40: Accountability
Concept 41: Advocacy
Concept 42: Ethics
Concept 43: Evidence-Based Practice
Concept 44: Health Care Systems
Concept 45: Health Policy
Concept 46: Informatics
Concept 47: Legal Issues
Concept 48: Quality Improvement
Concept 49: Safety
Appendix A: NANDA-Approved Nursing Diagnoses
Appendix B: Diagnostic Studies
Combined Glossary of Parts I, II, and III
Combined Index of Parts I, II, and III

Nursing
A Concept-Based
Approach to Learning

VOLUME 2

**North Carolina Concept-Based
Learning Editorial Board**

Pearson
Boston Columbus Indianapolis New York San Francisco Upper Saddle River
Amsterdam Cape Town Dubai London Madrid Milan Munich Paris Montreal Toronto
Delhi Mexico City Sao Paulo Sydney Hong Kong Seoul Singapore Taipei Tokyo

Library of Congress Cataloging-in-Publication Data

Nursing : A Concept-Based Approach to Learning / North Carolina Concept-Based Learning Editorial Board.
   p. ; cm.
Includes bibliographical references and index.
ISBN-13: 978-0-13-507806-8 (v.1)
ISBN-10: 0-13-507806-7 (v.1)
ISBN-13: 978-0-13-510351-7 (v. 2)
ISBN-10: 0-13-510351-7 (v.2)
1.   Nursing—Textbooks. I. North Carolina Concept-Based Learning Editorial Board.
[DNLM: 1. Nursing. 2. Nursing Care. WY 100 N9726 2011]
RT40.N87 2011
610.73—dc22

2009047837

Publisher: Julie Levin Alexander
Assistant to Publisher: Regina Bruno
Editor-in-Chief: Maura Connor
Assistant to the Editor-in-Chief: Deirdre MacKnight
Executive Acquisitions Editor: Kim Mortimer
Assistant to the Executive Acquisitions Editor: Marion Gottlieb
Assistant Editor: Sarah Wrocklage
Development Editor: Laura Horowitz, Hearthside Publishing Services
Director of Marketing: David Gesell
Marketing Specialist: Michael Sirinides
Managing Editor, Production: Patrick Walsh
Production Editor: GEX Publishing Services
Production Liaison: Anne Garcia
Media Project Manager: Rachel Collett
Manufacturing Manager: Ilene Sanford
Senior Art Director: Maria Guglielmo-Walsh
Interior Design: GEX Publishing Services
Cover Design: Mary Siener
Image Specialist: Annette Linder
Manager, Cover Visual Research & Permissions: Karen Sanatar
Composition: GEX Publishing Services
Printer/Binder: Courier Kendallville
Cover Printer: Lehigh-Phoenix Color/Hagerstown

10 9 8 7 6 5 4 3 2 1

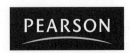

www.pearsonhighered.com

Volume 1:
ISBN-13: 978-0-13-507806-8
ISBN-10: 0-13-507806-7
Volume 2:
ISBN-13: 978-0-13-510351-7
ISBN-10: 0-13-510351-7

CONTRIBUTORS

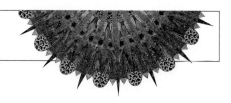

ADVISORY BOARD

Charlotte Blackwell, RN, BSN, MSEd
Wake Technical Community College

Carol Hardin Boles, RN, MSN
Surry Community College

Colleen Burgess, RN, MSN, APRN, BC, EdD
Healthcare Development, Community
Outreach and Research
Catawba Valley Community College

Delia Frederick, RN, MSNEd
Southwestern Community College

Robin Harris, RN, BSN, MSEd
College of the Albemarle

Barbara Knopp, RN, MSN
Manager – Education,
North Carolina Board of Nursing

Katherine K. Phillips, RN, MSN
Guilford Technical Community College

Linda Smith, RN, MSN
Johnston Community College

Renee Taylor, RN, BSN
Robeson Community College

Kathy Williford, MSN, RN
NEWH Nursing Consortium

Linda Wright, MSN, RN
Western Piedmont Community College

CONCEPT CONTRIBUTORS

Catherine Borysewicz, MSN, RN, BC, CNE
Carolinas College of Health Sciences

Colleen Burgess, RN, MSN, APRN, BC, EdD
Catawba Valley Community College

Barbara Callahan RN, NCC, BSN, MEd
Lenoir Community College

Sheryl Cornelius, MSN, RN
Mitchell Community College

Rachelle Denney, RN, BSN, MSNC
ECU 9/10
Fayetteville Technical Community College

Cathy L. H. Franklin-Griffin, RN, PhD
Surry Community College

Delia Frederick, RN, MSNEd
Southwestern Community College

Martha Freeze, MSN, ACNSBC
Rowan Cabarrus Community College

Barbara Knopp, RN, MSN
Manager – Education
North Carolina Board of Nursing

June Martin, RN, MSN
Forsyth Technical Community College

Debra S. McKinney, MSN, MBA/HCM, RN
University of Phoenix Online

Camille Reese, EdD, MSN, RNC
Mitchell Community College

Marilyn Springle, RN, MSN, FNPBC
Carteret Community College

Linda Wright, MSN, RN
Western Piedmont Community College

EDITORIAL CONSULTANTS

Bruce Goldfarb, BS
Writer

Laura S. Horowitz, BA
Editor
Hearthside Publishing Services

Adelaide R. McCulloch, BA
Editor

Debra S. McKinney, MSN, MBA/HCM, RN
Writer/Consultant

Nancy Peterson, BA
Editor

Kim Wyatt, BSN, MFA
Writer

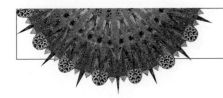

FOREWORD

During the years of 2006–2008, the Associate Degree Nursing faculty in 55 community colleges were involved in a Curriculum Improvement Project, a collaborative restructuring and revision of the Nursing Education curricula. The outcomes of the Curriculum Improvement Project included a multi-institutional effort that led to the adaptation and implementation of one Nursing Curriculum Standard, which met the standards of all the accrediting agencies and reflected the advances in nursing and health care practices.

Nurse educators across North Carolina investigated issues concerning the large volume of content included in their curricula. The educators agreed that the curriculum was experiencing content overload. After much research and consultation, the statewide team decided that a paradigm shift from a content-laden curriculum to a more conceptual approach to curriculum development and teaching was appropriate.

Much time and research was devoted to identifying and defining the specific concepts to be included in the statewide concept-based curriculum. Best examples of each concept, exemplars, were identified using research data derived from the *Healthy People 2010* report, the Institute of Medicine, the Centers for Disease Control and Prevention, the Joint Commission, the National Institute of Mental Health, the National Institute of Health, the NCLEX Test Plan, Quality & Safety Education for Nurses (QSEN), etc. Using data from these organizations, the statewide team identified exemplars that had high incidence and prevalence throughout the life span, across the health–illness continuum, and in various environmental settings.

The concepts were arranged into the classifications of Individual, Nursing, and Health Care Domains, and the exemplars were assigned to the most appropriate concepts. The statewide project representatives assigned the identified concepts and exemplars to specific courses. In each of the concept-based nursing courses, concepts are presented across the life span, the health–illness continuum, and environmental settings.

Providing a concept-based curriculum is only a single component of the complete curriculum restructuring process needed in order to implement conceptual learning. By shifting from teacher-centered instructional methods to facilitating learner-centered activities, the students emerge from an active, learner-centered environment able to identify the relationship among exemplars and concepts. Using exemplars to facilitate a deeper understanding of a concept facilitates abstract thinking, promotes schema construction, and allows the learner to transfer knowledge to various situations. Once a student is able to understand the connection between and among concepts, then, and only then, can conceptual learning and deep understanding occur.

Many nurse educators from North Carolina made important contributions to the concept-based curriculum. Sincere appreciation is extended to all my professional colleagues throughout the community college system, who have supported the efforts of this work. As project director, I gratefully acknowledge the tireless, unselfish efforts of the Curriculum Improvement Project Steering Committee members: Carol Boles, Colleen Burgess, Linda Smith, Kathy Williford, and Linda Wright. Sincere appreciation is extended to Barbara Knopp, Manager— Education for the North Carolina Board of Nursing, for her support of the project. Dr. Jean Giddens provided invaluable advice and consultation with the Curriculum Improvement Project Team, and I will always be grateful for her significant contributions.

The standardization of the Nursing curriculum at 55 colleges in North Carolina was a collaborative effort of many educators. The search for conceptually written texts and resources was important to the educators as they envisioned the implementation of the new conceptual curriculum and the student-centered learning activities. It is with great optimism that this conceptually written text will meet the needs of nurse educators and nursing students, not only in North Carolina, but across the United States as other states are developing concept-based, standardized curricula.

—Charlotte E. Blackwell

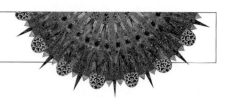

WELCOME!

Congratulations on your decision to enter the profession of nursing! While it will require much hard work, there is nothing more satisfying than making a positive difference in another person's life.

This textbook supports a brand new curriculum, which is the result of collaboration between the North Carolina Curriculum Improvement Project and Pearson Health Science, one of the nation's leaders in medical and educational publishing. Before beginning your journey in nursing, you'll want to know more about this textbook, which has been specially designed to meet the challenges facing nurses in the twenty-first century.

Nursing: A Concept-Based Approach to Learning represents the cutting edge in nursing education. North Carolina has designed the first concept-based nursing curriculum intended for use over the course of a Nursing program.

This curriculum offers a combination of traditional (text) and nontraditional (virtual) learning experiences. The textbooks to be used in the concept-based approach include the two volumes of concepts and a skills manual. The virtual learning opportunities include a computerized nursing kit with practical questions linking concepts together, case studies, and links to websites to further your learning. Individual schools also have the option to access Pearson's *The Neighborhood*, which is the brainchild of Dr. Jean Giddens. *The Neighborhood* is a virtual, web-based learning platform that presents a neighborhood of individuals from various professions and socioeconomic backgrounds with a variety of health alterations and concerns.

The goal of this textbook is to meet your needs and to help you learn and apply the knowledge you acquire to actual client care. This curriculum is dynamic and will be constantly revised to maintain evidenced-based practice. Those of you using the 1st edition have the unique opportunity to guide future editions. Students and professors working with this curriculum will have the opportunity to provide direct feedback to the NC Advisory Board and to Pearson Health Science. This feedback will help improve future versions of the curriculum and will be incorporated into the 2nd edition of this book—almost as soon as the first edition hits North Carolina classrooms. This is because both the NC advisory board and Pearson recognize that the curriculum and your textbooks must meet the changing needs of those using them.

Why Concept-Based Learning?

This curriculum began with a directive from the North Carolina community college presidents to design and implement a new curriculum for nursing programs. Nursing faculty from around the state, led by Charlotte Blackwell, RN, MSN, formed the North Carolina Curriculum Improvement Project (NCCIP). Together, project members examined a variety of resources, including:

- *Educational Rules for Nursing Programs*, 2007, which mandates conceptual teaching, improved utilization of technology, simulation, and evidence-based practice.
- The work of Dr. Jean Giddens, Associate Professor, the College of Nursing, University of New Mexico Health Science Center, an esteemed national nursing curriculum expert and the founder of concept-based learning in nursing.

Through extensive research, the NCCIP team realized the great benefit to students and faculty of a concept-based learning model. A concept-based curriculum sorts information into categories according to common characteristics and provides only the information and skills necessary for students to learn and apply the information when providing client care. For example, in one cohesive section, or exemplar, asthma is discussed within the oxygenation concept. In the exemplar you'll find information essential to providing culturally competent care to individuals with asthma across the life span: Pathophysiology, etiology, clinical manifestations, developmental and cultural considerations, and collaboration are all addressed. Older models addressed asthma separately in adult medical surgical classes, pediatric classes, and then again when studying geriatrics and obstetrics. Bringing all of the information together in one specific exemplar allows students to fully grasp the impact of asthma on a client in any stage of life and meet the nursing care needs of each unique individual.

How Is the Curriculum Organized?

After study and consultation with regional focus groups across the state, the NCCIP team decided on a shift in approach from the old medical model that emphasized the disease to a nursing approach that focused on active, collaborative learning. Through a workshop conducted by Dr. Giddens for nursing faculty from across the state, the team identified content for the new curriculum. Following agreement on the essential concepts, the team identified typical exemplars (the most

DOMAIN	COMPETENCIES
Individual (Volume 1 of text)	Developmentally appropriate client-centered care, collaboration, cultural competence, evidence-based practice, assessment, and communication
Nursing (Volume 2 of text)	Professional behavior, assessment, communication, clinical decision making, and other National League for Nursing Accreditation Committee (NLNAC) competencies for graduates of associate degree programs
Health Care (Volume 2 of text)	Quality improvement, evidence-based practice, informatics, and other elements essential to nursing within the health care system

important topics within the concept to focus on) that would facilitate the learning process for students. These were sorted into three domains of learning: individual, nursing, and health care. Each of these domains contains specific competencies and core elements that provide a comprehensive organizing framework for the curriculum.

Within each domain, the curriculum presents information that is critical to the practice of nursing. Each domain is divided into concepts, and each concept further organizes information into essential exemplars. Within the individual domain, the concept model delineates human systems of functioning, first describing the normal process of each system and then presenting common alterations from normal that are related to the system. These alterations are referred to as *exemplars*. For example, in the concept of oxygenation, the normal process of ventilation and gas exchange is presented, followed by five frequently seen alterations, or exemplars: asthma, acute respiratory distress syndrome, chronic obstructive pulmonary disease, respiratory syncytial virus/bronchiolitis, and sudden infant death syndrome. The information is provided in such a way that students will be able to apply information learned to other alterations in oxygenation in addition to those presented in the curriculum.

Further, the individual domain presents each concept with the underlying premise that no one concept functions without input from various other concepts. As such, this model provides opportunities for students to link concepts and their interactions together. For example, how does oxygenation link to the concept of perfusion? If I provide you with oxygen but your heart isn't beating to circulate the oxygen to the cells of the body, am I meeting your body's oxygen needs?

What Else Does This Curriculum Offer?

Nursing: A Concept-Based Approach to Learning offers a number of special features to help students acquire and use the information presented. These include the following:

- Assessment
- Alterations and Treatments
- Alternative Therapies
- Assessment Interview
- Care Settings

- Client Teaching
- Clinical Manifestations and Therapies
- Developmental Considerations
- Evidence-Based Practice
- Focus on Diversity and Culture
- Medications
- Multisystem Effects
- Nursing Care Plan
- Practice Alert.

Each of these features is further explained in the "User's Guide" section of Volumes 1 and 2 of this text.

The curriculum addresses traditional therapies and treatments as well as newer and alternative therapies. It provides information about diagnostic testing, assessment interviews, case studies and discussion questions, as well as critical thinking questions to promote linkage of concepts, helping students understand that no concept operates independently from other concepts.

SUPPLEMENTS

The following supplements are available for students and instructors.

Supplements for Instructors

INSTRUCTOR'S MANUAL AND RESOURCE GUIDE Each chapter in the Instructor's Manual is thoroughly integrated with the corresponding chapter in *Nursing: A Concept-Based Approach to Learning*, with detailed outlines and suggestions for classroom activities. The Instructor's Manual is available online on MyNursingKit.

TEST BANK Test Item Files with NCLEX®-style questions and complete rationales for correct and incorrect answers mapped to learning outcomes. *Available in TestGen and MS Word.*

Supplements for Students

NURSING: A CONCEPT-BASED APPROACH TO LEARNING SKILLS MANUAL With over 49 concepts, this skills book will ensure skills education is seamlessly integrated into the curriculum.

MYNURSINGKIT MyNursingKit is an online supplement that offers students book-specific learning objectives and practice tests as well as video clips and activities to aid student learning and comprehension.

MyNursingKit also provides instructors with easy and convenient access to important teaching resources, including detailed concepts for lecture and test banks.

Why the Inclusion of Virtual Learning Opportunities?

Nurses and clients alike are using technology more and more to gain access to information. In August 2009, the federal government announced $1.2 billion in grants to help hospitals transition medical records to electronic media. Today's nurses cannot function without advanced technological skills. In recognition of that, the NCCIP board and Pearson are designing new virtual learning opportunities to prepare students for the challenges they will face in the workplace.

Features to Help You Use This Book Successfully

Nursing students face challenges in their education—managing demands on their time, applying research findings, evaluating components of evidence-based practice, and developing their critical-thinking skills. Thus instructors and students alike value the in-text learning aids that we include in our textbooks to meet the challenges of nursing in today's world. We developed a textbook that is easy to learn from and easy to use as a professional reference. The following guide will help you use the text's features and resources to succeed in the classroom, in the clinical setting, on the NCLEX-RN® examination, and in nursing practice.

The **Concept Key Terms** and **Concept Learning Outcomes** at the beginning of each Concept highlight important terminology and provide an overview of topics that will be covered in the Concept.

Each Concept begins with an **"About"** section to give readers a foundational introduction to the concept.

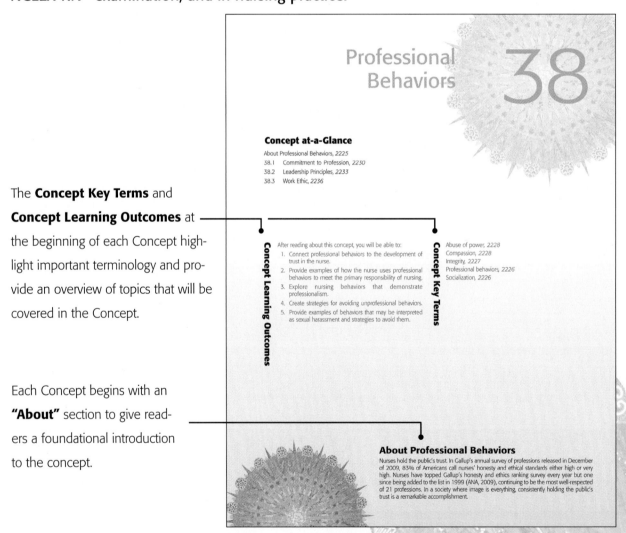

Professional Behaviors

38

Concept at-a-Glance

About Professional Behaviors, 2225
38.1 Commitment to Profession, 2230
38.2 Leadership Principles, 2233
38.3 Work Ethic, 2236

Concept Learning Outcomes

After reading about this concept, you will be able to:
1. Connect professional behaviors to the development of trust in the nurse.
2. Provide examples of how the nurse uses professional behaviors to meet the primary responsibility of nursing.
3. Explore nursing behaviors that demonstrate professionalism.
4. Create strategies for avoiding unprofessional behaviors.
5. Provide examples of behaviors that may be interpreted as sexual harassment and strategies to avoid them.

Concept Key Terms

Abuse of power, 2228
Compassion, 2228
Integrity, 2227
Professional behaviors, 2226
Socialization, 2226

About Professional Behaviors

Nurses hold the public's trust. In Gallup's annual survey of professions released in December of 2009, 83% of Americans call nurses' honesty and ethical standards either high or very high. Nurses have topped Gallup's honesty and ethics ranking survey every year but one since being added to the list in 1999 (ANA, 2009), continuing to be the most well-respected of 21 professions. In a society where image is everything, consistently holding the public's trust is a remarkable accomplishment.

Clinical Examples are used throughout the Health Care and Nursing domain concepts to provide real-world examples of the concepts.

CLINICAL EXAMPLE
Mark views himself as one of the smartest nurses on the unit because he belongs to several nursing organizations and works hard to maintain knowledge and competence by attending in-services, seminars, and regularly reading several nursing journals. However, when he enters clients' rooms wearing a wrinkled uniform and chewing gum, and then fails to answer clients' questions about their plan of care, the clients often discount what he is saying.

Appearance also affects how others within the medical community see the nurse. It is a form of nonverbal communication that evokes a response from others. Imagine a nurse approaching a doctor to question the validity of an order while talking on her cell phone. Will the doctor have enough confidence in the nurse to accept her concern and change the decision regarding the client's plan of care?

While simple rules of dress may seem obvious, some beginning nurses underestimate their importance. Nurses should take care to do the following:

■ Wear a clean uniform every day.
■ Keep hair contained and pulled back from the face to avoid it falling on a client or contaminating a sterile field.
■ Keep nails trimmed and filed to avoid scratching the client.
■ Shower daily and use deodorant or antiperspirant.
■ Avoid wearing jewelry that could injure the client (rings, bracelets, dangling earrings).
■ Avoid using perfumes or highly scented products (e.g., laundry detergent) that might irritate the allergic client or nauseate a client.
■ Avoid artificial fingernails, which harbor bacteria and increase the client's risk of infection.

Maintaining a professional appearance supports the nurse's credibility and increases the likelihood of gaining the trust of

Teamwork

How to work as a member of the team is discussed in detail in Concept 35, Collaboration. The nurse's skill in working as a team member contributes to others' opinions of the nurse as a professional and improves the quality of care delivered to the client. Consider the clinical example that follows.

CLINICAL EXAMPLE
Jose Guarez, 63 years old, is admitted to the unit with a medical diagnosis of angina, congestive heart failure, and left lower lobe pneumonia. Initially when Mr. Guarez is admitted, his condition is very unstable, with rapid respirations, hypoxia, and a weak productive cough. He requires endotracheal intubation and mechanical ventilation while receiving antibiotics and other medications. As his condition improves, Mr. Guarez is extubated and placed on oxygen, first by face mask and then by nasal cannula.

1. What members of the team would the nurse work with to provide care for Mr. Guarez?
2. How would nurse-to-nurse collaboration be important to the care of this client?
3. How would this client's care potentially suffer if the nurse preferred to function independently instead of as a member of the team?

Integrity

Integrity is the adherence to a strict moral or ethical code. Nurses adhere to the ANA Code of Ethics for Nurses (discussed in Concept 42, Ethics). Nurses demonstrate integrity by accepting feedback (positive or negative) as a tool for improving delivery of client care, by maintaining accountability for their actions and freely admitting when they make mistakes, and by following the nurse practice act and never working outside their scope of practice. Consider the clinical example that follows.

to respond to therapy, the team may agree that the social worker needs to intervene to help the client resolve his or her social needs before starting therapy. Nurses, by the nature of their holistic practice, are often able to help the team identify priorities and areas requiring further attention. Ideally, the collaborative team will ensure that the client is part of the decision-making process, even if the client is not able to be present. Decision-making processes are discussed in greater detail in Concept 34, Clinical Decision Making.

CLINICAL EXAMPLE
Betty Bradley, 87 years old, is a client in a long-term care facility. After fracturing her hip, Ms. Bradley is no longer stable on her feet and prefers to stay in bed for fear of falling. After speaking with Ms. Bradley to get a better understanding of her fears, the nurse consults with the physical therapist. Together they determine how they can help Ms. Bradley improve her mobility while reducing her risk of injury. After consulting with Ms. Bradley about their ideas and getting her agreement, the primary nurse and physical therapist develop a plan of care based on the nursing diagnoses of impaired mobility and risk for injury: falls. They list specific implementations including positioning, turning, and use of aids to prevent pressure ulcers. Once the plan of care is developed, it is posted on the wall by Ms. Bradley's bed so that all nurses can see it and administer care consistently. During the monthly team meeting, the plan of care for Ms. Bradley is evaluated. Both the physical therapist and the nurse report that Ms. Bradley has greatly improved both her strength and her mobility while reducing her risk for injury.

1. Why might collaborative care be of particular importance when caring for an elderly client who is a long-term resident in an extended care facility?
2. What other collaborative interventions might the team consider for this client?
3. How can the plan of care be posted on the client's wall without infringing on the client's right to confidentiality?

Increasingly, governments and society are working to reduce health risks, minimize the incidence of chronic illness, and improve the health and quality of life for all. Unfortunately, health and health care are not guaranteed. In the United States, the most pressing question for the health care system remains how to provide quality health care that is in line with the socioeconomic realities of society. A number of factors influence the provision of health care:

■ Although the diagnosis and treatment of illness are still critical, the focus of health care is changing. Health care consumers are demanding comprehensive, holistic, and compassionate health care that is also affordable. Clients expect that health care providers will view them as a biopsychosocial whole and respond to their needs as individuals while respecting them as collaborating members of the health care team.
■ Today's health care consumers have greater knowledge about their health than in previous years and, as a result, they increasingly are influencing health care delivery. Formerly, people expected a physician to make decisions about their care; today, however, consumers expect to be involved in making any decisions.
■ Health care consumers are assuming more responsibility for health and are more willing to participate in health-promoting activities. They are beginning to view health care professionals as a resource to guide these activities.

CLINICAL EXAMPLE
Nurses working in an outpatient surgical unit want to plan the on-call schedule at monthly staff meetings with their nurse manager. Currently, the staffing office for the entire surgical service plans that schedule. The nurses will need to negotiate the change and are planning a meeting to discuss strategy.

1. How might the nurses collaborate with the staffing office to increase their autonomy in creating a schedule?
2. How might the nurses approach the staffing office with their request to manage their own schedule?

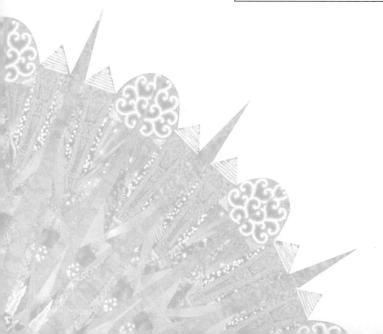

Care Settings boxes help readers apply the concepts to the many locations where nurses deliver health care.

Focus on Diversity and Culture boxes help students understand the broad range of clients they will work with in clinical practice.

The textbook highlights examples of **Evidence-Based Practice** throughout to provide students with the research-based rationales for their nursing care interventions.

Care across the life span is integrated throughout the text and featured in **Developmental Considerations** boxes.

DEVELOPMENTAL CONSIDERATIONS   **Communicating With Children and Adolescents**

The ability to communicate is directly related to the development of thought processes, the presence of intact sensory and motor systems, and the extent and nature of an individual's opportunities to practice communication skills. As children grow, their communication abilities change markedly.

INFANTS

- Infants communicate nonverbally, often in response to body feelings rather than in a conscious effort to be expressive.
- Infants' perceptions are related to sensory stimuli, so a gentle voice is soothing, for example, while tension and anger around them creates distress.

TODDLERS AND PRESCHOOLERS

- Toddlers and young children gain skills in both expressive (i.e., telling others what they feel, think, want, care about) and receptive (hearing and understanding what others are communicating to them) language.
- Toddlers need time to complete verbalizing their thoughts without interruption.
- Adults should provide simple responses to questions and simple, ~~short attention spans.~~
  ~~way for the child~~
  ~~eye level to help~~
  ~~bout a child's health~~
  ~~include the child in~~

ADOLESCENTS

- It takes time to build rapport with adolescents.
- Adults talking with adolescents should use active listening skills.
- Nurses working with adolescents should project a nonjudgmental attitude and nonreactive behaviors, even when an adolescent makes disturbing comments.

Nurses can use the following communication techniques to work effectively with children and their families:

- Play, the universal language, allows children to use other symbols, not just words, to express themselves.
- Drawing, painting, and other art forms can be used even by nonverbal children.
- Storytelling, in which the nurse and child take turns adding to a story or putting words to pictures, can help the child feel safer in expressing emotions and feelings.
- Word games that pose hypothetical situations or put the child in control, such as "What if ...?" "If you could ...," or "If a genie came and gave you a wish ...," can help a child feel more powerful or explore ideas about how to manage the illness.
- Read books with a theme similar to the child's condition or problem, and then discuss the meaning, characters, and feelings generated by the book. Movies or videos can also be used in this way.
- Writing can be used by older children to reflect on their situation, develop meaning, and gain a sense of control.

In all interactions with children, it is important to give them opportunities to be expressive, listen openly, and respond honestly, using words and concepts they understand.

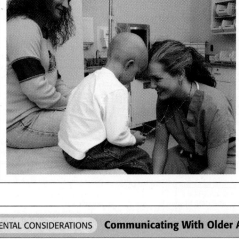

DEVELOPMENTAL CONSIDERATIONS   **Communicating With Older Adults**

Older adults may have physical or cognitive problems that necessitate nursing interventions for improvement of communication skills. Some of the common ones are as follows:

- Sensory deficits, such as vision and hearing
- Cognitive impairment, as in dementia
- Neurological deficits from strokes or other neurological conditions, such as aphasia (expressive and/or receptive) and lack of movement
- Psychosocial problems, such as depression.

Recognition of specific needs and obtaining appropriate resources for clients can greatly increase their socialization and quality of life. Interventions directed toward improving communication in clients with these special needs include the following:

- Assure that assistive devices, glasses, and hearing aids are being used and are in good working order.
- Make referrals to appropriate resources, such as speech therapy.
- Use communications aids, such as communication boards, computers, or pictures, when possible.

- Keep environmental distractions to a minimum.
- Speak in short, simple sentences, one subject at a time—reinforce or repeat what is said when necessary.
- Always face the person when speaking—coming up behind someone may be frightening.
- Include family and friends in conversation.
- Use reminiscing, either in individual conversations or in groups, to maintain memory connections and to enhance self-identity and self-esteem in the older adult.
- When verbal expression and nonverbal expression are incongruent, believe the nonverbal. Clarification of this and attentiveness to the client's feelings will help [...] caring and acceptance.
- Find out what has been important and has m[...] and try to maintain these things as much [...] things such as bedtime rituals become more [...] in a hospital or extended care setting.

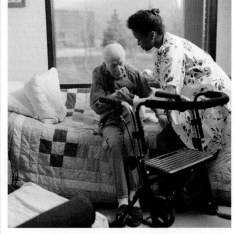

The **exemplars** in the Nursing and Health Care domains elaborate on topics within the concepts. For example, Exemplar 34.1 is a detailed discussion of the nursing process.

34.1 THE NURSING PROCESS

KEY TERMS

Actual diagnosis, 2065
Assessment, 2052
Assignment, 2092
Closed questions, 2056
Cognitive skills, 2096
Collaborative care plans, 2081
Collaborative interventions, 2090
Concept map, 2081
Critical pathways, 2081
Critical thinking, 2068
Cues, 2064
Database, 2052
Defining characteristics, 2066
Dependent functions, 2067
Dependent interventions, 2089
Diagnosis, 2065
Diagnostic label, 2065
Directive interview, 2056
Discharge planning, 2077
Etiology, 2065
Evaluation, 2098
Evaluation statement, 2099
Formal nursing care plan, 2077
Goals, 2085
Health promotion diagnosis, 2066
Implementation, 2096
Independent functions, 2067
Independent interventions, 2089
Indicator, 2086
Individualized care plan, 2077
Inferences, 2064
Informal nursing care plan, 2077
Interpersonal skills, 2096
Interview, 2056
Leading question, 2056
Multidisciplinary care plan, 2081
Neutral question, 2056
Nondirective interview, 2056
Norm, 2068
Nursing diagnosis, 2065
Nursing intervention, 2077
Nursing Interventions Classification (NIC), 2092
Nursing Outcomes Classification (NOC), 2086

Open-ended questions, 2056
PES format, 2072
Policies, 2079
Priority setting, 2083
Procedures, 2079
Protocols, 2079
Qualifiers, 2066
Rapport, 2056
Rationale, 2081
Risk factors, 2065
Risk nursing diagnosis, 2065
Signs, 2054
Standard, 2068
Standardized care plan, 2077
Standards of care, 2078
Standing order, 2080
Subjective data, 2054
Symptoms, 2054
Syndrome diagnosis, 2066
Technical skills, 2096
Validation, 2064
Wellness diagnosis, 2066

BASIS FOR SELECTION OF EXEMPLAR

NLN Competencies
Standards of Nursing Practice

LEARNING OUTCOMES

After reading about this exemplar, you will be able to:

1. Describe the purpose of the nursing process.
2. Define each phase of the nursing process.
3. Examine the interrelationship of each phase of the nursing process to one another.
4. Deconstruct the process of assessment to include collecting, organizing, and validating data.
5. Formulate nursing diagnostic statements appropriate to the client's priority needs.
6. Plan nursing care to include priorities of care, client goals, and selecting nursing interventions and activities.
7. Demonstrate the process of implementing nursing care.
8. Revise the nursing plan of care based on evaluation of client response.

...ing process in 1955, and ...iedenbach (1963) were ...eries of phases describ... ...en, various nurses have described the process of nursing and organized the phases in different ways.

The purpose of the nursing process is to identify a client's health status and actual or potential health care problems or needs, to establish plans to meet the identified needs, to deliver specific nursing interventions to meet those needs, and

REVIEW Professional Behaviors

RELATE: LINK THE CONCEPTS

Linking the concept of Professional Behaviors with the concept of Addiction Behaviors:

1. What impact does the nurse's use of substances (legal or illegal) have on the practice of nursing?
2. What is your professional responsibility when a nurse on your unit appears to be under the influence of a substance?

Linking the concept of Professional Behaviors with the concept of Clinical Decision Making:

3. How do professional behaviors result from clinical decision making and vice versa?
4. What conclusions would you draw, or have you drawn, about a nurse's ability to make clinical decisions on the basis of the nurse's professional or nonprofessional behaviors?

REFER: GO TO MYNURSINGKIT

REFLECT: CASE STUDY

Sally awakens suddenly, confused about her current surroundings. She looks around the dimly lit room, knowing only that this is not her bedroom. Where is she? The images start to form a pattern: a narrow bed with white sheets, a red "nurse" button glowing, a humming machine by her bedside, a tube in her nose, and, finally, the unmistakable pain in her back and hips. She is back in the hospital. The events of the day flood her memory: waking up on the floor at home; her husband standing over her calling 911, frantically describing her seizure; her two daughters, ages 10 and 12, crying as the ambulance takes her away; the repeat of scans, lab tests, and examinations she's had too many times before; the oncologist confirming that her breast cancer is back with a vengeance and saying words such as "palliative care" and "hospice referral." She is only 38, and it's been a long and hard fight for survival over the past 5 years.

Sally looks at the clock and reads 11:35 p.m. It's the night shift, and she needs something for pain. Yes, she needs medicine for her physical pain; but more than that, she needs something, someone, for her psychological pain. She wonders which nurse is assigned to her tonight. She knows all the regular staff on the oncology unit, having been a frequent visitor these past 5 years. She reaches for the red "nurse" light and pushes the button. "May I help you?" comes the response. "I want to see my nurse," she replies. "Can she bring you something?" comes the inevitable request to please be more specific. "I just need to see my nurse," she replies knowing that the response to her vague statement will give her lots of clues about the nurse who will be caring for her this night. She waits to see which door will open in response to her request.

Will it be Brittany Myers, who will roll her eyes as she instructs Sally to please be specific about her needs when asking for help so that fewer trips down the long hallway are required? Sally knows that if she tries to talk about her nightmare of a day, Brittany will interrupt to talk about her latest love interest and everything else going on in her own life. Will it be Marilyn Wiltshire, who will ask her about her pain level, location, description, and alleviating and aggravating factors; assess her IV site; check her infusion pump; and whisk away to get her pain medicine without ever really looking at her? Sally knows that Marilyn will provide her with competent care, will be quick to get her pain medication, and will even evaluate its response. She also knows that Marilyn is not comfortable with emotional discussions and will change the subject or mumble something about needing to see another client. Maybe, just maybe, it will be Lori Kauffman. Sally knows that if Lori comes in, she will really look at Sally and ask how she is doing. Lori will wait while Sally tries to find the words to express her extreme sadness and will understand if she needs to lash out at the unfairness of kno...

Each **Review** section includes a **Link the Concepts** section that provides critical-thinking questions to help students link the concepts from all three domains: Individual, Nursing, and Health Care.

In Volumes 1 and 2, many Review sections feature clients from The Neighborhood, Pearson's longitudinal case study that uses a conceptual approach, which complements the textbook.

REVIEW Documentation

RELATE: LINK THE CONCEPTS

Linking the exemplar of Documentation with the concept of Legal Issues:

1. How does proper documentation reduce the risk of lawsuits?
2. What components of nursing care must be included in the nurse's documentation to meet legal requirements?

Linking the exemplar of Documentation with the concept of Quality Improvement:

3. How is nursing documentation used to assess the quality of nursing care delivered?
4. How can incomplete documentation result in a negative evaluation of the quality of nursing care delivered?

REFER: GO TO MYNURSINGKIT

REFLECT: CASE STUDY

Kate Swanson is a 23-year-old nurse from a small, rural community. Kate graduated from nursing school a few months ago and took a job working on a general medical-surgical inpatient unit at Neighborhood Hospital. At some point, her goal is to work in an adult intensive care unit. She recently received a sign-on bonus and looks forward to buying her first new car.

Kate has a busy week because of increased client loads—she has seven to eight clients of her own. She has trouble managing her charting with all the client care she has to do. She ends up staying up to 2 hours after each shift to get it done. Kate's manager, Pat, talks with her about this and reviews the importance of point-of-care charting. The feedback he gives her is generally positive.

1. Why is Kate's manager trying to improve her point-of-care charting?
2. What are potential dangers of waiting until the end of the shift to document care?
3. What strategies might you suggest to Kate to help her improve point-of-care charting during a busy shift?

The content is **current** and includes information on the latest legislation, public health issues, and natural disasters around the world and how these incidents affect nurses. Current evidence is used to support assertions throughout the text.

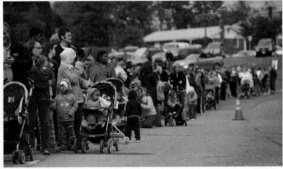

Box 44–1 **2010 Health Care and Education Reconciliation Act**

In 2010 Congress passed the Health Care and Education Reconciliation Act. The new law is intended to:

- Curb medical costs that are growing much faster than the rate of inflation
- Return insurance premiums to less costly rates so that more individuals and companies, especially small businesses, can afford to purchase insurance
- Remedy many unpopular insurance industry practices, such as denying coverage for clients with preexisting conditions or dropping coverage for clients who become ill
- Extend coverage to 32 million Americans, many of whom are working poor who do not qualify for public insurance programs and who work for employers who do not offer health insurance benefits.

Some of the provisions of the health care reform take effect immediately, while others will be implemented over several years.

Among provisions of the new law that take effect immediately:

- Children can no longer be denied health insurance coverage for preexisting conditions.
- Insurance companies can no longer drop clients when they become ill.
- Lifetime caps on coverage are eliminated. Annual caps on benefits are limited and will be eliminated in 2014. These measures help those who experience catastrophic illness or who live with costly chronic conditions such as hemophilia.
- Children will be allowed to remain on their parents' insurance plan until the age of 26.
- New health insurance plans must offer preventive care with no co-payment or deductible.
- Small employers that offer health insurance benefits to employees will receive a 35% tax credit for their share of premiums.
- Retirees aged 55-64 will be offered access to a re-insurance program.
- Medicare Part D recipients will receive a $250 credit.

BY 2011:

- Medicare must provide plans for preventive care with no copayment or deductible.
- Medicare Part D recipients in the "doughnut hole" of coverage will receive a 50% discount off prescription drugs.
- Health insurance companies will have to justify any premium increases or risk being taken out of state insurance exchange pools.

BY 2014:

- The uninsured and self-employed will be able to purchase insurance through state-based exchanges. Separate exchanges will be established for small companies.
- The IRS will impose a penalty of $750 per individual or 2% of income—whichever is greater—for those that choose not to purchase health insurance.
- Individuals and families who make between 100% to 400% of the Federal Poverty Level (FPL) and want to purchase their own health insurance on an exchange will be eligible for federal subsidies. In order to be eligible, these people cannot qualify for Medicare or Medicaid and cannot be covered by an employer. Eligible buyers will receive premium credits and there will be a limit to how much they have to contribute to their premiums.
- Private insurers will be required to accept all applicants without varying premiums on the basis of a person's health status. Insurance companies will not be able to deny coverage on the basis of preexisting conditions.
- Annual limits on benefits will be eliminated.
- The temporary high-risk pools for those unable to receive coverage prior to the law will be eliminated as people enroll in state insurance exchanges.

BY 2018:

- All insurance plans will be required to offer preventive care with no copayment or deductible.
- Insurance companies will pay a 40% excise tax on high-end benefit plans worth over $27,500 for families ($10,200 for individuals). Dental and vision plans will be exempt and will not be counted in the total cost of a family's plan.

Sources: Binckes J, Wing N. Health reform bill summary: The top 18 immediate effects. *Huffington Post*. Retrieved March 23, 2010, from http://www.huffingtonpost.com/2010/03/22/health-reform-bill-summary_n_508315.html#s75159. Jackson J, & Nolen J. Health care reform bill summary: A look at what's in the bill. *CBS News*, Retrieved March 23, 2010, from http://www.cbsnews.com/8301-503544_162-20000846-503544.html. Health care reform. *New York Times*, Retrieved March 26, 2010, from http://topics.nytimes.com/top/news/health/diseasesconditionsandhealthtopics/health_insurance_and_managed_care/health_care_reform/index.html. Health Care and Education Reconciliation Act of 2010. *Wikipedia*. Retrieved from http://en.wikipedia.org/wiki/Health_Care_and_Education_Reconciliation_Act_of_2010

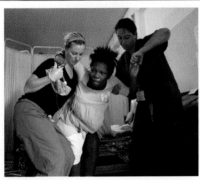

Figure 38–3 ■ Affective commitment leads nurses and other health care professionals to volunteer their services to help those in disasters, such as the January 2010 earthquake in Haiti. Here, Michele Shiel, an ER nurse from the U.S. Virgin Islands (left), helps to carry a woman from the hallway into a delivery room at the Haitian Community Hospital in Petionville, Haiti.

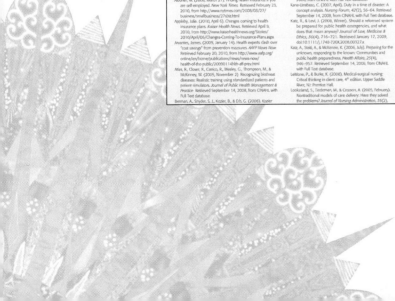

Figure 44–3 ■ Hundreds of county residents wait in a long line for the H1N1 vaccination shot at a clinic held by the Montgomery County Health and Human Services on October 14, 2009, at the Dennis Avenue County Health Center in Silver Spring, Maryland.

The content is supported by current evidence.

REFERENCES

Adams, M. P., Holland, L. N., Jr., & Bostwick, P. M. (2008). *Pharmacology for nurses* (2nd ed.). Upper Saddle River, NJ: Prentice Hall.

AHRQ (2007). *National healthcare disparities report*. Retrieved January 9, 2009, from http://www.ahrq.gov/qual/nhdr07/chap3a.htm#Ch3-Edv4

Alboher, M. (2008, March 27). Finding health insurance if you are self-employed. *New York Times*. Retrieved February 23, 2010, from http://www.nytimes.com/2008/03/27/business/smallbusiness/27cbiz.html

Appleby, Julie. (2010, April 6). Changes coming to health insurance plans. *Kaiser Health News*. Retrieved April 5, 2010, from http://www.kaiserhealthnews.org/Stories/2010/April/06/Changes-Coming-To-Insurance-Plans.aspx

Arvantes, James. (2009, January 14). Health experts clash over "cost savings" from prevention measures. *AAFP News Now*. Retrieved February 20, 2010, from http://www.aafp.org/online/en/home/publications/news/news-now/health-of-the-public/20090114hlth-all-prev.html

Atlas, R., Clover, R., Carrico, R., Wesley, G., Thompson, M., & McKinney, W. (2005, November 2). Recognizing biothreat diseases: Realistic training using standardized patients and patient simulators. *Journal of Public Health Management & Practice*. Retrieved September 14, 2008, from CINAHL with Full Text database.

Berman, A., Snyder, S. J., Kozier, B., & Erb, G. (2006). *Kozier*

Institute of Medicine (IOM). (2004). *Health literacy: A prescription to end confusion*. Retrieved October 3, 2009, from www.iom.edu/CMS/3775/3827/19723.aspx

Jones, K., & VanGilder, A. (2008, June 26). Bioterrorism agents: What the anesthesiologist needs to know. *Internet Journal of Anesthesiology*, *16*(2), 1-1. Retrieved September 14, 2008, from CINAHL with Full Text database.

Kane-Urrabazo, C. (2007, April). Duty in a time of disaster: A concept analysis. *Nursing Forum*, *42*(2), 56–64. Retrieved September 14, 2008, from CINAHL with Full Text database.

Katz, R., & Levi, J. (2008, Winter). Should a reformed system be prepared for public health emergencies, and what does that mean anyway? *Journal of Law, Medicine & Ethics*, *36*(4), 716–721. Retrieved January 17, 2009, doi:10.1111/j.1748-720X.2008.00327.x

Katz, A., Staiti, A., & McKenzie, K. (2006, July). Preparing for the unknown, responding to the known: Communities and public health preparedness. *Health Affairs*, *25*(4), 946–957. Retrieved September 14, 2008, from CINAHL with Full Text database.

LeMone, P., & Burke, K. (2008). *Medical-surgical nursing: Critical thinking in client care*, 4th edition. Upper Saddle River, NJ: Prentice Hall.

Lookisland, S., Tiedeman, M., & Crosson, A. (2005, February). Nontraditional models of care delivery: Have they solved the problems? *Journal of Nursing Administration*, *35*(2),

Richard, J., & Grimes, D. (2008, April). Bioterrorism: Class A agents and their potential presentations in immunocompromised patients. *Clinical Journal of Oncology Nursing*, *12*(2), 295–302. Retrieved September 14, 2008, from CINAHL with Full Text database.

Sage, W. (2007, November). Legislating delivery system reform: A 30,000-foot view of the 800-pound gorilla. *Health Affairs*, *26*(6), 1553–1556. Retrieved September 14, 2008, from CINAHL with Full Text database.

Shih, A. Davis, K. Schoenbaum, S. Gauthier, A. Nuzum, R. & McCarthy, D. (2008, August). *Organizing the U.S. health care delivery system for high performance*. The Commonwealth Fund.

Silenes, R., Akins, R., Parish, A., & Edwards, J. (2008, January). Developing disaster preparedness competence: An experiential learning exercise for multiprofessional education. *Teaching & Learning in Medicine*, *20*(1), 62–68. Retrieved January 17, 2009, doi:10.1080/10401330701798311

Tiedeman, M., & Lookinland, S. (2004, June). Traditional models of care delivery: What have we learned? *Journal of Nursing Administration*, *34*(6), 291–297. Retrieved September 3, 2008, from CINAHL with Full Text database.

The fire next time: Pandemic flu, bioterrorism, and ghost of SARS: Whether from man or nature, one calamity informs the next. (2007, March). *Bioterrorism Watch*. Retrieved September 14, 2008, from CINAHL with Full Text database.

Images and tables are used throughout to enhance student understanding of the topics.

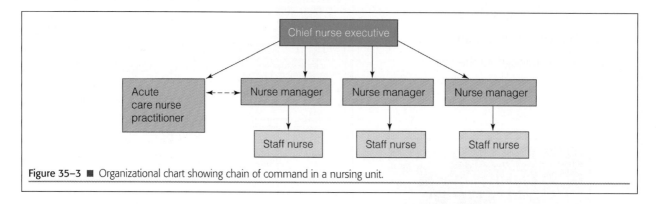

Figure 35–3 ■ Organizational chart showing chain of command in a nursing unit.

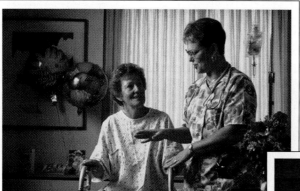

Figure 33–3 ■ The nurse helps her client learn to use a w
teaching her the appropriate technique for rising from the bed
standing nearby to encourage and support the client, ready t
in and provide assistance if necessary.

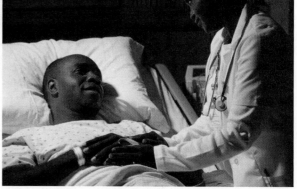

Figure 33–4 ■ This nurse is using touch and presence to help comfort her client.

TABLE 38–2 Description of Four Generations in the American Workforce

GENERATIONAL COHORT	LIFE EXPERIENCES	WORKFORCE ENTERED	WORK ETHIC
Veterans (born 1925–1944) Great Depression World War II	News came from newspapers and radio Long-distance phone calls were rare and expensive Shopping was mostly done at locally owned stores Movies were only seen in theaters Attitude toward children to be "seen and not heard"	End of depression and war Economic prosperity Emergence of middle class Able to thrive in a nice home on a single income Large, bureaucratic organizations Rules, policies, and procedures plainly outlined	Sacrifice and hard work are rewarded Seniority is important to advance career Value loyalty Respect authority Like working in teams with designated leaders Prefer personal forms of communication
Baby Boomers (born 1945–1960) Introduction of television Man landed on the moon Assassination of President Kennedy Vietnam War Civil Rights Movement Summer of Love Woodstock Watergate	Grew up in a healthy, flourishing economy Watched variety shows, movies, and sitcoms within their own home News became more visual and dramatic Raised in two-parent households in which father worked and mother was home caretaker Member of smaller families	Emphasis on freedom to be yourself—the "me" generation Heroes were those who questioned status quo People in positions of power were not to be trusted Raised to be independent, critical thinkers Many female college graduates went on to become secretaries, nurses, or teachers due to perception these were "primarily female professions"	Workaholics Embrace sense of professionalism Self-worth closely tied to work ethic Question authority Status quo can be transformed by working together Desire financial prosperity but long to make a significant contribution with their experience and expertise
Generation X (born 1961–1980) Rising divorce rates Microwaves Video games Computers Spaceship *Challenger* disaster Numerous scandals involving high-profile public figures	Lived in two-career households Many raised in single parent homes Watched parents work extremely long hours and sacrifice leisure time for success at work "Latch key" generation; learned to manage on their own; becoming adept, clever, and resourceful Allowed to be equal participants in family discussions, learned at an early age to participate in conversations, advocate for their point of view, and expect to have their opinions considered	Dramatic downsizing, reengineering, and layoffs seen with more senior colleagues, parents, and grandparents Hierarchical structures had begun to flatten, eliminating promotional opportunities for younger workers Large cohort of baby boomers remained in workforce filling limited managerial positions Assumed responsibility to keep themselves employable by constantly updating their skills	Seek challenges Self-directed Comfortable with technology Expect instant access to information Desire employment where they can create balance in work and personal life Prefer managers to be mentors and coaches Limited motivation to stay with same employer but loyal to their profession Desire more control over their own schedule Pragmatic focus on outcomes rather than process
Millennial Generation (born 1981–2000) Established infrastructure (childcare, preschool, after-school care) to assist dual-career parents Global generation Internet Bombing of federal building in Oklahoma City Columbine High School shootings Terrorist attack of September 11, 2001	Mostly children of baby boomers born to older mothers; "baby on board" signs in automobiles Live highly structured and scheduled with everything from soccer camp to piano lessons Parents heavily involved in their upbringing, often chaperoning or coaching extracurricular activities Accept multiculturalism Grew up using e-mail or the Internet more often than the telephone Raised enmeshed in digital technology with computer games at nursery school "Extreme sports" generation Mass consumption of television and pop culture	Economic downturn Job opportunities in many industries dried up Wall Street and banking industry crisis Believe education is the key to success Resurgence of heroism and patriotism Diversity a given Renewed sense of interest in contributing to collective good Volunteer for community service Joining organizations in record numbers	Social, confident, optimistic, talented, well-educated, collaborative, open-minded, achievement-oriented Expect daily feedback, high maintenance Potential to become the highest-producing workforce in history Thrive on the adrenaline rush of new challenges and new opportunities Consider personal cell phones a necessity for daily life and interpersonal communication

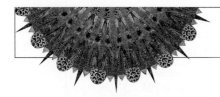

ACKNOWLEDGMENTS

The North Carolina Concept-Based Learning Editorial Board would like to thank the following people for their contributions to this project.

NORTH CAROLINA

The following groups and individuals working for organizations within North Carolina were instrumental in creating this product:
- The North Carolina Community College System (NCCCS)
- The North Carolina Board of Nursing
- The 52 CIP representatives, along with Dr. Jean Giddens.

PEARSON

The following staff from Pearson, our publisher, guided this project from conception through final production:
- Julie Alexander, publisher; Maura Connor, editor-in-chief; Kim Mortimer, executive acquisitions editor; Marion Gottlieb, assistant to the editor-in-chief; and Stephanie Klein, director of development, conceived of this project and provided the vision, staff, and budget to make it happen.
- Debra McKinney, RN, and Addy McCulloch gathered all of the content and put it in a consistent, readable format.
- Hearthside Publishing Services and GEX Publishing Services turned our thoughts and manuscript into a beautiful book.

SOURCE BOOKS

The following authors from Pearson generously allowed us to re-purpose their work for this project:
- Priscilla LeMone and Karen Burke, *Medical-Surgical Nursing: Critical Thinking in Client Care,* Fourth Edition
- Audrey Berman, Shirlee J. Snyder, Barbara Kozier, and Glenora Erb, *Kozier & Erb's Fundamentals of Nursing: Concepts, Process, and Practice,* Eighth Edition
- Jane W. Ball and Ruth C. Bindler, *Pediatric Nursing: Caring for Children,* Fourth Edition; and *Child Health Nursing,* Second Edition, along with Kay J. Cowen
- Patricia A. Tabloski, *Gerontological Nursing,* Second Edition
- Linda Eby and Nancy J. Brown, *Mental Health Nursing Care*, Second Edition
- Patricia A. Wieland Ladewig, Marcia L. London, and Michele R. Davidson, *Contemporary Maternal-Newborn Nursing Care,* Seventh Edition
- Donita D'Amico and Colleen Barbarito, *Health & Physical Assessment in Nursing*
- Karen Lee Fontaine, *Mental Health Nursing,* Sixth Edition
- Michael Patrick Adams, Leland Norman Holland, Jr., and Paula Manuel Bostwick, *Pharmacology for Nurses: A Pathophysiologic Approach,* Second Edition

- Kathleen Koerning Blais, Janice S. Hayes, Barbara Kozier, and Glenora Erb, *Professional Nursing Practice: Concepts and Perspectives,* Fifth Edition
- Mary Jo Clark, *Community Health Nursing: Advocacy for Population Health,* Fifth Edition
- Carol Ren Kneisl and Eileen Trigoboff, *Contemporary Psychiatric-Mental Health Nursing,* Second Edition
- Anita W. Finkelman, *Leadership and Management in Nursing*
- Eleanor J. Sullivan and Phillip J. Decker, *Effective Leadership and Management in Nursing*, Seventh Edition
- Sherry Makely, *Professionalism in Health Care: A Primer for Career Success*, Third Edition
- Toni Hebda and Patricia Czar, *Handbook of Informatics for Nurses & Healthcare Professionals*, Fourth Edition
- Rose Marie Nieswiadomy, *Foundations of Nursing Research*, Fifth Edition
- Audrey Berman, Shirlee J. Snyder, and Debra S. McKinney, *Nursing Basics for Clinical Practice*

REVIEWERS

The following nurse educators reviewed the concept and exemplar manuscripts. Their feedback was invaluable:
- Maureen Abraham, RNC, MSN, LCCE, Craven Community College
- Susan S. Barnes, RN, MSN, Guilford Technical Community College
- Charlotte Blackwell, RN, BSN, MSEd, Wake Technical Community College
- Catherine Borysewicz, MSN, RN, BC, CNE, Carolinas College of Health Sciences
- Colleen Burgess, EdD, RN, MSN, APRN, BC, Catawba Valley Community College
- Barbara Callahan, RN, NCC, BSN, MEd, Lenoir Community College
- Teresa Carnevale, RN, MSN, Lenoir-Rhyne University
- Sarah J. Clark, RN, MSN, CCRN, BC, Davidson County Community College
- Faye S. Cook, MSN, RN, Western Piedmont Community College
- Amy G. Crittendon, RN, MSN, CEN, Guilford Technical Community College
- Denise M. Davis, MA, BSN, RN, CMSRN, Brunswick Community College
- Dawn Day, MSN, RN, Johnston Community College
- Joyce Estes, RN, MSN, Catawba Community College
- Rhonda Evans, RN, BSN, MSN, Central Carolina Community College
- Amy L. Feaster, RN, MSN, Johnston Community College

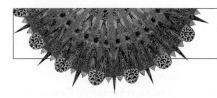
The education of professional nurses presents exciting opportunities for faculty and student learning. With the continual outburst of health care information and new technologies, faculty and students may feel they have entered a daily marathon without their best sneakers or a map of the route to help them reach the finish line. Tried and true teaching methods now seem antiquated as faculty compete for students' attention with a variety of new and engaging sources of information and entertainment. Add to this the overwhelming discovery of new knowledge in what has been known as the "information age" has resulted in nursing students feeling overwhelmed by the quantity of knowledge and skills they must gain in order to become practicing nurses.

Faced with these challenges, the 52 presidents in the North Carolina Community College System (NCCCS) appointed a team of nursing education experts to form the Associate Degree in Nursing Curriculum Improvement Project (CIP). The mission of the CIP was to develop a nursing curriculum to address contemporary nursing and workforce issues and to update the proverbial "paper map trail" into a "GPS system" to guide the future of nursing education within the community college system. Quickly the CIP embraced the idea of developing a concept-based nursing curriculum that utilizes today's multi-dimensional matrix of information, technology, communication, high fidelity simulation, and interactive virtual reality.

Recent education initiatives by the North Carolina Board of Nursing also reflect national initiatives and leadership. The Board of Nursing requires nurse educators in North Carolina to address current national trends, mandating conceptual teaching and improved utilization of technology, simulation, and the implementation of evidence-based practice in nursing. (*Education Rules for Nursing Programs, 2007*). An additional directive from the NCCCS was to design a curriculum that was learner-centered and allowed for the ready transfer of student credit from one college to another.

A final force behind the push for change came from North Carolina nursing workforce representatives and The Institute of Medicine's (2003) Task Force Workforce Committee. Both committees warned health educators that, due to the explosion of information and society's demand for technology, accountability, and responsibility, learning needs to be shifted to the learner.

The development of a new concept-based curriculum provides the impetus for educators to transition away from past, antiquated methods of faculty-centered teaching and passive learning and toward active, focused, participative, and collaborative teaching and learning. It offers the opportunity to equip nursing faculty and students with the knowledge and skills necessary to help them reach the finish line together—with the ultimate goal of increasing the competency and ability of nurses to serve the individuals seeking health care in the community.

THE PROCESS

In response to these multiple demands, the CIP Chair, Charlotte Blackwell, RN, MSN, in collaboration with the CIP Steering Committee and the 52 CIP representatives forged ahead to construct what is now known as the NC Concept-Based Nursing Curriculum. The CIP members set out to design a concept-based curriculum under the direction and consultation of Dr. Jean Giddens, an associate professor at the University of New Mexico Health Sciences Center, College of Nursing. Dr. Giddens is an esteemed national nursing curriculum expert and the original author and creator of concept-based learning in nursing education.

In addition, the CIP members consulted and worked collaboratively with Barbara Knopp, Manager—Education, from the North Carolina Board of Nursing Education, and Dr. Sharon Tanner, the National League for Nursing Accreditation Commission (NLNAC) consultant. The CIP members collected data about nursing, health care, and best practices at the national and state health levels. CIP members also conducted meetings and interviews with workforce representatives to elicit feedback about nursing and issues related to entry into practice for graduate nurses.

Faculty collected information from a variety of sources, including but not limited to the NLNAC competencies for Graduates of Associate Degree Nursing Programs, The Institute of Medicine publications, The PEW Commission, The Joint Commission public health reports, The Institute for Healthcare Improvement, *Healthy People 2010*, Chronic Disease Management IOM Centers for Disease Control, National Center for Health Statistics, Quality & Safety Education for Nurses; and the National Institute of Mental Health. These are just a few of the resources to which faculty turned to inform their decision-making for this project.

As the curriculum began to take shape, a unique opportunity was presented to the CIP Advisory Board. Attuned to national health care initiatives, representatives from Pearson Health Science volunteered their assistance and technology, providing access to their national publishing experts to facilitate the educational transition of this innovative curriculum. Together, CIP and Pearson representatives formed an advisory board for the publication of the NC Concept-Based Curriculum. The practical task of this board was to collaborate and navigate the complex information matrix, and to design, organize, and present the new curriculum in a meaningful manner for students and faculty.

As part of the exploration of concept-based learning, Dr. Giddens presented *The Neighborhood* to the CIP representatives and later to the ADN Council Members. Organized around concepts, *The Neighborhood* presents a variety of families from various professions and socioeconomic backgrounds who interact with their local health care system in a series of stories, which are essentially detailed case studies. Dr. Giddens' labor of love and degree of commitment to the profession of nursing were evident in the presentations. Audiences of nurse educators were enthralled and excited about the learning opportunities presented with this cognitive, experiential, and affective learning pedagogy.

Demonstrating commitment to the CIP project, Pearson representatives negotiated with Jean Giddens to launch *The Neighborhood* along with the new curriculum to enhance concept-based learning activities. *The Neighborhood* is now a virtual, web-based learning platform that gives students and faculty access to its compelling cast of characters with their various health alterations and concerns. This new learning platform adds an invaluable dimension to the construction of knowledge and creates meaning for students and faculty through a combination of cognitive, emotional, spiritual, and developmental stages for the acquisition of knowledge in the art and science of nursing.

THE FOUNDATION FOR THE NEW CURRICULUM

A basic understanding of the development of nursing education standards, curriculum, regulation, legislation and official mechanisms inherent in the process of curriculum development is necessary for both the student and faculty. Only those processes inherent in the development of this curriculum are presented here. The process of the development of the CIP is described within the context of national and state health care trends, the IOM, The National Academy of Science, The National League for Nursing (NLN), and the North Carolina Board of Nursing (NCBON). The National Academy of Science is a non-profit collaboration of scholars engaged in scientific research to advance science and technology for the general welfare of society. By congressional charter, the Institutes of Medicine act under the National Academy of Sciences to identify issues of medical care, research and education (IOM, 2003). The mission of the NLN is to advance quality nursing education and prepare the workforce within an ever-changing health care environment. This curriculum was developed and guided by the NLNAC core competencies for graduates of associate degree nurses.

National Initiatives

The IOM report *Crossing the Quality Chasm: A New Health System for the 21st Century* (2001) called for an interdisciplinary group of health care providers to be convened to reform health care education. As a result of this report, in 2002 a summit of professionals from health disciplines and occupations was assembled. The focus of this summit was to incorporate core competencies into health education. The five core competencies identified through these efforts are patient-centered care, interdisciplinary teams, evidence-based practice, quality improvement, and informatics.

In addition to the IOM reports, as early as the year 2000, the NLN published the *Educational Competencies for Graduates of Associate Degree Nursing Programs*. This document outlines consistent expectations of nursing programs. It challenges nurse educators in nursing programs to facilitate student learning though more effective simulation, virtual learning, and clinical and classroom design, as well as to develop a research base for teaching and learning. Other challenges addressed in this report include advanced technology, increased acuity levels, decreased length of stay, managed care, diverse and multifaceted client population, and diverse settings. The report outlines eight core competencies for graduates of nursing programs: professional behaviors, communication, assessment, clinical decision making, caring interventions, teaching and learning, collaboration, and managing care (NLN, 2000).

State Initiatives

In response to the IOM reports, the NC Institute of Medicine convened a task force on the NC Nursing Workforce in 2003. The Institute partnered with the North Carolina Area Health Education Centers, the North Carolina Center for Nursing, the North Carolina Hospital Association, and the North Carolina Nurses Association to address issues related to the nursing workforce in North Carolina. They analyzed the current and projected future demand for nursing professionals and paraprofessionals in the NC healthcare industry.

The task force focused on nursing faculty recruitment and retention, nursing education programs, transitions from school to work, and the nursing work environment. In addition, the task force identified that North Carolina needed to address retaining nurses in their jobs and the profession. The task force members agreed that *"all categories of nursing education programs need to produce more graduates, reduce attrition, and maintain current high pass rates on the NCLEX-RN® exam...."* Further suggestions included the development of a Comprehensive Articulation Agreement to improve transfer rates of nursing students from ADN to BSN programs.

The task force also identified nursing workforce goals including producing an adequate number of nurses to meet the state's needs, creating opportunities for nurses to advance education credentials, and elevating the overall level of education of the North Carolina workforce. Recent graduates, employers and supervisors expressed a need for transitional work experiences, such as clinical internships, for newly graduated nurses.

Concurrently, within the state of NC, the Associate Degree Nursing Deans/Directors expressed concerns that nursing courses were not easily transferable among all the community colleges and that some course descriptions did not reflect current nursing practice. The North Carolina Board of Nursing was in the process of revising the education rules for nursing education programs. The Board of Nursing mandated integration of the previously mentioned NC IOM "five practice competencies." At that point the Deans/Directors recommended that Wake Technical Community College in Raleigh, NC, request a grant to fund the Curriculum Improvement Project.

DESIGNING THE NEW CURRICULUM

The CIP grant was awarded to Wake Technical Community College. The Curriculum Improvement Project began with what Ralph Tyler in his classic text in 1949, *Basic Principles of Curriculum and Instruction,* suggested as imperative to curriculum development: a contemporary and current review of the literature. The CIP team's review included the documents previously mentioned, as well as other literature regarding nursing education and practice, education, and conceptual models. Tyler also emphasized (1969) the importance of developing curriculum that is relevant to the learner. The Project Director met with representatives of the North Carolina Board of Nursing to ensure that the curriculum would reflect current nursing practice. The CIP committee members reviewed the results of the state and national workforce initiative in nursing. The CIP Committee and Project Director formed Regional Workforce Focus Groups to identify industry, education, and learner needs.

Upon completion of the first review of current literature and direction from the North Carolina Board of Nursing Education Consultant, the CIP Project Director selected a concept- based model for designing the new curriculum. This concept-based model would incorporate the NLN's *Educational Competencies for Graduates of Associate Degree Nursing Programs.* Next, the CIP team hired a curriculum consultant with expertise in concept-based learning, Dr. Jean Giddens.

The committee embraced a theory of active learning and began with what Tyler (1969) refers to as "constructing." Concept-based learning is rooted in constructivist theory.

Constructivist Theory and Collaborative Learning

Constructivist educational theory is tied to cognitive psychology. This approach emphasizes learners actively constructing their own knowledge and meaning. Constructivism is the product of the work of numerous scholars, such as Jean Piaget, Jerome Bruner, Ernest van Glaserfeld, and Lev Vygotsky. Constructivism, which acknowledges that learning occurs in communities and groups, is the foundation of the collaborative learning movement.

Collaborative learning is at the core of any concept-based curriculum. Collaborative learning is also strongly based in constructivist theory. Learning is about making connections: Neuroscientists have discovered that the brain develops circuitry and grows as a result of experience and learning. Neurologists and cognitive scientists agree that humans build their minds by "constructing" mental structures and "hands-on" concrete application that connects and organizes information.

Andragogy

With this innovative curriculum design, a shift from pedagogy to andragogy is imperative. Knowles (2005) defines andragogy as "the art and science of helping adults learn." Basic assumptions of this theory include the following:

■ Belief in the learner's ability to learn

■ Learner control over objectives, strategies and evaluation
■ Helping students learn for themselves.

Andragogy assumes that the adult learner is qualitatively different from the child or adolescent learner, and educators need to understand those differences. Key differences are (1) the adult learner is self-directing; (2) the adult learner brings a different quality and greater volume of experience; (3) the adult learner approaches the learning activity on a need-to-know basis related to tasks associated with adult roles; (4) the adult learner is problem- and task-centered; and (5) the adult learner's motivations are internal and include self-esteem, recognition, and a better quality of life.

The Whole-Part-Whole (WPW) Learning Model by Knowles (2005) also informed the concept-based curriculum. Whole-Part-Whole learning is a three-stage process. In the first stage, a framework or landscape of learning provides context for and is connected to the learner. In this curriculum, the first stage—or Whole—is the concept. The second stage—the Part—introduces the students to skills, techniques, and processes that constitute new learning. In the NC concept-based curriculum, this stage will be achieved through learning the exemplars of each concept and the skills and techniques provided through the skills manual and clinical experiences. The last stage—the second Whole—links individual parts to allow the learner to comprehend the complete content. The second Whole involves piecing and organizing traces, active learning, repetition, and learning from simple to complex. This will be achieved through the examination of case studies and individual and group student learning projects. The learner must master each part of the framework in order to achieve learning goals.

THE DOMAINS, CONCEPTS, AND EXEMPLARS

The CIP representatives from the community colleges attended a workshop presented by Dr. Giddens and identified content that was considered a "must" for the new curriculum. Dr. Giddens held an additional workshop with the Concept Group Committee to sift through the comprehensive list of imperatives discussed in the previous workshop, and to review, categorize, and complete them. Upon agreement of the essential curriculum concepts, the group members developed typical exemplars for each concept to facilitate learning. CIP committee members also solicited feedback from faculty at their colleges about the prospective curriculum design and content. Their list of selected concepts and exemplars was presented to the CIP Steering Committee.

Upon receipt of the concepts and exemplars, the CIP Steering Committee sorted the concepts and categorized them under the domains of nursing to organize and frame the massive amount of information. As a result, three domains emerged: the individual domain, the nursing domain, and the health care domain, all of which operate within the broader context of environment (See Figure 1). Each of the domains contains specific competencies and core elements essential for nurses entering the work force.

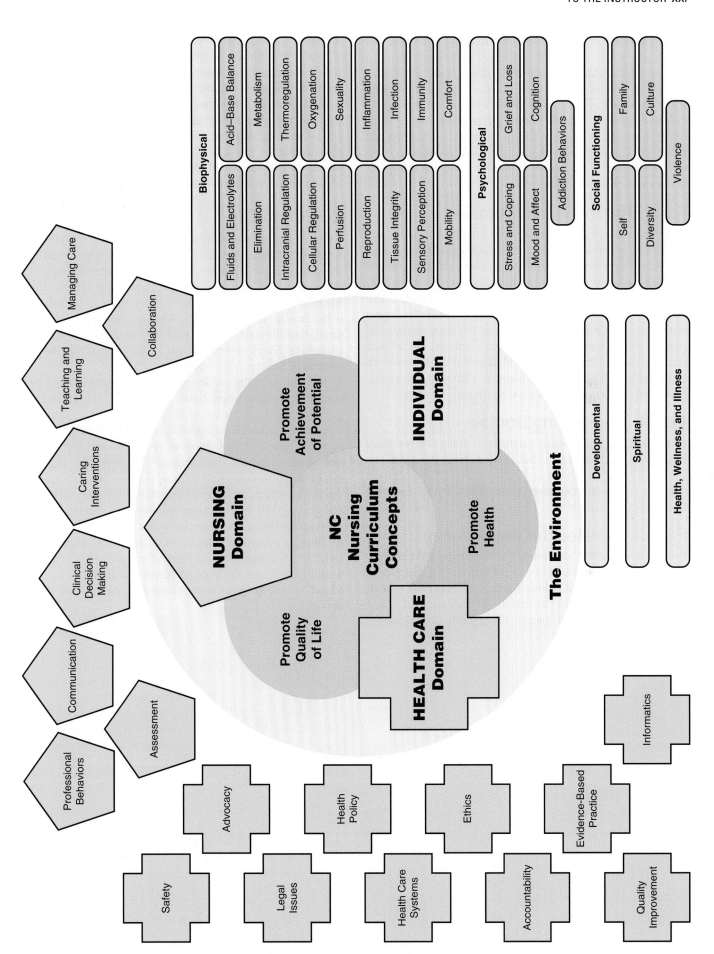

Biophysical
- Fluids and Electrolytes
- Acid–Base Balance
- Elimination
- Metabolism
- Intracranial Regulation
- Thermoregulation
- Cellular Regulation
- Oxygenation
- Perfusion
- Sexuality
- Reproduction
- Inflammation
- Tissue Integrity
- Infection
- Sensory Perception
- Immunity
- Mobility
- Comfort

Psychological
- Stress and Coping
- Grief and Loss
- Mood and Affect
- Cognition
- Addiction Behaviors

Social Functioning
- Self
- Family
- Diversity
- Culture
- Violence

- Developmental
- Spiritual
- Health, Wellness, and Illness

The Environment

NC Nursing Curriculum Concepts

NURSING Domain
- Promote Achievement of Potential
- Promote Quality of Life
- Promote Health

INDIVIDUAL Domain

HEALTH CARE Domain

- Managing Care
- Collaboration
- Teaching and Learning
- Caring Interventions
- Clinical Decision Making
- Communication
- Assessment
- Professional Behaviors

- Safety
- Advocacy
- Legal Issues
- Health Policy
- Health Care Systems
- Ethics
- Accountability
- Evidence-Based Practice
- Quality Improvement
- Informatics

An important decision made by the Steering Committee was to use the terms *individual* and *client* instead of the term *patient,* which is favored by the IOM, throughout the new curriculum. It was the consensus of the Steering Committee that the term *patient* elicits a more dependent view of those individuals entrusted to the care of nurses. It is the hope of the committee that nursing will not lose sight of the individual first and foremost. The term *individual* is intended to empower. The term *client* implies that nurses are working with the individual as a team to promote health.

Part I: The Individual Domain

All of the concepts related to the holistic individual, family, and community are presented in Part I: The Individual Domain. This addresses the biologic, physical, cognitive, and psychosocial processes and their alterations that most frequently bring the individual into contact with the nursing and health care domains. Each concept within the individual domain addresses the impact of that concept on individuals across the life span, inclusive of cultural, gender, and developmental considerations. Examples of concepts found in Part I include Acid–Base Balance (Concept 1); Culture (Concept 6); Health, Wellness, and Illness (Concept 13), Mood and Affect (Concept 20), and Spirituality (Concept 27).

Part II: The Nursing Domain

Part II, The Nursing Domain, contains all of the competencies required of graduate nurses such as Assessment (Concept 32), Clinical Decision Making (Concept 34), Collaboration (Concept 35), Communication (Concept 36), and Professional Behaviors (Concept 38).

Part III: The Health Care Domain

Part III, the Health Care Domain, contains the IOM competencies of Evidence-Based Practice (Concept 43), Informatics (Concept 46), and Quality Improvement (Concept 48), as well as additional elements essential to nursing: Advocacy (Concept 41), Ethics (Concept 42), Health Care Systems (Concept 44), Legal Issues (Concept 47), and Safety (Concept 49). Although advocacy is one of the competencies within the domain of nursing, the committee unanimously decided to highlight advocacy within the health care domain. Several years in a row, the Gallup polls (2005, 2006) have reported that Americans acknowledge nursing as the most ethical and trusted profession. In recognition and support of this perception, the CIP Steering Committee unanimously placed the competency of advocacy as a critical element to be highlighted in all curricula across the state.

CONCLUSION

Armed with a strong foundation in adult learning, this concept-based curriculum provides a focal point to direct learning through concepts, examples of alterations via exemplars, faculty and student activities, and collaborative group exercises. Modules were developed either directly by or in consultation with faculty members from various community colleges throughout the state of NC to ease the transition from teaching to learning. Faculty members from across the state provide peer reviews of concepts and exemplars.

In addition to the collaborative efforts made in the development of this concept-based curriculum, the curriculum provides many opportunities for student nurses to learn collaboratively through skill development, case studies and discussions, group examination of resources and technology, and student–faculty interactions. By working together, teachers and students will become partners in learning, promoting greater acquisition of knowledge and understanding, and greater skill development—all of which will produce the most successful, empathetic, informed, and skilled graduates of Nursing programs. Through the successful implementation of this concept-based curriculum, individuals seeking health care across the state of North Carolina will be comforted and cared for by more competent, caring, and skilled nursing professionals.

—*Colleen Burgess*

CONTENTS

PART II THE NURSING DOMAIN 1997

CONCEPT 32 Assessment 1999
Collecting Data Through Physical Examination 2000
Interpreting Findings From the Assessment Process 2006
Nursing Practice 2007
Holistic Health Assessment Across the Life Span 2008
Overview 2008
Special Considerations for Assessment of Children 2009
Assessment Specific to Stages of the Life Span 2012

CONCEPT 33 Caring Interventions 2027
Nursing Theories on Caring 2028
Types of Knowledge in Nursing 2031
Caring Encounters 2032
Maintaining Caring Practice 2034

CONCEPT 34 Clinical Decision Making 2037
Decision Making: A Response to Change 2038
The Decision-Making Process 2040
Problem-Solving Approaches 2043
Nursing Practice 2046
The Nursing Process 2047
Overview 2047
Phases of the Nursing Process 2050
Characteristics of the Nursing Process 2051
Collecting Data 2052
Data Collection Methods 2055
Organizing Data 2059
Validating Data 2064
Definitions 2065
Types of Nursing Diagnoses 2065
Components of a NANDA Nursing Diagnosis 2066
The Diagnostic Process 2068
Ongoing Development of Nursing Diagnoses 2074
Types of Planning 2077
Developing Nursing Care Plans 2077
The Planning Process 2083
Relationship of Implementing to Other Nursing Process Phases 2096
Skills Necessary for Implementation 2096
Process of Implementation 2096
Relationship of Evaluating to Other Nursing Process Phases 2098
Process of Evaluating Client Responses 2098
Applying Critical Thinking 2103
Critical Thinking 2104
Overview 2104
Skills in Critical Thinking 2105
Attitudes That Foster Critical Thinking 2106
Developing Critical Thinking Attitudes and Skills 2108
Standards of Critical Thinking 2109
Applying Critical Thinking to Nursing Practice 2110

CONCEPT 35 Collaboration 2113
The Nurse as Collaborator 2114
Collaborative Practice 2117
Benefits of Collaborative Care 2118
Competencies Basic to Collaboration 2118
Factors Leading to the Need for Increased Collegiality and Collaboration 2120
Nursing Practice 2120
Case Management 2121
Overview 2121
Critical Pathways 2123
Chain of Command 2126
Overview 2126
Conflict Resolution 2127
Overview 2127
Causes of Conflict 2128
Preventing Conflict 2129
Responding to Conflict 2129
Managing Conflict 2130
Gender Issues in Conflict 2130
Nurse–Physician Relationship 2131
Verbal Abuse 2131
Effects of Staff and Organizational Conflicts on Clients 2132
Conclusion 2132
Interdisciplinary Teams and Communication 2133
Overview 2133
Groups 2134
Management Theories 2142
Overview 2142
Leaders and Managers 2142
Management Functions 2143
Principles of Management 2144
Conclusion 2145

CONCEPT 36 Communication 2147
The Communication Process 2149
Modes of Communication 2149
Factors Influencing the Communication Process 2155
Barriers to Communication 2158
Nursing Practice 2163
Therapeutic Communication 2164
Overview 2164
Therapeutic Communication Techniques 2165
Barriers to Communication 2172
The Therapeutic Relationship 2172
Special Considerations When Working With Children and Families 2176
Conclusion 2178

Assertive Communication 2179
  Overview 2179
  Communication Styles 2179
  Assertive Communication 2180
Documentation 2182
  Overview 2182
  Ethical and Legal Considerations 2183
  Purposes of Client Records 2183
  Documentation Systems 2184
  Documenting Nursing Activities 2192
  Facility Specific Documentation 2194
  General Guidelines for Recording 2195
Reporting 2200
  Overview 2200

CONCEPT 37 Managing Care **2205**
  Managed Care 2206
  Case Management 2206
  Client-Focused Care 2206
  Differentiated Practice 2206
  Shared Governance 2206
  Case Method 2206
  Functional Method 2206
  Team Nursing 2206
  Primary Nursing 2207
  Nursing Practice 2207
Care Coordination 2208
  Overview 2208
  Barriers to Effective Coordination 2208
  Skills That Promote Effective Coordination 2208
  Application of Coordination 2209
Cost-Effective Care 2209
  Overview 2210
  Payment Sources in the United States 2210
  The International Perspective 2212
  Factors Influencing the Provision of Health Care 2213
  Cost-Containment Strategies 2214
  Nursing Economics 2215
Delegation 2217
  Overview 2217
  Principles of Delegation 2217
  Benefits of Delegation 2218
  The Delegation Process 2219
  Factors Affecting Delegation 2220
  Liability and Delegation 2222

CONCEPT 38 Professional Behaviors **2225**
  Components of Professionalism in Nursing 2226
  Unprofessional Behaviors 2228
  Conclusion 2229
Commitment to Profession 2230
  Overview 2230
  Factors of Professional Commitment 2230
  Types of Commitment 2231

  Stages of Commitment Development 2231
  Managing Stress 2232
Leadership Principles 2233
  Overview 2233
  Leadership Theories 2233
Work Ethic 2236
  Overview 2236
  Attendance and Punctuality 2236
  Reliability and Accountability 2237
  Attitude and Enthusiasm 2238
  Generational Differences in Work Ethic 2238

CONCEPT 39 Teaching and Learning **2243**
  The Art of Teaching 2244
  Learning 2245
  The Internet and Health Information 2251
Client Education 2253
  Overview 2254
  Teaching Clients and Their Families 2254
Mentoring 2269
  Overview 2269
  Mentoring 2269
  Precepting 2270
  Coaching 2270
  Networking 2271
Staff Education 2272
  Overview 2272
  Orientation 2272
  Staff Development Process 2273

PART III THE HEALTH CARE DOMAIN **2277**

CONCEPT 40 Accountability **2279**
  Criteria of a Profession 2280
  Socialization to Nursing 2281
  Factors Influencing Nursing Practice and Accountability 2282
  Nursing Practice 2284
Competence 2285
  Overview 2285
  Areas of Competency 2285
  Promoting Lifelong Competence 2286
  Nursing Practice 2286
Professional Development 2287
  Overview 2287
  Historical Perspectives 2287
  Contemporary Nursing Practice 2291
  Roles and Functions of the Nurse 2293
  Conclusion 2295

CONCEPT 41 Advocacy **2297**
  The Advocate's Role 2298
  Advocacy Interventions 2302
  Illegal, Immoral, or Unethical Activities of Professionals 2302
  Nursing Practice 2302

CONCEPT 42 Ethics 2305
    Values 2306
    Principles of Ethical Decision Making 2308
    Nursing Codes of Ethics 2308
    Models of Ethical Decision Making 2311
    Strategies to Enhance Ethical Decisions and Practice 2312
    Conclusion 2312
    Ethical Dilemmas 2312
        Overview 2312
        Bioethical Issues 2313
        Ethical Issues in Nursing Practice 2315
        Conclusion 2317
    Patient Rights 2318
        Overview 2218
        Protecting Patient Rights 2318
        Conclusion 2318

CONCEPT 43 Evidence-Based Practice 2323
    The Benefits of Evidence-Based Practice 2324
    Barriers to Evidence-Based Practice 2324
    Nursing Research 2325
    Ethical Considerations in Nursing Research 2332
    Developing Evidence-Based Practice 2334

CONCEPT 44 Health Care Systems 2339
    Types of Health Care Services 2340
    Types of Health Care Settings 2341
    Factors Affecting Delivery of Health Care 2341
    Frameworks for Providing Care 2343
    Nursing Practice 2344
    Access to Health Care 2345
        Overview 2345
        Barriers to Access 2345
        Solutions 2348
    Allocation of Resources 2349
        Overview 2349
        Examples of Resource Allocation 2349
        Nurses and Allocation of Resources 2350
    Emergency Preparedness 2351
        Overview 2351
        The Four Phases of Emergency Response 2351
        Responsibility for Emergency Management
          and Response 2355
        Triage 2356
        Site-Specific Disaster Zones 2356
        Bioterrorism 2357
        Collaboration 2358
        Nursing Practice 2358

CONCEPT 45 Health Policy 2361
    Developing Health Policies 2362
    Regulatory Agencies 2363
        Overview 2363
        Federal Agencies 2364
        State and Local Agencies 2365

    Accrediting Bodies 2366
        Overview 2366
        The Joint Commission 2366
        Nursing Education Program Accreditation Program 2366
    Professional Organizations 2366
        Overview 2366
        American Nurses Association 2366
        National Student Nurses Association 2366
        Specialty Practice Organizations 2367
        Sigma Theta Tau International 2367
        National League for Nursing 2367
        The American Association of Colleges of Nursing 2367
    Types of Reimbursement 2367
        Overview 2367
        Payment Sources 2367
        Conclusion 2369

CONCEPT 46 Informatics 2373
    Computer Terminology 2374
    Computer Information Systems 2375
    Trends in Informatics 2378
    Clinical Decision Support Systems 2385
        Overview 2385
        The Role of Uniform Languages 2386
        Utilizing Research 2386
        Computers in Nursing Research 2386
        Computers in Nursing Administration 2388
    Individual Information at Point of Care 2389
        Overview 2389
        Computer-Based Client Records 2390

CONCEPT 47 Legal Issues 2397
    Sources of Laws 2398
    Criminal and Civil Law 2398
    Tort Law 2399
    Strategies to Prevent Incidents of Professional
        Negligence 2401
    The Standard of Care 2402
    Selected Laws That Impact Nursing Practice 2402
    Conclusion 2406
    Nurse Practice Acts 2406
        Overview 2406
        Licensure 2407
        National Council of State Boards of Nursing 2408
        National Licensure Compact 2408
        Credentialing 2409
        Nursing Students 2409
        Standards of Practice 2410
    Advance Directives 2410
        Overview 2410
        Elements of an Advance Directive 2410
        Role of the Nurse 2412
    Health Insurance Portability and Accountability Act 2412
        Overview 2412

Protected Health Information 2412
Privacy Versus Confidentiality 2413
Mandatory Reporting 2413
Overview 2413
Abuse or Neglect of Minors and Older Adults 2413
Good Faith Immunity 2413
Mandatory Reporting of Nurses in Violation of the NPA 2414
Mandatory Reporting of Certain Injuries and Illnesses 2414
Other Examples of Mandatory Reporting 2415
Risk Management 2415
Overview 2415
Strategies for Risk Management 2415
Incident Reports 2417
Whistleblowing 2417
Overview 2417
Consequences of Whistleblowing 2418

CONCEPT 48 Quality Improvement 2421
The Need to Improve the Quality of Health Care 2422
National Initiatives 2423
Implementing Quality Improvement 2423
Components of Quality Management Programs 2424
Measuring Quality Improvement 2426
Improving the Quality of Care 2428
Risk Management 2429
Creating a Blame-Free Environment 2429
Nursing Practice 2430
Conclusion 2430

CONCEPT 49 Safety 2433
Factors Affecting Safety 2434
Hand-off Communication 2435
Standard Precautions 2435
Nursing Practice 2439
Anticipatory Guidance 2439
Overview 2439
Developmental Considerations 2440
Environmental Safety 2442
Overview 2442
Client Settings 2442
Health Care Settings 2443
Promoting Client Safety in the Health Care Setting 2444
Injury and Illness Prevention 2449
Overview 2450
Promoting Safety Across the Life Span 2454
Violence Hazards Across the Life Span 2458
National Patient Safety Goals 2459
Overview 2459
Responsible Sexual Behavior 2461
Overview 2461
Safer Sex 2461
Dating Violence 2461
Appendix A: NANDA-Approved Nursing Diagnoses A-1
Appendix B: Diagnostic Studies B-1
Combined Glossary G-1
Combined Index I-1

SPECIAL FEATURES

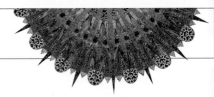

ASSESSMENT

Home Care Assessment Home Hazard Appraisal for Adults 2438

ASSESSMENT INTERVIEW

Learning Needs and Characteristics 2257

CARE SETTINGS

Advocacy in Home Care 2299
Assessing the Home Environment of Older Adults 2020
Preventing Medication Errors in the Home 2442

CLIENT TEACHING

Developing Written Teaching Aids 2258
Preventing Poisoning 2453
Reducing Electrical Hazards 2454
Safety Measures Throughout the Life Span 2455
Sample Teaching Plan for Wound Care 2261
Teaching Clients With Low Literacy Levels 2259
Teaching Tools for Children 2264

CONCEPT MAP

Ineffective Airway Clearance (Gas Exchange) 2095

DEVELOPMENTAL CONSIDERATIONS

Advocating for Safety 2298
Assessing the Pediatric Client 2012
Assessment of Children 2064
Communicating With Children and Adolescents 2155
Communicating With Older Adults 2160
Diagnosis 2076
Establishing Rapport With Children 2176
Evaluation 2101
Health Care Decisions 2042
Instruments for Use With Older Adults 2024
Long-Term Care 2194
Nursing Care Plan 2095

Reporting Abuse or Neglect of an Adult or Older Adult by a Caretaker 2414
Selected Hazards Throughout the Life Span 2434
Sleep Safety for Newborns and Infants 2440
Special Teaching Considerations 2256

EVIDENCE-BASED PRACTICE

Are Education, Experience, and Critical-Thinking Ability Related to Clinical Decision Making? 2044
Attitudes Toward Physician–Nurse Collaboration 2118
Bicycle Helmet Effectiveness and Use 2441
Can Animated Cartoons Increase Knowledge of Educational Information? 2259
Can Clients With Advanced Dementia Participate in a Social Conversation? 2161
Collaborative Health Care for Chronically Ill Older Adults 2117
Does Nursing Documentation Reflect Individualized Client Care? 2199
Does Point-of-Care Nursing Documentation Make a Difference? 2390
Do College Students Use the Internet to Obtain Health Information? 2252
Do the Types of Nurses and Delivery Models in Hospitals Influence Client Outcomes? 2207
How Do Nurses Feel About Abortion Based on the Reasons for Aborting? 2314
How Is Quality Improvement Being Conducted in Nursing Homes? 2430
The Impact of a Sharing Group on the Learning Process 2141
What Are New Nurses' Perceptions of Nursing Practice? 2281
What New Nursing Diagnoses Are Being Researched? 2076

FOCUS ON DIVERSITY AND CULTURE

Acceptable Child Behaviors 2010
Autonomy 2404
Culturally Sensitive Nursing 2029
Examples of Cultures That Value Family Inclusion in Client Teaching 2267
Variations in Applying Moral Principles 2315

The Nursing Domain

Part II contains concepts within the Nursing Domain. These are concepts essential to the practice of nursing and unique to the contributions nurses make to the health care team. Key among these concepts is clinical decision making and caring interventions. These concepts help to build the foundation of nursing practice with the client as the nurse's primary focus while meeting the NLNAC's competencies for nursing graduates.

Concept 32: Assessment

Concept 33: Caring Interventions

Concept 34: Clinical Decision Making

Concept 35: Collaboration

Concept 36: Communication

Concept 37: Managing Care

Concept 38: Professional Behaviors

Concept 39: Teaching and Learning

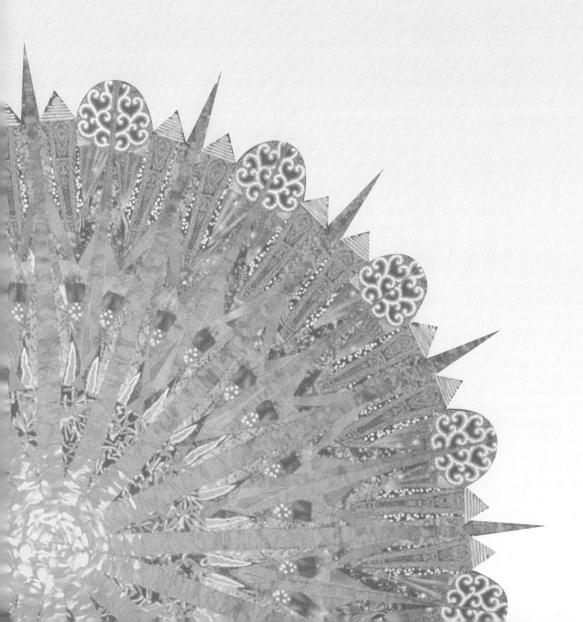

Assessment

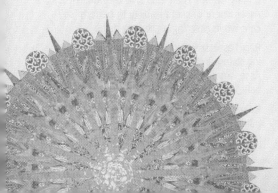

32

Concept at-a-Glance

About Assessment, *1999*

32.1   Holistic Health Assessment Across
        the Life Span, *2008*

Concept Learning Outcomes

After reading about this concept, you will be able to:

1. Describe different types of assessments, indicating the proper use of each.

2. Relate the purposes of conducting a physical examination.

3. Propose actions required when preparing to conduct a physical examination.

4. Discriminate among positions appropriate for examination of different areas of the body.

5. Demonstrate use of each method of examination: inspection, palpation, percussion, and ausculation.

6. Discuss factors required to properly interpret findings from the nursing assessment.

Concept Key Terms

Assessment, *1999*
Auscultation, *2004*
Communication, *2006*
Dullness, *2004*
Duration, *2005*
Flatness, *2004*
Holism, *2006*
Hyperresonance, *2004*
Inspection, *2002*
Intensity, *2005*

Palpation, *2002*
Percussion, *2003*
Pitch, *2004*
Pleximeter, *2004*
Plexor, *2004*
Quality, *2005*
Resonance, *2004*
Tympany, *2004*

About Assessment

Assessment may be defined as a systematic method of collecting data about a client for the purpose of determining the client's current and ongoing health status, predicting risks to health, and identifying health-promoting activities (D'Amico & Barbarito, 2007). The assessment's focus must include the problems presented by the client and the physical, social, cultural, environmental, and emotional factors that impact the overall well-being of the client in relation to the problems presented. Data gathered about the client's health status will include wellness behaviors, illness signs and symptoms, client strengths and weaknesses, and risk factors. The nurse will use a variety of sources to gather the data. Knowledge of the natural and social sciences is a strong foundation for the nurse. Effective communication techniques and use of critical thinking skills are essential in helping the nurse to gather detailed, complete, relevant data needed to formulate a plan of care to meet the needs of the client. Health assessment includes the interview and physical assessment, which must then be documented and interpreted. All future client care is directed by interpretation of findings from data collected throughout the assessment process.

While assessment techniques include observation, interviewing, and physical examination, this concept will focus primarily on physical assessment or examination of the client. Observations and client interviews are discussed in greater detail in Concept 34, Clinical Decision Making.

There are four different types of assessments: initial (or baseline) assessment, problem-focused (or system-specific) assessment, emergency assessment, and ongoing reassessment (see Table 32–1). ●

COLLECTING DATA THROUGH PHYSICAL EXAMINATION

The principal methods used to collect data are observing, interviewing, and examining. Observation occurs whenever the nurse is in contact with the client or support persons. Interviewing is used mainly while taking the nursing health history. Examining is the primary method used in the physical health assessment. All of the collected data must be documented accurately. Documentation is covered in Concept 36, Communication, Exemplar 36.2, Documentation.

The nurse uses all three methods simultaneously when assessing clients. For example, during the client interview the nurse observes, listens, asks questions, and mentally retains information to explore in the physical examination. This concept focuses on the physical examination, also referred to as the physical health assessment. Some nurses consider *assessment* to be the broad term used in applying the nursing process to health data and *examination* to be the physical process used to gather the data. A physical examination can be any of three types: (a) an initial assessment (e.g., when a client is admitted to a health care agency); (b) a system-specific examination (e.g., the cardiovascular system); or (c) an examination of a body area (e.g., the lungs, when difficulty with breathing is observed).

Physical examinations typically reveal normal and abnormal findings. The nurse must analyze both types of findings and make critical decisions regarding their meaning and importance. For example, when admitting the client with a diagnosis of appendicitis, the presence of pain in the right lower quadrant would be a normal finding, while absence of pain would be inconsistent with the diagnosis and might indicate the appendix has ruptured. When findings are different than anticipated, the nurse must make a decision regarding their importance and what to do with the information. If the nurse is unsure about the significance of a finding or to whom it should be reported, the nurse should consult with a more experienced nurse regarding the best course of action to follow. A complete physical examination may be conducted by starting at the head and proceeding in a systematic manner downward (head-to-toe assessment) or by systems (neurological system, respiratory system, etc). Whichever approach is used, the nurse must adapt the examination according to the age of the individual, the severity of the illness, the preferences of the nurse, the environment for the examination, and the agency's policies and procedures. The order of head-to-toe assessment is given in Box 32–1. Regardless of the procedure used, the client's energy level and time constraints need to be considered. The physical assessment is therefore conducted in a systematic and efficient manner that results in the fewest position changes for the client.

Frequently, nurses assess a specific body area instead of the entire body. These specific assessments are made in relation to client complaints, the nurse's observations, the client's presenting problem, nursing interventions provided, and medical therapies. Examples of these situations and assessments are provided in Table 32–2.

These are some of the purposes of the physical examination:
- To obtain baseline data about the client's functional abilities
- To supplement, confirm, or refute data obtained in the nursing history

TABLE 32–1 Types of Assessment

TYPE	TIME PERFORMED	PURPOSE	EXAMPLE
Initial (or baseline) assessment	Performed within specified time frame after admission to a health care agency (refer to agency policy and procedure)	To establish a complete baseline for problem identification, reference, and future comparison	Nursing admission assessment
Problem-focused (or system-specific) assessment	Ongoing process integrated with nursing care	To determine the status of a specific problem identified in an earlier assessment	Hourly assessment of client's fluid intake and urinary output in an intensive care unit (ICU) Assessment of client's ability to perform self-care while assisting a client to bathe
Emergency assessment	During any physiologic or psychologic crisis	To identify life-threatening problems To identify new or overlooked problems	Rapid assessment of a person's airway, breathing status, and circulation during a cardiac arrest Assessment of suicidal tendencies or potential for violence
Ongoing reassessment	Several months after initial assessment	To compare the client's current status to baseline data previously obtained	Reassessment of a client's functional health patterns in a home care or outpatient setting or, in a hospital, at shift change

Box 32–1 Head-to-Toe Framework

- General survey
- Vital signs
- Head
  - Hair, scalp, cranium, face
  - Eyes and vision
  - Ears and hearing
  - Nose and sinuses
  - Mouth and oropharynx
  - Cranial nerves
- Neck
  - Muscles
  - Lymph nodes
  - Trachea
  - Thyroid gland
  - Carotid arteries
  - Neck veins
- Upper extremities
  - Skin and nails
  - Muscle strength and tone
  - Joint range of motion
  - Brachial and radial pulses
  - Biceps tendon reflexes
  - Tendon reflexes
  - Sensation

- Chest and back
  - Skin
  - Chest shape and size
  - Lungs
  - Heart
  - Spinal column
  - Breasts and axillae
- Abdomen
  - Skin
  - Abdominal sounds
  - Specific organs (e.g., liver, bladder)
  - Femoral pulses
- Genitals
  - Testicles
  - Vagina
  - Urethra
- Anus and rectum
- Lower extremities
  - Skin and toenails
  - Gait and balance
  - Joint range of motion
  - Popliteal, posterior tibial, and pedal pulses
  - Tendon and plantar reflexes

- To obtain data that will help establish nursing diagnoses and plans of care
- To evaluate the physiologic outcomes of health care and thus the progress of a client in releation to health problems
- To make clinical judgments about a client's health status
- To identify areas for health promotion and disease prevention.

TABLE 32–2 Nursing Assessments Addressing Selected Client Situations

SITUATION	PHYSICAL ASSESSMENT
Client complains of abdominal pain.	Inspect, auscultate, and palpate the abdomen; assess vital signs.
Client is admitted with a head injury.	Assess level of consciousness using the Glasgow Coma Scale (discussed in Concept 17, Intracranial Regulation); assess pupils for reaction to light and accommodation; assess vital signs.
The nurse prepares to administer a cardiotonic drug to a client.	Assess apical pulse and compare with baseline data.
The client has just had a cast applied to the lower leg.	Assess peripheral perfusion of toes, capillary refill, pedal pulse if accessible, and vital signs.
The client's fluid intake is minimal.	Assess skin turgor, fluid intake and output, and vital signs.

Nurses use national guidelines and evidence-based practice while performing health assessments associated with various conditions. For example, when screening for cancer, nurses should keep in mind the American Cancer Society's guidelines for early detection (ACS, 2010a).

Preparing the Client

Most people need an explanation of the physical examination. Often clients are anxious about what the nurse will find. Nurses provide reassurance by explaining each step of the examination. The nurse should explain when and where the examination will take place, why it is important, and what will happen. The nurse should inform the client that all information gathered and documented during the assessment is kept confidential in accordance with the Health Insurance Portability and Accountability Act (HIPAA). This means that only those health care providers who have a legitimate need to know the client's information will have access to it.

Health examinations are usually painless; however, it is important to determine in advance any positions contraindicated for a particular client. For example, clients having difficulty breathing may experience increased difficulty when lying in a supine position. The nurse assists the client as needed to undress and put on a gown. Clients should empty their bladders before the examination. Doing so helps them feel more relaxed and facilitates palpation of the abdomen and pubic area. If a urinalysis is required, the urine should be collected in a container for that purpose.

Preparing the Environment

It is important to prepare the environment before starting the assessment. The time for the physical assessment should be convenient to both the client and the nurse. The environment should be well-lighted and the equipment organized for efficient use. A client who is physically relaxed will usually experience little discomfort. The room should be warm enough to be comfortable for the client.

Providing privacy is important. Most people are embarrassed if their bodies are exposed or if others can overhear or view them during the assessment. Culture, age, and gender of both the client and the nurse influence how comfortable the client will be and what special arrangements might be needed. For example, if the client and nurse are of different genders, the nurse should ask if it is acceptable to perform the physical examination or if a nurse of the same gender is preferred. Family and friends should not be present unless the client asks for someone.

Positioning

During the physical examination, it may be necessary to ask the client to maintain several positions. The nurse must consider the client's ability to assume each position. The client's physical condition, energy level, and age should also be taken into consideration. Some positions are embarrassing and uncomfortable and therefore should not be maintained for extended periods. By organizing the assessment so that several body areas can be assessed in one position, the nurse can minimize the number of position changes needed and maximize the client's comfort during the assessment (see Table 32–3).

TABLE 32–3 Client Positions and Body Areas Assessed

POSITION	DESCRIPTION	AREAS ASSESSED	CAUTIONS
Dorsal recumbent	Back-lying position with knees flexed and hips externally rotated; small pillow under the head; soles of feet on the surface	Female genitals, rectum, and female reproductive tract	May be contraindicated for clients who have cardiopulmonary problems.
Supine (horizontal recumbent)	Back-lying position with legs extended; with or without pillow under the head	Head, neck, axillae, anterior thorax, lungs, breasts, heart, vital signs, abdomen, extremities, peripheral pulses	Tolerated poorly by clients with cardiovascular and respiratory problems.
Sitting	A seated position, back unsupported and legs hanging freely	Head, neck, posterior and anterior thorax, lungs, breasts, axillae, heart, vital signs, upper and lower extremities, reflexes	Older adults and weak clients may require support.
Lithotomy	Back-lying position with feet supported in stirrups; the hips should be in line with the edge of the table	Female genitals, rectum, and female reproductive tract	May be uncomfortable and tiring for older adults and embarrassing for most clients.
Sims	Side-lying position with lowermost arm behind the body, uppermost leg flexed at hip and knee, upper arm flexed at shoulder and elbow	Rectum, vagina	Difficult for older adults and people with limited joint movement.
Prone	Lies on abdomen with head turned to the side, with or without a small pillow	Posterior thorax, hip joint movement	Often not tolerated by older adults and people with cardiovascular and respiratory problems.

Methods of Examining

Four primary techniques are used in the physical examination: inspection, palpation, percussion, and auscultation. Each requires practice to develop expertise.

INSPECTION Inspection is visual examination or assessing by using the sense of sight. The process should be deliberate, purposeful, and systematic. The nurse inspects with the naked eye and with a lighted instrument such as an otoscope (used to view the ear). In addition to visual observations, olfactory (smell) and auditory (hearing) cues are noted. Nurses frequently use visual inspection to assess moisture, color, and texture of body surfaces, as well as shape, position, size, color, and symmetry of the body. Lighting must be sufficient for the nurse to see clearly; either natural or artificial light can be used. When using the auditory senses it is important to have a quiet environment. Observation can be combined with the other assessment techniques.

PALPATION Palpation is the examination of the body using the sense of touch. The pads of the fingers are used because their concentration of nerve endings makes them highly sensitive to tactile discrimination. Palpation is used to determine the following characteristics:

- Texture (e.g., of the hair)
- Temperature (e.g., of a skin area)
- Vibration (e.g., of a joint)
- Position, size, consistency, and mobility of organs or masses
- Distention (e.g., of the urinary bladder)
- Pulsation
- The presence of pain upon touch or palpation.

There are two types of palpation: light and deep. *Light (superficial) palpation* should always precede *deep palpation* because heavy pressure on the fingertips can dull the sense of touch. For light palpation, the nurse extends the dominant hand's fingers parallel to the skin surface and presses gently

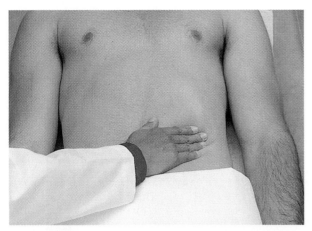

Figure 32–1 ■ The position of the hand for light palpation.

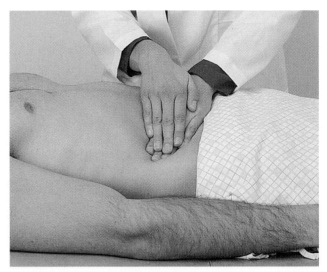

Figure 32–2 ■ The position of the hands for deep bimanual palpation.

while moving the hand in a circle (see Figure 32–1 ■). With light palpation, the skin is slightly depressed. If it is necessary to determine the details of a mass, the nurse presses lightly several times rather than holding the pressure. See Box 32–2 for the characteristics of masses.

Deep palpation is done with one hand or with two hands (bimanually). In deep bimanual palpation, the nurse extends the dominant hand as for light palpation, then places the finger pads of the nondominant hand on the dorsal surface of the distal interphalangeal joint of the middle three fingers of the dominant hand (Figure 32–2 ■). The top hand applies pressure while the lower hand remains relaxed to perceive the tactile sensations. For deep palpation using one hand, the finger pads of the dominant hand press over the area to be palpated. Often the other hand is used to support a mass or organ from below (Figure 32–3 ■). Deep palpation is usually not done during a routine examination and requires significant practitioner skill. It is performed with extreme caution because pressure can damage internal organs. Deep palpation is usually not indicated in clients who have acute abdominal pain or pain that is not yet diagnosed.

To test skin temperature, the nurse should use the dorsal aspect (back) of the hand and fingers where the skin is thinnest. To test for vibration, the nurse should use the palmar surface of the hand. General guidelines for palpation include the following:

- The nurse's hands should be clean and warm, and the fingernails short.
- Areas of tenderness should be palpated last.
- Deep palpation should be done after superficial palpation.

Box 32–2 **Characteristics of Masses**

Location—Site on the body, dorsal/ventral surface
Size—Length and width in centimeters
Shape—Oval, round, elongated, irregular
Consistency—Soft, firm, hard
Surface—Smooth, nodular
Mobility—Fixed, mobile
Pulsatility—Present or absent
Tenderness—Degree of tenderness to palpation

The effectiveness of palpation depends largely on the client's level of relaxation. Nurses can assist a client to relax by (a) gowning and/or draping the client appropriately, (b) positioning the client comfortably, and (c) ensuring that their own hands are warm before beginning. During palpation, the nurse should be sensitive to the client's verbal and nonverbal communication indicating discomfort.

PERCUSSION **Percussion** is the act of striking the body surface to elicit sounds that can be heard or vibrations that can be felt. There are two types of percussion: direct and indirect. In *direct percussion*, the nurse strikes the area to be percussed directly with the pads of two, three, or four fingers or with the pad of the middle finger. The strikes are rapid, and the movement is from the wrist (see Figure 32–4 ■).

Indirect percussion refers to the striking of an object (e.g., a finger) held against the body area to be examined. In this technique, the middle finger of the nondominant hand,

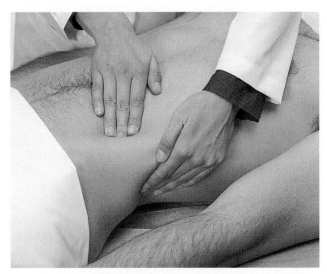

Figure 32–3 ■ Deep palpation using the lower hand to support the body while the upper hand palpates the organ.

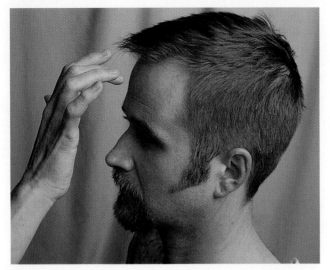

Figure 32–4 ■ Direct percussion. Using one hand to strike the surface of the body.

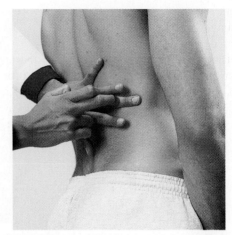

Figure 32–5 ■ Indirect percussion. Using the finger of one hand to tap the finger of the other hand.

referred to as the **pleximeter**, is placed firmly on the client's skin. Only the distal phalanx and joint of this finger should be in contact with the skin. Using the tip of the flexed middle finger of the other hand, called the **plexor**, the nurse strikes the pleximeter, usually at the distal interphalangeal joint (see Figure 32–5 ■). Some nurses may find a point between the distal and proximal joints to be a more comfortable pleximeter point. The motion comes from the wrist; the forearm remains stationary. The angle between the plexor and the pleximeter should be 90 degrees, and the blows must be firm, rapid, and short to obtain a clear sound.

Percussion is used to determine the size and shape of internal organs by establishing their borders. It indicates whether tissue is fluid filled, air filled, or solid. Percussion elicits five types of sound: flatness, dullness, resonance, hyperresonance, and tympany. **Flatness** is an extremely dull sound produced by very dense tissue, such as muscle or bone. **Dullness** is a thudlike sound produced by dense tissue such as the liver, spleen, or heart. **Resonance** is a hollow sound, such as that produced by lungs filled with air. **Hyperresonance** is not produced in the normal body. It is described as booming that can be heard over an emphysematous lung. **Tympany** is a musical or drumlike sound produced from an air-filled stomach. On a continuum, flatness reflects the most dense tissue (the least amount of air) and tympany the least dense tissue (the greatest amount of air). A percussion sound is described according to its intensity, pitch, duration, and quality (see Table 32–4).

AUSCULTATION **Auscultation** is the process of listening to sounds produced within the body. Auscultation may be direct or indirect. *Direct auscultation* is the use of the unaided ear, for example, to listen to a respiratory wheeze or the grating of a moving joint. *Indirect auscultation* refers to the use of a stethoscope, which transmits the sounds to the nurse's ears. A stethoscope is used primarily to listen to sounds from within the body, such as bowel sounds or valve sounds of the heart and blood pressure.

The stethoscope tubing should be 30–35 cm (12–14 in.) long, with an internal diameter of about 0.3 cm (1/8 in.). The earpieces of the stethoscope should fit comfortably into the nurse's ears, facing forward. The amplifier of the stethoscope is placed firmly but lightly against the client's skin.

PRACTICE ALERT

If the client has excessive hair, it may be necessary to dampen the hairs with a moist cloth so that they will lie flat against the skin and not interfere with clear sound transmission.

Auscultated sounds are described according to their pitch, intensity, duration, and quality. The **pitch** is the frequency of

TABLE 32–4 Percussion Sounds and Tones

SOUND	INTENSITY	PITCH	DURATION	QUALITY	EXAMPLE OF LOCATION
Flatness	Soft	High	Short	Extremely dull	Muscle, bone
Dullness	Medium	Medium	Moderate	Thudlike	Liver, heart
Resonance	Loud	Low	Long	Hollow	Normal lung
Hyperresonance	Very loud	Very low	Very long	Booming	Emphysematous lung
Tympany	Loud	High (distinguished mainly by musical timbre)	Moderate	Musical	Stomach filled with gas (air)

the vibrations (the number of vibrations per second). Low-pitched sounds, such as some heart sounds, have fewer vibrations per second than high-pitched sounds, such as bronchial sounds. The **intensity** (amplitude) refers to the loudness or softness of a sound. Some body sounds are loud, for example, bronchial sounds heard from the trachea; others are soft, for example, normal breath sounds heard in the lungs. The **duration** of a sound is its length (long or short). The **quality** of sound is a subjective description of a sound, for example, whistling, gurgling, or snapping.

Equipment

The physical examination requires use of common health care tools such as the stethoscope, penlight, gloves, or water-soluble lubricant. The nurse determines what equipment will be required for the specific examination to be performed, and collects the supplies in advance to avoid extending the length of time required of the client. Warm equipment that will touch the client's skin. All equipment should be cleaned according to the recommendations for each instrument after each use. Table 32–5 describes some of the most commonly used tools.

TABLE 32–5 Tools Used for a Health Examination

SUPPLIES		PURPOSE
Flashlight or penlight		To assist viewing of the pharynx and cervix or to determine the reactions of the pupils of the eye
Nasal speculum		To permit visualization of the lower and middle turbinates; usually, a penlight is used for illumination
Ophthalmoscope		A lighted instrument to visualize the interior of the eye
Otoscope		A lighted instrument to visualize the eardrum and external auditory canal (a nasal speculum may be attached to the otoscope to inspect the nasal cavities)
Percussion (reflex) hammer		An instrument with a rubber head to test reflexes
Tuning fork		A two-pronged metal instrument used to test hearing acuity and vibratory sense
Vaginal speculum		To assess the cervix and the vagina
Cotton applicators		To obtain specimens
Gloves		To protect the nurse and the client
Lubricant		To ease insertion of instruments (e.g., vaginal speculum)
Tongue blades (depressors)		To depress the tongue during assessment of the mouth and pharynx

INTERPRETING FINDINGS FROM THE ASSESSMENT PROCESS

Interpreting findings requires making determinations about all of the data collected in the health assessment process. The nurse must

- determine whether the findings fall within normal and expected ranges in relation to the client's age, gender, and race.
- determine the significance of the findings in relation to the client's health status and immediate and long-range health-related needs.

Interpretation of findings is influenced by a number of factors. These factors include the ability to obtain, recall, and apply knowledge; to communicate effectively; and to use a holistic approach.

Knowledge

Nurses obtain, recall, and apply knowledge from physical and social sciences, nursing theory, and all areas of research that impact current nursing practice. An example of nursing knowledge includes human anatomy and physiology and the differences that are associated with growth and development across the life span as well as characteristics specific to gender and race. Knowledge also reflects health-related and health care trends in groups and populations, such as the increased incidence of risk factors or actual illnesses in certain groups or populations. For example, in the United States one trend is the increased incidence of obesity in children and adults.

Nurses must be able to access and use reliable resources in interpretation of findings. Resources include research; scientific literature; and charts, scales, and graphs to indicate ranges of norms and expectations about physical and psychological development. Examples include Denver Developmental scores, mental status examinations, weight, body mass index, and growth charts prepared by centers for health statistics. Additionally, nurses must be able to communicate effectively, to think critically, to recognize and act on client cues, to incorporate a holistic perspective, and to determine the significance of data in meeting immediate and long-term client needs.

Expectations about interpretation of findings change as one gains skills and experience in nursing practice and with advanced practice education. The nurse must be able to recognize situations that require immediate attention, initiate care, and seek appropriate assistance.

A nursing student is expected to recall and apply knowledge to discriminate between normal and abnormal findings and use resources to understand the findings in relation to wellness or illness for a particular client. For example, consider the findings from the assessment of Julie Connor, a 12-year-old girl: asymmetrical shoulders and elevated right scapula on inspection of the posterior thorax, right lateral curvature of thoracic spine on palpation of vertebrae. Normally, scapulae should be symmetrical and the vertebrae should be aligned. The findings are interpreted as a deviation from the normal. They do not, however, give sufficient information for the purposes of making nursing diagnoses. More data is necessary to make diagnoses and design a plan of care for Julie.

The nurse gains confidence and ability to discriminate between normal and abnormal findings through experience and continuing education. With such experience, the nurse will learn to recognize patterns that predispose individuals to illness or are indicative of specific illnesses, and implement and evaluate appropriate nursing care. Consider the following findings from the assessment of James Long, a 46-year-old African American male: height 5'9", weight 220 lb, BP 156/94, mother died at age 62 from cerebrovascular accident (stroke), father died at age 42 from myocardial infarction (heart attack). Using knowledge of normal ranges of findings for vital signs, height, and weight, the nurse interprets his BP and weight results as abnormal findings: They indicate that Mr. Long has high blood pressure and is obese. The nurse applies knowledge of trends associated with health problems to interpret the significance of the findings for this client. The nurse knows that hypertension occurs more frequently in African American males than in Caucasians and that family history of coronary artery disease, hypertension, and obesity increase the risk of both acquiring hypertension and the complications associated with it. By combining knowledge of risk factors and complications with the findings themselves, the nurse working with Mr. Long can develop a plan of care in collaboration with other health care professionals to address Mr. Long's need to reduce his weight and blood pressure.

Communication

Effective communication is essential to the assessment process. **Communication** refers to the exchange of information, feelings, thoughts, and ideas. A variety of verbal techniques, such as open-ended or closed questions, statements, clarification, and rephrasing, are just a few of the techniques used to gather information. The communication techniques must incorporate regard for the individual in relation to the purposes of the data collection, the client's age, and the level of anxiety. In addition, the nurse must use techniques that accommodate language differences or difficulties, cultural influences, cognitive ability, affect, demeanor, and special needs. Communication is discussed in greater detail in Concept 36.

Holistic Approach

A holistic approach is an essential characteristic of nursing practice. **Holism** can best be defined as considering more than the physiological health status of a client. Holism includes all factors that impact the client's physical and emotional well-being. With a holistic approach, the nurse recognizes that developmental, psychological, emotional, family, cultural, and environmental factors will affect immediate and long-term actual and potential health goals, problems, and plans.

Developmental Factors

The client's developmental level impacts the health assessment. Sources of information may vary depending on the client's age and ability to communicate his or her symptoms. For clients with disabilities, findings must be interpreted according to the assessed developmental level, not the client's age. Parents or guardians are the primary sources for information about children and clients with disabilities or impairments that affect their ability to communicate. The developmental level of the client also influences the approach to assessment, including the words and terminology. For example, assessment of a pregnant adolescent would be different from that of a 38-year-old woman pregnant for the third time.

Psychological and Emotional Factors

Psychological and emotional factors impact physiological health and must be considered as predisposing or contributing factors when interpreting findings from a health assessment. One needs only to recall that anxiety triggers an autonomic response resulting in increased pulse and blood pressure to understand that relationship. Conversely, physical problems can impact emotional health. For example, childhood obesity can lead to problems with self-esteem and can impact socialization and development. Psychological problems such as anxiety and depression may interfere with the client's ability to fully participate in health assessment. Grieving may limit one's ability to carry out required health practices or recognize health problems.

Family Factors

Nurses must consider family history of illness or health problems in conducting a health assessment and interpreting findings. Individuals with a family history of some illnesses are considered at high risk for contracting those diseases. For example, having a first-degree relative (mother, sister, or daughter) with breast cancer about doubles a woman's risk of developing breast cancer herself (American Cancer Society, 2010b). Nurses must recognize that family dynamics may influence one's approach to health care. In some families, health-related decisions are not made independently, but rather by the family leader or by group consensus. Circumstances within families can impact both physical and emotional health and must be considered as part of health assessment. For example, children of alcoholics are not only at risk for alcoholism, but also at risk for emotional issues not encountered by other children; therefore, one must view and interpret unexpected physical or emotional behaviors in relation to the alcoholic family situation.

Cultural Factors

Cultural factors must be considered when collecting data and interpreting findings. Culture impacts language, expression, emotional and physical well-being, and health practices. Findings regarding physical and emotional health must be interpreted in relation to the cultural norms for the client. For example, many Asian cultures would not consider lack of eye contact during the interview as a lack of ability to interact, depression, or a problem with attention. Nurses must take care to provide clear explanations of abnormal findings, illnesses, and treatments because views of illness, causality, and treatment may have cultural influences. Refer to Concept 6, Culture, for more information on cultural considerations.

Environmental Factors

Internal and external environmental factors impact health assessment and interpretation of findings. Nurses must always consider data in relation to norms and expectation for age,

race, and gender, and in relation to factors impacting the individual client. The nurse should gather and record carefully all the information from the health history, focused interview, and physical assessment before beginning to interpret any of the data.

Data from the comprehensive health assessment provide cues about the client's internal environment, including emotional state, response to medication and treatment, and physiological or anatomical alterations that influence findings and interpretation. For example, the finding from the assessment of Mrs. Bernice Hall, a 49-year-old woman, is that she has dark, almost black, formed stools. This would be considered an abnormal finding since the normal finding would be brown-colored stools. During her health history, however, Mrs. Hall states that she has taken iron pills and eaten a lot of spinach and greens for years, and she reports that her stools are always dark and formed. Considering the internal environment of medication and diet, both of which darken the stool, the nurse interprets this as a normal finding for Mrs. Hall.

External environmental factors can also impact health, health assessment, and interpretation of findings. External factors may include any of the following:

- Inhaled toxins such as smoke, chemicals, and fumes
- Irritants that can be inhaled, ingested, or absorbed through the skin
- Noise, light, and motion
- Objects or substances encountered in the home, school, or workplace, such as animal dander or dust.

Consider the assessment of Martha Whitman, a 22-year-old woman complaining of back pain. The findings from the physical assessment are all within normal limits. Ms Whitman states that the pain started 2 weeks ago and has been getting worse with temporary relief from aspirin. Before referring this client for diagnostic studies, the nurse considers external environmental factors that may contribute to the back pain. The nurse asks about any activities or events associated with the onset of the pain. Ms Whitman reveals that she had taken up quilting about 2 weeks ago; she has been sitting and working with an embroidery hoop almost every day for an hour or so. The additional information assists the nurse in interpretation of the back pain. The nurse recommends ways to sit and perform the quilting without straining the muscles of the back and will follow up to see if this relieves the pain.

As another example, consider the assessment of a toddler with nausea and vomiting. The nurse must consider gathering information about the circumstances surrounding the onset of the problem. For example, was the child in a new environment in which he or she could have ingested medications, cleaning fluids, or other toxic substances?

NURSING PRACTICE

Nursing care always begins with assessment. Nurses should not develop a plan of care or initiate any intervention without first assessing the client. It is also essential that that nurse document findings in the client's medical record as soon as possible.

Nursing care is based on a strong knowledge base and the application of critical thinking. The knowledge base of the professional nurse is developed over time using information from the humanities and the biological, natural, and social sciences. Using evidence-based research data, standards of care, and the nursing process, the professional nurse provides competent care. Competent care includes promoting health and wellness, treating and caring for the ill, and caring for the dying individual while being supportive to family members. To perform these actions, the nurse works in a variety of settings including hospitals, clinics, nursing homes, clients' homes, schools, and workplaces.

Regardless of the setting, the role of the professional nurse is multifaceted. Each situation requires the professional nurse to use critical thinking and the nursing process. To provide care and utilize the nursing process, the professional nurse must develop strong assessment skills. The gathering of complete, accurate, and relevant data is required. While gathering the subjective and objective data from the client, the nurse must be attuned to the signs, symptoms, behaviors, and cues offered by the client. The collected data varies as the status of the client changes. The professional nurse functions as a teacher, caregiver, client advocate, and manager of client care.

REVIEW Assessment

RELATE: LINK THE CONCEPTS

Linking the concept of Assessment with the concept of Caring Interventions:

1. You are assigned to care for a client who has been receiving tube feedings via a nasogastric tube that has been in place for several days. Prior to administering the first tube feeding of the shift, what assessments would you perform?
2. Would the assessment performed be an initial assessment or a problem-focused assessment? Explain your answer.

Linking the concept of Assessment with the concept of Clinical Decision Making:

1. You are assigned care of a 46-year-old man admitted for status asthmaticus. His condition has stabilized and discharge is planned for tomorrow. When you enter his room for the first time you find he is short of breath and requesting you hand him his inhaler, which the doctor ordered to be kept at the bedside for self-administration as needed. What will you do first?
2. What critical thinking would you apply to the above situation?

READY: GO TO COMPANION SKILLS MANUAL

■ See all skills in Nursing Skills, Chapter 11

REFER: GO TO MYNURSINGKIT

REFLECT: CASE STUDY

Mary Wong is a 19-year-old college freshman living in the dormitory. She has come to the University Health Center with the following complaints: nausea, vomiting, abdominal pain increasing in severity, diarrhea, a fever, and dry mouth. She tells the nurse, "I have had abdominal pain for about 12 hours with nausea, vomiting, and diarrhea." She says that these symptoms "all started after supper in the student cafeteria on campus."

The nurse conducts an interview and follows it with a physical examination that reveals the following: symmetrical abdomen, bowel sounds in all quadrants, tender to palpation in the lower quadrants, guarding. Ms. Wong's skin is warm and moist, her lips and mucous membranes are dry.

1. Classify the findings as objective or subjective data.
2. Prepare a narrative nursing note from the data.
3. What factors must be considered in conducting the comprehensive health assessment of Ms. Wong?
4. Prior to developing a nursing diagnosis, what must the nurse do?

32.1 HOLISTIC HEALTH ASSESSMENT ACROSS THE LIFE SPAN

KEY TERMS

Centration, 2015
Hydrocephalus, 2014
Overnutrition, 2009
Undernutrition, 2010

BASIS FOR SELECTION OF EXEMPLAR

NLN Competencies
Standards of Nursing Practice

LEARNING OUTCOMES

After reading about this exemplar, you will be able to:

1. Correlate the role and impact of development on the nursing assessment, including the physical examination and interview for client history.
2. Differentiate how assessment of children varies from assessment of adults.
3. Propose differences in procedures when assessing a client in each stage of development.
4. Correlate specific health assessment needs with each stage of the life span.
5. Differentiate the needs of the older adult as related to the health assessment.

OVERVIEW

Nursing assessment requires the ability to interpret how the complex interactions of heredity; environment; and physiological, cognitive, and psychological development affect an individual at a particular time. By developing an image of what is usual or expected of children and adults of various ages, the nurse has a basis for a comparison with the norm. This knowledge and an understanding of individual variations provide a foundation for assessment that helps individuals attain their maximum level of wellness.

SPECIAL CONSIDERATIONS FOR ASSESSMENT OF CHILDREN

Children are not "little adults." Significant differences exist between infants, children, adolescents, and adults. These differences include variations in physiology, development, and cognition that must be incorporated into the nursing assessment.

The head-to-toe approach to physical assessment is useful in many situations and with different types of clients, but it may not work with young children. Adults and adolescents will usually sit on an examination table, wear a paper gown, and follow the nurse's instructions. However, infants and toddlers often refuse to sit still or cooperate.

Young children do not have the cognitive or verbal ability to describe symptoms or comply with complex instructions. Nurses must possess strong assessment skills in order to overcome the communication and situational challenges involved in pediatric physical assessment.

When assessing children, it may be helpful to conduct the nutrition history portion before the physical assessment in order to establish rapport and make the child more comfortable with the process. Rapport is essential, especially when assessing an adolescent. Infants and younger children need a caretaker present to assist with the assessment and to answer questions (Figure 32–6 ■). Adolescents may be more comfortable having privacy during the assessment. The nurse may discuss the assessment arrangement with the adolescent and caregiver separately to allow the adolescent to give an unpressured answer. A caregiver can be interviewed separately if appropriate.

The parameters of the physical assessment in children include anthropometric measurements and clinical observations appropriate for each child's age. Determination of developmental milestones provides critical information and is part of a complete assessment. Developmental milestones are covered in Concept 7, Development.

Anthropometric measurements in children should be obtained using equipment appropriate for the pediatric population. Recumbent length and weight measurements are needed in the infant and young child. Weight should be measured without a diaper. Older children can have their height and weight measured while standing. Skinfold measurements should be done using calipers calibrated to 0.2 mm since small changes in measurement can cause changes in assessment classification. The World Health Organization (WHO) recommends weight for height as the standard in measuring children since skinfold and circumference measurements are prone to errors that could result in misclassification of nutritional health. Head circumference is a measurement unique for assessing growth in children at or under 3 years of age. Beyond age 3, head circumference is not a valid tool to assess growth and nutritional status.

Anthropometric measurements have age-specific references established by the Centers for Disease Control (CDC) and WHO. In children under 20 years of age, references are described using charts with age-specific percentiles for height, weight, body mass index (BMI), and, for children under 36 months, head circumference. Percentiles are used to assess growth rate and health of weight for height. Percentile charts are derived from

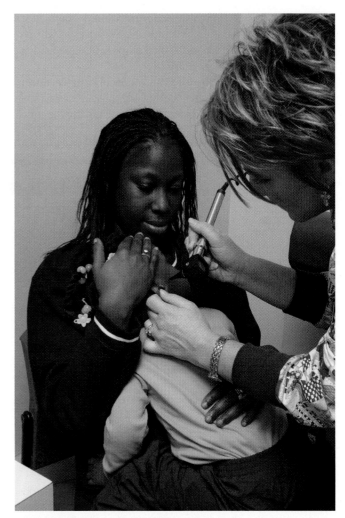

Figure 32–6 ■ It is often helpful to have a young child sit on his or her mother's lap when possible during the assessment.

the distribution of data from population studies and are age- and gender-specific descriptions of anthropometric measurements. Newer infant growth charts are more representative of the population-matched prevalence of breastfed infants compared to charts published before 2000. Breastfed infants normally grow at a slightly slower rate than formula-fed babies do.

Infants, children, and adolescents can be compared to their age-matched peers to determine their individual percentile within the population. A best use of percentile charts is in monitoring individual growth over time. Normally, children will remain within a narrow percentile range for each measurement over the course of childhood. For example, a child assessed sequentially in the 25th percentile for height (length) for age may have a small frame and parents with small stature and may not be at risk for poor nutritional health. A child sequentially in the 50th percentile for height for age who drops to the 25th percentile may be at risk for undernutrition. A significant drop or increase in percentile category is cause for further investigation to assess for undernutrition or overnutrition. Overweight and obesity (**overnutrition**) in children is defined as BMI for age greater than the 85th percentile and the

95th percentile, respectively. **Undernutrition** is defined as BMI for age less than the 5th percentile. Separate growth references exist for children with some chronic diseases and for knee-height estimates of stature.

Children are physically different from adults. Each concept in the individual domain (Concepts 1–31) discusses life span differences that can be anticipated when conducting the physical examination.

Nurses should use a caring, supportive, yet firm approach with children. Whenever possible, play should be incorporated into the assessment process. It is helpful to allow children to touch and manipulate equipment. Adhesive bandages or empty syringes can be provided for playacting with dolls. Nurses should encourage children to talk about their fears and concerns. Painful procedures should not be performed while a child is seated on a parent's lap. Children need to

---

FOCUS ON DIVERSITY AND CULTURE Acceptable Child Behaviors

Most of the world's cultures value children. However, there is significant variation among cultures with respect to what constitutes acceptable child behavior and expectations for health or caregiving. Nurses must be aware of the cultural influences on children and families. For example, European cultures encourage independence at an early age whereas other groups, such as Asians, Hispanics, and Arab Americans, stress a strong commitment to family. Commonly, children from these cultural groups are taught to respect elder family members and to place the needs of the family before their personal needs. Hispanics and Native Americans tend to be less strict with their children, especially with male children.

All of the dominant American cultures view mothers as the primary child caregivers. Overall, females are viewed as nurturers who are responsible for guiding and caring for children. It is common for mothers to make the decisions regarding home care of child illness and complaints. However, many groups, including Arab Americans, have patriarchal hierarchies where the father must be consulted prior to any professional health care decisions.

AFRICAN AMERICAN
- Newborns may have pustular melanosis, characterized by pustules that rupture to leave 2- to 3 mm brown macules. These brown marks will disappear spontaneously within 3–4 months.
- Hair texture will become coarser with tighter curls over the first 6 months of life.
- Mongolian spots are commonly located over the lower back and buttocks; they will begin to fade by age 2 or 3.
- Infants should be tested for sickle cell anemia at birth.
- Most are born with dark gray-brown eyes that will not change much as the baby gets older.
- Hypertension and insulin-resistant diabetes are more common in African American youth.

ASIAN
- As a sign of respect, many Asian parents may be reluctant to disagree with or displease a health care provider.
- Direct eye contact may be viewed as impolite.
- Mongolian spots are common.
- Most infants have dark gray eye color at birth.
- Vietnamese families believe the head is sacred. The nurse should avoid touching the head of the mother and baby without first asking permission.
- Chinese practice cupping, where a heated cup is placed over the skin to draw out illness. Vietnamese use coin rubbing, where a coin is rubbed on the trunk. Neither practice should be considered abuse.
- Many Asian families use the concept of hot and cold illnesses. Certain illnesses are considered to be hot or cold, and treatments should counter the effect of the illness. Therefore, hot illnesses should be treated with cold medicines and foods, whereas cold illnesses should be treated with hot medicines and foods.

HISPANIC
- Most infants have dark gray-brown eye color at birth.
- Mongolian spots are common.
- Infants should be tested for sickle cell anemia at birth.
- Many Mexican Americans consider it bad luck for a person to touch a child's head.
- Many Hispanic families use the concept of hot and cold illnesses. Certain illnesses are considered to be hot or cold, and treatments should counter the effect of the illness. Therefore, hot illnesses should be treated with cold medicines and foods, whereas cold illnesses should be treated with hot medicines and foods.
- Modesty may be important and should be respected.
- Some groups believe that complimenting a child without touching him or her can cause the "evil eye."
- Many consider fat to be healthy, especially in women and young children.

NATIVE AMERICAN
- Many Native Americans have strong beliefs that children should be allowed to develop at their own rate. Parents may be reluctant to force a child to stop bottle or pacifier use or to start toilet training.
- Mongolian spots are common.
- Hypothyroidism is more common in Native Americans (1 in 700). Newborn testing and vigilance for symptoms of hypothyroidism are recommended.
- It is taboo to purchase any clothing or items for the newborn prior to birth. This varies from the Western culture.
- Hypertension and insulin-resistant diabetes are more common in Native American youth.
- Direct eye contact may be avoided as a sign of respect.

MIDDLE EASTERN
- Direct eye contact may be viewed as impolite or improper, especially with members of the opposite sex.
- Physical examination by individuals of different gender is taboo after adolescence.
- Thalassemias are more common in children of Middle Eastern heritage than in children of European descent.
- Modesty may be important and should be respected.
- Females may defer to the male head of the family for health care decisions.

ALL RACES AND CULTURES
- Babies within all races and cultures are born with lighter, pinker skin. The true color of the baby will develop over the first year.
- All cultures and ethnic groups have folk beliefs that center around childbirth and child rearing. The nurse should assess for positive folk practices and incorporate them into nursing care.

know they are safe from painful experiences when they are with their parents.

When a child is ill, parents suffer from increased stress that results from interrupted sleep, concern for the child's well-being, and frustration at the inability to understand what is hurting or bothering their child. Each of these factors may impact a parent's ability to recall information or to follow complex instructions. Nurses can help parents by providing them with written instructions as appropriate and encouraging clients and families to journal their experiences or keep a notebook with information and details about the child's illness and treatment, including nutrition and activity levels. Nurses should consider parental stress levels when developing care plans.

The basic components of a health history are the same whether the nurse works with children or adults. However, a number of variations must be incorporated into the pediatric health history. It is essential that the nurse determine the relationship between the child who seeks health care and the adult who presents with the child. One must never assume legal or family ties between children and adults who accompany them. Nannies, babysitters, friends, siblings, and stepparents often transport children to health care appointments. State law determines which individuals can legally consent to medical treatment of a minor child. Federal privacy laws limit access to protected health information. Directly questioning relationships is the easiest way to ensure compliance with the legal and ethical concerns regarding the medical treatment of children.

Many children are nonverbal or possess limited language ability; therefore, nurses depend on parents and guardians for health history information. This can limit the specificity of the history information. However, it is important to ask preschoolers and older children about their chief complaint and symptoms even though the information they provide may not be as detailed as the information provided by their parents or guardians.

The nurse should determine if the parent is stressed or distracted prior to the health interview. Many parents of ill children are sleep deprived because of their child's altered sleep patterns. Sleep deprivation can result in altered recall, limited ability to follow complex questions, and diminished ability to remember verbal instructions. The presence of other children can be distracting, especially if the children are loud, active, or irritable. Nurses can distract energetic or fussy children with books, crayons, or toys.

The nurse should listen carefully to the parent or primary caregiver and use open-ended questions to elicit health information. Parents know their children better than anyone else. They are able to detect subtle differences in their child's behavior. It is essential to pay special attention to the chief complaints that parents describe. A thorough physical assessment is then conducted based on the issues and concerns raised in the health history.

The nurse should call the child by his or her name and use words that the child understands. For example, most preadolescents are not familiar with the word *abdomen*, but most children use the word *tummy* or *belly* from infancy. Instead of asking "Does your head hurt?" the nurse should ask the child to touch the head where it hurts. It is necessary to be patient. Children often pause between words or repeat phrases when they are excited or nervous.

Nurses should give children who are at least 10 years old the option of being examined without their parents present. The client is the child, not the parent. The nurse's legal and ethical responsibility is to the child first. The nurse must respect the confidentiality of the information provided by older children and be aware of state and federal laws regarding parental notification. The parent and the child should be told what the nurse can and cannot keep confidential. For example, statements like "What you and I talk about will be between the two of us, unless you tell me that you are thinking about harming yourself or someone else, or if you tell me that someone is hurting you" help establish rapport and boundaries to the nurse–child and nurse–parent relationship. If a nurse is required to report health interview information to others (e.g., public health departments or child protective service agents), the nurse should always inform the child of the need to share the information with others prior to actually doing so. Failure to do so can jeopardize the rapport between nurse and child.

There are many ways to make the examination tolerable. Allowing children to touch medical equipment is one (Figure 32–7 ■). For example, the nurse can ask a young child to put the otoscope's "hat" (i.e., speculum) on the light. Before examining the tympanic membrane, the nurse can ask toddlers and preschoolers if they have elephants or cartoon characters in their ear. Young children can be encouraged to take deep breaths by having them blow bubbles or blow out

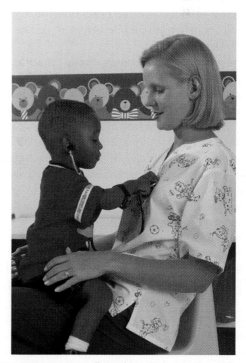

Figure 32–7 ■ A nurse allows her client to play with with her stethoscope before using it to assess his heart.

DEVELOPMENTAL CONSIDERATIONS **Assessing the Pediatric Client**

- Protect the modesty and privacy of children as you would for adults.
- Explain procedures and techniques in words that are understandable for children.
- Remember that young children are more comfortable and compliant when they sit on their parents' laps.
- Establish rapport with the parent and child before initiating any physical examination.
- Begin with the least threatening examinations; a flexible approach to assessment is essential.

- Perform painful or invasive procedures at the end of the assessment.
- Auscultate the thorax of the sleeping child.
- Allow children to touch equipment. Use games for examinations, such as asking children if they have elephants in their ears before examining the tympanic membrane.
- Use toys, for example, finger puppets, as distractions.
- Use standard precautions.

the light on the otoscope. Distracting children with toys is another way to make the assessment less frightening. Examples include finger puppets, small animals placed on the stethoscope, and whistles or small music boxes. Keep toys with small pieces out of the reach of infants, toddlers, and preschoolers.

ASSESSMENT SPECIFIC TO STAGES OF THE LIFE SPAN

A comprehensive assessment includes information about physical, cognitive, and emotional growth and development including both subjective and objective data. When conducting health assessments, the professional nurse must be able to obtain accurate data and interpret findings in relation to expectations and predicted norms and ranges for clients at various stages of physical and emotional development. Knowledge of anatomical and physiological changes as well as theoretical information about cognitive, psychoanalytic, and psychosocial events and expectations at each stage of human development are invaluable resources for the professional nurse. Further information about growth and development can be found in Concept 7, Development.

Physical growth and development change across the age span. Stages from infancy through adolescence are marked by spurts of rapid growth and development. Health assessment includes the use of clinical growth charts to index individual client measurements of height and weight (and head circumference in infants) as expected normal values for age and gender. Additional indicators for normal growth and development throughout these stages include eating, sleeping, elimination, and activity patterns. Neurologic and sensory functions are assessed by monitoring development of speech and language, muscular growth, strength and coordination, and tactile sensibility.

Puberty is a period of rapid physiological growth and development. Puberty occurs between the ages of 10 and 14 years in females and is marked by menarche, breast development, axillary and pubic hair growth, and a spurt in height. In males, puberty occurs between the ages of 12 and 16 years and is characterized by a spurt in height, development of the penis and testicles, and body hair growth (axillae, chest, facial) and presence of pubic hair. Young adulthood is the stage marked by completed growth in physical and mental structures. Physical development continues to be assessed by comparing individual findings to clinical growth charts and by assessing eating, sleeping, and activity patterns.

Middle age, occurring between the ages of 45 and 60 years, is another period in which dramatic changes in physical development occur. Primary changes are related to hormonal changes in both men and women, resulting in menopause in women. During middle age, changes occur in all systems and include decreases in basal metabolic rate, muscle size, nerve conduction, lung capacity, glomerular filtration, and cardiac output. The middle-aged client experiences increased adipose tissue deposit and skeletal changes leading to decreases in height, as well as changes in tactile sensibility, vision, and hearing. The physical changes continue into the stage of older adulthood. Middle and older adults are at risk for obesity and associated health problems. Health assessment will include use of BMI to assess weight and risk for disease. In addition, assessment will include the ability to carry out activities of daily living (ADLs) and regular testing of vision and hearing.

In addition to expectations about physical growth and development, there are also expectations about cognitive, psychosocial, and emotional development across the age span. For example, attachment is an essential element in infant development. Attachment refers to the tie between the infant and caregivers that promotes physical and psychosocial well-being. Assessment of attachment includes observing caregivers for eye contact, apparent interest in the child, talking or cooing to the child, response to infant needs, and communication.

Children are expected to develop language and cognitive abilities that enable them to learn and become independent over time. Young adults are expected to develop relationships with others and to become productive members of society. Maturity and aging lead individuals to contribute to the well-being of communities and their families and often to adapt to change and loss. Developmental milestones and crises occur in all stages of development and must be noted during assessment. A variety of instruments and scales can be used to identify developmental delays, behavioral patterns, and responses that indicate potential or actual problems with emotional, cognitive, and psychosocial development and adaptation in children and adults of all ages. Table 32–6 includes a list and description of some of the instruments available to measure aspects of growth and development.

TABLE 32–6 Instruments to Assess Growth and Development

Ages & Stages Questionnaire (ASQ)	A parent questionnaire that covers developmental areas of communication, gross motor, fine motor, problem solving, and personal-social in children.
Battelle Developmental Inventory	An inventory that tests developmental domains of cognition, motor, self-help, language, and social skills in children from birth through 8 years of age.
Brigance Screens	Screens that assess speech-language, motor, readiness, and general knowledge at younger ages and also reading and math. Used from 21 to 90 months of age.
Eyberg Child Behavior Inventory (ECBI)	The ECBI is a parent report scale of conduct problem behaviors in children ages 2–16 years.
Family Psychosocial Screening	A clinic intake form that identifies psychosocial risk factors associated with developmental problems including parental history of physical abuse as a child, parental substance abuse, and maternal depression.
Hassles and Uplifts Scale	Scale that measures adult attitudes about daily situations defined as "hassles" and "uplifts" and focuses on evaluation of positive and negative events in daily life rather than on life events.
Life Experiences Survey	Self-administered questionnaire that reviews life-changing events of a given year. Ratings are used to evaluate the level of stress one is experiencing.
McCarthy Scale of Children's Abilities	The McCarthy evaluates the general intelligence level of children ages 2½–8½ years. The scale identifies strengths and weaknesses in verbal, perceptual-performance, quantitative, memory, motor, and general cognitive skills.
Neonatal Behavioral Assessment Scale	Scale that is used to assess newborns and infants up to 2 months of age. It measures 28 behavioral and 18 reflex items and provides information about the baby's strengths, adaptive responses, and potential vulnerabilities.
Pediatric Symptom Checklist	Checklist of short statements that identifies conduct behaviors and behaviors associated with depression, anxiety, and adjustment in children ages 4–16 years. Item patterns determine the need for behavioral or mental health referrals.
Stanford-Binet Intelligence Scale: Fourth Edition	Test that measures general intelligence. The areas of verbal reasoning, quantitative reasoning, abstract/visual reasoning, and short-term memory can be tested from ages 2 to 23 years.
The Child Development Inventory	Scales that measure social, self-help, gross motor, fine motor, expressive language, language comprehension, letters, numbers, and general development in children from 15 months to 6 years of age.
The Denver II	Test that is administered to well children between birth and 6 years of age and is designed to test 20 simple tasks and items in four sectors: personal-social, fine motor adaptive, language, and gross motor.
The Mini-Mental Status Examination	This brief, quantitative measure of cognitive status in adults can be used to screen for cognitive impairment, to estimate the severity of cognitive impairment at a given point in time, to follow the course of cognitive changes in an individual over time, and to document an individual's response to treatment. It is used frequently to track cognitive changes in clients with dementia.
Wechsler Preschool and Primary Scale of Intelligence—Revised (WPPSI-R)	Standardized test of language and perception for children ages 4½–6 years.

Assessment of Infants

Frequent assessments during the first year provide opportunities to monitor the infant's rate of growth and development as well as to compare the infant with the norm for age. Height, weight, and head circumference measurements are plotted on an appropriate growth chart at each assessment. The three measurements should fall within two standard deviations of each other. More importantly, each measurement should follow the expected rate of growth, following the same percentile throughout infancy.

Accurate assessment combining information obtained by history, physical assessment, and knowledgeable observation allows early identification of common problems that may easily be resolved with early intervention. Often basic parent education and support remedy problems that, if left untreated, could result in significant health problems or disturbed parent–child interactions later.

Overnutrition and undernutrition are identified by weight that crosses percentiles. In *overnutrition*, the rate of weight gain is accelerated; in *undernutrition* the rate of weight gain diminishes. Overnutrition may occur when caregivers do not learn to read infants' cues but instead assume that every cry signals hunger. Cultural beliefs that a fat baby is a healthy baby may also lead parents and other caregivers to overfeed infants.

Undernutrition may be caused by inadequate caloric intake. This may result from lack of knowledge of normal infant feeding, a lack of financial resources to obtain formula, or inappropriate mixing of formula. Some quiet or passive infants do not demand feedings, and parents or caregivers may misinterpret this passivity as lack of hunger.

Head growth that crosses percentiles requires evaluation as it may indicate **hydrocephalus** (enlargement of the head caused by inadequate drainage of cerebrospinal fluid). Early diagnosis and intervention for rapid head growth prevents or diminishes serious neurologic effects.

Parents and caregivers generally enjoy relaying infants' new developmental milestones and can accurately describe infants' abilities. An infant who seems to be lagging behind on milestones may not be receiving appropriate stimulation. Assessment of caregivers' expectations and knowledge of infant development may reveal a knowledge deficit. Suggesting specific activities for caregivers to do with their infants may be the only intervention required. Infants who continue to lag further behind and are not achieving normal milestones require evaluation.

Healthy attachment is observed as a caregiver holds the infant closely in a manner that encourages eye contact (the *en face* position). The caregiver looks at the infant, smiles, talks, and interacts with the infant. The infant responds by fixing on the caregiver's face, smiling, and cooing. The caregiver stays close to the infant, providing support and reassurance during examinations or procedures (Figure 32–8 ■).

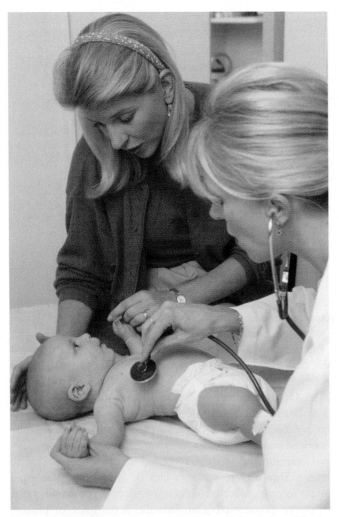

Figure 32–8 ■ This mother is interacting with her baby while the nurse performs the examination.

Failure to engage the infant through eye contact, talking, or a smile limits available opportunities for the caregiver to receive positive feedback from the infant. The infant, in turn, finds efforts to engage the parent frustrating, resulting in decreased attempts to interact. A negative pattern is quickly established, requiring more extensive intervention the longer it persists.

Assessment of Toddlers

Although the rate of growth of toddlers decreases, it proceeds in an expected manner. Height and weight continue to follow a percentile, although slight variations are often seen. Assessing caloric intake by obtaining a 24-hour recall provides clues to inappropriate feeding patterns. Toddlers generally feed themselves and begin to interact with the family at meals (Figure 32–9 ■). A favorite food one week may be refused the next, causing frustration and confusion in caregivers. Concern for the toddler's health may precipitate a power struggle as parents try to force the toddler to eat. Poor weight gain may result as the toddler exerts a newfound independence by refusing to eat. Excessive weight gain occurs when caregivers use food to quiet or bribe their toddlers. Discussing appropriate eating expectations and weight gain helps parents resolve eating problems.

Since cooperation of the young toddler is unlikely, a health history is often the best way to assess development. Older toddlers are more willing to play with developmental testing materials or explore the environment while in proximity to a caregiver, enabling direct observations of development. Because toddlers may not speak in a strange or threatening environment, language assessment can be difficult. Listening to the child talk in a playroom or waiting room increases the probability of assessing the toddler's language.

The toddler wanders a short distance from a caregiver to explore, returning periodically to "touch base." After receiving reassurance and encouragement, the child is ready for further exploration. Exploration provides learning opportunities but also places the toddler at risk for accidental injury or poisoning.

Toddlers have frequent tantrums, usually in response to unwanted limits or frustration. An attitude of calm understanding limits the duration of tantrums and keeps tantrums from becoming power struggles or attention-getting behavior.

Toddlers quickly turn to caregivers for comfort or when confronted with a stranger. Observing the adult–child interaction and listening to how the adult speaks to the child provides information on the quality of the relationship.

Continuous clinging of a toddler to a caregiver in a nonthreatening situation is unusual. Failure of the child to look to a caregiver for comfort and support may indicate that trust did not develop during infancy. Inappropriate caregiver expectations, such as expecting a toddler to sit quietly in a chair, may interfere with the normal progression of the toddler's development. Caregiver inattention to the activities of the child and failure to set limits result in the child's inability to develop self-control.

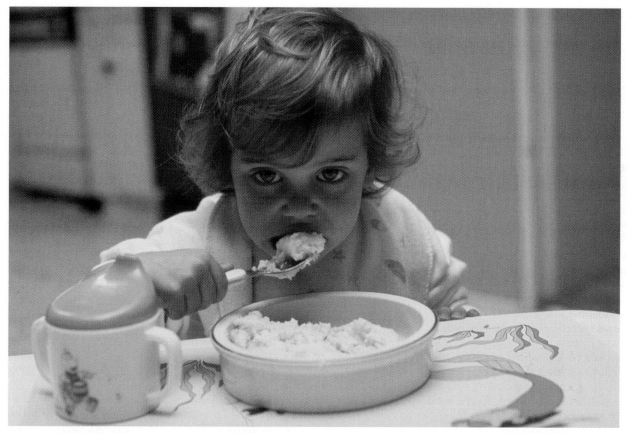

Figure 32–9 ■ Toddlers can generally feed themselves.

Assessment of Preschoolers

Preschoolers are generally pleasant, cooperative, and talkative. They are often less anxious if their caretaker is in view, but do not need to return to the caregiver for comfort except in threatening situations. Talking with preschoolers about favorite activities allows the nurse to assess language ability, cognitive ability, and development. The nurse evaluates the child's use of language to express thoughts, sentence structure, and vocabulary. It may be possible to identify **centration** (the ability to concentrate), magical thinking, and reality imitation as the child relays play activities. Lack of appropriate environmental stimulation may become evident, and the nurse may need to educate caregivers about age-appropriate activities for their children.

Preschoolers' slowed rate of growth is often of concern to caregivers. The nurse can allay anxiety by showing the preschooler's growth chart and discussing eating expectations.

A clinging, frightened preschooler in a nonthreatening situation may indicate a child who lacks a trusting relationship with his or her immediate caregivers. Lack of communication between caregiver and child limits the child's ability to learn appropriate social interaction and to practice language skills.

Children who do not exhibit appropriate achievement of developmental milestones should receive screenings and, if indicated, appropriate interventions. Periodic health assessments are necessary to ensure child well-being and to discuss child development with parents. See Box 32–3 for a detailed listing of interventions recommended during the periodic health examination for children ages birth to 10 years. Depending on the results of the examination, additional screenings or referrals to agencies that conduct developmental screenings may be warranted.

Assessment of School-Age Children

The slow, steady growth and changing body proportions of school-age children make them appear thin and gangly. Assessing children's intake of nutrients and calories and reviewing their growth charts reassures parents that their children are not too thin. By educating parents to evaluate objectively their children's diets during the early school-age years the nurse can help relieve family stress resulting from parents pushing children to eat and can help reinforce healthy eating habits that prevent obesity. Older school-age children have an increase in appetite as they enter the prepubertal growth spurt. During the growth spurt, height and weight increase and may normally cross percentiles.

School-age children are eager to talk about their hobbies, friends, school, and accomplishments. Increasing neurologic maturity allows them to master activities requiring gross and fine motor control, such as sports, dancing, playing a musical instrument, artistic pursuits, or building things. School-age

Box 32-3 Health Considerations: Birth to 10 Years

LEADING CAUSES OF DEATH
- Conditions originating in the perinatal period
- Congenital anomalies
- Sudden infant death syndrome (SIDS)
- Unintentional injuries (nonmotor vehicle)
- Motor vehicle injuries

INTERVENTIONS FOR THE GENERAL POPULATION

Screening
Height and weight
Blood pressure
Vision screen (age 3–4 years)
Hemoglobinopathy screen (birth)[1]
Phenylalanine level (birth)[2]
T_4 and/or TSH (birth)[3]

Counseling
- Injury prevention
  Child safety car seats (age <8 years or <80 lb)[4]
  Lap-shoulder belts (age ≥8 years or >80 lb)[4]
  Bicycle helmet; avoid bicycling near traffic
  Smoke detector, flame retardant sleepwear
  Hot water heater temperature <120–130°F
  Window/stair guards, pool fence
  Safe storage of drugs, toxic substances, firearms, and matches
  Syrup of ipecac, poison control phone number
  CPR training for parents/caretakers
- Diet and exercise
  Breastfeeding, iron-enriched formula and foods (infants and toddlers)

- Diet and Exercise
  Limit fat and cholesterol; maintain caloric balance; emphasize grains, fruits, vegetables (age ≥2 years)
  Regular physical activity
- Substance use
  Effects of passive smoking
  Antitobacco message
- Dental health
  Regular visits to dental care provider
  Floss, brush with fluoride toothpaste daily
  Advice about baby bottle tooth decay

Immunizations[5]
Diphtheria-tetanus-pertussis (DTP)
Oral poliovirus (OPV)
Measles-mumps-rubella (MMR)
H. influenzae type b (Hib) conjugate
Hepatitis B
Varicella

Chemoprophylaxis
Ocular prophylaxis (birth)

INTERVENTIONS FOR HIGH-RISK POPULATIONS

Population	Potential Interventions
Preterm or low birth weight	Hemoglobin/hematocrit
Infants of mothers at risk for HIV	HIV testing
Low income; immigrants	Hemoglobin/hematocrit; PPD
TB contacts	PPD
Native American/Alaska Native	Hemoglobin/hematocrit; PPD; hepatitis A vaccine; pneumococcal vaccine
Travelers to developing countries	Hepatitis A vaccine
Residents of long-term care facilities	PPD; hepatitis A vaccine; influenza vaccine
Certain chronic medical conditions	PPD; pneumococcal vaccine; influenza vaccine
Increased individual or community lead exposure	Blood lead level
Inadequate water fluoridation	Daily fluoride supplement
Family h/o skin cancer; nevi; fair skin, eyes, hair	Avoid excess/midday sun, use protective clothing

[1]Whether screening should be universal or targeted to high-risk groups will depend on the proportion of high-risk individuals in the screening area and other considerations. [2]If done during first 24 hours of life, repeat at age 2 weeks. [3]Optimally between day 2 and 6, but in all cases before newborn nursery discharge. [4]Child passenger safety laws differ among states. Nurses should know the laws in their state. [5]See Concept 14, Immunity, for information on immunizations.
CRP, Cardiopulmonary resuscitation; *HIV,* human immunodeficiency virus; *TB,* tuberculosis; *PPD,* purified protein derviative; *STDs,* sexually transmitted diseases; *BCG,* bacille Calmette-Guérin.
Source: Adapted from U.S. Preventive Services Task Force. (1996). *Guide to clinical preventive services* (2nd ed.). Baltimore: Williams & Wilkins.

---

children enjoy showing off newly acquired skills, and families display pride in their children's accomplishments.

School-age children frequently sort and classify collections of rocks, sports cards, dolls, coins, stamps, or almost anything (Figure 32–10 ■). They are industrious in school, feeling pride in their accomplishments as they master difficult concepts and skills. Families provide positive feedback and encouragement to their children and speak of their children's successes with pride.

Adult family members and school-age children communicate openly, with adults setting appropriate and much-needed limits. Although peer relationships are becoming more important, the family remains the major influence during most of the school-age years. As children approach adolescence, the relationship with family may become strained as the children are drawn closer to peer groups and seek greater independence.

Children who lack hobbies or cannot think of any accomplishments may be environmentally deprived. Caregivers

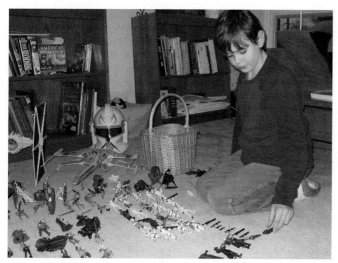

Figure 32–10 ■ This school-age child enjoys sorting his collection of action figures.

who are unable to think of anything positive to say about their children or who speak of them as a burden are likely to have a disturbed parent–child relationship. Children who lack encouragement and positive reinforcement at home for their achievements are at risk for gang recruitment. Gangs provide the "family" support children lack at home, increasing children's risk for violence, drug use, and illegal activity.

Problems in school may evolve at this time, and caregivers and children may have conflicts over grades and study time. The nurse can encourage the caregiver to help the child set a consistent place and time for homework. Caregivers should also be encouraged to communicate actively with the child's teacher. Teachers, adults, family members, and health care providers may identify learning disabilities at this time by careful observation.

Assessment of Adolescents

Parents and caregivers rarely express concern that their adolescents are not eating. The pubertal growth spurt requires adolescents to increase their caloric intake dramatically, causing parents concern that they eat constantly but never seem full. Despite this, adolescents (particularly women) are at risk for developing eating disorders. Information about eating disorders is included in Concept 24, Self.

Adolescents often communicate better with peers and adults outside of the family than with family members. Assessing adolescents with their parents and then one-on-one affords a more complete picture of their relationship and provides adolescents with an opportunity to express themselves and discuss concerns freely.

Most adolescents are able to hold an adult conversation and are often happy to discuss school, friends, activities, and plans for the future. They tend to be anxious about their bodies and the rapid changes occurring. Often adolescents are unsure if what is happening to them is normal, and they frequently express somatic complaints.

As adolescents become more independent, adult family members become anxious over their evolving lack of control.

Parents may be uncomfortable with adolescents' sexuality, rebellious dress and hairstyles, and developing values that may differ from those of the parents. Communication between parents and adolescents is often challenging at this stage.

Severely restricting the activities and freedom of adolescents inhibits their ability to progress toward independence. Adolescents who lack social contacts and spend much time alone may be depressed and at high risk for suicide. Acting out and risk-taking behaviors place adolescents at risk for serious injury from accidents or drug or alcohol use. Alliance with gangs places adolescents at risk for violence and participation in illegal activities.

See Box 32–4 for a detailed listing of health considerations for clients ages 11–24 years.

Assessment of Young Adults

Young adults are busy, productive, and healthy. At their maximum physical potential, young adults actively pursue sports and physical fitness activities. They refine their creative talents and enjoy activities with peers.

Young adults form intimate partnerships with others in mature, cooperative relationships. Traditionally, such intimate relationships involved marriage. Increasingly, these relationship are formed and maintained without a formal marriage or between two people of the same sex. Developmentally, the important concept is the formation of the mature, intimate relationship.

People deciding to have children in the twenty-first century have many more choices than their own parents and grandparents had: Surrogate motherhood, artificial insemination, in vitro fertilization, and other technological innovations make it possible for couples in a variety of situations to choose to become parents. Deciding not to have children or delaying having children is increasingly accepted, as is the decision of single women to have children.

Young adults have chosen an occupation, established their values, and adopted a lifestyle. Career advancement, quest for financial stability, and emotional investment characterize the young adult years (Figure 32–11 ■).

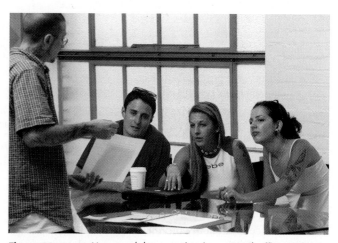

Figure 32–11 ■ Young adults, meeting in a casual office, strive to advance their careers.

Box 32–4 Health Considerations: Ages 11–24 Years

LEADING CAUSES OF DEATH
- Motor vehicle/other unintentional injuries
- Homicide
- Suicide
- Malignant neoplasms
- Heart diseases

INTERVENTIONS FOR THE GENERAL POPULATION

Screening
Height and weight
Blood pressure[1]
Papanicolaou (Pap) test[2] (females)
Chlamydia screen[3] (females <20 years)
Rubella serology or vaccination hx[4] (females >12 years)
Assess for problem drinking

Counseling
- Injury prevention
  Lap/shoulder belts
  Bicycle/motorcycle/ATV helmets
  Smoke detector
  Safe storage/removal of firearms
- Substance use
  Avoid tobacco use
  Avoid underage drinking and illicit drug use
  Avoid alcohol/drug use while driving, swimming, boating, etc.
- Sexual behavior
  STD prevention: abstinence; avoid high-risk behavior; use condoms, female barrier with spermicide
  Unintended pregnancy: contraception

- Diet and exercise
  Limit fat and cholesterol; maintain caloric balance; emphasize grains, fruits, vegetables
  Adequate calcium intake (females)
  Regular physical activity
- Dental health
  Regular visits to dental care provider
  Floss, brush with fluoride toothpaste daily

Immunizations[5]
Tetanus-diphtheria (Td) boosters (11–16 years)
Hepatitis B
MMR (11–12 years)
Varicella (11–12 years)
Rubella (females >12 years)

Chemoprophylaxis
Multivitamin with folic acid (females planning/capable of pregnancy)

INTERVENTIONS FOR HIGH-RISK POPULATIONS

Population	Potential Interventions
High-risk sexual behavior	RPR/VDRL; screen for gonorrhea (female), HIV, chlamydia (female); hepatitis A vaccine
Injection or street drug use	RPR/VDRL; HIV screen; hepatitis A vaccine; PPD; advice to reduce infection risk
TB contacts; immigrants; low income	PPD
Native Americans/Alaska Natives	Hepatitis A vaccine; PPD; pneumococcal vaccine
Travelers to developing countries	Hepatitis A vaccine
Certain chronic medical conditions	PPD; pneumococcal vaccine; influenza vaccine
Settings where adolescents and young adults congregate	Second MMR
Susceptible to varicella, measles, mumps	Varicella vaccine; MMR
Blood transfusion between 1978 and 1985	HIV screen
Institutionalized persons; health care/lab workers	Hepatitis A vaccine; PPD; influenza vaccine
Family h/o skin cancer; nevi; fair skin, eyes, hair	Avoid excess/midday sun, use protective clothing
Prior pregnancy with neural tube defect	Folic acid 4.0 mg
Inadequate water fluoridation	Daily fluoride supplement

[1]Periodic blood pressure for persons aged >21 years. [2]If sexually active at present or in the past: q ≤3 years. If sexual history is unreliable, begin Pap tests at age 18 years. [3]If sexually active. [4]Serologic testing, documented vaccination history, and routine vaccination against rubella (preferably with MMR) are equally acceptable alternatives. [5]See Concept 14, Immunity, for information on immunizations.
ATV, All-terrain vehicle; *STD,* sexually transmitted disease; *MMR,* measles-mumps-rubella; *TB,* tuberculosis; *HIV,* human immunodeficiency virus; *RPR,* rapid plasma reagin; *VDRL,* Venereal Disease Research Laboratories, *PPD,* purified protein derivative, *BCG,* bacille Calmette-Guérin.

The young adult without a steady job may lack direction and self-confidence. Marital discord may trigger feelings of failure and insecurity. Failing to achieve intimacy may place the young adult at risk for depression, alcoholism, or drug abuse.

Assessment of Middle-Aged Adults
Typically, the adult in the middle years of life is satisfied with past accomplishments and involved in activities outside the family. Healthy adjustment to the physical changes of

aging includes developing appropriate leisure activities in preparation for an active retirement. Good financial planning during the middle adult years helps financial security during retirement.

The middle adult years signal the end of childbearing and, most often, the end of child rearing. Individuals adjust to never having had children or to children leaving home. Couples may renew their relationships or find they have little in common and separate. Some women choose to delay childbearing until their late 30s or early 40s, after establishing their careers. They begin their child-rearing years as many of their peers are completing this phase of life. Older mothers must make the transition from career women to mothers, even if they continue their careers.

The dissatisfied middle adult is unhappy with the past and expresses little or no hope for the future. Sedentary and isolated, the individual complains about life, avoids involvement, and fails to plan appropriately for retirement.

Box 32–5 Health Considerations: Ages 25–64 Years

LEADING CAUSES OF DEATH
- Malignant
- Heart diseases
- Motor vehicle and other unintentional injuries
- Human immunodeficiency virus (HIV) infection
- Suicide and homicide

INTERVENTIONS FOR THE GENERAL POPULATION

Screening
Blood pressure
Height and weight
Total blood cholesterol (men ages 35–65, women ages 45–65)
Papanicolaou (Pap) test (women)[1]
Fecal occult blood test[2] and/or sigmoidoscopy (>50 years)
Mammogram ± clinical breast exam[3] (women 50–69 years)
Assess for problem drinking
Rubella serology or vaccination hx[4] (women of childbearing age)

Counseling
- Substance use
  Tobacco cessation
  Avoid alcohol/drug use while driving, swimming, boating, etc.
- Diet and exercise
  Limit fat and cholesterol; maintain caloric balance; emphasize grains, fruits, vegetables
  Adequate calcium intake (women)
  Regular physical activity

- Injury prevention
  Lap/shoulder belts
  Motorcycle/bicycle/ATV helmets
  Smoke detector
  Safe storage/removal of firearms
- Sexual behavior
  STD prevention: avoid high-risk behavior; use condoms/female barrier with spermicide
  Unintended pregnancy: contraception
- Dental health
  Regular visits to dental care provider
  Floss, brush with fluoride toothpaste daily

Immunizations
Tetanus-diphtheria (Td) boosters
Rubella[4] (women of childbearing age)

Chemoprophylaxis
Multivitamin with folic acid (women planning or capable of pregnancy)
Discuss hormone prophylaxis (peri- and postmenopausal women)

INTERVENTIONS FOR HIGH-RISK POPULATIONS

Population	Potential Interventions
High-risk sexual behavior	RPR/VDRL; screen for gonorrhea (female), HIV, chlamydia (female); hepatitis B vaccine; hepatitis A vaccine
Injection or street drug use	RPR/VDRL; HIV screen; hepatitis B vaccine; hepatitis A vaccine; PPD; advice to reduce infection risk
Low income: TB contacts; immigrants; alcoholics	PPD
Native Americans/Alaska Natives	Hepatitis A vaccine; PPD; pneumococcal vaccine
Travelers to developing countries	Hepatitis B vaccine; hepatitis A vaccine
Certain chronic medical conditions	PPD; pneumococcal vaccine; influenza vaccine
Blood product recipients	HIV screen; hepatitis B vaccine
Susceptible to measles, mumps, or varicella	MMR; varicella vaccine
Institutionalized persons	Hepatitis A vaccine; PPD; pneumococcal vaccine; influenza vaccine
Health care/lab workers	Hepatitis B vaccine; hepatitis A vaccine; PPD; influenza vaccine
Family h/o skin cancer; fair skin, eyes, hair	Avoid excess/midday sun, use protective clothing
Previous pregnancy with neural tube defect	Folic acid 4.0 mg

[1]Women who are or have been sexually active and who have a cervix: q ≤3 years. [2]Annually. [3]Mammogram q1–2 years, or mammogram q1–2 years with annual clinical breast examination. [4]Serologic testing, documented vaccination history, and routine vaccination (preferably with MMR) are equally acceptable alternatives.
ATV, All-terrain vehicles; *STD,* sexually transmitted disease; *TB,* tuberculosis; *RPR,* rapid plasma reagin; *VDRL,* Venereal Disease Research Laboratories; *HIV,* human immunodeficiency virus; *PPD,* purified protein derivative; *MMR,* measles-mumps-rubella.

Assessment of Older Adults

Comprehensive assessment is essential to understanding the health needs of the older adult. A key part of the geriatric evaluation is the functional assessment or systematic evaluation of the older person's level of function and self-care. As a result, the assessment is usually interdisciplinary and multidimensional and addresses function in the physical, social, and psychological domains.

Comprehensive geriatric assessment should be carried out on a regular basis, and

1. Following hospitalization for acute illness or injury.
2. When nursing home placement or a change in living status is being considered.
3. After any abrupt change in physical, social, or psychological function.
4. Yearly for the older person with complex health needs during the annual visit for routine health maintenance with the primary health care provider.
5. When the older client or family would like a second opinion regarding an intervention or treatment protocol recommended by the primary care provider.

Not all older adults will have need for, or access to, trained interdisciplinary teams; however, the careful clinician can incorporate holistic assessment techniques and standardized instruments into routine evaluations. Nurses are in an ideal position to advocate for older clients who would benefit from holistic assessment and to urge them to seek the services of specialized geriatric assessment teams.

Research evaluating the clinical outcomes of comprehensive geriatric evaluation with older clients reveals reduced hospital use, reduced mortality rates, improved mental status, lower health costs, improved functional ability, and lower hospital readmission rates (Engelhardt, Toseland, Gao, & Banks, 2006). The vision for the future is that every older adult will have access to appropriate interdisciplinary health care and that every health care organization and setting providing care to older adults will have financial support for an interdisciplinary geriatric service or program (Health Resources and Services Administration, 2003). The demand for nurses who can care for older clients is expected to increase 41% from 2 million in 2000 to 2.8 million in 2030. Not every older adult would receive care from an interdisciplinary team, but the team would be available for those older clients whose complex health needs require holistic assessment.

The nurse requires a different perspective during the geriatric assessment process and special instruments to gather appropriate data (see Developmental Considerations: Instruments for Use With Older Adults). The nurse must not only be knowledgeable in the content area of gerontology and geriatrics, but also be educated regarding the issues of team dynamics. Essential skills in team dynamics include the following:

- An awareness of the roles and contributions of all team members
- Excellent communication skills in order to share information
- Conflict resolution skills
- The ability to see that multiple disciplines can provide information critical to solving the problems of the older client.

CARE SETTINGS ▶ Assessing the Home Environment of Older Adults

Some geriatric assessment teams have the time and resources to visit the older client's home and conduct an assessment of the environment. While this direct observation is the best way to gather accurate and reliable data, it is time consuming and can be expensive. Therefore, many geriatric assessment teams question the older person and the family regarding the adequacy of the home environment and the available resources to maintain adequate levels of function.

Factors to be considered when assessing the home environment include the following:

- *Stairs.* Narrow stairs with poor lighting, inadequate railings, and uneven steps are fall risks. Does the older person have the strength and balance to climb stairs? If a wheelchair or walker is used, are there ramps present or space for them to be added?
- *Bathing and toileting.* Can the older client safely transfer on and off the toilet? Is a raised toilet seat needed? Are grab bars present? Is there an adequate bath mat in the tub? Is a shower seat needed? Is lighting adequate? Is the older client able to bathe without assistance?
- *Medications.* Where are medications stored? Are there grandchildren in the home who are at risk because of open storage or nonreplacement of caps? Are old and outdated medications disposed of to prevent accidents? Are medications refilled on time to prevent on–off dosing patterns? Is there a list of medications available for use in emergencies? Is the client responsible for taking his or her own medications, or does a family member help? Does the client use or need any reminders to help him or her remember to take medications?

- *Nutrition and cooking.* Is there adequate food in the home? Is there a stove or microwave to cook? Are any safety problems reported with the stove or microwave? If a gas stove, is it safe? Is the pilot light functioning properly? Are there gas leak detectors? Is food storage adequate? Is spoiled food present? Is the food preparation environment clean? Who does the grocery shopping? Who prepares the food? How are trash and garbage disposed?
- *Falls.* Are the floors free of cords, debris, and scatter rugs? Is there adequate lighting? Are there night-lights? Are there pets that dart around quickly? If there is a history of falls, would the older person consider wearing an emergency alert system around the neck?
- *Smoke detectors.* Are there functioning smoke detectors? Are batteries changed yearly?
- *Emergency numbers.* Are emergency phone numbers posted near or preprogrammed into the phone?
- *Temperature of home.* Is there adequate heat in the winter and cooling in the summer?
- *Temperature of water.* Is the hot water set below 120°F?
- *Safety of the neighborhood.* Can the older person venture outside without fear of becoming a crime victim? Are there adequate door locks and latches? How close is the nearest neighbor? Is there nearby help if it is needed?
- *Financial.* Are there stacks of unpaid bills? Are services such as phone and electricity in good working order? Are there large amounts of cash hidden or stored around the house? Is there adequate money to purchase nutritious food?

Despite variations in instruments, structure of the interdisciplinary team, and methods employed, several strategies have been proven to make the evaluation process more effective. These include the development of a close-knit interdisciplinary team with minimal redundancy in the assessments performed, the use of carefully designed questionnaires that reliable older clients or their caregivers can complete beforehand, and the effective use of assessment forms that are incorporated into computer databases (Kane, Ouslander, & Abrass, 2004).

There are three underlying principles of comprehensive geriatric assessment:

1. Physical, psychological, and socioeconomic factors interact in complex ways to influence the health and functional status of the older person.
2. Comprehensive evaluation of an older person's health status requires an assessment in each of these domains. The coordinated efforts of various health care professionals are needed to carry out the assessment.
3. Functional abilities should be a central focus of the comprehensive evaluation. Other more traditional measures of health such as medical diagnosis, nursing diagnosis, physical examination results, and laboratory findings form the basic foundation of the assessment in order to determine overall health, well-being, and the need for social services (Kane, Ouslander, & Abrass, 2004).

The interrelationships between the physical, social, and psychological aspects of aging and perhaps illness present a challenge to the nurse when beginning the geriatric evaluation. The nurse is often charged with the responsibility of obtaining the client's past health history and history of the present illness. The following contextual variables should be considered.

EVALUATION OF THE ENVIRONMENT Clear instructions should be provided to the client and family beforehand regarding the parking arrangements and registration process. In order to make the older client and family comfortable, environmental modifications should be made, if possible. Environmental modifications may include adequate lighting, decreased background noise, comfortable seating for the older client and family, easily accessible restrooms, examination tables that can be raised or lowered to assist clients with disabilities, and availability of water or juice for client use. Client comfort will ease communication and improve the data collection process.

ACCURACY OF THE HEALTH HISTORY Many assessment clinics mail an information packet in advance so that the older client can come prepared. This packet might include the following:

1. A past medical history form. This form can be completed at home and is helpful for clients with complicated medical histories. The dates of hospitalizations, operations, serious injuries or accidents, procedures, and so on can be ascertained beforehand to save time during the assessment appointment. The form would also include history of adverse drug effects or allergies.
2. Instructions to bring in all prescription and over-the-counter medications and herbal products/vitamins/mineral supplements for review by the nurse.

3. Instructions to bring any medical records, laboratory or x-ray reports, electrocardiograms, reports of vaccination, and other pertinent health records that the client or family may possess.
4. Instructions to write down and bring the names of all health care providers involved with the client's health care, including primary care providers, specialists, and alternative medicine practitioners (e.g., acupuncturists, massage therapists, chiropractors).

The more information that the client and family can organize ahead of time, the better and more efficiently the assessment can be performed. Patience is a virtue when obtaining a history, because many times the thought and verbal processes are slower in the older person. Clients should be allowed adequate time to answer questions and report information (Kane, Ouslander, & Abrass, 2004).

PRACTICE ALERT
When the older client is asked to bring all medications to the geriatric evaluation session and he or she arrives carrying a large bag of medication bottles, the nurse knows that the first notation on the problem list is likely to be "at risk for adverse drug reaction related to polypharmacy."

The history should include emphasis on the following:
- Review of acute and chronic medical problems
- Medications
- Disease prevention and health maintenance review: vaccinations, PPD (tuberculosis), cancer screenings
- Functional status (activities of daily living)
- Social supports (family, spiritual affiliations, caregiver stress, safety of living environment)
- Finances
- Driving status and safety record
- Geriatric review of symptoms (client/family perception of memory, dentition, taste, smell, nutrition, hearing, vision, falls, fractures, bowel and bladder function) (Stanford University Geriatric Education Resource Center, 2000).

Often, a standardized form is used to guide and direct the process of obtaining the health history. The nurse should be aware of potential difficulties in obtaining health histories from older persons, including the following:

- *Communication difficulties.* Decreased hearing or vision, slow speech, and use of English as a second language have an effect on communication.
- *Underreporting of symptoms.* Fear of being labeled as a complainer, fear of institutionalization, and fear of serious illness can influence symptom reporting.
- *Vague or nonspecific complaints.* These may be associated with cognitive impairment, drug or alcohol use or abuse, or atypical presentation of disease.
- *Multiple complaints.* Associated "masked" depression, presence of multiple chronic illnesses, and social isolation are often an older person's cry for help.

■ *Lack of time.* New clients scheduled for geriatric assessment should have the minimum of a 1-hour appointment with the gerontological nurse. Shorter appointments will result in a hurried interview with missed information (Kane, Ouslander, & Abrass, 2004).

SOCIAL HISTORY Holistic evaluation is not complete without an assessment of the social support system. Many frail older persons receive support and supervision from family members and significant others to compensate for functional disabilities.

Key elements of the social history include the following:

■ Past occupation and retirement status
■ Family history (helpful to construct a family genogram)
■ Present and former marital status, including quality of the relationship(s)
■ Identification of family members, with designation of level of involvement and place of residence
■ Current living arrangements
■ Family dynamics
■ Family and caregiver expectations
■ Economic status, including adequacy of health insurance
■ Social activities and hobbies
■ Mode of transportation
■ Community involvement and support
■ Religious involvement and spirituality.

Older persons who exhibit symptoms of sadness, social isolation, who question their existence, who feel they are being punished by God, or who ask about availability of religious or spiritual counseling should be asked if they would like help with their spiritual concerns. Religion and spirituality can be a great source of hope and strength in times of need and crisis. Many health care facilities and community agencies have access to religious and spiritual counselors who can meet with older persons and their families if there is need and the older person does not have an ongoing relationship with a priest, minister, rabbi, or spiritual counselor.

If there is a social worker on the assessment team, the nurse may collaborate with him or her closely to identify and address social problems. Older clients with inadequate health insurance can often be helped by accessing community services, hospital free care, hardship funds established for indigent clients by major drug companies, and referrals to community-based free clinics. This information is helpful to nurses working with older persons in many settings but is absolutely necessary for those being admitted to long-term care facilities and those expressing feelings of loneliness or absence of significant persons in their lives.

MINIMUM DATA SET Assessment of an older person for appropriate placement within the nursing home or within the long-term care system is done using the Minimum Data Set (MDS).

The MDS is a comprehensive multidisciplinary assessment that is used throughout the United States. It was devised and passed into law because of the belief that a more holistic client assessment would facilitate improved care. The Omnibus Budget Reconciliation Act of 1987 (OBRA 87) contained a provision mandating that all residents of facilities that collect funds from Medicare or Medicaid be assessed using the MDS. The MDS is used for validating the need for long-term care, reimbursement, ongoing assessment of clinical problems, and assessment of and need to alter the current plan of care.

The MDS consists of a core set of screening, clinical, and functional measures. It is used with the Resident Assessment Protocols (RAPs), the Resident Utilization Guidelines (RUGs), and the Resident Assessment Instrument (RAI):

■ RAPs are structured, problem-oriented guidelines that identify unique and relevant information about an older person. This information is needed for formulating an individualized nursing care plan.
■ RUGs determine the reimbursement the skilled nursing facility will receive for providing care to the older client. Factors considered include the need for supportive therapy (physical, occupational, and/or speech), ability of the older person to care for him- or herself, and the need for special treatments such as feeding tubes or skin care.
■ The RAI identifies medical problems and describes each older person's functional ability in a comprehensive and standardized format. This information is useful to the staff in formulating the plan of care and also helps to evaluate progress toward goals, indicating when a change in the care plan is needed.

Categories of data gathered for the MDS include the following:

■ Client demographics and background
■ Cognitive function
■ Communication and hearing
■ Mood and behavior patterns
■ Psychosocial well-being
■ Physical function and ADLs
■ Bowel and bladder continence
■ Diagnosed diseases
■ Health conditions (weight, falls, etc.)
■ Oral nutritional status
■ Oral and dental status
■ Skin condition
■ Activity pursuits
■ Medications
■ Need for special services
■ Discharge potential.

Certain information gathered for the MDS, such as functional decline or a poorly managed chronic disease, may trigger the need for further assessment using the RAPs. For instance, if information gathered for the MDS indicates that the nursing home resident has fallen, a RAP is triggered and indicates the need for direct gait assessment, medication review, and physical/occupational therapy evaluation.

LIFESTYLE AND HEALTH CONSIDERATIONS Well-adjusted older adults maintain an active lifestyle and involvement with others and often do not appear their age. Lifestyle changes occur in response to declining physical abilities and retirement. Participation in activities that promote the older adult's sense of self-worth and usefulness also provides opportunities for developing new friendships with others of similar abilities and interests. Intellectual function is maintained through continued intellectual pursuits. Content with their life review, well-adjusted older adults often enjoy their retirement years and accept death as the inevitable end of a productive life.

The older adult who has not successfully resolved developmental crises may feel that life has been unfair. Despair and hopelessness may be evident in the individual's lack of activity and bitter complaining. See Box 32–6 for a list of health considerations for adults ages 65 and older.

Each of the concepts within the individual domain contains information specific to assessment of the system represented within the concept. Also included are developmental considerations and common age-related disorders that may result in abnormal assessment findings. Concept 34 discusses assessment as a step in the nursing process and the interrelationship of each step of the process.

Box 32–6 Health Considerations: Ages 65 and Older

LEADING CAUSES OF DEATH
- Heart diseases
- Malignant neoplasms (lung, colorectal, breast)
- Cerebrovascular disease
- Chronic obstructive pulmonary disease
- Pneumonia and influenza

INTERVENTIONS FOR THE GENERAL POPULATION

Screening
Blood pressure
Height and weight
Fecal occult blood test[1] and/or sigmoidoscopy
Mammogram ± clinical breast exam[2] (women ≤69 years)
Papanicolaou (Pap) test (women)[3]
Vision screening
Assess for hearing impairment
Assess for problem drinking

Counseling
- Substance use
  Tobacco cessation
  Avoid alcohol/drug use while driving, swimming, boating, etc.
- Diet and exercise
  Limit fat and cholesterol; maintain caloric balance; emphasize grains, fruits, vegetables
  Adequate calcium intake (women)
  Regular physical activity

- Injury prevention
  Lap/shoulder belts
  Motorcycle and bicycle helmets
  Fall prevention
  Safe storage/removal of firearms
  Smoke detector
  Set hot water heater to <120–130°F
  CPR training for household members
- Dental health
  Regular visits to dental care provider
  Floss, brush with fluoride toothpaste daily
- Sexual behavior
  STD prevention; avoid high-risk sexual behavior; use condoms

Immunizations
Pneumococcal vaccine
Influenza[1]
Tetanus-dipththeria (Td) boosters

Chemoprophylaxis
Discuss hormone prophylaxis (women)

INTERVENTIONS FOR HIGH-RISK POPULATIONS

Population	Potential Interventions
Institutionalized persons	PPD; hepatitis A vaccine; amantadine/rimantadine
Chronic medical conditions; TB contacts; low income; immigrants; alcoholics	PPD
Persons ≥75 years; or ≥70 years with risk factors for falls	Fall prevention intervention
Cardiovascular disease risk factors	Consider cholesterol screening
Family h/o skin cancer; nevi; fair skin, eyes, hair	Avoid excess/midday sun, use protective clothing
Native Americans/Alaska Natives	PPD; hepatitis A vaccine
Travelers to developing countries	Hepatitis A vaccine; hepatitis B vaccine
Blood product recipients	HIV screen; hepatitis B vaccine
High-risk sexual behavior	Hepatitis A vaccine; HIV screen; hepatitis B vaccine; RPR/VDRL
Injection or street drug use	PPD; hepatitis A vaccine; HIV screen; hepatitis B vaccine; RPR/VDRL; advice to reduce infection risk
Health care/lab workers	PPD; hepatitis A vaccine; amantadine/rimantadine; hepatitis B vaccine
Persons susceptible to varicella	Varicella vaccine

[1]Annually. [2]Mammogram q1–2 years, or mammogram q1–2 years with annual clinical breast exam. [3]All women who are or have been sexually active and who have a cervix: q ≤3 years. Consider discontinuation of testing after age 65 years if previous regular screening with consistently normal results.
CPR, Cardiopulmonary resuscitation; *STD,* sexually transmitted disease; *TB,* tuberculosis; *PPD,* purified protein derivative; *HIV,* human immunodeficiency virus; *RPR,* rapid plasma reagin; *VDRL,* Venereal Disease Research Laboratories.

DEVELOPMENTAL CONSIDERATIONS Instruments for Use With Older Adults

The Hartford Institute recommends the following instruments for use when assessing the function of older adults. These instruments have been used clinically for many years, are commonly referred to in practice, and are validated on large client groups. Additional assessment tools that focus on specific problems can be found in the appropriate concepts within the individual domain. Recommended functional assessment tools include the following:

1. Katz Index of Independence in Activities of Daily Living (Katz et al., 1970)
2. Pulses Profile. Measures general functional performance in mobility and self-care, medical status, and psychosocial factors
   P = physical condition
   U = upper limb function
   L = lower limb function
   S = sensory components
   E = excretory functions
   S = support factors (Granger, Albrecht, & Hamilton, 1979)

3. SPICES. An overall assessment tool used to plan, promote, and maintain optimal function in older adults
   S = sleep disorders
   P = problems with eating and feeding
   I = incontinence
   C = confusion
   E = evidence of falls
   S = skin breakdown

Sources: Hartford Institute for Geriatric Nursing. (2007). *Best nursing practices in care for older adults: Incorporating essential gerontologic content into baccalaureate nursing education and staff development.* New York: New York University; Wallace, M., & Fulmer, T. (2007). Fulmer SPICES: An overall assessment tool for older adults. *Try this: Best Practices in Nursing Care to Older Adults.* Retrieved February 10, 2008, from http://www.hartfordign.org/publications/trythis

REVIEW Holistic Health Assessment Across the Life Span

RELATE: LINK THE CONCEPTS

Linking the exemplar of Holistic Health Assessment Across the Life Span with the concept of Communication:

1. What strategies would you use when communicating with an older adult with hearing loss when collecting information for a health history?
2. You are collecting information from the mother of a 3-year-old for a health history. The mother does not speak any English, but the 3-year-old does speak English. What communication strategies would you employ?

Linking the exemplar of Holistic Health Assessment Across the Life Span with the concept of Legal Issues:

3. You admit an adolescent to the adolescent unit of a local hospital and begin collecting data when you begin to suspect the adolescent may be abusing substances. With an understanding of your legal obligation to the adolescent, as well as the parents' desire to help their child, how would you handle your suspicions if the parents are in the room with the child?
4. You are assessing an older adult and discover bruises that you suspect may be the result of abuse. The client's son is in the room during the examination. What is the best legally appropriate action for you to take?

READY: GO TO COMPANION SKILLS MANUAL

■ See Nursing Skills, Chapter 11

REFER: GO TO MYNURSINGKIT

REFLECT: CASE STUDY

The nurse conducted a health history interview with Mrs. Martha Washburn, a 67-year-old African American. The following are excerpts from the health history.

"Mrs. Washburn, I am going to ask you a lot of questions before your physical. I need to have correct responses and I have to tell you, there will be a lot of them if we are to get to the root of your problem. I will use the information to develop a plan of care."

"What are you here for? Did someone come with you? I see on your chart that you have some problems with urination; are you incontinent? How long have you had the problem?"

The nurse included the following questions: "What is your economic status? Do you go to church? What do you do when you are ill?"

"We need information about your family, so let's start with your parents. Are they alive? Do you have siblings?"

The nurse completed a review of symptoms and prepared the client for the physical examination by showing her into a room and telling her to get undressed.

1. Critique the nurse's actions in the initial interview phase of the case study.
2. Identify the types of information sought in the questions in the case study.
3. Create alternative approaches to the interview and questioning techniques in the case study.
4. Describe your preparation for an interview of Mrs. Washburn.

EXPLORE PEARSON **mynursingkit**™

MyNursingKit is your one stop for online chapter review materials and resources. Prepare for success with additional NCLEX®-style practice questions, interactive assignments and activities, web links, animations and videos, and more!

Register your access code from the front of your book at
www.mynursingkit.com.

REFERENCES

American Cancer Society. (2010a). American Cancer Society guidelines for early detection of cancer. Retrieved May 10, 2010, from http://www.cancer.org/docroot/PED/content/PED_2_3X_ACS_Cancer_Early_Detection_Guidelines_36.asp

American Cancer Society (2010b). What causes breast cancer? Retrieved February 16, 2010, from http://www.cancer.org/docroot/CRI/content/CRI_2_2_2X_What_causes_breast_cancer_5.asp?sitearea=

D'Amico, D., & Barbarito, C. (2007). *Health & physical assessment in nursing*. Upper Saddle River, NJ: Pearson Prentice Hall.

Engelhardt, J., Toseland, R., Gao, J., & Banks, S. (2006). Long-term effects of geriatric outpatient evaluation and management on cost, health care utilization and survival. *Research on Social Work Practice, 16*(1), 20–27.

Granger, C., Albrecht, G., & Hamilton, B. (1979). Outcomes of comprehensive medical rehabilitation: Measures of PULSES profile and the Barthel index. *Archives of Physical Medicine and Rehabilitation, 60*, 145–154.

Hartford Institute for Geriatric Nursing. (2007). *Best nursing practices in care for older adults: Incorporating essential gerontologic content into baccalaureate nursing education and staff development*. New York: New York University.

Health Resources and Services Administration. (2003). *Changing demographics: Implications for physicians, nurses and other health workers*. U.S. Department of Health and Human Services, National Center for Health Workforce Analysis. Retrieved February 10, 2008, from http://hrsa.gov/bhpr

Kane, R., Ouslander, J., & Abrass, I. (2004). *Essentials of clinical geriatrics* (5th ed.). New York: McGraw-Hill.

Katz, S., Down, T. D., Cash, H. R., & Grotz, R. C. (1970). Progress in the development of the index of ADL. *The Gerontologist, 10*(1), 20–30.

Stanford University Geriatric Education Resource Center. (2000). *Geriatric pocket pare: Tools for geriatric care* (2nd ed.). Developed by John A. Hartford Foundation Consortium for Geriatrics Education in Residency Training. Palo Alto, CA: Stanford University Geriatric Education Resource Center.

Wallace, M., & Fulmer, T. (2007). Fulmer SPICES: An overall assessment tool for older adults. *Try this: Best Practices in Nursing Care to Older Adults*. Retrieved February 10, 2008, from http://www.hartfordign.org/publications/trythis

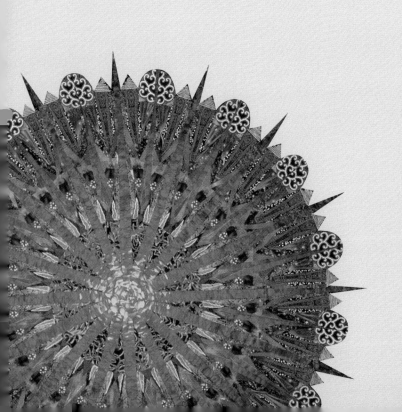

Caring Interventions

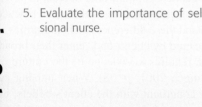

33

Concept at-a-Glance

About Caring Interventions, *2027*

Concept Learning Outcomes

After reading about this concept, you will be able to:

1. Discuss the meaning of caring.
2. Identify nursing theories focusing on caring.
3. Analyze the importance of different types of knowledge in nursing.
4. Describe how nurses demonstrate caring in practice.
5. Evaluate the importance of self-care for the professional nurse.

Concept Key Terms

Aesthetic knowing, *2031*
Caring, *2028*
Caring practice, *2028*
Empirical knowing, *2931*

Ethical knowing, *2032*
Personal knowing, *2032*
Presencing, *2032*

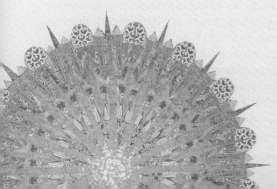

About Caring Interventions

The term *caring interventions* is a combination of two terms that are the heart of the nursing profession: *care*, which can be defined as "to feel interest or concern," and *intervention*, "an act that changes the outcome or course of a condition or process" (Merriam-Webster Online Dictionary, 2010). Throughout this book, a number of interventions are presented and discussed that enable nurses to act in order to change the course of clients' illness or injury or to help clients prevent illness or injury. Skills, techniques, methods, and instructions are provided that cover everything from how to teach a client to use an inhaler to how to assess a pregnant mother in her first trimester. What distinguishes nurses as professionals is both the skill necessary to provide these interventions and the *caring* manner in which nurses provide them. **Caring** means that people, relationships, and things matter. It is the *caring* facet of nursing that sets nursing apart as one of the most trusted professions.

Professionalization of Caring

Caring practice involves connection, mutual recognition, and involvement. Consider the following examples of caring taken from nursing situations:

- A client experiencing post-operative pain is given medication to control her symptoms, and then the nurse talks quietly and holds her hand for a few minutes as the pain resolves. The nurse's presence, in itself, provides comfort for the client.
- After the student nurse washes the hair of a client who is immobilized and assists the client with makeup application, the nurse helps the client to sit up in a wheelchair to greet her daughter and grandchildren. The client is extremely grateful just to be able to sit up after spending weeks in bed. The personal care provided by the student nurse enhances the client's sense of dignity.

Just as clients benefit from caring practices, the nurses involved in these situations experience benefits through knowing that they have made a difference in their clients' lives. Consider, for example, one nurse's feeling of satisfaction: "It is not something that can be defined but . . . [it's] the feeling that you've made a difference to an individual, and had I not been there at that time, that would never have occurred" (Pask, 2003, p. 169).

Caring as "Helping the Other Grow"

Milton Mayeroff (1990), a noted philosopher, has proposed that to care for another person is to help him or her grow and achieve self-actualization. Recognizing that the other person has the potential and the need for growth, the caregiver does not impose direction, but allows the direction of the other person's growth to help determine the caregiver's response.

Aspects of caring identified by Mayeroff include:

- *Knowing* means understanding the other's needs and how to respond to the needs
- *Alternating rhythms* means moving back and forth between the immediate and long-term meanings of behavior, while taking the past into consideration
- *Patience* enables the other to grow in his or her own way and time;
- *Honesty* includes an awareness and openness to one's own feelings as well as genuine caring for the other
- *Trust* involves letting go, to allow the other to grow in his or her own way and own time
- *Humility* means acknowledging that there is always more to learn, and that learning may come from any source
- *Hope* is belief in the possibilities of the other's growth
- *Courage* is the sense of going into the unknown, informed by insight from past experiences.

Mayeroff proposes that the caring process also has benefits for the one providing care. By helping the other person grow, the caregiver moves toward self-actualization. Through caring and being cared for, each person "finds his place" in the world. •

NURSING THEORIES ON CARING

Caring is a multidimensional concept. In a comprehensive review of the concept of caring, Morse, Solberg, Neander, Battorff, and Johnson (1990) identified different definitions of caring, which were summarized as the following five viewpoints:

- Caring as a moral imperative
- Caring as an affect
- Caring as a human trait
- Caring as an interpersonal relationship
- Caring as a therapeutic intervention.

Nurse scholars have reviewed the literature, conducted research, and analyzed nurses' experiences, resulting in the development of theories and models of caring. These theories and models are grounded in humanism and the idea that caring is the basis for human science. Several nursing theorists focus on caring: Leininger, Ray, Roach, Boykin and Schoenhofer, Watson, and Benner and Wrubel.

Culture Care Diversity and Universality (Leininger)

Based on studies in nursing and anthropology, Madeleine Leininger noted that caring, as nurturing behavior, has been present throughout history and is one of the most critical factors in helping people maintain or regain health. Leininger proposes that "caring is the essence of nursing, and the distinct, dominant, central, and unifying focus of nursing" (Leininger, 2001, p. 35). Her theory of culture care diversity and universality is based on the assumption that nurses must understand different cultures in order to function effectively.

Transcultural nursing focuses on both the differences and similarities among persons in diverse cultures. While cultures have different ways of caring for others, there are also universal behaviors among all cultures of the world. In order to provide care that is congruent with cultural values, beliefs, and practices, the nurse must understand these differences and similarities. To understand the care desired by clients and "enter their broader worldview," the nurse requires knowledge of the culture and local language (Leininger, 2001, p. 58). When nursing care fails to be reasonably congruent with the client's beliefs, lifeways, and values, there may be signs of conflict, noncompliance, and stress.

Culturally congruent care is provided in three major ways: (a) by preserving the client's familiar ways of life, (b) by making accommodations in care that are satisfying to clients, and (c) by structuring nursing care to help the client move toward wellness (Leininger, 2001). Leininger defines caring as "assisting, supporting, or enabling another individual or group with evident or anticipated needs to ameliorate or improve a human condition or lifeway, or to face death" (2001, p. 46).

Theory of Bureaucratic Caring (Ray)

Marilyn Anne Ray's theory of bureaucratic caring focuses on caring in organizations (e.g., hospitals). Ray suggests that caring in nursing is contextual and is influenced by the organizational structure. Her research found that the meaning of caring varied in the emergency department, intensive care unit, oncology unit, and other areas of the hospital. For example, an intensive care unit had a dominant value of technological caring (i.e., monitors, ventilators, treatments, and pharmacotherapeutics), and an oncology unit had a value of a more intimate,

FOCUS ON DIVERSITY AND CULTURE Culturally Sensitive Nursing

The primary focus of nursing care is the client as he or she relates to the environment and experiences events or situations related to health or illness. The client's culture and beliefs give shape and personal meaning to the client's experiences. In order to provide caring interventions and a caring environment that promotes health and wellness for all clients, nurses must increase their cultural competence.

The 1992 American Academy of Nursing Expert Panel on Culturally Competent Nursing Care identified several reasons why it has become increasingly important for nurses to plan culturally sensitive care:

■ The demographic and ethnic composition of the population of the world in general, and the United States in particular, has changed markedly. Ethnic representation among health care professionals has yet to reflect the changes occurring in the population. Information and knowledge about values, beliefs, experiences, and health care needs of various populations is limited.

■ Among the larger population and among health care professionals, there is a growing awareness and acceptance of diversity and an increased willingness to maintain and support ethnic and cultural heritage.

■ In the United States, people from all cultures are facing increasing unemployment, decreasing opportunity, and limited access to health care.

■ The international focus on providing health care for all people (within the context of inequality, barriers, and lack of access) has made health care professionals more aware of the inequities inherent in health care systems in both developing countries and developed countries.

■ Nurses comprise the largest force in the delivery of health care and therefore have the potential to contribute to promoting equality and accessibility in the health care system

■ Consumers are becoming increasingly aware of what is competent and sensitive health care.

This same panel of experts proposed general principles for nurses to become sensitive to cultural diversity and to provide culturally sensitive care:

■ Nurses must learn to appreciate cultural diversity and commonalties in racial/ethnic minority populations.

■ Nurses must understand how socioeconomic factors shape health behaviors and practices among members of racial/ethnic minorities.

■ Nurses must confront their own prejudices.

■ Nurses must examine and evaluate services provided to people in their community from different cultures.

People of every culture have the right to have their cultural values known, respected, and addressed appropriately within nursing and other health care services (Leininger, 1991). To provide nursing care that is culturally sensitive, nurses must develop a sensitivity to personal values about health and illness; must accept the existence of differing values; and must be respectful of, interested in, and understanding of other cultures without being judgmental.

---

spiritual caring (i.e., family-focused, comforting, compassionate). The meaning of caring was further influenced by the role and position a person held. Staff nurses valued caring in terms of how it related to clients, while administrators valued caring as more system-related, such as safeguarding the economic well-being of the hospital (Coffman, 2006).

As depicted in Figure 33–1 ■, spiritual-ethical caring influences each of the aspects of the organization's bureaucratic system (political, legal, economic, educational, physiologic, social-cultural, and technological). Each of these aspects is different, but collectively they make up an entire system (e.g., a hospital). Nurses influence client care by making choices about each of these aspects (Ray, 2001). Nurses make these choices with the interest of the client at heart and use ethical principles as the foundation for the basis of professional decision making.

Caring, the Human Mode of Being (Roach)

M. Simone Roach focuses on caring as a philosophical concept and proposes that caring is the human mode of being, or the "most common, authentic criterion of humanness" (Roach, 2002, p. 28). Roach identifies ways in which caring is common among people in general, but examines how caring is unique to nursing, since it is at the center of all the attributes used to describe nursing. Roach defines these attributes as the six Cs of caring: compassion, competence, confidence, conscience, commitment, and comportment. See Box 33–1 for definitions of each characteristic. The six Cs are used as a broad framework, suggesting categories of behavior that describe professional caring. Each category reflects specific values and includes virtuous actions by which a nurse can demonstrate caring.

Box 33–1 The Six Cs of Caring in Nursing

COMPASSION
Awareness of one's relationship to others, sharing their joys, sorrows, pain, and accomplishments. Participation in the experience of another.

COMPETENCE
Having the knowledge, judgment, skills, energy, experience, and motivation to respond adequately to others within the demands of professional responsibilities.

CONFIDENCE
The quality that fosters trusting relationships. Comfort with self, client, and family.

CONSCIENCE
Morals, ethics, and an informed sense of right and wrong. Awareness of personal responsibility.

COMMITMENT
Convergence between one's desires and obligations and the deliberate choice to act in accordance with them.

COMPORTMENT
Appropriate demeanor, dress, and language, that are in harmony with a caring presence. Presenting oneself as someone who respects others and in turn demands respect.

Source: Adapted fbbrom Roach, M. S. (2002) *Caring, the human mode of Being* (2nd ed.). CHA Press. Reprinted with permission.

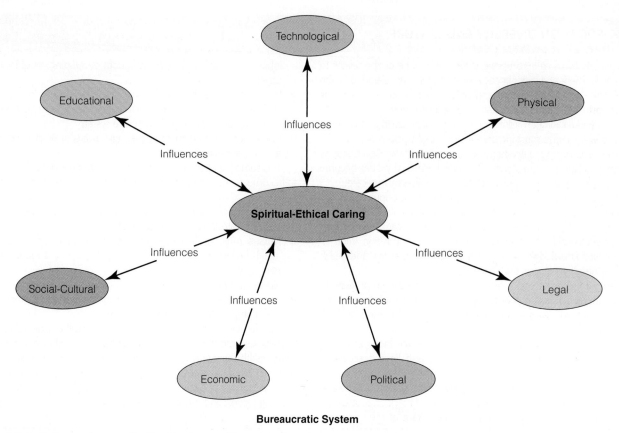

Figure 33-1 ■ Concept map reflecting the theory of bureaucratic caring.

Nursing as Caring (Boykin and Schoenhofer)

Boykin and Schoenhofer suggest that the purpose of the discipline and profession of nursing is to know individuals and nurture them as individuals in a caring environment (Purnell, 2006). Respect for individuals and what matters to them is at the core of the theory of nursing as caring. Boykin and Schoenhofer emphasize the importance of the nurse knowing him- or herself as a caring person. Maintaining this approach may be difficult in practice environments that depersonalize the nurse and view nursing care only as tasks that need to be completed. However, caring is a lifetime process, and not confined to any one environment or situation. Self awareness allows the nurse to authentically care for others in nursing practice.

Caring in nursing is "an altruistic, active expression of love, and is the intentional and embodied recognition of value and connectedness" (Boykin & Schoenhofer, 2001, p. 393). From the perspective of the theory of nursing as caring, the nurse approaches each client as a caring person, whole and complete in the moment. The idea of wholeness includes the understanding that people are not perfect, but are constantly growing and changing. By living nursing as caring, the nurse establishes a mutual relationship of trust and respect with the client. Through fully appreciating the lifeworld of others, the nurse energizes him- or herself and others to grow as caring persons.

Theory of Human Care (Watson)

Watson's theory of human care views caring as the essence and the moral ideal of nursing. Human care is the basis for nursing's role in society; indeed, nursing's contribution to society lies in its moral commitment to human care. Nursing as human care goes beyond the realm of ethics, as described by Watson (1999, p. 29):

> Human caring in nursing, therefore, is not just an emotion, concern, attitude, or benevolent desire. Caring is the moral ideal of nursing whereby the end is protection, enhancement, and preservation of human dignity. Human caring involves values, a will and a commitment to care, knowledge, caring action, and consequences. All of human caring is related to intersubjective human responses to health-illness conditions; a knowledge of health-illness, environmental-personal interactions; a knowledge of the nurse caring process; self-knowledge, knowledge of one's power and transaction limitations.

Watson emphasizes nursing's commitment to care of the whole person as well as a concern for the health of individuals and groups. The nurse and client are coparticipants in the client's movement toward health and wholeness. Watson labels this process transpersonal human caring through which the nurse enters into the experience of the client, and the client can enter into the nurse's experience. By identifying with each other, the nurse and client gain self-knowledge and keep alive their common humanity, avoiding reducing the other to an object.

The Primacy of Caring (Benner and Wrubel)

As Benner and Wrubel listened to expert nurses' stories and analyzed their meanings, caring emerged as the essence of excellence in nursing. Nursing is described as a relationship in which caring is primary because it sets up the possibility of giving and receiving help (Benner & Wrubel, 1989). Caring practice requires attending to the client over time, determining what matters to the client, and using this knowledge in making clinical judgments. As nurses gain expertise, they become more effective in determining client needs. Caring facilitates the nurse's ability to problem solve and to implement individualized solutions.

A caring relationship requires a certain amount of openness and capacity to respond to care on the part of the client. In caring practice, being with someone may be just as important as doing something for that person, if not more so. As nurses gain expertise, they learn how to be with people, and to respect who they are and where they are at that moment. Thus, caring practice involves providing the conditions necessary to help the client grow and develop (Gordon, Benner, & Noddings, 1996).

TYPES OF KNOWLEDGE IN NURSING

Nursing involves different types of knowledge that are integrated into nursing practice. Nurses require scientific competence (empirical knowing), therapeutic use of self (personal knowing), moral/ethical awareness (ethical knowing), and creative action (aesthetic knowing). These four types of knowledge were identified by Carper (1978) from her observations of nurses' activities. An understanding of each type of knowledge is important for the nursing student because only by integrating all ways of knowing can the nurse develop a professional practice. Figure 33–2 ■ illustrates the interconnection of these different types of knowledge.

Empirical Knowing: The Science of Nursing

Knowledge about the empirical world is systematically organized into laws and theories for the purpose of describing, explaining, and predicting events of concern to the discipline of nursing. **Empirical knowing** ranges from factual, observable events (e.g., anatomy, physiology, chemistry) to theoretical analysis (e.g., developmental theory, adaptation theory).

Aesthetic Knowing: The Art of Nursing

Aesthetic knowing is the art of nursing as expressed by the individual nurse through his or her creativity and style in meeting the needs of clients. The nurse uses aesthetic knowing to provide care that is both effective and satisfying. Empathy, compassion, holism, and sensitivity are important modes in the aesthetic pattern of knowing.

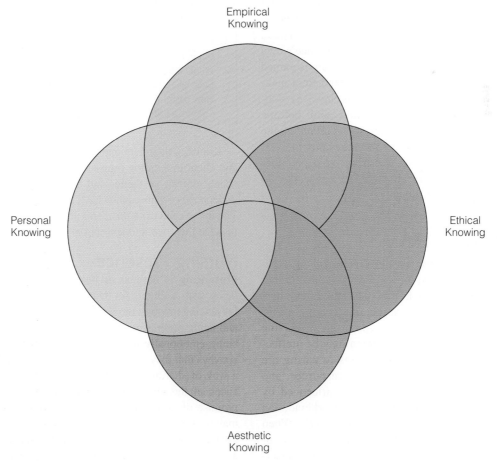

Figure 33–2 ■ The four ways of knowing.

Personal Knowing: The Therapeutic Use of Self

Personal knowledge is concerned with the knowing, encountering, and actualizing of the concrete, individual self. Because nursing is an interpersonal process, the way in which nurses view themselves and the client is of primary concern in any therapeutic relationship. **Personal knowing** promotes wholeness and integrity in the personal encounter, achieves engagement rather than detachment, and denies the manipulative or impersonal approach.

Ethical Knowing: The Moral Component

Goals of nursing include the conservation of life, alleviation of suffering, and promotion of health. **Ethical knowing** focuses on matters of obligation or what ought to be done, and goes beyond simply following the ethical codes of the discipline. Nursing care involves a series of deliberate actions or choices that are subject to the judgment of right or wrong. Occasionally, the principles and norms that guide choices may be in conflict. The more sensitive and knowledgeable the nurse is regarding these issues, the more "ethical" he or she will be.

Developing Ways of Knowing

The methods for developing each type of knowledge are unique (Chinn & Kramer, 2004). The methods that are required for developing one pattern cannot be used to develop knowledge within another pattern. For example, personal knowing is developed through critical reflection on one's own actions and feelings in practice. Empirical knowing is gained from studying scientific models and theories, and from making objective observations. Ethical knowing involves confronting and resolving conflicting values and beliefs. Aesthetic knowing arises from a deep appreciation of the uniqueness of each individual and the meanings that individual ascribes to a given situation. The nurse who practices effectively is able to integrate all types of knowledge to understand situations more holistically.

CARING ENCOUNTERS

How does a nurse demonstrate caring? Given similar situations, why is one nurse judged to be "caring" while another is said to be "uncaring"? Nurse theorists and researchers have studied this question and have identified caring attributes and behaviors. Because caring is contextual, a nursing approach used with a client in one situation may be ineffective in another situation. Clients' responses to caring are as varied as clients' needs, environmental resources, and nurses' imaginations. Caring encounters are influenced by the diversity of human responses, the nurse's workload, and the preferences of the nurse and client (Cooper, 2001). When clients perceive the encounter to be caring, their sense of dignity and self-worth is increased, and feelings of connectedness are expressed.

Knowing the Client

Caring requires understanding the client as a whole person. The nurse asks, "Who is this person? What is his or her history? Needs? Desires? Dreams? Spiritual beliefs? Who loves and cares for this person at home? Where is home and what resources are available there? What does this person need today, from me, right now? Can he or she communicate to me what is needed?" Personal knowledge of the client is a key in the caring relationship between nurse and client. The nurse aims to know who the client is, his or her *uniqueness*. This knowledge is gained by using listening and communication skills while observing and talking with the client and family. The nurse cannot remain detached, but is actively engaged with the client. Consider the following example:

CLINICAL EXAMPLE

Shameka Weaver is an 18-year-old female who is experiencing post-operative pain following reconstructive surgery of her knee after a motor vehicle accident. The nurse assesses Shameka's pain, using an appropriate pain scale. The nurse also assesses Shameka's positioning, hygiene, amount of rest, and other physiological variables for their effect on her pain. The nurse considers other factors that affect the client's perception of pain, including how likely it is that Shameka will be able to return to playing soccer: Shameka has been offered a scholarship to play at the local university. During the assessment, the nurse discovers that Shameka lost her mother to cancer last year. Shameka's older sister provides primary support. The nurse discusses with Shameka's sister how they can make Shameka more comfortable.

1. How might the loss of her mother affect Shameka's perception of pain?
2. What caring interventions could the nurse provide to help Shameka manage her pain?
3. How might the nurse determine other people of significance in Shameka's life and why would this be important to know?

Knowing the client and family ultimately involves the nurse and client in a caring transaction. By attending broadly to personal, ethical, aesthetic, and empirical knowledge, the nurse understands events as they have meaning in the life of the client. The nurse's *knowing the client* ultimately increases the possibilities for therapeutic interventions to be perceived as relevant.

Nursing Presence

Presencing is defined as being present, being there, or just being with a client. As discussed in Concept 27, Spirituality, presencing involves the nurse being fully present in the moment and being present in a way that is meaningful to the client. By being emotionally present for the client and family, the nurse conveys that they and their experiences matter. Being present is a way of sharing in the meanings, feelings, and lived experiences of the client. Physical presence is combined with the promise of availability, especially during a time of need. This may be as simple as responding promptly to a call bell in a hospital unit, or as complex as sitting with a parent who has just lost a child in a neonatal intensive care unit. In an account by the parent of a newborn with a serious heart defect, Schroeder

(1998) described how a nurse periodically sat with her. "Her words and presence began to fill some of the emptiness inside me," (p. 19) she said. Quietly talking with the nurse helped this mother find meaning in her current situation, as she "began to see that perhaps this experience wasn't just meaningless destruction, torture and death: regardless of outcome, we were all growing in ways denied ordinary people" (p. 20).

Covington (2003) defines caring presence as an "interpersonal, intersubjective human experience of connection within a nurse-client relationship that makes it safe for sharing oneself with another" (p. 312). The nurse brings conscious awareness (intentionality), and is open to opportunities for connection with the client. Through this sharing, both client and nurse attempt to discover meaning in the experience of health and illness. A possible outcome is transformation and growth of both the client and the nurse.

Empowering the Client

Through knowing the client and engaging in a mutual relationship, the nurse is able to identify and build upon client/family strengths. By empowering the client and family to see strengths and act on them, the nurse models a healthy coping mechanism and provides a measure of hope for the client and family. The nurse also offers an environment in which the client can feel safe to try the next step, and to ask for help when needed (Figure 33–3 ■).

Compassion

Universally, clients equate compassion with caring. The caring nurse is described as warm and empathic, compassionate and concerned. In order to demonstrate empathy, the nurse must be able to identify with the client, appreciating the pain and discomfort of illness, or imagining "walking in his shoes," in regard to some part of the client's life experience.

Roach (2002) defines compassion as "a way of living born out of an awareness of one's relationship to all living creatures" (p. 50). Like empathy, compassion involves participating in the client's experience with sensitivity to the client's pain or discomfort, and a willingness to share in the client's experience. Compassion becomes part of the caring relationship, as the nurse shares the client's joys, sorrows, pain, and accomplishments. Compassion is a gift from the heart, rather than an advanced skill or technique.

Attention to spiritual needs is part of compassionate care, particularly in the face of death and bereavement. The nurse is aware that spiritual and religious beliefs are important coping mechanisms in dealing with issues of mortality (see Exemplar 5.2, End-of-Life Care). The nurse does not impose his or her own spiritual beliefs, but rather assists the client and family in drawing upon their own beliefs as spiritual resources.

Comfort is often associated with compassionate care, and many nursing interventions are carried out to provide comfort. For example, bathing, positioning, talking, touching, and listening are often performed to increase the client's comfort level (Figure 33–4 ■). Just like pain or discomfort, comfort is subjective and is defined as "whatever

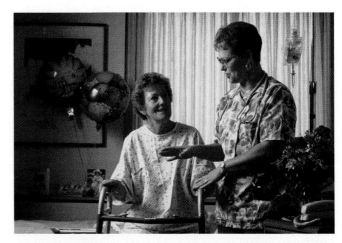

Figure 33–3 ■ The nurse helps her client learn to use a walker, teaching her the appropriate technique for rising from the bed, and standing nearby to encourage and support the client, ready to step in and provide assistance if necessary.

the client says it is," based on the individual's perceptions. Despite this subjectivity, comfort care is often the basis for nursing in settings ranging from intensive care to hospice, and serves as a motivator for nursing interventions. Nurses are challenged to be creative and innovative, basing interventions on knowledge of the client's preferences, in order to provide comfort care.

Competence

The competent nurse employs the necessary knowledge, judgment, skills, and motivation to respond adequately to the client's needs. Just as competence without compassion is cold and inhumane, compassion without competence is meaningless and dangerous. The competent nurse, as described by Roach (2002), understands the client's condition, its treatment, and associated care. The nurse is able to provide the necessary care, while guiding the client and family through the process. The nurse's abilities to assess, plan, implement, and evaluate a plan of care are focused on

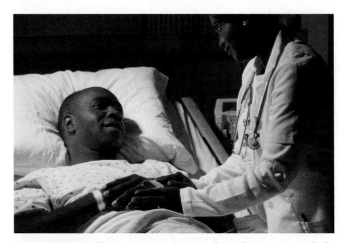

Figure 33–4 ■ This nurse is using touch and presence to help comfort her client.

meeting the client/family needs. Practice of these skills requires a high level of cognitive, affective, technical, and administrative skills.

Jacob Martinez, 4 years old, speaks no English and was admitted to the hospital with multiple injuries, the result of abuse at the hands of his father. His mother was admitted to the intensive care unit with severe trauma to the head and chest, also the result of his father's physical abuse. His siblings were placed in foster care and there are no other relatives living in the United States.

Jacob is frightened and withdrawn, and will not speak even when a gentle interpreter is brought in to talk with him in his native language. He lies quietly in his bed and curls into the fetal position when the nurse enters his room. He shrinks away when anyone reaches out to touch him and cries quietly during procedures without making a sound.

1. Develop a nursing plan of care for Jacob addressing his fear and withdrawal.
2. What actions can the nurse take to help Jacob feel safe?
3. Looking toward Jacob's eventual discharge and potential placement in foster care, how might the nurse advocate for Jacob to make the transition less fearful?

MAINTAINING CARING PRACTICE

The concept of caring for self seems almost foreign to many nurses and nursing students, because of the professional emphasis on meeting the needs of others. Yet, as nurses take on multiple commitments to family, work, school, and community, they risk exhaustion, burnout, and stress. Obstacles to self-care may be professional, related to the demands of a particular work setting, or may be personal, such as poor health habits or unrealistic expectations of self (see Concept 28 for more information on stress and coping). Despite these challenges, it is imperative that nurses attend to their own needs because caring for self is central to caring for others.

Caring for Self

Mayeroff (1990) describes caring for self as helping oneself grow and actualize one's possibilities. Caring for self means taking the time to nurture oneself. This involves initiating and maintaining behaviors that promote healthy living and well-being. Although different activities may be helpful to different people, some examples of these activities are:

- A balanced diet
- Regular exercise
- Adequate rest and sleep
- Recreational activities
- Meditation and prayer.

Self-care focuses on care of the self in the deepest sense. Self-awareness and self-esteem are intimately connected to self-care. In its code of ethics, the American Holistic Nurses Association states that "the nurse has a responsibility to model healthcare behaviors. Holistic nurses strive to achieve harmony in their own lives and to assist others who are striving to do the same" (American Holistic Nurses Association, 2010). Individuals with high self-esteem can critically problem solve and tackle obstacles more effectively. Self-care practices build self-esteem, leading to feelings of comfort and accomplishment. The self-esteem questionnaire in Box 33–2 is a measure to assess self-esteem. The more "yes" answers on the tool, the more opportunity exists for improving self-esteem.

The death of a client, particularly a child, can be a very difficult time in the life of a nurse. Nurses who work with the terminally ill and their families require special training and preparation to meet the needs of these clients and to manage their own personal stress. Nurses caring for dying clients should take advantage of support systems that help them balance the stresses that they face at work. These may include discussions with peers, group counseling sessions in the work place, and other types of support. Continuing education courses may help nurses identify coping strategies for personal care (Meadors & Lamson, 2008).

A Healthy Lifestyle

Everyone needs to pay attention to nutrition and exercise, and to avoid unhealthy lifestyle practices. Key words for a healthy lifestyle are *balance* and *moderation*. Nurses in particular need to engage in healthy habits in order to maintain a healthy immune system and model for their families, clients, and communities. Healthy lifestyle practices should be supplemented by regular physical examinations and health screenings. Healthy lifestyle practices include the following:

- Adequate nutrition
- Activity and exercise
- Recreation
- Avoiding unhealthy practices.

Appropriate nutrition and sufficient activity and exercise are lifetime endeavors that are essential for healthy living (see Figure 33–5 ■). A balanced diet provides more energy,

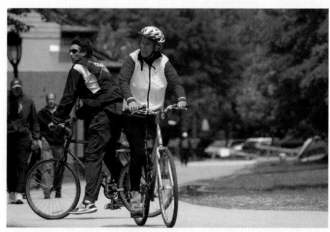

Figure 33–5 ■ Regular activity and exercise is an effective self-care practice.

Box 33-2 Self-Esteem Questionnaire

Answer Yes or No to the following questions. Check the box appropriate for how you feel the majority of time.

	Yes	No
Do you have a hard time nurturing yourself?		
Have you ever turned down an invitation to a party or function because of the way you felt about yourself?		
Do you get your sense of self-worth from the approval of others?		
Are you supportive of others but berate yourself?		
Whenever things go wrong in life do you blame yourself?		
Do you react to disappointment by blaming others?		
Do you begin each day with a negative attitude?		
Do you feel undeserving?		
Do you ever feel like an impostor and that soon your deficiencies will be exposed?		
Do you have an inner-critic who is disparaging or demeaning?		
Do you believe that being hard on yourself is the best motivation for change?		
Do your good points seem ordinary and your failings all-important?		
Do you feel unattractive?		
Have you ever felt your accomplishments are due to luck, but your failures due to incompetence or inadequacy?		
Have you ever felt that if you are not a total success, then you are a failure, and that there is no middle ground with no points for effort?		
Do you feel unappreciated?		
Do you feel lonely?		
Do you struggle with feelings of inferiority?		
Do other people's opinions count more to you than your own?		
Do you criticize yourself often?		
Do others criticize you often?		
Do you hesitate to do things because of what others might think?		
TOTALS		

Source: © Martin, Catherine A. (1998) *The Positive Way.* Retrieved from www.positive-way.com. Used with permission.

builds endurance for carrying out daily activities, and reduces risks for certain health problems. Exercises promotes healthy physiologic and psychologic responses. The Centers for Disease Control recommend that healthy adults engage in a combination of moderate-intensity aerobic activity and muscle strengthening activities for a total of 2 hours and 30 minutes over a period of 2 or more days every week. Recommendations regarding the amount of exercise and total time of exercise vary depending on age, health status, and the type of exercise (CDC, 2009).

Self-care also includes taking time to do the things that bring joy and stimulate creativity. Nurses need to reward themselves, experience spontaneity, and even take downtime (time to do nothing). Nurses must also avoid activities or thought patterns that contribute to negative health outcomes. Negative thinking can create a stress response, affecting physiological, mental, and emotional outcomes. Practices such as identifying negative feelings, refocusing on the positive, and using humor are helpful to avert the stress response by changing thought patterns. It is also important to avoid destructive lifestyle choices such as smoking, abuse of alcohol or drugs, and misusing medications.

REVIEW Caring Interventions

RELATE: LINK THE CONCEPTS

Linking the concept of Caring Interventions with the concept of Violence:

1. You are working in the Emergency Department of a local hospital when the police bring in a 16-year-old girl whom they found naked and beaten in an alley. What caring interventions will you provide to her immediately upon arrival?

2. Her mother is summoned from work to come to the hospital and be with her daughter. The first words the mother says to the client are "How did you let this happen?!" How would you, as the nurse, respond to the mother?

Linking the concept of Caring Interventions with the concept of Fluids and Electrolytes:

1. You are caring for a client with acute nausea and vomiting. What caring interventions could you provide to make this client more comfortable?
2. What would you do to determine how to make a client with acute renal failure more comfortable?

REFER: GO TO MYNURSINGKIT

REFLECT: CASE STUDY

After morning report, the nurse, Megan, approaches Robbie James, a 10-year-old boy lying quietly in his hospital bed. She introduces herself and writes her name on the white board in the room so that when Robbie's mother arrives, she will know the name of Robbie's nurse. Megan's client assignment today consists of four acutely ill children of different ages. As Megan makes her initial rounds, she assesses the immediate needs of each child and begins to prioritize her nursing activities.

Megan has her own needs. She is tired from the night before because her own daughter was up late with coughing and a fever. She is comfortable with her arrangements for child care, and she is able to focus on her care of the clients on the pediatric unit.

When Megan returns with intravenous morphine, Robbie barely speaks and has a pinched look of discomfort on his face. Using the FACES pain scale, Robbie has identified his pain as the "worst possible pain," which is confirmed prior to administration of medication by the nurse This is his first day postoperative after removal of a ruptured appendix. He has a nasogastric (NG) tube in place connected to low wall suction. She checks patency and placement of the NG tube and assesses Robbie's vital signs. Megan administers the medication according to unit protocol and continues her assessment, rechecking vital signs after the medication begins to take effect.

Megan notes a "walking chart" on the wall beside Robbie's bed. The walking chart includes spaces to place a sticker each time Robbie walks in the hall. Robbie knows that after three stickers, he can choose a prize from the treasure box. Before Megan leaves the room, she suggests to Robbie, "When you feel better from this medicine, I'll help you walk, and we'll put another sticker on that chart!"

1. Describe which aspect of the nurse's approach relates to each of the following six Cs of caring in nursing as outlined by Roach: compassion, competence, confidence, conscience, commitment, comportment.
2. In analyzing this case study and reflecting on the four ways of knowing (e.g., personal, empirical, aesthetic, and ethical), describe how each type of knowing prepared the nurse, Megan, for her caring approach.

EXPLORE PEARSON mynursingkit™

MyNursingKit is your one stop for online chapter review materials and resources. Prepare for success with additional NCLEX®-style practice questions, interactive assignments and activities, web links, animations and videos, and more!

Register your access code from the front of your book at www.mynursingkit.com.

REFERENCES

American Holistic Nurses Association. (2010). Position statements. Retrieved May 10, 2010, from http://www.ahna.org/Resources/Publications/PositionStatements/tabid/1926/Default.aspx#P2

Benner, P., & Wrubel, J. (1989). The primacy of caring: Stress and coping in health and illness. Menlo Park, CA: Addison-Wesley.

Boykin, A., & Schoenhofer, S. (2001). Nursing as caring: An overview of a general theory of nursing. In M. Parker (Ed.), Nursing theories and nursing practice (pp. 391–402). Philadelphia: F. A. Davis.

Cameron, J. (2002). The artist's way. New York: Jeremy P. Tarcher/Putnam.

Carper, B. (1978). Fundamental patterns of knowing in nursing. Advances in Nursing Science, 1(1), 13–23.

Centers for Disease Control and Prevention. (2009). How much physical activity do adults need? Retrieved February 25, 2010, from http://www.cdc.gov/physicalactivity/everyone/guidelines/adults.html

Chinn, P., & Kramer, M. (2004). Integrated knowledge development in nursing (6th ed.). St. Louis, MO: Mosby.

Coffman, S. (2006). Marilyn Anne Ray: Theory of bureaucratic caring. In A. Tomey & M. Alligood (Eds.), Nursing theorists and their work (6th ed., pp. 116–139). St. Louis, MO: Mosby.

Cooper, C. (2001). The art of nursing. Philadelphia: W. B. Saunders.

Covington, H. (2003). Caring presence. Journal of Holistic Nursing, 21(3), 301–317.

Gordon, S., Benner, P., & Noddings, N. (1996). Caregiving. Philadelphia: University of Pennsylvania Press.

Leininger, M. (1991). Transcultural care principles, human rights, and ethical considerations. Journal of Transcultural Nursing, 3(1), 21–23.

Leininger, M. M. (2001). Culture care diversity & universality: A theory of nursing. Sudbury, MA: Jones & Bartlett.

Mayeroff, M. (1990). On caring. New York: Harper Collins.

Meadors, P., & Lamson, A. (2008). Compassion fatigue and secondary traumatization: Provider self care on intensive care units for children. Journal of Pediatric Health Care, 22(1), 24–34.

Merriam-Webster Online Dictionary. (2010). Caring. Retrieved March 1, 2010, from http://www.merriam-webster.com/dictionary/caring

Morse, J., Solberg, S., Neander, W., Battorff, J., & Johnson, J. (1990). Concepts of caring and caring as a concept. Advances in Nursing Science, 13(1), 1–14.

Pask, E. (2003). Moral agency in nursing: Seeing value in the work and believing that I make a difference. Nursing Ethics, 10(2), 165–174.

The Positive Way. (2006) Self-esteem questionnaire. Retrieved June 7, 2006, from http://www.positive-way.com/self-est1.htm

Purnell, M. (2006). Nursing as caring: A model for transforming practice. In A. Tomey & M. Alligood (Eds.), Nursing theorists and their work (6th ed.). St. Louis, MO: Mosby.

Ray, M. (2001). The theory of bureaucratic caring. In M. Parker (Ed.), Nursing theories and nursing practice (pp. 422–431). Philadelphia: F. A. Davis.

Roach, M. S. (2002). Caring, the human mode of being (2nd ed.). Ottawa, Ontario, Canada: CHA Press.

Schroeder, C. (1998). So this is what it's like: Struggling to survive in pediatric intensive care. Advances in Nursing Science, 10(4), 13–22.

Watson, J. (1999). Nursing: Human science and human care. A theory of nursing. Boston: Jones & Bartlett.

Clinical Decision Making

34

Concept at-a-Glance

About Clinical Decision Making, *2037*

34.1   The Nursing Process, *2047*

34.2   Critical Thinking, *2104*

 Concept Learning Outcomes

After reading about this concept, you will be able to:

1. Discuss the need for decision making in the nursing process in order to maintain safe nursing practice.

2. Describe the relationships among the nursing process, critical thinking, the problem-solving process, and the decision-making process.

3. Illustrate the impact of change on the need for decision making.

4. Identify essential decisions made by nurses in their daily practice.

5. Predict potential barriers to decision making in nursing practice and strategies to overcome them.

6. Using a client scenario, analyze each step in the decision-making process.

7. Integrate decision making and problem solving in all phases of the nursing process.

 Concept Key Terms

Chief complaint, *2045*

Critical thinking, *2038*

Decision making, *2037*

Evaluation, *2046*

Implementation, *2045*

Intuition, *2044*

Nonprogrammed decisions, *2040*

Problem, *2039*

Problem-solving process, *2038*

Programmed decisions, *2040*

Research process, *2044*

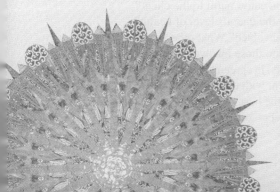

About Clinical Decision Making

Decision making is a critical-thinking process for choosing the best actions to meet a desired goal. Decisions must be made whenever several mutually exclusive choices are available or when there is an option to act or not. For example, individuals who wish to become nurses in the United States have several possible courses of action: a diploma program, an associate degree program, or a baccalaureate program. Prospective students must choose which to pursue. Therefore, they must evaluate the different types of programs, as well as personal circumstances, to make a decision appropriate to their situations. In order to make a decision, they use critical thinking and employ the problem-solving process to determine available options and the best choice of the alternatives.

Critical thinking is a cognitive process during which an individual reviews data and considers potential explanations and outcomes before forming an opinion or making a decision. The term **problem-solving process** refers to "a process whereby a dilemma is identified and corrected" (Sullian & Decker, 2001, p. 153). Nurses are expected to use critical thinking to solve client problems and make better decisions. Thus, critical thinking, problem solving, and decision making are interrelated processes, with creativity enhancing the result. Decisions that nurses must make about client care and about the distribution of limited resources force them to think and act in areas where neither clear answers nor standard procedures exist and where conflicting forces turn decision making into a complex process.

Nurses make decisions in the course of solving problems. Decision making, however, is also used in situations that do not involve problem solving. Nurses make value decisions (e.g., to keep client information confidential), time management decisions (e.g., taking clean linens to the client's room at the same time as the medication in order to save steps), scheduling decisions (e.g., to bathe the client before visiting hours), and priority decisions (e.g., which interventions are most urgent and which can be delegated).

Nurses must make decisions and assist clients to make decisions. When faced with several client needs at the same time, the nurse must prioritize and decide which client to assist first. The nurse may (a) look at advantages and disadvantages of each option, (b) apply Maslow's hierarchy of needs, (c) consider which tasks can be delegated to others, or (d) use another priority-setting framework. When a client is trying to make a decision about what course of treatment to follow, the nurse may need to provide information or resources the client can use in making a decision (Figure 34–1 ■). Nurses also must make decisions in their own personal and professional lives. For example, nurses must decide whether to work in a hospital or community setting, whether to join a professional association, and whether to carry professional liability insurance.

Another factor that promotes the need for strong clinical decision-making skills is the constantly changing health care environment. New technology, the need for cost containment, client and staff diversity, clients' varying responses to care, and the ever-expanding body of knowledge that nurses manage lead to constant change within the profession. Change impacts the decision-making process.

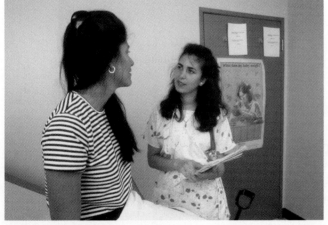

Figure 34–1 ■ Nurses provide information to clients to assist them in making decisions about their health care.

"In the 21st century, the demand for change and innovation is challenging and enormous. Nurses need to do far more than simply manage change; they need to passionately champion both change and innovation" (Gebelein et al., 2000, p. 24). Nurses tend to think that leaders and managers will save the day by helping them cope with the ever-changing health care environment. The truth is that most managers will not be able to do this, as many are not prepared to cope with this rate of change themselves (Bennis & Goldsmith, 1997). What does this mean? Nurses at all levels must make a commitment to the change process and take active roles. Change that comes from, and is totally managed by, a manager will not be successful. Nurses who pull back and wait for the manager to make the difference will often find that changes will occur without their input. They will also miss opportunities to gain experience that comes with participating in the change process as well as miss opportunities to make themselves heard. Nurses must embrace and participate in decision making processes in order to improve both the quality of client care and that of their workplace environment. ●

DECISION MAKING: A RESPONSE TO CHANGE

Decision making is, above all else, a response to change. As such, it is "a process that begins with the identification of a problem and ends with the evaluation of the choices and taking a course of action" (Bernard & Walsh, 1990, as cited in Krairiksh & Anthony, 2001, p. 16). In order to take a course of action, individuals and group invoke the planning process. "The planning process parallels the decision-making process; this makes sense, since developing plans involves deciding today what you'll do tomorrow. Both involve establishing objectives or criteria, developing and analyzing alternatives based on information obtained, evaluating the alternatives, and then making a choice" (Dessler, 2002, p. 93). This section of the concept focuses on decision making, a function that every nurse uses in the practice of nursing. Any response to change requires decisions, and many of these decisions require careful planning.

Decisions are a means rather than ends. They are used to achieve a goal. When decisions are made, the goal is usually related to both tasks and relationships. Some decisions may focus more on one than the other (Gebelein et al., 2000). Those who make decisions must learn to cope with being right some of the time and also learn to live with the consequences when they are wrong or when a perfect solution cannot be found. The most important consideration in making a sound decision is the criteria one uses to make that decision. Some examples of criteria that nurses might use can be framed in the following questions:

- Will the decision cause harm to the client?
- Will it improve the client's level of health?
- What risks are involved? What other benefits?
- Are the client and those involved with the client's care (e.g., spouse or parents) in agreement with the decision? Is the decision in agreement with the client's values or spiritual beliefs?
- Is the decision the best option given existing time restraints, current resources, or other priorities (Gebelein et al., 2000, p. 114)?

How is decision making related to planning? Nurses actively use decision making in a variety of situations, particularly during planning—client care planning, planning the work day, and planning to whom tasks can be delegated. "Planning is setting goals and deciding on courses of action, developing rules and procedures, developing plans" (Dessler, 2002, p. 3.). Planning activities apply both to the client and to those providing care for the client. Planning also includes consideration of how the client's needs may change based on the plan of care. Planning may also include accounting for a variety of future possibilities, such as preventing a problem or anticipating a change. Planning is often necessary to resolve a problem.

"A **problem** is a discrepancy between a desirable and an actual situation" (Dessler, 2002, p. 68). Decisions are required to resolve this discrepancy. Typically, decision making and problem solving are used interchangeably though decisions do not always focus on problems. Decisions, however, are also made when problems are solved. For example, after changing the treatment plan for a client with asthma, the nurse determines the new treatment works best but the client is more comfortable with the old regimen. A decision must now be made about when, or if, the new treatment regimen will be used.

Decision-Making Styles

In addition to planning, creativity is an important part of the decision-making process. Stepping "outside the box" is a phrase frequently used in all types of organizations. Decision making that routinely results in similar outcomes and does not consider diversity in client needs and innovative outcomes will not be as effective in the long run. Nurses, managers, and other health care providers must employ creativity to achieve effective solutions for both clients and organizations.

Decisions can be made by individuals or groups. Decision-making styles have been identified for both.

INDIVIDUAL DECISION MAKING Individual styles of decision making are affected by creativity or innovation. There are several common individual decision-making styles. In *unilateral decision making* one person makes decisions for another without input from others, such as when the nurse decides how to intervene for a client without the client's input. *Individual decision making* refers to one person making decisions on his or her own behalf, such as the nurse making a decision about what job to accept. In *authoritarian decision making* one person makes a decision requiring others to conform, such as when the employer decides on a policy that the nurse is expected to follow. In each of these processes one person makes the decision with limited or no input from others. The opposite of these styles is *participative* or *consensus decision making*. Here the emphasis is on including others in the decision making, even if an individual must make the final decision. The individual who uses this style pays close attention to feedback from others and uses that feedback when making the final decision.

Other decision-making styles that have been described are decisive, integrative, hierarchic, and flexible (Milgram, Spector, & Treger, 1999). These styles apply to managers and to staff. The difference in these four styles is in the amount of data that is used to make a decision and the options that are considered:

- The decisive style depends on less data to arrive at one decision.
- The integrative style uses all available data and identifies multiple alternatives.
- The hierarchic style focuses on a large amount of information but arrives at one alternative or solution.
- The flexible style uses a small amount of data while generating multiple alternatives and may change as information is reinterpreted.

It is typical for individuals to use one style primarily, though some use mixed styles or may switch styles depending upon the situation. For example, when a situation changes, different factors become more important, and the nurse may change styles to adjust. A nurse may encourage client participation in decisions and allow time for this, but if the client's condition deteriorates rapidly then the nurse may need to step in and make decisions quickly.

Dessler identifies two additional approaches to decision making: systematic vs. intuitive (Dessler, 2002). *Systematic decision makers* form their decisions more logically and use a structured approach. *Intuitive decision makers* are at the other end of the spectrum; here the focus is on a trial-and-error approach. They may ignore information and change their alternatives if it does not feel right. This is the "gut" approach. A nurse will say, "I just had a feeling about it." Again, the situation can make a difference. When a nurse has expertise in an area, decisions may appear to be more intuitive because the nurse may feel more confident and can rely more on a "gut feeling," though the decision is probably supported by expertise.

GROUP DECISION MAKING Many organizations use group decision making in various situations. *Group decision making* allows people with multiple ideas and experiences to come together to form a decision. The primary advantage of this method is that ideas from more than one person tend to improve other ideas and the final decision. As group members discuss an issue, ideas tend to bounce off of each other, which stimulate further ideas. The major disadvantage is that it takes longer to make a decision. Futhermore, some issues or problems may be made worse by group decision making. For example, during an emergency, decisions must be made quickly and clearly so that all can follow them. Employing a group process that lengthens the time it takes to make a decision can cause unnecessary delay that may compromise the health of the client.

The group decision-making process emphasizes that ideas and suggestions of all participants are important. By providing feedback to each other, group members can improve the process over the long term. It is important that group leaders provide feedback to group members equally, and that no member feels left out or feels that his or her time has been wasted. Recognition goes a long way to improve morale, encourage others to increase participation, and improve group decision making.

Dessler (2002) identifies additional advantages and disadvantages for using group decision making. The generally accepted advantage of "two heads are better than one" allows for more points of view and develops more acceptance and commitment from those who participate. The result usually is a greater effort to make the decision work during implementation. Why would there be disadvantages to group decision making? There may be greater pressure for consensus when members may not actually agree. Some groups experience dominance by one individual, diluting the effect of group input. Also, group members can believe so much in their own ideas that they are unable to openly consider other ideas. Group decisions can also take longer, which for some situations may be a disadvantage.

CLINICAL EXAMPLE

Care plan meetings are an example of group decision making and involve multiple team members using their unique expertise to resolve client care issues. This is discussed in more detail in Concept 36, Communication.

Groups can, of course, be quite successful in making decisions, but decision making does not just happen. There usually must be some guidance or facilitation. Brainstorming requires that all members are clear about what the issue is about and what it is not about. Setting a reasonable time limit pushes group members to move toward a result. Ground rules should make clear that the following are not helpful: (a) digression into details, (b) focusing on reasons about why an idea will not work or the constraints, and (c) criticism of ideas or evaluation of alternatives (Gebelein et al., 2000).

There are methods other than brainstorming that also facilitate group decision making, such as idea-generating questions (for example, "If we had enough time, what would we do?" and "If we had the correct equipment, how would we solve the problem?"). It is helpful to stimulate the group so that the group considers how similar problems were solved in the past, and then the group compares and contrasts the past with the present problem. Taking a different point of view than what would normally be taken may help the group understand the problem or issue from another perspective, which may lead to different alternatives, moving the decision making "out-of-the-box."

Nurses use a type of group decision-making process when they collaborate about how best to resolve a problem. Even the most experienced nurses will encounter situations that puzzle them or leave them unsure of how best to respond. Collaboration allows nurses to consult those who may have expertise in a different area or to engage in discussion that brings up possibilities that otherwise may not be considered.

Types of Decisions

There are two major types of decisions that most nurses must make. **Programmed decisions** are repetitive and routine. They are typically related to a policy or procedure and don't take much time to make. For example, if a client leaves the hospital against medical advice (AMA), there is a procedure for an AMA discharge. Similarly, if a nurse misses an order for a medication, there is a procedure to follow such as whom to notify, what to document, and so on. Most decisions that a nurse needs to make are programmed decisions. **Nonprogrammed decisions** are not so routine. Situations that require nonprogrammed decisions typically require more time, data collection, critical thinking and analysis, and may require consultation with others. Situations requiring nonprogrammed decisions frequently represent new experiences for the nurse. They require more judgment or the "cognitive or thinking aspects of the decision-making process" (Dessler, 2002, p. 68).

An alternate view of the types of decisions considers the focus of the decision (Anthony, 1997, 1999; Blegen et al., 1993; Krairiksh & Anthony, 2001). Client care decisions are one type of decision that nurses make in their practice. As the name implies, these decisions directly affect client care. The second type is decisions about the condition of work. This type affects the work environment, groups of clients, and how work is conducted. Most nurses tend to participate more in decisions with direct care implications (Krairiksh & Anthony, 2001). However, nurses are becoming more involved as leaders in the health care delivery system, and therefore have greater opportunities to make decisions about the conditions in which they work.

THE DECISION-MAKING PROCESS

The decision-making process is a dynamic process. The most effective decisions are made in collaboration with others in the organization. Collaboration between nurses and physicians provides greater opportunities for nurses to participate in making decisions. When collaboration is used, nurses and physicians share responsibility and respect one another more. They also share knowledge, ideas, and skills. This type of relationship can only improve decision making. Critical thinking should be part of problem-solving process and is discussed in more detail in Exemplar 34.2. It is important, however, to note that critical thinking is not the same as problem solving or decision making. Nurses who develop critical-thinking skills will relieve their own stress, solve problems, and make more effective decisions. Table 34–1 provides a comparison of critical thinking, decision making, and problem solving.

Identify the Need for Decision Making: What Is the Problem?

After a review of related issues, the need to make a decision should be carefully identified. A solution cannot be found for something that is truly unknown or poorly understood. Clarifying the problem is not always easy. Nurses may have different perspectives on an issue. For example, one nurse may believe that a client's behavior is an indication of a mental

TABLE 34–1 Comparison of Critical Thinking, Decision Making, and Problem Solving

CRITICAL THINKING	DECISION MAKING	PROBLEM SOLVING
Definition: A process of reviewing, interpreting, and evaluating data, and exploring possible explanations and outcomes before forming an opinion or making a decision. ■ Seeks no single solution. ■ Focuses on creativity and innovation. ■ Purposeful and constantly reevaluating. ■ May be used in both decision making and problem solving. ■ Allows the person to "think outside the box" and consider many ideas without prejudice.	Definition: "A process whereby appropriate alternatives are weighed and one is ultimately selected" (Sullivan & Decker, 2001, p. 153). ■ Decisions are made daily by nurses: care decisions, management decisions, and professional decisions. ■ Decisions may not involve a problem. ■ Ideally, critical thinking is used when decisions are made. ■ Decisions require a choice between alternatives.	Definition: "A process whereby a dilemma is identified and corrected" (Sullivan & Decker, 2001, p. 153). ■ A problem is a gap in how things are and how they might be. ■ Problem solving requires that the problem is identified or diagnosed. ■ There may not be the need to select a correct solution—for example, there may be no response to the problem. This in itself is a form of a decision. ■ Resolving a problem may include critical thinking—and the best resolutions include critical thinking. ■ Resolving a problem includes many decisions, typically some minor and some major. ■ Problem-solving process: define the problem, gather information, analyze the information, develop solutions, make a decision or choose the solution, implement the decision (solution), and evaluate the decision (solution). ■ The problem-solving process corresponds to the nursing process.

Source: Author. Adapted from Sullivan E., & Decker P. (2001). *Effective leadership and management in nursing.* Upper Saddle River, NJ: Prentice Hall.

health issue while another may believe there is a physiological issue. The questions found in Box 34–1 should be considered in this step of the process.

Decision-Making Conditions

When discussing decision-making conditions, the first major issue is who is responsible for making the decision. Nurses who take on decisions that are not theirs to make or who do not make decisions they are responsible for making can cause further difficulty for the client and create problems for their colleagues. How does one find out about who is responsible for a decision? Position descriptions and agency organizational charts typically clarify which staff members are responsible for decisions at various levels.

If the decision is the client's to make, a number of factors may impact the client's ability or willingness to make the decision. Does the client have the mental ability, energy, or knowledge required to make an informed decision? Is the client willing to make a decision about care or would he or she prefer to have the nurse or health care team make the decision? Is it necessary to collaborate or consult another member of the health care team, such as the physician, in order to make a decision? Has the client been fully informed of his or her options, following the requirements for obtaining informed consent? (See Concept 47, Legal Issues.) Clients who feel uncomfortable may avoid decision making, let others make the decision, execute the decision-making process poorly, or arrive at poor decisions that fail to meet their immediate needs. Those who work with this type of client will also feel uncomfortable about the decisions that are made. This, in

turn, affects morale, client outcomes, safety and quality, and the overall client care.

Box 34–1 Identifying the Need for Decision Making: Questions to Ask

■ What is the issue or problem? State the issue or problem in terms of need rather than a solution, using terms that are understood.

■ What important, critical facts are known? Describe these as clearly as possible.

■ What is unknown? How important is the unknown? Who might know the information or how can it be obtained? Be willing to identify factors that might be negative or different.

■ When does the problem occur? When is it absent? Consider days of week, time of day, and factors that might affect timing.

■ What is the consequence of the problem or issue? This step should include negative and positive consequences.

■ What has been tried in the past to deal with the situation? This may be an action that occurred within the organization or was externally considered (literature review, network with others, and so on). What happened as a result of these actions?

■ How do people feel about the situation and changes to it?

■ What related problems are present? If something changes, what else will likely change as a result of the initial change?

■ What assumptions—about people, technology, systems, funding—have been made that might need to be challenged?

Source: Author content and some summarized content from Gebellin, S., et al. (2000). *Successful manager's handbook.* Minneapolis, MN: Personnel Decisions International Corporation; Marrelli, T. (1997). *The nurse manager's guide.* St. Louis, MO: Mosby-Year Book, Inc.

If there is discomfort with decision making, nurses should investigate the key reasons for this discomfort (Gebelein et al., 2000). When a person feels that there is a lack of knowledge about the true risk of the alternatives, there is an increase in discomfort. For this person, whether it's a client or health care professional, further data collection and analysis are important. Some people are uncomfortable with the possible consequences of risk taking. When this occurs, a typical question might be, "What is the worst thing that could happen?" It is important to consider impact and strategies to reduce risks. Maybe the person is focusing too much on the negative aspects. Others feel uncomfortable when the risk factors are unknown. Again, there needs to be more data collection, analysis, and talking to others who may help clarify the issue.

Some nurses are uncomfortable when certain types of decisions must be made such as those dealing with spirituality, grief and loss, or sexuality. If this is the case, it is important to learn more about these areas and gain some expertise and confidence. For example, the nurse working in the intensive care unit may need to make a personal decision about participating in the discontinuation of life support, particularly if the client is a child.

Improving decision-making competency is important for all nurses. Increasing knowledge, researching to gain more information, and getting additional experience helps to improve decision making. Discussing concerns with colleagues is another important strategy for every nurse to use.

Barriers to Decision Making

Barriers to decision making are similar to barriers to change. Barriers can be conditions that exist within an organization or those that are beyond the control of an organization, such as whether or not a client has health insurance. Whenever barriers are considered, it is critical to be clear about the barriers that exist within the organization. Examples of typical organizational barriers include organizational dysfunction, poor communication among staff or health care team members, lack of participation by one or more essential members of the health care team, the organization's own internal policies and procedures, and poor relationships with the community and consumers.

In addition, other barriers exist that focus more on the individuals who make the decisions (Dessler, 2002). Some individuals, for example, may have a tendency to take decision-making shortcuts. This can be an advantage, but it can also be a barrier to success when the shortcut limits data collection, analysis, and the quantity and quality of alternatives that are considered. If a member of the health care team or even the client fails to give an accurate description of an issue, this can be a barrier to the decision making process. A frequent error in describing an issue or problem occurs when the person unconsciously considers some information to be important when it is not (Dessler, 2002, p. 76). An individual's psychological set, which is a rigid strategy or point-of-view, is another major barrier. When a nurse enters the decision-making process with a rigid idea about possible cause(s) or strategies, there is an immediate block to success.

Barriers to decision making can change throughout the client's treatment process, thereby affecting the client's needs and conditions for treatment. A client with a chronic illness may lose his or her health insurance benefits during the course of treatment. A nurse who has a particularly good rapport with an unusually difficult client may be reassigned. Because barriers can change, they need to be considered throughout the decision-making process.

 DEVELOPMENTAL CONSIDERATIONS **Health Care Decisions**

CHILDREN

Parents most often make decisions about the health care of children. Growing children can participate in those decisions in age-appropriate ways. As described by Piaget, the ability of children to reason and critically think about themselves and their situation develops gradually. At each stage, nurses should be aware of the ways children think and be sensitive to how they can be involved in health care decisions:

- Infants progress from reflexive behavior to simple, repetitive behavior and then to imitative behaviors, learning the concepts of cause and effect and object permanence. Though not involved in making decisions, they need to be comforted and secure as care is given.
- Toddlers and preschoolers are very egocentric and engage in magical thinking. They cannot reason out the implications of care, but need explanations in language they can understand. Play therapy and use of dolls and toys can help them adjust to care, and they can sometimes be given options (e.g., do you want your dressing changed before breakfast or after?).
- School-age children tend to be concrete thinkers. They benefit from simple, direct explanations; hands-on exploration of equipment and materials; and helping the care provider as appropriate

during procedures. Involving these children in care can increase cooperation and decrease anxiety.
- Adolescents are increasingly able to think abstractly and may make many of their own health care decisions. They should be actively consulted as a part of the family system.

OLDER ADULTS

It is important to include all adult clients in decision making and planning nursing care, but it is especially difficult to do this when working with older adults who have impaired cognitive abilities such as Alzheimer's disease. The nurse should allow them as much control and input as possible, keeping things simple and direct so they understand. Older adults with impairments are usually unable to perform multiple tasks or even to think of more than one step at a time. The nurse must have patience and be willing to calmly repeat instructions if necessary. Presenting and discussing issues in basic terms helps to maintain respect and dignity and allows older adults to participate in their own care for as long as possible. If the older adult is unable to perform self-care activities such as bathing or health-related activities such as a dressing change, the nurse seeks appropriate alternative methods for assisting the elder with these.

Steps in the Decision-Making Process

A solid decision-making process follows a series of sequential steps. More experienced nurses will do this instinctively. Health care professionals who operate in emergency settings, such as emergency medical services personnel and emergency department staff, will be aided by numerous protocols that dictate how decisions are made under urgent circumstances. Nursing students and less experienced health care personnel will benefit by employing the following steps in a sequential, thoughtful manner:

1. *Identify the purpose.* The nurse identifies why a decision is needed and what needs to be determined.
2. *Set the criteria.* When the nurse sets the criteria for decision making, three questions must be answered: What is the desired outcome, what needs to be preserved, and what needs to be avoided? For example, for a client with pain, the criteria would be as follows:
   a. *What is the desired outcome?* Relief of pain.
   b. *What needs to be preserved?* Physical functioning, cognitive functioning, psychologic functioning.
   c. *What needs to be avoided?* Central nervous system depression, respiratory depression, nausea.
3. *Weight the criteria.* In this step, the decision maker sets priorities or ranks activities or services from least important to most important as they relate to the specific situation. Because the weighting is specific to the situation, an activity may be ranked as most important in one situation and less important in another situation. For example, the nurse avoids medication that can cause sedation of a client with a head injury; for a client with terminal cancer, pain relief may be more important than avoiding the sedative side effects of the pain medication.
4. *Seek alternatives.* The decision maker identifies possible ways to meet the criteria. In clinical situations, the alternatives may be selected from a range of nursing interventions or client care strategies. Pain may be treated with oral or injectable medications, as needed (p.r.n.) or on a schedule, or without pharmacologic intervention at all, instead using complementary and alternative therapies such as acupuncture.
5. *Examine alternatives.* The nurse analyzes the alternatives to ensure that there is an objective rationale in relation to the established criteria for choosing one strategy over another. For pain that results from a procedure (such as removal of a foreign object), complementary and alternative medicine (CAM) may not provide strong enough relief, and oral medication may be effective but act too slowly, so an intravenous narcotic might be the better choice.
6. *Project.* The nurse applies creative thinking and skepticism to determine what might go wrong as a result of a decision and develops plans to prevent, minimize, or overcome any problems. If the intravenous narcotic is selected, what safety procedures need to be in place—for example, a narcotic antidote and supplemental oxygen?
7. *Implement.* The decision plan is enacted and pain treatment begins.

TABLE 34–2 Comparison Between the Nursing Process and the Decision-Making Process

NURSING PROCESS	DECISION-MAKING PROCESS*
Assess	Identify the purpose.
Diagnose	
Plan	Set the criteria.
	Weight the criteria.
	Seek alternatives.
	Examine alternatives.
	Project.
Implement	Implement.
Evaluate	Evaluate the outcome.

*The decision-making process parallels the nursing process but is also used during each phase of the process.

8. *Evaluate the outcome.* As with all nursing care, the nurse evaluates the client's responses to determine the effectiveness of the plan and whether the initial purpose was achieved. For example, how does the client rate the level of pain following the procedure?

The decision-making process and the nursing process share similarities, and the nurse uses decision making in all phases of the nursing process. Table 34–2 compares these processes. It is essential that the nurse use critical thinking in each step or phase of these processes so that decisions and care are well considered and delivered with the highest possible quality.

PROBLEM-SOLVING APPROACHES

When a problem arises, the nurse uses the problem-solving process to determine what possible solutions may be appropriate. In problem solving, the nurse obtains information that clarifies the nature of the problem and suggests possible solutions. The nurse then carefully evaluates the possible solutions and chooses the best one to implement, after which he or she monitors the situation over time to ensure its initial and continued effectiveness. The nurse does not discard the other solutions but holds them in reserve in the event that the first solution is not effective. The nurse may also encounter a similar problem in a different client situation where an alternative solution is determined to be the most effective. Therefore, problem solving for one situation contributes to the nurse's body of knowledge for problem solving in similar situations. Commonly used approaches to problem solving include trial and error, intuition, the research process, and the scientific/modified scientific method.

Trial and Error

One way to solve problems is through trial and error, in which a number of approaches are tried until a solution is found. However, without considering alternatives systematically, one cannot know why the solution works. Trial-and-error methods in nursing care can be dangerous because the client might suffer harm if an approach is inappropriate. However, nurses often use trial and error in the home setting where, due to logistics, equipment, and client lifestyle, hospital procedures cannot work as effectively (e.g., there may be no pole from which to hang an IV bag or no electricity to plug in a device).

Intuition

Intuition is the understanding or learning of things without the conscious use of reasoning. It is also known as a sixth sense, hunch, instinct, feeling, or suspicion. As a problem-solving approach, intuition is viewed by some people as a form of guessing and, as such, an inappropriate basis for nursing decisions. However, others view intuition as an essential and legitimate aspect of clinical judgment acquired through knowledge and experience. The nurse must first have the knowledge base necessary to practice in the clinical area and then use that knowledge in clinical practice. Clinical experience allows the nurse to recognize cues and patterns and begin to reach correct conclusions.

Experience is important in improving intuition because the rapidity of the judgment depends on the nurse having seen similar client situations many times before. Sometimes nurses use the words "I had a feeling" to describe the critical-thinking element of considering evidence. These nurses are able to judge quickly which evidence is most important and to act on that limited evidence. Nurses in critical care often pay closer attention than usual to a client when they sense that the client's condition could change suddenly.

Although the intuitive method of problem solving is gaining recognition as part of nursing practice, it is not recommended for novices or students, because they usually lack the knowledge base and clinical experience on which to make a valid judgment.

Research Method and Scientific/Modified Scientific Method

The **research process** is a formalized, logical, systematic approach to solving problems. The classic scientific method is most useful when the researcher is working in a controlled

TABLE 34–3 Comparison Between the Research Process and the Modified Scientific Method

RESEARCH PROCESS (SCIENTIFIC METHOD)	MODIFIED SCIENTIFIC METHOD
State a research question or problem.	Define the problem.
Define the purpose of or the rationale for the study.	
Review related literature.	Gather information.
Formulate hypotheses and defining variables.	Analyze the information.
Select a method to test hypotheses.	Develop solutions.
Select a population, sample, and setting.	
Conduct a pilot study.	Make a decision.
Collect the data.	Implement the decision.
Analyze the data.	Evaluate the decision.
Communicate conclusions and implications.	

situation. Health professionals, often working with people in uncontrolled situations, require a modified approach to the scientific method for solving problems. For example, unlike experiments with animals, the effects of diet on health are complicated by a person's genetic variations, lifestyle, and personal preferences.

Table 34–3 compares the research process or scientific method with the modified scientific method. Critical thinking is important in all problem-solving processes as the nurse evaluates potential solutions to a given problem and makes a decision to select the most appropriate solution for that situation.

Nursing research entails developing and expanding knowledge about human responses to actual or potential health

---

EVIDENCE-BASED PRACTICE Are Education, Experience, and Critical-Thinking Ability Related to Clinical Decision Making?

This pilot study investigated the premise that there would be relationships between the education and experience of critical care nurses and their ability to make consistent clinical decisions. Critical-thinking ability, as measured by skills and dispositions tests, was also expected to correlate with decision making. Fifty-four nurses with a BSN or MSN working in adult critical care units in teaching hospitals were included in the study. Results showed that, overall, the more complex the clinical situation, the less consistent the nurses were in their decisions. Intuition, as a decision-making strategy, was most related to consistent decisions. No correlation was found between education or total years of experience and consistency in decision making. There was an association between years of experience in critical care and decision consistency.

Implications

This study reinforces that decision making and critical thinking are complex when applied in real clinical situations. That the results showed greater consistency in decisions when intuition was used and when the nurse had more years of critical care nursing experience (not just overall nursing experience) suggests that there is a type of nurse thinking in clinical specialty that does not necessarily evolve with more global exposure to client care. It also suggests that the method of thinking used by nurses who choose critical care practice may be an inherent characteristic.

Note: From Hicks, F. D., Merritt, S. L., & Elstein, A. S. (2003). Critical thinking and clinical decision making in critical care nursing: A pilot study. *Heart & Lung, 32,* pp. 169–180.

problems and investigating the effects of nursing actions on those responses. The major goal of nursing research is to improve client care. Nursing research and evidenced-based practice are discussed in greater detail in Concept 43, Evidenced-Based Practice.

NURSING PROCESS

Nurses make decisions at every step in the nursing process. Watch an experienced nurse as care is delivered and it is entirely possibly the decision making that occurs within the nurse's head may not be visible, despite the fact that he or she follows the nursing process, using critical thinking to guide decision making and problem solving. The experienced nurse also bases decisions on past experiences, knowledge, nursing research findings, and skills. As the student nurse's knowledge and skills improve, he or she will be able to make better decisions faster using the nursing process as a decision-making tool.

Assessment

During the assessment process, nurses makes decisions regarding what data to collect, the meaning of both normal and abnormal findings, and what data is relevant to the client's problem. For example, the nurse admits a client who is suspected of having appendicitis. During the assessment, the nurse determines it is important to assess for pain severity, location, and type as well as temperature and results of lab studies such as the white blood count (WBC) with differential. The nurse collects other data that may be relevant, such as the client's past history, support systems, and coping patterns. The nurse may also collect data that may not be relevant to the client's current condition but that may have relevance at a later date.

The nurse makes decisions about how to react to assessment findings. For example, the nurse may interpret the findings that a client, whose heart rate is falling quickly, requires immediate notification of the physician and initiation of appropriate interventions. Apart from a life-threatening circumstance such as absence of circulation or breathing, no action should ever be taken without first performing a thorough assessment to collect enough data to make the best possible decision regarding how to react to a situation. For detailed information regarding the assessment process, please see Concept 32, Assessment.

Diagnosis

When developing nursing diagnoses, the nurse reviews all the data collected and makes decisions regarding the client's priorities for care. (For a detailed explanation of the diagnosis phase, please see the Nursing Process exemplar that follows.) Clients with multiple problems require a higher degree of decision making. For example, the nurse admits a client with a history of congestive heart failure, chronic renal failure, pulmonary edema, diabetes, and prostate cancer. The client's **chief complaint** (symptoms causing the need for admission or contact with the health care team) is shortness of breath secondary

to pulmonary edema caused by both the congestive heart failure and chronic renal failure. The client is anxious secondary to hypoxia, has an elevated potassium level secondary to renal failure, and is tachycardic. The nurse must decide which of these symptoms is the priority of care. Remembering the ABCs (airway, breathing, and circulation), the nurse prioritizes care with the following nursing diagnoses in this order:

- Ineffective Airway Clearance
- Ineffective Breathing Pattern
- Impaired Gas Exchange
- Decreased Cardiac Output
- Electrolyte Imbalance.

The nurse does not choose anxiety as a nursing diagnosis because this will resolve as oxygenation improves. Reduced cardiac output is impacting perfusion and causing tachycardia and these will also resolve by improving cardiac output. The decision-making process helps the nurse to choose the priorities of nursing care and choose the best nursing diagnoses.

Plan

During the planning phase, the nurse must make decisions regarding client goals and the best interventions to address the chosen nursing diagnoses. The nurse uses the data collected during the assessment to make the best selections while considering all factors impacting the client's condition. The nurse, when caring for the client described in the diagnosis section, decides that an important priority of care for this client is to monitor oxygen saturation, vital signs, and breath sounds. Goals for the client are designed with the client's participation and include the following:

- Client will reduce weight gain secondary to fluid retention to baseline weight following hemodialysis.
- Breath sounds will clear following hemodialysis.
- Oxygen saturation will be maintained greater than 90% at all times.

Once goals are decided upon, interventions can be chosen to help the client work toward meeting them.

Implementation

Implementation is the phase of the nursing process in which the nursing care plan is put into action. Choosing how to react to a client scenario involves a great deal of critical thinking and decision making. Consider the following:

CLINICAL EXAMPLE
The nurse is working on the cardiac step-down unit and sees on the monitor that the client in room 214 is in ventricular tachycardia (rapid, life-threatening rhythm). The nurse runs down to the room and administers a medication to improve the client's rhythm and the client becomes unconscious, stops breathing, and loses pulse.

What did the nurse do wrong? The nurse failed to gather data and acted on the decision that the client was in ventricular tachycardia without determining if the conclusion was correct. Part of decision making and implementing actions is to verify data—especially data obtained from machinery that can be inaccurate or incorrect. A loose lead, the client scratching the chest, or an action as simple as the client shaking a bottle of juice can all give the impression of ventricular tachycardia. However, had the nurse checked the client's pulse rate and found it strong, regular, and at a rate of 72 beats per minute, the nurse might have taken a different course of action. This demonstrates the importance of always making clinical decisions based on sound data and verified for accuracy, and never acting without making sure the data collected is still current and valid.

Decision making during the implementation phase of the nursing process often involves consideration of a number of different factors including a client's development, culture, support systems, and socioeconomic status. For example, consider this case study:

CLINICAL EXAMPLE

Mrs. Barnes, 65 years old, has experienced a small stroke that has reduced the functionality of her left hand. She lives alone in a small first-floor apartment. The physician suggests she consider inpatient rehabilitation but the client prefers to be discharged to her own home and receive outpatient rehabilitation care. The physician reminds her she will be unable to drive, which will make attending rehabilitation therapy difficult, but Mrs. Barnes is adamant she can work things out if she is discharged to her home. The home care nurse assesses Mrs. Barnes' home care environment, social support system, and socioeconomic status and learns the client has a large support system with numerous friends who will gladly drive her to her appointments and grocery shop for her. Mrs. Barnes has the financial resources to hire home help as needed, and feels she will improve faster in her own home.

Evaluation

Evaluation is a planned, ongoing, purposeful activity in which clients and health care professionals determine (a) the client's progress toward achievement of goals/outcomes and (b) the effectiveness of nursing interventions. Evaluating the effectiveness of care requires collecting further data and comparing it to data collected during the assessment phase in order to decide if the client's condition has improved, stayed the same, or worsened. Based on these findings, the nurse makes decisions about whether to continue the plan of care as developed or alter the plan to improve client outcomes. If the decision is made to alter the plan of care, the nurse must decide what parts of the plan are effective and what parts are not working, and how the plan should be amended to improve the client's outcomes.

NURSING PRACTICE

Every aspect of nursing practice involves decision making. Any time a client's condition changes, decisions must be made about how to properly respond. This requires initiating the problem-solving process. While some actions are performed routinely, such as measuring vital signs at the beginning of the shift or introducing oneself when meeting a new client, other actions require careful consideration, critical thinking, problem solving, and decision making in order to provide the highest quality nursing care and assure the safety of clients and staff.

Exemplar 34.1 will introduce the nursing process as a problem-solving tool used by all nurses. Each step of the nursing process will be explained. Exemplar 34.2 discusses the skill of critical thinking and offers guidelines for developing or improving critical thinking skills.

REVIEW About Clinical Decision Making

RELATE: LINK THE CONCEPTS

Linking the concept of Clinical Decision Making with the concept of Legal Issues:
1. What legal actions occur if the nurse fails to make prudent clinical decisions? Explain your answer.
2. What role regarding sound clinical decision making is expected as a result of licensure as a nurse?

Linking the concept of Clinical Decision Making with the concept of Ethics:
3. What ethical obligation does the nurse hold toward the client related to clinical decision making?
4. What ethical obligation does the nurse hold toward the hiring facility related to clinical decision making?

REFER: GO TO MYNURSINGKIT

REFLECT: CASE STUDY

The nurse is caring for a client who was admitted 3 days ago with acute abdominal pain. Following extensive diagnostic testing the client has received a medical diagnosis of stomach cancer with suspected metastasis to the liver and pancreas. The physician has

informed the client that there are several options related to treatment. Option 1 is to have as much of the tumor surgically removed as possible followed by chemotherapy and radiation therapy. This is the most aggressive approach with the best odds for survival but the doctor has told the client that with the amount of metastasis that has already occurred, the odds for survival are still not very good (less than 10%). The second option is to do nothing, allowing the client to remain as comfortable as possible until death, which will likely occur in 3–6 months. The third option is the most moderate option and involves chemotherapy to slow cancer growth, which can prolong the client's life but will result in side effects that often include hair loss, vomiting, weakness, anemia, and other discomforts depending on the medications used. After the physician leaves the room the client looks to the nurse and asks, "What do you think I should do? What would you do if you were me?"

1. What nursing diagnosis would be most appropriate for this client?
2. What ethical, legal, and moral duties guide the nurse when responding to this client's questions?
3. How would you respond to each of the client's questions?

34.1 THE NURSING PROCESS

KEY TERMS

Actual diagnosis, *2065*
Assessment, *2052*
Assignment, *2092*
Closed questions, *2056*
Cognitive skills, *2096*
Collaborative care plans, *2081*
Collaborative interventions, *2090*
Concept map, *2081*
Critical pathways, *2081*
Critical thinking, *2068*
Cues, *2064*
Database, *2052*
Defining characteristics, *2066*
Dependent functions, *2067*
Dependent interventions, *2089*
Diagnosis, *2065*
Diagnostic label, *2065*
Directive interview, *2056*
Discharge planning, *2077*
Etiology, *2065*
Evaluation, *2098*
Evaluation statement, *2099*
Formal nursing care plan, *2077*
Goals, *2085*
Health promotion diagnosis, *2066*
Implementation, *2096*
Independent functions, *2067*
Independent interventions, *2089*
Indicator, *2086*
Individualized care plan, *2077*
Inferences, *2064*
Informal nursing care plan, *2077*
Interpersonal skills, *2096*
Interview, *2056*
Leading question, *2056*
Multidisciplinary care plan, *2081*
Neutral question, *2056*
Nondirective interview, *2056*
Norm, *2068*
Nursing diagnosis, *2065*
Nursing intervention, *2077*
Nursing Interventions Classification (NIC), *2092*
Nursing Outcomes Classification (NOC), *2086*
Objective data, *2054*

Open-ended questions, *2056*
PES format, *2072*
Policies, *2079*
Priority setting, *2083*
Procedures, *2079*
Protocols, *2079*
Qualifiers, *2066*
Rapport, *2056*
Rationale, *2081*
Risk factors, *2065*
Risk nursing diagnosis, *2065*
Signs, *2054*
Standard, *2068*
Standardized care plan, *2077*
Standards of care, *2078*
Standing order, *2080*
Subjective data, *2054*
Symptoms, *2054*
Syndrome diagnosis, *2066*
Technical skills, *2096*
Validation, *2064*
Wellness diagnosis, *2066*

BASIS FOR SELECTION OF EXEMPLAR

NLN Competencies
Standards of Nursing Practice

LEARNING OUTCOMES

After reading about this exemplar, you will be able to:

1. Describe the purpose of the nursing process.
2. Define each phase of the nursing process.
3. Examine the interrelationship of each phase of the nursing process to one another.
4. Deconstruct the process of assessment to include collecting, organizing, and validating data.
5. Formulate nursing diagnostic statements appropriate to the client's priority needs.
6. Plan nursing care to include priorities of care, client goals, and selecting nursing interventions and activities.
7. Demonstrate the process of implementing nursing care.
8. Revise the nursing plan of care based on evaluation of client response.

OVERVIEW

Lydia E. Hall originated the term *nursing process* in 1955, and Johnson (1959), Orlando (1961), and Wiedenbach (1963) were among the first to use it to refer to a series of phases describing the practice of nursing. Since then, various nurses have

described the process of nursing and organized the phases in different ways.

The purpose of the nursing process is to identify a client's health status and actual or potential health care problems or needs, to establish plans to meet the identified needs, to deliver specific nursing interventions to meet those needs, and to evaluate the success of those interventions. The client may be an individual, a family, or a group.

The use of the nursing process in clinical practice gained additional legitimacy in 1973 when the phases were included in the American Nurses Association (ANA) *Standards of Nursing Practice*. The standards of practice within the most current *Scope and Standards of Nursing Practice* include the five phases of the nursing process: assessment, diagnosis, plan, implementation, and evaluation (ANA, 2004). Virtually every state has since revised its nursing practice acts to reflect the nursing process. See Figure 34–2 ■ for an illustration of the nursing process in action.

THE NURSING PROCESS IN ACTION

The nursing process is a systematic, rational method of planning and providing nursing care. Its purpose is to identify a client's health care status, and actual or potential health problems, to establish plans to meet the identified needs, and to deliver specific nursing interventions to address those needs. The nursing process is cyclical; that is, its components follow a logical sequence, but more than one component may be involved at one time. At the end of the first cycle, care may be terminated if goals are achieved, or the cycle may continue with reassessment, or the plan of care may be modified.

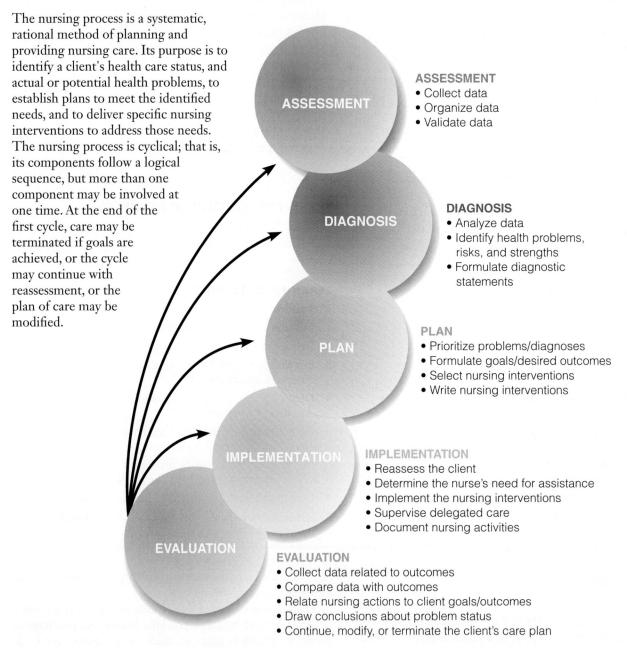

Figure 34–2 ■ The nursing process in action.

Amanda Aquilini, a 28-year-old married attorney, was admitted to the hospital with an elevated temperature, a productive cough, and rapid, labored respirations. In taking a nursing history, Nurse Mary Medina, RN, finds that Amanda has had a "chest cold" for two weeks, and has been experiencing shortness of breath upon exertion. Yesterday she developed an elevated temperature and began to experience "pain" in her "lungs."

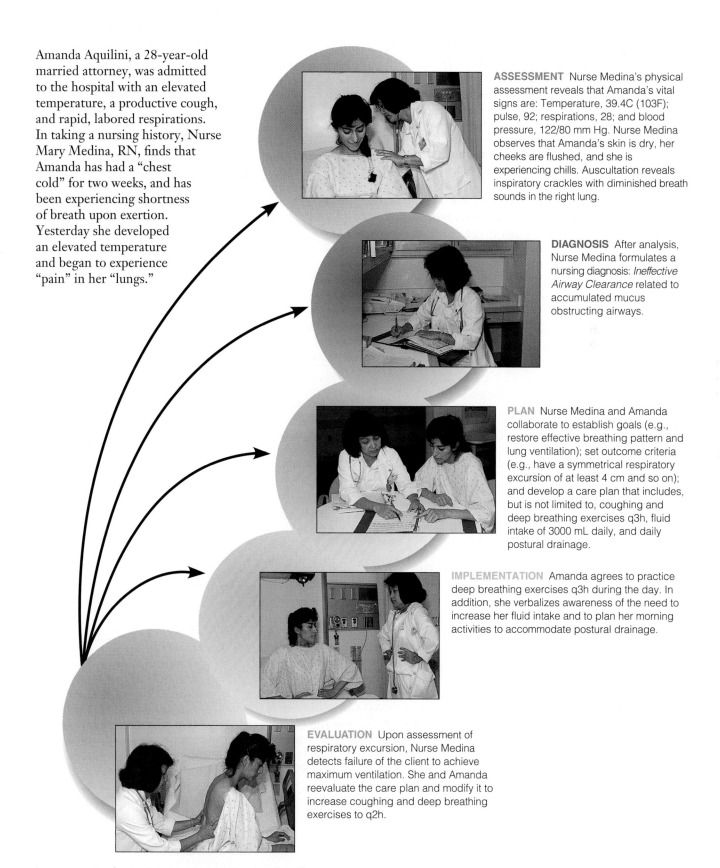

ASSESSMENT Nurse Medina's physical assessment reveals that Amanda's vital signs are: Temperature, 39.4C (103F); pulse, 92; respirations, 28; and blood pressure, 122/80 mm Hg. Nurse Medina observes that Amanda's skin is dry, her cheeks are flushed, and she is experiencing chills. Auscultation reveals inspiratory crackles with diminished breath sounds in the right lung.

DIAGNOSIS After analysis, Nurse Medina formulates a nursing diagnosis: *Ineffective Airway Clearance* related to accumulated mucus obstructing airways.

PLAN Nurse Medina and Amanda collaborate to establish goals (e.g., restore effective breathing pattern and lung ventilation); set outcome criteria (e.g., have a symmetrical respiratory excursion of at least 4 cm and so on); and develop a care plan that includes, but is not limited to, coughing and deep breathing exercises q3h, fluid intake of 3000 mL daily, and daily postural drainage.

IMPLEMENTATION Amanda agrees to practice deep breathing exercises q3h during the day. In addition, she verbalizes awareness of the need to increase her fluid intake and to plan her morning activities to accommodate postural drainage.

EVALUATION Upon assessment of respiratory excursion, Nurse Medina detects failure of the client to achieve maximum ventilation. She and Amanda reevaluate the care plan and modify it to increase coughing and deep breathing exercises to q2h.

Figure 34–2 ■ The nursing process in action, continued.

PHASES OF THE NURSING PROCESS

Although nurse theorists may use different terms to describe the phases of the nursing process, the activities of the nurse using the process are similar. For example, *diagnosis* may also be called *analysis*, and *implementation* may be called *intervention* or *intervening*.

An overview of the five-phase nursing process is shown in Table 34–4. Each of the five phases is discussed in depth within this exemplar and is used throughout both volumes of this text. The phases of the nursing process are not separate entities—they are overlapping, continuing subprocesses (see Figure 34–3 ■). For example, assessment, which may be considered the first phase of the nursing process, is also carried out during the implementing and evaluating phases. For instance, while actually administering medications (implementation), the nurse continuously assesses the client to determine continued need for the medication, response to the medication, and appearance of potential side-effects.

Each phase of the nursing process affects the others; they are closely interrelated. For example, if inadequate data are obtained during assessment, the nursing diagnoses will be incomplete or incorrect; inaccuracy will also be reflected in the planning, implementation, and evaluation phases. Because the nursing process is the problem-solving tool that guides the

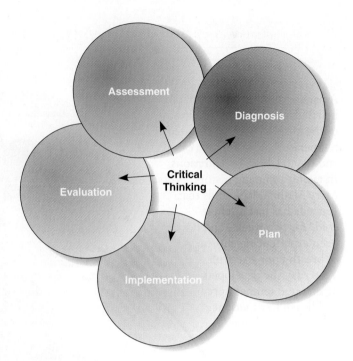

Figure 34–3 ■ The five overlapping phases of the nursing process. Each phase depends on the accuracy of the other phases. Each phase involves critical thinking.

TABLE 34–4 Overview of the Nursing Process

PHASE AND DESCRIPTION	PURPOSE	ACTIVITIES
Assessment		
Collecting, organizing, validating, and documenting client data	To establish a database about the client's response to health concerns or illness and the ability to manage health care needs	Establish a database: ■ Obtain a nursing health history. ■ Conduct a physical assessment. ■ Review client records. ■ Review nursing literature. ■ Consult support persons. ■ Consult health professionals. Update data as needed. Organize data. Validate data. Communicate/document data.
Diagnosis		
Analyzing and synthesizing data	To identify client strengths and health problems that can be prevented or resolved by collaborative and independent nursing interventions To develop a list of nursing and collaborative problems	Interpret and analyze data: ■ Compare data against standards. ■ Cluster or group data (generate tentative hypotheses). ■ Identify gaps and inconsistencies. Determine client's strengths, risks, diagnoses, and problems. Formulate nursing diagnoses and collaborative problem statements. Document nursing diagnoses on the care plan.

TABLE 34–4 **Overview of the Nursing Process** (continued)

PHASE AND DESCRIPTION	PURPOSE	ACTIVITIES
Plan Determining how to prevent, reduce, or resolve the identified priority client problems; how to support client strengths; and how to implement nursing interventions in an organized, individualized, and goal-directed manner	To develop an individualized care plan that specifies client goals/desired outcomes, and related nursing interventions	Set priorities and goals/outcomes in collaboration with client. Write goals/desired outcomes. Select nursing strategies/interventions. Consult other health professionals. Write nursing interventions and nursing care plan. Communicate care plan to relevant health care providers.
Implementation Carrying out (or delegating) and documenting the planned nursing interventions	To assist the client to meet desired goals/outcomes; promote wellness; prevent illness and disease; restore health; and facilitate coping with altered functioning	Reassess the client to update the database. Determine the nurse's need for assistance. Perform planned nursing interventions. Communicate what nursing actions were implemented: ■ Document care and client responses to care. ■ Give verbal reports as necessary.
Evaluation Measuring the degree to which goals/outcomes have been achieved and identifying factors that positively or negatively influence goal achievement	To determine whether to continue, modify, or terminate the plan of care	Collaborate with client and collect data related to desired outcomes. Judge whether goals/outcomes have been achieved. Relate nursing actions to client outcomes. Make decisions about problem status. Review and modify the care plan as indicated or terminate nursing care. Document achievement of outcomes and modification of the care plan.

nurse's approach to client care and decision making, the process begins with accurate data collection.

CHARACTERISTICS OF THE NURSING PROCESS

The nursing process has distinctive characteristics that enable the nurse to respond to the changing health status of the client. These characteristics include its cyclic and dynamic nature, client centeredness, focus on problem solving and decision making, interpersonal and collaborative style, universal applicability, and use of critical thinking:

■ Data collected during each phase inform the next phase. Findings from evaluation feed back into assessment. Hence, the nursing process is a regularly repeated event or sequence of events (a cycle) that is continuously changing (dynamic) rather than staying the same (static).

■ The nursing process is client-centered. The nurse organizes the plan of care according to client problems rather than nursing goals. In the assessment phase, the nurse collects data to determine the client's habits, routines, and needs, enabling the nurse to incorporate client routines into the care plan as much as possible.

■ The nursing process is an adaptation of problem solving and systems theory. It can be viewed as parallel to but separate

from the process used by physicians (the medical model). Both processes (a) begin with data gathering and analysis, (b) base action (intervention or treatment) on a problem statement (nursing diagnosis or medical diagnosis), and (c) include an evaluative component. However, the medical model focuses on physiological systems and the disease process, whereas the nursing process is directed toward a client's responses to disease and illness.

■ Decision making is involved in every phase of the nursing process. Nurses can be highly creative in determining when and how to use data to make decisions. They are not bound by standard responses and may apply their repertoire of skills and knowledge to assist clients. This facilitates the individualization of the client's plan of care.

■ The nursing process is interpersonal and collaborative. It requires the nurse to communicate directly and consistently with clients and families to meet their needs. It also requires that nurses collaborate with other members of the health care team in a joint effort to provide quality client care.

■ The universally applicable characteristic of the nursing process means that it is used as a framework for nursing care in all types of health care settings and with clients of all age groups.

■ Nurses must use a variety of critical-thinking skills to carry out the nursing process. Table 34–5 provides examples of critical thinking in the nursing process.

TABLE 34-5 **Examples of Critical Thinking in the Nursing Process**

NURSING PROCESS PHASE	CRITICAL-THINKING ACTIVITIES
Assessment	■ Making reliable observations ■ Distinguishing relevant from irrelevant data ■ Distinguishing important from unimportant data ■ Validating data ■ Organizing data ■ Categorizing data according to a framework ■ Recognizing assumptions ■ Identifying gaps in the data
Diagnosis	■ Finding patterns and relationships among cues ■ Making inferences ■ Suspending judgment when lacking data ■ Stating the problem ■ Examining assumptions ■ Comparing patterns with norms ■ Identifying factors contributing to the problem
Plan	■ Forming valid generalizations ■ Transferring knowledge from one situation to another ■ Developing evaluative criteria ■ Hypothesizing ■ Making interdisciplinary connections ■ Prioritizing client problems ■ Generalizing principles from other sciences
Implementation	■ Evaluating ■ Applying knowledge to perform interventions
Testing hypotheses	■ Deciding whether hypotheses are correct ■ Making criterion-based evaluations

Note: From Wilkinson, J. M., (2007). *Nursing process & critical thinking* (4th ed.). Upper Saddle River, NJ: Pearson Prentice Hall, pp. 66–69. Adapted with permission.

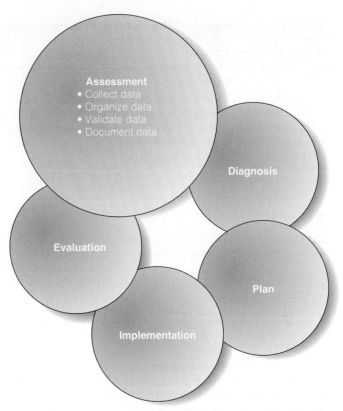

Figure 34–4 ■ Assessment: The assessment process involves four closely related activities.

are outlined in Concept 32, Assessment, and summarized in Table 32–1, Types of Assessment. Assessments vary according to their purpose, timing, time available, and client status.

Nursing assessments focus on a client's responses to a health problem. A nursing assessment should include the client's perceived needs, health problems, related experience, health practices, values, and lifestyles. To be most useful, the data collected should be relevant to a particular health problem. Therefore, nurses should think critically about what to assess. The assessment process involves four closely related activities: collecting data, organizing data, validating data, and documenting data (see Figure 34–4 ■).

COLLECTING DATA

Data collection is the process of gathering information about a client's health status. It must be both systematic and continuous to prevent the omission of significant data and reflect a client's changing (in other words, not static) health status.

A **database** is all the information about a client; it includes the nursing health history (see Box 34–2), physical assessment, primary care provider's history and physical examination, results of laboratory and diagnostic tests, and material contributed by other health personnel.

Client data should include past history as well as current problems. For example, a previous allergic reaction to penicillin is a vital piece of historical data. Past surgical procedures, folk healing practices, and chronic diseases are also

Assessment

Assessment is the systematic and continuous collection of data about a client for the purpose of determining the client's current and ongoing health status, predicting the client's risks to health, and identifying appropriate health-promoting activities. Assessment is a continuous process carried out during all phases of the nursing process. For example, in the evaluation phase, assessment is done to determine the outcomes of the nursing strategies and to evaluate goal achievement. All phases of the nursing process depend on the accurate and complete collection of data. There are four different types of assessments: initial assessment, problem-focused assessment, emergency assessment, and time-lapsed reassessment. The types

Box 34–2 **Components of a Nursing Health History**

BIOGRAPHIC DATA
Client's name, address, age, sex, marital status, occupation, religious preference, health care financing, and usual source of medical care.

CHIEF COMPLAINT OR REASON FOR VISIT
The chief complaint is the answer given to the question "What is troubling you?" or "Can you tell me the reason you came to the hospital or clinic today?" It should be recorded in the client's own words.

HISTORY OF PRESENT ILLNESS
- When the symptoms started
- Whether the onset of symptoms was sudden or gradual
- How often the problem occurs
- Exact location of the distress
- Character of the complaint (e.g., intensity of pain or quality of sputum, emesis, or discharge)
- Activity in which the client was involved when the problem occurred
- Phenomena or symptoms associated with the chief complaint
- Factors that aggravate or alleviate the problem

PAST HISTORY
- *Childhood illnesses*, such as chickenpox, mumps, measles, rubella (German measles), rubeola (red measles), streptococcal infections, scarlet fever, rheumatic fever, and other significant illnesses
- *Childhood immunizations* and the date of the last tetanus shot
- *Allergies* to drugs, animals, insects, or other environmental agents; the type of reaction that occurs; and how the reaction is treated
- *Accidents and injuries*: how, when, and where the incident occurred, type of injury, treatment received, and any complications
- *Hospitalization for serious illnesses*: reasons for the hospitalization, dates, surgery performed, course of recovery, and any complications
- *Medications*: all currently used prescription and over-the-counter medications, such as aspirin, nasal spray, vitamins, or laxatives

FAMILY HISTORY OF ILLNESS
To ascertain risk factors for certain diseases, the ages of siblings, parents, and grandparents and their current state of health or, if they are deceased, the cause of death are obtained. Particular attention should be given to disorders such as heart disease, cancer, diabetes, hypertension, obesity, allergies, arthritis, tuberculosis, bleeding, alcoholism, and any mental health disorders.

LIFESTYLE
- *Personal habits.* The amount, frequency, and duration of substance use (tobacco, alcohol, coffee, cola, tea, and illicit or recreational drugs)
- *Diet.* Description of a typical diet on a normal day or any special diet, number of meals and snacks per day, who cooks and shops for food, ethnically distinct food patterns, and allergies
- *Sleep/rest patterns.* Usual daily sleep/wake times, difficulties sleeping, and remedies used for difficulties
- *Activities of daily living (ADLs).* Any difficulties experienced in the basic activities of eating, grooming, dressing, elimination, and locomotion

- *Instrumental ADLs.* Any difficulties experienced in food preparation, shopping, transportation, housekeeping, laundry, and ability to use the telephone, handle finances, and manage medications
- *Recreation/hobbies.* Exercise activity and tolerance, hobbies and other interests, and vacations

SOCIAL DATA
- *Family relationships/friendships.* The client's support system in times of stress (who helps in time of need?), what effect the client's illness has on the family, and whether any family problems are affecting the client
- *Ethnic affiliation.* Health customs and beliefs; cultural practices that may affect health care and recovery
- *Educational history.* Data about the client's highest level of education attained and any past difficulties with learning
- *Occupational history.* Current employment status, the number of days missed from work because of illness, any history of accidents on the job, any occupational hazards with a potential for future disease or accident, the client's need to change jobs because of past illness, the employment status of spouses or partners and the way child care is handled, and the client's overall satisfaction with the work
- *Economic status.* Information about how the client is paying for medical care (including what kind of medical and hospitalization coverage the client has), and whether the client's illness presents financial concerns
- *Home and neighborhood conditions.* Home safety measures and adjustments in physical facilities that may be required to help the client manage a physical disability, activity intolerance, and ADLs; the availability of neighborhood and community services to meet the client's needs

PSYCHOLOGIC DATA
- *Major stressors* experienced and the client's perception of them
- *Usual coping pattern* with a serious problem or a high level of stress
- *Communication style*, or the ability to verbalize appropriate emotion; nonverbal communication—such as eye movements, gestures, use of touch, and posture; interactions with support persons; and the congruence of nonverbal behavior and verbal expression

PATTERNS OF HEALTH CARE
Patterns of health care are all health care resources the client is currently using and has used in the past. These include the primary care provider, specialists (e.g., ophthalmologist or gynecologist), dentist, folk practitioners (e.g., herbalist or curandero), health clinic, or health center; whether the client considers the care being provided adequate; and whether access to health care is a problem.

examples of historical data. Current data relate to present circumstances, such as pain, nausea, sleep patterns, and religious practices. To ensure accuracy, both the client and nurse must participate actively in the data collection process. Data can be subjective or objective, and may be constant or variable. Data can come from a primary or secondary source.

Types of Data

Subjective data, also referred to as **symptoms** or covert data, are apparent only to the client affected and can be described or verified only by that client. Itching, pain, and feelings of worry are examples of subjective data. Subjective data include the client's sensations, feelings, values, beliefs, attitudes, and perception of personal health status and life situation.

Objective data, also referred to as **signs** or overt data, are detectable by an observer or can be measured or tested against an accepted standard. They can be seen, heard, felt, or smelled, and they are obtained by observation or physical examination. Examples of objective data include a discoloration of the skin and a blood pressure reading. During the physical examination, the nurse obtains objective data to validate subjective data and to complete the assessment phase of the nursing process.

Constant data is information that does not change over time such as race or blood type. Variable data can change quickly, frequently, or rarely and include data such as blood pressure, age, and level of pain.

A complete database provides a baseline for comparing the client's responses to nursing and medical interventions. Examples of subjective and objective data are shown in Table 34–6.

Sources of Data

Sources of data are primary or secondary. The client is the primary source of data. Family members or other support persons, other health care professionals, records and reports, laboratory and diagnostic analyses, and relevant literature are secondary or indirect sources. In fact, all sources other than the client are considered secondary sources. All data from secondary sources should be validated if possible.

CLIENT The best source of data is usually the client, unless the client is too ill, young, or confused to communicate clearly. The client can provide subjective data that no one else can offer. Most often, primary data refers to statements made by the client but also include those objective data that can be directly obtained by the nurse from the client, such as gender. Some clients cannot or do not wish to provide accurate data. These include young children and clients who are confused, afraid, embarrassed, or distrustful, or who do not speak the nurse's language (D'Amico & Barbarito, 2007).

SUPPORT PEOPLE Family members, friends, and caregivers who know the client well often can supplement or verify information provided by the client. They might convey information about the client's response to illness, the stresses the client was experiencing before the illness, family attitudes on illness and health, and the client's home environment.

Support people are an especially important source of data for a client who is very young, unconscious, or confused. In some cases—a client who is physically or emotionally abused, for example—the person giving information may wish to remain anonymous. Before eliciting data from support people, the nurse should ensure that the client, if mentally able, accepts such input. The nurse should also indicate on the nursing history that the data were obtained from a support person.

Information supplied by family members, significant others, or other health care professionals is considered subjective if it is not based on fact. If the client's daughter says, "Dad is very confused today," that is secondary subjective data because it is an interpretation of the client's behavior by the daughter. The nurse should attempt to verify the reported confusion by interviewing the client directly. However, if the daughter says, "Dad said he thought it was the year 1941 today," that may be considered secondary objective data since the daughter heard her father state this directly.

The presence or absence of support people in a client's life can itself be a significant assessment finding. A young child who is brought in for a clinic visit by foster parents will require a different combination of assessment tools than a child who is brought in by his or her own parent. Similarly, an older client who lives alone and is suspected of having dementia will require an assessment that differs somewhat from a healthy older client who lives an active life with his or her spouse.

TABLE 34–6 Examples of Subjective and Objective Data

SUBJECTIVE	OBJECTIVE
"I feel weak all over when I exert myself."	Blood pressure 90/50* Apical pulse 104 Skin pale and diaphoretic
Client states he has a cramping pain in his abdomen: "I feel sick to my stomach."	Vomited 100 mL green-tinged fluid Abdomen firm and slightly distended Active bowel sounds auscultated in all four quadrants
"I'm short of breath."	Lung sounds clear bilaterally; diminished in right lower lobe
Wife states, "He doesn't seem so sad today." (This is subjective and secondary source data.)	Client cried during interview
"I would like to see the chaplain before surgery."	Holding open Bible Has small silver cross on bedside table

*Blood pressure obtained using an external cuff and manometer may be considered secondary or indirect data since it does not directly measure the pressure within the arteries.

CLIENT RECORDS Client records include information documented by various health care professionals. Client records also contain data regarding the client's occupation, religion, and marital status. By reviewing such records before interviewing the client, the nurse can avoid asking questions for which answers have already been supplied. Repeated questioning can be stressful and annoying to clients and cause concern about the lack of communication among health professionals. Types of client records include medical records, records of therapies, and laboratory records.

Medical records (e.g., medical history, physical examination, operative report, progress notes, and consultations done by primary care providers) provide information about a client's present and past health and illness patterns. These records also can provide nurses with information about the client's coping behaviors, health practices, previous illnesses, and allergies.

Records of therapies provided by other health professionals, such as social workers, nutritionists, dietitians, or physical therapists, help the nurse obtain relevant data not expressed by the client. For example, a social agency's report on a client's living conditions or a home health care agency's report on a client's self-care abilities can also inform the nurse's assessment of the client.

Laboratory records are another source of pertinent health information. For example, the determination of blood glucose level allows health care professionals to monitor the administration of oral hypoglycemic medications. Any laboratory data about a client must be compared to the agency or performing laboratory's norms for that particular test and for the client's age, sex, and other significant client data. (Descriptions of diagnostic studies with normal values can be found in Appendix B).

The nurse must always consider the information in client records in light of the present situation. For example, if the most recent medical record is 10 years old, the client's health practices and coping behaviors are likely to have changed. Older clients may have numerous previous records. These are very useful and contribute to a full understanding of the health history, especially if the client's memory is impaired.

HEALTH CARE PROFESSIONALS Because assessment is an ongoing process, verbal reports from other health care professionals serve as other potential sources of information about a client's health. Nurses, social workers, primary care providers, and physiotherapists, for example, may have information from either previous or current contact with the client. Sharing of information among professionals is especially important to ensure continuity of care when clients are transferred to and from home and health care agencies.

LITERATURE Nursing and related literature, such as professional journals and reference texts, can provide additional information that can assist the nurse in developing or interpreting the assessment. The nurse may review literature to gather additional information on one or more of the following:

- Standards or norms against which to compare findings (e.g., height and weight tables, normal developmental tasks for an age group)
- Cultural and social health practices
- Spiritual beliefs
- Assessment data needed for specific client conditions
- Nursing interventions and evaluation criteria relevant to a client's health problems
- Medical diagnoses, treatment, and prognoses
- Current methodologies and research findings.

DATA COLLECTION METHODS

The principal methods used to collect data are observing, interviewing, and examining. Observation occurs whenever the nurse is in contact with the client or support persons. Interviewing is used mainly while taking the nursing health history. Examining is the major method used in the physical health assessment.

In reality, the nurse uses all three methods simultaneously when assessing clients. For example, during the client interview the nurse observes, listens, asks questions, and mentally retains information to explore in the physical examination. These topics are covered further in Concepts 32, Assessment, and Concept 36, Communication.

Observing

To *observe* is to gather data by using the senses. Observation is a conscious, deliberate skill that is developed through effort and with an organized approach. Although nurses observe mainly through sight, most of the senses are engaged during careful observations. Examples of client data observed through the senses are shown in Table 34–7.

TABLE 34–7 Using the Senses to Observe Client Data

SENSE	EXAMPLE OF CLIENT DATA
Vision	Overall appearance (e.g., body size, general weight, posture, grooming); signs of distress or discomfort; facial and body gestures; skin color and lesions; abnormalities of movement; nonverbal demeanor (e.g., signs of anger or anxiety); religious or cultural artifacts (e.g., books, icons, candles, beads)
Smell	Body or breath odors
Hearing	Lung and heart sounds; bowel sounds; ability to communicate; language spoken; ability to initiate conversation; ability to respond when spoken to; orientation to time, person, and place; thoughts and feelings about self, others, and health status
Touch	Skin temperature and moisture; muscle strength (e.g., hand grip); pulse rate, rhythm, and volume; palpatory lesions (e.g., lumps, masses, nodules)

Observation has two aspects: (a) noticing the data and (b) selecting, organizing, and interpreting the data. A nurse who observes that a client's face is flushed must relate that observation to findings such as body temperature, activity, environmental temperature, and blood pressure. Errors can occur in selecting, organizing, and interpreting data. For example, a nurse might not notice certain signs, either because they are unexpected or because they do not conform to preconceptions about a client's illness. Nurses often need to focus on specific data in order not to be overwhelmed by a multitude of data. Observing, therefore, involves distinguishing data in a meaningful manner. For example, nurses caring for newborns learn to ignore the usual sounds of machines in the nursery but respond quickly to an infant's cry or movement.

The experienced nurse is often able to attend to an intervention (e.g., give a bed bath or monitor an intravenous infusion) and at the same time make important observations (e.g., note a change in respiratory status or skin color). The beginning student must learn to make observations and complete tasks simultaneously.

PRACTICE ALERT

Learn to incorporate multiple activities at the same time. For example, while changing the client's linen use the time to talk with the client to assess response to treatments, or while bathing the client assess for skin integrity or wound healing. This helps to improve the efficiency of nursing care.

Nursing observations must be organized so that nothing significant is missed. Most nurses develop a particular sequence for observing events, usually focusing on the client first. For example, a nurse walks into a client's room and observes, in the following order:

1. Clinical signs of client distress (e.g., pallor or flushing, labored breathing, and behavior indicating pain or emotional distress)
2. Threats to the client's safety, real or anticipated (e.g., a lowered side rail)
3. The presence and functioning of associated equipment (e.g., intravenous equipment and oxygen)
4. The immediate environment, including the people in it.

Interviewing

An **interview** is a planned communication or a conversation with a purpose. Interviews may be used to:
- Get or give information
- Identify problems of mutual concern
- Evaluate change
- Teach
- Provide support, counseling, or therapy.

One example of the interview is the nursing health history, which is a part of the nursing admission assessment.

There are two approaches to interviewing: directive and nondirective. The **directive interview** is highly structured and elicits specific information. The nurse establishes the purpose of the interview and controls the interview, at least at the outset. The client responds to questions but may have limited opportunity to ask questions or discuss concerns. Nurses frequently use directive interviews to gather and to give information when time is limited (e.g., in an emergency situation).

During a **nondirective interview**, or rapport-building interview, the nurse allows the client to control the purpose, subject matter, and pacing. **Rapport** is an understanding between two or more people.

A combination of directive and nondirective approaches is usually appropriate during the information-gathering interview. The nurse begins by determining areas of concern for the client. If, for example, a client expresses worry about surgery, the nurse pauses to explore the client's worry and to provide support. Simply noting the worry, without dealing with it, can leave the impression that the nurse does not care about the client's concerns or dismisses them as unimportant.

TYPES OF INTERVIEW QUESTIONS Questions are often classified as closed or open ended, and neutral or leading. **Closed questions**, used in the directive interview, are restrictive and generally require only "yes" or "no" or short factual answers giving specific information. Closed questions often begin with "when," "where," "who," "what," "do (did, does)," or "is (are, was)." Examples of closed questions are "What medication did you take?" "Are you having pain now? Show me where it is." "How old are you?" "When did you fall?" The highly stressed person and the person who has difficulty communicating will find closed questions easier to answer than open-ended questions.

Open-ended questions, associated with the nondirective interview, invite clients to discover and explore, elaborate, clarify, or illustrate their thoughts or feelings. An open-ended question specifies only the broad topic to be discussed, and invites answers longer than one or two words. Such questions give clients the freedom to divulge only the information that they are ready to disclose. The open-ended question is useful at the beginning of an interview or to change topics and to elicit attitudes.

Open-ended questions may begin with "what" or "how." Examples of open-ended questions are "How have you been feeling lately?" "What brought you to the hospital?" "How did you feel in that situation?" "Would you describe more about how you relate to your child?" "What would you like to talk about today?"

The type of question a nurse chooses depends on the needs of the client at the time. Nurses often find it necessary to use a combination of closed and open-ended questions throughout an interview to accomplish the goals of the interview and obtain needed information. See Box 34–3 for advantages and disadvantages of open-ended and closed questions.

A **neutral question** is a question the client can answer without direction or pressure from the nurse, is open-ended, and is used in nondirective interviews. Examples are "How do you feel about that?" and "Why do you think you had the operation?" A **leading question**, by contrast, is usually closed, used in a directive interview, and thus directs the client's

---

Box 34–3 Selected Advantages and Disadvantages of Open-Ended and Closed Questions

OPEN-ENDED QUESTIONS

Advantages

1. They let the interviewee do the talking.
2. The interviewer is able to listen and observe.
3. They are easy to answer and nonthreatening.
4. They reveal what the interviewee thinks is important.
5. They may reveal the interviewee's lack of information, misunderstanding of words, frame of reference, prejudices, or stereotypes.
6. They can provide information the interviewer may not ask for.
7. They can reveal the interviewee's degree of feeling about an issue.
8. They can convey interest and trust because of the freedom they provide.

Disadvantages

1. They take more time.
2. Only brief answers may be given.
3. Valuable information may be withheld.
4. They often elicit more information than necessary.
5. Responses are difficult to document and require skill in recording.
6. The interviewer requires skill in controlling an open-ended interview.
7. Responses require psychologic insight and sensitivity from the interviewer.

CLOSED QUESTIONS

Advantages

1. Questions and answers can be controlled more effectively.
2. They require less effort from the interviewee.
3. They may be less threatening, since they do not require explanations or justifications.
4. They take less time.
5. Information can be asked for sooner than it would be volunteered.
6. Responses are easily documented.
7. Questions are easy to use and can be handled by unskilled interviewers.

Disadvantages

1. They may provide too little information and require follow-up questions.
2. They may not reveal how the interviewee feels.
3. They do not allow the interviewee to volunteer possibly valuable information.
4. They may inhibit communication and convey lack of interest by the interviewer.
5. The interviewer may dominate the interview with questions.

Note: From Stewart, C. J., & Cash, Jr., W. B. (2006). *Interviewing: Principles and practices* (11th ed.). McGraw-Hill. Reprinted with permission from The McGraw-Hill Companies.

---

answer. Examples are "You're stressed about surgery tomorrow, aren't you?" "You will take your medicine, won't you?" The leading question gives the client less opportunity to decide whether the answer is true or not. Leading questions create problems if the client, in an effort to please the nurse, gives inaccurate responses. This can result in inaccurate data.

PLANNING THE INTERVIEW AND SETTING Before beginning an interview, the nurse reviews available information, for example, the operative report, information about the current illness, or literature about the client's health problem. The nurse also reviews the agency's data collection form to identify which data must be collected and which data are within the nurse's discretion to collect based on the specific client. If a form is not available, most nurses prepare an interview guide to help them remember areas of information and determine what questions to ask. The guide includes a list of topics and subtopics rather than a series of questions.

Both nurses and clients are made comfortable in order to encourage an effective interview by balancing several factors. Each interview is influenced by time, place, seating arrangement or distance, and language.

Time Nurses need to plan interviews with clients when the client is physically comfortable and free of pain, and when interruptions by friends, family, and other health professionals are minimal. Nurses should schedule interviews with clients in their homes at a time selected by the client.

Place A well-lighted, well-ventilated room that is relatively free of noise, movements, and distractions encourages communication. In addition, a place where others cannot overhear or see the client is desirable.

Seating Arrangement Standing and looking down at a client who is in bed or in a chair, the nurse risks intimidating the client. When a client is in bed, the nurse can sit at a 45-degree angle to the bed. This position is less formal than sitting behind a table or standing at the foot of the bed. During an initial admission interview, a client may feel less confronted if there is an overbed table between the client and the nurse. Sitting on a client's bed hems the client in and makes staring difficult to avoid. A seating arrangement with the nurse behind a desk and the client seated across creates a formal setting that suggests a business meeting between a superior and a subordinate. In contrast, a seating arrangement in which the parties sit on two chairs placed at right angles to a desk or table or a few feet apart, with no table between, creates a less formal atmosphere, and the nurse and client tend to feel on equal terms. In groups, a horseshoe or circular chair arrangement can avoid a superior or head-of-the-table position.

Distance The distance between the interviewer and interviewee should be neither too small nor too great, because people feel uncomfortable when talking to someone who is too close or too far away. Proxemics is the study of use of space. As a species, humans are highly territorial but we are rarely aware of it unless our space is somehow violated. Most people feel comfortable maintaining a distance of 2–3 feet during an interview. Some clients require more or less personal space, depending on their cultural and personal needs. See Box 34–4.

Language   Failure to communicate in language the client can understand is a form of discrimination. The nurse must convert complicated medical terminology into common English usage, and interpreters or translators are needed if the client and the nurse do not speak the same language or dialect (a variation in a language spoken in a particular geographic region). Translating medical terminology is a specialized skill because not all persons fluent in the conversational form of the language are familiar with anatomic or other health terms. Interpreters, however, may make judgments about precise wording but also about subtle meanings that require additional explanation or clarification according to the specific language and ethnicity. They may edit the original source to make the meaning clearer or more culturally appropriate.

If giving written documents to clients, the nurse must determine that the client can read in his or her native language. Live translation is preferred since the client can then ask questions for clarification. Nurses must be cautious when asking family members, client visitors, or agency nonprofessional staff to assist with translation. Issues of confidentiality or gender mismatch can interfere with effective communication. Services such as AT&T Language Line are available 24 hours a day in about 140 languages or a fee paid by the health care provider. Many large agencies possess their own on-call translator services for the languages or dialects commonly spoken in their area.

PRACTICE ALERT
Avoid use of family members for translation whenever possible. Family members may insert their own advice or alter information to reduce anxiety in the client.

Even among clients who speak English, there may be differences in understanding terminology. Clients from different parts of the country may have strong accents, or clients less well educated and teen clients may ascribe different meanings to words. For example, "cool" may imply something good to one client and something not warm to another. The nurse must always confirm accurate understandings.

Box 34–4 Personal Space Variables

■ Accepted distance between individuals in conversation varies with ethnicity. It is about 8–12 inches in Arab countries, 18 inches in the United States, 24 inches in Britain, and 36 inches in Japan.
■ Men of all cultures usually require more space than women.
■ Anxiety increases the need for space.
■ Direct eye contact increases the need for space.
■ Physical contact is used only if it has a therapeutic purpose. Touch, even a simple hand on the shoulder, can be misinterpreted—especially between persons of opposite gender.

STAGES OF AN INTERVIEW   An interview has three major stages: the opening or introduction, the body or development, and the closing.

The Opening   The opening can be the most important part of the interview because it sets the tone for the remainder of the interview. What the nurse says, how he or she says it, and the attitude the nurse projects to the client can make a huge difference in the client's attitude. The purposes of the opening are to establish rapport and orient the interviewee.

Establishing rapport is a process of creating goodwill and trust. It can begin with a greeting ("Good morning, Mr. Johnson") or a self-introduction ("Good morning. I'm Becky James, a nursing student") accompanied by nonverbal gestures such as a smile, a handshake, and a friendly manner. The nurse must be careful not to overdo this stage; too much superficial talk can arouse anxiety and may appear insincere.

In orientation, the nurse explains the purpose and nature of the interview, for example, what information is needed, how long it will take, and what is expected of the client. The nurse tells the client how the information will be used and usually states that the client has the right not to provide information.

The following is an example of an interview introduction:

Step 1—Establish Rapport

Nurse: Hello, Ms. Goodwin, I'm Ms. Fellows. I'm a nursing student, and I'll be assisting with your care here today.
Client: Hi. Are you a student from the college?
Nurse: Yes, I'm in my final year. Are you familiar with the campus?
Client: Oh, yes! I'm an avid basketball fan. My nephew graduated in 2004, and I often attend basketball games with him.
Nurse: That's great! Sounds like fun.
Client: Yes, I enjoy it very much.

Step 2—Orientation

Nurse: May I sit down with you for about 10 minutes to talk about how I can help you while you're here?
Client: All right. What do you want to know?
Nurse: To help plan your care after your operation, I'd like to get some information about your usual daily activities and what you expect here in the hospital. I'll take notes while we talk to get the important points and have them available to the other staff who will also look after you.
Client: OK. That's all right with me.
Nurse: If there is anything you don't want to talk about, please feel free to say so. Everything you tell me will be confidential and only be shared with others who have the legal right to know it.
Client: Sure, that will be fine.

The Body   In the body of the interview, the client communicates what he or she thinks, feels, knows, and perceives in response to questions from the nurse. Effective development of the interview demands that the nurse use communication techniques that make both parties feel comfortable and serve the purpose of the interview. For communicating during an interview, follow these guidelines:

- Listen attentively, using all your senses, and speak slowly and clearly.
- Use language the client understands, and clarify points that are not understood.
- Plan questions to follow a logical sequence.
- Ask only one question at a time. Multiple questions limit the client to one choice and may confuse the client.
- Acknowledge the client's right to look at things the way they appear to him or her and not the way they appear to the nurse or someone else.
- Do not impose your own values on the client.
- Avoid using personal examples, such as saying, "If I were you...."
- Nonverbally convey respect, concern, interest, and acceptance.
- Be aware of the client's and your own body language.
- Be conscious of the client's and your own voice inflection, tone, and affect.
- Sit down to talk with the client (be at an even level).
- Use and accept silence to help the client search for more thoughts or to organize them.
- Use eye contact and be calm, unhurried, and sympathetic.

The Closing The nurse terminates the interview when the necessary information has been obtained. In some cases, however, a client terminates the interview. For example, the client may decide not to give any more information or may be unable to offer more information for some other reason—fatigue, for example. The closing is important for maintaining the rapport and trust and for facilitating future interactions. The following techniques are commonly used to close an interview:

1. Offer to answer questions: "Do you have any questions?" "I would be glad to answer any questions you have." Be sure to allow time for the person to answer, or the offer will be regarded as insincere.
2. Conclude by saying "Well, that's all I need to know for now" or "Well, those are all the questions I have for now." Preceding a remark with the word "well" generally signals that the end of the interaction is near.
3. Thank the client: "Thank you for your time and help. The questions you have answered will be helpful in planning your nursing care." You may also shake the client's hand.
4. Express concern for the person's welfare and future: "Take care of yourself. I hope all goes well for you."
5. Plan for the next meeting, if there is to be one, or state what will happen next. Include the day, time, place, topic, and purpose: "Let's get together again here on the fifteenth at 9:00 a.m. to see how you are managing then." Or "Ms. Cho, I will be responsible for giving you care three mornings per week while you are here. I will be in to see you each Monday, Tuesday, and Wednesday between eight o'clock and noon. At those times, we can adjust your care as needed."

6. Provide a summary to verify accuracy and agreement. Summarizing serves several purposes, such as helping to terminate the interview, reassuring the client that the nurse has listened, checking the accuracy of the nurse's perceptions, clearing the way for new ideas, and helping the client to note progress and a forward direction: "Let's review what we have just covered in this interview." Summaries are particularly helpful for clients who are anxious or who have difficulty staying with the topic: "Well, it seems to me that you are especially worried about your hospitalization and chest pain because your father died of a heart attack five years ago. Is that correct? ... I'll discuss this with you again tomorrow, and we'll decide what plans need to be made to help you."

Examining

The physical examination or physical assessment is a systematic data collection method that uses observation (i.e., the senses of sight, hearing, smell, and touch) to detect health problems. To conduct the examination the nurse uses techniques of inspection, auscultation, palpation, and percussion (see Concept 32, Assessment, for more information on the physical examination).

ORGANIZING DATA

The nurse uses a written or digital format that organizes the assessment data systematically. This is often referred to as a nursing health history, nursing assessment, or nursing database form. The format may be modified according to the client's physical status, such as one focused on musculoskeletal data for orthopedic clients.

Conceptual Models/Frameworks

Most schools of nursing and health care agencies have developed their own structured assessment format. Many of these are based on selected nursing models or frameworks. Three examples are Gordon's functional health pattern framework, Orem's self-care model, and Roy's adaptation model.

Gordon (2006) provides a framework of 11 functional health patterns (see Box 34–5). Gordon uses the word *pattern* to signify a sequence of recurring behavior. The nurse collects data about dysfunctional as well as functional behavior. Thus, by using Gordon's framework to organize data, nurses are able to discern emerging patterns.

Orem (2001) delineates eight universal self-care requisites of humans (see Box 34–6), such as maintaining sufficient food intake and maintaining a balance between activity and rest. Roy and Andrews (1998) outline the data to be collected according to the Roy adaptation model and classify observable behavior into four categories: physiologic, self-concept, role function, and interdependence (see Box 34–7).

Box 34–5 Gordon's Typology of 11 Functional Health Patterns

1. *Health-perception/health-management pattern.* Describes the client's perceived pattern of health and well-being and how health is managed.
2. *Nutritional-metabolic pattern.* Describes the client's pattern of food and fluid consumption relative to metabolic need and pattern indicators of local nutrient supply.
3. *Elimination pattern.* Describes the patterns of excretory function (bowel, bladder, and skin).
4. *Activity-exercise pattern.* Describes the pattern of exercise, activity, leisure, and recreation.
5. *Sleep-rest pattern.* Describes patterns of sleep, rest, and relaxation.
6. *Cognitive-perceptual pattern.* Describes sensory-perceptual and cognitive patterns.
7. *Self-perception/self-concept pattern.* Describes the client's self-concept pattern and perceptions of self (e.g., self-conception/worth, comfort, body image, feeling state).
8. *Role-relationship pattern.* Describes the client's pattern of role participation and relationships.
9. *Sexuality-reproductive pattern.* Describes the client's patterns of satisfaction and dissatisfaction with sexuality pattern; describes reproductive patterns.
10. *Coping/stress-tolerance pattern.* Describes the client's general coping pattern and the effectiveness of the pattern in terms of stress tolerance.
11. *Value-belief pattern.* Describes the patterns of values, beliefs (including spiritual), and goals that guide the client's choices or decisions.

Note: From Gordon, M. (2006). *Manual of nursing diagnosis* (11th ed.). Boston: Jones & Bartlett, pp. 2–5. Reprinted with permission.

Figure 34–5 ■ is a concise data collection tool that is organized according to body systems and specific nursing concerns (e.g., screening for falls and allergies); it does not use one particular nursing model. In Box 34–8, the data for the case study of Amanda Aquilini, the client in Figure 34–5, are shown after being organized according to 11 functional health patterns. Note how the categories in the box differ from those in Figure 34–5. As a rule, the nurse organizes the data using the same model on which the data collection tool is based. However, different models are provided here to demonstrate differences in organizing frameworks, and to show that the nurse is not limited to the exact framework provided by the data collection tool.

Wellness Models

Nurses use wellness models to assist clients to identify health risks and to explore lifestyle habits and health behaviors, beliefs, values, and attitudes that influence levels of wellness. Such models generally include the following:
- Health history
- Physical fitness evaluation
- Nutritional assessment
- Life-stress analysis
- Lifestyle and health habits

Box 34–6 Orem's Self-Care Model

UNIVERSAL SELF-CARE REQUISITES
1. The maintenance of a sufficient intake of air.
2. The maintenance of a sufficient intake of water.
3. The maintenance of a sufficient intake of food.
4. The provision of care associated with elimination processes and excrement.
5. The maintenance of a balance between activity and rest.
6. The maintenance of a balance between solitude and social interaction.
7. The prevention of hazards to human life, human functioning, and human well-being.
8. The promotion of human functioning and development within social groups in accord with human potential, known human limitations, and human desire to be normal. (Normalcy is used in the sense of that which is essentially human and that which is in accord with the genetic and constitutional characteristics and the talents of individuals.)

Note: Adapted from Orem, D. E. (2001). *Nursing: Concepts of practice* (6th ed.), p. 225, with permission from Elsevier.

- Health beliefs
- Sexual health
- Spiritual health
- Relationships
- Health risk appraisal.

Non-nursing Models

Frameworks and models from other disciplines may also be helpful for organizing data. These frameworks are narrower than the model required in nursing; therefore, the nurse usually needs to combine these with other approaches to obtain a complete history.

BODY SYSTEMS MODEL The body systems model focuses on abnormalities of the following anatomic systems:
- Integumentary system

Box 34–7 Roy's Adaptation Model

ADAPTIVE MODES
1. Physiologic needs
   - Activity and rest
   - Nutrition
   - Elimination
   - Fluid and electrolytes
   - Oxygenation
   - Protection
   - Regulation: temperature
   - Regulation: the senses
   - Regulation: endocrine system
2. Self-concept
   - Physical self
   - Personal self
3. Role function
4. Interdependence

Note: Adapted from Roy, C., & Andrews, H. A. (1999). *The Roy adaptation model: The definitive statement* (2nd ed.). Upper Saddle River, NJ: Prentice-Hall.

Box 34–8 Example of Data Organized According to Functional Health Patterns

HEALTH PERCEPTION/HEALTH MANAGEMENT
- Aware/understands medical diagnosis
- Gives thorough history of illnesses and surgeries
- Complies with Synthroid regimen
- Relates progression of illness in detail
- Expects to have antibiotic therapy and "go home in a day or two"
- States usual eating pattern "3 meals a day"

NUTRITIONAL/METABOLIC
- 158 cm (5 ft, 2 in.) tall; weighs 56 kg (125 lb)
- Usual eating pattern "3 meals a day"
- "No appetite" since having "cold"
- Has not eaten today; last fluids at noon
- Nauseated
- Oral temperature 39.4°C (103°F)
- Decreased skin turgor

ELIMINATION
- Usually no problem
- Decreased urinary frequency and amount × 2 days
- Last bowel movement yesterday, formed, states was "normal"

ACTIVITY/EXERCISE
- No musculoskeletal impairment
- Difficulty sleeping because of cough
- "Can't breathe lying down"
- States, "I feel weak"
- Short of breath on exertion
- Exercises daily

COGNITIVE/PERCEPTUAL
- No sensory deficits
- Pupils 3 mm, equal, brisk reaction
- Oriented to time, place, and person
- Responsive, but fatigued
- Responds appropriately to verbal and physical stimuli
- Recent and remote memory intact
- States "short of breath" on exertion
- Reports "pain in lungs," especially when coughing
- Experiencing chills
- Reports nausea

ROLES/RELATIONSHIPS
- Lives with husband and 3-year-old daughter
- Husband out of town; will be back tomorrow afternoon
- Child with neighbor until husband returns
- States "good" relationships with friends and coworkers
- Working mother, attorney

SELF-PERCEPTION/SELF-CONCEPT
- Expresses "concern" and "worry" over leaving daughter with neighbors until husband returns
- Well-groomed, says, "Too tired to put on makeup"

COPING/STRESS
- Anxious, says, "I can't breathe"
- Facial muscles tense; trembling
- Expresses concerns about work, says, "I'll never get caught up"

VALUE/BELIEF
- Catholic
- No special practices desired except anointing of the sick
- Middle-class, professional orientation
- No wish to see chaplain or priest at present

MEDICATION/HISTORY
- Synthroid 0.1 mg per day
- Client has history of appendectomy, partial thyroidectomy

NURSING PHYSICAL ASSESSMENT
- 28 years old
- Height 158 cm (5 ft, 2 in.); weight 56 kg (125 lb)
- TPR 39.4°C, 92, 28
- Radial pulses weak, regular
- Blood pressure 122/80 sitting
- Skin hot and pale, cheeks flushed
- Mucous membranes dry and pale
- Respirations shallow; chest expansion < 3 cm
- Cough productive of small amounts of pale pink sputum
- Inspiratory crackles auscultated throughout right upper and lower chest
- Diminished breath sounds on right side
- Abdomen soft, not distended
- Old surgical scars: anterior neck, RLQ abdomen
- Diaphoretic

- Respiratory system
- Cardiovascular system
- Nervous system
- Musculoskeletal system
- Gastrointestinal system
- Genitourinary system
- Reproductive system
- Immune system.

MASLOW'S HIERARCHY OF NEEDS Maslow's hierarchy of needs (see Box 34–13 for more information about Maslow's hierarchy) clusters data pertaining to the following:
- Physiologic needs (survival needs)
- Safety and security needs

- Love and belonging needs
- Self-esteem needs
- Self-actualization needs.

DEVELOPMENTAL THEORIES Several physical, psychosocial, cognitive, and moral developmental theories may be used by the nurse in specific situations (see Concept 7, Development). Examples include the following:
- Havighurst's age periods and developmental tasks
- Freud's five stages of development
- Erikson's eight stages of development
- Piaget's phases of cognitive development
- Kohlberg's stages of moral development.

ADMISSION DATA

Date 4-16-07 Time 3:15 p.m Primary Language English
Arrived Via: ☐ Wheelchair ☐ Stretcher ☑ Ambulatory
From: ☐ Admitting ☐ ER ☑ Home ☐ Nursing Home ☐ Other
Admitting M.D. R. Katz   Time Notified 5 p.m.

ORIENTATION TO UNIT

	YES	NO		YES	NO
Arm Band Correct	☒	☐	Visiting Hours	☒	☐
Allergy Band	☒	☐	Smoking Policy	☒	☐
Telephone	☒	☐	TV, Lights, Bed Controls,		
Electrical Policy	☒	☐	Call Lights, Side Rails	☒	☐
Educational Mat©l	☒	☐	Nurses Station	☒	☐
(TV Brochure)	☒	☐			

Family M.D. R. Katz
Weight 125 lb. Height 5 ft. 2 in.   BP:R — L 122/80
Temp. 103F Pulse 92, weak Resp 28, shallow
Source Providing Information ☑ Patient ☐ Other
Unable to Obtain History ☐
Reason for Admission (Onset, Duration, Pt.'s Perception) ("Chest cold" X2 weeks S.O.B on exertion. "Lung pain, fever." "Dr. says I have pneumonia.")

ALLERGIES & REACTIONS

Drugs Penicillin
Food/Other
Signs & Symptoms rash, nausea
Blood Reaction ☐ Yes ☑ No Dyes/Shellfish ☐ Yes ☑ No

MEDICATIONS

Current Meds	Dose/Freq.	Last Dose
Synthroid	0.1 mg. daily	4-16, 8 a.m.

Disposition of Meds: ☒ Home ☐ Pharmacy ☐ Safe *At Bedside

MEDICAL HISTORY

☑ No Major Problems   ☐ Gastro
☐ Cardiac   ☐ Arthritis
☐ Hyper/Hypotension   ☐ Stroke
☐ Diabetes   ☐ Seizures
☐ Cancer   ☐ Glaucoma
☐ Respiratory   ☑ Other Childbirth-2000

Surgery/Procedures	Date
Appendectomy	1985
Partial thyroidectomy	2000

SPECIAL ASSISTIVE DEVICES

☐ Wheelchair   ☐ Contacts   ☐ Venous   ☐ Dentures
☐ Braces   ☐ Hearing Aid Access   ☐ Partial
☐ Cane/Crutches ☐ Prosthesis Device   ☐ Upper
☐ Walker   ☐ Glasses   ☐ Epidural Catheter ☐ Lower
☐ Other None

VALUABLES

Patient informed Hospital not responsible for personal belongings.
Valuables Disposition: ☐ Patient ☐ Safe ☐ Given to
Patient/SO Signature None

PSYCHOSOCIAL HISTORY

Recent Stress None
Coping Mechanism Not assessed because of fatigue
Support System Husband, coworkers, friends
Calm: ☑ Yes ☐ No
Anxious: ☐ Yes ☐ No Facial muscles tense; trembling
Religion Catholic. Would want Last Rites
Tobacco Use: ☐ Yes ☑ No
Alcohol Use: ☐ Yes ☑ No
Drug Use: ☐ Yes ☑ No

NEUROLOGICAL

Oriented: ☑ Person ☑ Place ☑ Time ☐ Confused ☐ Sedated
         ☐ Alert ☐ Restless ☑ Lethargic ☐ Comatose
Pupils: ☑ Equal ☐ Unequal ☑ Reactive ☐ Sluggish
        ☐ Other 3mm.
Extremity Strength: ☑ Equal ☐ Unequal
Speech: ☑ Clear ☐ Slurred ☐ Other

MUSCULO-SKELETAL

Normal ROM of Extremities ☑ Yes ☐ No
☑ Weakness ☐ Paralysis ☐ Contractures ☐ Joint Swelling ☑ Pain
☐ Other ↓ related to fatigue   when coughing

RESPIRATORY

Pattern: ☐ Even ☐ Uneven ☑ Shallow ☑ Dyspnea
         ☑ Other diminished breath sounds
Breathing Sounds: ☐ Clear ☑ Other inspiratory crackles
Secretions: ☐ None ☑ Other pink, thick sputum
Cough: ☐ None ☑ Productive ☐ Nonproductive

CARDIOVASCULAR

Pulses: Apical Rate 92-W ☑ Reg. ☐ Irregular ☐ Pacemaker
        S = Strong W = Weak A = Absent D = Doppler
Radial R 92 L ___ Pedal R ___ L ___
Edema: ☑ Absent ☐ Present Site
Perfusion: ☐ Warm ☐ Dry ☑ Diaphoretic ☐ Cool (Hot)

GASTROINTESTINAL

Oral Mucosa ☐ Normal ☑ Other pale and dry
Bowel Sounds: ☑ Normal ☐ Other Abd. soft
Wt. Change: ☐ ☑ N/V Stool Frequency/Character 1/day; soft
Last B/M 4-15-07   ☐ Ostomy (type)
Equip.

GENITOURINARY

Urine: Last Voided This morning
☐ Normal ☐ Anuria ☐ Hematuria ☐ Dysuri ☐ Incontinent
☒ Other ↓ amount & frequency since ill
☐ Catheter (type)   Other
LMP 4-1-07   ☐ Vaginal/Penile Discharge
Other

SELF CARE

Need Assist with: ☐ Ambulating ☐ Elimination
                  ☐ Meals ☒ Hygiene ☐ Dressing
                  While fatigued

Amanda Aquilini [F. age 28]
#4637651

★ NORTH BROWARD HOSPITAL DISTRICT
NURSING ADMINISTRATION ASSESSMENT

Figure 34–5 ■ Assessment for Amanda Aquilini.

Source: Nursing assessment tool courtesy of North Broward Hospital District, Broward County, Florida. Reprinted with permission.

NUTRITION

General Appearance: ☑ Well Nourished ☐ Emaciated
☐ Other _____
Appetite: ☐ Good ☐ Fair ☑ Poor -x 2 days
Diet _Liquid_ Meal Pattern _3/day_
☐ Feeds Self ☐ Assist ☐ Total Feed

SKIN ASSESSMENT

Color: ☐ Normal ☐ Flushed ☑ Pale ☐ Dusky ☐ Cyanotic
☐ Jaundiced ☑ Other _Cheeks flushed, hot_
General Description _Surgical scars:_
RLQ abdomen; anterior neck
_____
_____
_____
Note Cultures Obtained _____
_____
_____

PRESSURE SORE ™AT RISK☐ SCREENING CRITERIA

OVERALL SKIN CONDITION

Grade
	0	Turgor (elasticity adequate, skin warm and moist)
✓	1	Poor turgor, skin cold & dry
	2	Areas mottled, red or denuded
	3	Existing skin ulcer/lesions

BOWEL AND BLADDER CONTROL

Grade
✓	0	Always able to ask for bedpan
	1	Incontinence of urine
	2	Incontinence of feces
	3	Totally incontinent Confined to bed

REHABILITATIVE STATE

Grade
	0	Fully ambulatory
✓	1	Ambulated with assistance
	2	Chair to bed ambulation only
	3	Confined to bed
	4	Immobile in bed

NUTRITIONAL STATE

Grade
	0	Eats all
✓	1	Eats very little
	2	Refuses food often
	3	Tube feeding
	4	Intravenous feeding

MENTAL STATE

Grade
✓	0	Alert and clear
	1	Confused
	2	Disoriented/senile
	3	Stuporous
	4	Unconcious

CHRONIC DISEASE STATUS
(i.e. COPD, ASCVD. Peripheral Vascular Disease, Diabetes, or Renal Disease, Cancer, Motor or Sensory Deficits, Elderly, Other)

Grade
✓	0	Absent
	1	One Present
	2	Two Present
	3	Three or more Present

TOTAL _____ Refer to Skin Care Protocol

FALLS SCREENING

If one or more of the following are checked institute fall precautions/plan of care
☐ History of Falls ☐ Unsteady Gait ☐ Confusion/Disorientation ☐ Dizziness

If two or more of the following are checked institute fall precautions/plan of care
☐ Age over 80
☐ Impaired vision
☐ Multiple Diagnoses
☐ Inability to understand or follow directions
☐ Utilizes cane, walker, w/c
☐ Impaired hearing
☐ Sleeplessness
☐ Urgency/frequency in elimination
☐ Medication/Sedative /Diuretic etc.

NURSE SIGNATURE/TITLE	DATE	TIME
Mary Medina, RN	_4-16-07_	_3:30pm_
NURSE SIGNATURE/TITLE	DATE	TIME

EDUCATION/DISCHARGE PLANNING

1. What do you know about your present illness? _"Dr. says I have pneumonia." "I will have an I.V."_
2. What information do you want or need about your illness? _____
3. Would you like family/SO involved in your care? _Husband, Michael_
4. How long do you expect to be in the hospital? _"1-2 days"_
5. What concerns do you have about leaving the hospital? ____

CHECK APPROPRIATE BOX

Will patient need post discharge assistance with ADLs/physical functioning? ☐ Yes ☑ No ☐ Unknown
Does patient have family capable of and willing to provide assistance post discharge?
☑ Yes ☐ No ☐ Unknown ☐ No family
Is assistance needed beyond that which family can provide?
☐ Yes ☑ No ☐ Unknown
Previous admission in the last six months?
☐ Yes ☑ No ☐ Unknown
Patient lives with _Husband and 1 child_
Planned discharge to _Home_
Comments: _Fatigue and anxiety may have interfered with learning. Re-teach anything covered at admission, later._

Social Services Notified ☐ Yes ☑ No

NARRATIVE NOTES

S--c/o sharp chest pain when coughing and dyspnea on exertion. States unable to carry out regular daily exercise for past week. Coughing relieved "if I sit up and sit still." Nausea associated with coughing. Having occasional "chills." Occasionally becomes frightened, stating, "I can't breathe." Well groomed but "too tired to put on make-up." O--Chest expansion < 3cm, no nasal flaring or use of accessory muscles. Breath sounds and insp. crackles in ℞ upper and lower chest. Assesses own supports as "good" (eg, relationship c husband). Is "worried" about daughter. States husband will be out of town until tomorrow. Left 3-year-old daughter with neighbor. Concerned too about her work (is attorney). "I'll never get caught up." Had water at noon—no food today. Agrees to save urine for 24 hr. specimen. IV D₅W LR 1000 mL started in ℞ arm, 100 mL/hr. Slow capillary refill. Keeping head of bed≠ to facilitate breathing.

✷ **NORTH BROWARD HOSPITAL DISTRICT**
NURSING ADMINISTRATION ASSESSMENT

Figure 34–5 ■ Assessment for Amanda Aquilini, continued.

DEVELOPMENTAL CONSIDERATIONS   Assessment of Children

Consider this example: A 4-year-old girl is admitted following emergency surgery for a ruptured appendix. She is awake and alert, but refuses to talk. Her parents have had little sleep for over 24 hours and are extremely anxious.

■ Gathering assessment data in this situation requires the nurse to be sensitive to the parents' needs for rest and assurance; at the same time, the nurse must collect information to compile an adequate database for appropriate nursing care decisions. Assessment will be problem-focused, monitoring the condition of the child as she recovers from surgery and being alert to potential problems.

■ The parents become the major source of subjective data, although the child should be encouraged to tell the nurse how she is feeling.

■ Objective data collected include vital signs; level of and response to pain (often called the fifth vital sign); bleeding or discharge from the incision; mobility; integrity of dressings, intravenous lines, catheters, nasogastric tubes, or other medical devices; and affect.

■ Since children are a part of families, assessment will include observation of family dynamics and questions that could lead to care of the family system.

VALIDATING DATA

The information gatheredduring the assessment phase must be complete, factual, and accurate because the nursing diagnoses and interventions are based on this information. **Validation** is the act of "double-checking" or verifying data to confirm that it is accurate and factual. Validating data helps the nurse do the following:

■ Ensure that assessment information is complete.

■ Ensure that objective and related subjective data agree.

■ Obtain additional information that may have been overlooked.

■ Differentiate between cues and inferences. **Cues** are subjective or objective data that can be directly observed by the nurse, that is, what the client says or what the nurse can see, hear, feel, smell, or measure. For example, the asthmatic client might say, "My chest feels tight," and on auscultation the nurse hears wheezing. **Inferences** are the nurse's

interpretation or conclusions made based on the cues (e.g., a nurse observes the cues that an incision is red, hot, and swollen; the nurse makes the inference that the incision is infected).

■ Avoid jumping to conclusions and focusing in the wrong direction to identify problems.

Not all data require validation. For example, data such as height, weight, birth date, and most laboratory studies that can be measured with an accurate scale can be accepted as factual. As a rule, the nurse validates data when there are discrepancies between data obtained in the nursing interview (subjective data) and the physical examination (objective data), or when the client's statements differ at different times in the assessment. Guidelines for validating data are shown in Table 34–8.

To collect data accurately, nurses need to be aware of their own biases, values, and beliefs, and to separate fact from inference, interpretation, and assumption. For example, a

TABLE 34–8 Validating Assessment Data

GUIDELINES	EXAMPLE
Compare subjective and objective data to verify the client's statements with your observations.	Client's perceptions of "feeling hot" need to be compared with measurement of the body temperature.
Clarify any ambiguous or vague statements.	*Client:* "I've felt sick on and off for 6 weeks." *Nurse:* "Describe what your sickness is like. Tell me what you mean by 'on and off.'"
Be sure your data consist of cues and not inferences.	*Observation:* Dry skin and reduced tissue turgor *Inference:* Dehydration *Action:* Collect additional data that are needed to make the inference in the diagnosing phase. For example, determine the client's fluid intake, amount and appearance of urine, and blood pressure.
Double-check data that are extremely abnormal.	*Observation:* A resting pulse of 30 beats per minute or a blood pressure of 210/95 *Action:* Repeat the measurement. Use another piece of equipment as needed to confirm abnormalities, or ask someone else to collect the same data.
Determine the presence of factors that may interfere with accurate measurement.	A crying infant will have an abnormal respiratory rate and will need quieting before accurate assessment can be made.
Use references (textbooks, journals, research reports) to explain phenomena.	A nurse considers tiny purple or bluish black swollen areas under the tongue of an elderly client to be abnormal until reading about physical changes of aging. Such varicosities are common.

nurse seeing a man holding his arm to his chest might assume that he is experiencing chest pain, when in fact he has a painful hand.

To build an accurate database, nurses must validate assumptions regarding the client's physical or emotional behavior. In the previous example, the nurse should ask the client why he is holding his arm to his chest. The client's response may validate the nurse's assumptions or prompt further questioning. Figure 34–5 indicates that the nurse auscultated the client's heart and lungs to validate her statement that she had "lung pain" and "shortness of breath" on exertion. Failure to validate assumptions can lead toan inaccurate or incomplete nursing assessment and could compromise client safety.

Diagnosis

Diagnosis is the second phase of the nursing process. In this phase, nurses use critical-thinking skills to interpret assessment data and identify client strengths and problems. Diagnosis is a pivotal step in the nursing process. Assessment activities preceding this phase are directed toward formulating the nursing diagnoses; the care-planning activities following this phase are based on the nursing diagnoses (see Figure 34–6 ■) developed by the North American Nursing Diagnosis Association (NANDA).

In order to identify nursing diagnoses effectively and then create and complete a nursing care plan, the nurse must be familiar with the definitions of terms used, the types, and the components of nursing diagnoses.

DEFINITIONS

A **diagnosis** is a statement or conclusion regarding the nature of a phenomenon. The standardized NANDA names for the diagnoses are called **diagnostic labels**; the client's problem statement, consisting of the diagnostic label plus **etiology** (causal relationship between a problem and its related or risk factors), is called a **nursing diagnosis**. **Risk factors** are factors that cause a client to be vulnerable to developing a health problem. The term *diagnosing* refers to the reasoning process the nurse uses to formulate the nursing diagnosis.

In 1990, NANDA first adopted an official working definition of nursing diagnosis, which is maintained today as "... a clinical judgment about individual, family, or community responses to actual and potential health problems/life processes. A nursing diagnosis provides the basis for selection of nursing interventions to achieve outcomes for which the nurse is accountable" (as cited in NANDA International, 2009, p. 41). This definition implies the following:

- Professional nurses (registered nurses) are responsible for making nursing diagnoses, even though other nursing personnel may contribute data to the process of diagnosing and may implement specified nursing care. The ANA's *Nursing: Scope and Standards of Practice* (2004) states that nurses are accountable for this phase of the nursing process. The Joint Commission requires evidence of nursing diagnoses in clients' medical records as well (Joint Commission, 2005).
- The domain of nursing diagnosis includes only those health states that nurses are educated and licensed to treat. For example, generalist nurses are not educated to diagnose or treat diseases such as diabetes mellitus; this task is defined legally as within the practice of medicine. Yet nurses can diagnose and treat deficient knowledge, ineffective coping, or imbalanced nutrition, all of which are the human responses to the medical diagnosis of diabetes mellitus.
- A nursing diagnosis is a judgment made only after thorough, systematic data collection.
- Nursing diagnoses describe a continuum of health states: deviations from health, presence of risk factors, and areas of enhanced personal growth.

TYPES OF NURSING DIAGNOSES

NANDA International has identified five types of nursing diagnoses. However, it is important to note that the organization is constantly reviewing existing diagnoses, retiring those that no long remain functional and incorporating new diagnoses as the body of knowledge on which they are based grows. Both graduate and student nurses can contribute to the development of diagnoses by joining the organization and becoming involved in committees. The existing types of diagnoses include actual, risk, health promotion, wellness, and syndrome.

1. An **actual diagnosis** is a client problem that is present at the time of the nursing assessment. Examples are ineffective breathing pattern and anxiety. An actual nursing diagnosis is based on the presence of associated signs and symptoms.
2. A **risk nursing diagnosis** is a clinical judgment that a problem does not exist, but the presence of risk factors indicates a problem is likely to develop unless the nurse intervenes. For example, all people admitted to a hospital

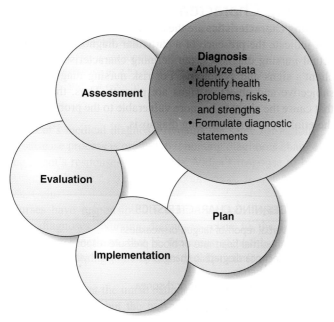

Figure 34–6 ■ Diagnosis. The pivotal second phase of the nursing process.

TABLE 34–11 Comparison of Nursing Diagnoses, Medical Diagnoses, and Collaborative Problems

	NURSING DIAGNOSES	MEDICAL DIAGNOSES	COLLABORATIVE PROBLEMS
Example	Activity Intolerance related to decreased cardiac output	Myocardial infarction	Potential complication of myocardial infarction: congestive heart failure
Description	Describe human responses to disease process or health problem; consist of a one-, two-, or three-part statement, usually including problem and etiology	Describe disease and pathology; do not consider other human responses; usually consist of not more than three words	Involve human responses—mainly physiologic complications of disease, tests, or treatments; consist of a two-part statement of situation/pathophysiology and the potential complication
Orientation and responsibility for diagnosing	Oriented to the individual; nurses responsible for diagnosing	Oriented to pathology; physician responsible for diagnosing; diagnosis not within the scope of nursing practice	Oriented to pathophysiology; nurses responsible for diagnosing
Nursing focus	Treat and prevent	Implement medical orders for treatment and monitor status of condition	Prevent and monitor for onset or status of condition
Nursing actions	Independent	Dependent (primarily)	Some independent actions, but primarily for monitoring and preventing
Duration	Can change frequently	Remains the same while disease is present	Present when disease or situation is present
Classification system	Classification system is developed and being used but is not universally accepted	Well-developed classification system accepted by the medical profession	No universally accepted classification system

THE DIAGNOSTIC PROCESS

The diagnostic process uses the critical-thinking skills of analysis and synthesis. **Critical thinking** is a cognitive process during which a person reviews data and considers potential explanations before forming an opinion or making a decision. Analysis is the separation into components, that is, the breaking down of the whole into its parts (deductive reasoning). Synthesis is the opposite, that is, the putting together of parts into the whole (inductive reasoning). See Exemplar 34.2, Critical Thinking, in this concept for more information on types of reasoning.

The diagnostic process is used continuously by most nurses. An experienced nurse may enter a client's room and immediately observe significant data and draw conclusions about the client. As a result of attaining knowledge, skill, and expertise in the practice setting, the expert nurse may seem to perform these mental processes automatically. Novice nurses, however, need guidelines to understand and formulate nursing diagnoses. The diagnostic process has three steps:

1. Analyzing data
2. Identifying health problems, risks, and strengths
3. Formulating diagnostic statements.

Analyzing Data

In the diagnostic process, analyzing involves the following steps:

1. Comparing data against standards (identify significant cues)
2. Clustering cues (generate tentative hypotheses)
3. Identifying gaps and inconsistencies.

For experienced nurses, these activities occur continuously rather than sequentially.

COMPARING DATA WITH STANDARDS Nurses draw on knowledge and experience to compare client data to standards and norms and identify significant and relevant cues. A **standard** or **norm** is a generally accepted measure, rule, model, or pattern. The nurse uses a wide range of standards, such as growth and development patterns, normal vital signs, and laboratory values. A cue is considered significant if it does any of the following:

- *Points to negative or positive change in a client's health status or pattern.* For example, the client states, "I have recently experienced shortness of breath while climbing stairs" or "I have not smoked for 3 months."
- *Varies from norms of the client population.* The client's pattern may fit within cultural norms but vary from norms of the general society. The client may consider a pattern—for example, eating very small meals and having little appetite—to be normal. This pattern, however, may not be healthy and may require further exploration.
- *Indicates a developmental delay.* To identify significant cues, the nurse must be aware of the normal patterns and changes that occur as the person grows and develops. For example, by age 9 months an infant is usually able to sit alone without support. The infant who has not accomplished this task needs further assessment for possible developmental delays.

Table 34–12 lists specific examples of client cues and norms to which they may be compared.

CLUSTERING CUES Data clustering or grouping cues is a process of determining the relatedness of facts and determining whether any patterns are present, whether the data represent isolated incidents, and whether the data are significant.

TABLE 34-12 Comparing Cues to Standards and Norms

TYPE OF CUE	CLIENT CUES	STANDARD/NORM
Deviation from population norms	Height is 158 cm (5 ft, 2 in.). Woman with small frame. Weighs 109 kg (240 lb).	Height and weight tables indicate that the "ideal" weight for a woman 158 cm (5 ft, 2 in.) with a small frame is 49–53 kg (108–121 lb).
Developmental delay	Child is 17 months old. Parents state child has not yet attempted to speak. Child laughs aloud and makes cooing sounds.	Children usually speak their first word by 10–12 months of age.
Changes in client's usual health status	States, "I'm just not hungry these days." Ate only 15% of food on breakfast tray. Has lost 13 kg (30 lb) in past 3 months.	Client usually eats three balanced meals per day. Adults typically maintain stable weight.
Dysfunctional behavior	Amy's mother reports that Amy has not left her room for 2 days. Amy is 16 years old. Amy has stopped attending school and has withdrawn from social contact.	Adolescents usually like to be with their peers; the social group is very important. Functional behavior includes school attendance.
Changes in client's usual behavior	Mrs. Stuart reports that lately her husband angers easily. "Yesterday he even yelled at the dog." "He just seems so tense."	Mr. Stuart is usually relaxed and easygoing. He is friendly and kind to animals.

The nurse may cluster data inductively (as in Table 34–13) by combining data from different assessment areas to form a pattern, or the nurse may begin with a framework, such as Gordon's functional health patterns, and organize the subjective and objective data into the appropriate categories (see Box 34–5). The latter is a deductive approach to data clustering.

Experienced nurses may cluster data as they collect and interpret it, as evidenced in remarks or thoughts such as "I'm getting a sense of ... " or "This cue doesn't fit the picture." The novice nurse does not have the knowledge base or the clinical experience that aids in recognizing cues. Thus, the novice must take careful assessment notes, search data for abnormal cues, and use textbook resources for comparing the client's cues with the defining characteristics and etiologic factors of the accepted nursing diagnoses.

Data clustering involves making inferences about the data. The nurse interprets the possible meaning of the cues and labels the cue clusters with tentative diagnostic hypotheses. Data clustering or grouping for the client is illustrated in Table 34–13, in which data are clustered according to standardized diagnosis labels.

IDENTIFYING GAPS AND INCONSISTENCIES IN DATA
Skillful assessment minimizes gaps and inconsistencies in data. However, data analysis should include a final check to ensure that data are complete and correct.

TABLE 34-13 Formulating Nursing Diagnoses

FUNCTIONAL HEALTH PATTERN	CLIENT CUE CLUSTERS	INFERENCES (TENTATIVE IDENTIFICATION OF PROBLEMS)	FORMULATING DIAGNOSTIC STATEMENTS
Health perception/health management			No problem *Client strength:* Shows healthy lifestyle, understanding of and compliance with treatment regimens
Nutritional/metabolic (includes hydration)	"No appetite" since having "cold"; has not eaten today; last fluids at noon today Nauseated × 2 days	Imbalanced Nutrition: Less Than Body Requirements	Imbalanced Nutrition: Less Than Body Requirements related to decreased appetite and nausea and increased metabolism (secondary to disease process) *Client strength:* Normal weight for height

(continued)

TABLE 34–13 Formulating Nursing Diagnoses (continued)

FUNCTIONAL HEALTH PATTERN	CLIENT CUE CLUSTERS	INFERENCES (TENTATIVE IDENTIFICATION OF PROBLEMS)	FORMULATING DIAGNOSTIC STATEMENTS
	Last fluids at noon today Oral temp 39.4°C (103°F) Skin hot and pale, cheeks flushed Mucous membranes dry Poor skin turgor *Cues from elimination pattern:* Decreased urinary frequency and amount × 2 days	Deficient Fluid Volume	Deficient Fluid Volume related to intake insufficient to replace fluid loss secondary to fever, diaphoresis, anorexia
Elimination	Decreased urinary frequency and amount × 2 days	Cues consist of elimination data but are actually symptoms of a fluid volume problem in the nutritional/metabolic functional health pattern	No elimination problem
Activity/exercise	Difficulty sleeping because of cough "Can't breathe lying down"	Disturbed Sleep Pattern	Disturbed Sleep Pattern related to cough, pain, orthopnea, fever, and diaphoresis
	States, "I feel weak" Short of breath on exertion *Cues from cognitive/perceptual pattern:* Responsive but fatigued "I can think OK, just weak" *Cues from cardiovascular pattern:* Radial pulses weak, regular Pulse rate 92	Activity Intolerance	Activity Intolerance related to general weakness, imbalance between oxygen supply/demand *Client strength:* No musculoskeletal impairment, normal energy level is satisfactory, exercises regularly
Cognitive/perceptual	Reports pain in chest, especially when coughing	Acute Pain	Acute Pain (Chest) related to cough secondary to pneumonia
	Responsive but fatigued "I can think OK, just weak"	These are cognitive/perceptual data, but they reflect symptoms of problems in the activity/exercise pattern	*Client strength:* No cognitive or sensory deficits
Roles/relationships	Husband out of town; will be back tomorrow afternoon Child with neighbor until husband returns	Interrupted Family Processes related to mother's illness and temporary unavailability of father to provide child care	Risk for Interrupted Family Processes related to mother's illness and temporary unavailability of father to provide child care *Client strength:* Neighbors available and willing to help
Self-perception/self-concept	Expresses "concern" and "worry" over leaving daughter with neighbors until husband returns	Cues also related to a problem in the coping/stress pattern Cue is a symptom of a problem in the coping/stress pattern	No self-perception/self-concept problem
Coping/stress	Anxious: "I can't breathe" Facial muscles tense; trembling Expresses concerns about work: "I'll never get caught up" *Cues from role/relationship pattern:* Husband out of town; will be back tomorrow afternoon Child with neighbor until husband returns *Cues from self-perception/self-concept patterns:* Expresses "concern" and "worry" over leaving daughter with neighbors	Anxiety related to difficulty breathing, inability to work, and child care	Anxiety related to difficulty breathing and concerns over work and parenting roles
Medication/history	No significant cues	No problem	No problem

(continued)

TABLE 34–13 **Formulating Nursing Diagnoses** (continued)

FUNCTIONAL HEALTH PATTERN	CLIENT CUE CLUSTERS	INFERENCES (TENTATIVE IDENTIFICATION OF PROBLEMS)	FORMULATING DIAGNOSTIC STATEMENTS
Physical assessment			
Cardiovascular	Radial pulses weak, regular Pulse rate 92	Cues are symptoms only; symptoms of exercise/rest and oxygenation problems	No cardiovascular problem
Oxygenation	Skin hot, pale, and moist Respirations shallow; chest expansion, 3 cm Cough productive of small amounts of thick pale pink sputum Inspiratory crackles auscultated throughout right upper and lower lungs Diminished breath sounds on right side Mucous membranes pale, dry	Ineffective Airway Clearance related to disease process	Ineffective Airway Clearance related to viscous secretions and shallow chest expansion secondary to pain, fluid volume deficit, and fatigue
Skin	Old surgical scars, anterior neck, RLQ abdomen	No problem now	Old problems; resolved

Inconsistencies are conflicting data. Possible sources of conflicting data include measurement error, expectations, and inconsistent or unreliable reports. For example, a nurse may learn from the nursing history that the client reports not having seen a doctor in 15 years, yet during the physical health examination he or she states, "My doctor takes my blood pressure every year." All inconsistencies must be clarified before a valid pattern can be established.

IDENTIFYING HEALTH PROBLEMS, RISKS, AND STRENGTHS
After data are analyzed, the nurse and client can together identify strengths and problems. This is primarily a decision-making process.

Determining Problems and Risks   After grouping and clustering the data, the nurse and client together identify problems that support tentative actual, risk, and possible diagnoses. In addition the nurse must determine whether the client's problem is a nursing diagnosis, medical diagnosis, or collaborative problem. See Figure 34–7 ■ and Table 34–11.

Significant cues and data clusters for the client that were extracted from Figure 34–5 and Box 34–8 are shown in Table 34–13. In this example, the nurse and client identified eight tentative problems:
- Imbalanced Nutrition: Less Than Body Requirements
- Deficient Fluid Volume
- Disturbed Sleep Pattern
- Activity Intolerance
- Acute Pain (Chest)
- Interrupted Family Processes
- Anxiety
- Ineffective Airway Clearance.

Note that some data may indicate a possible problem but when clustered with other data, the possible problem disappears. For example, the following data for the client discussed in this exemplar, "Decreased urinary frequency and amount × 2 days,"

suggests a possible urinary elimination problem. However, when these data are considered along with data associated with deficient fluid volume, the nurse eliminates urinary elimination as a problem.

Determining Strengths   At this stage, the nurse and client also establish the client's strengths, resources, and abilities to cope. Most people have a clearer perception of their problems or weaknesses than of their strengths and assets, which they often take for granted. By taking an inventory of strengths, the client can develop a more well-rounded self-concept and self-image. Strengths can be an aid to mobilizing health and regenerative processes.

A client's strengths might include weight that is within the normal range for age and height, thus enabling the client to cope better with surgery. Another client's strengths might be absence of allergies and being a nonsmoker.

A client's strengths can be found in the nursing assessment record (health, home life, education, recreation, exercise, work, family and friends, religious beliefs, and sense of humor, for example), the health examination, and the client's records. See Table 34–13 for the strengths identified for a client.

Formulating Diagnostic Statements
Most nursing diagnoses are written as two-part or three-part statements, but there are variations of these.

BASIC TWO-PART STATEMENTS   The basic two-part statement includes the following:
1. *Problem (P):* statement of the client's response (NANDA label)
2. *Etiology (E):* factors contributing to or probable causes of the responses

The two parts are joined by the words *related to* rather than *due to*. The phrase *due to* implies that one part causes or is responsible for the other part. By contrast, the phrase *related*

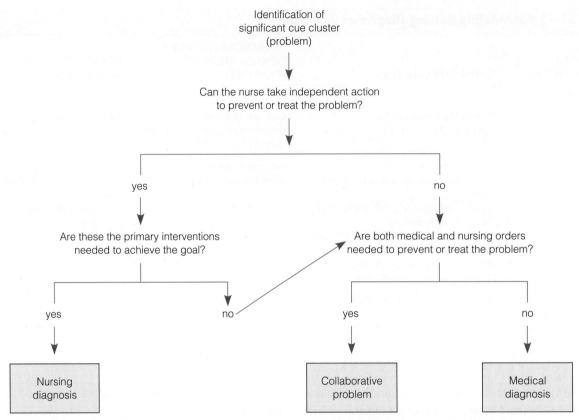

Figure 34–7 ■ Decision tree for differentiating among nursing diagnoses, collaborative problems, and medical diagnoses.

to merely implies a relationship. Some examples of two-part nursing diagnoses are shown in Box 34–9.

For NANDA labels that contain the word *specify*, the nurse must add words to indicate the problem more specifically. The format is still a two-part statement. For example, *noncompliance (specify)* would be noncompliance (diabetic diet) related to denial of having disease. For ease in alphabetizing, many NANDA lists are arranged with qualifying words after the main word (e.g., infection, risk for). Avoid writing diagnostic statements in that manner; instead, write them as they would be stated in normal conversation (e.g., risk for infection).

BASIC THREE-PART STATEMENTS The basic three-part nursing diagnosis statement is called the **PES format** and includes the following:

1. *Problem (P):* statement of the client's response (NANDA label)
2. *Etiology (E):* factors contributin g to or probable causes of the response
3. *Signs and symptoms (S):* defining characteristics manifested by the client

Box 34–9 **Basic Two-Part Diagnostic Statement**		
PROBLEM	RELATED TO	ETIOLOGY
Constipation	related to	prolonged laxative use
Severe Anxiety	related to	threat to physiologic integrity: possible cancer diagnosis

Actual nursing diagnoses can be documented by using the three-part statement (see Box 34–10) because the signs and symptoms have been identified. This format cannot be used for risk diagnoses because the client does not have signs and symptoms of the diagnosis.

The PES format is especially recommended for beginning diagnosticians because the signs and symptoms validate why the diagnosis was chosen and make the problem statement more descriptive. The PES format can create very long problem statements, sometimes making the problem and etiology unclear. To minimize long problem statements, the nurse can record the signs and symptoms in the nursing notes instead of on the care plan. Another possibility, recommended for students, is to list the signs and symptoms on the care plan below the nursing diagnosis, grouping the subjective (S) and objective (O) data. The signs and symptoms are easily accessible, and the problem and etiology stand out clearly. For example:

Noncompliance (diabetic diet) related to unresolved anger about diagnosis as manifested by

S— "I forget to take my pills."
 "I can't live without sugar in my food."
O— Weight 98 kg (215 lb) (gain of 4.5 kg [10 lb])
 Blood pressure 190/100

ONE-PART STATEMENTS Some diagnostic statements, such as wellness diagnoses and syndrome nursing diagnoses, consist of a NANDA label only. As the diagnostic labels are refined, they tend to become more specific so that nursing interventions can be derived from the label itself. Therefore, an

Box 34–10 **Basic Three-Part Diagnostic Statement**

PROBLEM	RELATED TO	ETIOLOGY	AS MANIFESTED BY	SIGNS AND SYMPTOMS
Situational Low Self-Esteem	related to (r/t)	feelings of rejection by husband	as manifested by (a.m.b.)	hypersensitivity to criticism; states, "I don't know if I can manage by myself," and rejects positive feedback

etiology may not be needed. For example, adding an etiology to the label Rape-Trauma Syndrome does not make the label any more descriptive or useful.

NANDA has specified that any new wellness diagnoses will be developed as one-part statements beginning with the words *readiness for enhanced* followed by the desired higher level wellness (for example, readiness for enhanced parenting).

Currently the NANDA list includes several wellness diagnoses. Some of these are spiritual well-being, effective breastfeeding, health-seeking behaviors, and anticipatory grieving. These are usually accepted as one-part statements but may be made more explicit by adding a descriptor, for example, health-seeking behaviors (low-fat diet).

VARIATIONS OF BASIC FORMATS Variations of the basic one-, two-, and three-part statements include the following:

1. Writing *unknown etiology* when the defining characteristics are present but the nurse does not know the cause or contributing factors. One example is noncompliance (medication regimen) related to unknown etiology.
2. Using the phrase *complex factors* when there are too many etiologic factors or when they are too complex to state in a brief phrase. The actual causes of chronic low self-esteem, for instance, may be long term and complex, as in the following nursing diagnosis: chronic low self-esteem related to complex factors.
3. Using the word *possible* to describe either the problem or the etiology. When the nurse believes more data are needed about the client's problem or the etiology, the word *possible* is inserted. Examples are possible low self-esteem related to loss of job and rejection by family; altered thought processes possibly related to unfamiliar surroundings.
4. Using *secondary to* to divide the etiology into two parts, thereby making the statement more descriptive and useful. The part following *secondary to* is often a pathophysiologic or disease process or a medical diagnosis, as in risk for impaired skin integrity related to decreased peripheral circulation secondary to diabetes.
5. Adding a second part to the general response or NANDA label to make it more precise. For example, the diagnosis

impaired skin integrity does not indicate the location of the problem. To make this label more specific, the nurse can add a descriptor as follows: impaired skin integrity (left lateral ankle) related to decreased peripheral circulation.

COLLABORATIVE PROBLEMS Carpenito-Moyet (2006) has suggested that all collaborative (multidisciplinary) problems begin with the diagnostic label *Potential Complication* (PC). Nurses should include in the diagnostic statement both the possible complication they are monitoring and the disease or treatment that is present to produce it. For example, if the client has a head injury and could develop increased intracranial pressure, the nurse should write the following:

Potential Complication of Head Injury:
Increased intracranial pressure

When monitoring for a group of complications associated with a disease or pathology, the nurse states the disease and follows it with a list of the complications:

Potential Complication of Pregnancy-Induced Hypertension: seizures, fetal distress, pulmonary edema, hepatic/renal failure, premature labor, CNS hemorrhage

In some situations, an etiology might be helpful in suggesting interventions. Nurses should write the etiology when (a) it clarifies the problem statement, (b) it can be concisely stated, and (c) it helps to suggest nursing actions. See the examples in Box 34–11.

EVALUATING THE QUALITY OF THE DIAGNOSTIC STATEMENT In addition to using the correct format, nurses must consider the content of their diagnostic statements. The statements should, for example, be accurate, concise, descriptive, and specific. The nurse must always validate the diagnostic statements with the client and compare the client's signs and symptoms to the NANDA defining characteristics. For risk problems, the nurse compares the client's risk factors to NANDA risk factors. After writing nursing diagnoses, the nurse checks them against the criteria in Table 34–14.

Box 34–11 **Collaborative Problems**

DISEASE/SITUATION	COMPLICATION	RELATED TO	ETIOLOGY
Potential complication of childbirth:	hemorrhage	related to	uterine atony retained placental fragments bladder distention
Potential complication of diuretic therapy:	arrhythmia	related to	low serum potassium

TABLE 34–14 Guidelines for Writing a Nursing Diagnostic Statement

GUIDELINE	CORRECT STATEMENT	INCORRECT OR AMBIGUOUS STATEMENT
1. State in terms of a problem, not a need.	Deficient Fluid Volume (problem) related to fever	Fluid Replacement (need) related to fever
2. Word the statement so that it is legally advisable.	Impaired Skin Integrity related to immobility (legally acceptable)	Impaired Skin Integrity related to improper positioning (implies legal liability)
3. Use nonjudgmental statements.	Spiritual Distress related to inability to attend church services secondary to immobility (nonjudgmental)	Spiritual Distress related to strict rules necessitating church attendance (judgmental)
4. Make sure that both elements of the statement do not say the same thing.	Risk for Impaired Skin Integrity related to immobility	Impaired Skin Integrity related to ulceration of sacral area (response and probable cause are the same)
5. Be sure that cause and effect are correctly stated (i.e., the etiology causes the problem or puts the client at risk for the problem).	Pain: Severe Headache related to fear of addiction to narcotics	Pain related to severe headache
6. Word the diagnosis specifically and precisely to provide direction for planning nursing intervention.	Impaired Oral Mucous Membrane related to decreased salivation secondary to radiation of neck (specific)	Impaired Oral Mucous Membrane related to noxious agent (vague)
7. Use nursing terminology rather than medical terminology to describe the client's response.	Risk for Ineffective Airway Clearance related to accumulation of secretions in lungs (nursing terminology)	Risk for Pneumonia (medical terminology)
8. Use nursing terminology rather than medical terminology to describe the probable cause of the client's response.	Risk for Ineffective Airway Clearance related to accumulation of secretions in lungs (nursing terminology)	Risk for Ineffective Airway Clearance related to emphysema (medical terminology)

AVOIDING ERRORS IN DIAGNOSTIC REASONING Some error is inherent in any human undertaking, and diagnosis is no exception. However, it is important that nurses make nursing diagnoses with a high level of accuracy. Nurses can avoid some common errors of reasoning by recognizing them and applying the appropriate critical-thinking skills. Error can occur at any point in the diagnostic process: data collection, data interpretation, and data clustering.

Nurses should do the following to minimize diagnostic error:

- *Verify.* Hypothesize possible explanations of the data, but realize that all diagnoses are only tentative until they are verified. Begin and end the diagnostic process by talking with the client and family. When collecting data, ask them what their health problems are and what they believe the causes to be. At the end of the process, ask them to confirm the accuracy and relevance of your diagnoses.
- *Build a good knowledge base and acquire clinical experience.* Nurses must apply knowledge from many different areas to recognize significant cues and patterns and generate hypotheses about the data. To name only a few, principles from chemistry, anatomy, and pharmacology each help the nurse understand client data in a different way.
- *Have a working knowledge of what is normal.* Nurses need to know the population norms for vital signs, laboratory tests, speech development, breath sounds, and so on. In addition, nurses must determine what is usual for a particular person, taking into account age, physical makeup, lifestyle, culture, and the person's own perception of what his or her normal status is. For example, normal blood pressure for adults is in the range of 110/60 to 140/80. However, a nurse might obtain

a reading of 90/50 that is perfectly normal for a particular client. The nurse should compare actual findings to the client's baseline when possible.

- *Consult resources.* Both novices and experienced nurses should consult appropriate resources whenever in doubt about a diagnosis. Professional literature, nursing colleagues, and other professionals are all appropriate resources. The nurse should use a nursing diagnosis handbook to determine whether the client's signs and symptoms truly fit the NANDA label chosen.
- *Base diagnoses on patterns—that is, on behavior over time—rather than on an isolated incident.* For example, even though the client is concerned today about needing to leave her child with a neighbor, it is likely that this concern will be resolved without intervention by the next day. Therefore, the admitting nurse should not diagnose interrupted family processes.
- *Improve critical-thinking skills.* These skills help the nurse to be aware of and avoid errors in thinking, such as overgeneralizing, stereotyping, and making unwarranted assumptions.

ONGOING DEVELOPMENT OF NURSING DIAGNOSES

The first taxonomy of nursing diagnoses was alphabetical. This ordering was considered unscientific by some, and a hierarchic structure was sought. In 1982, NANDA accepted the "nine patterns of unitary man" (based on the nursing models of Sr. Callista Roy and Martha Rogers) as an organizing principle. In 1984, NANDA renamed the "patterns of unitary man" as "human response patterns" based more on the work of Marjorie Gordon (Kim, McFarland, & McLane, 1984), as listed in Box 34–12.

Having undergone refinements, revisions, and acceptance of new diagnoses, the taxonomy is now called Taxonomy II (NANDA International, 2009). Taxonomy II has three levels: domains, classes, and nursing diagnoses (Figure 34–8 ■). The diagnoses are no longer grouped by Gordon's patterns but coded according to seven axes: diagnostic concept, time, unit of care, age, health status, descriptor, and topology. In addition, diagnoses are now listed alphabetically by concept, not by first word.

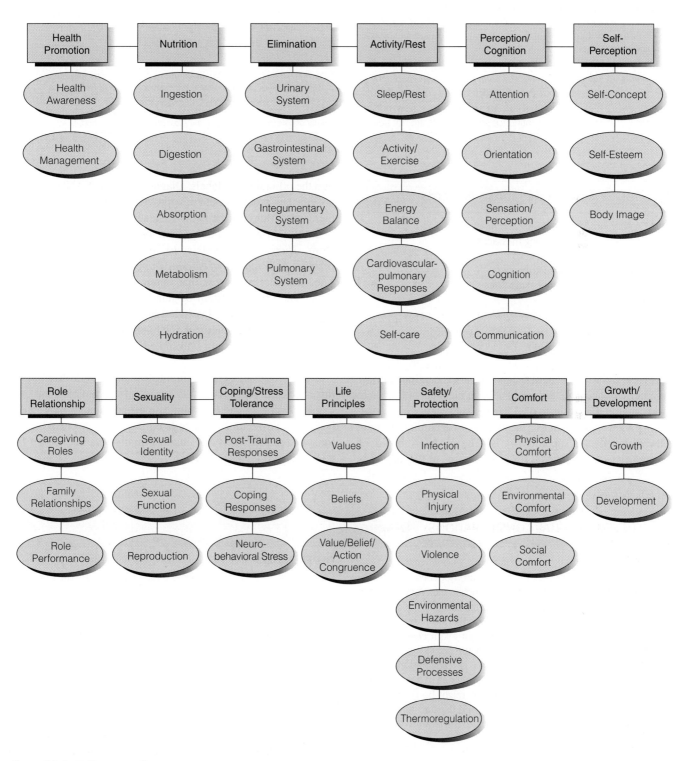

Figure 34–8 ■ Taxonomy II.

Source: From NANDA International. (2003). *Definitions and classifications, 2003–2004.* Philadelphia, PA. Adapted with permission.

EVIDENCE-BASED PRACTICE What New Nursing Diagnoses Are Being Researched?

The *International Journal of Nursing Terminologies and Classifications* is a public forum for the publication of work currently conducted worldwide on the development of nursing diagnoses, outcomes, and interventions. In the paper by Lamont, the author reviewed published literature with the goal of establishing *discomfort* as a separate nursing diagnosis from *pain*. However, his review failed to provide clear evidence for this discrimination. He suggests that research be conducted to attempt to determine if pain and discomfort can be usefully separated.

Lopes and Higa conducted interviews with 148 women who had complaints of urinary incontinence. Over half the women (57%) described incontinence with characteristics of both urge and stress incontinence. They suggest that this should lead to a new nursing diagnosis of mixed urinary incontinence so that clients are not treated for urge or stress incontinence when they truly require a plan related to both types.

Implications

Many nursing diagnoses are being studied in a variety of settings. This is important work to determine the reliability and validity of existing diagnoses, identify gaps in the current list, and establish usefulness of the diagnoses in everyday practice. Nurses should be familiar with the direction of this work as it progresses.

Note: From Lamont, S. C. (2003). Discomfort as a potential nursing diagnosis: A concept analysis and literature review. *International Journal of Nursing Terminologies and Classifications, 14*(4 Suppl), p. 5; and Lopes, M. H. B., & Higa, R. (2003). Mixed incontinence in women: A new nursing diagnosis. *International Journal of Nursing Terminologies and Classifications, 14*(4 Suppl), p. 49.

Box 34–12 Human Response Patterns

1. *Exchanging:* mutual giving and receiving
2. *Communicating:* sending messages
3. *Relating:* establishing bonds
4. *Valuing:* assigning relative worth
5. *Choosing:* selection of alternatives
6. *Moving:* activity
7. *Perceiving:* reception of information
8. *Knowing:* meaning associated with information
9. *Feeling:* subjective awareness of information

Review and refinement of diagnostic labels continue as new and modified labels are discussed at each biannual conference. Nurses submit diagnoses to the Diagnostic Review Committee, which reviews and "stages" the diagnosis according to how well-developed and supported it is. The NANDA board of directors gives final approval for incorporation of the diagnosis into the official list of labels. Diagnoses on the NANDA list are not finished products but are approved for clinical use and further study. Many on the list have been studied only minimally.

In 1997, NANDA changed the name of its official journal from *Nursing Diagnosis* to *Nursing Diagnosis: The International Journal of Nursing Language and Classification.* The subtitle emphasizes that nursing diagnosis is part of a larger, developing system of standardized nursing language. This system includes classifications of nursing interventions (NIC) and nursing outcomes (NOC) that are being developed by other research groups and linked to the NANDA diagnostic labels.

Research groups are examining what nurses do from these three different perspectives (diagnoses, interventions, and outcomes) to clarify and communicate the role nurses play in the health care system. A standardized language will also enable nurses to implement a Nursing Minimum Data Set needed for computerized client records.

DEVELOPMENTAL CONSIDERATIONS Diagnosis

CHILDREN

Many developmental issues in pediatrics are not considered problems or illnesses, yet can benefit from nursing intervention. When applied to children and families, nursing diagnoses may reflect a condition or state of health. For example, parents of a newborn infant may be excited to learn all they can about infant care and child growth and development. Assessment of the family system might lead the nurse to conclude that the family is ready and able, even eager, to take on the new roles and responsibilities of being parents. An appropriate diagnosis for such a family might be readiness for enhanced family processes, with nursing care directed to educating and providing encouragement and support to the parents.

OLDER ADULTS

Older adults tend to have multiple problems with complex physical and psychosocial needs when they are ill. If the nurse has done a thorough, accurate assessment, nursing diagnoses can be selected to cover all problems and, at the same time, prioritize the special needs. For example, if a client is admitted with severe congestive heart failure, prompt attention will be focused on decreased cardiac output and excess fluid volume, with interventions selected to improve these areas quickly. As these conditions improve, then other nursing diagnoses, such as activity intolerance and deficient knowledge related to a new medication regimen, might require more attention. They are all part of the same medical problem of congestive heart failure, but each nursing diagnosis has specific expected outcomes and nursing interventions. The client's strengths should be an essential consideration in all phases of the nursing process.

Plan

The planning process is a deliberative, systematic phase of the nursing process during which the nurse develops the client's plan of care. This phase involves decision making and problem solving. While planning, the nurse refers to the client's assessment data and diagnostic statements for direction in formulating client goals and designing the nursing interventions required to prevent, reduce, or eliminate the client's health problems (see Figure 34–9 ■). A **nursing intervention** is "any treatment, based upon clinical judgment and knowledge, that a nurse performs to enhance patient/client outcomes" (Dochterman & Bulechek, 2004, p. xxiii). The client care plan is the end product of this process.

Although planning is basically the nurse's responsibility, input from the client and support persons is essential if a plan is to be effective. Nurses do not plan for the client, but encourage the client to participate actively to the extent possible. In a home setting, the client's support people and caregivers are the ones who implement the plan of care; thus, its effectiveness depends largely on them.

TYPES OF PLANNING

Planning begins with the first client contact and continues until the nurse–client relationship ends, usually when the client is discharged from the health care agency. All planning is multidisciplinary (involves all health care providers interacting with the client) and includes the client and family to the fullest extent possible in every step.

Initial Planning

The nurse who performs the admission assessment usually develops the initial comprehensive plan of care. This nurse has the benefit of the client's body language as well as some intuitive kinds of information that are not available solely from the written database. Planning should be initiated as soon as possible after the initial assessment, especially because of the trend toward shorter hospital stays.

Ongoing Planning

Ongoing planning is done by all nurses who work with the client. As nurses obtain new information and evaluate the client's responses to care, they can individualize the initial care plan further. Ongoing planning also occurs at the beginning of a shift as the nurse plans the care to be given that day. Using ongoing assessment data, the nurse carries out daily planning for the following purposes:

1. To determine whether the client's health status has changed
2. To set priorities for the client's care during the shift
3. To decide which problems to focus on during the shift
4. To coordinate the nurse's activities so that more than one problem can be addressed at each client contact.

Discharge Planning

Discharge planning, the process of anticipating and planning for needs after discharge, is a crucial part of comprehensive health care and should be addressed in each client's care plan. Because the average client stay in acute care hospitals has become shorter, people are sometimes discharged still needing care. Although many clients are discharged to other agencies (e.g., long-term care facilities), such care is increasingly being delivered in the home. Effective discharge planning begins at first client contact and involves comprehensive and ongoing assessment to obtain information about the client's ongoing needs.

DEVELOPING NURSING CARE PLANS

The end product of the planning phase of the nursing process is a formal or informal plan of care. An **informal nursing care plan** is a strategy for action that exists in the nurse's mind. For example, the nurse may think, "Mrs. Phan is very tired. I will need to reinforce her teaching after she is rested." A **formal nursing care plan** is a written or computerized guide that organizes information about the client's care. The most obvious benefit of a formal written care plan is that it provides for continuity of care.

A **standardized care plan** is a formal plan that specifies the nursing care for groups of clients with common needs (e.g., all clients with myocardial infarction). An **individualized care plan** is tailored to meet the unique needs of a specific client—needs that are not addressed by the standardized plan. It is important that all caregivers work toward the same outcomes and, if available, use approaches shown to be effective with a particular client. Nurses also use the formal care plan for direction about what needs to be documented in client progress notes and as a guide for delegating and assigning staff to care for clients. When nurses use the client's nursing diagnoses to develop goals and nursing interventions, the result is a holistic, individualized plan of care that will meet the client's unique needs.

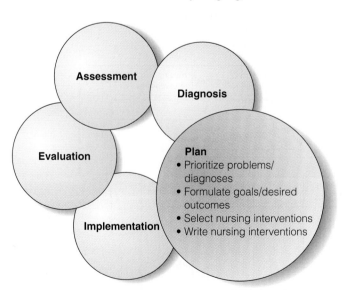

Figure 34–9 ■ Plan. The third phase of the nursing process, in which the nurse and client develop client goals/desired outcomes and nursing interventions to prevent, reduce, or alleviate the client's health problems.

Care plans include the actions nurses must take to address the client's nursing diagnoses and produce the desired outcomes. The nurse begins the plan when the client is admitted to the agency and constantly updates it throughout the client's stay in response to changes in the client's condition and evaluations of goal achievement. During the planning phase, the nurse must (a) decide which of the client's problems need individualized plans and which problems can be addressed by standardized plans and routine care, and (b) write individualized desired outcomes and nursing interventions for client problems that require nursing attention beyond preplanned, routine care.

The complete plan of care for a client is made up of several different documents that (a) describe the routine care needed to meet basic needs (e.g., bathing, nutrition), (b) address the client's nursing diagnoses and collaborative problems, and (c) specify nursing responsibilities in carrying out the medical plan of care (e.g., keeping the client from eating or drinking before surgery; scheduling a laboratory test). A complete plan of care integrates dependent and independent nursing functions into a meaningful whole and provides a central source of client information. Figure 34–10 ■ illustrates the various documents that may be included in a nursing care plan.

Standardized Approaches to Care Planning

Most health care agencies have devised a variety of preprinted, standardized plans for providing essential nursing care to specified groups of clients who have certain needs in common (e.g., all clients with pneumonia). Standards of care, standardized care plans, protocols, policies, and procedures are developed and accepted by the nursing staff in order to (a) ensure that minimally acceptable standards are met and (b) promote efficient use of nurses' time by removing the need to author common activities that are done over and over for many of the clients on a nursing unit.

Standards of care describe nursing actions for clients with similar medical conditions rather than individuals, and they describe achievable rather than ideal nursing care. They define the interventions for which nurses are held accountable; they do not contain medical interventions. Standards of care are

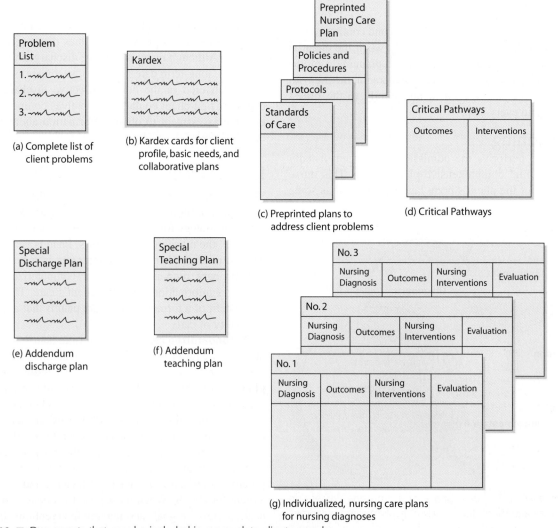

(a) Complete list of client problems

(b) Kardex cards for client profile, basic needs, and collaborative plans

(c) Preprinted plans to address client problems

(d) Critical Pathways

(e) Addendum discharge plan

(f) Addendum teaching plan

(g) Individualized, nursing care plans for nursing diagnoses

Figure 34–10 ■ Documents that may be included in a complete client care plan.

Source: From Wilkinson, J. M. (2007). *Nursing process & critical thinking* (4th ed.). Upper Saddle River, NJ: Prentice Hall, p. 452. Adapted with permission.

usually agency records and not part of the client's care plan, but they may be referred to in the plan (e.g., a nurse might write "See unit standards of care for cardiac catheterization"). Standards of care may or may not be organized according to problems or nursing diagnoses. They are written from the perspective of the nurse's responsibilities. Figure 34–11 ■ shows unit standards of care for the client with thrombophlebitis.

Standardized care plans are preprinted guides for the nursing care of a client who has a need that arises frequently in the agency (e.g., a specific nursing diagnosis or all nursing diagnoses associated with a particular medical condition). They are written from the perspective of what care the client can expect. They should not be confused with standards of care. Although the two have some similarities, they have important differences. Figure 34–12 ■ shows a standardized care plan for deficient fluid volume. Standardized care plans

■ are kept with the client's individualized care plan on the nursing unit. When the client is discharged, they become part of the permanent medical record.

■ provide detailed interventions and contain additions or deletions from the standards of care of the agency.

■ typically are written in the nursing process format:

Problem → Goals/Desired Outcomes → Nursing Interventions → Evaluation

■ frequently include checklists, blank lines, or empty spaces to allow the nurse to individualize goals and nursing interventions.

The use of standardized care plans is supported by the Joint Commission standards for nursing care, which no longer require a handwritten care plan for every client.

Like standards of care and standardized care plans, **protocols** are preprinted to indicate the actions commonly required for a particular group of clients. For example, an agency may have a protocol for admitting a client to the intensive care unit or for caring for a client receiving continuous epidural analgesia. Protocols may include both the physician's orders and nursing interventions. Depending on the agency, protocols may or may not be included in the client's permanent record.

Policies are rules developed to govern the handling of frequently occurring situations. **Procedures** are the steps used to carry out a given policy. For example, a hospital may have a policy specifying the number of visitors a client may have.

STANDARDS OF CARE: Patient with thrombophlebitis

Goal: **1.** To monitor for early signs and symptoms of compromised respiratory status
 2. To report any abnormal signs and/or symptoms promptly to the medical staff
 3. To initiate appropriate nursing actions when signs and/or symptoms of compromised respiratory status occur
 4. To institute protocol for emergency intervention should the client develop cardiopulmonary dysfunction

SUPPORTIVE DATA: The purpose of these standards of care is to prevent, monitor, report, and record the client's response to a diagnosis of thrombophlebitis. Thrombophlebitis places the client at risk for pulmonary embolism. The hemodynamic consequences of embolic obstruction to pulmonary blood flow involve increased pulmonary vascular resistance, increased right ventricular workload, decreased cardiac output, and development of shock and pulmonary arrest.

CLINICAL MANIFESTATIONS: Nursing assessments performed q3–4h should monitor for the following signs/symptoms:

- Dyspnea
- Sudden substernal pain
- Rapid/weak pulse
- Syncope
- Anxiety
- Fever
- Cough/hemoptysis
- Accelerated respiratory rate
- Pleuritic type chest pain
- Cyanosis

PREVENTIVE NURSING MEASURES:

- Encourage increased fluid intake to prevent dehydration.
- Maintain anticoagulant intravenous therapy as prescribed (see Protocol for Anticoagulant Administration).
- Maintain prescribed bedrest.
- Prevent venous stasis from improperly fitting elastic stockings; check q3–4h.
- Encourage dorsiflexion exercises of the lower extremities while on bedrest.

INDIVIDUALIZED PLANS/ADDITIONAL NURSING/MEDICAL ORDERS

 Do not massage lower extremities.
 Intake and output q8h.

Initiated by: _S. Ibarra, RN_ Date: _4-9-07_

Figure 34–11 ■ Standards of care for thrombophlebitis.

Source: From Wilkinson, J. M. (2007). *Nursing process & critical thinking* (4th ed.). Upper Saddle River, NJ: Prentice Hall, p. 461. Adapted with permission.

Etiology	Desired Outcomes	Nursing Interventions (Identify Frequency)
✓ Decreased oral intake	✓ Urinary output > 30 mL/hr	✓ Monitor intake and output q _1_ h
✓ Nausea	✓ Urine specific gravity 1.005–1.025	✓ Weigh daily
__ Depression	✓ Serum Na⁺ within normal limits	✓ Monitor serum electrolyte levels X 1 or until normal
✓ Fatigue, weakness	✓ Mucous membranes moist	✓ Assess skin turgor and mucous membranes q _8_ h
__ Difficulty swallowing	✓ Skin turgor elastic	✓ Monitor temperature q _4_ h
__ Other:_____	✓ No weight loss	✓ Administer prescribed IV therapy (Monitor according to protocol for Intravenous Therapy) 1000 mL D₅ LR at 100 mL/hr
✓ Excess fluid loss	✓ 8-hour intake = _400 mL oral_	✓ Offer 8 oz. oral liquids q _1_ h
✓ Fever or increased metabolic rate	Other:	Type _clear, cold_
✓ Diaphoresis		✓ Instruct client regarding amount, type, and schedule of fluid intake.
✓ Vomiting		✓ Assess understanding of type of fluid loss; teach accordingly
__ Diarrhea		✓ Mouth care prn with _mouthwash_
__ Burns		✓ Institute measures to reduce fever (e.g., lower room temperature, remove bed covers, offer cold liquids.)
__ Other_____		Other Nursing Orders:_____
		Monitor urine specific gravity
Defining Characteristics		_q shift_
✓ Insufficient intake		_____
✓ Negative balance of intake and output		_____
✓ Dry mucous membranes		_____
✓ Poor skin turgor		_____
__ Concentrated urine		_____
__ Hypernatremia		
✓ Rapid, weak pulse		
__ Falling B/P		
__ Weight loss		

Plan initiated by:_ M. Medina RN _____ Date _4–15–07_____

Plan/outcomes evaluated_____ Date_____

Plan/outcomes evaluated_____ Date_____

Client:___ Amanda Aquilini _____

Figure 34–12 ■ A standardized care plan for the nursing diagnosis of deficient fluid volume.

Some policies and procedures are similar to protocols and specify what is to be done, for example, in the case of cardiac arrest. If a policy covers a situation pertinent to client care, it is usually noted on the care plan (e.g., "Make Social Service referral according to policy manual"). Policies are institutional records and do not become a part of the care plan or permanent record.

A **standing order** is a written document about policies, rules, regulations, or orders regarding client care. Standing orders give nurses the authority to carry out specific actions under certain circumstances, often when a physician is not immediately available. In a hospital critical care unit, a common example is the administration of emergency antiarrhythmic medications when a client's cardiac monitoring pattern changes. In a home care setting, a physician may write a standing order for the nurse to obtain blood tests for a client who has been on a certain therapy for a prescribed amount of time.

Regardless of whether care plans are handwritten, computerized, or standardized, nursing care must be individualized to fit the unique needs of each client. In practice, a care plan usually consists of both preprinted and nurse-created sections. The nurse uses standardized care plans for predictable, commonly occurring problems, and creates an individual plan for unusual problems or problems needing special attention. For example, a standardized care plan for all "clients with a medical diagnosis of pneumonia" would probably include a nursing diagnosis of deficient fluid volume and direct the nurse to assess the client's hydration status. On a respiratory or medical unit this would be a common nursing diagnosis; therefore, the client's nurse was able to obtain a standardized plan directing care commonly needed by clients with efficient fluid volume (see Figure 34–12). However, the nursing diagnosis risk for interrupted family processes would not be common to all clients with pneumonia; it is specific to the client. Therefore, the goals and nursing interventions for that diagnosis would need to be created by the nurse.

Formats for Nursing Care Plans

Although formats differ from agency to agency, the care plan is often organized into four columns or categories: (a) nursing diagnoses, (b) goals/desired outcomes, (c) nursing interventions, and (d) evaluation. Some agencies use a three-column plan in which evaluation is done in the goals column or in the nurses' notes; others have a five-column plan that adds a column for assessment data preceding the nursing diagnosis column.

STUDENT CARE PLANS Because student care plans are a learning activity as well as a plan of care, they may be more lengthy and detailed than care plans used by working nurses. To help students learn to write care plans, educators may require that more of the plan be handwritten. They may also modify the three-, four-, or five-column plan by adding a column for "Rationale" after the nursing interventions column. A **rationale** is the scientific principle given as the reason for selecting a particular nursing intervention. Students may also be required to cite supporting literature for their stated rationale. Another method of organizing and representing care plan information is the use of a concept map. An example of a nursing care plan can be found later in this exemplar.

A **concept map** is a visual tool in which ideas or data are enclosed in circles or boxes of some shape and relationships between these are indicated by connecting lines or arrows. Concept maps are creative endeavors. They can take many different forms and encompass various categories of data, according to the creator's interpretation of the client or health condition. The concept map for the client discussed in this exemplar is another way of depicting the nursing care plan and

includes unique boxes that enclose assessment, nursing diagnosis, outcomes, and interventions. The arrows represent the flow of the phases of the nursing process. Concept maps other than care plans are often used to depict complex relationships among ideas, processes, actions, and so on. Some are referred to as mind maps. Students are often asked to complete pathophysiology flow sheets or concept maps as a method of learning and demonstrating the linkages among disease processes, laboratory data, medications, signs and symptoms, risk factors, and other relevant data (Figure 34–13 ■).

COMPUTERIZED CARE PLANS Many health care agencies use computers to create and store nursing care plans. The computer can generate both standardized and individualized care plans. Nurses access the client's stored care plan from a centrally located terminal at the nurses' station or from terminals in client rooms. For an individualized plan, the nurse chooses the appropriate diagnoses from a menu suggested by the computer. The computer then lists possible goals and nursing interventions for those diagnoses; the nurse chooses those appropriate for the client and types in any additional goals and interventions or nursing actions not listed on the menu. The nurse can read the plan on the computer screen or print out an updated working copy. This topic is covered further in Concept 46, Informatics.

MULTIDISCIPLINARY (COLLABORATIVE) CARE PLANS A **multidisciplinary care plan** is a standardized plan that outlines the care required for clients with common, predictable—usually medical—conditions. Such plans, also referred to as **collaborative care plans** and **critical pathways**, sequence the care that must be given on each day during the projected length of stay for the specific type of condition. Like the traditional nursing care plan, a multidisciplinary care plan can specify outcomes and nursing interventions to address client problems (including nursing diagnoses). However, it includes medical treatments to be performed by other health care providers as well.

The plan is usually organized with a column for each day, listing the interventions that should be carried out and the client outcomes that should be achieved on that day. There are as many columns on the multidisciplinary care plan as the preset number of days allowed for the client's diagnosis-related group (DRG). Multidisciplinary care plans do not include detailed nursing activities. They should be drawn from but do not replace standards of care and standardized care plans.

Guidelines for Writing Nursing Care Plans

The nurse should use the following guidelines when writing nursing care plans:

1. Date and sign the plan. The date the plan is written is essential for evaluation, review, and future planning. The nurse's signature demonstrates accountability to the client and to the nursing profession, since the effectiveness of nursing actions can be evaluated.

2. Use category headings. "Nursing Diagnoses," "Goals/ Desired Outcomes," "Nursing Interventions," and "Evaluation." Include a date for the evaluation of each goal.

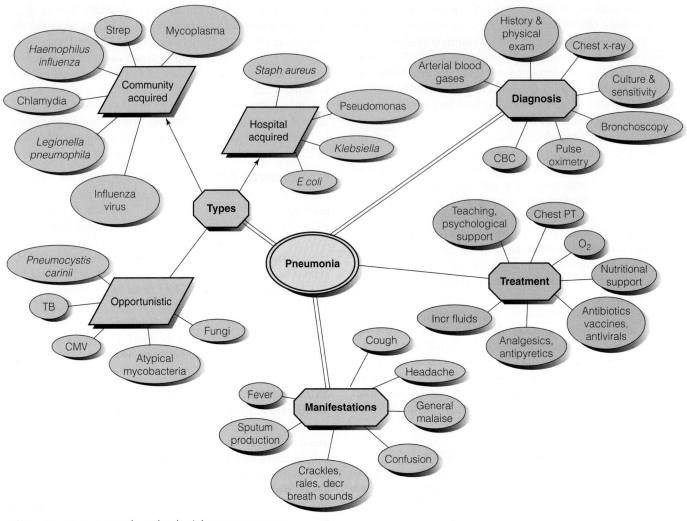

Figure 34–13 ■ A sample pathophsyiology concept map.

3. Use standardized/approved medical or English symbols and key words rather than complete sentences to communicate your ideas unless the agency policy dictates otherwise. For example, write "Turn and reposition q2h" rather than "Turn and reposition the client every two hours." Or, write "Clean wound c̄ H₂O₂ bid" rather than "Clean the client's wound with hydrogen peroxide twice a day, morning and evening." See Table 36–4 in Concept 36 on page 2174 for a list of standard medical abbreviations.

4. Be specific. Because nurses are now working shifts of different lengths, some working 12-hour shifts and some working 8-hour shifts, it is even more important to be specific about expected timing of an intervention. If the intervention reads "change incisional dressing q shift," it could mean either twice in 24 hours, or three times in 24 hours, depending on the shift time. This miscommunication becomes even more serious when medications are ordered to be given "q shift." Writing down specific times during the 24-hour period will help clarify.

5. Refer to procedure books or other sources of information rather than including all the steps on a written plan. For

example, write "See unit procedure book for tracheostomy care," or attach a standard nursing plan about such procedures as radiation-implantation care and preoperative or postoperative care.

6. Tailor the plan to the unique characteristics of the client by ensuring that the client's choices, such as preferences about the times of care and the methods used, are included. This reinforces the client's individuality and sense of control. For example, the written nursing intervention "Provide prune juice at breakfast rather than other juice" indicates that the client was given a choice of beverages.

7. Ensure that the nursing plan incorporates preventive and health maintenance aspects as well as restorative ones. For example, carrying out the intervention "Provide active-assistance ROM (range-of-motion) exercises to affected limbs q2h" prevents joint contractures and maintains muscle strength and joint mobility.

8. Ensure that the plan contains interventions for ongoing assessment of the client (e.g., "Inspect incision q8h").

9. Include collaborative and coordination activities in the plan. For example, the nurse may write interventions to

ask a nutritionist or physical therapist about specific aspects of the client's care.

10. *Include plans for the client's discharge and home care needs.* The nurse begins discharge planning as soon as the client has been admitted. It is often necessary to consult and make arrangements with the community health nurse, social worker, and specific agencies that supply client information and needed equipment. Add teaching and discharge plans as addenda if they are lengthy and complex.

THE PLANNING PROCESS

In the process of developing client care plans, the nurse engages in the following activities:

■ Setting priorities
■ Establishing client goals/desired outcomes
■ Selecting nursing interventions
■ Writing individualized nursing interventions on care plans.

Setting Priorities

Priority setting is the process of establishing a preferential sequence for addressing nursing diagnoses and interventions. The nurse and client begin planning by deciding which nursing diagnosis requires attention first, which second, and so on. Instead of rank-ordering diagnoses, nurses can group them as having high, medium, or low priority. Life-threatening problems, such as loss of respiratory or cardiac function, are designated as high priority. Health-threatening problems, such as acute illness and decreased coping ability, are assigned medium priority because they may result in delayed development or cause destructive physical or emotional changes. A low-priority problem is one that arises from normal developmental needs or that requires only minimal nursing support.

Nurses frequently use Maslow's hierarchy of needs when setting priorities (see Figure 34–14 ■). In Maslow's hierarchy, physiologic needs such as air, food, and water are basic to life and receive higher priority than the need for security

---

Box 34-13 **Maslow's Needs Theory**

In *Motivation and Personality* (1970), Abraham Maslow ranks human needs on five levels (see Figure 34–14). The five levels in ascending order are as follows:

■ *Physiologic needs.* Needs such as air, food, water, shelter, rest, sleep, activity, and temperature maintenance are crucial for survival.

■ *Safety and security needs.* The need for safety has both physical and psychologic aspects. The person needs to feel safe, both in the physical environment and in relationships.

■ *Love and belonging needs.* The third level of needs includes giving and receiving affection, attaining a place in a group, and maintaining the feeling of belonging.

■ *Self-esteem needs.* The individual needs both self-esteem (i.e., feelings of independence, competence, and self-respect) and esteem from others (i.e., recognition, respect, and appreciation).

■ *Self-actualization.* When the need for self-esteem is satisfied, the individual strives for self-actualization, the innate need to develop one's maximum potential and realize one's abilities and qualities.

---

or activity (see Box 34–13). Growth needs, such as self-esteem, are not perceived as "basic" in this framework. Thus, nursing diagnoses such as ineffective airway clearance and impaired gas exchange would take priority over nursing diagnoses such as anxiety or ineffective coping.

It is not necessary to resolve all high-priority diagnoses before addressing others. The nurse may partially address a high-priority diagnosis and then deal with a diagnosis of lesser priority. Furthermore, because the client may have several problems, the nurse often deals with more than one diagnosis at a time. Table 34–15 lists the priorities assigned to the client's nursing diagnoses.

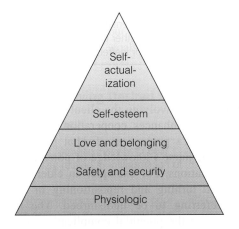

Maslow's hierarchy of needs

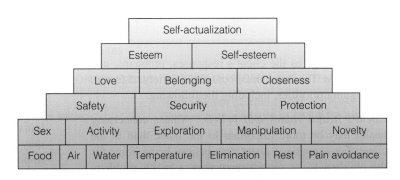

Maslow's hierarchy of needs, as adapted by Kalish

Figure 34–14 ■ Maslow's hierarchy of needs.

TABLE 34–18 Components of Goals/Desired Outcomes

SUBJECT	VERB	CONDITIONS/MODIFIERS	CRITERION OF DESIRED PERFORMANCE
Client	drinks	2500 mL of fluid	daily (time)
Client	administers	correct insulin dose	using aseptic technique (quality standard)
Client	lists	three hazards of smoking (after reading literature)	(accuracy indicated by "three hazards")
Client	recalls	five symptoms of diabetes before discharge	(accuracy indicated by "five symptoms")
Client	walks	the length of the hall without a cane	by date of discharge (time)
Client's ankle	measures	less than 10 inches in circumference	in 48 hours (time)
Client	performs	leg ROM exercises as taught	every 8 hours (time)
Client	identifies	foods high in salt from a prepared list	before discharge (time)
Client	states	the purposes of his or her medications	before discharge (time)

TABLE 34–19 Desired Outcomes for the Client

NURSING DIAGNOSIS*	GOAL STATEMENTS (NOC)/DESIRED OUTCOMES
Ineffective Airway Clearance related to viscous secretions and shallow chest expansion secondary to fluid volume deficit, pain, and fatigue	Respiratory Status: Gas exchange [0402], as evidenced by the following: ■ Absence of pallor and cyanosis (skin and mucous membranes) ■ Use of correct breathing/coughing technique after instruction ■ Productive cough ■ Symmetric chest excursion of at least 4 cm Within 48–72 hours: ■ Lungs clear to auscultation ■ Respirations 12–22/minute, pulse <100 beats/minute ■ Inhales normal volume of air on incentive spirometer
Deficient Fluid Volume: Intake Insufficient to Replace Fluid Loss related to vomiting, fever, and diaphoresis	Fluid balance [0601], as evidenced by the following: ■ Urine output greater than 30 mL/h ■ Urine specific gravity 1.005–1.025 ■ Good skin turgor ■ Moist mucous membranes ■ Stating the need for oral fluid intake
Anxiety related to difficulty breathing and concerns about work and parenting roles	Anxiety control [1402], as evidenced by the following: ■ Listening to and following instructions for correct breathing and coughing technique, even during periods of dyspnea ■ Verbalizing understanding of condition, diagnostic tests, and treatments (by end of day) ■ Decrease in reports of fear and anxiety; none within 12 hours ■ Voice steady, not shaky ■ Respiratory rate of 12–22/minute ■ Freely expressing concerns and possible solutions about work and parenting roles
Risk for Interrupted Family Processes related to mother's illness and temporary unavailability of father to provide child care	Family coping [2600], as evidenced by the following: ■ Report of satisfactory child care arrangements having been made ■ Client and husband communicating effectively and working together to solve problems ■ Family members expressing feelings and providing mutual support
Imbalanced Nutrition: Less Than Body Requirements related to decreased appetite, nausea, and increased metabolism secondary to disease process	Nutritional status: Nutrient intake [1009], as evidenced by the following: ■ Eating at least 85% of each meal ■ Maintaining present weight ■ Verbalizing importance of adequate nutrition ■ Verbalizing improved appetite
Bathing/Hygiene Self-Care Deficit related to activity intolerance secondary to airway clearance and sleep pattern disturbance	Self-care: Activities of daily living [0300], as evidenced by the following: ■ Ambulates to bathroom without dyspnea, fatigue, ineffective or shortness of breath ■ Within 24 hours, bathes with assistance in bed; within 48 hours, bathes with assistance at sink; within 72 hours, bathes in shower without dyspnea ■ Reports satisfaction and comfort with hygiene needs
Disturbed Sleep Pattern related to cough, pain, orthopnea, and diaphoresis	Sleep [0004], as evidenced by the following: ■ Observed sleeping at night rounds ■ Reports feeling rested ■ Does not experience orthopnea

*The nursing diagnoses are listed in priority order.

GUIDELINES FOR WRITING GOALS/DESIRED OUTCOMES

The following guidelines can help nurses write useful goals and desired outcomes:

1. Write goals and outcomes in terms of client responses, not nurse activities. Beginning each goal statement with *the client will* may help focus the goal on client behaviors and responses. Avoid statements that start with *enable, facilitate, allow, let, permit,* or similar verbs followed by the word *client*. These verbs indicate what the nurse hopes to accomplish, not what the client will do.
   Correct: Client will drink 100 mL of water per hour (client behavior).
   Incorrect: Maintain client hydration (nursing action).

2. Be sure that desired outcomes are realistic for the client's capabilities, limitations, and designated time span, if it is indicated. *Limitations* refers to finances, equipment, family support, social services, physical and mental condition, and time. For example, the outcome "Measures insulin accurately" may be unrealistic for a client who has poor vision due to cataracts.

3. Ensure that the goals and desired outcomes are compatible with the therapies of other professionals. For example, the outcome "Will increase the time spent out of bed by 15 minutes each day" is not compatible with a primary care provider's prescribed therapy of bed rest.

4. Make sure that each goal is derived from only one nursing diagnosis. For example, the goal "The client will increase the amount of nutrients ingested and show progress in the ability to feed self" is derived from two nursing diagnoses: feeding self-care deficit and impaired nutrition: less than body requirements. Keeping the goal statement related to only one diagnosis facilitates evaluation of care by ensuring that planned nursing interventions are clearly related to the diagnosis.

5. Use observable, measurable terms for outcomes. Avoid words that are vague and require interpretation or judgment by the observer. For example, phrases such as *increase daily exercise* and *improve knowledge of nutrition* can mean different things to different people. If used in outcomes, these phrases can lead to disagreements about whether the outcome was met. These phrases may be suitable for a broad client goal but are not sufficiently clear and specific to guide the nurse when evaluating client responses.

6. Make sure the client considers the goals/desired outcomes important and values them. Some outcomes, such as those for problems related to self-esteem, parenting, and communication, involve choices that are best made by the client or in collaboration with the client.

   Some clients may know what they wish to accomplish with regard to their health problem; others may not know all the outcome possibilities. The nurse must actively listen to the client to determine personal values, goals, and desired outcomes in relation to current health concerns. Clients are usually motivated and expend the necessary energy to reach goals they consider important.

Selecting Nursing Interventions and Activities

Nursing interventions and activities are the actions that a nurse performs to achieve client goals. The specific interventions chosen should focus on eliminating or reducing the etiology of the nursing diagnosis, which is the second clause of the diagnostic statement.

When it is not possible to change the etiologic factors, the nurse chooses interventions to treat the signs and symptoms or the defining characteristics in NANDA terminology. Examples of this situation would be pain related to surgical incision and anxiety related to unknown etiology.

Interventions for risk nursing diagnoses should focus on measures to reduce the client's risk factors, which are also found in the second clause.

Correct identification of the etiology during the diagnosing phase provides the framework for choosing successful nursing interventions. For example, the diagnostic label activity intolerance may have several etiologies: pain, weakness, sedentary lifestyle, anxiety, or cardiac arrhythmias. Interventions will vary according to the cause of the problem.

TYPES OF NURSING INTERVENTIONS Nursing interventions are identified and written during the planning step of the nursing process; however, they are actually performed during the implementing step. Nursing interventions include both direct and indirect care, as well as nurse-initiated, physician-initiated, and other provider-initiated treatments. Direct care is an intervention performed through interaction with the client. Indirect care is an intervention performed away from but on behalf of the client, such as interdisciplinary collaboration or management of the care environment.

Independent interventions are those activities that nurses are licensed to initiate on the basis of their knowledge and skills. They include physical care, ongoing assessment, emotional support and comfort, teaching, counseling, environmental management, and making referrals to other health care professionals. Recall that nursing diagnoses are client problems that can be treated primarily by independent nursing interventions. In performing an autonomous activity, the nurse determines that the client requires certain nursing interventions, either carries these out or delegates them to other nursing personnel, and is accountable or answerable for the decision and the actions. An example of an independent action is planning and providing special mouth care for a client after diagnosing impaired oral mucous membranes.

Dependent interventions are activities carried out under the physician's orders or supervision, or according to specified routines. Physicians' orders commonly direct the nurse to provide medications, intravenous therapy, diagnostic tests, treatments, diet, and activity. The nurse is responsible for assessing the need for, explaining, and administering the medical orders. Nursing interventions may be written to individualize the medical order based on the client's status. For example, for a medical order of

"Progressive ambulation, as tolerated," a nurse might write the following:

1. Dangle for 5 min, 12 h postop.
2. Stand at bedside 24 h postop; observe for pallor, dizziness, and weakness.
3. Check pulse before and after ambulating. Do not progress if pulse >110.

Collaborative interventions are actions the nurse carries out in collaboration with other health care team members, such as physical therapists, social workers, dietitians, and physicians. Collaborative nursing activities reflect the overlapping responsibilities of, and collegial relationships between, health care personnel. For example, the physician might order physical therapy to teach the client crutch-walking. The nurse would be responsible for informing the physical therapy department and for coordinating the client's care to include the physical therapy sessions. When the client returns to the nursing unit, the nurse would assist with crutch-walking and collaborate with the physical therapist to evaluate the client's progress.

The amount of time the nurse spends in an independent versus a collaborative or dependent role varies according to the clinical area, type of institution, and specific position of the nurse.

CONSIDERING THE CONSEQUENCES OF EACH INTERVENTION Usually several possible interventions can be identified for each nursing goal. The nurse's task is to choose those that are most likely to achieve the desired client outcomes. The nurse begins by considering the risks and benefits of each intervention. An intervention may have more than one consequence. For example, "Provide accurate information" could result in the following client behaviors:

- Increased anxiety
- Decreased anxiety
- Wish to talk with the primary care provider
- Desire to leave the hospital
- Relaxation.

Determining the consequences of each intervention requires nursing knowledge and experience. For example, the nurse's experience may suggest that providing information the night before the client's surgery may increase the client's worry and tension, whereas maintaining the usual rituals before sleep is more effective. The nurse might then consider providing information several days before surgery.

CRITERIA FOR CHOOSING NURSING INTERVENTIONS After considering the consequences of the alternative nursing interventions, the nurse chooses one or more that are likely to be most effective. Although the nurse bases this decision on knowledge and experience, the client's input is important.

The following criteria can help the nurse choose the best nursing interventions. The plan must be

- Safe and appropriate for the individual's age, health, and condition.
- Achievable with the resources available. For example, a home care nurse might wish to include an intervention for an elderly client to "Check blood glucose daily," but in order for that to occur either the client must have intact sight, cognition, and memory to carry this out independently, or daily visits from a home care nurse must be available and affordable.
- Congruent with the client's values, beliefs, and culture.
- Congruent with other therapies (e.g., if the client is not permitted food, the strategy of an evening snack must be deferred until health permits).
- Based on nursing knowledge and experience or knowledge from relevant sciences (i.e., based on a rationale).
- Within established standards of care as determined by state laws, professional associations (ANA), and the policies of the institution. Many agencies have policies to guide the activities of health professionals and to safeguard clients. Rules for visiting hours and procedures to follow when a client has cardiac arrest are examples. If a policy does not benefit clients, nurses have a responsibility to bring this to the attention of the appropriate people.

Writing Individualized Nursing Interventions

After choosing the appropriate nursing interventions, the nurse writes them on the care plan. See examples of nursing interventions for the client in Table 34–20.

TABLE 34–20 Identifying Nursing Diagnoses, Outcomes, and Interventions

Nursing Diagnosis: Ineffective airway clearance related to viscous secretions and shallow chest expansion secondary to deficient fluid volume, pain, and fatigue.

DESIRED OUTCOMES*/INDICATORS	NURSING INTERVENTIONS	RATIONALE
Respiratory Status: Gas exchange [0402], as evidenced by the following: ■ Absence of pallor and cyanosis (skin and mucous membranes) ■ Use of correct breathing/coughing technique after instruction	Monitor respiratory status q4h: rate, depth, effort, skin color, mucous membranes, amount and color of sputum. Monitor results of blood gases, chest x-ray studies, and incentive spirometer volume as available. Monitor level of consciousness.	To identify progress toward or deviations from goal. Ineffective airway clearance leads to poor oxygenation, as evidenced by pallor, cyanosis, lethargy, and drowsiness.

*The NOC # for desired outcomes is listed in brackets following the appropriate outcome. Outcomes, interventions, and activities selected are only a sample of those suggested by NOC and Nursing Interventions Classification (NIC) and should be further individualized for each client.

TABLE 34–20 Identifying Nursing Diagnoses, Outcomes, and Interventions (continued)

■ Productive cough ■ Symmetric chest excursion of at least 4 cm	Auscultate lungs q4h. Vital signs q4h (TPR, BP, pulse oximetry).	Inadequate oxygenation causes increased pulse rate. Respiratory rate may be decreased by narcotic analgesics. Shallow breathing further compromises oxygenation.
Within 48–72 hours		
■ Lungs clear to auscultation ■ Respirations 12–22/minute; pulse, 100 beats/minute	Instruct in breathing and coughing techniques. Remind to perform, and assist q3h.	To enable client to cough up secretions. May need encouragement and support because of fatigue and pain.
■ Inhales normal volume of air on incentive spirometer	Administer prescribed expectorant; schedule for maximum effectiveness. Maintain Fowler's or semi-Fowler's position. Administer prescribed analgesics. Notify physician if pain not relieved.	Helps loosen secretions so they can be coughed up and expelled. Gravity allows for fuller lung expansion by decreasing pressure of abdomen on diaphragm. Controls pleuritic pain by blocking pain pathways and altering perception of pain, enabling client to increase thoracic expansion. Unrelieved pain may signal impending complication.
	Administer oxygen by nasal cannula as prescribed. Provide portable oxygen if client goes off unit (e.g., for x-ray examination).	Supplemental oxygen makes more oxygen available to the cells, even though less air is being moved by the client, thereby reducing the work of breathing.
	Assist with postural drainage daily at 0930.	Gravity facilitates movement of secretions upward through the respiratory passage.
	Administer prescribed antibiotic to maintain constant blood level. Observe for rash and GI or other side effects.	Resolves infection by bacteriostatic or bactericidal effect, depending on type of antibiotic used. Constant level required to prevent pathogens from multiplying. Allergies to antibiotics are common.

Nursing Diagnosis: Deficient fluid volume: intake insufficient to replace fluid loss (see standardized care plan for nursing diagnosis of deficient fluid volume, Figure 34–12).

Nursing Diagnosis: Anxiety related to difficulty breathing and concern about work and parenting roles.

DESIRED OUTCOMES*/INDICATORS	NURSING INTERVENTIONS	RATIONALE
Anxiety control [1402], as evidenced by the following:	When client is dyspneic, stay with her; reassure her you will stay.	Presence of a competent caregiver reduces fear of being unable to breathe.
■ Listening to and following instructions for correct breathing and coughing technique, even during periods of dyspnea	Remain calm; appear confident. Encourage slow, deep breathing.	Control of anxiety will help client to maintain effective breathing pattern.
■ Verbalizing understanding of condition, diagnostic tests, and treatments (by end of day)	When client is dyspneic, give brief explanations of treatments and procedures.	Reassures client the nurse can help her. Focusing on breathing may help client feel in control and decrease anxiety.
■ Decrease in reports of fear and anxiety ■ Voice steady, not shaky ■ Respiratory rate of 12–22/minute	When acute episode is over, give detailed information about nature of condition, treatments, and tests.	Anxiety and pain interfere with learning. Knowing what to expect reduces anxiety.
■ Freely expressing concerns and possible solutions about work and parenting roles; exploring alternatives as needed	As client can tolerate, encourage to express and expand on her concerns about her child and work.	Awareness of source of anxiety enables client to gain control over it. Husband's continued absence would constitute a defining characteristic for this nursing diagnosis.

Note whether husband returns as scheduled. If not, institute care plan for actual interrupted family processes.

APPLYING CRITICAL THINKING

1. What assumptions does the nurse make when deciding that using a standardized care plan for deficient fluid volume is appropriate for this client?
2. Identify an outcome in the care plan and its nursing intervention that contributes to discharge care planning. What evidence supports your choice?
3. Consider how the nurse shares the development of the care plan and outcomes with the client.
4. Not every intervention has a time frame or interval specified. It may be implied. Under what circumstances is this acceptable practice?
5. In Table 34–15, ineffective airway clearance is the client's highest priority nursing diagnosis. Under what conditions might this diagnosis be of only moderate priority?

*The NOC # for desired outcomes is listed in brackets following the appropriate outcome. Outcomes, interventions, and activities selected are only a sample of those suggested by NOC and NIC and should be further individualized for each client.

Nursing interventions on the care plan are dated when they are written and reviewed regularly at intervals that depend on the individual's needs. In an intensive care unit, for example, the plan of care will be continually monitored and revised. In a community clinic, weekly or biweekly reviews may be indicated.

The format of written interventions is similar to that of outcomes: verb, conditions, and modifiers, plus time element. The action verb starts the intervention and must be precise. For example, "Explain (to the client) the actions of insulin" is a more precise statement than "Teach (the client) about insulin." "Measure and record ankle circumference daily at 0900 h" is more precise than "Assess edema of left ankle daily." Sometimes a modifier for the verb can make the nursing intervention more precise. For example, "Apply spiral bandage firmly to left lower leg" is more precise than "Apply spiral bandage to left leg."

The time element answers when, how long, or how often the nursing action is to occur. Examples are "Assist client with tub bath at 0700 daily" and "Administer analgesic 30 minutes prior to physical therapy."

In some settings, the intervention (and other segments of the nursing care plan) is signed. The signature of the nurse prescribing the intervention shows the nurse's accountability and has legal significance.

RELATIONSHIP OF NURSING INTERVENTIONS TO PROBLEM STATUS
Depending on the type of client problem, the nurse writes interventions for observation, prevention, treatment, and health promotion.

Observations include assessments made to determine whether a complication is developing, as well as observation of the client's responses to nursing and other therapies. The nurse should write observations for both real problems and those for which the client is at risk. Some examples are "Auscultate lungs q8h," "Observe for redness over sacrum q2h," and "Record intake and output hourly."

Prevention interventions prescribe the care needed to avoid complications or reduce risk factors. They are needed mainly for potential nursing diagnoses and collaborative problems. Examples are "Turn, cough, and deep breathe q2h" (to prevent respiratory complications) and "Keep bed rails raised and bed in low position" (to minimize chances of client falling out of bed).

Treatments include teaching, referrals, physical care, and other care needed for an actual nursing diagnosis. Some interventions may accomplish either prevention or treatment functions, depending on the status of the problem. In the preceding examples, "Turn, cough, and deep breathe q2h" can also be intended to treat an existing respiratory problem.

Health promotion interventions are appropriate when the client has no health problems or when the nurse makes a wellness nursing diagnosis. Such nursing interventions focus on helping the client identify areas for improvement that will lead to a higher level of wellness and actualize the client's overall health potential. Examples are "Discuss the importance of daily exercise" and "Explore infant stimulation techniques."

DELEGATING IMPLEMENTATION
Delegating is another activity that occurs during the planning phase of the nursing process. While choosing and writing nursing interventions on the client's care plan, the nurse must also determine who should actually perform the activity. The ANA defines delegation as "the transfer of responsibility for the performance of an activity from one person to another while retaining accountability for the outcome." This differs from **assignment**, which is a "downward or lateral transfer of both the responsibility *and accountability* [emphasis added] of an activity from one individual to another" (ANA, 1997, Attachment I, #5–6). The ability to delegate client care and assign tasks is a vital skill for registered nurses because many health care institutions use assistive personnel (e.g., licensed practical nurses and unlicensed nursing assistants). To delegate appropriately, the nurse must match the needs of the client and family with the skills and knowledge of the available caregivers. This requires knowing the background, experience, knowledge, skills, and strengths of each person, and understanding which tasks are and are not within their legal scope of practice (ANA, 2010).

The nurse has two responsibilities in delegating and assigning: (1) appropriate delegation of duties (that is, giving people duties within their scope of practice) and (2) adequate supervision of personnel to whom work is delegated or assigned. The RN can delegate certain tasks to an unlicensed person but cannot assign responsibility for total nursing care. The RN is responsible for seeing that delegated tasks are carried out properly. Assistive personnel may perform tasks such as measuring intake and output, but the RN is still responsible for analyzing data, planning care, and evaluating outcomes. Because there are no universal standards for the training of unlicensed personnel, nurses often must assume responsibility for supplementing the training those staff members have received.

THE NURSING INTERVENTIONS CLASSIFICATION
In addition to the efforts of NANDA to standardize the language for describing problems that require nursing care and to create a taxonomy of standardized client outcome labels, nurse researchers also recognized the need for a standardized language to describe the interventions that nurses perform. A taxonomy of nursing interventions referred to as the **Nursing Interventions Classification (NIC)** taxonomy, developed by the Iowa Intervention Project, was first published in 1992 and has been updated every 4 years since then. This taxonomy consists of three levels: (a) level 1, domains; (b) level 2, classes; and (c) level 3, interventions. Table 34–21 shows the seven domains and 30 classes of interventions within the taxonomy.

More than 514 interventions (level 3) have been developed. Similar to NANDA diagnoses, each broadly stated intervention includes a label (name), a definition, and a list of activities that outline the key actions of nurses in carrying out the intervention. For example, the level 3 intervention Touch is one of several interventions developed within the

TABLE 34–21 **NIC Taxonomy**

LEVEL 1: DOMAINS	LEVEL 2: CLASSES (LETTERED FOR CROSS-REFERENCING)
Domain 1 Physiological: Basic Care that supports physical functioning	A. Activity and Exercise Management: Interventions to organize or assist with physical activity and energy conservation and expenditure B. Elimination Management: Interventions to establish and maintain regular bowel and urinary elimination patterns and manage complications due to altered patterns C. Immobility Management: Interventions to manage restricted body movement and the sequelae D. Nutrition Support: Interventions to modify or maintain nutritional status E. Physical Comfort Promotion: Interventions to promote comfort using physical techniques F. Self-Care Facilitation: Interventions to provide or assist with routine activities of daily living
Domain 2 Physiological: Complex Care that supports homeostatic regulation	G. Electrolyte and Acid–Base Management: Interventions to regulate electrolyte/acid–base balance and prevent complications H. Drug Management: Interventions to facilitate desired effects of pharmacological agents I. Neurologic Management: Interventions to optimize neurologic functions J. Perioperative Care: Interventions to provide care before, during, and immediately after surgery K. Respiratory Management: Interventions to promote airway patency and gas exchange L. Skin/Wound Management: Interventions to maintain or restore tissue integrity M. Thermoregulation: Interventions to maintain body temperature within a normal range N. Tissue Perfusion Management: Interventions to optimize circulation of blood and fluids to the tissue
Domain 3 Behavioral Care that supports psychosocial functioning and facilitates lifestyle changes	O. Behavior Therapy: Interventions to reinforce or promote desirable behaviors or alter undesirable behaviors P. Cognitive Therapy: Interventions to reinforce or promote desirable cognitive functioning or alter undesirable cognitive functioning Q. Communication Enhancement: Interventions to facilitate delivering and receiving verbal and non-verbal messages R. Coping Assistance: Interventions to assist another to build on own strengths, to adapt to a change in function, or to achieve a higher level of function S. Patient Education: Interventions to facilitate learning T. Psychological Comfort Promotion: Interventions to promote comforts using psychological techniques
Domain 4 Safety Care that supports protection against harm	U. Crisis Management: Interventions to provide immediate short-term help in both psychological and physiological crises
Domain 5 Family Care that supports the family unit	V. Risk Management: Interventions to initiate risk-reduction activities and continue monitoring risks over time W. Childbearing Care: Interventions to assist in understanding and coping with the psychological and physiological changes during the childbearing period Z. Childrearing Care: Interventions to assist in child rearing X. Life Span Care: Interventions to facilitate family unit functioning and promote the health and welfare of family members throughout the lifespan
Domain 6 Health System Care that supports effective use of the health care delivery system	Y. Health System Mediation: Interventions to facilitate the interface between patient/family and the health care system
Domain 7 Community Care that supports the health of the community	a. Health System Management: Interventions to provide and enhance support services for the delivery of care b. Information Management: Interventions to facilitate communication among health care providers c. Community Health Promotion: Interventions that promote the health of the whole community d. Community Risk Management: Interventions that assist in detecting or preventing health risks to the whole community

Note: From Dochterman, J. C., & Bulechek, G. M. (Eds.). (2004). *Nursing interventions classification (NIC)* (4th ed.). St. Louis, MO: Mosby, pp. 112–113. Reprinted with permission.

Behavioral domain and its class entitled Coping Assistance (see Box 34–15).

All NIC interventions have been linked to NANDA nursing diagnostic labels. The nurse can look up a client's nursing diagnosis to see which nursing interventions are suggested. However, each nursing diagnosis contains suggestions for several interventions, so nurses need to select the appropriate interventions based on their judgment and knowledge of the client. For example, the nursing diagnostic label disturbed sleep pattern has 10 NIC interventions listed for problem resolution and 18 additional optional interventions (see Box 34–16).

When planning and documenting care in an agency that uses the NIC taxonomy, the nurse chooses the broad intervention label (e.g., Touch). Not all activities suggested for the

Box 34–15 Example of an NIC Nursing Intervention Label

INTERVENTION: TOUCH [5460]
DEFINITION: Providing comfort and communication through purposeful tactile contact
ACTIVITIES:

- Observe cultural taboos about touch.
- Give a reassuring hug, as appropriate.
- Put arm around patient's shoulders, as appropriate.
- Hold patient's hand to provide emotional support.
- Apply gentle pressure at wrist, hand, or shoulder of seriously ill patient.
- Rub back in synchrony with patient's breathing, as appropriate.
- Stroke body part in slow, rhythmical fashion, as appropriate.
- Massage around painful area, as appropriate.
- Elicit from parents common actions used to soothe and calm their child.
- Hold infant or child firmly and snugly.
- Encourage parents to touch newborn or ill child.

- Surround premature infant with blanket rolls (nesting).
- Swaddle infant snugly in a blanket to keep arms and legs close to the body.
- Place infant on mother's body immediately after birth.
- Encourage mother to hold, touch, and examine the infant while umbilical cord is being severed.
- Encourage parents to hold infant.
- Encourage parents to massage infant.
- Demonstrate quieting techniques for infants.
- Provide appropriate pacifier for nonnutritional sucking in newborns.
- Provide oral stimulation exercises before tube feedings in premature infants.

Note: From Dochterman, J. C., & Bulechek, G. M. (Eds.). (2004). *Nursing interventions classification (NIC)* (4th ed.). St. Louis, MO: Mosby, p. 738. Reprinted with permission.

---

intervention would be needed for every client, so the nurse chooses the activities appropriate for the client and individualizes them to fit the supplies, equipment, and other resources available in the agency. When writing individualized nursing interventions on a care plan, the nurse should record customized activities rather than the broad intervention labels.

The NIC taxonomy provides many benefits to nurse practitioners, nurse educators, nurse administrators, and the nursing profession as a whole (see Box 34–17).

Box 34–16 Examples of NIC Interventions Linked to the NANDA Nursing Diagnosis of Disturbed Sleep Pattern

DISTURBED SLEEP PATTERN
Definition: Time limited disruption of sleep (natural, periodic suspension of consciousness) amount and quality

SUGGESTED NURSING INTERVENTIONS
FOR PROBLEM RESOLUTION

Dementia Management	Medication Prescribing
Environmental Management	Security Enhancement
Environmental Management: Comfort	Simple Relaxation Therapy
Medication Administration	Sleep Enhancement
Medication Management	Touch

ADDITIONAL OPTIONAL INTERVENTIONS

Anxiety Reduction	Meditation
Autogenic Training	Music Therapy
Bathing	Nutrition Management
Calming Technique	Pain Management
Coping Enhancement	Positioning
Energy Management	Progressive Muscle Relaxation
Exercise Promotion	Self-Care Assistance: Toileting
Exercise Therapy: Ambulation	Simple Massage
Kangaroo Care	Urinary Incontinence Care: Enuresis

Note: From Dochterman, J. C., & Bulechek, G. M. (Eds.). (2004). *Nursing interventions classification (NIC)* (4th ed.). St. Louis, MO: Mosby, p. 877. Reprinted with permission.

Box 34–17 Benefits of the Nursing Interventions Classification

- Helps demonstrate the impact that nurses have on the health care delivery system.
- Standardizes and defines the knowledge base for nursing curricula and practice.
- Facilitates the appropriate selection of a nursing intervention.
- Facilitates communication of nursing treatments to other nurses and other providers.
- Enables researchers to examine the effectiveness and cost of nursing care.
- Assists educators to develop curricula that better articulate with clinical practice.
- Facilitates the teaching of clinical decision making to novice nurses.
- Assists administrators in planning more effectively for staff and equipment needs.
- Promotes the development of a reimbursement system for nursing services.
- Facilitates the development and use of nursing information systems.
- Communicates the nature of nursing to the public.

Note: From Dochterman, J. C., & Bulechek, G. M. (Eds.). (2004). *Nursing interventions classification (NIC)* (4th ed.). St. Louis, MO: Mosby, p. vi. Reprinted with permission.

DEVELOPMENTAL CONSIDERATIONS **Nursing Care Plan**

OLDER ADULTS

When a client is in an extended-care facility or a long-term care facility, interventions and medications often remain the same day after day. It is important to review the care plan on a regular basis because changes in the condition of older adults may be subtle and go unnoticed. This applies to both changes of improvement or deterioration. Either one should receive attention so that appropriate revisions can be made in expected outcomes and interventions. Outcomes need to be realistic with consideration given to the client's physical condition, emotional condition, support systems, and mental status. Outcomes for older clients often have to be stated and expected to be completed in very small steps. For instance, a client who has had a cerebrovascular accident may spend weeks learning to brush her own teeth or dress herself. When these small steps are successfully completed, it gives the client a sense of accomplishment and motivation to continue working toward increasing self-care. This particular example also demonstrates the need to work collaboratively with other departments, such as physical and occupational therapy, to develop the nursing care plan.

CONCEPT MAP **Ineffective Airway Clearance (Gas Exchange)**

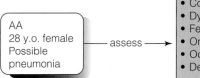

AA
28 y.o. female
Possible pneumonia

→ assess →

- Cold x 2 weeks
- Dyspnea on exertion
- Fever
- Orthopnea
- Occasional chills
- Decreased oral intake x 2 days

- T: 103F P: 92 R: 22, shallow BP: 122/80
- Dry mucous membranes; skin hot, pale
- Cheeks flushed
- Decreased breath sounds
- Inspiratory crackles RUL and RLL
- Ineffective cough—small amount thick, pale pink sputum
- Lethargic, c/o being weak, fatigued

generate nursing diagnosis

Ineffective Airway Clearance r/t viscous secretions, & shallow chest expansion, secondary to deficient fluid volume, pain, & fatigue

outcome

Respiratory status: Gas Exchange aeb
- Absent of pallor & cyanosis
- Use of correct breathing/coughing technique after instruction
- Productive cough
- Symmetric chest excursion

Within 24 hours

- Lungs clear to auscultation
- Respirations 12-22/min; pulse <100 bpm
- Inhales normal volume air on incentive spirometer

nursing intervention

Respiratory Monitoring

activity

Monitor results of blood gases, x-rays & incentive spirometry

activity

Auscultate breath sounds q4h

activity

Monitor level of consciousness

activity

Monitor rate, depth, effort, skin color, mucous membranes, amount & color of sputum of respirations q4h

nursing intervention

Respiratory Monitoring

activity

Administer antibiotics

activity

Instruct in breathing & coughing techniques. Remind & assist q3h

activity

Administer expectorants

activity

Administer analgesics

activity

Administer O₂ per NC

activity

Assist with postural drainage @ 9:30 AM

Implementation

The nursing process is action oriented, client centered, and outcome directed. After developing a plan of care based on the assessing and diagnosing phases, the nurse implements the interventions written during the planning process.

In the nursing process, implementing is the action phase in which the nurse performs the nursing interventions. **Implementation** consists of doing and documenting the specific nursing actions needed to carry out the interventions. The nurse performs or delegates the nursing activities for the interventions that were developed in the planning step and then concludes the implementing step by recording nursing activities and the resulting client responses.

Although the nurse may act on the client's behalf (e.g., referring the client to a community health nurse for home care), professional standards support client and family participation in all phases of the nursing process. The degree of participation depends on the client's health status. For example, an unconscious man is unable to participate in his care and therefore needs to have care given to him. By contrast, an ambulatory client may require very little care from the nurse and carry out health care activities independently.

RELATIONSHIP OF IMPLEMENTING TO OTHER NURSING PROCESS PHASES

The first three nursing process phases—assessing, diagnosing, and planning—provide the basis for the nursing actions performed during the implementing step. In turn, the implementing phase provides the actual nursing activities and client responses that are examined in the final phase, the evaluating phase. Using data acquired during assessment, the nurse can individualize the care given in the implementing phase, tailoring the interventions to fit a specific client rather than applying them routinely to categories of clients (e.g., all clients with pneumonia).

While implementing nursing care, the nurse continues to reassess the client at every contact, gathering data about the client's responses to the nursing activities and about any new problems that may develop. A nursing activity on the client's care plan for the NIC intervention airway management might read "Auscultate breath sounds q4h." When performing this activity, the nurse is both carrying out the intervention (implementing) and performing an assessment. Some routine nursing activities are themselves assessments. For example, while bathing an elderly client, the nurse observes a reddened area on the client's sacrum. Or, when emptying a urinary catheter bag, the nurse measures 200 mL of offensive smelling, brown urine.

SKILLS NECESSARY FOR IMPLEMENTATION

To implement the care plan successfully, nurses need cognitive, interpersonal, and technical skills. Although these skills are distinct from one another, in practice nurses use them in various combinations and with different emphasis, depending on the activity. For instance, when inserting a urinary catheter the nurse needs cognitive knowledge of the principles and steps of the procedure, interpersonal skills to inform and reassure the client, and technical skill in draping the client and manipulating the equipment.

Cognitive skills (intellectual skills) include problem solving, decision making, critical thinking, and creativity. They are crucial to safe, intelligent nursing care.

Interpersonal skills are all of the activities, verbal and nonverbal, people use when interacting directly with one another. The effectiveness of a nursing action often depends largely on the nurse's ability to communicate with others. The nurse uses therapeutic communication to understand the client and, in turn, be understood. A nurse also needs interpersonal skills to work effectively with others as a member of the health care team.

Interpersonal skills are necessary for all nursing activities: Caring, comforting, advocating, referring, counseling, and supporting are just a few. Interpersonal skills include conveying knowledge, attitudes, feelings, interest, and appreciation of the client's cultural values and lifestyle. Before nurses can be highly skilled in interpersonal relations, they must have self-awareness and sensitivity to others.

Technical skills are purposeful, "hands-on" skills such as manipulating equipment, giving injections, bandaging, moving, lifting, and repositioning clients. These skills are also called tasks, procedures, or psychomotor skills. The term *psychomotor* refers to physical actions that are controlled by the mind, not reflexive.

Technical skills require knowledge and, frequently, manual dexterity. The number of technical skills expected of a nurse has greatly increased in recent years because of the pervasive use of technology, especially in acute-care hospitals.

PROCESS OF IMPLEMENTATION

The process of implementation (see Figure 34–16 ■) normally includes the following:

- Reassessing the client
- Determining the nurse's need for assistance
- Implementing the nursing interventions
- Supervising the delegated care
- Documenting nursing activities.

Reassessing the Client

Just before implementing an intervention, the nurse must reassess the client to make sure the intervention is still needed. Even though an order is written on the care plan, the client's condition may have changed. For example, a client has a nursing diagnosis of disturbed sleep pattern related to anxiety and unfamiliar surroundings. During rounds, the nurse discovers that the client is sleeping and therefore defers the back massage that had been planned as a relaxation strategy.

New data may indicate a need to change the priorities of care or the nursing activities. For example, a nurse begins to teach a client who has diabetes how to give himself insulin injections. Shortly after beginning the teaching, the nurse realizes that the client is not concentrating on the lesson. Subsequent discussion reveals that he is worried about his eyesight and fears he is going blind. Realizing that the client's level of stress is interfering with his learning, the nurse ends

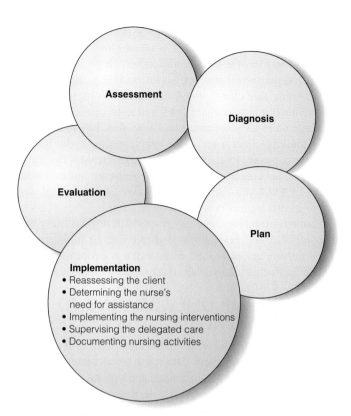

Figure 34–16 ■ Implementation. The fourth phase of the nursing process, in which the nurse implements the nursing interventions and documents the care provided.

the lesson and arranges for a primary care provider to examine the client's eyes. The nurse also provides supportive communication to help alleviate the client's stress.

Determining the Nurse's Need for Assistance

When implementing some nursing interventions, the nurse may require assistance for one or more of the following reasons:

- The nurse is unable to implement the nursing activity safely or efficiently alone (e.g., ambulating an unsteady obese client).
- Assistance would reduce stress on the client (e.g., turning a person who experiences acute pain when moved).
- The nurse lacks the knowledge or skills to implement a particular nursing activity (e.g., a nurse who is not familiar with a particular model of traction equipment needs assistance the first time it is applied).

Implementing the Nursing Interventions

It is important to explain to the client what interventions will be done, what sensations to expect, what the client is expected to do, and what the expected outcome is. For many nursing activities, it is important to ensure the client's privacy, for example by closing doors, pulling curtains, or draping the client. The number and kind of direct nursing interventions are almost unlimited and include coordination of client care. This activity involves scheduling client contacts with other departments (e.g., laboratory and x-ray technicians, physical and respiratory therapists) and serving as a liaison among the members of the health care team.

When implementing interventions, nurses should follow these guidelines:

- Base nursing interventions on scientific knowledge, nursing research, and professional standards of care (evidence-based practice) when these exist. The nurse must be aware of the scientific rationale, as well as possible side effects or complications, of all interventions. For example, a client prefers to take an oral medication after meals; however, this medication is not absorbed well in the presence of food. Therefore, the nurse will need to explain why this preference cannot be honored.
- Clearly understand the interventions to be implemented and question any that are not understood. The nurse is responsible for intelligent implementation of medical and nursing plans of care. This requires knowledge of each intervention, its purpose in the client's plan of care, any contraindications (e.g., allergies), and changes in the client's condition that may affect the order.
- Adapt activities to the individual client. A client's beliefs, values, age, health status, and environment are factors that can affect the success of a nursing action. For example, the nurse determines that a client chokes when swallowing pills, so he or she consults with the physician to change the order to a liquid form of the medication. Or, the nurse recognizes that many Asian persons prefer to drink hot water rather than ice water and, after confirming it with a specific client, supplies this at the bedside.
- Implement safe care. For example, when changing a sterile dressing, the nurse practices sterile technique to prevent infection; when giving a medication, the nurse administers the correct dosage by the ordered route.
- Provide teaching, support, and comfort. See Box 39–5 in Concept 39, Teaching and Learning, for examples of verbs used in writing learning outcomes. The nurse should always explain the purpose of interventions, what the client will experience, and how the client can participate. The client must have sufficient knowledge to agree to the plan of care and to be able to assume responsibility for as much self-care as possible. These independent nursing activities enhance the effectiveness of nursing care plans (see Figure 34–17 ■).
- Respect the client's ethnic background and cultural preferences. The nurse must always view the client as a whole and consider the client's responses in that context. For example, whenever possible, the nurse honors the client's expressed preference that interventions be planned for times that fit with the client's usual schedule of visitors, work, sleep, or eating.
- Respect the dignity of the client and enhance the client's self-esteem. Providing privacy and encouraging clients to make their own decisions are ways of respecting dignity and enhancing self-esteem.
- Encourage clients to participate actively in implementing the nursing interventions. Active participation enhances the client's sense of independence and control. However, clients vary in the degree of participation they desire. Some want total involvement in their care, whereas others prefer little involvement. The amount of desired involvement may be related to the severity of the illness; the client's culture; or the client's fear, understanding of the illness, and understanding of the intervention.

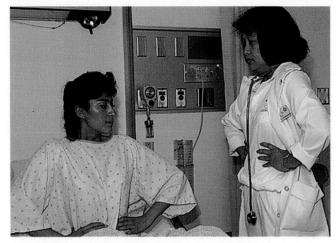

Figure 34–17 ■ Ms Aquilini agrees to practice deep-breathing exercises q3h during the day. In addition, she verbalizes awareness of the need to increase her fluid intake.

Supervising Delegated Care

If care has been delegated to other health care personnel, the nurse responsible for the client's overall care must ensure that the activities have been implemented according to the care plan. Other caregivers may be required to communicate their activities to the nurse by documenting them on the client record, reporting verbally, or filling out a written form. The nurse validates and responds to any adverse findings or client responses. This may involve modifying the nursing care plan.

Documenting Nursing Activities

After carrying out the nursing activities, the nurse completes the implementing phase by recording the interventions and client responses in the nursing progress notes. Documentation is discussed in Concept 36, Communication. Nursing activities are communicated verbally as well as in writing. When a client's health is changing rapidly, the charge nurse and/or the physician may want to be kept up-to-date with verbal reports. Nurses also report client status at a change of shift and on a client's discharge to another unit or health agency in person, via a voice recording, or in writing.

Evaluation

After implementing nursing care the nurse evaluates the desired outcomes. On the basis of this evaluation, the plan of care is either continued, modified, or terminated. As in all phases of the nursing process, clients and support persons are encouraged to participate as much as possible.

To evaluate means to judge or to appraise. Evaluating is the fifth and last phase of the nursing process. In this context, **evaluation** is a planned, ongoing, purposeful activity in which clients and health care professionals determine (a) the client's progress toward achievement of goals/outcomes and (b) the effectiveness of the nursing care plan. Evaluation is an important aspect of the nursing process because conclusions drawn from the evaluation determine whether the nursing interventions should be terminated, continued, or changed.

Evaluation is continuous. Evaluation done during or immediately after implementation of a nursing order enables the nurse to make on-the-spot modifications in an intervention. Evaluation performed at specified intervals (e.g., once a week for the home care client) shows the extent of progress toward goal achievement and enables the nurse to correct any deficiencies and modify the care plan as needed. Evaluation continues until the client achieves the health goals or is discharged from nursing care. Evaluation at discharge includes the status of goal achievement and the client's self-care abilities with regard to follow-up care. Most agencies have a special discharge record for this evaluation.

Through evaluating, nurses demonstrate responsibility and accountability for their actions, indicate interest in the results of the nursing activities, and demonstrate a desire not to perpetuate ineffective actions but to adopt more effective ones.

RELATIONSHIP OF EVALUATING TO OTHER NURSING PROCESS PHASES

Successful evaluation depends on the effectiveness of the steps that precede it. Assessment data must be accurate and complete so that the nurse can formulate appropriate nursing diagnoses and desired outcomes. The desired outcomes must be stated concretely in behavioral terms if they are to be useful for evaluating client responses. And finally, without the implementing phase in which the plan is put into action, there would be nothing to evaluate.

The evaluating and assessing phases overlap. As previously stated, assessment (data collection) is ongoing and continuous at every client contact. However, data are collected for different purposes at different points in the nursing process. During the assessment phase, the nurse collects data for the purpose of making diagnoses. During the evaluation step, the nurse collects data for the purpose of comparing it to preselected goals and judging the effectiveness of the nursing care. The act of assessing (data collection) is the same; the differences lie in (a) when the data are collected and (b) how the data are used.

PROCESS OF EVALUATING CLIENT RESPONSES

Before evaluation, the nurse identifies the desired outcomes (indicators) that will be used to measure client goal achievement. (This is done in the planning step.) Desired outcomes serve two purposes: They establish the kind of evaluative data that need to be collected and provide a standard against which the data are judged. For example, given the following expected outcomes, any nurse caring for the client would know what data to collect:

■ Daily fluid intake will not be less than 2500 mL
■ Urinary output will balance with fluid intake
■ Residual urine will be less than 100 mL.

The evaluation process has five components (see Figure 34–18 ■):

1. Collecting data related to the desired outcomes (NOC indicators)
2. Comparing the data with outcomes

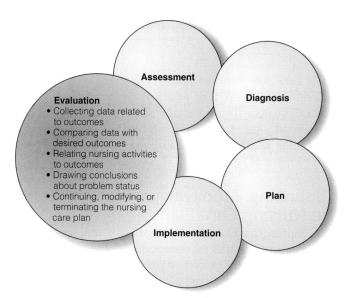

Figure 34–18 ■ Evaluation. The final phase of the nursing process, in which the nurse determines the client's progress toward goal achievement and the effectiveness of the nursing care plan. The plan may be continued, modified, or terminated.

3. Relating nursing activities to outcomes
4. Drawing conclusions about problem status
5. Continuing, modifying, or terminating the nursing care plan.

Collecting Data

Using the clearly stated, precise, and measurable desired outcomes as a guide, the nurse collects data so that conclusions can be drawn about whether goals have been met. It is usually necessary to collect both objective and subjective data.

Some data may require interpretation. Examples of objective data requiring interpretation are the degree of tissue turgor of a dehydrated client or the degree of restlessness of a client with pain. Examples of subjective data needing interpretation include complaints of nausea or pain by the client. When interpreting subjective data, the nurse must rely upon either (a) the client's statements (e.g., "My pain is worse now than it was after breakfast") or (b) objective indicators of the subjective data, even though these indicators may require further interpretation (e.g., decreased restlessness, decreased pulse and respiratory rates, and relaxed facial muscles as indicators of pain relief). Data must be recorded concisely and accurately to facilitate the next part of the evaluating process.

Comparing Data With Outcomes

If the first two parts of the evaluation process have been carried out effectively, it is relatively simple to determine whether a desired outcome has been met. Both the nurse and client play an active role in comparing the client's actual responses with the desired outcomes. Did the client drink 3000 mL of fluid in 24 hours? Did the client walk unassisted the specified distance per day? When determining whether a goal has been achieved, the nurse can draw one of three possible conclusions:

1. The goal was met; that is, the client response is the same as the desired outcome.

2. The goal was partially met; that is, either a short-term goal was achieved but the long-term goal was not, or the desired outcome was only partially attained.

3. The goal was not met.

After determining whether a goal has been met, the nurse writes an evaluative statement (either on the care plan or in the nurse's notes). An **evaluation statement** consists of two parts: a conclusion and supporting data. The *conclusion* is a statement that the goal/desired outcome was met, partially met, or not met. The *supporting data* are the list of client responses that support the conclusion, for example:

Goal met: Oral intake 300 mL more than output; skin turgor resilient; mucous membranes moist

See the nursing care plan at the end of this exemplar for evaluation statements for the client discussed in this exemplar. Data in the Evaluation Statements column on this table represent the client's responses to care as observed by the night nurse on the morning after the client's admission to the unit. In practice, care plans usually do not have a column for evaluation statements; rather, these are recorded in the nurse's notes. If NOC indicators are being used with the outcomes, scores on the scales after intervention would be compared with those measured at baseline to determine improvement. See Table 34–17 for an example of the NOC rating scales used for indicators of mobility. The column explaining rationale for continuing or modifying the plan is included in a student care plan.

Relating Nursing Activities to Outcomes

The fourth aspect of the evaluating process is determining whether the nursing activities had any relation to the outcomes. It should never be assumed that a nursing activity was the cause of or the only factor in meeting, partially meeting, or not meeting a goal.

CLINICAL EXAMPLE

For example, Ruth Horowitz, an obese client, needed to lose 14 kg (30 lb). When the nurse and Mrs. Horowitz drew up a care plan, one goal was "Lose 1.4 kg (3 lb) in 4 weeks." A nursing strategy in the care plan was "Explain how to plan and prepare a 1200-calorie diet." Four weeks later, Mrs. Horowitz weighed herself and had lost 1.8 kg (4 lb). The goal had been met—in fact, exceeded. It is easy to assume that the nursing strategy was highly effective. However, it is important to collect more data before drawing that conclusion. On questioning Mrs. Horowitz, the nurse might find any of the following: (a) She planned a 1200-calorie diet and prepared and ate the food; (b) she planned a 1200-calorie diet but did not prepare the correct food; (c) she did not understand how to plan a 1200-calorie diet, so she did not bother with it.

If the first possibility is found to be true, the nurse can safely judge that the nursing strategy "Explain how to plan and prepare a 1200-calorie diet" was effective in helping Mrs. Horowitz lose weight. However, if the nurse learns that either the second or third possibility actually happened, then it must be assumed that the nursing strategy did not affect the outcome. The next step for the nurse is to collect data about what Mrs. Horowitz actually did to lose weight. It is important to establish the relationship (or lack thereof) of the nursing actions to the client responses.

Drawing Conclusions About Problem Status

The nurse uses the judgments about goal achievement to determine whether the care plan was effective in resolving, reducing, or preventing client problems. When goals have been met, the nurse can draw one of the following conclusions about the status of the client's problem:

- The actual problem stated in the nursing diagnosis has been resolved, or the potential problem is being prevented and the risk factors no longer exist. In these instances, the nurse documents that the goals have been met and discontinues the care for the problem.
- The potential problem stated in the nursing diagnosis is being prevented, but the risk factors are still present. In this case, the nurse keeps the problem on the care plan.
- The actual problem still exists even though some goals are being met. For example, a desired outcome on a client's care plan is "Will drink 3000 mL of fluid daily." Even though the data may show this outcome has been achieved, other data (dry oral mucous membranes) may indicate that there is deficient fluid volume. Therefore, the nursing interventions must be continued even though this one goal was met.

When goals have been partially met or when goals have not been met, two conclusions may be drawn:
- The care plan needs to be revised, since the problem is only partially resolved. The revisions may need to occur during assessing, diagnosing, or planning phases, as well as implementing.

OR

- The care plan does not need revision because the client merely needs more time to achieve the previously established goal(s). To make this decision, the nurse must assess why the goals are being only partially achieved, including whether the evaluation was conducted too soon (see Figure 34–19 ■).

Continuing, Modifying, and Terminating the Nursing Care Plan

After drawing conclusions about the status of the client's problems, the nurse modifies the care plan as indicated. Depending on the agency, modifications may be made by drawing a line through portions of the care plan; marking portions using a highlighting pen; or writing "Discontinued" (dc'd), "goal met," or "problem resolved" and the date.

Whether or not goals were met, a number of decisions need to be made about continuing, modifying, or terminating nursing care for each problem. See Table 34–22 for a checklist to use when reviewing a care plan. Although the checklist uses a closed, yes/no format, its only intent is to identify areas that require the nurse's further examination.

Before making modifications, the nurse must determine if the plan as a whole was not completely effective. This requires

---

TABLE 34–22 Evaluation Checklist

ASSESSMENT	DIAGNOSIS	PLAN	IMPLEMENTATION
_____ Are data complete, accurate, and validated? _____ Do new data require changes in the care plan?	_____ Are nursing diagnoses relevant and accurate? _____ Are nursing diagnoses supported by the data? _____ Has problem status changed (i.e., potential, actual, risk)? _____ Are the diagnoses stated clearly and in correct format? _____ Have any nursing diagnoses been resolved?	**Desired Outcomes** _____ Do new nursing diagnoses require new goals? _____ Are goals realistic? _____ Was enough time allowed for goal achievement? _____ Do the goals address all aspects of the problem? _____ Does the client still concur with the goals? _____ Have client priorities changed? **Nursing Interventions** _____ Do nursing interventions need to be written for new nursing diagnoses or new goals? _____ Do the nursing interventions seem to be related to the stated goals? _____ Is there a rationale to justify each nursing order? _____ Are the nursing interventions clear, specific, and detailed? _____ Are new resources available? _____ Do the nursing interventions address all aspects of the client's goals? _____ Were the nursing interventions actually carried out?	_____ Was client input obtained at each step of the nursing process? _____ Were goals and nursing interventions acceptable to the client? _____ Did the caregivers have the knowledge and skill to perform the interventions correctly? _____ Were explanations given to the client prior to implementing?

DEVELOPMENTAL CONSIDERATIONS Evaluation

Evaluation of goals, selected outcomes, and interventions needs to be continuous, with ongoing assessment and reassessment of the situation. Priority needs can change quickly and must be reprioritized when problems occur. Infants and young children are vulnerable to rapid change in their condition due to their small body size, disproportionate size of organs, and immaturity of body systems. Also, they may not be able to verbalize how they are feeling. Older adults may have conditions that impair communication, such as aphasia from a cerebrovascular accident, dementia, multiple sclerosis, or other neurological conditions. In such cases, the nurse needs to be even more astute in performing nonverbal assessments, being alert to potential problems, and detecting changes in the client's condition. If evaluations are done often and thoroughly, changes can be made quickly to intervene more effectively and improve outcomes. Constant assessment, communication, and interpersonal skills are as essential in the evaluation phase as they are in the initial assessment.

a review of the entire care plan and a critique of each step of the nursing process involved in its development.

ASSESSMENT   An incomplete or incorrect database influences all subsequent steps of the nursing process and care plan. If data are incomplete, the nurse needs to reassess the client and record the new data. In some instances, new data may indicate the need for new nursing diagnoses, new goals, and new nursing interventions.

DIAGNOSIS   If the database was incomplete, new diagnostic statements may be required. If the database was complete, the nurse needs to analyze whether the problems were identified correctly and whether the nursing diagnoses were relevant to that database. After making judgments about problem status, the nurse revises or adds new diagnoses as needed to reflect the most recent client data.

PLAN: REVISING CLIENT OUTCOMES   If a nursing diagnosis was inaccurate, obviously the goal statement(s) will need revision. If the nursing diagnosis was appropriate, the nurse then checks if the goals were realistic and attainable. Unrealistic goals require correction. The nurse should also determine whether priorities have changed and whether the client still agrees with the priorities. For example, the amount of time delineated for a specific amount of weight loss was possibly too short and should be extended. Goals must also be written for any new nursing diagnoses.

PLAN: REDESIGNING NURSING INTERVENTIONS   The nurse investigates whether the nursing interventions were related to goal achievement and whether the best nursing interventions were selected. Even when diagnoses and goals were appropriate, the nursing interventions selected may not have been the best ones to achieve the goal. New nursing interventions may reflect changes in the amount of nursing care the client needs, scheduling changes, or rearrangement of nursing activities to group similar activities or to permit longer rest or activity periods for the client. For example, for a client who wishes to stop smoking, there are many potential interventions. If medication was prescribed but the client is still smoking, a behavioral intervention such as group counseling may need to be added. If new nursing diagnoses have been written, then new nursing interventions will also be necessary.

IMPLEMENTATION   Even if all sections of the care plan appear to be satisfactory, the manner in which the plan was implemented may have interfered with goal achievement. Before selecting new interventions, the nurse should confirm whether they were carried out. Other personnel may not have carried them out, either because the interventions were unclear or because they were unreasonable in terms of external constraints such as money, staff, time, and equipment.

After making the necessary modifications to the care plan, the nurse implements the modified plan and begins the nursing process cycle again. Refer to the Table 34–23 to see how the plan for the client in the care plan throughout this exemplar was modified after evaluation of goal achievement and review of the nursing process. A line has been drawn through portions the nurse wished to delete; additions to the care plan are shown in italics.

In addition to evaluating the client's response to the nursing plan of care, nurses also evaluate nursing care. This evaluation process is known as quality improvement and is discussed in Concept 48.

Figure 34–19 ■ Upon assessment of respiratory excursion, Nurse Medina detects failure of the client to achieve maximum ventilation. She and Ms. Aquilini reevaluate the care plan and modify it to increase coughing and deep-breathing exercises to q2h.

TABLE 34–23 Identifying Nursing Diagnoses, Outcomes, and Interventions, Modified Following Implementation and Evaluation

Nursing Diagnosis: Ineffective airway clearance related to viscous secretions and shallow chest expansion secondary to deficient fluid volume, pain, and fatigue.

DESIRED OUTCOMES*/INDICATORS	EVALUATION STATEMENTS	NURSING INTERVENTIONS**	EXPLANATION FOR CONTINUING OR MODIFYING NURSING INTERVENTIONS
Respiratory status: gas exchange [0402], as evidenced by the following:			
■ Absence of pallor and cyanosis (skin and mucous membranes)	Partially met. Skin and mucous membranes not cyanotic, but still pale.	Monitor respiratory status q4h; rate, depth, effort, skin color, mucous membranes, amount and color of sputum.	Retain nursing interventions to continue to identify progress. Goal status indicates problem not resolved.
■ Use of correct breathing/coughing technique after instruction	Partially met. Uses correct technique when pain well controlled by narcotic analgesics.	Monitor results of blood gases, chest x-ray studies, pulse oximetry, and incentive spirometer volume as available.	
■ Productive cough	Met. Cough productive of moderate amounts of thick, yellow, pink-tinged sputum.	Monitor level of consciousness.	
■ Symmetric chest excursion of at least 4 cm	Not met. Chest excursion = 3 cm.	Auscultate lungs q4h.	
■ Lungs clear to auscultation within 48–72 hours	Not met. Scattered inspiratory crackles auscultated throughout right anterior and posterior chest.	Vital signs q4h (TPR, BP, pulse oximetry).	Does not need to be reinstructed as client demonstrates correct techniques. May still need support and encouragement because of fatigue and pain of breathing.
■ Respirations 12–22/minute, pulse, <100 beats/minute	Partially met. Respirations 26/minute, pulse 96.	Instruct in breathing and coughing techniques. Remind to perform and assist q3h. *Support and encourage. (4/17/07, JW)*	
■ Inhaling normal volume of air on incentive spirometer	Not met. Tidal volume only 350 mL. *(Evaluated 4/17/07, JW)*	Administer prescribed expectorant; schedule for maximum effectiveness. Maintain Fowler's or semi-Fowler's position. Administer prescribed analgesics. Notify primary care provider if pain not relieved. Administer oxygen by nasal cannula as prescribed. Provide portable oxygen if client goes off unit (e.g., for x-ray examination). Assist with postural drainage daily at 0930. *On 4/17 teach to continue prn at home. (4/17/07, JW)* Administer prescribed antibiotic to maintain constant blood level. Observe for rash and GI or other side effects.	As soon as client is hydrated and fever is controlled, she will probably be discharged to self-care at home.
Anxiety control [1402], as evidenced by the following:			
■ Listening to and following instructions for correct breathing and coughing technique, even during periods of dyspnea	Met. Performed coughing techniques as instructed during periods of dyspnea.	When client is dyspneic, stay with her; reassure her you will stay. Remain calm, appear confident.	

TABLE 34–23 Identifying Nursing Diagnoses, Outcomes, and Interventions, Modified Following Implementation and Evaluation (continued)

■ Verbalizing understanding of condition, diagnostic tests, and treatments (by end of day)	Met. See nurse's notes for 3–11 shift. Stated, "I know I need to try to breathe deeply even when it hurts." Demonstrated correct use of incentive spirometer and stated understanding of the need to use it. Understands IV is for hydration and antibiotics. *(Evaluated 4/17/07, JW)*	Encourage slow, deep breathing. When client is dyspneic, give brief explanations of treatments and procedures.	
■ Decrease in reports of fear and anxiety	Met. Stated, "I know I can get enough air, but it still hurts to breathe."		
■ Voice steady, not shaky	Met. Speaks in steady voice.		
■ Respiratory rate of 12–22 minute	Not met. Rate 26–36/minute.	~~When acute episode is over, give detailed information about nature of condition, treatments, and tests.~~ *Reassess whether client needs any information on condition, treatments, or tests. (4/17/07, JW).*	Detailed information has been given. Because client shows understanding, there is no need to repeat information.
■ Freely expresses concerns and possible solutions about work and parenting roles	Partially met. Discussed only briefly on 3–11 shift. Not done on 11–7 shift because of client's need to rest. *(Evaluated 4/17/07, JW)*	As client can tolerate, encourage to express and expand on her concerns about her child and her work. Explore alternatives as needed. Note whether husband returns as scheduled. If not, institute care plan for actual interrupted family process. *(Do on 4/17, day shift) (4/17/07, JW)*	It is important that this assessment be made right away so child care can be arranged if needed.

*The NOC # for desired outcomes is listed in brackets following the appropriate outcome. Outcomes are only a sample of those suggested by NOC and should be further individualized for each client.

**In this care plan, a line has been drawn through portions the nurse wished to delete; additions to the care plan are shown in italics.

APPLYING CRITICAL THINKING

1. From reviewing this nursing care plan, what general conclusions can you make about the desired outcomes for ineffective airway clearance and anxiety?
2. Despite some of the outcomes being only partially met or not met, no new interventions were written for several outcomes. What reasons might there be for this?
3. For the nursing diagnosis of anxiety, most of the outcomes are fully met. Would you delete this diagnosis from the care plan at this time? Why or why not?
4. Since the Evaluation Statements column is generally not used on written care plans, where would auditors or persons conducting quality assessments find these data?

REVIEW The Nursing Process

RELATE: LINK THE CONCEPTS

Linking the exemplar of the Nursing Process with the concept of Communication:
1. How does the nurse communicate the use of the nursing process when documenting?
2. The nurse is caring for a client with postoperative pain and administers an analgesic 10 minutes before the end of the shift. How does the nurse communicate the need for evaluation of effectiveness of pain management to the oncoming shift?

Linking the exemplar of the Nursing Process with the concept of Legal Issues:
3. How does use of the nursing process in providing care and documenting care reduce the nurse's risk of malpractice claims?

4. What legal obligations does the nurse have related to use of the nursing process?

REFER: GO TO MYNURSINGKIT

REFLECT: CASE STUDY

Dr. Danilo Ocampo is a 74-year-old retired pathologist. He lives in his home with Lydia, his wife of 51 years. Their only child, a son, was killed at age 22 in an automobile accident. Dr. Ocampo was born and raised in the Philippines and came to the United States when he was 23. He is the last living member of his immediate family. He has a few nephews and nieces in the Philippines, but no relatives live nearby.

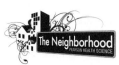

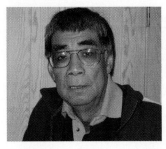

Dr. Ocampo's health has been declining for the past few years. He has a medical history that includes hypertension, myocardial infarction, angina, and class 2 heart failure. Because of these cardiovascular disorders, he takes multiple medications, including metoprolol, lisinopril, Aldactone, furosemide off and on, K+ when taking furosemide, aspirin, isosorbide dinitrate, and nitroglycerin. He has a good understanding of the pharmaceutical properties of the medications. At times, he is not sure he gets good health care because of all the medications he takes. He often does not believe they are helpful because he experiences many side effects, and he has required multiple admissions to the hospital. He usually feels better after a few days in the hospital but typically checks himself out of the hospital before his physicians are ready to discharge him.

Because Lydia has dementia, most of Dr. Ocampo's time and energy are spent managing their household and taking care of her. He has been resistant to outside help, believing he can care for her better than anyone else does. He maintains a very consistent schedule, and they get along quite well. Although at one time in their lives they were very socially active, at this point, they rarely go out.

Dr. Ocampo has become increasingly short of breath and is very fatigued. He notices his legs have become edematous. He goes to the neighborhood drugstore to use the "self-serve" blood pressure machine and finds his blood pressure to be 152/106 mm Hg. He is resistant to the idea of seeing his physician or going to the emergency department for fear of being admitted. Instead, he increases the dose of furosemide and lisinopril by 1 tablet per day and tries to get a bit more rest. A week later when his symptoms fail to improve and seem to worsen slightly, Dr. Ocampo visits his provider's office and reports his symptoms and increase in medication dosages.

1. What are the priorities of care for Dr. Ocampo?
2. What data would you collect from Dr. Ocampo on initial examination?
3. Develop a nursing plan of care for this client.

34.2 CRITICAL THINKING

KEY TERMS

Creativity, 2105
Critical analysis, 2105
Critical thinking, 2104
Deductive reasoning, 2106
Inductive reasoning, 2106
Socratic questioning, 2105

BASIS FOR SELECTION OF EXEMPLAR

NLN Competencies
Standards of Nursing Practice

LEARNING OUTCOMES

After reading about this exemplar, you will be able to:

1. Define critical thinking in terms of its importance to nursing practice.
2. Predict uses of critical thinking in nursing practice.
3. Apply attitudes that foster critical thinking to events that commonly occur in nursing practice.
4. Construct a plan to improve critical thinking skills and attitudes.

OVERVIEW

Critical thinking has many definitions. In the About Clinical Decision Making section of this concept, critical thinking is appropriately defined as a cognitive process during which an individual reviews data and considers potential explanations and outcomes before forming an opinion or making a decision. Another definition that is specifically designed for nursing practice comes from the National League for Nursing (2000): "Critical thinking in nursing practice is a discipline specific, reflective reasoning process that guides a nurse in generating, implementing, and evaluating approaches for dealing with client care and professional concerns" (p. 2). Nurses are expected to use critical thinking to solve client problems and make better decisions. Thus, critical thinking, problem solving, and decision making are interrelated processes, with creativity enhancing the result.

Critical thinking is essential to safe, competent, skillful nursing practice. The amount of knowledge that nurses must use and the continuing rapid growth of this knowledge prevent nurses from being effective practitioners if they attempt to function with only the information acquired in school or outlined in books. Decisions that nurses must make about client care and about the distribution of limited resources force them to think and act in areas where there are neither clear answers nor standard procedures and where conflicting forces turn decision making into a complex process. Nurses therefore need to embrace the attitudes that promote critical thinking and master critical-thinking skills in order to process and evaluate both previously learned and new information. Box 34–18 lists some reasons supporting the importance of critical thinking.

Nurses use critical-thinking skills in a variety of ways:

■ *Nurses use knowledge from other subjects and fields.* Because nurses deal holistically with human responses, they must draw meaningful information from other subject areas (i.e., make interdisciplinary connections) in order to understand the meaning of client data and to plan effective interventions. Nursing students take courses in the biologic and social sciences and in the humanities so that they can acquire a strong foundation on which to build their nursing knowledge and skill. For example, the nurse might use knowledge from nutrition, physiology, and physics to promote wound healing and prevent further injury to a client with a pressure ulcer.

Box 34–18 Top 10 Reasons to Improve Thinking

10. Things aren't what they used to be or what they will be.

9. Clients are sicker, with multiple problems.

8. More consumer involvement (clients and families).

7. Nurses must be able to move from one setting to another.

6. Rapid change and information explosion requires us to develop new learning and workplace skills.

5. Consumers and payers demand to see evidence of benefits, efficiency, and results.

4. Today's progress often creates new problems that can't be solved by old ways of thinking.

3. Redesigning care delivery and nursing curricula is useless if students and nurses don't have the thinking skills required to deal with today's world.

2. It can be done—it doesn't have to be that difficult.

1. **Your ability to focus your thinking to get the results you need can make the difference between whether you succeed or fail in this fast-paced world.**

Note: Reprinted from Alfaro-LeFevre, R. (2004). *Critical thinking in nursing: A practical approach* (3rd ed.) with permission from Elsevier.

- *Nurses deal with change in stressful environments.* Nurses work in rapidly changing situations. Treatments, medications, and technology change constantly, and a client's condition may change from minute to minute. Routine actions are not always adequate to deal with the situation at hand. Familiarity with the routine for giving medications, for example, does not help the nurse deal with a client who is frightened of injections or with one who does not wish to take a medication. When unexpected situations arise, critical thinking enables the nurse to recognize important cues, respond quickly, and adapt interventions to meet specific client needs.

- *Nurses make important decisions.* During the course of a workday, nurses make vital decisions of many kinds. These decisions determine the well-being and, often, the very survival of clients, so it is important that the decisions be sound. Nurses use critical thinking to collect and interpret the information needed to make decisions. Nurses must use good judgment, for example, to decide which observations must be reported to the primary care provider immediately and which can be noted in the client record for the primary care provider to address later, during a routine visit with the client.

Creativity is a major component of critical thinking. When nurses incorporate creativity into their thinking, they are able to find unique solutions to unique problems. **Creativity** can be defined as thinking that results in the development of new ideas and products. Creativity in problem solving and decision making is the ability to develop and implement new and better solutions.

Creativity is required when the nurse encounters a new situation or a client situation in which traditional interventions are not effective.

CLINICAL EXAMPLE

For example, a pediatric home health nurse is caring for a 9-year-old girl who has ineffective respirations following abdominal surgery. The primary care provider has ordered incentive spirometry (a treatment device that promotes alveolar expansion). The child is frightened by the equipment and tires quickly during the treatments. The nurse offers her a bottle of blow bubbles and a blowing wand. She is delighted with blowing bubbles. The nurse knows that the respiratory effort in blowing bubbles will promote alveolar expansion and suggests that she blow bubbles between incentive spirometry treatments.

Creative thinkers must have knowledge of the problem. They must have assessed the present problem and be knowledgeable about the underlying facts and principles that apply. For example, in the previous situation, the nurse knows the anatomy and physiology of respiratory function and is aware of the purpose of incentive spirometry. The nurse also understands pediatric growth and development. In trying to assist the child, the nurse builds on this knowledge and comes up with a creative solution. Using creativity, nurses

- Generate many ideas rapidly
- Are generally flexible and natural; that is, they are able to change viewpoints or directions in thinking rapidly and easily
- Create original solutions to problems
- Tend to be independent and self-confident, even when under pressure
- Demonstrate individuality.

SKILLS IN CRITICAL THINKING

Complex mental processes such as analysis, problem solving, and decision making require the use of cognitive critical-thinking skills. These skills include critical analysis, inductive and deductive reasoning, making valid inferences, differentiating facts from opinions, evaluating the credibility of information sources, clarifying concepts, and recognizing assumptions.

Critical analysis is the application of a set of questions to a particular situation or idea to determine essential information and ideas and discard superfluous information and ideas. The questions are not sequential steps; rather, they are a set of criteria for judging an idea. Not all questions will need to be applied to every situation, but one should be aware of all the questions in order to choose those questions appropriate to a given situation. Socrates (born about 470 B.C.) was a Greek philosopher who developed the Socratic method of posing a question and seeking an answer. Box 34–19 lists Socratic questions to use in critical analysis. **Socratic questioning** is a technique one can use to look beneath the surface, recognize and examine assumptions, search for inconsistencies, examine multiple points of view, and differentiate what one knows from what one merely believes. Nurses should employ Socratic questioning when listening to an end-of-shift report, reviewing a history or progress notes, planning care, or discussing a client's care with colleagues.

Box 34–19 Socratic Questions

QUESTIONS ABOUT THE QUESTION (OR PROBLEM)
- Is this question clear, understandable, and correctly identified?
- Is this question important?
- Could this question be broken down into smaller parts?
- How might _____ state this question?

QUESTIONS ABOUT ASSUMPTIONS
- You seem to be assuming _____; is that so?
- What could you assume instead? Why?
- Does this assumption always hold true?

QUESTIONS ABOUT POINT OF VIEW
- You seem to be using the perspective of _____. Why?
- What would someone who disagrees with your perspective say?
- Can you see this any other way?

QUESTIONS ABOUT EVIDENCE AND REASONS
- What evidence do you have for that?
- Is there any reason to doubt that evidence?
- How do you know?
- What would change your mind?

QUESTIONS ABOUT IMPLICATIONS AND CONSEQUENCES
- What effect would that have?
- What is the probability that will actually happen?
- What are the alternatives?
- What are the implications of that?

Two other critical-thinking skills are inductive and deductive reasoning. In **inductive reasoning**, generalizations are formed from a set of facts or observations. When viewed together, certain bits of information suggest a particular interpretation. Inductive reasoning moves from specific examples (premises) to a generalized conclusion—for example, after touching several hot flames (premise), we conclude that *all* flames are hot. A nurse who observes a client who has dry skin, poor turgor, sunken eyes, and dark amber urine and who is otherwise determined to be dehydrated (premise) concludes that the presence of those signs indicate that other clients are dehydrated.

Deductive reasoning, by contrast, is reasoning from the general premise to the specific conclusion. If you begin with the premise that the sum of the angles in any triangle is always 180 degrees, you can then conclude that the sum of the angles in the triangle you happen to have is also 180 degrees. A nurse might start with a premise that all children love peanut butter sandwiches. If the client is a child, then the child will love peanut butter sandwiches. This is an example in which the premise is not always valid and, thus, the conclusion also may not be valid. Nurses use critical thinking to help analyze situations and establish which premises are valid.

In critical thinking, the nurse also differentiates statements of fact, inference, judgment, and opinion. Table 34–24 shows how these may be applied to a client. Evaluating the credibility of information sources is an important step in critical thinking. Unfortunately, we cannot always believe what we read or are told. The nurse may need to ascertain the accuracy of information by checking other documents or with other informants.

To comprehend a client situation clearly, the nurse and the client must agree on the meaning of terms. For example, if the client says to the nurse, "I think I have a tumor," the nurse needs to clarify what this word means to the client—the medical definition of tumor (a solid mass) or the common lay meaning of cancer—before responding.

Persons also live their lives under certain assumptions. Some people view humans as having a basically generous nature whereas others believe that the human tendency is to act in their own best interest. The nurse may believe that life should be considered worth living no matter what the condition whereas the client believes that quality of life is more important than quantity of life. If they recognize that they make choices based on these assumptions, they can still work together toward an acceptable plan of care. Difficulty arises when people do not take the time to consider what assumptions underlie their beliefs and actions.

ATTITUDES THAT FOSTER CRITICAL THINKING

Certain attitudes are crucial to critical thinking. These attitudes are based on the assumption that a rational person is motivated to develop, learn, and grow. A critical thinker works to develop the following attitudes or traits: independence, fair-mindedness, insight, intellectual humility, intellectual courage, integrity, perseverance, confidence, and curiosity.

Independence

Critical thinking requires that individuals think for themselves. People acquire many beliefs as children that provide an explanation that they understand but that may not necessarily be

TABLE 34–24 Differentiating Types of Statements

STATEMENT	DESCRIPTION	EXAMPLE
Facts	Can be verified through investigation	Blood pressure is affected by blood volume.
Inferences	Conclusions drawn from the facts, going beyond facts to make a statement about something not currently known	If blood volume is decreased (e.g., in hemorrhagic shock), the blood pressure will drop.
Judgments	Evaluation of facts or information that reflect values or other criteria; a type of opinion	It is harmful to the client's health if the blood pressure drops too low.
Opinions	Beliefs formed over time and include judgments that may fit facts or be in error	Nursing intervention can assist in maintaining the client's blood pressure within normal limits.

based on reason. As they mature and acquire knowledge and experience, critical thinkers examine their beliefs in the light of new evidence. Critical thinkers consider seriously a wide range of ideas, learn from them, and then make their own judgments about them. Nurses are open-minded about considering different methods of performing technical skills—not just the single way they may have been taught in school. They are not easily swayed by the opinions of others but take responsibility for their own views (Catalano, 2003).

Fair-Mindedness

Critical thinkers are fair-minded, assessing all viewpoints with the same standards and not basing their judgments on personal or group bias or prejudice (Catalano, 2003). Fair-mindedness helps one to consider opposing points of view and to try to understand new ideas fully before rejecting or accepting them. Critical thinkers strive to be open to the possibility that new evidence could change their minds. The nurse listens to opinions of all the members of a family, young and old.

Insight Into Egocentricity

Critical thinkers are open to the possibility that their personal biases or social pressures and customs could unduly affect their thinking. They actively try to examine their own biases and bring them to awareness each time they think or make a decision.

CLINICAL EXAMPLE

Kyle Keller, an RN working at an HIV/AIDS clinic, spends extensive time trying to teach Shaun Moore, a 35-year-old HIV positive client, how to prevent future recurrence of opportunistic infection. Mr. Keller is mystified when Mr. Moore appears uninterested and does not follow his advice. Mr. Keller's tendency to assume that all clients are motivated and interested in preventive care (as Mr. Keller is) resulted in an inaccurate assessment of Mr. Moore's desire to learn. As a result, both the nurse's and the client's time was wasted. Had Mr. Keller assessed Mr. Moore's background and beliefs about the problem and collected sufficient evidence, Mr. Keller might have identified a problem more relevant to the client's priorities and, thus, developed a better care plan.

Intellectual Humility

Intellectual humility means having an awareness of the limits of one's own knowledge. Critical thinkers are willing to admit what they do not know; they are willing to seek new information and to rethink their conclusions in light of new knowledge. They never assume that what everybody believes to be right will always be right, because new evidence may emerge. A hospital nurse might be unable to imagine how the elderly wife will care for her husband who has recently had a stroke. However, the nurse also recognizes that it is not really possible to know what the couple can achieve.

Intellectual Courage to Challenge the Status Quo and Rituals

With an attitude of courage, one is willing to consider and examine fairly one's own ideas or views, especially those to which one may have a strongly negative reaction. This type of

courage comes from recognizing that beliefs are sometimes false or misleading. Values and beliefs are not always acquired rationally. Rational beliefs are those that have been examined and found to be supported by solid reasons and data. After such examination, it is inevitable that some beliefs previously held to be true will be found to contain questionable elements and that some truth will emerge from ideas considered dangerous or false. Courage is needed to be true to new thinking in such cases, especially if social penalties for nonconformity are severe. As an example, previously many nurses believed that allowing family members to observe an emergency (such as cardiopulmonary resuscitation) would be psychologically harmful to the family and that members would get in the health care team's way. Others felt that blanket exclusion of family members was unnecessary and extremely stressful for some of them. As a result, nurses initiated research that has demonstrated that family presence can be accomplished without detrimental effects to the nurse, the client, or the family.

Integrity

Intellectual integrity requires that individuals apply the same rigorous standards of proof to their own knowledge and beliefs as they apply to the knowledge and beliefs of others. Critical thinkers question their own knowledge and beliefs as quickly and thoroughly as they challenge those of another. They are readily able to admit and evaluate inconsistencies within their own beliefs and between their own beliefs and those of another. A nurse might believe that wound care always requires sterile technique. Reading a new article on the use and outcomes of clean technique for some wounds leads the critically thinking nurse to reconsider.

Perseverance

Nurses who are critical thinkers show perseverance in finding effective solutions to client and nursing problems. This determination enables them to clarify concepts and sort out related issues, in spite of difficulties and frustrations. Confusion and frustration are uncomfortable, but critical thinkers resist the temptation to find a quick and easy answer. Important questions tend to be complex and confusing and therefore often require a great deal of thought and research to arrive at an answer. The nurse needs to continue to address the issue until it is resolved. For example, the nurses on a unit have tried to establish a policy for selected clients to leave the hospital on a pass rather than to be discharged and readmitted in the same day. The need for involvement of nursing, medical, administrative, and accounting staff gradually generates solutions to obstacles. The development of the policy moves forward, although very slowly.

Confidence

Critical thinkers believe that well-reasoned thinking will lead to trustworthy conclusions. Therefore, they cultivate an attitude of confidence in the reasoning process and examine emotion-laden arguments using the standards for evaluating thought by asking questions such as these: Is that argument fair? Is it based on sufficient evidence? Consider nurses attempting to determine the best way to allocate holiday time off for staff. Should they go by seniority, use random selection (lottery), give preference to those who have children, use "first-come, first-served," or use another method?

The critical thinker develops skill in both inductive reasoning and deductive reasoning. As the nurse gains greater awareness of the thinking process and more experience in improving such thinking, confidence in the process will grow. This nurse will not be afraid of disagreement and indeed will be concerned when others agree too quickly. Such a nurse can serve as a role model to colleagues, inspiring and encouraging them to think critically as well.

Curiosity

The mind of a critical thinker is filled with questions: Why do we believe this? What causes that? Does it have to be this way? Could something else work? What would happen if we did it another way? Who says that is so? The curious nurse may value tradition but is not afraid to examine traditions to be sure they are still valid. The nurse may, for example, apply these questions to the issue of moving responsibility for a procedure such as the drawing of arterial blood samples among the nursing, respiratory therapy, or laboratory department staff.

DEVELOPING CRITICAL THINKING ATTITUDES AND SKILLS

After gaining an idea of what it means to think critically, solve problems, and make decisions, nurses need to become aware of their own thinking style and abilities. Acquiring critical-thinking skills and a critical attitude then becomes a matter of practice. Critical thinking is not an "either-or" phenomenon; people develop and use it more or less effectively along a continuum. Some people make better evaluations than others do, some people believe information from nearly any source, and still others seldom believe anything without carefully evaluating the credibility of the information. Critical thinking is not easy. Solving problems and making decisions is risky. Sometimes the outcome is not what was desired. With effort, however, everyone can achieve some level of critical thinking to become an effective problem solver and decision maker.

Self-Assessment

The nurse should consider some of the attitudes discussed earlier that facilitate critical thinking, such as curiosity, fair-mindedness, humility, courage, and perseverance. A nurse might benefit from a rigorous personal assessment to determine which attitudes he or she already possesses and which need to be cultivated. This could also be done with a partner or as a group. The nurse first determines which attitudes he or she holds strongly and form a base for thinking and which attitudes he or she holds minimally or not at all. The nurse also needs to reflect on situations where he or she made decisions that were later regretted, and analyze thinking processes and attitudes or ask a trusted colleague to assess him or her. Identifying weak or vulnerable skills and attitudes is also important.

Reflection, at every step of critical thinking and nursing care, helps examine the ways in which the nurse gathers and analyzes data, makes decisions, and determines the effectiveness of interventions. Reflection requires the nurse to pause in order to consider his or her beliefs, knowledge, values, and abilities in the particular situation at hand. The purpose of this reflection is to determine if the current course of action is the best one and to improve future actions. Figure 34–20 ■, the Mind Map for Critical Thinking in Nursing, is a visual depiction of the interactive loops of concepts used in critical thinking. Note that the action of reflection appears as part of three of the steps shown: the starting points, processes, and outcomes.

Tolerating Dissonance and Ambiguity

The nurse needs to take deliberate efforts to cultivate critical-thinking attitudes. For example, to develop fair-mindedness, the nurse may deliberately seek out information that is in opposition to his or her own views; this provides practice in understanding and learning to be open to other viewpoints.

It is a human tendency to seek out information that corresponds to one's previously held beliefs and to ignore evidence that may contradict cherished ideas. This perspective is true for both the nurse and the client. Older adults may have great difficulty accepting the pervasiveness of technology, that people don't stay in the hospital as long as they did in the 1970s, or that having a diagnosis of cancer doesn't always mean that one is going to die. On the other hand, older adults have a wealth of knowledge and experience and often know better than the health care provider what will work well and be acceptable to them. Nurses should increase their tolerance for ideas that contradict previously held beliefs, and they should practice suspending judgment.

Suspending judgment means tolerating ambiguity for a time. If an issue is complex, it may not be resolved quickly or neatly, and judgment should be postponed. For a while, the nurse will need to say, "I don't know" and be comfortable with that answer until more is known. Although postponing judgment may not be feasible in emergency situations where fast action is required, it is usually feasible in other situations.

Seeking Situations Where Good Thinking Is Practiced

Nurses will find it valuable to attend conferences in clinical or educational settings that support open examination of all sides of issues and respect for opposing viewpoints. Cultivating a questioning attitude, using either Socratic questioning or another technique, is vital. Nurses need to review the standards for evaluating thinking and apply them to their own thinking. If nurses are aware of their own thinking—while they are doing the thinking—they can detect thinking errors.

Creating Environments That Support Critical Thinking

A nurse cannot develop or maintain critical-thinking attitudes in a vacuum. Nurses in leadership positions must be particularly aware of the climate for thinking that they establish, and they must actively create a stimulating environment that

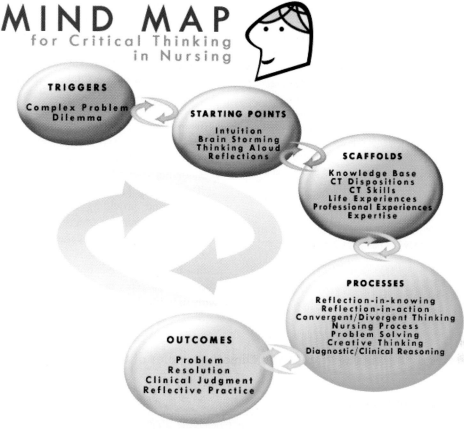

Figure 34–20 ■ Mind Map for Critical Thinking in Nursing.

Source: Duphorne, P., & Giddens, J. (2004). *Critical thinking in nursing.* Resource funded by intramural grant of College of Nursing, University of New Mexico.

encourages differences of opinion and fair examination of ideas and options. Nurses must embrace exploration of the perspectives of persons from different ages, cultures, religions, socioeconomic levels, and family structures. As leaders, nurses should encourage colleagues to examine evidence carefully before they come to conclusions, and to avoid "group think," the tendency to defer unthinkingly to the will of the group.

STANDARDS OF CRITICAL THINKING

How can one know whether one's thinking is critical thinking? Paul and Elder (2005) proposed that thinkers can use universal standards, shown in Table 34–25. Explicitly stating the standards for critical thinking promotes the reliability and validity of the thinking and thus makes appropriate action more likely. Forneris (2004) described core attributes of critical thinking: reflection, context, dialogue, and time. *Reflection* involves determining what data are relevant and making connections between that data and the decisions reached. *Context* is an essential consideration in nursing since care must always be individualized, taking knowledge and applying it to real people. *Dialogue*, which need not involve other persons, refers to the process of serving as both teacher and student in learning

from situations, questioning, making connections, and determining motivation. Finally, the attribute of *time* emphasizes the value of using past learning in current situations that then guide future actions.

TABLE 34–25 Universal Intellectual Standards

STANDARD	SAMPLE QUESTION
Clarity	What is an example of this?
Accuracy	How can I find out if that is true?
Relevance	How does that help me with the issue?
Logicalness	Does that follow from the evidence?
Breadth	Do I need to consider another point of view?
Precision	Can I be more specific?
Significance	Which of these facts is most important?
Completeness	Have I missed any important aspects?
Fairness	Am I considering the thinking of others?
Depth	What makes this a difficult problem?

Source: From Paul, R., Elder, L. (2005). *A guide for educators to critical thinking competency standards.* Foundation for Critical Thinking. Adapted with permission. www.criticalthinking.org

CLINICAL EXAMPLE

Martina Amarino, 62 years old, is admitted to the acute care facility with a medical diagnosis of pulmonary edema secondary to left-sided heart failure. Ms. Amarino has a history of type 2 diabetes requiring insulin injections in addition to oral hypoglycemic medications, hypertension, and early stage chronic renal failure. She is married, has no children, and lives with her husband in a high-rise apartment building that has a functioning elevator.

Within 12 hours of admission Ms. Amarino has lost 8 pounds, is breathing more comfortably, breath sounds are mostly clear with some fine rales in the bases, and vital signs have returned to within normal range. The next day when you return to the unit and are again assigned to her care you receive report from the previous shift that she has been confused and disoriented for the past two hours, her blood sugar last checked 30 minutes ago was within normal limits, and her husband has been notified and plans to come in and sit with her today but has not yet arrived.

Using critical thinking, answer the following questions:
1. What would you do first?
2. What data would you want to collect?
3. What factors could be contributing to Ms. Amarino's confusion?

APPLYING CRITICAL THINKING TO NURSING PRACTICE

Nurses function effectively some part of every day without thinking critically. Many small decisions are based primarily on habit with minimal thinking involved; examples include selecting what uniform to wear, choosing which route to take to work, and deciding what to eat for lunch. Psychomotor skills in nursing often involve minimal thinking, such as operating a familiar piece of equipment. However, the higher order skills of critical thinking are put into play as soon as a new idea is encountered or a less-than-routine decision must be made.

The nursing process is a systematic, rational method of planning and providing individualized nursing care. The phases of the nursing process—assessing, diagnosing, planning, implementing, and evaluating—are discussed in detail in Exemplar 34.1. The phases of the nursing process and application to a clinical example of critical thinking are shown in Table 34–26. This demonstrates the use of critical thinking with individual clients. In addition, a nurse employs critical

TABLE 34–26 Phases of the Nursing Process and Clinical Examples of Critical Thinking

NURSING PROCESS	CLINICAL APPLICATION
Assessment	*Data*: A 45-year-old male Latino complains of severe headache; 20 lb overweight; blood pressure 180/95 mm Hg. States he has been taking high blood pressure pills only when he has a headache. Is self-employed as a gardener; lives with wife, mother-in-law, and four children. Given these data, a critical thinker is aware that more data must be obtained about the client's cultural health values and reasons for stated behavior. Failure to think critically and to obtain additional data leads to inaccurate goals, diagnosis, and interventions.
Diagnosis	A critical thinker will defer identifying the client's diagnosis until more data are obtained and the client's priorities are known. This prevents a premature diagnosis based on insufficient data.
Diagnosis	As a critical thinker, the nurse is aware that the client's point of view may differ from the nurse's. Although the nurse may support the Western medical belief system that puts high priority on preventing disease, the critical thinker is also aware that the client may hold diverse views of health and illness, therapy, and preventive measures.
Diagnosis	The critical thinker recognizes that the client's erratic use of the prescribed medication may have multiple causes (e.g., troublesome side effects, or belief that illness is due to God's will and is not preventable) and will not infer a diagnosis with etiology until more data are obtained. Failure to think critically can lead to interpretations that are irrelevant, inadequate, and superficial (e.g., an erroneous interpretation that the client's problem is lack of sufficient knowledge).
Diagnosis	The critical thinker makes assumptions in accordance with a broad, unbiased database and mutually set client goals. The critical thinker avoids making unverified assumptions, such as that an increase in knowledge will increase this client's compliance or that this client is motivated to prevent a cerebrovascular accident (CVA).
Plan	*Goal:* To increase compliance with medication regimen in order to relieve headaches and prevent a CVA. Thinking critically, a nurse will try to determine the client's goals and to agree to mutual goals.
Plan	The critical thinker uses concepts about motivation, change theory, and multicultural nursing to understand the client's behavior and motivation to change. Failure to think critically can lead to exclusive reliance on a simplistic concept, such as "knowledge creates change." Plans of care, including goals and outcomes, are based on ongoing assessment of the client's cultural values, beliefs, and needs.
Implementation	The critical thinker considers the implications and consequences of selected nursing strategies before implementing plans of care. Failure to think critically may lead to ineffective interventions, such as client teaching that focuses only on resolving a knowledge deficit about the prescribed medication. The critical thinker recognizes that a knowledge deficit may or may not be one of several problems.
Evaluation	The critical thinker bases evaluation of client outcomes and the effectiveness of nursing interventions on well-developed, measurable criteria and considers rationally whether outcomes have been validated. Failure to think critically may lead to client noncompliance and an inference that the client did not learn effectively and needs further instruction.

thinking when setting priorities for the day. When analyzing a situation and planning strategies for conflict resolution or change, the nurse manager uses critical-thinking attitudes and skills. The nurse clinician and nurse manager seek awareness of their thinking as they are thinking, as they apply standards for thinking, and as their thinking progresses.

Nurses use critical thinking in nursing practice primarily when solving problems and making decisions. These two processes are described in more detail.

REVIEW Critical Thinking

RELATE: LINK THE CONCEPTS

Linking the exemplar of Critical Thinking with the concept of Accountability:

1. How is the use of critical thinking related to the nurse's accountability to the client?
2. How is the use of critical thinking related to the nurse's accountability to the employer?

Linking the exemplar of Critical Thinking with the concept of Evidenced-Based Practice:

3. The nurse with strong critical thinking maintains an evidenced based practice by _____.
4. The nurse reads a peer reviewed article that recommends changing currently accepted practice. What critical thinking will the nurse perform before accepting the article's recommendations?

REFER: GO TO MYNURSINGKIT

REFLECT: CASE STUDY

Doniette McEverson, 31 years old, was born with cerebral palsy and is profoundly mentally retarded. She has very limited mobility and uses a wheelchair when she is out of bed. She has no control over the chair's movement and is pushed by an attendant. She lives in a group home with other mentally retarded adults and spends weekends at home with her family. She is brought to the emergency department during one of her weekend visits after falling down a flight of stairs and losing consciousness for "about 5 minutes" according to her mother. When asked for more detail about the accident, her mother reports that the door to the basement was left open and her sister forgot to lock the wheels when Doniette was dressed and brought into the living area this morning. Mrs. McEverson assumes that Doniette somehow managed to move the chair toward the door and fell but says she didn't witness the fall, only heard the crash and ran to see what had happened, finding Doniette at the bottom of the stairs.

Using critical thinking, answer the following questions:

1. What is your priority action at this time?
2. What is your interpretation of what Mrs. McEverson related regarding the accident?
3. What interview questions would you ask and of whom would you ask them?

REFERENCES

Agency for Healthcare Research and Quality. (2004). *Mission statement: Center for Quality Improvement and Patient Safety*. Rockville, MD. Retrieved April 16, 2006, from http://www.ahrq.gov/about/cquips/cquipsmiss.htm

Alfaro-LeFevre, R. (2004). *Critical thinking in nursing: A practical approach* (3rd ed.). Philadelphia: W. B. Saunders.

American Nurses Association. (1973). *Standards of nursing practice*. Kansas City, MO: Author.

American Nurses Association. (2004). *Nursing: Scope and standards of nursing practice*. Kansas City, MO: Author.

American Nurses Association. (2010). Unlicensed assistive personnel. Retrieved February 19, 2010, from http://www.nursingworld.org/MainMenuCategories/HealthcareandPolicyIssues/ANAPositionStatements/uap.aspx

Anthony, M. (1999). The relationship of authority to decision-making behavior, implications for redesign. *Research Nursing Health, 22,* 388–398.

Bennis, W., & Goldsmith, G. (1997). *Learning to lead.* Reading, MA: Perseus Books.

Berlowitz, D. R., Young, G. J., Hickey, E. C., Saliba, D., Mittman, B. S., Czarnowski, E., et al. (2003). Quality improvement implementation in the nursing home. *Health Services Research, 38*(1 Part 1), 65–83.

Bernhard, L., & Walsh, M. (1990). Leadership: The key to the profession of nursing (2nd ed.). St. Louis, MO: C. V. Mosby.

Blegen, M., et al. (1993). Preferences for decision-making autonomy. *Image Journal of Nursing Scholarship, 25,* 339–344.

Carpenito-Moyet, L. J. (2006). *Nursing diagnosis: Application to clinical practice* (11th ed.). Philadelphia: Lippincott Williams & Wilkins.

Catalano, J. T. (2003). *Nursing now! Today's issues, tomorrow's trends* (3rd ed.). Philadelphia: F. A. Davis.

D'Amico, D., & Barbarito, C. (2007). *Health & physical assessment in nursing.* Upper Saddle River, NJ: Pearson Prentice Hall.

Dessler, G. (2002). *Management.* Upper Saddle River, NJ: Prentice Hall.

Dochterman, J., & Bulechek, G. B. (Eds.). (2004). *Nursing interventions classification (NIC)* (4th ed.). St. Louis, MO: Mosby.

Finkelman, A. (2001). *Managed care: A nursing perspective.* Upper Saddle River, NJ: Prentice Hall.

Forneris, S. G. (2004). Exploring the attributes of critical thinking: A conceptual basis. *International Journal of Nursing Education Scholarship, 1* (1), Article 9, 1–19. Retrieved June 18, 2006, from http://www.bepress.comlijnes/vol1/iss1/art9

Gebelein, S., et al. (2000). *Successful manager's handbook.* Minneapolis, MN: Personnel Decisions International Corporation.

Gordon, M. (2006). *Manual of nursing diagnosis* (11th ed.). Boston: Jones & Bartlett.

Hall, L. (1955, June). Quality of nursing care. *Public Health News.* Newark, NJ: State Department of Health.

Hendry, C., & Walker, A. (2004). Priority setting in clinical nursing practice: Literature review. *Journal of Advanced Nursing, 47,* 427–436.

Hicks, F. D., Merritt, S. L., & Elstein, A. S. (2003). Critical thinking and clinical decision making in critical care nursing: A pilot study. *Heart & Lung, 32,* 169–180.

Johnson, D. E. (1959). A philosophy of nursing. *Nursing Outlook, 7,* 198–200.

Joint Commission on Accreditation of Healthcare Organizations. (2005). *2005 Comprehensive accreditation manual for hospitals.* Chicago: Author.

Kim, M. J., McFarland, G. K., & McLane, A. M. (Eds.). (1984). *Classification of nursing diagnoses: Proceedings of the fifth national conference.* St. Louis, MO: Mosby.

Kohn, L. T., Corrigan, J. M., & Donaldson, M. S. (Eds.). (2000). *To err is human: Building a safer health system.* Washington, DC: Committee on Quality of Health Care in America, Institute of Medicine National Academy Press. Retrieved June 21, 2006, from http://books.nap.edu/books/0309068371/html/index.html

Krairiksh, M., & Anthony, M. (2001). Benefits and outcomes of staff nurses' participation in decisionmaking. *Journal of Nursing Administration, 31*(1), 16–23.

Lamont, S. C. (2003). Discomfort as a potential nursing diagnosis: A concept analysis and literature review. *International Journal of Nursing Terminologies and Classifications, 14*(4 Suppl), 5.

Leape, L. L., & Berwick, D. M. (2005). Five years after To Err Is Human: What have we learned? *Journal of the American Medical Association, 293,* 2384–2390.

Lopes, M. H. B., & Higa, R. (2003). Mixed incontinence in women: A new nursing diagnosis. *International Journal of Nursing Terminologies and Classifications, 14*(4 Suppl), 49.

Milgram, L., Spector, A., & Treger, M. (1999). *Managing smart.* Houston, TX: Cashman Dudley.

Moorhead, S., Johnson, M., & Maas, M. (Eds.). (2004). *Nursing outcomes classification (NOC)* (3rd ed) St. Louis, MO: Mosby.

NANDA International. (2009). *NANDA nursing diagnoses: Definitions and classification 2009–2011.* Wiley-Blackwell, Chichester, West Suffix, Great Britain.

National League for Nursing. (2000). *Think tank on critical thinking.* New York: Author.

Orem, D. E. (2001). *Nursing: Concepts of practice* (6th ed.). St. Louis, MO: Mosby.

Orlando, I. (1961). *The dynamic nurse–patient relationship.* New York: Putnam.

Paul, R., & Elder, L. (2005). *A guide for educators to critical thinking competency standards.*

Roy, C., & Andrews, H. A. (1998). *The Roy adaptation model* (2nd ed.). Upper Saddle River, NJ: Prentice Hall.

Stewart, C. J., & Cash, Jr., W. B. (2006). *Interviewing principles and practices* (11th ed.). New York: McGraw-Hill.

Wiedenbach, E. (1963). The helping art of nursing. *American Journal of Nursing, 63*(11), 54–57.

Wilkinson, J. M. (2007). *Nursing process & critical thinking* (4th ed.). Upper Saddle River, NJ: Prentice Hall Health. Dillon Beach, CA: Foundation for Critical Thinking.

Collaboration

35

Concept at-a-Glance

About Collaboration, *2113*

35.1   Case Management, *2121*

35.2   Chain of Command, *2126*

35.3   Conflict Resolution, *2127*

35.4   Interdisciplinary Teams
        and Communication, *2133*

35.5   Management Theories, *2142*

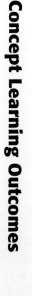

Concept Learning Outcomes

After reading about this concept, you will be able to:

1. Expand upon the essential aspects of collaborative nursing practice.

2. Analyze factors that affect collaboration in health care.

3. Analyze the purpose and need for a chain of command within an organization.

4. Expand upon strategies for conflict prevention, response, and management.

5. Differentiate between different types of interdisciplinary and intradisciplinary groups in nursing and health care delivery.

6. Describe characteristics of effective groups using the essential characteristics of group dynamics.

7. Contrast leaders and managers.

8. Categorize various leadership styles, behaviors, and theories.

Concept Key Terms

Collaboration, *2113*
Communicator style, *2119*
Feedback, *2119*
Mutual respect, *2119*

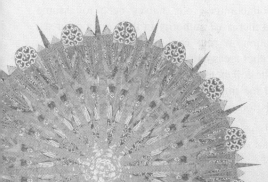

About Collaboration

The nature of health care today is so complex that it is impossible for any single provider or professional to provide quality client care without working with others. The best care is delivered in a collaborative environment with all members of the health care team working to improve client health outcomes. **Collaboration** is defined as two or more people working toward a common goal by combining their skills, knowledge, and resources while avoiding duplication of effort. In a health care environment, the common goal of each collaborative

---

Box 35–1 Characteristics and Beliefs Basic to Collaborative Health Care

- Clients have a right to self-determination—that is, the right to choose to participate or not to participate in health care decision making.
- Clients and health care professionals interact in a reciprocal relationship. Instead of making decisions about the client's health care, health care professionals engage in joint decision making with the client.
- Equality among human beings is desired in collaborative health care relationships. The ideas of both clients and health care professionals receive an equal hearing.

- Responsibility for the client's health falls on the client rather than on health care professionals.
- Each individual's concept of health is important and legitimate for that individual. Although clients lack expert knowledge, they have their own ideas about health and illness. Health care professionals need to understand these ideas to be able to effectively help the client.
- Collaboration involves negotiating and seeking consensus rather than questioning and ordering.

---

team is to improve client outcomes, whether the client is an individual, a group, or a community.

Changing models of health care have created a need for modification of traditional roles. Nurses and physicians have been especially affected by these changes and work more collaboratively as colleagues. According to the American Nurses Association (ANA) (1995),

The boundaries of each health care professional are constantly changing, and members of various professions cooperate by exchanging knowledge and ideas about how to deliver high-quality health care. Collaboration among health care professionals involves recognition of the expertise of others within and outside one's profession and referral to those providers when appropriate. Collaboration also involves some shared functions and common focus on the same overall mission.

During the early years, the nurse was seen as providing assistance to the physician in caring for clients, except during wars and times of crisis when nurses worked in a more collegial (friendly) and autonomous manner. As early as the American Civil War, there is documentation of a more independent approach to nursing practice (ANA, 1998). The emergence of advanced practice nursing roles led to an increasing focus on collaboration.

In 1992, the ANA held a Congress on Nursing Practice and adopted the following operational definition of collaboration:

Collaboration means a collegial working relationship with another health care provider in the provision of (to supply) patient care. Collaborative practice requires (may include) the discussion of patient diagnosis and cooperation in the management and delivery of care. Each collaborator is available to the other for consultation either in person or by communication device, but need not be physically present on the premises at the time the actions are performed. The patient-designated health care provider is responsible for the overall direction and management of patient care. (ANA, 1992)

Virginia Henderson (1991, p. 44), one of the pioneers of nursing, defines collaborative care as "a partnership relationship between doctors, nurses, and other health care providers with patients and their families." Mutual respect and a true sharing of both power and control are essential elements. Ideally, collaboration becomes a dynamic, interactive process in which clients (individuals, groups, or communities) work together with physicians,

nurses, and other health care providers to meet their health objectives. Effective collaboration requires cooperation and coordination between client(s) and various health care providers across the continuum of care (see Box 35–1). ●

THE NURSE AS COLLABORATOR

A published executive summary from the ANA (1998) released in *Nursing Trends and Issues* described collaboration as intrinsic to nursing, as follows:

- Collaboration involves nurses and physicians working together and independently assessing, diagnosing, and caring for consumers by preparing client histories, conducting physical and psychosocial assessments, and reviewing and discussing their cases with other health professionals to determine the changing health status of each client.
- To provide effective and comprehensive care, nurses, physicians, and other health care professionals must collaborate with each other. No group can claim total authority over the other.
- The different areas of professional competence exhibited by each profession, when combined, provide a continuum of care that the consumer has come to expect.

The ANA *Nursing: Scope and Standards of Practice* (2004) includes collaboration by the registered nurse with clients and families as well as other health care providers. See Box 35–2.

Nurses collaborate with clients, peers, and other health care professionals. They frequently collaborate about client care but may also be involved in collaborating on bioethical issues, on legislation, on health-related research, and with professional organizations. Box 35–3 outlines selected aspects of the nurse's role as a collaborator.

To fulfill a collaborative role, nurses need to assume accountability and increased authority in their practice areas. Continuing education in role exploration, communication, group work, and other areas helps members of the health care team understand the collaborative nature of their roles, specific contributions, and the importance of working together. Each professional needs to understand how an integrated delivery

Box 35–2 ANA Standard of Professional Nursing Performance

Standard 11. Collaboration

THE REGISTERED NURSE COLLABORATES WITH PATIENT, FAMILY, AND OTHERS IN THE CONDUCT OF NURSING PRACTICE.

Measurement Criteria

The registered nurse:

- Communicates with the patient, family, and other health care providers regarding patient care and the nurse's role in the provision of that care.
- Collaborates in creating a documented plan focused on outcomes and decisions related to care and delivery of services, that indicates communication with patients, families, and others.
- Partners with others to effect change and generate positive outcomes through knowledge of the patient or situation.
- Documents referrals, including provisions for continuity of care.

Additional Measurement Criteria for the Advanced Practice Registered Nurse:

The advanced practice registered nurse:

- Partners with other disciplines to enhance patient care through interdisciplinary activities, such as education, consultation, management, technological development, or research opportunities.
- Facilitates an interdisciplinary process with other members of the health care team.
- Documents plan of care communications, rationales for plan of care changes, and collaborative discussions to improve patient care.

Additional Measurement Criteria for Nursing Role Specialty:

The registered nurse in a nursing role specialty:

- Partners with others to enhance health care and, ultimately, patient care through interdisciplinary activities, such as education, consultation, management, technological development, or research opportunities.
- Documents plans, communications, rationales for plan changes, and collaborative discussions.

Source: From American Nurses Association. (2004). *Nursing: Scope and standards of practice.* Washington, DC: ANA. Used by Permission.

---

system centers on the client's health care needs rather than on the particular care given by any one group. Table 35–1 lists a number of professionals who may serve as members of the health care team and their respective roles.

In addition to collaborating with other members of the health care team, nurses must collaborate with clients. Kim's theory of collaborative decision making in nursing practice (1983, 1987) describes and explains collaborative interactions between clients and nurses in making health care decisions and how these affect client outcomes. Dalton (2003)

expanded the theory to include the client, nurse, and family caregiver. In this theory, all three enter into the collaboration from their own context of role expectations and attitudes, knowledge, personal traits, and definition of the situation. The three combine to form a coalition with opportunities for collaboration within the context of the situation. Dalton's theory proposes that level of collaboration achieved and the nature of the decision are the primary outcomes leading to secondary outcomes of goal attainment, autonomy, and satisfaction.

Box 35–3 The Nurse as a Collaborator

WITH CLIENTS:

- Acknowledges, supports, and encourages clients' active involvement in health care decisions.
- Encourages a sense of client autonomy and an equal position with other members of the health care team.
- Helps clients set mutually agreed-upon goals and objectives for health care.
- Provides the client with consultation in a collaborative fashion.

WITH PEERS:

- Shares personal expertise with other nurses and elicits the expertise of others to ensure quality client care.
- Develops a sense of trust and mutual respect with peers that recognizes their unique contributions.

WITH OTHER HEALTH CARE PROFESSIONALS:

- Recognizes the contribution that each member of the interdisciplinary team can make by virtue of his or her expertise and view of the situation.
- Listens to each individual's views.

- Shares health care responsibilities with other members of the team in order to explore care options, set realistic and attainable goals, and make decisions about the plan of care with clients and their families.
- Participates in collaborative interdisciplinary research to increase knowledge of a clinical problem or situation.

WITH PROFESSIONAL NURSING ORGANIZATIONS:

- Seeks out opportunities to collaborate with and within professional organizations.
- Serves on committees in state (or provincial), national, and international nursing organizations or specialty groups.
- Supports professional organizations in political action to create solutions for professional and health care concerns.

WITH LEGISLATORS:

- Offers expert opinions on legislative initiatives related to health care.
- Collaborates with other health care providers and consumers on health care legislation to best serve the needs of the public.

TABLE 35-1 Members of the Health Care Team

HEALTH CARE PROFESSIONAL	ROLE
Nurse	The role of the nurse varies with the needs of the client, the nurse's credentials, and the type of employment setting. A registered nurse (RN) assesses a client's health status, identifies health problems, and develops and coordinates care. A licensed vocational nurse (LVN), in some states known as a licensed practical nurse (LPN), provides direct client care under the direction of a registered nurse, physician, or other licensed practitioner.
Unlicensed assistive personnel	Unlicensed assistive personnel (UAP) are health care staff who assume delegated aspects of basic client care. These tasks include bathing, assisting with feeding, and collecting specimens. UAP titles include certified nurse assistants, hospital attendants, nurse technicians, patient care technicians, and orderlies. Some of these categories of provider may have standardized education and job duties (e.g., certified nurse assistants), while others do not. The parameters regarding nurse delegation to UAP are delineated by the state boards of nursing.
Alternative (complementary) care provider	Alternative or complementary health care refers to those practices not commonly considered part of Western medicine. Chiropractors, herbalists, acupuncturists, massage therapists, reflexologists, holistic health healers, and other health care providers are playing increasing roles in the contemporary health care system. These providers may practice alongside Western health care providers, or clients may use their services in conjunction with, or instead of, Western therapies.
Case manager	The case manager's role is to ensure that clients receive fiscally sound, appropriate care in the best setting. This role is often filled by the member of the health care team who is most involved in the client's care. Depending on the nature of the client's concerns, the case manager may be a nurse, a social worker, or any other member of the health care team.
Dentist	Dentists diagnose and treat dental problems. Dentists are also actively involved in preventive measures to maintain healthy oral structures (e.g., teeth and gums). Many hospitals, especially long-term care facilities, have dentists on staff.
Dietician or nutritionist	A dietitian, often a registered dietitian, has special knowledge about the diets required to maintain health and to treat disease. Dietitians in hospitals generally are concerned with therapeutic diets, may design special diets to meet the nutritional needs of individual clients, and supervise the preparation of meals to ensure that clients receive the proper diet. A nutritionist is a person who has special knowledge about nutrition and food. The nutritionist in a community setting recommends healthy diets and gives broad advisory services about the purchase and preparation of foods. Community nutritionists often function at the preventive level. They promote health and prevent disease, for example, by advising families about balanced diets for growing children and pregnant women.
Occupational therapist	An occupational therapist (OT) assists clients with impaired function to gain the skills to perform activities of daily living. For example, an occupational therapist might teach a man with severe arthritis in his arms and hands how to adjust his kitchen utensils so that he can continue to cook. The occupational therapist teaches skills that are therapeutic and at the same time provide some fulfillment. For example, weaving is a recreational activity but also exercises the arthritic man's arms and hands.
Paramedical technologist	Laboratory technologists, radiological technologists, and nuclear medicine technologists are just three kinds of paramedical technologists in the expanding field of medical technology. *Paramedical* means having some connection with medicine. Laboratory technologists, for example, examine specimens such as urine, feces, blood, and discharges from wounds to provide exact information that facilitates the medical diagnosis and the prescription of a therapeutic regimen.
Pharmacist	A pharmacist prepares and dispenses medications in hospital and community settings. The role of the pharmacist in monitoring and evaluating the actions and effects of medications on clients is becoming increasingly prominent. A clinical pharmacist is a specialist who guides physicians in prescribing medications.
Physical therapist	The licensed physical therapist (PT) assists clients with musculoskeletal problems. Physical therapists treat movement dysfunctions by means of heat, water, exercise, massage, and electric current. The physical therapist's functions include assessing client mobility and strength, providing therapeutic measures (e.g., exercises and heat applications to improve mobility and strength), and teaching new skills (e.g., how to walk with an artificial leg). Some physical therapists provide their services in hospitals; however, independent practitioners establish offices in communities and serve clients either at the office or in the home.
Physician	The physician is responsible for medical diagnosis and for determining the therapy required by a person who has a disease or injury. The physician's role has traditionally been the treatment of disease and trauma (injury); however, many physicians are now including health promotion and disease prevention in their practice. Some physicians are general practitioners (also known as primary care or family practitioners), while others are dermatologists, neurologists, oncologists, orthopedists, pediatricians, psychiatrists, radiologists, or surgeons—to name a few.

TABLE 35–1 **Members of the Health Care Team** (continued)

HEALTH CARE PROFESSIONAL	ROLE
Physician assistant	Physician assistants (PAs) perform certain tasks under the direction of a physician. They diagnose and treat certain diseases, conditions, and injuries. In many states, nurses are not legally permitted to follow a PA's orders unless they are cosigned by a physician. In some settings, PAs and nurse practitioners have similar job descriptions.
Respiratory therapist	A respiratory therapist is skilled in therapeutic measures used in the care of clients with respiratory problems. These therapists are knowledgeable about oxygen therapy devices, intermittent positive pressure breathing respirators, artificial mechanical ventilators, and accessory devices used in inhalation therapy. Respiratory therapists administer many of the pulmonary function tests.
Social worker	A social worker counsels clients and their support persons regarding problems, such as finances, marital difficulties, and adoption of children. It is not unusual for health problems to produce problems in day-to-day living and vice versa. For example, an elderly woman who lives alone and has a stroke resulting in impaired walking may find it impossible to continue to live in her third-floor apartment. Finding a more suitable living arrangement can be the responsibility of the social worker if the client has no support network in place.

COLLABORATIVE PRACTICE

The overall objectives of collaborative initiatives are high-quality client care and client satisfaction. In addition, many health care professionals believe that a multidisciplinary, collaborative framework can limit costs as well as enhance quality. Collaborative practice models attempt to achieve the following objectives:

- Provide client-directed and client-centered care using a multidisciplinary, integrated, participative framework.
- Enhance continuity of care across the continuum of health, from wellness and prevention, through acute illness, to recovery or rehabilitation.
- Improve client(s) and family satisfaction with care.
- Provide quality, cost-effective, research-based care that improves client outcomes.
- Promote mutual respect, communication, and understanding between the client(s) and members of the health care team.
- Create a synergy among clients and providers, in which the sum of their efforts is greater than the parts.
- Provide opportunities to address and solve system-related issues and problems.
- Develop interdependent relationships and understanding among providers and clients.

Collaborative practice can include nurse–physician interaction in joint practice, nurse–physician collaboration in caregiving, or interdisciplinary collaboration in planning and care by a number of health care providers working on behalf of the same client or community. Interdisciplinary teams may include nurses, physicians, therapists, and social workers.

Collaborative health care teams provide comprehensive care by providing a full range of expertise. They can manage care with less redundancy, more efficiency, and fewer omissions (Patel, Cytryn, Shortliffe, & Safran, 2000). These interdisciplinary health care teams have been particularly effective in outpatient services where clients are seen by a primary care physician or by a nurse practitioner and consultations are implemented as needed. The ability to collaborate becomes particularly important when nurses implement advanced-practice roles; it has been designated as a core competency for advanced-practice nurses.

This increased emphasis on collaboration is a result of changes in certification and practice standards as well as changes in health care reform, such as group practice and managed care. A continuum of collaboration, as illustrated in Figure 35–1 ■, reflects the following levels of communication

---

EVIDENCE-BASED PRACTICE **Collaborative Health Care for Chronically Ill Older Adults**

An interdisciplinary, collaborative practice intervention for community-dwelling seniors with a chronic illness included a primary care physician, a nurse, and a social worker. A cohort study of 543 patients in 18 private offices was conducted, with half the group receiving care from the collaborative practice team and the other half receiving care from the primary care physician only. Before the start of the study, both groups were determined to be equivalent in service use and self-reported health status. During the study the control group (physician only) increased their hospitalization rate while the intervention group stayed at baseline. Readmission in the intervention group decreased over a year and the control group readmission rate

increased. Visits to the physician increased in the control group and decreased in the intervention group. Further, the seniors in the intervention group reported that they engaged in an increased number of social activities compared to the control group. This model of primary care collaborative practice supports the effectiveness in reducing utilization of service and maintaining health status for seniors with chronic illness.

Source: Sommers, L., Marton, K., Barbaccia, J., & Randolph, J. (2000). Physician, nurse, and social worker collaboration in primary care for chronically ill seniors. *Archives of Internal Medicine, 160*(12), 1825–1833.

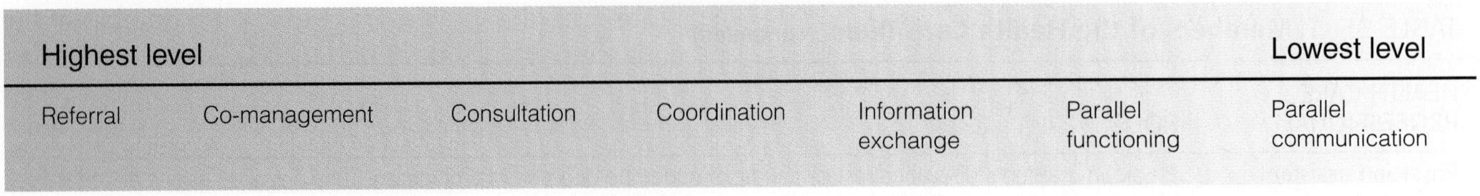

Highest level						Lowest level
Referral	Co-management	Consultation	Coordination	Information exchange	Parallel functioning	Parallel communication

Figure 35–1 ■ Continuum of collaboration.

and action, beginning with parallel communication and progressing toward co-management and referral:

■ Parallel communication is when each professional communicates with the client independently and asks the same or similar questions.
■ Parallel functioning is when communication may be more coordinated, but each professional has separate interventions and a separate plan of care.
■ Information exchange involves planned communication, but decision making is unilateral, involving little, if any, collegiality.
■ Coordination and consultation represent midrange levels of collaboration seeking to maximize the efficiency of resources.
■ Co-management and referral represent the upper levels of collaboration, where providers retain responsibility and accountability for their own aspects of care and clients are directed to other providers when the problem is beyond the initial provider's expertise.

Characteristics of effective collaboration include the following:

1. Common purpose and goals identified at the outset
2. Clinical competence of each provider
3. Interpersonal competence
4. Humor
5. Trust
6. Valuing and respecting diverse, complementary knowledge.

Processes associated with these characteristics include recurring interactions that develop connections and, therefore, mutual respect and trust among the health care professionals. Interpersonal skills and respect for the competence of all collaborators are essential to achieving greater health outcomes for clients.

BENEFITS OF COLLABORATIVE CARE

A collaborative approach to health care ideally benefits clients, professionals, and the health care delivery system. Care becomes client centered and, most important, client directed. Clients become informed consumers and actively participate with the health care team in the decision-making process. When clients are empowered to participate actively and professionals share mutually set goals with clients, quality of care improves and everyone—including the organization and health care system—ultimately benefits. When quality improves, adherence to therapeutic regimens increases, lengths of stay decrease, and overall costs to the system decline. When professional interdependence develops, collegial relationships emerge and overall satisfaction increases. A collegial relationship is characterized by cooperation and shared authority. The work environment becomes more supportive and acknowledges the contributions of each team member: "Because authority is shared, this effort results in more integrated and comprehensive care, as well as shared control of costs and liability" (Miccolo & Spanier, 1993, p. 447).

COMPETENCIES BASIC TO COLLABORATION

Key features necessary for collaboration include effective communication skills, mutual respect, trust, giving and receiving feedback, decision making, and conflict management.

Communication Skills

Collaborating to solve complex problems requires effective communication skills. Initially, the health care team needs to define collaboration clearly, establish its goals and objectives, and specify each team member's role.

EVIDENCE-BASED PRACTICE **Attitudes Toward Physician–Nurse Collaboration**

The purpose of this study was to test three hypotheses about attitudes toward collaboration across genders, disciplines, and cultures.
1. U.S. physicians and nurses would both express more positive attitudes toward physician–nurse collaboration than their Mexican counterparts.
2. Nurses would express more positive attitudes toward physician–nurse collaboration than physicians regardless of the country in which they practice.
3. Female physicians would express more positive attitudes toward physician–nurse collaboration than their male counterparts.
An attitude scale was administered to a total of 639 physicians and nurses working in the United States and Mexico. A three-way analysis

of variance confirmed the first two hypotheses and did not confirm the third. Based upon these findings, the researchers recommend that medical and nursing schools in both countries teach the importance of collaboration in their curricula to facilitate an understanding of the complementary nature of the roles and to encourage an interdependent relationship. This collaborative education is needed to promote positive attitudes toward collaborative practice.

Source: Hojat, M., Nasca, T., Cohen, M., Fields, S., Rattner, S., Griffiths, M., Ibarra, D., de Gonzalez, A., Torres-Ruiz, A., Ibarra, G., & Garcia, A. (2001). Attitudes toward physician-nurse collaboration: A cross-cultural study of male and female physicians and nurses in the United States and Mexico. *Nursing Research, 50*(2), 123–128.

Effective communication can occur only if each team member is committed to understanding each member's professional role and appreciating each member as an individual. Additionally, each member must be sensitive to differences among communication styles. Instead of focusing on distinctions among members, each team must center on his or her common purpose: to meet the client's needs.

Communication styles are especially important to successful collaboration. Norton's theory of **communicator style** (1983) defines style as the manner in which one communicates and includes the way in which one interacts. Therefore, what is said and how it is said are both important. This theory describes nine specific communicator styles that commonly are used and influence the nature of the relationship between communicants. Three of these communicator styles (dominant, contentious, and attentive) have been used in a nursing study of collaboration styles as they relate to degree of collaboration and improved quality of care (Van Ess Coeling & Cukr, 2000). This study found that using attentive style and avoiding contentious (argumentative) and dominant styles made a significant difference in nurse–physician collaboration, positive client outcomes, and nurse satisfaction. The researchers assert that attentive style can be taught by modeling the behavior of obvious listening, such as making eye contact while communicating and refraining from participating in other activities while someone is trying to communicate. Verbal feedback and the act of repeating back what is said offer the listener the opportunity to reflect on what the speaker said and to correct misunderstanding. Questioning provides an opportunity to share concerns and initiate dialogue. To prevent conflict, an individual must develop the judgment to recognize when it is necessary to stop a conversation and ask for clarification of an important point and when it is better to ignore a comment that is not essential to the goal, even if the individual finds the comment disagreeable. To avoid developing a dominant style of communication, the individual must avoid monopolizing conversations or speaking so forcefully that others become too intimidated to respond. Role-playing followed by discussion and role modeling have been identified as effective strategies for developing positive communicator styles.

Mutual Respect and Trust

Mutual respect occurs when two or more people show or feel honor or esteem toward one another. Trust occurs when a person is confident in the actions of another person. Both mutual respect and trust imply a mutual process and outcome. They must be expressed both verbally and nonverbally. Sometimes professionals may verbalize respect or trust of others but demonstrate a lack of trust and respect through their actions. The health care system itself has not always created an environment that promotes respect or trust of the various health care providers. Although progress has been made toward creating more trusting relationships, past attitudes may continue to impede efforts toward collaborative practice. Magnet hospitals are an example of successful efforts by health care organizations to foster respect among professionals. They have found that placing the head of the nursing department (previously

known as the Director of Nursing) on an equal managerial level with the chief of physicians (usually called the Chief Medical Officer) improves mutual respect between physicians and nurses, thereby improving their relationships.

Giving and Receiving Feedback

One of the most difficult challenges for professionals is giving and receiving timely, relevant, and helpful **feedback** (the response the receiver of a message gives to the message's sender) to and from each other and their clients. When professionals work closely together, it may be appropriate to address attitudes or actions that affect the collaborative relationship. Giving and receiving feedback may be affected by each person's perceptions, personal space, roles, relationships, self-esteem, confidence, beliefs, emotions, environment, and time. For example, a supervisor who chooses to give feedback to an employee the day after the employee returns from funeral leave is a) likely not to have the employee's full attention during the meeting and b) likely to invite responses from the employee that the employee might not normally make.

Negative feedback implies not negative content but rather a negative communication style, such as an attitude of condescension. Positive feedback is characterized by a communication style that is warm, caring, and respectful. A review of basic communication skills and an opportunity to practice listening and giving and receiving feedback can enhance any professional's ability to communicate effectively (Ferguson, Howell, & Batalden, 1993, p. 5). Giving and receiving feedback helps individuals acquire self-awareness, while assisting the collaborative team to develop an understanding and effective working relationship. It is important that each nurse and health care provider learn to accept feedback in a professional manner without becoming defensive. Communication techniques are discussed in greater detail in Concept 36, Communication.

Decision Making

Collaboration involves shared responsibility for the outcome. Obviously, to create a solution, the team must follow each step of the decision-making process, beginning with a clear definition of the problem. Team decision making must be directed at the objectives of the specific effort. As previously discussed, factors that enhance the process include mutual respect and constructive and timely feedback (Mariano, 1989, p. 287).

Decision making at the team level requires full consideration and respect of diverse viewpoints. Members must be able to verbalize their perspectives in a nonthreatening environment. Group members effectively use communication skills and give and receive feedback in the decision-making process. Interdependent relationships are actualized as members focus on client care issues (Velianoff, Neely, & Hall, 1993, p. 28).

Sound decision making regarding the client's care requires that the interdisciplinary team focus on the client's priority needs and organize interventions accordingly. The discipline best able to address the client's needs is identified, given priority in planning, and is held responsible for providing its interventions in a timely manner. For example, when social needs (such as loss of a home or job) interfere with the client's ability to respond to therapy, the team may agree that the social worker needs to intervene to help the client resolve his or her social needs before starting therapy. Nurses, by the nature of their holistic practice, are often able to help the team identify priorities and areas requiring further attention. Ideally, the collaborative team will ensure that the client is part of the decision-making process, even if the client is not able to be present. Decision-making processes are discussed in greater detail in Concept 34, Clinical Decision Making.

CLINICAL EXAMPLE

Betty Bradley, 87 years old, is a client in a long-term care facility. After fracturing her hip, Ms. Bradley is no longer stable on her feet and prefers to stay in bed for fear of falling. After speaking with Ms. Bradley to get a better understanding of her fears, the nurse consults with the physical therapist. Together they determine how they can help Ms. Bradley improve her mobility while reducing her risk of injury. After consulting with Ms. Bradley about their ideas and getting her agreement, the primary nurse and physical therapist develop a plan of care based on the nursing diagnoses of impaired mobility and risk for injury: falls. They list specific implementations including positioning, turning, and use of aids to prevent pressure ulcers. Once the plan of care is developed, it is posted on the wall by Ms. Bradley's bed so that all nurses can see it and administer care consistently. During the monthly team meeting, the plan of care for Ms. Bradley is evaluated. Both the physical therapist and the nurse report that Ms. Bradley has greatly improved both her strength and her mobility while reducing her risk for injury.

1. Why might collaborative care be of particular importance when caring for an elderly client who is a long-term resident in an extended care facility?
2. What other collaborative interventions might the team consider for this client?
3. How can the plan of care be posted on the client's wall without infringing on the client's right to confidentiality?

FACTORS LEADING TO THE NEED FOR INCREASED COLLEGIALITY AND COLLABORATION

Collaboration is necessary to address the current problems facing the health care system, including the following:

■ The unmet health care needs of the older adult
■ The increased number of people who have chronic illnesses
■ Poverty and homelessness.

These health problems are complex and involve diverse needs requiring expertise across multiple disciplines.

Worldwide, there are a number of significant influences on health and health care that require international collaboration. The World Health Organization (WHO) set an objective that it hoped all persons would achieve by the year 2000, a level of health that would permit them to lead socially and economically productive lives. *Healthy People 2010* (USDHHS, 2000) identified a set of leading health indicators that reflect major public health concerns in the United States. These indicators can be found in Box 13–3 on page 640 in Volume 1.

Increasingly, governments and society are working to reduce health risks, minimize the incidence of chronic illness, and improve the health and quality of life for all. Unfortunately, health and health care are not guaranteed. In the United States, the most pressing question for the health care system remains how to provide quality health care that is in line with the socioeconomic realities of society. A number of factors influence the provision of health care:

■ Although the diagnosis and treatment of illness are still critical, the focus of health care is changing. Health care consumers are demanding comprehensive, holistic, and compassionate health care that is also affordable. Clients expect that health care providers will view them as a biopsychosocial whole and respond to their needs as individuals while respecting them as collaborating members of the health care team.
■ Today's health care consumers have greater knowledge about their health than in previous years and, as a result, they increasingly are influencing health care delivery. Formerly, people expected a physician to make decisions about their care; today, however, consumers expect to be involved in making any decisions.
■ Health care consumers are assuming more responsibility for health and are more willing to participate in health-promoting activities. They are beginning to view health care professionals as a resource to guide these activities.

CLINICAL EXAMPLE

Nurses working in an outpatient surgical unit want to plan the on-call schedule at monthly staff meetings with their nurse manager. Currently, the staffing office for the entire surgical service plans that schedule. The nurses will need to negotiate the change and are planning a meeting to discuss strategy.

1. How might the nurses collaborate with the staffing office to increase their autonomy in creating a schedule?
2. How might the nurses approach the staffing office with their request to manage their own schedule?

As clients become more informed health care consumers, nurses must increase their efforts to collaborate with their clients. Parents of ill children, especially those with chronic illnesses, are often the best source of information regarding changes in the child's condition, history of illness, and treatment options that have worked best in the past. Caregivers and clients can contribute to the plan of care by sharing their past experiences and responses to treatment, as well as participating in planning care that meets their needs.

NURSING PRACTICE

Collaboration is becoming more important as the complexity of medicine continues to increase with each new discovery. For example, the information technology expert has become a valued member of the team in many organizations. Each team member has specialized knowledge from which the nurse can learn and that can contribute to client care. Failure to collaborate can result in serious consequences for the client.

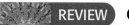 **REVIEW** **Collaboration**

RELATE: LINK THE CONCEPTS

Linking the concept of Collaboration with the concept of Communication:

1. How does the nurse's communication skills impact his or her ability to collaborate?
2. How does communication style impact the process of collaboration? Give some examples.

Linking the concept of Collaboration with the concept of Oxygenation:

3. How would the care of a client with chronic obstructive pulmonary disease (COPD) benefit from a nurse who collaborates well with other members of the health care team?
4. When caring for the client with COPD, what aspects of care would require collaboration?

REFER: GO TO MYNURSINGKIT

REFLECT: CASE STUDY

Josiah Elliot, 72 years old, is admitted to the hospital with medical diagnoses of congestive heart failure, chronic renal failure, hypertension, and benign prostatic hypertrophy. The nurse admits him and develops his plan of care, including the nursing diagnoses of fluid volume excess, urinary retention, altered gas exchange, and anxiety related to hypoxia. Three days later Mr. Elliot has lost 18 lb, is breathing more easily, and the nursing diagnoses of fluid volume excess, altered gas exchange, and anxiety are all marked as resolved. During morning rounds, the nurse provides the physician with an update on the client's condition and questions the need to continue administering the large doses of diuretics ordered when the client was admitted. The physician agrees and reduces the dosage of the medications. The physician raises concerns regarding the client's nutritional status and suitability for discharge to home. After some discussion, the physician and nurse agree to consult with a dietician and a social worker for further evaluation of the client's care.

1. Describe the impact of the team's collaborative approach on Mr. Eliot's outcomes.
2. How might Mr. Eliot's care have differed if the team had failed to collaborate?
3. What further collaboration is indicated in providing care for Mr. Eliot?

35.1 CASE MANAGEMENT

KEY TERMS

Care management model, *2121*
Care map, *2123*
Case management, *2121*
Critical pathway, *2121*

BASIS FOR SELECTION OF EXEMPLAR

IOM Compentency
NLN Competencies
Standards of Nursing Practice

LEARNING OBJECTIVES

After reading about this exemplar, you will be able to:

1. Describe the purpose of case management and the role of the case manager.
2. Correlate the need for critical pathways in the case management process.

OVERVIEW

Case management describes a range of models for integrating health care services for individuals or groups. Generally, case management involves multidisciplinary teams that assume collaborative responsibility for assessing needs, planning and coordinating, implementing, and evaluating care for groups of clients from preadmission to discharge or transfer and recuperation. A case manager may be a nurse, social worker, or other appropriate professional. In some areas of the United States, case managers may be referred to as discharge planners. Key responsibilities for case managers are shown in Box 35–4.

The **care management model** focuses on the needs of the integrated delivery system. It has many similarities to case management, in that it includes planning, assessment, and coordination of health services. The client focus is population-based instead of based on an individual client. The population might be the entire population, members of a managed care plan, or could be a specific group with similarities, such as clients with diabetes. The goal of the care managed model is to integrate a continuum of clinical services. Care management is not only concerned with medical care but also with health promotion, disease prevention, costs, and use of resources. Case management is often used within the care management model. Typical tools used to facilitate care management are clinical pathways, disease management programs, and benchmarking.

Case management may be used as a cost-containment strategy in managed care. Both case management and managed care systems often use critical pathways to track the client's progress. A **critical pathway** is a standardized plan that helps track care provided to clients with similar, predictable medical

Box 35–4 Responsibilities of Case Managers

- Assessing clients and their homes and communities
- Coordinating and planning client care
- Collaborating with other health professionals
- Monitoring clients' progress
- Evaluating client outcomes

conditions. Critical pathways are also called critical paths, interdisciplinary plans, anticipated recovery plans, interdisciplinary action plans, and action plans.

Nursing case management organizes client care by major diagnoses or *diagnosis-related groups* (DRGs). DRGs allow nurses to work toward predetermined client outcomes within specific time frames and resources.

Nursing case management requires the following:

- Collaboration of all members of the health care team
- Identification of expected client outcomes within specific time frames
- Use of principles of continuous quality improvement (CQI) and variance analysis
- Promotion of professional practice.

Case management has been particularly successful with disability management, especially when applied to helping injured employees to return to work (Salazar, 2000). Likewise, home care and ambulatory settings lend themselves to case management (Figure 35–2 ■). The case manager, who may be called a care coordinator, usually does not provide direct client care but rather coordinates and monitors the care provided by licensed and unlicensed care providers. Client involvement and participation is key to successful case management (Aliotta, 2002).

In an acute care setting, the case manager has a caseload of 10–15 clients and follows clients' progress through the system from admission to discharge, accounting for variances from expected progress. Nursing case managers on a client care unit may coordinate, communicate, collaborate, problem solve, and facilitate client care for a group of clients. Ideally, nursing case managers have advanced degrees and considerable clinical experience in nursing.

CLINICAL EXAMPLE

Martha Ellison is an RN with 10 years experience and a master's degree in nursing. She is the case manager on the orthopedic unit of the city hospital. She is currently managing 10 clients on the unit: 4 with injuries that resulted from car accidents; 2 older adults, each with a fractured hip; and 4 adolescent clients who required placement of pins and traction to stabilize fractures. Martha compares their progress to the critical pathway for each client and makes recommendations to the physician managing their care related to meeting specific needs.

One of the clients under Martha's care is a 22-year-old client who experienced significant head injuries and multiple fractures as a result of a motor vehicle accident. Martha works with the hospital physical therapy department to optimize the client's mobility and range of motion in order to prepare him for rehabilitation. She collaborates with a rehabilitation center that will continue his care following discharge. Martha also collaborates with the neurologist and family care providers in order to assure the client's other needs are met and he is able to be discharged as soon as possible.

To initiate case management, specific client diagnoses that represent high-volume, high-cost, and high-risk cases are selected. High-volume cases are those that occur frequently, such as total hip replacements on an orthopedic floor. High-risk cases include clients or case types who have complications,

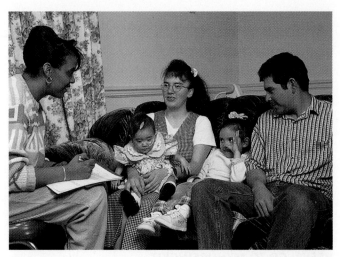

Figure 35–2 ■ A nurse case manager works with families to evaluate care being provided to a child with a complex health condition at home. The case manager coordinates specialty services, such as respiratory therapy, as well as providing client and family education.

stay in a critical care unit longer than 2 days, or require ventilatory support. Clients also may be selected because they are treated by a physician who supports case management. Whatever client population is selected, baseline data must be collected and analyzed. These data provide the information necessary to measure the effectiveness of case management. Essential baseline data include length of stay, cost of care, and complication information.

Five elements are essential to successful implementation of case management:

1. Support by key members of the organization (administrators, physicians, nurses)
2. A qualified nurse case manager
3. Collaborative practice teams
4. A quality management system
5. Established critical pathways (see next section).

When a specific client population is selected to be "case managed," a collaborative practice team is established. The team, which includes clinical experts from appropriate disciplines (e.g., nursing, medicine, physical therapy) needed for the selected client population, defines the expected outcomes of care for the client population. Based on expected client outcomes, each member of the team, using his or her discipline's contribution, helps determine appropriate interventions within a specified time frame.

In case management, all professionals are equal members of the team; thus, one group does not determine interventions for other disciplines. All members of the collaborative practice team agree on the final draft of the critical pathways, take ownership of client outcomes, and accept responsibility and accountability for the interventions and client outcomes associated with their discipline. The emphasis must be on managing client outcomes and building consensus among team members. Outcomes must be specified in measurable terms.

CRITICAL PATHWAYS

Successful case management relies on critical pathways to guide care. The term critical pathway, also called a **care map**, refers to the expected outcomes and care strategies developed through collaboration by the health care team. Again, the inter-disciplinary team must reach consensus regarding client care and determine specific, measurable outcomes.

Critical paths provide direction for managing the care of a specific client during a specified time period. Critical paths are useful because they accommodate the unique characteristics of the client and the client's condition while making use of the predictable characteristics of the course of the client's disease or injury. Critical paths use resources appropriate to the care needed, thereby reducing cost and length of stay. Critical paths are used in every setting where health care is delivered.

A critical path quickly orients the nurse to the outcomes that should be achieved for the client for that day. Nursing diagnoses identify the outcomes needed. If client outcomes are not achieved, the case manager is notified and the situation is analyzed to determine how to modify the critical path.

Altering time frames or interventions is categorized as a variance, and the case manager tracks all variances. After a time, the appropriate collaborative practice teams analyze the variances, note trends, and decide how to manage them. Teams may then revise the critical pathway or decide to gather additional data before making changes.

Some features are included on all critical paths. These include specific medical diagnosis, the expected length of stay, client identification data, appropriate time frames (in days, hours, minutes, or visits) for interventions, and client outcomes. Interventions are presented in modality groups (medications, nursing activity, and so on). The critical path must include a means to identify variances easily and to determine whether outcomes are met.

Table 35–2 is an example of a collaborative critical path for clients having a total hip replacement. Normally a client would be expected to be discharged on the sixth day after surgery. This path describes expectations for days 1–3.

A recent evolution of critical paths is the inclusion of actual and potential nursing diagnoses with specific time frames into the critical pathway (the lower section of Table 35–2). Education paths are also excellent tools for planning client and family education (Table 35–3). A copy of the client's education plan is given to the client and the family, and the nurse reviews the information with them. Thus, both the client and the family know what to expect during an anticipated, uncomplicated hospitalization.

TABLE 35–2 **Critical Path With Actual/Potential Nursing Diagnoses for Total Hip Replacement**

Collaborative Critical Path

Case Type: Total Hip Replacement

Client Name: _____   DRG: <u>209</u>

Record Number: _____   Expected LOS: <u>6 days</u>

	DAY 1 / OR	Y/N	DAY 2 / POST-OPERATIVE DAY 1	Y/N	DAY 3 / POST-OPERATIVE DAY 2	Y/N
Client Activity	Bed rest	—	Begin mobility plan	—	Continue mobility plan	—
	T-DB q2h	—	T-DB q2h	—	T-DB q2h	—
	Initiate skin protection		Continue skin protection		Continue skin protection	
	protocol	—	protocol	—	protocol	—
Nursing	VS qh × 4,	—	VS q4h	—	VS q8h	—
	then q4h	—				
	Assess cir/neuro		Assess cir/neuro q4h		D/C assessment	—
	legs qh × 4,	—				
	then q4h;	—			D/C Hemovac;	
	Check drainage/		Check drainage/		Check drainage	
	Hemovac qh × 4,	—	Hemovac q4h	—	q8h	—
	then q4h;	—			I & O q8h	
	I & O (Foley/		I & O (Foley/		D/C Foley; urinates	
	Hemovac) q8h;	—	Hemovac) q8h	—	within 8h	—
	Thigh-high elastic hose	—	Continue elastic hose	—	Continue elastic hose	—
Medications	Antibiotic	—	Continue antibiotic	—	Continue antibiotic	—

(continued)

TABLE 35–2 Critical Path With Actual/Potential Nursing Diagnoses for Total Hip Replacement (continued)

	Pain control:		Continue pain control	—	PO pain control	—
	PCA pump	—				
	Stool softener	—	Continue stool softener	—	Continue stool softener	—
	Continue home Rx;	—	Continue home Rx	—	Continue home Rx	—
	IVs	—	IVs continue	—	IV to heparin lock	—
			Coumadin	—	Cont coumadin	—
			Sleeping Rx	—	Sleeping Rx	—
Physical Therapy	Preop instructions	—	Evaluate mobility		Evaluate mobility	
			progress	—	progress	—
Diagnostic Tests	H & H 2h post-op	—	H & H	—	Prothrombin time	—
			Prothrombin time	—		
Nutrition	NPO—Cl liq as tol	—	Diet as tolerated	—	Diet as tolerated	—
Teaching	*Pre-op:* Pain control	—	Repeat teaching		Repeat teaching	
	Use of assist devices	—	if nec	—	if nec	—
	Gait control	—				
	Incentive spirometry	—				
	Mobility plan	—				
	Pt/family crit plan		Review pt/family		Review pt/family	
	given & reviewed	—	crit plan if nec	—	crit plan if nec	—
Discharge Plan	SNU evaluation	—			Review transfer	
	Home Health				discharge needs	—
	evaluation	—				

Client Problems and Outcomes for Total Hip Replacement

NURSING DIAGNOSIS	DAY 1 / OR	Y/N	DAY 2 / POST-OPERATIVE DAY 1	Y/N	DAY 3 / POST-OPERATIVE DAY 2	Y/N
Knowledge deficit: medications; use of assistive devices; treatments	Appropriately uses:		Uses all devices appropriately	—	Verbalizes additions to care	—
	PCA pump,	—				
	incentive spirometry,					
	assistive devices;	—				
	Verbalizes mobility plan	—				
Pain related to surgery, physical injury	Pain managed	—	Pain managed	—	Pain managed	—
Risk for infection related to invasive procedures, immobility	Remains afebrile	—	Remains afebrile	—	Remains afebrile	—
	No skin breakdown	—	No skin breakdown	—		
Impaired physical mobility related to surgery, prosthesis	Verbalizes mobility plan	—	Meeting mobility expectations	—	Participates in transfer/ discharge plans, decisions	—
	Verbalizes role of staff providing assistance	—				
Risk for injury related to altered tissue perfusion, altered mobility, and prosthesis	Explains need for frequent assessments	—	Circulation to extremities good	—	Circulation to extremities normal	—
	Verbalizes need for early mobility and hose	—	Leg maintained in proper alignment		Leg in proper alignment	

TABLE 35–3 Patient/Family Education Path for Total Hip Replacement

	DAY 1 / OR	DAY 2 / POSTOPERATIVE DAY 1	DAY 3 / POST-OPERATIVE DAY 2
Unit	Admission process; surgery and recovery areas; then Orthopedic Unit	Orthopedic Unit	Orthopedic Unit (Possible transfer next day to SNU or Rehab Unit)
Patient Activity and Safety Issues	Bed rest first 24 hr; leg exercises qh (q4h); T-DB q2h; explain skin protection plan; give copy of mobility plan; assist c̄ bath; thigh-high elastic support hose	Up in chair c̄ help; Leg exercises q2h; T-DB q2h; cont skin protect plan; cont mobility plan; assist c̄ bath; cont thigh-high elastic support hose	Up in chair and walking as outlined in mobility plan; T-DB q2h; cont skin protection plan; assist c̄ bath; cont thigh-high elastic support hose
Nursing Care	Frequency of taking vital signs (BP-P-R-T); check drainage on dressing; check circulation and sensations to legs; intake and output measured q8h; Foley and Hemovac in for 48 hr	Vital sign checks q4h; dressing, circulation, and sensation checks to legs q4h; I & O (Foley and Hemovac) measured q8h	Vital sign checks q8h; D/C Foley and Hemovac; I & O q8h; urinate with in 8 hr; D/C dressing, circulation, and sensation checks to legs
Medications	Verify list of home Rx so physician can order; pain medication and PCA pump; IVs and need for arm restraint; other drugs that will be ordered (e.g., antibiotics; stool softener)	Cont pain management c̄ PCA pump; IVs; cont arm restraint; cont antibiotic and other drugs (sleeping assistance)	Oral pain management; IV to heparin lock; cont antibiotic and other drugs
Diet	NPO before OR; clear liquids, ice chips	Diet as tolerated	Diet as tolerated
Tests	Blood test: Hemoglobin and hematocrit 2 hr after OR	Blood tests: H & H and prothrombin time	Blood test: prothrombin time
Teaching	Pain management; use of assistive devices (trapeze, walker) and incentive spirometry; mobility plan reviewed: how to transfer from bed to chair, and so on	Clarify questions	Clarify questions
Discharge Plan	Discuss purpose of Skilled Nursing Unit and Rehab Unit; identify need for Home Health Service after discharge	Cont with discussion of SNU, Rehab, and Home Health Services	Clarify questions and needs with transfer/discharge plans

REVIEW Case Management

RELATE: LINK THE CONCEPTS

A neonate is born with a severe congenital heart defect that will require numerous open heart surgeries and regular follow-up with cardiology and pediatrics. The parents, who carry comprehensive medical insurance, will require assistance paying for medical bills because the cost of care is expected to exceed the child's life-time maximum coverage within a few years.

Linking the exemplar of Case Management with the concept of Perfusion:
1. How might this family benefit from case management?
2. What would the case manager do for this family?

Linking the exemplar of Case Management with the concept of Oxygenation:
3. The nurse is caring for two clients: one client has pneumonia that is resolving with IV antibiotics; the other client has had asthma for many years. Which client would benefit most from case management? Explain your answer.
4. The nurse is caring for a client with a chronic alteration in oxygenation requiring many different medications, frequent doctor visits, and a history of 2–3 hospital admissions per year. How might case management help this client?

REFER: GO TO MYNURSINGKIT

REFLECT: CASE STUDY

Mrs. Covana is a 92-year-old client who lives alone in an assisted living facility. While she has many friends in the area, she has no family. Her husband died more than 20 years ago, and her only daughter died at age 65.

Mrs. Covana takes medications for congestive heart failure, chronic renal failure, hypertension, chronic obstructive pulmonary disease, glaucoma, and osteoporosis. She is admitted to the hospital with a fractured hip following a fall in her apartment. While admitted, she developed a hospital-acquired pneumonia requiring intubation and mechanical ventilation. She has remained in the ICU for the past 6 weeks with a tracheostomy because she has not tolerated extubation and cannot breathe adequately without mechanical support. She is awake, but cannot communicate due to the tube in her trachea. Her condition has stabilized, but she remains in the ICU because she requires mechanical ventilation; she will require 24-hour care upon discharge. The nurses in the ICU report that Mrs. Covana is confused and requires restraints to prevent her from pulling at central lines, indwelling catheter, and trach tube.
1. How might this client benefit from case management?
2. What priorities of care would be identified by the case manager?
3. Develop a critical pathway for this client.

35.2 CHAIN OF COMMAND

KEY TERMS
Authority, *2126*
Chain of command, *2126*
Line authority, *2126*
Organizational chart, *2126*
Responsibility, *2126*
Staff authority, *2126*

LEARNING OUTCOMES
After reading about this exemplar, you will be able to:
1. Differentiate between line authority and staff authority.
2. Explain how the organizational chart contributes to chain of command.
3. Expand upon the nurse's responsibility related to chain of command.

BASIS FOR SELECTION OF EXEMPLAR
Nursing Practice

OVERVIEW

The term **chain of command** refers to the hierarchy of authority and responsibility within an organization. **Authority** is defined as the right to direct others and their activities, whereas **responsibility** is the obligation to meet objectives or perform tasks. The line of authority is such that higher levels of management delegate work to those below them in the organization.

One type of authority is **line authority**, in which the supervisor directs the activities of the employees that he or she supervises. Another type of authority, **staff authority**, consists of an advisory relationship in which the person in authority recommends or offers advice to the employee but is not responsible for assigning work activities. In Figure 35–3 ■, the relationships among the chief nurse executive, nurse manager, and staff nurse are examples of line authority. The relationship between the acute care nurse practitioner and the nurse manager illustrates staff authority. Neither the acute care nurse practitioner nor the nurse manager is responsible for the work of the other; instead, they collaborate to improve the efficiency and productivity of the unit for which the nurse manager is responsible.

A chain of command provides structure necessary for employees to understand how to perform their tasks and how to manage supervisory relationships within the organization. It also provides a structure for reporting issues that need management's attention. Any nurse who identifies a problem requiring management intervention should follow the chain of command for the organization in which the nurse is employed. Generally, the problem is first reported to the charge nurse, then the unit manager, and, if resolution is still not obtained, the nurse may approach someone in middle or upper management.

The student nurse should also follow the chain of command, with the nursing instructor acting as the first link in that chain. When the student identifies a problem, whether in the clinical area or in the classroom, the student should first discuss the problem with the instructor. If the instructor is unable to resolve the issue to the student's satisfaction, the student should then approach the program director. Failure to follow the chain of command is considered unprofessional and slows the resolution process. In some organizations, failure to follow chain of command may result in disciplinary action.

Most agencies have an organizational chart that outlines the various divisions and units of the agency and the chain of command that each unit or division follows: "An **organizational chart** is a graphical representation of an organization's hierarchical structure and the flow of responsibility within the organization. It should reflect the chain of command and illustrate the relationships between staff members" (Milgram, Spector, & Treger, 1999, p. 29). It provides a visual presentation of the chain of command, centralization/decentralization approach, departments, and span of control.

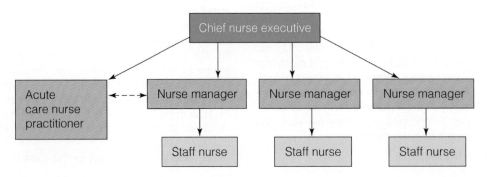

Figure 35–3 ■ Organizational chart showing chain of command in a nursing unit.

When assessing an organization's structure, it is important to remember that each organization has a formal and an informal aspect. The organization's organizational chart describes the formal positions and hierarchy, but does not reflect the informal structure. Nurses and others who are leaders who do not hold a formal title in the hierarchy would not be indicated in the structure described in the organizational chart. Similarly, organizational charts do not provide information about which managers are more powerful, although they all have the same authority due to their position as manager.

REVIEW Chain of Command

RELATE: LINK THE CONCEPTS

Link the exemplar on Chain of Command with the concept of Addiction Behaviors:

1. You report to work one morning and discover one of your coworkers exhibiting behavior that causes you to believe the coworker is substance impaired. Following the chain of command, to whom would you report your suspicions? Explain your answer.
2. You report your coworker's behavior to the proper person who replies, "Oh, she and I are good friends. Don't worry about it. She probably just stayed out partying too late last night." What would you do next?

Link the exemplar on Chain of Command with the concept of Managing Care:

3. How does the proper use of chain of command reduce the cost of health care?
4. How does chain of command impact proper delegation?

REFER: GO TO MYNURSINGKIT

REFLECT: CASE STUDY

Brittany Miller, RN, reports to work at 6:45 a.m. and is preparing for change of shift report. When she greets one of her coworkers, she smells alcohol on the coworker's breath. Brittany notices her coworker lacks coordination and seems to be unable to focus. Brittany reports her observation to the charge nurse who says, "Oh, she's probably just not awake yet. I'm sure she's fine!"

1. What should Brittany do next? Who would be next in the chain of command?
2. Would it be wrong for Brittany to go against what the charge nurse decided?
3. Would it have been better if Brittany had gone to the unit director or director of nursing first? What would the unit director or director of nursing have said if Brittany came to them before talking to the charge nurse?

35.3 CONFLICT RESOLUTION

KEY TERMS

Conflict, *2127*
Covert conflict, *2128*
Individual conflict, *2127*
Intergroup conflict, *2128*
Interpersonal conflict, *2127*
Organizational conflict, *2128*
Overt conflict, *2128*
Role conflict, *2127*
Verbal abuse, *2131*
Workplace bullying, *2131*

BASIS FOR SELECTION OF EXEMPLAR

NLN Competencies
Standards of Nursing Practice

LEARNING OUTCOMES

After reading about this exemplar, you will be able to:

1. Contrast different forms of conflict.
2. Explain factors that can initiate conflict.
3. Demonstrate appropriate conflict management strategies in the work place.

OVERVIEW

Conflict is defined as tension that arises when "the action of one person frustrates the ability of the other to achieve a goal" (Boggs, 2003, p. 366). Although conflict in an organization can never be eliminated, it can be managed. Conflicts can take place between individual nurses, within a unit, or within a department. They can be inter-unit and interdepartmental, affect the entire organization, or even occur between multiple organizations, between or within teams or units, or between an organization and the community.

There are three types of conflict: individual, interpersonal, and intergroup/organizational (Dessler, 2002).

- The most common type of **individual conflict**—conflict that takes place within a single individual—is **role conflict**, which occurs when there is incompatibility between one or more role expectations. The most obvious example may be that of the single working parent, who experiences conflicts of time, energy, and expectations between his or her role as a parent and as a working professional.
- **Interpersonal conflict** occurs between people. Sometimes this is due to differences and/or personalities, competition, or concern about territory, control, or loss. Interpersonal conflict may arise in the workplace when one staff member misunderstands the roles or responsibility of another. For example, a nurse may feel that another is not doing his or her job because the person is neglecting to perform an activity that is really the responsibility of another nurse. Other interpersonal conflicts can arise as the result of bullying, when a

member of the team belittles another or attempts to coerce others into behaving in ways that cause frustration, guilt or other types of conflict.

- When conflict occurs between groups, it is called **intergroup** or **organizational conflict** (e.g., units, services, teams, health care professional groups, agencies, community and a health care provider organization, and so on). One example of this conflict is the debate that is occurring between physician groups who want to bring control of nurse practitioners under the medical board, while nurses feel strongly that their practice should remain under the control of the board of nursing.

"Conflict is merely individuals or groups experiencing differences in views, goals, or facts that place them at opposite poles. It usually involves areas of differing expertise, practice, or authority" (Cesta, Tahan, & Fink, 1998, p. 68). This can be particularly true when one or more individuals misunderstands others' roles and responsibilities.

Covert and Overt Conflict

Conflict can be overt or covert; both can lead to problems as well as opportunities. In **overt conflict**, the individuals or group members who are in conflict address the conflict openly. In **covert conflict**, the conflict is not discussed openly. It may be avoided or ignored. Covert conflict may be exhibited in reactive, repressive, and avoidant behaviors. Reactive behaviors include whining, complaining, agreeing with others without really listening to them, and passive-aggressive behavior. Gossip is another form of reactive behavior, and rumor mills are common in workplaces in which covert conflict thrives. Repressive behaviors include absenteeism and tardiness. Avoidance behaviors include avoiding contact with others (including withholding information) and "disappearing" from work, e.g., taking extended breaks (Clement, 2001).

Everyone has experienced covert conflict. Cover conflict results in increased stress, distress, and confusion about how to address the conflict. Acknowledging covert conflict is not easy, and nurses will have different perceptions of the conflict since it operates below the surface. Overt conflict is obvious, at least to most people, and thus coping with it is usually easier. It is easier to arrive at an agreement that conflict is present and easier to arrive at a description of the conflict. Most people have had an experience with a friend or loved one who is acting differently, but when one asks the person what's wrong he or she says "Nothing!" How much easier would it be to resolve the conflict if it were overt and the person explained exactly what was bothering him or her?

The common assumption about conflict is that it is destructive, and it certainly can be. There is, however, another view of conflict: "Despite its adverse effects, conflict is viewed by most experts today as potentially useful because it can, if properly channelled, be an engine of innovation and change. This view explicitly encourages a certain amount of controlled conflict in organizations because lack of active debate can permit the status quo or mediocre ideas to prevail" (Dessler, 2002, p. 315). In reality, nurses really cannot avoid conflict because some conflict is inevitable.

If nurses were asked if they wanted to experience conflict, they would say "no." Behind this response may lie a lack of understanding on how to handle conflict, which can create anxiety. Avoiding conflict, however, usually results in the conflict continuing and becoming more difficult to resolve. The longer conflict goes unchecked, the more individuals may attach emotions to it, making it even more difficult to resolve.

CAUSES OF CONFLICT

In order to resolve conflict effectively, it is necessary to understand its cause. Some conflicts have more than one cause. Typical causes of conflict between individuals and between groups include the following:

- Inadequate communication
- Incorrect facts
- Lack of trust
- Unclear position descriptions
- Misunderstanding of roles and responsibilities
- Unclear or conflicted goals and objectives
- Inadequate action plans
- Directions
- Unstable leadership
- Receiving direction from two or more "bosses"
- Inability to accept change
- Lack of leadership
- Lack of or limited staff participation in decision making
- Power issues (Finkelman, 1996, p. 1–1:17).

Dessler (2002) discusses three additional major causes of intergroup conflict found in the literature that are relevant to health care settings:

- The first view is that groups that must work interdependently and compete for scarce resources will experience more conflict (Walton & Dutton, 1969). For example, if units or services are competing for staff, a scarce resource, conflict may arise as each unit tries to "prove" to administration that it needs the staff more than another unit or service.
- The second cause focuses on differences in goals, which can include content of goals as well as issues of flexibility, performance measurement, and differences between the goals and societal needs (Dutton & Walton, 1966). This can certainly be seen in individuals, but groups that need to work together will find tension rising if they do not agree on the goals.
- The third cause is related to the amount of differentiation of authority between coworkers (Lawrence & Lorsch, 1961). A common example in nursing is conflict between professional nursing staff and nonprofessional nursing staff such as UAPs or LPNs.

These causes are highlighted in Box 35–5.

Competition for resources and inadequate communication often lead to conflict. For example, it is rare that a major change on a unit or in a health care organization does not result in competition for resources (staff, financial, space, supplies). Consequently, conflicts will arise between units or between those who may or may not receive the resources or may lose resources. As has been demonstrated in some of the examples, causes of conflict can be varied. An understanding of a conflict requires as thorough an assessment as possible, with the goal of determining what is occurring and how the problem is perceived by all parties involved.

PREVENTING CONFLICT

Nurses as individuals and as members of an organization need to take steps to prevent conflicts. Clear communication is essential to prevent misunderstandings, which can lead to conflicts. Understanding and recognizing causes of conflict can assist individuals and organizations to develop strategies to prevent conflict. Clear understanding of roles and responsibilities also helps prevent conflict. Other strategies that help prevent conflict include the following:

- Allocating resources fairly
- Clearly stating expectations (at all levels)
- Avoiding sudden unexplained changes in processes
- Addressing staff fears (Milgram, Spector, & Treger, 1999, p. 297).

Nurses must be able to identify potential barriers that can either act as barriers to conflict resolution or that increase the likelihood that a situation will turn into a conflict. First and foremost, nurses need to recognize their own tension or stress level in the work place: Taking steps to decrease or manage their stress levels help them prevent and resolve conflict. Nurses should also:

- Deal with difficult issues as they occur. Do not put off interventions as this will only make the tension rise.
- Avoid behavior that might lead to defensiveness or counteractions. Examples of this behavior include threats, limited patience, and use of hot-button or demoralizing words (for example, "never").
- Observe nonverbal communication that might indicate staff are upset (e.g., sarcasm, body posture, raising voice or tone of voice, hand movements).
- Treat others with respect, which will decrease defensiveness.
- Avoid arguments. Sometimes people do need to vent, and as long as it is done appropriately and in a private place, it may be helpful in decreasing tension.
- Listen to each other.
- Consider the other person's point of view, including cultural beliefs and values.
- Consider the phases of conflict resolution (Milgram, Spector, & Treger, 1999, p. 296).

RESPONDING TO CONFLICT

Not everyone responds to conflict in the same way, and individuals vary in how they respond in different circumstances. The nurse who can recognize the types of responses to conflict will be better equipped to predict and manage conflict. Four typical responses to conflict are avoidance, accommodation, competition, and collaboration (Boggs, 2003).

- *Avoidance* occurs when a person withdraws from a stressful situation due to extreme levels of discomfort and an inability to cope. There are times when this may be the most appropriate response, particularly when the situation may lead to negative results, but in many situations this increases conflict over the long term. Avoidance might occur when a nurse is in conflict with a manager and disagrees with the manager. The nurse must consider whether it is worth it to disagree publicly. Typically, avoidance occurs when one side is perceived as more powerful than the other. Avoidance is a helpful approach when more information is needed or when the issue just is not worth risking further conflict or a loss of opportunity or consideration.
- *Accommodation* occurs when one person tries to make the situation better by cooperating with the individual with whom he or she is in conflict. The goal of accommodation is to eliminate the conflict as quickly as possible, despite the fact that it will not resolve the conflict. Accommodation works best when one person or group is less interested in the issue than the other. It can be advantageous in that it serves to develop harmony. It also can provide power in future conflict since one party was more willing to let the conflict deflate.
- A third response is *competition*, in which power is used to stop the conflict. A manager might say, "This is the way it will be." This prevents further efforts by others who may be in conflict with the manager.
- *Collaboration* is a positive approach, with all parties attempting to reach an acceptable solution, and in the end both sides feel that they won something. Collaboration often involves some compromise, which is a method used to respond to conflict.

When conflict occurs, each individual involved has a personal perspective of the issue and conflict. Nurses need to avoid taking things that a client or coworker says or does personally; doing so interferes with thoughtful problem solving. When the nurse gets defensive or emotional, interventions taken to resolve a conflict may not be effective. Conflict in the health care delivery environment combined with inherent workplace stress may lead to misunderstandings, ineffective communication, and reduced productivity (Iacono, 2000). The strategies outlined in Box 35–6 were developed by a specific health care organization (the St. Joseph Hospital Health Center in Syracuse, New York) to assist staff with conflict resolution. These strategies demonstrate how serious this organization considers the problem of conflict in the workplace. Conflict resolution is much like the nursing process: Assess to determine the problem, involve the people who have the conflict in developing a plan to reduce tension, implement the plan, and evaluate its effectiveness.

Box 35–6 Strategies for Conflict Resolution

1. Identify the problem behaviors. It is important to focus on behaviors, not personalities.
2. Collect facts about the problem behaviors. Clear and specific description of the problem behaviors is critical. Problems should be kept separate so that the focus is clear.
3. Document the facts and their sources.
4. Ensure privacy when the behaviors and related issues are discussed.
5. Explore the different perspectives. In this discussion make sure that understanding of the issue and expectations is present.
6. Use counseling sessions as a learning opportunity for growth, which requires objective feedback and encourages active participation.
7. Document both the manager's and employee's personal reactions to the counseling and the results.
8. Document employee's response to counseling and the corrective action.
9. Clarify with the employee who has access to the documentation, who will be told about the counseling session and action plan, and the timeline for change.
10. Report the results to the appropriate supervisor, if required (Iacono, 2000, p. 261).

MANAGING CONFLICT

Nurses in every health care setting need to know how to manage conflict, whether the conflict is with a coworker, a client or family member, or another individual with whom the nurse comes in contact during the course of a shift.

Managing Conflict in the Workplace

Aggressive behavior can be described as hostile behavior and can lead to conflict. Hostile behavior by even a single person in the workplace can increase the anxiety of many others. The first response toward a hostile staff member should be to communicate control to that staff member and to insert calm into the situation. When the nurse manager or team leader is the one who is hostile, the situation carries greater complexity and requires assistance from higher level management. Regardless of who is exhibiting hostility, someone should gain control and try to move the hostile staff member to a private place. Demonstrations of open conflict with hostility should not take place in client or public areas. If the suggestion to move to a private area does not work and the situation continues to escalate, simply walking away may help set some boundaries. This allows time for all parties to take a breath, calm down, and revisit the situation at a more appropriate time.

Managing Conflict With Clients and Families

When conflict occurs with clients or their families, what is the best way to cope? In addition to the strategies already presented, setting limits can be an effective way to manage conflict with clients and families. Nurses set limits when they provide instructions such as, "I can see you are upset and I want to help you, but I will not tolerate abusive language." Setting limits can help anxious clients monitor their own behaviors and keep the nurse from being interrupted too frequently.

It is never appropriate to allow clients or families to demonstrate anger inappropriately. When this occurs, the nurse needs to set reasonable limits that are based on an assessment of the situation. There may be many reasons for anger and inappropriate behavior, such as pain, medications, fear and anxiety, psychosis, dysfunctional communication, and so on. If a different culture is involved, then this factor needs to be considered (for example, some cultures consider it appropriate to be very emotional while others do not). In the long term, active listening and clear communication are critical to prevent and manage conflict.

GENDER ISSUES IN CONFLICT

Are there differences in the way that women and men negotiate or handle conflict? Wyatt (2000) discusses factors related to these differences. In general, men tend to negotiate to win while women focus more on fairness. Women will make an effort to reach win-win solutions. Men will test the limits that have been set more overtly than women, so it is important for women to set and maintain limits. It also is important, despite the differences described, to avoid stereotyping.

How can women participate more positively in negotiating conflict? The key is in planning: "Negotiation is 80% planning, and 20% action" (Wyatt, 2000, p. 45). How do the differences in women and men affect this process?

■ During the first step of preparation and planning, women tend to take things more personally. By refusing to take things personally and focusing on the task at hand, women will be better able to identify opportunities to succeed. In the planning stage, women should assess the power bases—which people in the room or in the discussions have real power and which have perceived power. Women also should come to the negotiation table dressed appropriately for the occasion: Appearance can make a difference in how one's own power is perceived (Figure 35–4 ■).

■ During the second step, defining the ground rules, parties set rules and boundaries. Issues such as the time and place for meeting become important, as some people may be more or less comfortable at the negotiation table depending on where discussions are held. Body language that displays confidence is important. This includes good posture, looking at the person who is speaking, and looking at others while speaking rather speaking with one's head down.

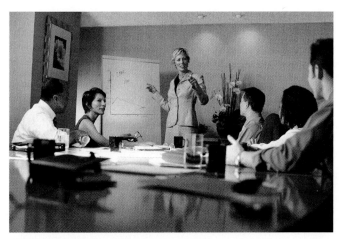

Figure 35–4 ■ A professional appearance can help women perceive their own power in a negotiation.

- Clarifying and justifying is the third step in the process. During this step, both sides educate one another about the issue: "Sex differences become readily apparent during this step because when a women states her proposal, she often characterizes her explanation using adjectives, adverbs, and expletives less powerful than those commonly used by males. This manner of speech conveys triviality by male standards. When women use these patterns of communication, they are perceived as incompetent, whereas if men use them, they are perceived as polite" (Lenz, 1990, as cited in Wyatt, 2000, p. 44). Using assertiveness skills is important. For example, women tend to apologize more than men saying things such as, "Excuse me for interrupting but..." or "I'm sorry to bother you but..." whereas men are more likely to say, "I need to interrupt you" or "I need to talk to you." When a woman uses an apology to begin communicating, it weakens her position and increases others' perceptions that she is less competent or less powerful.
- During the fourth step, the focus is on bargaining and problem solving. Both parties make compromises and concessions. Communication skills are critical in this stage. When men and women have similar expertise, men tend to talk longer than women and therefore are seen as being more dominant. Men also interrupt more when they want to demonstrate their dominance. Women need to be assertive and not give up their time to express their views or allow the interruptions to occur (Lenz, 1990). "Women have to be active listeners and interrupters–but when you interrupt you have to know what your talking about" asserts former U.S. Secretary of State Madeleine Albright (*Time Magazine*, 2008). During this fourth step, emotions tend to increase, and all parties, women and men, must keep their emotions in check.
- The final step is closure and implementation. Afterward, an agreement is formalized. Women should be as polite as necessary, but no more polite or courteous than the men in the room. "Over thanking" someone for his or her help can show weakness.

THE NURSE–PHYSICIAN RELATIONSHIP

The nurse–physician relationship should be the strongest relationship that nurses have in order to meet the needs of the client. Unfortunately, it frequently is not. Both sides can contribute to inadequacies in this relationship. When conflict does occur, it can act as a barrier to effective client care.

Literature about magnet hospitals distinguishes between collegial and collaborative relationships between nurses and physicians (Kramer & Schmalenberg, 2002). *Collegial relationships* are those where there is equality of power. Magnet hospitals equalize power between nurses and physicians, making power different but equal. In contrast, collaborative relationships between nurses and physicians focus on mutual power, but the physician's power is greater. The nurse's power is based on the nurse's extended time with clients, experience, and knowledge. In addition to power, this relationship requires respect and trust between the nurse and physician. Due to these factors, it is a complex relationship.

Positive professional communication is critical. Both sides should initiate positive dialogue rather than adversarial positions. Cooperation and collaboration are also integral to the success of this relationship. A frequent question discussed in the literature is, "Why is there conflict between nurses and physicians?" One approach suggests that the conflict exists because the two professions structure their work differently (Finkelman, 1996; Sheard, 1980). This perspective identifies the key elements that are important in the work structure: sense of time, sense of resources, understanding of care delivery, and type of rewards.

- The physician's sense of time focuses on the course of illness. The nurse typically focuses on shorter periods of time.
- Physicians frequently exhibit a lack of understanding of the nurse's work structure. This can create conflict when a physician fails to understand why an order cannot be completed within a certain period of time.
- Physicians often are less concerned with resources, though this is certainly changing as physicians do recognize that there is a shortage of staff as well as issues about costs and reimbursement for care. There are, of course, other resources such as equipment availability, supplies, and funds that can cause problems and conflicts. Nurses are typically more aware of the effect that resource availability has on daily care.
- Physicians also do not have an understanding of nursing delivery models such as team nursing or primary nursing, and often nurses themselves are not clear about them. This affects nurses' ability to explain how they work.
- Clearly, the sense of reward is different. Nurses work in a task-oriented environment and typically get paid an hourly rate. Most physicians are not salaried; instead, they work as independent practitioners and bill for procedures performed or number of clients treated.

VERBAL ABUSE

Conflict and verbal abuse are related. **Verbal abuse** or **workplace bullying** is defined as malicious, repeated, harmful mistreatment of an individual with whom one works, regardless of whether that person is an equal, a superior, or a subordinate. Behaviors that constitute verbal abuse include berating, humiliating, ridiculing, blaming, and threatening. Verbal abuse occurs in health care settings between clients and staff, nurses and other nurses, physicians and nurses, and all other staff relationships. This abuse can consist of statements made directly to a staff member or about a staff member to others. A recent study of staff nurses revealed that the greatest sources of hostility were senior nurses (24%) followed by charge nurses (17%) and nurse managers (14%) (Vessey, et al., 2009).

Another common complaint from nurses regards verbal abuse from physicians: "Some nurses, particularly new ones, allow physicians to verbally abuse them because they are insecure about their knowledge base" (Parks, 2001, p. 20MW). Verbal abuse affects turnover rates and contributes to the nursing shortage so it is has serious consequences (Stringer, 2001). Verbal abuse among health care professionals negatively affects their interactions, and, therefore, may compromise client care.

How can verbal abuse in the workplace be eliminated? A critical step is for all staff members (regardless of their profession or position within the organization) to gain better understanding of each profession's viewpoint and demonstrate less automatic acceptance of inappropriate behavior. This requires that management become proactive in eliminating negative communication and behavior. Health care organizations should implement strategies to deal with verbal abuse including encouraging all staff to report abuse by allowing anonymity and encouraging all staff—nurses, physicians, unlicensed assistive professionals, and others—to speak firmly and address abuse as soon as it occurs (Stringer, 2001).

What can nurses do about this? One suggestion is that they improve their own knowledge base to increase their self-confidence: "Remind yourself that you have many valuable skills, and you don't deserve to be verbally abused. These efforts will help decrease the feelings of intimidation" (Parks, 2001, p. 20MW). Another problem is that nurses think they must resolve all problems and "make things" work correctly. This thinking can lead to nurses becoming scapegoats. Verbal abuse, no matter who is doing it, physician or nurse, or under what circumstances should not be tolerated. Those involved need to be approached in private to identify the need for a change in behavior. All staff need to be respected.

EFFECTS OF STAFF AND ORGANIZATIONAL CONFLICTS ON CLIENTS

Clients should not become part of staff or organizational conflicts, and there is risk that this may occur. These conflicts need to be resolved or client care may suffer negative consequences. Consider these examples:

- The interdisciplinary team cannot agree on a treatment approach and must do this by the end of the team meeting.
- A client's managed care organization or health plan refuses to allow the client to stay two more days in the hospital. The hospital's nurse case manager must work with the managed care representative to reach a compromise.

- Staffing in a hospital is being reduced, and the nurses are convinced that the new staffing level will be unsafe for clients. Something must be done to resolve this issue.
- A home care agency has learned that the Medicare contract has decided that specific clients will receive fewer visits.

How can these examples be resolved satisfactorily so that the quality of care does not suffer? When approaching conflict resolution, it is important to recognize that both sides contributed to the conflict. Another critical issue is to carefully consider if this is the time and place to address the conflict. They can also agree by defining "the conflict in terms of needs, not solutions. People may disagree about the right solution, but they can agree on needs and thus focus on creative problem solving and looking at alternatives" (Gebelein, 2000, p. 469). When the environment is too emotional, conflict resolution will be difficult. Stepping back or taking a break may be the best position to take. Professionals who find themselves in conflict with each other will do well to remember the following strategies:

- Separate people from positions.
- Establish mutual trust and respect.
- Avoid one-sided or personal gains.
- Allow time for expressing the interests of each side/party.
- Listen actively during the process, and acknowledge what is being said; avoid defending or explaining yourself.
- Use data/evidence to strengthen your position.
- Focus on client care interests.
- Always remember that the process is a problem-solving one, and the benefit is for the client and family.
- Clearly identify the priority and arrive at common goal(s).
- Avoid using pressure.
- Identify and understand the real reasons underlying the problem.
- Be knowledgeable about organizational policies, procedures, systems, standards, and the law, applying this knowledge as needed.
- Try to understand the other side, and ask questions and seek clarification when unsure or uncertain; understanding the other side first before explaining yours increases effectiveness.
- Avoid emotional outbursts and overreacting if the other party exhibits such behavior; depersonalize the conflict.
- Avoid premature judgments, blame, and inflammatory comments.
- Be concrete and flexible when presenting your position.
- Be reasonable and fair (Cesta, Tahan, & Fink, 1998; Gebelein et al., 2000).

CONCLUSION

Conflict is unavoidable in nursing. Family members become angry with care providers, physicians and nurses disagree about priorities or treatment plans, and disagreements arise between coworkers. Conflict that is ignored or mishandled can lead to greater stress and lower morale in the unit. While conflict is never comfortable or easy to deal with, nurses can and must learn to deal with it effectively, thereby reducing stress in the workplace and creating an environment for providing safe client care.

REVIEW Conflict Resolution

RELATE: LINK THE CONCEPTS

Linking the exemplar of Conflict Management with the concept of Stress and Coping:

1. How do different levels of stress impact both the occurrence of conflict and the management of conflict that arises?
2. How can an understanding of different people's coping mechanisms improve the ability to manage conflict?

Linking the exemplar of Conflict Management with the concept of Advocacy:

3. How does the nurse's role of client advocate compel the nurse to manage conflict appropriately?
4. The client and his spouse disagree on the client's choice of treatment plan. As the client's advocate, what is the nurse's role regarding this conflict?

REFER: GO TO MYNURSINGKIT

REFLECT: CASE STUDY

Dee Johnston has worked in pediatric intensive care for the past 5 years. She decides to leave her current position because she feels her coworkers still see her as the inexperienced nurse who first took the job and do not see how her practice, knowledge, and skill have improved over time. She accepts a position as a staff nurse in the pediatric ICU at another facility and spends three weeks in orientation. Her preceptor quickly recognizes her expertise and feels additional orientation is unnecessary. Dee likes her new job and loves caring for the children, but begins to notice one of her coworkers seems to be watching her all the time. At first, Dee wonders why this coworker, Joan, keeps watching her, and eventually Dee starts to feel nervous. Every time she turns around and sees Joan watching, Dee feels like she's all thumbs, drops things, and forgets what she is doing. The situation worsens when Joan begins to say things to Dee like, "If you don't know what you're doing you should ask for help" or "It might be better if you let someone with more experience perform that procedure."

1. How is Dee interpreting Joan's watchful behavior?
2. Why might Joan be watching Dee as closely as she is?
3. If you were Dee, how might you handle this conflict?

35.4 INTERDISCIPLINARY TEAMS AND COMMUNICATION

KEY TERMS

Apathy, *2139*
Brainstorming, *2136*
Cohesiveness, *2138*
Delphi technique, *2137*
Formal group, *2135*
Group, *2133*
Groupthink, *2139*
Informal group, *2135*
Monopolizing, *2139*
Nominal group technique, *2136*
Primary group, *2134*
Scapegoat, *2139*
Secondary group, *2134*
Self-help group, *2141*
Semiformal group, *2135*
Transference, *2139*

BASIS FOR SELECTION OF EXEMPLAR

NLN Competencies
Standards of Nursing Practice

LEARNING OUTCOMES

After reading about this exemplar, you should be able to:

1. Describe and contrast different types of groups and their functions.
2. Analyze group dynamics within the classroom or clinical setting.

OVERVIEW

A **group** is defined by Adams and Galanes (2003, p. 11) as "three or more individuals who have a common purpose, interact with each other, influence each other, and are interdependent." Nurses belong to a variety of professional groups, ranging from small groups of a few people, to large professional associations. The nurse may fill a variety of roles within a group, including leader, advisor, elaborator, and encourager.

Groups are important in people's lives. People are usually born into a family group and interact with other groups at all stages of their lives through cultural, religious, and professional socialization. The family provides for initial socialization, whereas other groups (e.g., peer, social, religious, work, political) are vehicles for continued learning and socialization. *Group dynamics*, or group processes, refers to the ways in which groups function. For group work to be accomplished and group goals to be achieved, group dynamics must be effective.

The changing health care system presents challenges for health care professionals if they are to be actively involved in decisions about health care policy and health care practice. Such decisions are made by groups of people at all levels of society: think tanks, advocacy groups, professional groups, and politicians at local, regional, state, national, and international levels.

These challenges provide opportunities for nurses to participate as active members of the various decision-making groups. To be effective members of these groups, nurses must be knowledgeable about the dynamics of group work.

GROUPS

Groups exist to help people achieve goals that might be unattainable by individual effort alone. By pooling the ideas and expertise of several individuals, groups often can solve problems more effectively than one person acting alone. Information can be disseminated to groups more quickly and with more consistency than to individuals. In addition, groups often take greater risks than do individuals as they support each other in decision making. Just as group members share responsibilities for the group's actions, they also share the consequences of those actions.

In the clinical setting, nurses work in groups as they collaborate with other nurses, other health care professionals, clients, and family members when planning and providing care. Nurses also work in groups in professional and specialty organizations and civic and community groups. Within these organizations nurses promote the goals of nursing on professional, civic, and political levels. Group skills are therefore important for nurses in all settings.

Types of Groups

Groups are classified as either primary or secondary, according to their structure and type of interaction. A **primary group** is a small, intimate group in which the relationships among members are personal, spontaneous, sentimental, cooperative, and inclusive. Examples are the family, a play group of children, informal work groups, and friendship groups. Members of a primary group communicate with each other largely in face-to-face interactions and develop a strong sense of unity, or "oneness." What belongs to one person is often seen as belonging to the group. For example, a success achieved by one member is shared by all and is seen as a success of the group.

Primary groups set standards of behavior for the members. They also support and sustain each member in stressful situations that he or she would otherwise not be able to withstand. Expectations are informally administered and involve primarily internal constraints imposed by the group itself. To its members, the primary group has a value in itself, not merely as a means to some other goal. The group has a sense of "we" and "our" to it, in contrast to "I" and "mine."

The role of the primary group, particularly the family, in health care is increasingly recognized. Most people turn to their primary group for help and support when they have health problems. For this reason, health care providers and organizations are expanding their focus to include the family.

A **secondary group** is generally larger, more impersonal, and less sentimental than a primary group. Examples are professional associations, task groups, ad hoc committees, political parties, and business groups. Members view these groups simply as a means of getting things done. Interactions do not necessarily occur in face-to-face contact and do not require that the members know each other personally. Thus, there is little sentiment attached to these relationships. Expectations of members are formally administered through impersonal controls and external restraints. Once the goals of the group are achieved or change, the interaction is discontinued.

Functions of Groups

Sampson and Marthas (1990, pp. 3–21) describe eight functions of groups (see Table 35–4). Any one group generally has more than one function, and it may serve different

---

TABLE 35–4 Functions of Groups

FUNCTION	DESCRIPTION
Socialization	■ Primary socialization in growth and development. ■ Professional socialization into nursing or to a change in position. ■ Socialization into the culture of an organization (i.e., new customs and beliefs), as when a hospital is taken over by a corporate organization.
Support	■ Provision of social support for the members, a source of collegiality, and a source of help when needed.
Task completion	■ Complete tasks that are beyond the scope of any one individual. ■ Each person may bring specialized knowledge and skills. ■ Cooperation is important in task completion.
Camaraderie	■ Provision of goodwill among the members, which provides moments of pleasure.
Information	■ Provide a context for defining social reality, for setting performance goals, for establishing priorities, and for sharing special knowledge.
Normative function	■ Develop definitions and standards and enforce those standards, thereby encouraging compliance and discouraging deviations.
Empowerment	■ Empowering people and thereby encouraging change. A group often has more power than any individual.
Governance	■ Groups are often active in making decisions and serving as a source of governance within an organization.

Source: Adapted from Marthas, M. & Sampson, E. E. (1990). *Group process for health professions* (3rd ed.). Albany, NY: Delmar.

functions for different group members. For example, for one member a group may provide support; for another, it may provide information.

Levels of Group Formality

There are three levels of group formality: formal, semiformal, and informal.

FORMAL GROUPS The most common example of the **formal group** is the work organization. People become familiar with many different formal work groups during their lifetimes and spend a major part of their working hours in such groups. Formal groups usually exist to carry out a task or goal rather than to meet the needs of group members (Figure 35–5 ■). An example of a formal group is the staff of a nursing unit where the nurse manager provides the authority and structure through staff meetings. Traditional features of formal groups are shown in Box 35–7.

SEMIFORMAL GROUPS Examples of **semiformal groups** include churches, lodges, social clubs, parent–teacher organizations, and some labor unions. Many aspects of an individual's social and ego needs are often satisfied by membership in these groups. Semiformal groups are similar in form to formal groups, but exhibit slight differences. Characteristics of semiformal groups are shown in Box 35–8.

INFORMAL GROUPS From childhood on, most people belong to numerous **informal groups**. Informal groups are described by Crenshaw (2003) as groups "that provide much of a person's education and contribute greatly to his or her cultural values; members do not depend on one another." Examples of informal groups include the following:

■ *Friendship groups.* The first groups formed in life are friendship groups. In early childhood, they are often formed on the basis of proximity—children who live in the same neighborhood or go to the same preschool. Later, friendship groups are often formed on the basis of common interests. Many arise out of semiformal group interactions (e.g., playing on the same sports team) or form spontaneously from work organizations.

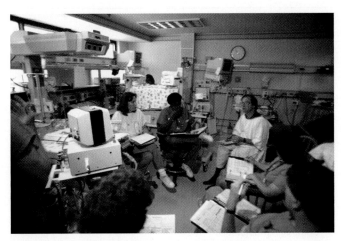

Figure 35–5 ■ A health care team gathers to discuss issues affecting client care.

Box 35–7 **Characteristics of Formal Groups**

- Authority is imposed from above.
- Leadership selection is assigned from above and made by an authoritative and often arbitrary order or decree.
- Managers are symbols of power and authority.
- The goals of the formal group are normally imposed at a much higher level than the direct leadership of the group.
- Management is endangered by its aloofness from the members of the work group.
- Behavioral norms (expected standards of behavior), regulations, and rules are usually superimposed. The larger the turnover rate of members, the greater the structuring of rules.
- Membership in the group is only partly voluntary.
- Rigidity of purpose is often a necessity for protection of the formal group in the pursuit of its objectives.
- Interactions within the group as a whole are limited, but informal subgroups often are formed.

■ *Hobby groups.* Hobby groups bring together people from all walks of life. Differences in members' personalities and backgrounds are largely ignored in the interests of the hobby itself.

■ *Convenience groups.* Many examples of convenience groups are found both in and out of the work setting. Two examples are carpool and the childcare groups often organized by groups of parents.

■ *Work groups.* Informal work groups can make or break an organization. Managers need to be sensitive to such groups and cultivate their cooperation and goodwill. Informal work groups may consist of nurses who work the same shift or share similar duties (Figure 35–6 ■).

■ *Self-protective groups.* Self-protective groups can be found anywhere but are particularly common in work organizations. They arise spontaneously out of a real or perceived threat. For example, a supervisor may approach a worker too strongly and find a group of workers organizing a united front against the supervisor. Such groups dissipate as soon as the conflict subsides.

Box 35–8 **Characteristics of Semiformal Groups**

- The structure is formal.
- The hierarchy is carefully delineated.
- Membership is voluntary but selective.
- Prestige and status are often accrued from membership.
- Structured, deliberate activities absorb a large part of the group's meeting time.
- Objectives and goals are rigid; change is not recognized as desirable.
- In many cases, the leader has direct control over the choice of a successor.
- The day-to-day operating standards and methods (group norms) are negotiable. Because most people become bored at quibbling about norms, people can often "railroad" acceptance of a list of norms they desire.

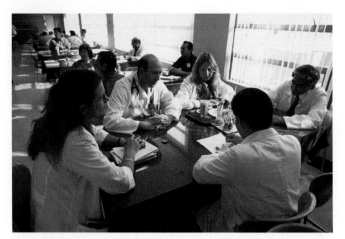

Figure 35–6 ■ Nurses and doctors chat during their lunch break.

The main characteristics of informal groups are shown in Box 35–9.

Characteristics of Effective Groups

To be effective, a group must achieve three main functions:

1. Accomplish its goals
2. Maintain its cohesion
3. Develop and modify its structure to improve its effectiveness.

Many factors can promote or inhibit a group's ability to achieve these functions. These include atmosphere, ability to set goals, and intergroup communication. These and other factors are compared in Table 35–5.

Group Dynamics

Group dynamics, or group processes, are related to how the group functions, communicates, sets goals, and achieves objectives (Marriner-Tomey, 2000). Every group has its own characteristics and ways of functioning. Five aspects of group dynamics follow.

COMMITMENT The members of effective groups are committed to the goals and output of the group. Because groups demand time and attention, members must give up some autonomy and self-interest. Inevitably, conflicts arise between the interests of individual group members and those of the group as a whole. However, members who are committed to the group feel close to each other and willingly work for the achievement of the group's goals and objectives. Some indications of group commitment are shown in Box 35–10.

DECISION-MAKING METHODS The ability to make sound decisions is essential to effective group functioning. Effective decisions are made when the following things occur:

1. The group determines which decision method to adopt.
2. The group listens to all the ideas of members.
3. Members feel satisfied with their participation.
4. The expertise of group members is well used.
5. The problem-solving ability of the group is facilitated.
6. The group atmosphere is positive.
7. Time is used well; that is, the discussion focuses on the decision to be made.
8. Members feel committed to the decision and responsible for its implementation.

Three decision-making aids are described by McMurray (1994, pp. 62–65): brainstorming, the nominal group technique, and the Delphi technique. In **brainstorming**, several people in a group generate ideas about a subject for the group as a whole to comment on, discuss, improve upon, select, or reject. For brainstorming to succeed, (1) the individuals in the group must have a level of trust, (2) there must be a criticism-free atmosphere that allows ideas to flow freely, and (3) all ideas receive initial approval and are critically examined thereafter.

Nominal group technique (NGT) is also an aid to decision making. It is especially useful when multiple ideas from group members may result in difficulty reaching a decision. Adams and Galanes (2003, p. 246) describe **nominal group technique** as the process of alternating "between individual work and group

---

Box 35–9 **Characteristics of Informal Groups**

- The group is not bound by any set of written rules or regulations.
- Usually there is a set of unwritten laws and a strong code of ethics.
- The group is purely functional and has easily recognized basic objectives.
- Rotational leadership is common. The group recognizes that only rarely are all leadership characteristics found in one person.
- The group assigns duties to the members best qualified for certain functions. For example, the person who is recognized as outgoing and sociable will be assigned responsibilities for planning parties.
- Judgments about the group's leader are made quickly and surely. Leaders are replaced when they make one or more mistakes or do not get the job done.
- The group is an ideal testing ground for new leadership techniques, but there is no guarantee that such techniques can be transferred effectively to a large, formal organization.

- Behavioral norms are developed either by group effort or by the leader and adopted by the group.
- Deviance by one member from the group's behavioral norms is more threatening to the perpetuation of small, informal groups than to large, formal, heterogeneous groups. Conformity and group solidarity are important for the protection and preservation of small groups.
- Group norms are enforced by sanctions (punishments) imposed by the group on those who violate a norm. Different values are placed on norms in accordance with the values of the leader. One leader may regard the action as a gross violation, whereas another leader may find it quite acceptable.
- Interpersonal interactions are spontaneous.

TABLE 35–5 Comparative Features of Effective and Ineffective Groups

FACTOR	EFFECTIVE GROUPS	INEFFECTIVE GROUPS
Atmosphere	Informal, comfortable, and relaxed. It is a working atmosphere in which people demonstrate their interest and involvement.	Obviously tense. Signs of boredom may appear.
Goal setting	Goals, tasks, and objectives are clarified, understood, and modified so that members of the group can commit themselves to cooperatively structured goals.	Unclear, misunderstood, or imposed goals may be accepted by members. The goals are competitively structured.
Leadership and member participation	Shift from time to time, depending on the circumstances. Different members assume leadership at various times, because of their knowledge or experience.	Delegated and based on authority. The chairperson may dominate the group, or the members may defer unduly. Members' participation is unequal, with high-authority members dominating.
Goal emphasis	All three functions of groups are emphasized—goal accomplishment, internal maintenance, and developmental change.	One or more functions may not be emphasized.
Communication	Open and two-way. Ideas and feelings are encouraged, both about the problem and about the group's operation.	Closed or one-way. Only the production of ideas is encouraged. Feelings are ignored or taboo. Members may be tentative or reluctant to be open and may have "hidden agendas" (personal goals at cross purposes with group goals).
Decision making	By consensus, although various decision-making procedures appropriate to the situation may be instituted.	By the higher authority in the group, with minimal involvement by members; or an inflexible style is imposed.
Cohesion	Facilitated through high levels of inclusion, trust, liking, and support.	Either ignored or used as a means of controlling members, thus promoting rigid conformity.
Conflict tolerance	High. The reasons for disagreements or conflicts are carefully examined, and the group seeks to resolve them. The group accepts unresolvable basic disagreements.	Low. Attempts may be made to ignore, deny, avoid, suppress, or override controversy by premature group action. The group may choose to live with conflict rather than attempt to resolve it.
Power	Determined by the members' abilities and the information they possess. Power is shared. The issue is how to get the job done.	Determined by position in the group. Obedience to authority is strong. The issue is who controls.
Problem solving	High. Constructive criticism is frequent, frank, relatively comfortable, and oriented toward removing an obstacle to problem solving.	Low. Criticism may be destructive, taking the form of either overt or covert personal attacks. It prevents the group from getting the job done.
Self-evaluation of the group	Frequent. All members participate in evaluation and decisions about how to improve the group's functioning.	Minimal. What little evaluation there is may be done by the highest authority in the group rather than by the membership as a whole.
Creativity	Encouraged. There is room within the group for members to become self-actualized and interpersonally effective.	Discouraged. People are afraid of appearing foolish if they put forth a creative thought.

Source: From Kneisl, C. R. & H. S. Wilson (1996). *Psychiatric nursing* (5th ed., p. 736). Redwood City, CA: Addison-Wesley Nursing.

Box 35–10 Indications of Group Commitment

- Members feel a strong sense of belonging.
- Members enjoy each other.
- Members seek each other for counsel and support.
- Members support each other in difficulty.
- Members value the contributions of other members.
- Members are motivated by working in the group and want to do their tasks well.
- Members express good feelings openly and identify positive contributions.
- Members feel that the goals of the group are achievable and important.

work to help a group hear from every member when discussing a controversial issue." In this instance the individuals meet as a group, but they write their responses without discussion. The ideas are then collected and an open discussion proceeds. The steps used for conducting nominal group technique are shown in Figure 35–7 ■.

The **Delphi technique** was originally used for technologic forecasting. It has been used for decisions that require more time or need responses from people in disparate locations. The Delphi technique requires participants to maintain their anonymity, which eliminates peer pressure. Data are gathered through interviews or questionnaires in a series of rounds in which an initial question is posed. Once the responses are

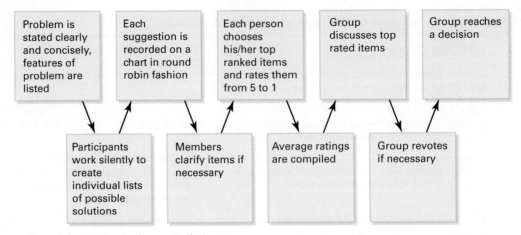

Figure 35–7 ■ Steps for conducting nominal group technique.

Source: From Adams, K. & Galanes, G.J. (2003). *Communicating in groups: Applications and skills* (9th ed., p. 247). Boston: McGraw-Hill. Reprinted with permission.

returned, they are compiled and redistributed. The participants do not know who said what: The comments or ratings are gathered for a compiled listing and are rated through averaging or statistical analysis. With the Delphi technique, agreement is reached as the process continues, either by consensus, voting, or mathematical average (McMurray, 1994, p. 64). See Table 35–6 for a comparison of brainstorming, nominal group technique, and the Delphi technique.

MEMBER BEHAVIORS The degree of input by members into goal setting, decision making, problem solving, and group evaluation is related to the group structure and leadership style, but members are responsible for their own behavior and participation. Each member participates in a wide range of roles (assigned or assumed functions) during group interactions. Individuals may perform different roles during interactions in the same group or may vary roles in different groups. Various roles that have been identified include *information givers*, who provide factual information; *information seekers*,

who seek factual information about tasks at hand; and *opinion givers*, who care more about values and beliefs than facts (Marriner-Tomey, 2000, and Adams and Galanes, 2003).

COHESIVENESS Groups that have the characteristic of cohesiveness possess a certain group spirit, a sense of being "we," and a common purpose. Adams and Galanes (2003, p. 187) define **cohesiveness** as the "attachment members feel toward each other, the group, and the task." When there is a high level of cohesiveness, group members feel greater satisfaction. Groups lacking cohesiveness are unstable and more prone to disintegration. See Box 35–11 for some of the attitudes and behaviors that reflect group cohesiveness.

POWER Patterns of behavior in groups are greatly influenced by the force of power. Power can be defined as the ability to influence another person in some way or the ability to do something, whether it is to decide the fate of a nation or to decide that a certain change in policy or practice is necessary. For example,

TABLE 35–6 **Comparison of Brainstorming, Nominal Group Technique, and Delphi Technique**

BRAINSTORMING	NOMINAL GROUP TECHNIQUE	DELPHI TECHNIQUE
Group activity, open discussion.	Group activity; initial silent interaction with later discussion.	No personal interaction; input is anonymous.
Can be conducted in one session.	Can be conducted in one session.	Takes place over three to four rounds of data collection and analysis.
Relaxed, noncritical atmosphere is essential.	Noncritical atmosphere desirable in discussion stage.	No interaction; responses are anonymous.
Largely unstructured format.	Structured format; sequential steps or stages to be followed.	Structured format; requires "rounds" of interaction.
Easy to conduct; requires little preparation or understanding.	Easy to conduct; requires little preparation or understanding.	Requires coordination of responses, can be time-consuming.
Promotes more ideas than do individuals acting alone.	Promotes more and better quality ideas than does brainstorming.	Promotes many high-quality ideas.
Possible influence of results by peer pressure.	Peer influence likely only in discussion phase.	Little peer pressure noted.

Source: From McMurray, A. R. (March/April 1994). Three decision-making aids: Brainstorming, nominal group and delphi technique. *Journal of Nursing Staff Development, 10,* 62–65. Used with permission.

Box 35–11 Attributes of Group Cohesiveness

MEMBERS' ATTITUDES AND BEHAVIORS
- Like each other, trust one another, and are friendly and willing to interact.
- Receive support from the group and praise one another for accomplishments.
- Have similar attitudes and beliefs.
- Are loyal to the group and defend it against outside criticism.
- Readily accept assigned roles and tasks.
- Influence each other and value being influenced by others.
- Feel satisfied and secure.
- Stay in the group and value group goals.

GROUP CHARACTERISTICS
- Goals are valued and are consistent with the goals of individuals.
- Activities are handled by group action.
- Actions are interdependent and cooperative.
- Goals that are difficult to achieve are met by persistent efforts.
- Participation is high.
- Commitment is high.
- Communication is high.
- "We" is frequently heard in discussions.
- Productivity is high.
- Norms are adhered to and protected.

a new member of a group may be more influenced by the group member who asked him or her to enter into membership than by other members. Similarly, group members may afford power to those group members who most closely share their interests.

Many people have a negative concept of power, likening it to control, domination, and even coercion of others by muscle and clout. However, power can be viewed as a vital, positive force that moves people toward the attainment of individual or group goals. The overall purpose of power is to encourage cooperation and collaboration in accomplishing a task.

Group Problems

Problems that occur in groups include monopolizing, conflict, groupthink, scapegoating, silence and apathy, and transference and countertransference. Nurses need to be able to recognize and avoid these behaviors when working in collaborative groups. These behaviors are described in the following sections.

MONOPOLIZING **Monopolizing** is the domination of a discussion by one member of a group. Because most group meetings have time restraints, monopolizing seriously deprives others of their chances to participate. A sense of injustice among members develops, and ultimately some members may direct their frustration and anger toward the group leader, whom they expect to do something to stop the monopolizer's behavior.

Monopolizing behavior may be motivated by anxiety or a need for attention, recognition, and approval. Often, compulsive talkers are unaware of their behavior and its effect on others and need help to recognize their behavior and its consequences.

Strategies for dealing with monopolizing include the following:
- *Interrupt simply, directly, and supportively.* This strategy is an initial attempt to get the person to hear others.
- *Reflect the person's behavior.* This strategy is an attempt to help the person become aware of the monopolizing behavior.
- *Reflect the group's feelings.* This strategy is an attempt to help the person become aware of the effects of his or her behavior on others.
- *Confront the person and/or the group.* This strategy can be directed toward the individual or toward the group to help members realize their own responsibility for the problem.

GROUPTHINK **Groupthink** is a type of decision making characterized by a group's failure to critically examine their own processes and practices. Groupthink may also occur when members of a group fail to recognize and respond to change. It may occur in highly cohesive groups when group members do not want to disagree or criticize group thinking for fear of being considered disloyal. For example, the administrators of a local urgent care center fail to recognize that an influx of Latino clients signifies a change in its local population, and refuse to hire Spanish-speaking staff or engage the services of a full-time interpreter. Symptoms of groupthink are shown in Table 35–7.

SCAPEGOATING A **scapegoat** is an individual who has been selected to take the blame for another individual or for a group. Individuals and groups who engage in scapegoating minimize their own feelings of ineptitude by focusing on the weakness of others. For leaders to deal with scapegoating, they must be alert to its development and be prepared to accept anger when they confront the scapegoaters. Scapegoating is a grossly unprofessional behavior that has no place within the profession of nursing, which emphasizes responsibility and accountability.

SILENCE AND APATHY Nonparticipation or **apathy** (lack of interest or enthusiasm) of one or more group members is sometimes best handled without intervention. Sometimes such silences are not a reflection of something in the immediate group setting but rather of some past experience. For example, after expressing an idea previously, this person may have been told, "That was a stupid thing to say." Having been hurt once in a group, such persons feel insecure about their views and are reluctant to express themselves again in groups.

Continued nonparticipation or apathy, however, needs to be dealt with by the leader after a careful assessment of whether the apathy is a reflection of leadership style, task issues, or interpersonal conflicts.

TRANSFERENCE AND COUNTERTRANSFERENCE **Transference** in the group setting is defined as the transfer of feelings that were originally evoked by one's parents or significant others to people in the present setting. An example is a group member who acts toward the leader as she or he

TABLE 35-7 Symptoms of Groupthink

THE GROUP OVERESTIMATES ITS POWER AND MORALITY	THE GROUP BECOMES CLOSED-MINDED	GROUP MEMBERS EXPERIENCE PRESSURE TO CONFORM
■ Group believes its cause is right. ■ Members convince themselves they cannot fail.	■ Group is selective in gathering information: chooses only information that supports its predisposition. ■ Group is biased in evaluating information. ■ Group excludes or ignores members and outsiders who seem to hold opposing views.	■ Members censor their own remarks. ■ Members who voice contradictory opinions receive pressure from other members to conform. ■ Members have the illusion that the group opinion is unanimous.

Source: From Adams, K. A. & Galanes, G. J. (2003) *Communicating in groups: Applications and skills* (5th ed., p. 234). Boston: McGraw Hill. Reprinted with permission.

would act toward a parent. In addition, members of a group can transfer to others in the group personal feelings of love, guilt, or hate.

When leaders respond to group members because of reactions from earlier relationships, they are engaging in *countertransference.* For example, if a group member reminds a leader of a teacher who was menacing and demanding, the leader is likely to react with anxiety and may become unreasonably fearful. It is therefore important that group members and leaders recognize the possibility of overreaction because of countertransference and that it is not an unusual reaction among nurses who are highly involved in helping others.

Types of Health Care Groups

Much of a nurse's professional life is spent in a wide variety of groups. As a participant in a group, the nurse may be required to fulfill different roles as member or leader, teacher or learner, adviser or advisee. Common types of health care groups include committees, teams, teaching groups, self-help groups, self-awareness/growth groups, therapy groups, work-related social support groups, and professional nursing organizations. There are similarities and differences among the characteristics of these various types of groups and the roles of nurses participating in them.

COMMITTEES OR TEAMS Committees are "relatively stable and formally composed" (Huber, 2000, p. 253). These are the most common types of work-related groups. They usually have a specific purpose that is part of their organizational structure and meet at defined intervals. Examples are policy committees, quality improvement committees, health care planning committees, nursing organization committees, and governmental affairs committees. Committees may also be referred to as teams, such as nursing care teams or wound-care teams. Teams are defined as "a small number of consistent people committed to a relevant shared purpose, with common performance goals, complementary and overlapping skills, and a common approach to their work" (Manion, Lorimer, & Leander, 1996, p. 6).

The leader of a committee or team, usually called the chairperson, must be accepted by the members as an appropriate

leader and, therefore, should be an expert in the area of the committee's focus. The chairperson's role is to identify the specific task, clarify communication, and assist in expressing opinions and offering solutions. Within a single organization, committee or team members are generally selected in terms of their individual functional roles and employment status rather than in terms of their personal characteristics. If a committee or team is composed of representatives from multiple organizations, the members are generally assigned by the member organizations. Committee members may reflect diverse expertise in order to assist the committee to achieve its purpose. In some cases, membership may be designated by rule or law. For example, membership in county child fatality review teams typically is designated by law and includes representatives of local hospitals, emergency medical systems, law enforcement, community health nurses, etc. Additional member positions called "at large" positions may be designated to enable local committees to add members from organizations whose membership would be helpful but are not on the list of those designated by rule or law. Regardless of the type of committee or team, members are accountable for the group's results or outcomes.

TASK FORCES Task forces or ad hoc committees are work groups that usually have a defined task that is limited in duration. In other words, the task force is brought together to perform a specific activity, such as preparation for a Joint Commission visit or Nurse Week. When the activity is accomplished, the task force is dissolved. Task forces and ad hoc committees function in the same way as committees or work teams. The difference is in the duration of their work.

TEACHING GROUPS The major purpose of teaching groups is to impart information to the participants. Examples of teaching groups include group continuing education and client health care groups. Numerous subjects are often handled using a group teaching format: childbirth techniques, exercise for middle-aged and older adults, and instructions to family members about follow-up care for discharged clients. A nurse who leads a group in which the primary purpose is to teach or learn must be skilled in the teaching-learning process discussed in Concept 39, Teaching and Learning.

SELF-HELP GROUPS A **self-help group** is composed of individuals who come together to face a common problem or difficulty (Frisch & Frisch, 2002, p. 721). These groups are based on the helper-therapy principle: Those who help are helped most. A central belief of the self-help movement is that persons who experience a particular social or health problem have an understanding of that condition which those without it do not. Alcoholics Anonymous (AA) is an example of a self-help group. Other support groups may consist of individuals who have specialized knowledge to help individuals who have the problem or who have experienced it. Reach for Recovery (a support group to assist women with breast cancer) is an example of this type of group in which members may be victims of breast cancer or they may be other individuals who have the ability to help, such as oncology nurses. Positive aspects of these groups are outlined in Box 35–12.

SELF-AWARENESS/GROWTH GROUPS The purpose of self-awareness/growth groups is to develop or use interpersonal strengths. The overall aim is to improve the person's functioning in the group to which he or she returns, whether the group is a job, family, or community. From the beginning, broad goals are usually apparent—for example, to study communication patterns, group process, or problem solving. Because the focus of these groups is interpersonal concerns around current situations, the work of the group is oriented to reality testing with a here-and-now emphasis. Members are responsible for correcting inefficient patterns of relating and communicating with each other. They learn group process through participation and involvement in guided exercises.

THERAPY GROUPS Therapy groups are composed of people coming together to receive psychotherapy through which they work toward self-understanding, more satisfactory ways of relating or handling stress, and changing patterns of behavior toward health. Members are referred to as clients, participants, or, in some settings, as patients. They are selected by health professionals after extensive selection interviews that consider the pattern of personalities, behaviors, needs, and identification of group therapy as the treatment of choice. Duration of

---

Box 35–12 Positive Aspects of Self-Help Groups

- Members can experience almost instant kinship, because the essence of the group is the idea that "you are not alone."
- Members can talk about their feelings and listen to the concerns of others, knowing they all share this experience.
- The group atmosphere is generally one of acceptance, support, encouragement, and caring.
- Many members act as role models for newer members and can inspire them to attempt tasks they might consider impossible.
- The group provides the opportunity for people to help as well as to be helped—a critical component in restoring self-esteem.

Source: From Gilbey, V. J. (April 1987) Self-Help. *Canadian Nurse, 83,* 25.

---

therapy groups is not usually set. A termination date is usually mutually determined by the therapist and members. Therapy groups are characterized by different approaches to psychotherapy—for example, interpersonal groups, existential groups, cognitive-behavioral groups, and psychodrama.

WORK-RELATED SOCIAL SUPPORT GROUPS Many nurses, such as hospice, emergency, and critical care nurses, experience high levels of vocational stress. Social support groups can help reduce stress if various types of support are provided to buffer the stress. Group members who know about the work of others can encourage and challenge members to be more creative and enthusiastic about their work. For example, a nurse may help another group member consider alternative strategies for intervention. Members also can share the joys of success and the frustration of failure through active listening without giving advice or making judgments. This type of social support is best given outside the work-related support group.

PROFESSIONAL NURSING ORGANIZATIONS Professional nursing organizations function as groups, and through smaller groups composed of organization members promote quality health care for all and support the needs of nurses. Professional nursing organizations can serve as task groups, teaching groups, self-help groups, and support groups. The effectiveness of professional nursing organizations is related to the commitment and effectiveness of their members.

EVIDENCE-BASED PRACTICE The Impact of a Sharing Group on the Learning Process

Lin, Chang, and Wang (2000) performed a qualitative study to explore the learning process in a sharing group during nursing students' clinical practice and to determine its implications for interpersonal learning. The sample consisted of 14 senior baccalaureate nursing students in China. The students were invited to discuss their experiences in clinical practice during a focus interview process. All the interviews were recorded and transcribed. Narrative analysis was used to summarize the context of the learning process in the sharing group. Four categories were identified: (1) yielding to an open mind, (2) reflecting real self, (3) learning with regard for others, and (4) taking pleasure in learning. The interaction between the students in the sharing group provided a mechanism for self-understanding and change.

Using a sharing group process encourages more in-depth introspection and self-accommodation, which could help students better perform their professional roles. The findings may have implications for nurses working in stressful work areas, who may use the sharing group process to gain greater awareness and understanding about themselves and their co-workers.

Source: Lin, M., Chang, Y., & Wang, C. (2000). The power of sharing groups: An exploration of nurse students' learning process in the clinical practice. *Journal of Nursing Research (China), 8*(5), 503–514.

REVIEW Interdisciplinary Teams and Communication

RELATE: LINK THE CONCEPTS

Linking the exemplar of Interdisciplinary Teams and Communication with the concept of Managing Care:

1. How does an understanding of interdisciplinary teams improve the nurse's ability to manage care?
2. How does an understanding of interdisciplinary teams improve the nurse's ability to delegate?

Linking the exemplar of Interdisciplinary Teams and Communication with the concept of Advocacy:

3. How does knowledge of interdisciplinary teams impact the nurse's role as an advocate?
4. Why is membership in a professional organization important to the nurse's role as an advocate?

REFER: GO TO MYNURSINGKIT

REFLECT: CRITICAL THINKING

1. Identify teams, teaching groups, self-help groups, self-awareness groups, therapy groups, and work-related groups in your practice setting. What are the purposes of these various groups? In what way are nurses actively involved in these groups? If nurses are not involved in the various groups, how might the lack of their participation affect the perception of professional nursing? How might nurses become involved in these groups?

2. Identify the various health care groups in your community. Identify specific task groups, teaching groups, self-help groups, self-awareness groups, therapy groups, and work-related groups in your community. What are the purposes of these various groups? In what way are nurses actively involved in these groups? If nurses are not involved in the various groups, how might that affect the perception of professional nursing? How might nurses become involved in these groups?

3. Identify the various professional nursing organizations in your community, state, and region. How effective are these organizations in promoting quality health care for the community, state, region, and nation? What is your own involvement in these organizations?

35.5 MANAGEMENT THEORIES

KEY TERMS

Accountability, *2144*
Authority, *2144*
Contingency planning, *2143*
Controlling, *2144*
Directing, *2143*
Effectiveness, *2144*
Efficiency, *2144*
Leader, *2142*
Manager, *2142*
Organizing, *2143*
Planning, *2143*
Productivity, *2144*

Responsibility, *2144*
Strategic planning, *2143*

LEARNING OUTCOMES

After reading about this exemplar, you will be able to:

1. Differentiate between managers and leaders.
2. Describe the duties of a manager based on management theory.

BASIS FOR SELECTION OF EXEMPLAR

NLN Competencies
Standards of Nursing Practice

OVERVIEW

Managers are essential to any organization. A manager's responsibilities are enormous and difficult. In any health care organization, a manager must balance the needs of clients, the organization itself, professional and nonprofessional staff and contractors, and self. Nurse managers need a body of knowledge and skills distinctly different from those needed for nursing practice, yet few nurses have the education or training necessary to be managers (Grossman & Valiga, 2005). Frequently, managers depend on experiences with former supervisors, who also learned supervisory techniques on the job. Often a gap exists between what managers know and what they need to know. A master's degree in nursing, with emphasis on management, is increasingly being required for nurse managers to eliminate this gap in knowledge.

Today, all nurses are managers, not in the formal organizational sense but in practice. They direct the work of nonprofessionals and professionals in order to achieve desired outcomes in client care. Acquiring the skills to be both a leader and a manager will help the nurse become more effective and successful in any position.

LEADERS AND MANAGERS

Manager, leader, supervisor, and administrator are often used interchangeably, yet they are not the same. A **leader** is anyone who uses interpersonal skills to influence others to accomplish a specific goal. The leader exerts influence by using a flexible combination of personal behaviors and strategies. The leader creates connections among an organization's members to promote high levels of performance and quality outcomes. Leadership is discussed in detail in Concept 38, Professional Behaviors.

A **manager**, in contrast, is an individual employed by an organization who is responsible and accountable for efficiently accomplishing the goals of the organization. Managers focus on coordinating and integrating resources, using the functions of planning, organizing, supervising, staffing, evaluating, negotiating, and representing. Interpersonal skill is important, but a manager also has authority, responsibility, accountability, and power defined by the organization. The manager's job is to do the following:

- Clarify the organizational structure
- Choose the means by which to achieve goals
- Assign and coordinate tasks, developing and motivating as needed
- Evaluate outcomes and provide feedback.

All good managers are also good leaders—the two go hand in hand. However, one may be a good manager of resources and lack skills necessary to lead people. Likewise, a person who is a good leader may not manage well. Both roles can be learned; skills gained can enhance either role.

MANAGEMENT FUNCTIONS

In 1916, French industrialist Henri Fayol first described the functions of management as planning, organizing, directing, and controlling. These are still relevant today.

Planning

Planning is a four-stage process:

1. Establish objectives (goals)
2. Evaluate the present situation and predict future trends and events
3. Formulate a planning statement (means)
4. Convert the plan into an action statement.

Planning is important on both an organizational and a personal level. It may be an individual or group process that addresses the questions of what, why, where, when, how, and by whom. Decision making and problem solving are inherent in planning. Numerous computer software programs and databases are available to help facilitate planning.

Organization-level plans, such as determining organizational structure and staffing or operational budgets, evolve from the mission, philosophy, and goals of the organization. The nurse manager plans and develops specific goals and objectives for his or her area of responsibility.

CLINICAL EXAMPLE

Antonio, the nurse manager of a home care agency, plans to establish an in-home phototherapy program, knowing that part of the agency's mission is to meet the health care needs of the child-rearing family. To effectively implement this program, he would need to address the following:

- How the program supports the organization's mission
- Why the service would benefit the community and the organization
- Who would be candidates for the program
- Who would provide the service
- How staffing would be accomplished
- How charges would be generated
- What those charges should be.

Planning can be contingent or strategic. Using **contingency planning** the manager identifies and manages the many problems that interfere with getting work done. Contingency planning may be *reactive*, in response to a crisis, or *proactive*, in anticipation of problems or in response to opportunities. Examples of these problems include the following:

- Two registered nurses call in sick for the 12-hour night shift
- The manager of a specialty unit receives a call for an admission, but all the unit's beds are taken
- The manager of a pediatric oncology clinic discovers that a client's sibling exposed a number of other immunocompromised clients to chickenpox.

Planning for crises such as these are examples of contingency planning.

Strategic planning refers to the process of continual assessment, planning, and evaluation to guide the future. Its purpose is to create an image of the desired future and design ways to make those plans a reality. A nurse manager might be charged, for example, with developing a business plan to add a time-saving device to commonly-used equipment, presenting the plan persuasively, and developing operational plans for implementation, such as acquiring devices and training staff.

ORGANIZING **Organizing** is the process of coordinating the work to be done. Formally, it involves identifying the work of the organization, dividing the labor, developing the chain of command, and assigning authority. It is an ongoing process that systematically reviews the use of human and material resources. In health care, the mission, formal organizational structure, delivery systems, job descriptions, skill mix, and staffing patterns form the basis for the organization.

CLINICAL EXAMPLE

In organizing the home phototherapy project, Antonio develops job descriptions and protocols, determines how many positions are required, selects a vendor, and orders supplies.

DIRECTING **Directing** is the process of getting the organization's work done. Power, authority, and leadership style are intimately related to a manager's ability to direct. Communication abilities, motivational techniques, and delegation skills also are important. In today's health care organization, professional staff are autonomous, requiring guidance rather than direction. The manager is more likely to sell the idea, proposal, or new project to staff members rather than tell them what to do. The manager coaches and counsels to achieve the organization's objectives. In fact, it may be the nurse who assumes the traditional directing role when working with unlicensed personnel.

CLINICAL EXAMPLE

In directing the home phototherapy project, Antonio assembles the team of nurses to provide the service, explains the purpose and constraints of the program, and allows the team members to decide how they will staff the project, giving guidance and direction when needed.

CONTROLLING **Controlling** involves comparing actual results with projected results, similar to the evaluation step in the nursing process. Controlling includes establishing standards of performance, determining the means to be used in measuring performance, evaluating performance, and providing feedback. The efficient manager constantly attempts to improve productivity by incorporating techniques of quality management, evaluating outcomes and performance, and instituting change as necessary.

Today, managers share many of the control functions with the staff. In organizations using a formal quality improvement process, such as continuous quality improvement (CQI), staff members participate in and lead the teams. Some organizations use peer review to control quality of care.

> **CLINICAL EXAMPLE**
> When Antonio introduces the home phototherapy program, the team of nurses involved in the program identifies standards regarding phototherapy and the members individual performances. A subgroup of the team routinely reviews monitors designed for the program and identifies ways to improve the program.

Planning, organizing, directing, and controlling reflect a systematic, proactive approach to management. This approach is used widely in all types of organizations, health care included. Timmereck (2000) found that health care managers used these classic functions extensively.

PRINCIPLES OF MANAGEMENT

A manager has authority, accountability, and responsibility. **Authority** is defined as the right to direct others and their activities. It is an integral component of managing. Authority is conveyed through leadership actions; it is determined largely by the situation, and it is always associated with responsibility and accountability. The manager must accept the authority granted.

Accountability is the ability and willingness to assume responsibility for one's actions and to accept the consequences of one's behavior. Accountability can be viewed as hierarchic, starting at the individual level, then the institutional or professional level, and finally the societal level. At the individual or client level, accountability is reflected in the nurse's ethical integrity. At the institutional level, it is reflected in the statement of philosophy and objectives of the nursing department and nursing audits. At the professional level, it is reflected in standards of practice developed by national or provincial nursing associations. At the societal level, it is reflected in legislated nurse practice acts.

Responsibility is an obligation to obtain objectives or perform tasks. Managers are responsible for the utilization of resources, communication to subordinates, and implementation of organizational goals and objectives.

Managing Resources

One of the greatest responsibilities of managers is their accountability for human, fiscal (financial), and material resources. Budgeting and determining variances between the actual and budgeted expenses are crucial skills for any manager. Allocation of resources is discussed in Concept 44, Health Care Systems.

Enhancing Employee Performance

Managers are responsible for ensuring that employees develop through appropriate learning opportunities, whether through in-service education, facilitating attendance at professional workshops and conventions, or encouraging achievement of advanced education such as higher degrees or certifications. The nurse manager who empowers other nurses by providing information, support, resources, and opportunities to participate will find that those nurses have greater commitment to the institution, are more effective in their role, have increased self-esteem, and are better able to meet their goals.

Building and Managing Teams

The manager is responsible for building and managing the work team. Familiarity with group processes facilitates the manager's ability to lead the group and enhances the development of the group into a work team. The purposes of the team as a whole and the role of each member must be clear. Each member must feel that the manager and the other members recognize his or her contributions. In health care, the team may consist of any health care providers: nurses, therapists, unlicensed personnel, clergy, and so on. All members of the team need to use effective communication skills.

Evaluating the group's work is another responsibility of the manager. Effectiveness, efficiency, and productivity are three outcome measures that are frequently used. In health care, **effectiveness** is a measure of the quality or quantity of services provided. **Efficiency** is a measure of the resources used in the provision of nursing services. In nursing, **productivity** is a performance measure of both the effectiveness and efficiency of nursing care. Productivity is frequently measured by the amount of nursing resources used per client or in terms of required versus actual hours of care provided.

Managing Conflict

Nurse managers are frequently in a position to manage conflict among people, groups, or teams. The conflict may arise from differing values, philosophies, or personalities. In health care, it can also arise due to competition for resources.

There are many methods the nurse can use to manage conflict and each has its advantages and disadvantages (see Exemplar 35.3, Conflict Resolution). The new nurse manager may require training to become proficient in the use of these methods.

Managing Time

The effective nurse manager uses time effectively and assists others to do the same. Many factors inhibit good use of time such as preference for doing things the nurse likes to do before things the nurse prefers not to have to do, emergencies or crises that divert one's attention, and unrealistic demands from others. Strategies that the manager, and all nurses, can use in order to use time well involve setting goals and priorities, delegating appropriately, examining how time is used, minimizing paperwork (automating whenever possible), and using regular schedules that avoid interruptions and set time limits on activities (Sullivan & Decker, 2005).

CONCLUSION

An understanding of management theory and principles will increase nurses' ability to succeed when collaborating with their nurse manager. Every employee has a responsibility to put his or her best face forward when working with managers and coworkers. A collaborative rather than combattive relationship with one's manager promotes efficiency and productivity, but also makes it possible for both parties to enjoy and thrive in their working environment.

REVIEW Management Theories

RELATE: LINK THE CONCEPTS

Linking the exemplar of Management Theories with the concept of Quality Improvement:

1. How does principle of accountability impact the quality improvement process?
2. How does the nurse manager's role in enhancing employee performance impact an organization's quality improvement process?

Linking the exemplar of Management Theories with the concept of Managing Care:

3. How might strategic planning help to reduce the cost of health care?
4. How does managing resources affect managing care?

REFER: GO TO MYNURSINGKIT

REFLECT: CASE STUDY

The newly graduated nurse accepts a position working in a small community hospital on the medical/surgical unit. The unit has 32 beds and is usually staffed on the night shift, when the nurse works, with two RNs, two LPN/LVNs, and two nursing assistants. After a few months the nurse is surprised to notice how often staff members sit and complain about their nurse manager during their free time. The staff members describe the manager as "uncaring" and report that whenever they take a problem to her, she always responds by asking "How do you suggest correcting this problem?"

1. Why might the nurse manager ask for the staff nurses' input when they report a problem? Is this an effective approach?
2. What is the new graduates best action when staff sit and complain about the manager?
3. You are elected to take the staff's concerns to the nurse manager. What will you say to the manager?

PEARSON

EXPLORE mynursingkit™

MyNursingKit is your one stop for online chapter review materials and resources. Prepare for success with additional NCLEX®-style practice questions, interactive assignments and activities, web links, animations and videos, and more!

Register your access code from the front of your book at
www.mynursingkit.com.

REFERENCES

10 questions for Madeleine Albright. (2008, January). *Time Magazine.* Retrieved January 27, 2010 from http://www .time.com/time/magazine/article/0,9171,1702358,00.html

Abrams, W. B., Beers, M. H., & Berkow, R. (Eds.). (2000). *The Merck manual of geriatrics* (3rd ed.). Whitehouse Station, NJ: Merck.

Adams, K., & Galanes, G. J. (2003). *Communicating in groups: Applications and skills.* Boston: McGraw-Hill.

Adler, C. L., & Zarchin, Y. R. (2002). The "virtual focus group": Using the Internet to reach pregnant women on home bed rest. *JOGNN: Journal of Obstetric, Gynecologic, and Neonatal Nursing, 31*(4), 418–427.

Aliotta, S. (2002). Direct outcomes of case management: Involvement/participation, empowerment, and knowledge. *Case Manager, 13*(4), 67–71.

American Nurses Association. (1992). *House of delegates report: 1992 convention, Las Vegas, Nevada.* Kansas City, MO: ANA, 104–120.

American Nurses Association. (1995). *Nursing's policy statement.* Washington, DC: ANA.

American Nurses Association. (1998). Collaboration and independent practice: Ongoing issues for nursing. *Nursing Trends and Issues, 3*(5).

American Nurses Association. (2004). *Nursing: Scope and standards of practice.* Washington, DC: ANA.

Benson, L., & Ducanis, A. (1995). Nurses' perceptions of their role and role conflicts. *Rehabilitation Nursing, 20,* 204–211.

Bradford, L. P., Stock, D., & Horwitz, M. (1974). How to diagnose group problems. In L. P. Bradford (Ed.), *Group development.* La Jolla, CA: University Associates.

Centers for Disease Control and Prevention. (2004). *Basic statistics.* Division of HIV/AIDS Prevention. http://www .hivmail@cdc.gov.

Cohen, E. L., & Cesta, T. G. (2005). Dimensions of nursing case management. In E. L. Cohen & T. G. Cesta *Nursing case management* (4ᵗʰ ed.). St. Louis, MO: Elsevier.

Crenshaw, B. G. T. (2003). Working with groups. In W. K. Mohr (Ed.), *Johnson's psychiatric mental health nursing* (5ᵗʰ ed.). Philadelphia: Lippincott.

Dalton, J. M. (2003). Development and testing of the theory of collaborative decision-making in nursing practice for triads. *Journal of Advanced Nursing, 41*(1), 22–33.

Ferguson, S., Howell, T., & Batalden, P. (1993). Knowledge and skills needed for collaborative work. *Quality Management in Health Care, 1,* 1–11.

Foley, B. J., Minick, P., & Kee, C. (2000). Nursing advocacy during a military operation. *Western Journal of Nursing Research, 22*(4), 492–507.

Frisch, N. C., & Frisch, L. E. (2002). *Psychiatric mental health nursing* (2ⁿᵈ ed.). Albany, NY: Delmar.

Gilby, V. J. (1987, April). Self-help. *Canadian Nurse, 83,* 23, 25.

Hamric, A. B. (2000). What is happening to advocacy? *Nursing Outlook, 48*(3), 103–104.

Henderson, V. A. (1991). *The nature of nursing: Reflections after 25 years.* New York: National League for Nursing.

Huber, D. (2000). *Leadership and nursing care management* (2ⁿᵈ ed.). Philadelphia: W. B. Saunders.

Kim, H. S. (1983). Collaborative decision-making in nursing practice: A theoretical framework. In P.L. Chinn, (Ed.), *Advances in nursing theory development* (pp. 271–283). Rockville, MD: Aspen.

Kim, H.S. (1987). Collaborative decision-making with clients. In K. Hannah, M. Reimer, W. Mills, & S. Letourneau (Eds.), *Clinical judgment and decision making: The future with nursing diagnosis* (pp. 58–62). New York: Wiley.

Kneisl, C. R., Wilson, H. S., & Trigoboff, E. (2004). *Contemporary psychiatric-mental health nursing.* Upper Saddle River, NJ: Prentice Hall.

Lin, M., Chang, Y., & Wang, C. (2000). The power of sharing groups: An exploration of nurse students' learning process in the clinical practice. *Journal of Nursing Research (China), 8*(5), 503–514.

Manion, J., Lorimer, W., & Leander, W. J. (1996). *Team-based health care organizations: Blueprint for success.* Gaithersburg, MD: Aspen.

Mariano, C. (1989). The case for interdisciplinary collaboration. *Nursing Outlook, 37,* 285–288.

Marriner-Tomey, A. (2000). *Guide to nursing management and leadership* (6ᵗʰ ed.). St. Louis: Mosby.

McMurray, A. R. (1994, March/April). Three decision-making aids: Brainstorming, nominal group and Delphi technique. *Journal of Nursing Staff Development, 10,* 62–65.

Miccolo, M. A., & Spanier, A. H. (1993). Critical care management in the 1990s. *Critical Care Unit Management, 9*(3), 443–453.

Milgram, L., Spector, A., & Treger, M. (1999). *Managing smart.* Houston, TX: Cashman Dudley.

Mohr, W. K. (2003). *Johnson's psychiatric mental health nursing,* (5ᵗʰ ed.). Philadelphia: Lippincott.

Mok, E., & Martinson, I. (2000). Empowerment of Chinese clients with cancer through self-help groups in Hong Kong. *Cancer Nursing, 23*(3), 206–213.

National Coalition for the Homeless. (2002a). *NCH fact sheet #1: Why are people homeless?* Washington, DC: NCH.

National Coalition for the Homeless. (2002b). *NCH fact sheet #2: How many people experience homelessness?* Washington, DC: NCH.

Norton, R. W. (1983). *Communicator style: Theory, applications, and measures.* Beverly Hills, CA: Sage Publications.

Patel, V. L., Cytryn, K. N., Shortliffe, E. H., & Safran, C. (2000). The collaborative health care team: The role of individual and group expertise. *Teaching and Learning in Medicine, 12*(3), 117–132.

Salazar, M. K. (2000). Maximizing the effectiveness of case management service delivery. *Case Manager, 11*(3), 58–63.

Sampson, E. E., & Marthas, M. S. (1990). *Group process for the health professions* (3ʳᵈ ed.). New York: Delmar.

Smith, G. B., & Hukill, E. (1994, July). Quality work improvement groups: From paper to reality. *Journal of Nursing Care Quality, 8,* 1–12.

Smith-Love, J., & Carter, C. (1999, Fall). Collaboration, problem-solving reevaluation: Foundation for the Heart Center of Excellence. *Progress in Cardiovascular Nursing,* 143–149.

Tuckman, B. W., & Jensen, M. A. (1977). Stages of small group development revisited. *Group and Organization Studies, 2,* 419–427.

U.S. Bureau of the Census. (2003). *Health insurance coverage in the United States: 2002.* Washington, DC: Current Population Reports.

U.S. Department of Health and Human Services, Public Health Service. (1990). *Healthy People 2000: National Health Promotion and Disease Prevention Objectives.* DHHS Pub no. (PHS) 91–50212. Washington, DC: U.S. Government Printing Office.

U.S. Department of Health and Human Services, Public Health Service. (2000). *Healthy People 2010 Goals.* http://www .healthypeople.gov/.

Van Ess Coeling, H., & Cukr, P. L. (2000). Communication styles that promote perceptions of collaboration, quality, and nurse satisfaction. *Journal of Nursing Care Quality, 14*(2), 63–74.

Velianoff, G. D., Neely, C., & Hall, S. (1993). Development levels of interdisciplinary collaborative practice committees. *Journal of Nursing Administration, 23,* 26–29.

Vessey, Judith A., DeMarco, Rosanna F., Gaffrey, Donna A., Budin, Wendy C. (2009) Bullying of staff registered nurses in the workplace: a preliminary study for developing personal and organizational strategies for the transformation of hostile to healthy workplace environments. *Journal of Professional Nursing, 29*(5), 299-306.

Wilson, H. S., & Kneisl, C. R. (1996). *Psychiatric nursing* (5ᵗʰ ed.). Redwood City, CA: Addison-Wesley Nursing.

Communication

36

Concept at-a-Glance

About Communication, *2147*

36.1   Therapeutic Communication, *2164*

36.2   Assertive Communication, *2179*

36.3   Documentation, *2182*

36.4   Reporting, *2200*

Concept Learning Outcomes

After reading about this concept, you will be able to:

1. Describe the various modes of communication.

2. Justify when a specific mode of communication may be most useful.

3. Propose advantages and disadvantages to each mode of communication.

4. Analyze the components of each mode of communication.

5. Describe barriers to successful communication and suggest strategies to reduce the risk of each barrier.

6. Predict the impact of each factor influencing the communication process.

7. Compare and contrast different communication techniques aimed at preventing communication barriers.

8. Diagram the need for strong communication skills in each phase of the nursing process.

9. Recommend strategies the nurse may implement to improve communication with a client who has communication deficits.

10. Recommend strategies that the nurse may implement to improve communication with a client of limited English proficiency.

Concept Key Terms

Channel, *2149*

Communication, *2148*

Congruent communication, *2157*

Credibility, *2150*

Decode, *2149*

Elderspeak, *2158*

Electronic communication, *2150*

Encoding, *2149*

Feedback, *2149*

Intimate distance, *2156*

Message, *2149*

Nonverbal communication, *2149*

Personal distance, *2156*

Personal space, *2156*

Proxemics, *2156*

Public distance, *2157*

Receiver, *2149*

Response, *2149*

Sender, *2149*

Social distance, *2156*

Territoriality, *2157*

Values, *2156*

Verbal communication, *2149*

About Communication

Nursing involves interactions between nurses and clients, nurses and other health professionals, and nurses and the community. The process of human interaction occurs through communication: verbal and nonverbal, written and unwritten, planned and unplanned. Communication between people conveys thoughts, ideas, feelings, and information. For nurses to be effective in their interactions, they must have effective verbal and written communication skills. They must be aware of what their words and body language say to others. Nurses also must have effective computer and electronic communication skills.

The term *communication* has various meanings, depending on the context in which it is used. To many people, communication is the interchange of information between two or more people; in other words, the exchange of ideas or thoughts. This kind of communication uses methods such as talking and listening or writing and reading. However, painting, dancing, and storytelling are also methods of communication. Thoughts and ideas can be conveyed to others not only through spoken or written words but also through gestures or body actions.

Communication can also be a transmission of feelings or a more personal and social interaction between people. Within personal contexts, people frequently do not comment on communication unless their skills are lacking in some way. Consider one spouse complaining that the other does not communicate, or a teenager complaining that his parents don't understand.

In the health care professions, sometimes a nurse or doctor is said to be lacking in something called "bedside manner." A failure on the part of a health-care professional to communicate successfully with a client or other health-care professional can result in poor health outcomes for the client. This concept provides nurses with essential information that they need to communicate successfully with clients, colleagues, and other health-care professionals. For the purposes of this text, **communication** is any means of exchanging information or feelings between two or more people. It is a basic component of human relationships, including nursing.

The intent of any communication is to elicit a response. Thus, communication is a process that has two main purposes: to influence others to respond and to obtain information. Communication can be described as helpful or unhelpful. Helpful communication encourages a sharing of information, thoughts, or feelings between two or more people. Unhelpful communication hinders or blocks the transfer of information and feelings. In nursing, any form or failure of communication that prevents the sharing of information and feelings can have negative consequences for the client.

Nurses who communicate effectively are better able to collect assessment data, develop care plans in collaboration with clients, initiate interventions, evaluate outcomes of interventions, initiate change that promotes health, and prevent legal problems associated with nursing practice. The communication process is built on a trusting relationship with a client and support persons. Effective communication is essential for the establishment of a nurse–client relationship.

Communication also occurs on an intrapersonal level—that is, a person's thoughts are a form of communication. Intrapersonal communication is also called *self-talk* and describes the thoughts or communication an individual keeps to him- or herself. When any two people are talking with each other, each of them will usually be engaging in intrapersonal communication at the same time. Each will be thinking his or her own thoughts before, during, and after sending a message to the other person. This intrapersonal communication occurs constantly. Consequently, it can interfere with a person's ability to hear a message as the sender intended (see Figure 36–1 ■).

Clear communication is essential to both the safety of the client and the ability of the nurse to collaborate with an increasingly diverse health care team. Other factors complicating the communication process include the client's short stay in the acute care facility, the complexity of his or her illnesses, and the need to quickly prepare him or her for complex care requirements after discharge. Communicating is essential to collaboration, professional communication, and avoiding cultural misunderstandings.

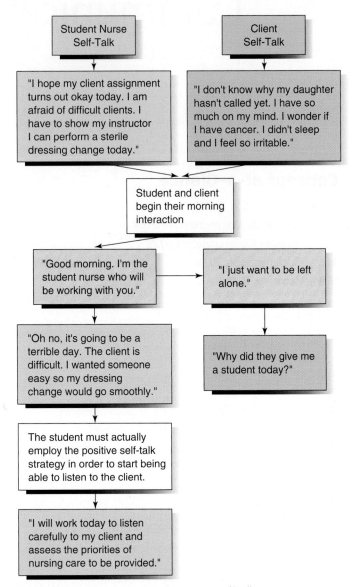

Figure 36–1 ■ Improving student nurse self-talk.

Clear and appropriate communication can pose a unique challenge in the current health care environment. Overcoming barriers to communication is necessary in a society in which many languages are spoken and the population is multicultural. Individual nurses cannot be fluent in each language they will encounter, nor can they be fully informed of the cultural contexts of words and phrases that may have multiple meanings. Nonverbal communication also has cultural meaning that must be understood to avoid barriers.

Professional communication and collaboration can be a challenge when working with colleagues from diverse cultures and languages. Clear communication about care and about client information is equally important, whether it is in the form of verbal interactions, written recordings, or computerized documentation. A challenge for nurses in the twenty-first century is to become proficient in communicating via technology, including telephone communication such as telephone triage and communication using computers such as nursing-documentation systems, personal data information systems, and e-mail.

Finding effective ways to overcome communication barriers provides the opportunity for nurses to bridge cultural gaps in delivering health care. Nurses who can use available resources and solve problems when there are communication difficulties will be better able to assist clients and families to access care and benefit from health care services. Clear communication will help the health care team provide effective care. It is essential in interdisciplinary teams. When nurses are able to communicate well in verbal and written form, the quality of professional communication benefits and nurses can provide better care to the client. Nurses can use technology to enhance communication with clients and other health care providers, to improve access to care for people in remote areas, and to increase their own knowledge using the information resources available on the Internet. ●

THE COMMUNICATION PROCESS

Face-to-face communication involves a sender, a message, a receiver, and a response, or feedback (see Figure 36–2 ■). In its simplest form, communication is a two-way process involving the sending and the receiving of a message. Because the intent of communication is to elicit a response, the process is ongoing; the receiver of the message then becomes the sender of a response, and the original sender then becomes the receiver.

Sender

The **sender**, a person or group who wishes to convey a message to another, can be considered the *source-encoder*. This term suggests that the person or group sending the message must have an idea or reason for communicating (source) and must put that idea or reason into a form that can be transmitted. **Encoding** involves the selection of specific signs or symbols (codes) to transmit the message, such as which language and words to use, how to arrange the words, and what tone of voice and gestures to use. For example, if the receiver speaks English, the sender usually selects English words. If the message is "Mr. Johnson, you have to wait another hour for your pain medication," the tone of voice selected and a shake of the head can reinforce it. Nurses must not only deal with dialects and foreign languages but also cope with two language levels—the client's and the health professional's.

Message

The next component of the communication process is the **message** itself—what is actually said or written, the body language that accompanies the words, and how the words are transmitted. The medium used to convey the message is the

channel, and it can target any of the receiver's senses. It is important for the channel to be appropriate for the message and it should help make the intent of the message clearer. In some instances, for example, talking face to face with a person may be more effective than telephoning or writing a message. Recording messages on tape or communicating by radio or television may be more appropriate for larger audiences. Written communication is often appropriate for long explanations or for a communication that needs to be preserved. The nonverbal channel of touch is often highly effective. Some of the most effective communications use more than one sensory channel.

Receiver

The **receiver**, the third component of the communication process, is the listener, who must listen, observe, and attend. This person is the *decoder*, who must perceive what the sender intended (interpretation). Perception uses all of the senses to receive verbal and nonverbal messages. To **decode** means to relate the message perceived to the receiver's storehouse of knowledge and experience and to sort out the meaning of the message. Whether the receiver accurately decodes the message according to the sender's intent depends largely on their similarities in knowledge and experience and sociocultural background. If the meaning of the decoded message matches the intent of the sender, then the communication has been effective. Ineffective communication occurs when the sender's message is misinterpreted by the receiver. For example, when the nurse prepares to feed the client who requires assistance and repeatedly glances at the clock, the client may interpret this behavior as indicating the nurse is in a hurry, which may make the client feel rushed and like a burden. It is important for nurses to consider the unplanned message their behavior may be sending.

Response

The **response**, the fourth component of the communication process, is the message that the receiver returns to the sender. It is also called **feedback**. A response can be either verbal, nonverbal, or both. Nonverbal examples are a nod of the head or a yawn. Either way, feedback allows the sender to correct or reword a message. In the case of Mr. Johnson, the receiver may appear irritated or say, "Well, the nurse on the other shift gives me my pain medication early if I need it." The sender then knows the message was interpreted accurately. However, now the original sender becomes the receiver, who is required to decode and respond.

MODES OF COMMUNICATION

Communication is generally carried out in two different modes: verbal and nonverbal. **Verbal communication** uses the spoken or written word; **nonverbal communication** uses other forms, such as gestures or facial expressions, and touch. Although both kinds of communication occur concurrently, the majority of communication is nonverbal. Learning about nonverbal communication helps nurses develop effective communication patterns and relationships with clients. Another

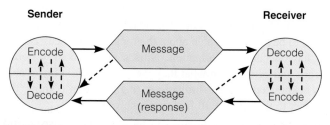

Figure 36–2 ■ The communication process. The dashed arrows indicate intrapersonal communication (self-talk). The solid lines indicate interpersonal communication.

mode of communication has evolved with technology—**electronic communication**. E-mail is the most common form of electronic communication, although social networking and text messaging are used frequently outside the workplace. It is important for nurses to know when it is appropriate and not appropriate to use e-mail to communicate with clients.

Verbal Communication

Because people choose the words they use, verbal communication is a largely conscious and purposeful activity. Words and phrasing used vary among individuals according to culture, socioeconomic background, age, and education. An abundance of words can be used to form messages. In addition, a wide variety of feelings can be conveyed when people talk. As a result, countless possibilities exist for the way ideas and information are exchanged.

When choosing what words to say or write, nurses need to consider pace and intonation, simplicity, clarity and brevity, timing and relevance, adaptability, credibility, and humor.

PACE AND INTONATION The manner of speech, as in the pace or rhythm and intonation, will modify the feeling and impact of the message. The intonation can express enthusiasm, joy, sadness, anger, or amusement. The pace of speech may indicate interest, anxiety, boredom, or fear. For example, speaking slowly and softly may help calm an excited client.

SIMPLICITY Simplicity of speech refers to the use of commonly understood words, brevity, and completeness. Many complex technical terms become natural to nurses. However, clients who are laypersons often misunderstand these terms. Words such as *vasoconstriction* or *cholecystectomy* are meaningful to the nurse and may be easy to use but are ill advised when communicating with clients. Nurses need to learn to select appropriate, understandable terms based on the age, knowledge, culture, and education of the client. For example, instead of saying to a client, "The nurses will be catheterizing you tomorrow for a urine analysis," it may be more appropriate and understandable to say, "Tomorrow we need to get a sample of your urine, so we will collect it by putting a small tube into your bladder." The latter statement is more likely to elicit a response from the client as to why it is needed and whether it will be uncomfortable; the statement is simpler and therefore easier to understand.

CLARITY AND BREVITY A message that is direct and simple will be more effective. Clarity is saying precisely what is meant, and brevity is using the fewest words necessary. Using clarity and brevity results in a message that is simple and clear. An aspect of this is congruence, or consistency, where the nurse's behavior or nonverbal communication matches the words spoken. When the nurse tells the client, "I am interested in hearing what you have to say," the nurse should use nonverbal behavior that includes facing the client, making eye contact (if culturally appropriate), and leaning forward. The goal is to communicate clearly so that all aspects of a situation or circumstance are understood. To ensure clarity in communication, nurses also need to speak slowly and enunciate carefully.

PRACTICE ALERT
Careful enunciation does not require speaking loudly. Speaking loudly to a client, even if he or she is hard of hearing, especially in a quiet setting, may be viewed by the client as patronizing or aggressive and often undermines the nurse–client relationship.

TIMING AND RELEVANCE Nurses need to be aware of both relevance and timing when communicating with clients. No matter how clearly or simply words are stated or written, the timing needs to be appropriate to ensure that the words are heard. Moreover, the message needs to relate to the person or to the person's interests and concerns.

This requires the nurse to be sensitive to the client's needs and concerns. For example, a client who is enmeshed in fear of cancer may not hear the nurse's explanations about the upcoming gallbladder surgery. In this situation, it is better for the nurse first to encourage the client to express concerns, and then to deal with those concerns. The necessary explanations can be provided at another time when the client is able to listen or after the client's primary fears have been addressed.

Another problem of poor timing results from asking several questions at once. For example, a nurse enters a client's room and says in one breath, "Good morning, Mrs. Brody. How are you this morning? Did you sleep well last night? Your husband is coming to see you before your surgery, isn't he?" The client no doubt wonders which question to answer first, if any. Asking a question without waiting for an answer before making another comment is another example of poor timing. Research shows that by allowing the client to respond to social talk or chat, as well as to questions regarding the client's condition, the nurse develops a rapport with the client (Fenwick, Barclay, & Schmeid, 2001). This rapport can help facilitate effective therapeutic communication.

ADAPTABILITY Spoken messages need to be altered in response to behavioral cues from the client. This adjustment is referred to as *adaptability*. What the nurse says and how it is said must be individualized and carefully considered. This requires astute assessment and sensitivity on the part of the nurse. For example, a nurse who usually smiles, appears cheerful, and greets his or her client with an enthusiastic "Hi, Mrs. Brown!" notices that the client is not smiling and appears distressed. It is important that the nurse modify his or her tone of speech and express concern in his or her facial expression while moving toward the client.

CREDIBILITY **Credibility** is the quality of being truthful, trustworthy, and reliable. Credibility may be the most important criterion of effective communication. Nurses foster credibility by being consistent, dependable, and honest. Nurses need to be knowledgeable about the topic being discussed and to have accurate information. Nurses should convey confidence and certainty in what they are saying, while being able to acknowledge their limitations (e.g., "I don't know the answer to that, but I will find someone who does").

HUMOR The use of humor can be a positive and powerful tool in the nurse–client relationship, but it must be used with care. Humor can be used to help clients adjust to difficult and painful situations. The physical act of laughter can be an emotional and physical release, reducing tension by providing a different perspective and promoting a sense of well-being.

When using humor, it is important to consider the client's perception of what is considered humorous. Timing is also important. MacDonald (2004) states that while humor and laughter can help reduce stress and anxiety in the early and recovery stages of a crisis, it may be considered offensive or distracting at a peak crisis period (p. 23).

Nonverbal Communication

Nonverbal communication is sometimes called *body language*. It includes gestures, body movements, use of touch, and physical appearance, including adornment. Nonverbal communication often tells others more about what a person is feeling than what is actually said, because nonverbal behavior is controlled less consciously than verbal behavior (see Figure 36–3 ■). Nonverbal communication either reinforces or contradicts what is said verbally. For example, if a nurse says to a client, "I'd be happy to sit here and talk to you for a while," yet glances nervously at a watch every few seconds, the actions contradict the verbal message. The client is more likely to believe the nonverbal behavior, which conveys "I am very busy and need to leave." On the other hand, when the nurse enters the client's room and finds the client crying, if the nurse pulls a chair close to the bed and touches the forearm gently saying, "I can see how upset you are, what is bothering you?" the nurse conveys the message that she cares and has the time and willingness to listen to the client.

Observing and interpreting the client's nonverbal behavior is an essential skill that nurses must develop. To observe nonverbal behavior efficiently requires a systematic assessment of the person's overall physical appearance, posture, gait, facial expressions, and gestures. Nurses should exercise caution in interpretation, always clarifying any observation with the client.

Clients who have altered thought processes, such as in schizophrenia or dementia, may experience times when expressing themselves verbally is difficult or impossible. During these times, the nurse needs to be able to interpret the feeling or emotion that the client is expressing nonverbally. An attentive nurse who clarifies observations very often portrays caring and acceptance to the client. This can be a beginning for establishing a trusting relationship between the nurse and the client, even in clients who have difficulty communicating appropriately.

PRACTICE ALERT

Clients who are on the autistic spectrum will likely have difficulty understanding nonverbal communication. Many people with autism find eye contact difficult, so they avoid eye contact when communicating. When speaking to an autistic client, the nurse's communication should be direct and specific. The nurse should select words carefully, keeping in mind that the client will not understand any nonverbal messages that may be communicated with the words. Offering the client handouts or brochures can help convey the message.

Nonverbal communication varies widely among cultures. Even for behaviors such as smiling and handshaking, cultures differ. For example, many Hispanics feel that smiling and handshaking are an integral part of an interaction and essential to establishing trust. The same behavior might be perceived by a Russian as insolent and frivolous. Refer to Concept 6, Culture, for more information on cultural differences.

The nurse cannot always be sure of the correct interpretation of the feelings expressed nonverbally. The same feeling can be expressed nonverbally in more than one way, even within the same cultural group. For example, anger may be communicated by aggressive or excessive body motion, or it may be communicated by frozen stillness. In some cultures, a smile may be used to conceal anger. Therefore, the interpretation of such observations requires validation with the client.

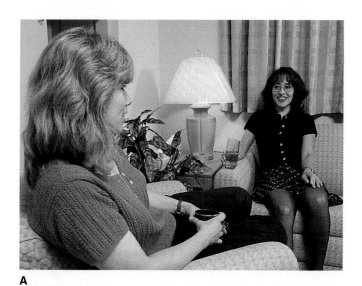

A

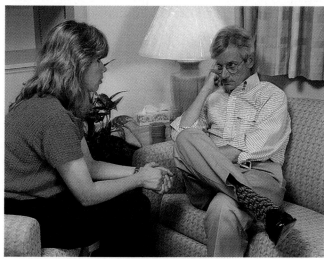

B

Figure 36–3 ■ Nonverbal communication sometimes conveys meaning more effectively than words. *A,* The postures of these women indicate openness to communication. *B,* The listener's posture suggests resistance to communication.

For example, the nurse might say, "You look like you have been crying. Is something upsetting you?"

PERSONAL APPEARANCE   Clothing and accessories can be sources of information about a person. Although choice of apparel is highly personal, it may convey social and financial status, culture, religion, group association, and self-concept. Charms and amulets may be worn for decorative or for health protection purposes. When the symbolic meaning of an object is unfamiliar, the nurse can inquire about its significance. This may foster rapport with the client and help the nurse gain a better understanding of the client's beliefs.

How a person dresses is often an indicator of how the person feels. Someone who is tired or ill may not have the energy or the desire to maintain his or her normal grooming. When a person known for immaculate grooming becomes lax about appearance, the nurse may suspect a loss of self-esteem or a physical illness. The nurse must validate these observed nonverbal data by asking the client. For acutely ill clients in hospital or home care settings, a change in grooming habits may signal that the client is feeling better. A man may request a shave, or a woman may request a shampoo and some makeup.

POSTURE AND GAIT   The ways people walk and carry themselves are often reliable indicators of self-concept, current mood, and health. Erect posture and an active, purposeful stride suggest a feeling of well-being. Slouched posture and a slow, shuffling gait suggest depression or physical discomfort. Tense posture and a rapid, determined gait suggest anxiety or anger. The posture of people when they are sitting or lying can also indicate feelings or mood. Again, the nurse clarifies the meaning of the observed behavior by describing to the client what the nurse sees and then asking what it means or whether the nurse's interpretation is correct. For example, "You look like it really hurts you to move. I'm wondering how your pain is and if you might need something to make you more comfortable?"

FACIAL EXPRESSION   No part of the body is as expressive as the face (see Figure 36–4 ■). Feelings of surprise, fear, anger, disgust, happiness, and sadness can be conveyed by facial expressions. Although the face may express the person's genuine

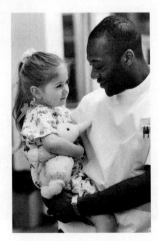

Figure 36–4 ■ The nurse's facial expression communicates warmth and caring.

emotions, it is also possible to control these muscles so the emotion expressed does not reflect what the person is feeling. When the message is not clear, it is important to get feedback to be sure of the intent of the expression. Many facial expressions convey a universal meaning. The smile expresses happiness. Contempt is conveyed by the mouth turned down, the head tilted back, and the eyes directed down the nose. No single expression can be interpreted accurately, however, without considering other reinforcing physical cues, the setting in which it occurs, the expression of others in the same setting, and the cultural background of the client.

Nurses need to be aware of their own expressions and what they are communicating to others. Clients are quick to notice the nurse's facial expression, particularly when the client feels unsure or uncomfortable. The client who questions the nurse about a feared diagnostic result will watch whether the nurse maintains eye contact or looks away when answering. The client who has had disfiguring surgery will examine the nurse's face for signs of disgust. It is impossible to control all facial expression, but the nurse must learn to control expressions of feelings such as fear or disgust in some circumstances.

Eye contact is another essential element of facial communication. In many cultures, mutual eye contact acknowledges recognition of the other person and a willingness to maintain communication. (See Concept 6, Culture.) Often a person initiates contact with another person with a glance, capturing the person's attention prior to communicating. A person who feels weak or defenseless often averts the eyes or avoids eye contact; the communication received may be too embarrassing or too dominating.

GESTURES   Hand and body gestures may emphasize and clarify the spoken word, or they may occur without words to indicate a particular feeling or to give a sign. A father awaiting information about his daughter in surgery may wring his hands, tap his foot, pick at his nails, or pace back and forth. A gesture may more clearly indicate the size or shape of an object. A wave good-bye and the motioning of a visitor toward a chair are gestures that have relatively universal meanings. Some gestures, however, are culture specific. The Anglo American gesture meaning "shoo" or "go away" means "come here" or "come back" in some Asian cultures. In the Hmong culture it is considered rude to point at something with your toe.

For people with special communication problems, such as the deaf, the hands are invaluable in communication. Many people who are deaf learn sign language. Ill persons who are unable to reply verbally can similarly devise a communication system using the hands. The client may be able to raise an index finger once for "yes" and twice for "no." Other signals can often be devised by the client and the nurse to denote other meanings.

Electronic Communication

Nurses are increasingly using e-mail to communicate with other nurses, other departments in their employment setting, and resources outside the employment setting. It is important for nurses to follow standard guidelines for the use of e-mail, and to understand its advantages and disadvantages.

ADVANTAGES E-mail has many positive advantages. It is a fast, efficient way to communicate and it is legible. It provides a record of the date and time of the message that was sent or received. Some health care facilities provide information to their clients on how they can reach specified staff members by e-mail. This improves communication and continuity of client care. E-mail provides better access.

DISADVANTAGES The disadvantage or negative aspect of e-mail is the risk to client confidentiality. The Health Insurance Portability and Accountability Act (HIPAA) requires organizations to apply "reasonable and appropriate safeguards" when e-mailing protected health information (PHI) (Anonymous, 2005). Each health care agency needs to have an e-mail encryption system to ensure security. An agency may use its own system or outsource an encryption service.

Another disadvantage is one of socioeconomics. Not everyone has a computer. While there may be available access to a computer, not everyone has the necessary computer skills. E-mail may enhance communication with some clients, but others will not have access to it at all. Alternate forms of communication will be needed for clients who have limited abilities with speaking English, reading, writing, or using a computer.

WHEN NOT TO USE E-MAIL Austin (2006) lists the following situations when it is best to avoid using e-mail:

- When the information is urgent and the client's health could be in jeopardy if he or she doesn't read the e-mail message immediately.
- Highly confidential information (e.g., HIV status, mental health, chemical dependency).
- Abnormal lab data. If the information is confusing and could prompt many questions by the client, it is better to either see or telephone the person.

OTHER GUIDELINES Agencies usually develop standards and guidelines for the use of e-mail in health care. It is important for nurses to know their employer's guidelines regarding using e-mail to communicate with clients. Usually there is an e-mail consent form that the client signs. This form provides information about the risks of e-mail and authorizes the health agency to communicate with the client at a specified e-mail address.

Austin (2006) cautions the nurse to be sure to identify that the e-mail is "confidential" in the subject line. She advises including a disclaimer that the message is to be read only by the person to whom it is addressed and that no one else is authorized to read the message. Additionally, the disclaimer should state that if the e-mail is sent to anyone else by mistake, they should contact the sender.

Information sent to a client via e-mail is considered part of the client's medical record. Therefore, a copy of the e-mail needs to be put in the client's chart. E-mails, like other documentation in the client's record, may be used as evidence during litigation. Rules for written communication (below) also apply to e-mail communication.

E-mail is another form of communication that can enhance effective relationships with clients. It is not, however, a substitute for effective verbal and nonverbal communication. Nurses need to use their professional judgment about what form of communication(s) will best meet their client's health needs.

Written Communication

Written communication can be considered a form of verbal communication, and electronic communication is a form of written communication, but for the purpose of this text it will be considered separately because written communication does not convey nonverbal cues to help the reader understand the context of the message. For example, you may receive a text message from a friend that says, "GET OUT OF HERE!!" Without an understanding of context, this message could be interpreted as shock and disbelief at something you told your friend, anger and the wish for you to vacate the friend's life, or it could be interpreted as a request to stop bothering the person because he or she is busy. Only by hearing tone of voice and seeing body language can context be relayed. As a result, rules for written communication differ from rules for other forms of communicating.

Nurses have many requirements as well as opportunities for written communication. The most common form of written communication in nursing is the notes nurses make in the medical record about a client's status, which will be discussed in Exemplar 36.3, Documentation. Nurses also write discharge instructions for clients and their families, memos to nursing colleagues and other health care professionals, and client educational materials. Nurse-managers write employee evaluations; policies and procedures; and other communications to administrators, colleagues, and nursing staff. Nurse-educators write educational handouts and course syllabi. An important consideration in written communication is that decoding often occurs when the writer is not present and may occur long after the document is written. Therefore, clarity is important because it may not be possible to ask questions or clarify areas of confusion.

CHARACTERISTICS OF EFFECTIVE WRITTEN COMMUNICATION In addition to simplicity, brevity, clarity, relevance, credibility, and humor (characteristics of effective oral communication), written communication must contain (1) appropriate language and terminology; (2) correct grammar, spelling, and punctuation; (3) logical organization; and (4) appropriate use and citation of resources.

1. *Appropriate language and terminology.* Language and terminology must be appropriate for the age, education and reading level, and culture of the reader. Health education materials written for children should be different than materials written for adults. For people whose primary language is not English, it may be more effective to have written materials translated into their primary language by a professional translator. Appropriate lay terminology may be substituted for medical terminology; for example, high blood pressure may be used instead of hypertension. See Box 36–1 for national standards on culturally and linguistically appropriate services.

2. *Correct grammar, spelling, and punctuation.* Using correct grammar, spelling, and punctuation provides clarity for the reader. Misspelled words, misplaced punctuation, or incorrect grammar can change the intended meaning and lead to

confusion on the part of the reader. They can also undermine the reader's confidence in the sender. Most computer word-processing programs have spelling- and grammar-checking features that assist writers in improving their writing.

3. *Logical organization.* Written materials are well organized when they are logical and easy for readers to follow. Consider what the reader needs to know first. Simple and foundational information is usually provided first, followed by more complex information. Using examples can also assist readers.

4. *Appropriate use and citation of resources.* Information taken from other sources must always be credited to the original source. Failure to reference work taken from another writer is called plagiarism, is considered unethical, and may violate copyright laws. There are various styles of referencing, including the Modern Language Association (MLA) and the American Psychological Association (APA). Another benefit of citing references is that readers who want additional information have other references to read.

Box 36–1 National Standards on Culturally and Linguistically Appropriate Services (CLAS)

STANDARD 1

Health care organizations should ensure that patients/consumers receive from all staff member's effective, understandable, and respectful care that is provided in a manner compatible with their cultural health beliefs and practices and preferred language.

STANDARD 2

Health care organizations should implement strategies to recruit, retain, and promote at all levels of the organization a diverse staff and leadership that are representative of the demographic characteristics of the service area.

STANDARD 3

Health care organizations should ensure that staff at all levels and across all disciplines receive ongoing education and training in culturally and linguistically appropriate service delivery.

STANDARD 4

Health care organizations must offer and provide language assistance services, including bilingual staff and interpreter services, at no cost to each patient/consumer with limited English proficiency at all points of contact, in a timely manner during all hours of operation.

STANDARD 5

Health care organizations must provide to patients/consumers in their preferred language both verbal offers and written notices informing them of their right to receive language assistance services.

STANDARD 6

Health care organizations must assure the competence of language assistance provided to limited English proficient patients/consumers by interpreters and bilingual staff. Family and friends should not be used to provide interpretation services (except on request by the patient/consumer).

STANDARD 7

Health care organizations must make available easily understood patient-related materials and post signage in the languages of the commonly encountered groups and/or groups represented in the service area.

STANDARD 8

Health care organizations should develop, implement, and promote a written strategic plan that outlines clear goals, policies, operational plans, and management accountability/oversight mechanisms to provide culturally and linguistically appropriate services.

STANDARD 9

Health care organizations should conduct initial and ongoing organizational self-assessments of CLAS-related activities and are encouraged to integrate cultural and linguistic competence-related measures into their internal audits, performance improvement programs, patient satisfaction assessments, and outcomes-based evaluations.

STANDARD 10

Health care organizations should ensure that data on the individual patient's/consumer's race, ethnicity, and spoken and written language are collected in health records, integrated into the organization's management information systems, and periodically updated.

STANDARD 11

Health care organizations should maintain a current demographic, cultural, and epidemiological profile of the community as well as a needs assessment to accurately plan for and implement services that respond to the cultural and linguistic characteristics of the service area.

STANDARD 12

Health care organizations should develop participatory, collaborative partnerships with communities and utilize a variety of formal and informal mechanisms to facilitate community and patient/consumer involvement in designing and implementing CLAS-related activities.

STANDARD 13

Health care organizations should ensure that conflict and grievance resolution processes are culturally and linguistically sensitive and capable of identifying, preventing, and resolving cross-cultural conflicts or complaints by patients/consumers.

STANDARD 14

Health care organizations are encouraged to regularly make available to the public information about their progress and successful innovations in implementing the CLAS standards and to provide public notice in their communities about the availability of this information.

Source: U.S. Department of Health and Human Services. The Office of Minority Health. National Standards on Culturally and Linguistically Appropriate Services (CLAS). Retrieved March 7, 2010, from http://raceandhealth.hhs.gov/templates/browse.aspx?lvl=2&lvlID=15

FACTORS INFLUENCING THE COMMUNICATION PROCESS

Many factors influence the communication process. Some of these are development, gender, values and perceptions, personal space, territoriality, roles and relationships, environment, congruence, and attitudes.

Development

As individuals grow and develop, language and communication skills develop through various stages. It is important for a nurse to understand the developmental processes related to speech, language, and communication skills. Knowledge of the client's developmental stage enables the nurse to select appropriate communication strategies. For example, when communicating with infants and toddlers whose language skills are not well developed, the nurse may rely more on the child's nonverbal communications to assess comfort and pain. The nurse may hold the child and use touch to provide comfort and demonstrate caring. For older children, nurses may use pictures as an adjunct to verbal language to communicate. For adolescents and adults, nurses are more able to rely on verbal language for communication. With older adults,

physical changes associated with the aging process may affect communication. For example, it may be more effective to use visual communication methods for clients who are hearing impaired or aural communication methods for clients who are visually impaired. Also, intellectual processes develop across the life span as people acquire knowledge and experience. The knowledge and experiences that people have influence their understanding and acceptance of transmitted information and feelings.

Gender

From an early age, females and males communicate differently. They may give different meanings to transmitted information or feelings. Boys use communication to establish independence and negotiate status within a group, whereas girls use communication to seek confirmation, minimize differences, and establish or reinforce intimacy. These differences may result from psychosocial development and can continue into adulthood so that the same communication may be interpreted differently by a man and a woman. It is important that nurses, when working with clients or colleagues of the opposite gender, be aware that the same communication may be interpreted differently by a man and a woman.

DEVELOPMENTAL CONSIDERATIONS Communicating With Children and Adolescents

The ability to communicate is directly related to the development of thought processes, the presence of intact sensory and motor systems, and the extent and nature of an individual's opportunities to practice communication skills. As children grow, their communication abilities change markedly.

INFANTS
- Infants communicate nonverbally, often in response to body feelings rather than in a conscious effort to be expressive.
- Infants' perceptions are related to sensory stimuli, so a gentle voice is soothing, for example, while tension and anger around them creates distress.

TODDLERS AND PRESCHOOLERS
- Toddlers and young children gain skills in both expressive (i.e., telling others what they feel, think, want, care about) and receptive (hearing and understanding what others are communicating to them) language.
- Toddlers need time to complete verbalizing their thoughts without interruption.
- Adults should provide simple responses to questions and simple, one-step directions because toddlers have short attention spans.
- Drawing a picture can provide another way for the child to communicate.

SCHOOL-AGE CHILDREN
- Adults should talk to a child at his or her eye level to help decrease intimidation.
- When communicating with a child's parents about a child's health status, if the child is present, the nurse should include the child in the conversation.

ADOLESCENTS
- It takes time to build rapport with adolescents.
- Adults talking with adolescents should use active listening skills.
- Nurses working with adolescents should project a nonjudgmental attitude and nonreactive behaviors, even when an adolescent makes disturbing comments.

Nurses can use the following communication techniques to work effectively with children and their families:
- Play, the universal language, allows children to use other symbols, not just words, to express themselves.
- Drawing, painting, and other art forms can be used even by nonverbal children.
- Storytelling, in which the nurse and child take turns adding to a story or putting words to pictures, can help the child feel safer in expressing emotions and feelings.
- Word games that pose hypothetical situations or put the child in control, such as "What if ...?" "If you could ...," or "If a genie came and gave you a wish ...," can help a child feel more powerful or explore ideas about how to manage the illness.
- Read books with a theme similar to the child's condition or problem, and then discuss the meaning, characters, and feelings generated by the book. Movies or videos can also be used in this way.
- Writing can be used by older children to reflect on their situation, develop meaning, and gain a sense of control.

In all interactions with children, it is important to give them opportunities to be expressive, listen openly, and respond honestly, using words and concepts they understand.

Sociocultural Characteristics

Culture, education, or economic level can influence communication. Nonverbal communication characteristics such as body language, eye contact, and touch are influenced by cultural beliefs about appropriate communication behavior. Some cultures may believe direct eye contact is disrespectful, whereas other cultures believe that direct eye contact shows trustworthiness. In some cultures, touch would be appropriate to communicate caring and concern, but in other cultures physical touch would be offensive. Verbal communication may be difficult for the receiver whose primary language is not that of the sender. More information about the influence of culture on communication can be found in Concept 6, Culture.

People's level of education may affect the extent of their vocabulary or their ability to read written communication. Economic level may affect a person's ability to access written communication. While many people are using e-mail to communicate or the Internet to obtain health information, people who cannot afford a computer or who do not have access to one are not able to communicate using that means.

Values and Perceptions

Values are the standards that influence behavior, and *perceptions* are the personal views of an event. Because each person has unique personality traits, values, and life experiences, each will perceive and interpret messages and experiences differently. For example, if the nurse draws the curtains around a crying woman and leaves her alone, the woman may interpret this as "The nurse thinks that I will upset others and that I shouldn't cry" or "The nurse respects my need to be alone." It is important for the nurse to be aware of a client's values and to validate or correct perceptions to avoid creating barriers in the nurse–client relationship.

Personal Space

Personal space is the distance people prefer in interactions with others. **Proxemics** is the study of distance between people in their interactions. Middle-class North Americans use definite distances in various interpersonal relationships, along with specific voice tones and body language. Communication thus alters in accordance with four distances, each with a close and a far phase. Tamparo and Lindh (2000, p. 31) list the following examples:

1. *Intimate:* Touching to 1 ½ feet
2. *Personal:* 1 ½ to 4 feet
3. *Social:* 4 to 12 feet
4. *Public:* 12 to 15 feet

Intimate distance communication is characterized by body contact, heightened sensations of body heat and smell, and vocalizations that are low. Vision is intense, is restricted to a small body part, and may be distorted. Intimate distance is frequently used by nurses. Examples include cuddling a baby, touching the sightless client, positioning clients, observing an incision, and restraining a toddler for an injection. It is a natural protective instinct for people to maintain a certain amount of space immediately around them. That amount varies with individuals and cultures. When someone who wants to communicate steps too close, the receiver automatically steps back a pace or two. In their therapeutic roles, nurses often are required to violate this personal space. However, it is important for them to be aware when this will occur and to forewarn the client. In many instances, the nurse can respect (not come as close as) a person's intimate distance. In other instances, the nurse may come within intimate distance to communicate warmth and caring.

Personal distance is less overwhelming than intimate distance. At personal distance, voice tones are moderate, and body heat and smell are less noticeable. Physical contact such as a handshake or touching a shoulder is possible. More of the person is perceived at a personal distance, so that nonverbal behaviors such as body stance or full facial expressions are seen with less distortion. Much communication between nurses and clients occurs at this distance. Examples occur when nurses are sitting with a client, giving medications, or establishing an intravenous infusion. Communication at a close personal distance can convey involvement by facilitating the sharing of thoughts and feelings. On the other hand, it can also create tension if the distance encroaches upon the other's personal space (Figure 36–5 ■). At the outer extreme of 4 feet, however, less involvement is conveyed. Bantering and some social conversations usually take place at this distance.

Social distance is characterized by a clear visual perception of the whole person. Body heat and odor are imperceptible, eye contact is increased, and vocalizations are loud enough to be overheard by others. Communication is therefore more formal and is limited to seeing and hearing. The person is protected and out of reach for touch or personal sharing of thoughts or feelings. Social distance allows more activity and movement back and forth. It is expedient in communicating with several people

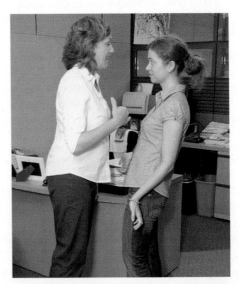

Figure 36–5 ■ Personal space influences communication in social and professional interactions. Encroachment into another individual's personal space creates tension.

at the same time or within a short time. Examples occur when nurses make rounds or wave a greeting to someone. Social distance is important in accomplishing the business of the day. However, it is frequently misused. For example, the nurse who stands in the doorway and asks a client, "How are you today?" will receive a more noncommittal reply than the nurse who moves to a personal distance to make the same inquiry.

Public distance requires loud, clear vocalizations with careful enunciation. Although the faces and forms of people are seen at public distance, individuality is lost. Instead, the perception is of the group of people or the community.

Territoriality

Territoriality is a concept of the space and things that an individual considers as belonging to the self. Territories marked off by people may be visible to others. For example, clients in a hospital often consider their territory as bounded by the curtains around the bed unit or by the walls of a private room. This human tendency to claim territory must be recognized by all health care workers. Clients often feel the need to defend their territory when it is invaded by others; for example, when a visitor or nurse removes a chair to use at another bed, the visitor has inadvertently violated the territoriality of the client whose chair was removed. Nurses need to obtain permission from clients to remove, rearrange, or borrow objects in their hospital area.

Roles and Relationships

The roles and the relationships between sender and receiver affect the communication process. Roles such as nursing student and instructor, client and primary care provider, or parent and child affect the content and responses in the communication process. Choice of words, sentence structure, message content and channel, body language, and tone of voice vary considerably from role to role. In addition, the specific relationship between the communicators is significant. The nurse who meets with a client for the first time communicates differently from the nurse who has previously developed a relationship with that client. Nurses may choose a more informal or comfortable stance when communicating with clients or colleagues and a more formal stance when communicating with

physicians or administrators. The length of the relationship may also affect communication. For example, nurses may use more formal language and a more formal stance when meeting clients or colleagues for the first time but use a more relaxed posture when interacting with those with whom they have an established relationship.

Environment

People usually communicate most effectively in a comfortable environment. Temperature extremes, excessive noise, and a poorly ventilated environment can all interfere with communication. Also, lack of privacy may interfere with a client's communication about matters the client considers private. For example, a client who is worried about the ability of his wife to care for him after discharge from the hospital may not wish to discuss this concern with a nurse within hearing of other clients in the room. Environmental distraction can impair and distort communication.

Congruence

In **congruent communication**, the verbal and nonverbal aspects of the message match. Clients more readily trust the nurse when they perceive the nurse's communication as congruent. This also helps prevent miscommunication. Congruence between verbal expression and nonverbal expression is easily seen by both the nurse and the client. Nurses are taught to assess clients, but clients are often just as adept at reading a nurse's expression or body language. If there is an incongruence, the sender's true meaning is usually conveyed by his or her body language. For example, when teaching a client how to care for a colostomy, the nurse might say, "You won't have any problem with this." However, if the nurse looks worried or disgusted while saying this, the client is less likely to trust the nurse's words. Guidelines for improving nonverbal awareness can be found in Box 36–2.

Interpersonal Attitudes

Attitudes convey beliefs, thoughts, and feelings about people and events. Attitudes are communicated convincingly and rapidly to others. Attitudes such as caring, warmth, respect, and acceptance facilitate communication, whereas condescension, lack of interest, and coldness inhibit communication.

Box 36–2 Guidelines for Improving Nonverbal Communication

- **Relax.** The simple act of relaxing makes it easier for others to be relaxed and more open. Remember, anxiety is interpersonally communicated. Taking some deep breaths, doing a quick body scan, and allowing the tension to flow out of the body can make a positive impact on the communication process.
- **Use facial, hand, and body gestures judiciously.** Nonverbal gestures that are used indiscriminately lose their effectiveness. By overdoing a gesture—constantly smiling, constantly nodding your head—the nurse may unintentionally undermine his or her own sincerity, annoy the client, and make the communication process more difficult.

- **Get feedback on nonverbal communication.** Classmates and instructors are wonderful sources of feedback. Students can ask each other and instructors to comment on the facial expressions and body gestures they use during conversations. Videotaping can assist students in determining if they possess any mannerisms or gestures that intrude on their ability to be effective communicators.
- **Practice.** Once students have identified any intrusive facial expressions or body gestures, they should practice blending verbal messages with appropriate nonverbal cues such as hand gestures, body posture, facial expression, and tone of voice. Role playing with classmates and asking them to comment on effectiveness of communication is one way to do this.

TABLE 36-1 Features of Elderspeak and Alternative Strategies

ELDERSPEAK	ALTERNATIVE STRATEGY
Diminutives (inappropriately intimate terms of endearment, imply parent–child relationship). Examples: honey, sweetie, dearie, grandma	Refer to clients by their full name (i.e., Mrs. Robinson) or by their preferred name.
Inappropriate plural pronouns (substituting a collective pronoun, e.g., *we*, when referring to an independent older adult). Example: "Are *we* ready for *our* medicine?"	"Are *you* ready for *your* medicine?"
Tag questions (prompts the answer to the questions and implies the older adult can't act alone). Example: "You would rather wear the blue socks, *wouldn't you?*"	"Would you like to wear the blue socks?"
Shortened sentences, slow speech rate, and simple vocabulary (sounds like baby talk)	Use usual sentence structure, speech rate, and vocabulary.

Note: From Williams, K., Kemper, S., & Hummert, M. L. (2004). Enhancing communication with older adults: Overcoming elderspeak. *Journal of Gerontological Nursing.* Copyright © 2004 *SLACK,* Inc. Reprinted with permission.

Haskard, DiMatteo, and Heritage (2009) conducted a research study that found that effective nursing communication is significantly related to client satisfaction with care. Key in nursing communication, both verbal and nonverbal, is communicating warmth, positivity, energy, and capability, which improves client satisfaction with both competence and interpersonal care. Caring involves giving feelings, thoughts, skill, and knowledge. It requires psychologic energy and poses the risk of gaining little in return; yet by caring, people usually reap the benefits of greater communication and understanding.

Respect is an attitude that emphasizes the other person's worth and individuality. It conveys that the person's hopes and feelings are special and unique even though similar to others in many ways. People have a need to be different from—and at the same time similar to—others. Being too different can be isolating and threatening. A nurse conveys respect by listening open-mindedly to what the other person is saying, even if the nurse disagrees. Nurses can learn new ways of approaching situations when they conscientiously listen to another person's perspective.

Health care providers may unknowingly use speech that they believe shows caring but that the client perceives as demeaning or patronizing. This frequently happens in settings that provide health care to older adults and/or individuals with obvious physical or mental disabilities (Williams, Kemper, & Hummert, 2004). **Elderspeak** is a speech style similar to babytalk, which gives the message of dependence and incompetence to older adults. It does not communicate respect. Many health care providers are not aware that they use elderspeak or that it can have negative meanings to the client. The characteristics of elderspeak include diminutives (inappropriate terms of endearment), inappropriate plural pronoun use, tag questions, and slow, loud speech, and they should not be used with any age group (Williams et al., 2004, p. 22). See Table 36–1 for features of elderspeak and alternative strategies to use.

Acceptance emphasizes neither approval nor disapproval. The nurse willingly receives the client's honest feelings. An accepting attitude allows clients to express personal feelings freely and to be themselves. The nurse may need to restrict acceptance in situations where clients' behaviors are harmful to themselves or to others. Helping the client to find appropriate behaviors for feelings is often part of client teaching.

BARRIERS TO COMMUNICATION

Just as there are characteristics of effective communication, there are identified barriers to effective communication. Nurses need to be cognizant of these barriers and avoid them. Nurses also need to recognize them when they occur so that they can change to more effective communication. Failure to listen, improperly decoding the client's intended message, and placing the nurse's needs above the client's needs are major barriers to communication. Additional barriers to effective communication are given in Table 36–2.

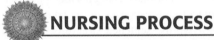

NURSING PROCESS

Communication is an integral part of the nursing process. Nurses use communication skills in each phase of the nursing process. Communication skills take on greater importance when caring for the client with sensory, language, developmental, or cognitive deficits.

Assessment

To assess the client's communication, the nurse determines communication impairments or barriers and communication style. When doing so, the nurse should remember that culture may influence when and how a client speaks. Obviously, language varies according to age and development. With children, the nurse observes sounds, gestures, facial expressions, and vocabulary.

Throughout the process of collecting data, the nurse uses communication skills to increase the nurse–client rapport, put the client at ease when discussing personal matters, and interpret the client's nonverbal communication. Exemplar 36.1 discusses the role of therapeutic communication in creating a helping relationship with the client.

Various barriers may alter a client's ability to send, receive, or comprehend messages. These include language deficits, sensory deficits, cognitive impairments, structural deficits, and paralysis. The nurse must assess for the presence of each.

TABLE 36–2 Barriers to Communication

TECHNIQUE	DESCRIPTION	EXAMPLES
Stereotyping	Offering generalized and oversimplified beliefs about groups of people that are based on experiences too limited to be valid. These responses categorize clients and negate their uniqueness as individuals.	"Two-year-olds are brats." "Women are complainers." "Men don't cry." "Most people don't have any pain after this type of surgery."
Agreeing and disagreeing	Akin to judgmental responses, agreeing and disagreeing imply that the client is either right or wrong and that the nurse is in a position to judge this. These responses deter clients from thinking through their position and may cause a client to become defensive.	*Client:* "I don't think Dr. Broad is a very good doctor. He doesn't seem interested in his clients." *Nurse:* "Dr. Broad is head of the department of surgery and is an excellent surgeon."
Being defensive	Attempting to protect a person or health care service from negative comments. These responses prevent the client from expressing true concerns. The nurse is saying, "You have no right to complain." Defensive responses protect the nurse from admitting weaknesses in the health care services, including personal weaknesses.	*Client:* "Those night nurses must just sit around and talk all night. They didn't answer my light for over an hour." *Nurse:* "I'll have you know we literally run around on nights. You're not the only client, you know."
Challenging	Giving a response that makes clients prove their statement or point of view. These responses indicate that the nurse is failing to consider the client's feelings, making the client feel it necessary to defend a position.	*Client:* "I felt nauseated after that red pill." *Nurse:* "Surely you don't think I gave you the wrong pill?" *Client:* "I feel as if I am dying." *Nurse:* "How can you feel that way when your pulse is 60?" *Client:* "I believe my husband doesn't love me." *Nurse:* "You can't say that; why, he visits you every day."
Probing	Asking for information chiefly out of curiosity rather than with the intent to assist the client. These responses are considered prying and violate the client's privacy. Asking "why" is often probing and places the client in a defensive position.	*Client:* "I was speeding along the street and didn't see the stop sign." *Nurse:* "Why were you speeding?" *Client:* "I didn't ask the doctor when he was here." *Nurse:* "Why didn't you?"
Testing	Asking questions that make the client admit to something. These responses permit the client only limited answers and often meet the nurse's need rather than the client's.	"Who do you think you are?" (forces people to admit their status is only that of client) "Do you think I am not busy?" (forces the client to admit that the nurse really is busy)
Rejecting	Refusing to discuss certain topics with the client. These responses often make clients feel that the nurse is rejecting not only their communication but also the clients themselves.	"I don't want to discuss that. Let's talk about. . . . " "Let's discuss other areas of interest to you rather than the two problems you keep mentioning." "I can't talk now. I'm on my way for coffee break."
Changing topics and subjects	Directing the communication into areas of self-interest rather than considering the client's concerns is often a self-protective response to a topic that causes anxiety. These responses imply that what the nurse considers important will be discussed and that clients should not discuss certain topics.	*Client:* "I'm separated from my wife. Do you think I should have sexual relations with another woman?" *Nurse:* "I see that you're 36 and that you like gardening. This sunshine is good for my roses. I have a beautiful rose garden."
Unwarranted reassurance	Using clichés or comforting statements of advice as a means to reassure the client. These responses block the fears, feelings, and other thoughts of the client.	"You'll feel better soon." "I'm sure everything will turn out all right." "Don't worry."
Passing judgment	Giving opinions and approving or disapproving responses, moralizing, or implying one's own values. These responses imply that the client must think as the nurse thinks, fostering client dependence.	"That's good (bad)." "You shouldn't do that." "That's not good enough." "What you did was wrong (right)."
Giving common advice	Telling the client what to do. These responses deny the client's right to be an equal partner. Note that giving expert rather than common advice is therapeutic.	*Client:* "Should I move from my home to a nursing home?" *Nurse:* "If I were you, I'd go to a nursing home, where you'll get your meals cooked for you."

Language Deficits

Determine whether the client speaks another language or has an impairment that affects his or her ability to communicate verbally. When assessing for the need for an interpreter, remember that some clients who use English as a second language may have language skills that are inadequate to meet their needs in a health care environment.

Sensory Deficits

The ability to hear, see, feel, and smell are important adjuncts to communication. Deafness can significantly alter the message the client receives; impaired vision alters the ability to observe nonverbal behavior, such as a smile or a gesture; and inability to feel and smell can impair the client's capabilities to report injuries or detect smoke from a fire. For clients with severe hearing impairments, follow these steps:

- Look for a Medic-Alert bracelet (or necklace or tag) indicating hearing loss.
- Determine whether the client wears a hearing aid and whether it is functioning.
- Observe whether the client is attempting to see your face to read lips.
- Observe whether the client is attempting to use hands to communicate with sign language.

Cognitive Impairments

Any disorder that impairs cognitive functioning (e.g., cerebrovascular disease, Alzheimer's disease, and brain tumors or injuries) may affect a client's ability to use and understand language. These clients may develop total loss of speech, impaired articulation, or the inability to find or name words. Certain medications such as sedatives, antidepressants, and neuroleptics may also impair speech, causing the client to use incomplete sentences or to slur words.

The nurse assesses whether these clients respond when asked a question and, if so, assesses the following: Is the client's speech fluent or hesitant? Does the client use words correctly? Can the client comprehend instructions as evidenced by following directions? Can the client repeat words or phrases? In addition, the nurse assesses the client's ability to understand written words: Can the client follow written directions? Can the client respond correctly by pointing to a written word? Can the client read aloud? Can the client recognize words or letters if unable to read whole sentences? The nurse uses large, clearly written words when trying to establish abilities in this area.

PRACTICE ALERT

When the client is unconscious, the nurse looks for any indication that suggests comprehension of what is communicated (e.g., tries to arouse the client verbally and through touch). Ask a closed question like "Can you hear me?" and watch for a nonverbal response such as a nod of the head for yes or a shake for no, or ask for a hand squeeze or blink of the eye once for yes or twice for no. The nurse may ask the client to grip the hand or move a finger if the client hears and understands. Because damage to the spinal cord may preclude movement, attempts to determine comprehension must be specific to the needs of the client.

Structural Deficits

Structural deficits of the oral and nasal cavities and respiratory system can alter a person's ability to speak clearly and spontaneously. Examples include cleft palate, artificial airways such as an endotracheal tube or tracheostomy, and laryngectomy (removal of the larynx). Extreme dyspnea (shortness of breath) can also impair speech patterns.

Paralysis

If verbal impairment is combined with paralysis of the upper extremities that impairs the client's ability to write, the nurse should determine whether the client can point, nod, shrug, blink, or squeeze a hand. Any of these could be used to devise a simple communication system.

Style of Communication

In assessing communication style, the nurse considers both verbal and nonverbal communication. In addition to physical barriers, some psychologic illnesses (e.g., depression or psychosis) influence the ability to communicate. The client may demonstrate constant verbalization of the same words or phrases, a loose association of ideas, or flight of ideas.

DEVELOPMENTAL CONSIDERATIONS   Communicating With Older Adults

Older adults may have physical or cognitive problems that necessitate nursing interventions for improvement of communication skills. Some of the common ones are as follows:

- Sensory deficits, such as vision and hearing
- Cognitive impairment, as in dementia
- Neurological deficits from strokes or other neurological conditions, such as aphasia (expressive and/or receptive) and lack of movement
- Psychosocial problems, such as depression.

Recognition of specific needs and obtaining appropriate resources for clients can greatly increase their socialization and quality of life. Interventions directed toward improving communication in clients with these special needs include the following:

- Assure that assistive devices, glasses, and hearing aids are being used and are in good working order.
- Make referrals to appropriate resources, such as speech therapy.
- Use communications aids, such as communication boards, computers, or pictures, when possible.

- Keep environmental distractions to a minimum.
- Speak in short, simple sentences, one subject at a time—reinforce or repeat what is said when necessary.
- Always face the person when speaking—coming up behind someone may be frightening.
- Include family and friends in conversation.
- Use reminiscing, either in individual conversations or in groups, to maintain memory connections and to enhance self-identity and self-esteem in the older adult.
- When verbal expression and nonverbal expression are incongruent, believe the nonverbal. Clarification of this and attentiveness to the client's feelings will help promote a feeling of caring and acceptance.
- Find out what has been important and has meaning to the person and try to maintain these things as much as possible. Simple things such as bedtime rituals become more important, especially in a hospital or extended care setting.

Verbal Communication

When assessing verbal communication, the nurse focuses on three areas: the content of the client's message, the themes, and verbalized emotions. In addition, the nurse considers the following:

- Whether the client's communication pattern is slow, rapid, quiet, spontaneous, hesitant, evasive, etc.
- The client's vocabulary, particularly any changes from the vocabulary normally used (for example, a person who normally never swears may indicate increased stress or illness by an uncharacteristic use of profanity)
- The presence of hostility, aggression, assertiveness, reticence, hesitance, anxiety, or loquaciousness (incessant verbalization) in communication
- Difficulties with verbal communication, such as slurring, stuttering, inability to pronounce a particular sound, lack of clarity in enunciation, inability to speak in sentences, loose association of ideas, flight of ideas, or the inability to find or name words or identify objects
- Refusal or inability to speak.

PRACTICE ALERT

Changes in the client's ability to put words together to form sentences, proper naming of an item, or struggling to find the right word for common objects may be an indication of neurological impairment. Assessment of the client's communication, especially following any type of head trauma, is an important tool in detecting alterations in the client's condition.

Diagnosis

Impaired verbal communication may be used as a nursing diagnosis when "an individual experiences a decreased, delayed, or absent ability to receive, process, transmit, and use a system of symbols—anything that has meaning (i.e., transmits meaning)" (Wilkinson, 2005, p. 80). Communication problems may be *receptive* (e.g., difficulty hearing) or *expressive* (e.g., difficulty speaking).

Wilkinson (2005) points out that the impaired verbal communication diagnosis may not be useful when an individual's communication problems are caused by a psychiatric illness or a coping problem. In those instances, the diagnoses of fear or anxiety may be more appropriate. Other nursing diagnoses (NANDA International, 2007) used for clients experiencing communication problems that involve impaired verbal communication as the *etiology* could include the following:

- Anxiety related to impaired verbal communication
- Powerlessness related to impaired verbal communication
- Situational Low Self-Esteem related to impaired verbal communication
- Social Isolation related to impaired verbal communication
- Impaired Social Interaction related to impaired verbal communication.

Plan

When a nursing diagnosis related to impaired verbal communication has been made, the nurse and client determine outcomes and begin planning ways to promote effective communication. Establishing communication with the client may require creativity or technology. New devices are being developed, ranging from thought-activated computers that verbalize for the client to devices that can be operated with a stylus in the mouth to verbalize needs.

Specific nursing interventions will be planned from the stated etiology and may include the following:

- Establish an effective means for the client to communicate needs.
- Maximize the client's ability to perceive messages accurately.
- Obtain resources as needed to optimize the client's ability to communicate.

Implementation

Nursing interventions to facilitate communication with clients who have problems with speech or language include manipulating the environment, providing support, employing measures

EVIDENCE-BASED PRACTICE **Can Clients With Advanced Dementia Participate in a Social Conversation?**

The nursing literature provides general principles to use when communicating with clients with dementia. However, there is little research that documents the effectiveness of the principles or strategies. The purpose of this study by Perry, Galloway, Bottorff, and Nixon (2005) was to describe the communication strategies used by expert nurses in communicating with residents with advanced dementia and to assess the effectiveness of the strategies in supporting participation in social conversations.

The researchers used a descriptive study design. Two of the researchers led a weekly socialization group over a 10-week period for eight women with dementia. The socialization group sessions were audiotaped and transcribed verbatim. These data resulted in the formation of two taxonomies: one represented the nurses' communication and the other represented the participants' communication repertoire.

The research supported the use of a greater number of conversational strategies than what is often stated in the nursing literature. The findings also suggested that clients with advanced dementia are able to engage in social conversation beyond what was expected given their Mini-Mental State Examination (MMSE) score.

Implications

This study suggests that individuals with advanced dementia are able to participate in a conversation when nurses use a broad range of conversational strategies. Moreover, the use of socialization groups to allow clients with advanced dementia to interact with others is a cost-effective way of enhancing their quality of life.

Note: From Perry, J., Galloway, S., Bottorff, J., & Nixon, S. (2005). Nurse-patient communication in dementia. Improving the odds. *Journal of Gerontological Nursing.* Copyright © 2005 *SLACK*, Inc. Reprinted with permission.

to enhance communication, and educating the client and support person.

Manipulate the Environment

A quiet environment with limited distractions will make the most of the communication efforts of both the client and the nurse and increase the possibility of effective communication. Sufficient light will help in conveying nonverbal messages, which is especially important if visual or auditory acuity is impaired. Initially, the nurse needs to provide a calm, relaxed environment, which will help reduce any anxiety the client may have. Remember that any factor that affects communication can create feelings of frustration, anxiety, depression, or hostility in the client. Communication normally contributes to a client's sense of security and feelings that he or she is not alone, so communication problems may cause some clients to feel isolated and confused. To further reduce these emotions, the nurse should acknowledge and praise the client's attempts at communication.

Provide Support

The nurse should convey encouragement to the client and provide nonverbal reassurance, perhaps by touch if appropriate. If the nurse does not understand, it is critical to let the client know so that he or she can provide clarification with other words or through some other means of communication. When speaking with a client who has difficulty understanding, the nurse should check frequently to determine what the client has heard and understood. Using open-ended questions will assist the nurse in obtaining accurate information about the effectiveness of communication.

CLINICAL EXAMPLE

Maria Perez, who has limited English skills, is being taught about diet related to her Crohn's disease. The nurse asks, "Do you understand what to eat?" Ms. Perez nods her head yes. The nurse realizes that her question really did not elicit an answer that sufficiently confirms that Ms. Perez understood. The nurse asks a follow up question: "What do you think will be good for you to eat when you go home?" At the same time, the nurse's body language (e.g., gestures, posture, facial expression, and eye contact) conveys acceptance and approval. When Ms. Perez begins to explain what foods she should avoid, the nurse is confident that she communicated the information to Ms. Perez successfully.

Employ Measures to Enhance Communication

First determine how the client can best receive messages: by listening, by looking, through touch, or through an interpreter. Ways to help communication include keeping words simple and concrete and discussing topics of interest to the client. It is often helpful to use alternative communication strategies such as word boards, pictures, or paper and pencil.

Nurses will also need to implement measures to enhance communication with individuals who are hard of hearing. It is important that nurses be considerate and respectful when a client is hard of hearing. Here are some suggestions based on the work of Dreher (2001) for communicating with a client who is hard of hearing:

1. Speak from a distance of 3–6 feet from the client.
2. Determine if the client hears better through one ear than the other. If so, speak into the good ear.
3. Choose an environment that is free of competing noise and turn off television sets, radios, etc.
4. Place yourself so that the client can see you clearly, preferably with light on your face.
5. Make sure the client can see your lips and be careful not to obscure them with gestures or articles of clothing.
6. Speak at a natural rate. Since people comprehend faster than they speak, it is not necessary to speak slowly unless the client does not understand.

Also see Table 25–5 in Exemplar 25.1, Hearing Impairment, in Volume 1 for more communication techniques.

Failing to recognize and compensate for a client's hearing problem risks miscommunication and can undermine the nurse–client relationship.

Avoid Potential Cultural Barriers to Communication

When English is not the client's primary language, the nurse should select words to use carefully, avoiding buzz words, slang, and technical jargon. Show respect to the client by speaking clearly and directly to the client, and by speaking at a normal pace. Words that are slurred, have many syllables in them, or are too technical make communication more difficult. Speaking too fast may overload the client and make it difficult for the client to follow. Speaking too slowly may lose the client's attention.

Select gestures with care, using nonverbal behavior to underscore words and actions. The proper use of gestures can clarify a message; drawings can sometimes be helpful. However, be careful; not all gestures mean the same thing in all cultures and some body language may be offensive or misunderstood.

Listen to the client's words and watch the client's gestures carefully. The nurse should try to understand and validate the meaning that the client's actions have for the nurse. Listening carefully to the client helps the nurse avoid focusing on what to say or do next and demonstrates genuine concern for the client's distress.

If the client attempts to speak English, his or her thoughts may appear distorted when language is the real problem. There have been a number of documented instances in which people have been diagnosed as mentally disordered and confined to a mental hospital because mental health professionals erroneously diagnosed a language problem or value difference as disordered thinking or psychosis. Use open-ended questions and rephrase them in several ways to obtain accurate information.

An interpreter may be necessary if language is a barrier. In August 2000, the federal Office for Civil Rights (OCR) of the Department of Health and Human Services mandated that any entities that receive federal funds, including health care organizations (e.g., through Medicaid or the Children's Health

Insurance Program), "must communicate effectively with patients, family members, and visitors who are deaf or hard-of-hearing and must take reasonable steps to provide meaningful access to their programs for persons who have limited English proficiency" (OCR, 2010). This is not a new law, but rather a clarification of Title VI of the Civil Rights Act of 1964. Essentially, service providers who fail to provide meaningful access to individuals with LEP are considered to be discriminating. If the client does not have his or her own interpreter, the nurse may be able to enlist the aid of a bilingual staff member. Using family members as interpreters raises issues of client confidentiality and privacy. Clients may not want family members privy to personal information (Martin & Nakayama, 2006), for example, sexual preference, drug or alcohol use, or content of hallucinations (what the voices say). Health and social services departments, international institutes, college language departments, neighborhood houses, or cultural centers will often know of people who are willing to volunteer as interpreters. When working with an interpreter, remember to always speak directly to the client and not to the interpreter.

Being aware of cultural phenomena that affect etiquette will be appreciated by the client. Spector (2006) suggests the following strategies:

1. Use the proper form of address for a given culture.
2. Know the ways by which people from that culture welcome one another, that is, when a handshake or embrace is expected as well as when physical contact is prohibited.
3. Be aware of when smiling indicates friendliness or is taboo, and when eye contact is a sign of respect or aggression.
4. Remember that gestures do not have universal meaning.

Emphasizing similarities can help to form a therapeutic relationship. Differences may serve as topics for discussion. An open, ongoing dialogue is beneficial for both parties because it promotes understanding.

Educate the Client and Support Persons

Sometimes clients and support people can be prepared in advance for communication problems, for example, before an intubation or throat surgery. By explaining anticipated problems, the client is often less anxious when problems arise and a means of communicating can be practiced in advance.

Evaluation

Evaluation is useful for both client and nurse communication. Evaluation of nurse communication is discussed in greater detail in Exemplar 36.1, Therapeutic Communication.

PRACTICE ALERT

Nodding, smiling, or agreeing are inadequate means of evaluating client understanding and often result in misunderstandings or misinterpretation of client learning. Instead, ask the client to explain in his or her own words what was said, which allows the nurse to truly evaluate the client's understanding of communications. If medical terminology is relayed by the client, ask him or her to define what is meant by the term to assure understanding.

To establish whether client outcomes have been met in relation to communication, the nurse must listen actively and observe nonverbal cues. The overall client outcome for persons with impaired verbal communication is to reduce or resolve the factors impairing the communication. Examples of statements indicating outcome achievement include "Using picture board effectively to indicate needs" or "The client stated, 'I listened more closely to my daughter yesterday and found out how she feels about our divorce.'" Examples of outcome criteria to evaluate the effectiveness of nursing interventions and achievement of client goals include the following:

The client

- Communicates that needs are being met.
- Begins to establish a method of communication:
  a. Signals yes/no to direct questions using vocalization or agreed-on physical cue (i.e., eye blink, hand squeeze)
  b. Uses verbal or nonverbal techniques to indicate needs.
- Perceives the message accurately, as evidenced by appropriate verbal and/or nonverbal responses.
- Communicates effectively:
  a. Using dominant language
  b. Using translator/interpreter
  c. Using sign language
  d. Using word board or picture board
  e. Using a computer.
- Regains maximum communication abilities.
- Expresses minimum fear, anxiety, frustration, and depression.
- Uses resources appropriately.

NURSING PRACTICE

Communication is a critical skill for nursing. It is the process by which humans meet their survival needs, build relationships, and experience emotions. In nursing, communication is a dynamic process used to gather assessment data, to teach and persuade, to collaborate with other health-care professionals, to advocate for clients, to express caring, and to provide comfort. It is an integral part of the helping relationship.

Four specific types of communication are explored in the remainder of this concept. Each of these is essential to successful nursing practice. Therapeutic communication is an essential tool for developing the nurse–client helping relationship. Assertive communication improves the student's ability to advocate for the client by improving collaborative communication. Documentation is the primary form of written communication used by nurses in all aspects of health care. Finally, reporting is the process of nurse-to-nurse communication that ensures continuity of care for the client from one shift change or visit to another.

REVIEW About Communication

RELATE: LINK THE CONCEPTS

Linking the concept of Communication with the concept of Culture:

1. How can misunderstanding the client's culture act as a barrier to communication when the nurse's culture differs?
2. The nurse is studying a culture different from the one in which the nurse was raised. What aspects of the culture would the nurse wish to learn about in order to understand how that culture's communication style may differ?

Linking the concept of Communication with the concept of Professional Behaviors:

3. How do the nurse's communication skills impact other's (both clients and other members of the health care team) perceptions regarding the nurse's professionalism?
4. The client asks the nurse a question. The nurse is very knowledgeable about the subject questioned. While answering the client the nurse stumbles over words, repeatedly starts sentences over again, uses words like "ahh" and "umm" a number of times, and gives the impression of weighing each word carefully. What impact will this delivery have on the client's perception of the nurse's professionalism and knowledge of the subject matter being explained?

REFER: GO TO MYNURSINGKIT

REFLECT: CASE STUDY

Madeline McCormick, 24 years old, is an RN who has worked in the local acute care hospital on the medical floor for the past 3 years. Last night her boyfriend proposed. She accepted and is so thrilled she can't wait to show her new diamond ring to all of her coworkers and tell them the good news. She arrives at work early to share the good news and they all congratulate her and shower her with questions about her ideas for the wedding.

You are a student nurse assigned to Ms. McCormick's floor today. As you walk by one of the client rooms you hear Madeline, who is providing a.m. care to a client, talking to the client and telling her all about how her boyfriend proposed, her wedding plans, and how happy she is.

1. Is it appropriate for Ms. McCormick to share her good news with her coworkers? Why or why not?
2. Is it appropriate for Ms. McCormick to share her news with her client? Why or why not?
3. How does Ms. McCormick's excitement over her engagement impact the nurse–client communication process?

36.1 THERAPEUTIC COMMUNICATION

KEY TERMS

Attentive listening, *2165*
Physical attending, *2166*
Therapeutic communication, *2164*
Therapeutic relationships, *2172*

BASIS FOR SELECTION OF EXEMPLAR

NCLEX Test Plan
NLN Competencies
Standards of Nursing Practice

LEARNING OUTCOMES

After reading about this exemplar, you will be able to:

1. Differentiate between attentive listening and physical attending as it applies to therapeutic communication and the therapeutic relationship.
2. Demonstrate therapeutic communication techniques, indicating when each might be of particular use when providing client care.
3. Contrast methods of delivering feedback to clients versus members of the health care team.
4. Explain the phases of the therapeutic relationship and provide examples of behaviors that occur in each phase.
5. Relate the importance of therapeutic communication to the development of a therapeutic relationship.
6. Contrast the type of communication used in the therapeutic relationship versus the communication of the nurse in health care groups.

OVERVIEW

Therapeutic communication is defined as "an interactive process between nurse and client that helps the client overcome temporary stress, to get along with other people, to adjust to the unalterable, and to overcome psychological blocks which stand in the way of self-realizations" (Kozier et al., 2004, p. 1467). Therapeutic communication promotes understanding and can help establish a constructive relationship between the nurse and the client. Unlike the social relationship, where there may not be a specific purpose or direction, the nurse establishes a therapeutic helping relationship with the purpose of helping the client achieve health goals.

In therapeutic communication, the nurse responds not only to the content of a client's verbal message but also to the feelings expressed and nonverbal cues. It is important to understand how the client views the situation and feels about it before responding. The content of the client's communication is the words or thoughts, as distinct from the feelings. Sometimes people can convey a thought in words while their emotions contradict the words; that is, their words and feelings are incongruent. For example, a client says, "I am glad he has left me; he was very cruel." However, the nurse observes that the client has tears in her eyes as she says this. To respond to the client's *words*, the nurse might simply rephrase, saying, "You are pleased that he has left you." To respond to the client's *feelings*, the nurse would need to acknowledge the tears in the client's eyes, saying, for example, "You seem saddened by all this." Such a response helps the client to focus on her feelings. In some instances, the nurse may need to know more about the client and her resources for coping with these feelings.

Sometimes clients need time to deal with their feelings, especially before coping with other matters such as learning new skills or planning for the future. This is most evident in hospitals when clients learn that they have a terminal illness. Some require hours, days, or even weeks before they are ready to start other tasks. Some need only time to themselves, others need someone to listen, others need assistance identifying and verbalizing feelings, and others need assistance in identifying alternatives about future courses of action (nurses should not assist in the clients decision making, but should help them explore alternatives). Nurses can employ a number of different techniques to support clients as they deal with their feelings related to their health and health care.

THERAPEUTIC COMMUNICATION TECHNIQUES

A number of techniques, presented here, foster effective communication. Nurses must embrace and adapt them to improve each encounter with a client. No set of communication skills is a "magic" potion that will guarantee a successful encounter with any client. People, and the relationships they develop, are unique and much too complex for any communication formula to be applied consistently and in every instance. A holistic approach is essential and is inconsistent with the rigid, inflexible application of communication techniques.

Empathizing

Nursing students are taught the skills of active listening. But listening without empathy is not enough. Empathetic understanding not only increases the nurse's grasp of the client's difficulties but also helps the nurse offer feedback on how the client affects others. *Empathy* can best be understood as a process through which people feel with one another. The person empathizing is able to embrace the attitude of the person who is speaking.

Central to learning to empathize with clients is learning to grasp the idea that what the client has to say or what the client feels is important (to the client) and deserves acknowledgment. A recent study of what it means to individuals with mental illness to be understood revealed three predominant themes: "I was important," "It really made us connect," and "They got on my level" (Shatell, McAllister, Hogan, & Thomas, 2006). Being empathetic helps nurses connect with clients and validates the importance of the client's message.

The term *empathy* is often mistakenly used synonymously with *sympathy*. Empathy contains no elements of condolence, agreement, or pity. When nurses sympathize rather than empathize, they assume that there is a parallel between their feelings and those of the client. The perceived similarity makes professional judgment and objectivity difficult. When nurses empathize, they interpret the client's feelings and do not insert their own feelings into the experience.

Empathetic involvement with troubled clients can have a number of stressful consequences. Problems can arise at any phase in the empathy process. The obstacles to achieving an empathetic concern for clients can be understood as a failure to cope with one of the four phases of achieving empathy. These four phases are discussed in Box 36–3. Nurses should take care not to identify too closely with the client and lapse into sympathy. By doing so, nurses may fail to incorporate the client's feelings and instead project personal ones. Bypassing the reverberation phase and substituting gut-level intuitions for rational problem solving can be another problem. Nurses should guard against overdistancing or burnout.

Attentive Listening

Attentive listening, also called *mindful listening*, is listening actively, using all the senses, as opposed to listening passively with just the ear. It is probably the most important technique in nursing and is the basis of all other techniques. Attentive listening is an active process that requires energy and concentration. It is more than being quiet while the other person talks: It involves paying attention to the total message, both verbal and nonverbal, and noting whether these communications are congruent. Attentive listening means absorbing both the content and the feeling the person is conveying, without selectivity. The listener does not select or listen solely to what the listener wants to hear; the nurse focuses not on the nurse's own needs but rather on the client's needs. Attentive listening conveys an attitude of caring and interest, thereby encouraging the client to talk (see Figure 36–6 ■).

Attentive listening also involves listening for key themes in the communication. The nurse must be careful not to react quickly to the message. The speaker should not be interrupted and the nurse (the responder) should take time to think about the message before responding. As a listener, the nurse also should ask questions either to obtain additional information or to clarify.

Box 36–3 Four Phases of Therapeutic Empathizing

The process of empathetic understanding has four phases:
1. *Identification.* Through the relaxation of conscious controls, we allow ourselves to become absorbed in contemplating the client and the client's experiences.
2. *Incorporation.* We take in the experiences of the client rather than attribute our own experiences and feelings to the client.
3. *Reverberation.* We interplay the internalized feelings of the client and our own experiences or fantasies. While fully absorbed in the identity of the client, we still experience ourselves as separate personalities.
4. *Detachment.* We withdraw from subjective involvement and totally resume our own identity. We use the insight gained from the reverberation phase as well as reason and objectivity to offer responses that are useful to the client.

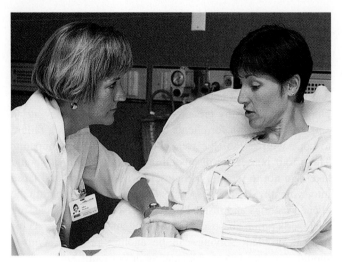

Figure 36–6 ■ The nurse conveys attentive listening through a posture of involvement.

Nurses need to be aware of their own biases. A message that reflects different values or beliefs should not be discredited for that reason. According to Rondeau (1992), the message sender (i.e., the client) should decide when to close a conversation. When the nurse closes the conversation, the client may assume that the nurse considers the message unimportant.

There are several blocks to listening that may prevent the nurse from hearing what the client says and may convey the message that what the client says is not very important (see Box 36–4).

In summary, attentive listening is a highly developed skill, which can be learned with practice. A nurse can listen attentively to clients in various ways. Common responses are nodding the head, uttering "uh huh" or "mmm," repeating the words that the client has used, or saying "I see what you mean." Each nurse has characteristic ways of responding, and the nurse must take care not to sound insincere or phony.

Box 36–4 Blocks to Attentive Listening

- *Rehearsing.* When the nurse is busy planning what he or she will say next
- *Being concerned with oneself.* When the nurse is focusing on his or her own intelligence, level of competence, feelings, or accomplishments
- *Assuming.* The nurse assumes what the client "really means"
- *Judging.* The nurse frames the message in terms of his or her judgment of the client as being wrong, immature, anxious, paranoid, or depressed
- *Identifying.* The nurse focuses on his or her own similar experiences, feelings, or beliefs when what the client says triggers the nurse's memories or concerns
- *Getting off track.* Changing the subject or making light of it when the nurse becomes uncomfortable, bored, or tired
- *Filtering.* Tuning out certain topics or hearing only certain things, perhaps because of anxiety, regardless of what else is said.

Physical Attending

Egan (1998) has outlined five specific ways to convey **physical attending**, which he defines as the manner of being present to another or being with another. Listening, in his frame of reference, is what a person does while attending. The five actions of physical attending, which convey a "posture of involvement," are described in Box 36–5.

Therapeutic communication techniques facilitate communication and focus on the client's concerns (see Table 36–3).

Using Silence

It is not necessary to respond after every statement a client makes. *Using silence* goes beyond attentive listening and can be a very effective therapeutic technique. A nurse who uses silence will sit or walk quietly with a client with the goal of providing a therapeutic purpose, such as the following:

- Encouraging the client to communicate
- Allowing the client time to ponder what has been said or a connection that the client has made
- Allowing the client time to collect his or her thoughts
- Allowing the client time to consider alternatives.

Looking interested while maintaining an open posture or a questioning look will encourage the client to use the time effectively.

Uncomfortable silences should be broken and analyzed. Do not allow the client to become increasingly anxious or resistive. Remember, silence is an effective communication technique

---

Box 36–5 Actions of Physical Attending

- *Face the other person squarely.* This position says, "I am available to you." Moving to the side lessens the degree of involvement.
- *Adopt an open posture.* The nondefensive position is one in which neither arms nor legs are crossed. It conveys that the person wishes to encourage the passage of communication, as the open door of a home or an office does.
- *Lean toward the person.* People move naturally toward one another when they want to say or hear something—by moving to the front of a class, by moving a chair nearer a friend, or by leaning across a table with arms propped in front. The nurse conveys involvement by leaning forward, closer to the client.
- *Maintain good eye contact.* Mutual eye contact, preferably at the same level, recognizes the other person and denotes willingness to maintain communication. Eye contact neither glares at nor stares down another but is natural.
- *Try to be relatively relaxed.* Total relaxation is not feasible when the nurse is listening with intensity, but the nurse can show relaxation by taking time in responding, allowing pauses as needed, balancing periods of tension with relaxation, and using gestures that are natural.

These five attending postures need to be adapted to the specific needs of clients in a given situation. For example, leaning forward may not be appropriate at the beginning of an interview. It may be reserved until a closer relationship grows between the nurse and the client. The same applies to eye contact, which is generally uninterrupted when the communicators are very involved in the interaction.

TABLE 36–3 **Therapeutic Communication Techniques**

TECHNIQUE	DESCRIPTION	EXAMPLES
Using silence	Accepting pauses or silences that may extend for several seconds or minutes without interjecting any verbal response.	Sitting quietly (or walking with the client) and waiting attentively until the client is able to put thoughts and feelings into words.
Providing general leads	Using statements or questions that (a) encourage the client to verbalize, (b) choose a topic of conversation, and (c) facilitate continued verbalization.	"Can you tell me how it is for you?" "Perhaps you would like to talk about...." "Would it help to discuss your feelings?" "Where would you like to begin?" "And then what?"
Being specific and tentative	Making statements that are specific rather than general, and tentative rather than absolute.	"Rate your pain on a scale of 0–10." (specific statement) "Are you in pain?" (general statement) "You seem unconcerned about your diabetes." (tentative statement) "You don't care about your diabetes and you never will." (absolute statement)
Using open-ended questions	Asking broad questions that lead or invite the client to explore (elaborate, clarify, describe, compare, or illustrate) thoughts or feelings. Open-ended questions specify only the topic to be discussed and invite answers that are longer than one or two words.	"I'd like to hear more about that." "Tell me about.... " "How have you been feeling lately?" "What brought you to the hospital?" "What is your opinion?" "You said you were frightened yesterday. How do you feel now?"
Using touch	Providing appropriate forms of touch to reinforce caring feelings. Because tactile contacts vary considerably among individuals, families, and cultures, the nurse must be sensitive to the differences in attitudes and practices of clients and self.	Putting an arm over the client's shoulder. Placing your hand over the client's hand.
Restating or paraphrasing	Actively listening for the client's basic message and then repeating those thoughts and/or feelings in similar words. This conveys that the nurse has listened and understood the client's basic message and also offers clients a clearer idea of what they have said.	Client: "I couldn't manage to eat any dinner last night—not even the dessert." Nurse: "You had difficulty eating yesterday." Client: "Yes, I was very upset after my family left." Client: "I have trouble talking to strangers." Nurse: "You find it difficult talking to people you do not know?"
Seeking clarification	A method of making the client's broad overall meaning of the message more understandable. It is used when paraphrasing is difficult or when the communication is rambling or garbled. To clarify the message, the nurse can restate the basic message or confess confusion and ask the client to repeat or restate the message. Nurses can also clarify their own message with statements.	"I'm puzzled." "I'm not sure I understand that." "Would you please say that again?" "Would you tell me more?" "I meant this rather than that." "I'm sorry that wasn't very clear." Let me try to explain another way."
Perception checking or seeking consensual validation	A method similar to clarifying that verifies the meaning of specific words rather than the overall meaning of a message.	Client: "My husband never gives me any presents." Nurse: "You mean he has never given you a present for your birthday or Christmas?" Client: "Well—not never. He does get me something for my birthday and Christmas, but he never thinks of giving me anything at any other time."
Offering self	Suggesting one's presence, interest, or wish to understand the client without making any demands or attaching conditions that the client must comply with to receive the nurse's attention.	"I'll stay with you until your daughter arrives." "We can sit here quietly for a while; we don't need to talk unless you would like to." "I'll help you to dress to go home, if you like."

(continued)

TABLE 36–3 Therapeutic Communication Techniques (continued)

TECHNIQUE	DESCRIPTION	EXAMPLES
Giving information	Providing, in a simple and direct manner, specific factual information the client may or may not request. When information is not known, the nurse states this and indicates who has it or when the nurse will obtain it.	"Your surgery is scheduled for 11 a.m. tomorrow." "You will feel a pulling sensation when the tube is removed from your abdomen." "I do not know the answer to that, but I will find out from Mrs. King, the nurse in charge."
Acknowledging	Giving recognition, in a nonjudgmental way, of a change in behavior, an effort the client has made, or a contribution to a communication. Acknowledgment may be with or without understanding, verbal or nonverbal.	"You trimmed your beard and mustache and washed your hair." "I notice you keep squinting your eyes. Are you having difficulty seeing?" "You walked twice as far today with your walker."
Clarifying time or sequence	Helping the client clarify an event, situation, or happening in relationship to time.	Client: "I vomited this morning." Nurse: "Was that after breakfast?" Client: "I feel that I have been asleep for weeks." Nurse: "You had your operation Monday, and today is Tuesday."
Presenting reality	Helping the client to differentiate the real from the unreal.	"That telephone ring came from the program on television." "I see shadows from the window coverings." "Your magazine is here in the drawer. It has not been stolen."
Focusing	Helping the client expand on and develop a topic of importance. It is important for the nurse to wait until the client finishes stating the main concerns before attempting to focus. The focus may be an idea or a feeling; however, the nurse often emphasizes a feeling to help the client recognize an emotion disguised behind words.	Client: "My wife says she will look after me, but I don't think she can, what with the children to take care of, and they're always after her about something—clothes, homework, what's for dinner that night." Nurse: "Sounds like you are worried about how well she can manage."
Reflecting	Directing ideas, feelings, questions, or content back to clients to enable them to explore their own ideas and feelings about a situation.	Client: "What can I do?" Nurse: "What do you think would be helpful?" Client: "Do you think I should tell my husband?" Nurse: "You seem unsure about telling your husband."
Summarizing and planning	Stating the main points of a discussion to clarify the relevant points discussed. This technique is useful at the end of an interview or to review a health teaching session. It often acts as an introduction to future care planning.	"During the past half hour we have talked about...." "Tomorrow afternoon we may explore this further." "In a few days I'll review what you have learned about the actions and effects of your insulin." "Tomorrow, I will look at your feeling journal."

only when it is used as an appropriate and purposeful therapeutic intervention. Nurses who are silent because they are uncomfortable or because they lack the knowledge or the skill to communicate effectively must seek an experienced clinical supervisor to help them analyze their own personal and professional growth needs.

Reflecting

Reflecting is repeating the client's verbal or nonverbal message for the client's benefit. It encourages the client to become more actively involved. Reflecting also actively acknowledges what you have heard or seen.

REFLECTING CONTENT Reflecting the *content* of the message basically repeats the client's statement. This gives clients the opportunity to hear and mull over what they have told you.

Content reflection is perhaps one of the most misused and overused methods in mental health counseling. Because content reflection loses its effectiveness when used for lack of other choices, nurses should use it judiciously.

CLINICAL EXAMPLE

Mr. Jackson, a 58-year-old man admitted to the hospital with a diagnosis of acute inferior myocardial infarction, says to the nurse, "I can't believe I had a heart attack. Those are for old people! I still feel young, but I guess now I'm going to slow down." The nurse reflects back to the client by stating, "You feel that, as a result of having had a heart attack, you can no longer lead an active life?" This statement, made by the nurse, will encourage the client to continue sharing his thoughts and explain why he believes this is true. This will allow the nurse to correct any misunderstandings about recovery post-MI.

REFLECTING FEELINGS Reflecting *feelings* is verbalizing the implied feelings in the client's comment. Nurses should respect the client's right to his or her opinion and feelings even when they disagree with them.

- "Sounds like you're really angry at your brother."
- "You're feeling anxious about being discharged from the hospital."

In reflecting feelings, nurses attempt to identify latent and connotative meanings that may either clarify or distort the content. Reflection is useful because it encourages the client to make additional clarifying comments.

Imparting Information

Imparting information is helping the client by supplying additional data. This encourages further clarification based on new or additional input.

- "Group therapy will be held on Tuesday evening from 6:30 until 8:00."
- "I am a psychiatric nursing student."

It is not constructive to withhold useful information from the client or to reply "What do you think?" to a straightforward, information-seeking question. However, nurses must be careful not to cross the line between giving information and giving advice, or giving information as a way of avoiding an area of interpersonal difficulty. Also, by giving personal, social information nurses move out of the realm of therapeutic intervention (see the information on avoiding self-disclosure that follows). Information that is important to disclose to the client to protect the client's rights includes the nurse's title and position. A nurse who is new to the organization or to the field should resist the temptation to avoid disclosing that information, as it may only cause mistrust.

Remember that clients' participation in decision making begins when they take in and understand information about their own condition. The goal of imparting information should be to provide effective education that empowers clients and their families. Studies have shown that an educated, empowered client is more likely to achieve positive mental health outcomes and less likely to need admission or readmission to an acute care facility.

Avoiding Self-Disclosure

From time to time a client may ask the nurse personal questions, such as those that inquire about the nurse's marital status, home address, religious affiliation, or a pressing personal problem. Auvil and Silver (1984) offer these ways to deflect a request for self-disclosure:

- *Use honesty.* "I don't want to share my home address with you."
- *Use benign curiosity.* "I wonder why you're asking me this today?"
- *Use refocusing.* "You were talking about how your father treats you. I wonder why you changed the topic? You were saying that...."
- *Use interpretation.* "I notice that every time you talk about your father, you change the subject and ask me a question." (pause)
- *Seek clarification.* "You keep asking me my home address. I wonder what concerns you might have about me today."
- *Respond with feedback and limit setting.* "I'm really uncomfortable when you ask me who pays my tuition. Talking about my finances isn't part of our agreement to work together." Adding "The last time we met, you were deciding if you were going to call your boss on the phone...." helps restructure the situation.

Nurses should use these communication techniques in the context of the therapeutic relationship, and assess and evaluate client responses in an ongoing manner with an instructor or clinical supervisor.

PRACTICE ALERT
Remember that therapeutic communication revolves around the needs of the client. Talking with the client about your experiences, what you did last night, or your thoughts on a given subject wastes time that could be used learning more about the client's needs, thoughts, concerns, or problems. Maintain a client focus in all client communications.

Clarifying

Sometimes, even though the nurse has listened carefully, the nurse may need to ask the client to clarify information. *Clarifying* is an attempt to understand the basic nature of a client's statement.

- "I'm confused about exactly what is upsetting to you. Could you go over that again, please?"
- "You say you're feeling anxious now. What's that like for you?"

Asking the client to give an example to clarify a meaning helps the nurse understand the client's intended message better. The need for clarification can occur as the result of terminology the client uses, such as the adolescent who uses fad language, or because the nurse is not certain the message is being adequately interpreted. A person who describes a concrete incident is more likely to see the connections between it and similar occurrences. Illustrations or examples are also very useful qualifiers.

CLINICAL EXAMPLE
The nurse is caring for a 36-year-old man recently diagnosed with testicular cancer. The physician has informed him his chance of full recovery is excellent and has recommended a course of treatment to include removal of the involved testi followed by chemotherapy. While the nurse is providing preoperative instructions, the client says, "I'll sign the consent form but I'll be dead before the date for surgery." The nurse is not sure if the client is fearful of dying from cancer or if this may be a statement of an intent to attempt suicide. The nurse seeks clarification by asking, "Why do you think you'll be dead before the date for surgery arrives?"

Paraphrasing

In *paraphrasing*, the nurse assimilates or restates in his or her own words what the client has said.

- "In other words, you're fed up with being treated like a child."
- "I hear you saying that when people compliment you, you feel embarrassed. If they knew the real you, they'd stay away."

Paraphrasing gives the nurse the opportunity to test his or her understanding of what a client is attempting to communicate. It is reflective in nature, in that it lets the client know what the nurse heard and how the nurse understands what has been said. It also gives the client the opportunity to clarify content or feelings.

Checking Perceptions

Checking perceptions means sharing how one person perceives and hears another. After sharing perceptions of the client's behaviors, thoughts, and feelings, ask the client to verify the perception.

■ "Let me know if this is how you see it too."
■ "I get the feeling that you're uncomfortable when we're silent. Does that seem to fit?"

Using perception checks helps the nurse make sure that he or she understands the client. An effective perception check conveys the message, "I want to understand...." It gives the other person the opportunity to correct inaccurate perceptions. It also allows the nurse to avoid actions based on false assumptions about the client.

Questioning

Questioning is a very direct way of speaking with clients. It can be useful when the nurse is seeking specific information. When the intent is to engage the client in meaningful dialogue, however, questions should be limited because too many questions may control the nature and range of the client's responses.

Open-ended questions elicit more information than closed-ended questions. An *open-ended question* focuses the topic but allows freedom of response.

■ "How were you feeling when your mother said that to you?"
■ "What's your opinion about...?"

The *closed question* limits the client's choice of responses, generally to "yes" or "no" ("Were you feeling angry when your mother said that?"). Closed questions limit therapeutic exploration. However, the client whose thinking is disorganized may need to be guided by closed questions.

"Why" questions generally are less helpful than open-ended questions. They are often impossible to answer and rarely lead to a clearer understanding of the situation. However, "who," "what," "when," and "how" questions may be helpful when used judiciously.

Nurses should be careful when questioning not to steer the client to answer in a certain way. For example, "You don't drink alcohol to excess, do you?" suggests that the client should answer "no."

Structuring

Structuring is an attempt to create order or establish guidelines. It helps the client become aware of problems and the order in which the client might deal with them.

■ "You've mentioned that you want to improve your relationships with your wife, your sister, and your boss. Let's put them in order of priority."
■ "No, I won't be giving you advice, but we can discuss some possible solutions together."

Structuring is particularly useful when clients introduce a number of concerns in a brief period and have little idea of where to begin. The nurse can use structuring not only to explore content but also to define the parameters of the nurse–client relationship and how the nurse will participate with the client in the problem-solving process.

Pinpointing

Pinpointing calls attention to certain kinds of statements and relationships. For example, the nurse may point to inconsistencies among statements; to similarities and differences in the points of view, feelings, or actions of two or more people; or to differences between what one says and what one does.

■ "So, you and your wife don't agree about how many children you want."
■ "You say you're sad, but you're smiling."

Linking

In *linking*, the nurse responds to the client in a way that ties together two events, experiences, feelings, or people. Nurses can use linking to connect past experiences with current behaviors. Another example is linking the tension between two people with current life stress.

■ "You felt depressed after the birth of both of your children."
■ "So, the arguments didn't really begin until after you got your promotion."

Giving Feedback

Giving *feedback* occurs when the nurse shares his or her reaction to what the client has said. It helps clients become aware of how their behavior affects others and how others perceive their actions. Responding with feedback can be therapeutic self-disclosure on the nurse's part. It allows the nurse to offer clients constructive information that makes them aware of their effect on others. However, total self-disclosure by the nurse (as discussed previously) is inappropriate in the nurse–client relationship. It places a burden of interdependence on the client and limits the time and energy available to work on the client's concerns. Reciprocal self-disclosure is more appropriate in friend and colleague relationships.

Effective feedback should be immediate (given as soon as possible), honest (giving one's true reaction), and supportive (given in ways that are tolerable to hear and not hurtful or brutal).

■ "When you wring your hands, I feel your anxiety."
■ "Sometimes when you turn your head away from me, I think you're angry."

It is important to give feedback in a way that does not threaten the client and result in increased defensiveness. The more defensive the client, the less likely the client will hear and understand the feedback. Clients may feel offended if they perceive the nurse as rejecting them (Hem & Heggen, 2004). Feedback that is harsh, hurtful, or cruel, or appears to reject the client, creates boundaries between the nurse and the client. The nurse should try to prevent the client from experiencing the nurse's feedback as a personal rejection. Box 36–6 lists strategies and rationales for giving helpful, nonthreatening feedback.

Clients not only express information about themselves when they interact with the nurse, but also information about how they perceive the nurse. Nurses should be open and receptive to unsolicited cues—the client's feedback to the nurse—that can help them become more effective in working with

Box 36–6 **Giving Helpful, Nonthreatening Feedback**

STRATEGY	RATIONALE
■ Focus feedback on behavior rather than on client.	Refer to what client actually does rather than how you imagine client to be.
■ Focus feedback on observations rather than inferences.	Refer to what you actually see or hear client do; inferences refer to conclusions or assumptions you make about client.
■ Focus feedback on description rather than judgment.	Report what occurred rather than evaluating it in terms of good or bad, right or wrong.
■ Focus feedback on "more or less" rather than "either/or" descriptions of behavior.	"More or less" descriptions stress quantity rather than quality (which may be value-laden).
■ Focus feedback on here-and-now behavior rather than there-and-then behavior.	The most meaningful feedback is given as soon as it is appropriate to do so.
■ Focus feedback on sharing of information and ideas rather than advice.	Sharing ideas and information helps client make decisions about own well-being; giving advice takes away client's freedom to be self-determining.
■ Focus feedback on exploration of alternatives rather than answers or solutions.	Focusing on a variety of alternatives for accomplishing a particular goal prevents premature acceptance of answers or solutions that may not be appropriate.
■ Focus feedback on its value to the client rather than on catharsis it provides you.	Feedback should serve client's needs, not your own.
■ Limit feedback to amount of information client is able to use rather than amount you have available to give.	Overloading will decrease effectiveness of feedback.
■ Limit feedback to appropriate time and place.	Excellent feedback presented at an inappropriate time may be ineffective or harmful.
■ Focus feedback on what is said rather than why it is said.	Focusing on why things are said or done moves away from observations and toward motive or intent (which can only be assumed, unless verified).

their clients. Box 36–7 provides strategies to help nurses reflect on feedback from clients.

Confronting

Constructive confrontations often lead to productive change. *Confronting* is a deliberate invitation to examine some aspect of personal behavior that indicates a discrepancy between what the person says and what the person does. Confrontation requires careful attention to nonverbal communication and the discrepancies between nonverbal and verbal messages.

Confrontations may be informational or interpretive, and they may be directed toward both the resources and the limitations of the client. An *informational confrontation* describes the visible behavior of another person.

■ "You look sad and say you're 'the dummy in the family,' yet none of your brothers or sisters made the honor roll like you did."

An *interpretive confrontation* expresses thoughts and feelings about the other's behavior and draws inferences about the meaning of the behavior.

■ "Ever since Sally and Joe criticized the way you conducted the meeting, you haven't spoken to them. It looks like you're feeling angry."

Six skills to be incorporated in constructive confrontations are the following:

1. Use of personal statements with the words *I*, *my*, and *me*

2. Use of relationship statements expressing what you think or feel about the client in the here and now

3. Use of behavior descriptions (statements describing the visible behavior of the client)

Box 36–7 **Reflecting on Feedback From Your Clients**

Input—both positive and negative—from clients, classmates, instructors, staff, and family members and friends can help you to become aware of your "blind spots," the characteristics about yourself that you ignore, deny, or defend. Protecting oneself through self-deception interferes with both relating and communicating. To become more self-aware, do the following:

■ Think about a recent interaction with a client and how that client responded to you.

■ Identify the positive/negative elements in the interaction.

■ Try to determine what the client was telling you about yourself in this interaction, that is: What characteristic(s) do you have that enables clients to openly express their thoughts and feelings? What characteristic(s) do you have that prevents clients from openly expressing their thoughts and feelings?

■ Discuss the interaction and your interpretation of it with an instructor.

■ Ask for feedback on your behavior from others—family members, classmates, staff, friends.

4. Use of description of personal feelings, specifying the feeling by name
5. Use of responses aimed at understanding, such as paraphrasing and perception checking
6. Use of constructive feedback skills.

Summarizing

Summarizing is the highlighting of the main ideas expressed in an interaction. It conveys understanding to the client and allows the nurse and the client to benefit by reviewing the main themes of the conversation. Summarizing is also useful in focusing the client's thinking and aiding conscious learning.

- "The last time we were together you were concerned about...."
- "You had three main concerns today."

Nurses can use this technique appropriately at different times during an interaction. In the first few minutes of an interaction with the client, it is useful to summarize what happened at the time of the previous interaction. Early summarizing helps the client recall the areas discussed and gives the client the opportunity to see how the nurse has synthesized the content of a previous session. Summarizing is useful because it keeps the participants directed toward a goal.

Injudicious use of summarizing is a common pitfall. For example, the nurse may rush to summarize despite other, more pressing and immediate client concerns. In this instance, summarizing may meet the nurse's need for structure, but does nothing to address the client's here-and-now concerns.

Processing

Processing is a complex and sophisticated technique. Process comments direct attention to the interpersonal dynamics of the nurse–client experience—in the content, feelings, and behavior being expressed.

- "It seems that important things that need to be taken care of come up in the last 5 minutes we have together."
- "Today is the first day our time together has started out with silence. Last week it seemed there wouldn't be enough time."

As you can see, processing is an advanced skill. Processing is most useful when therapeutic intimacy has been achieved.

CLINICAL EXAMPLE
The nurse is conducting a home visit to Michael Bardinovich, a 78-year-old man who has lived in an assisted living apartment for the past 10 years. Mr. Bardinovich was recently discharged back to his apartment following a diagnosis of pneumonia. The nurse has cared for Mr. Bardinovich for many years and knows him as a friendly, outgoing man with a great sense of humor who loves to tease people. Today, the nurse finds him quiet and reserved with little to say and comments, "You're very quiet today; you haven't teased me at all," to which he responds, "I'm not in a teasing mood." By processing the client's behavior the nurse has helped the client to begin talking about how he is feeling, which will promote a better assessment of his mood and thoughts.

Common Mistakes

It can be difficult to empathize and to communicate with clients in a therapeutic way when the nurse is experiencing discomfort or strong negative feelings. Some common mistakes to guard against are:

- *Giving advice.* Giving advice ("You should...," "Why don't you...," "It would be better if you...") carries the implicit message that the client is incapable of solving his or her own problem.
- *Minimizing or discounting feelings.* Telling a client that he or she is overreacting, that there is nothing to be afraid of, or not to worry are attempts at reassurance that minimize and discount the client's feelings.
- *Deflecting.* Hearing clients express their pain can be anxiety-provoking. Changing the subject or making a joke are attempts to move to something less painful. This is not a positive shift of focus—rather, it gives the client the message that you cannot or do not want to cope with the pain the client is feeling.
- *Interrogating.* Asking a barrage of questions implies that you are more interested in gathering information than you are in listening to the client.
- *Sparring.* No matter what the client says, you know better. Debating or disagreeing with the client prevents you from listening to the client.

BARRIERS TO COMMUNICATION

Nurses need to recognize barriers or nontherapeutic responses to effective communication (see Table 36–2). Failure to listen, improperly decoding the client's intended message, and placing the nurse's needs above the client's needs are major barriers to communication. Barriers to communication are discussed in the About Communication section of this concept.

THE THERAPEUTIC RELATIONSHIP

Nurse–client relationships are referred to by some as interpersonal relationships, by others as **therapeutic relationships**, and by still others as helping relationships. Helping is a growth-facilitating process that strives to achieve two basic goals (Egan, 1998):

1. Help clients manage their problems in living more effectively and develop unused or underused opportunities more fully.
2. Help clients become better at helping themselves in their everyday lives.

A therapeutic relationship may develop over weeks of working with a client, or within minutes. The keys to the therapeutic relationship are (a) the development of trust and acceptance between the nurse and the client and (b) an underlying belief that the nurse cares about and wants to help the client.

The therapeutic relationship is influenced by the personal and professional characteristics of the nurse and the client. Age, sex, appearance, diagnosis, education, values, ethnic and cultural background, personality, expectations, and setting can all affect the development of the nurse–client relationship. Consideration of all of these factors, combined with good communication skills and sincere interest in the client's welfare, enables the nurse to create a therapeutic relationship. Characteristics of therapeutic relationships are named in Box 36–8.

Phases of the Therapeutic Relationship

The therapeutic relationship process can be described in terms of four sequential phases, each characterized by identifiable tasks and skills. The relationship must progress through the stages in succession because each builds on the one before. Nurses can identify the progress of a relationship by understanding these phases: preinteraction phase, introductory phase, working (maintaining) phase, and termination phase. Table 36–4 summarizes the tasks and skills required.

PREINTERACTION PHASE The preinteraction phase is similar to the planning stage before an interview. In most situations, the nurse has information about the client before the first face-to-face meeting. Such information may include the client's name, address, age, medical history, and/or social history. Planning for the initial visit may generate some anxious feelings in the nurse. If the nurse recognizes these feelings and identifies specific information to be discussed, positive outcomes can evolve.

INTRODUCTORY PHASE The introductory phase, also referred to as the orientation phase or the pretherapeutic phase, is important because it sets the tone for the rest of the relationship. During this initial encounter, the client and the nurse closely observe each other and form judgments about the other's behavior. The three stages of this introductory phase are opening the relationship, clarifying the problem, and structuring and formulating the contract (Brammer, 1988). Other important tasks of the introductory phase include getting to know each other and developing a degree of trust.

After introductions, the nurse may initially engage in some social interaction to put the client at ease. For example, the nurse and client may talk about what a nice day it is or a local news or sports event.

During the initial parts of the introductory phase, the client may display some resistive behaviors. *Resistive behaviors* are those that inhibit involvement, cooperation, or change. These behaviors may arise from the client's difficulty in acknowledging the need for help, fear of exposing and facing feelings, anxiety about the discomfort involved in changing problem-causing behavior patterns, and fear or anxiety in response to the nurse's approach, which may, in the client's opinion, be inappropriate.

The nurse can overcome a client's resistive behaviors by conveying a caring attitude, genuine interest in the client, and competence. Using these techniques help the nurse foster the development of trust in the relationship. *Trust* can be described as a reliance on someone without doubt or question, or the belief that the other person is capable of assisting in times of distress and in all likelihood will do so. To trust another person involves risk; clients become vulnerable when they share thoughts, feelings, and attitudes with the nurse. Trust, however, enables the client to express thoughts and feelings openly.

By the end of the introductory phase, clients should begin to

- Develop trust in the nurse.
- View the nurse as a competent professional capable of helping.
- View the nurse as honest, open, and concerned about their welfare.
- Believe the nurse will try to understand and respect their cultural values and beliefs.
- Believe the nurse will respect client confidentiality.
- Feel comfortable talking with the nurse about feelings and other sensitive issues.
- Understand the purpose of the relationship and the roles.
- Feel that they are active participants in developing a mutually agreeable plan of care.

Box 36–8 **Characteristics of a Therapeutic Relationship**

A THERAPEUTIC RELATIONSHIP
- Is an intellectual and emotional bond between the nurse and the client and is focused on the client.
- Respects the client as an individual, including the following:
  a. Maximizing the client's abilities to participate in decision making and treatments.
  b. Considering the client's ethnic background and cultural practices.
  c. Considering family relationships and values.
- Respects client confidentiality.
- Focuses on the client's well-being.
- Is based on mutual trust, respect, and acceptance.

CLINICAL EXAMPLE

While working in an ambulatory care setting the nurse is asked by the provider to talk with a client and explain the need for phlebotomy secondary to the client's diagnosis of polycythemia. The female client's hemoglobin is 17.4 mg/dl; it has been steadily increasing since 1 year ago when it was 16.2 mg/dl. The nurse enters the room and says, "Hello, my name is Mikela Mathews. I'm an RN working for Dr. Shah. He asked me to speak with you about the need to remove blood to lower your hemoglobin." The client says, "I'm just not sure I want to do that, but I'll call you after I have time to think about it." The nurse responds by stating, "Good for you! You have every right to make a decision in your own best interest. What if I just give you some information while you're here so you can make your decision based on all the details. I can explain the risks of polycythemia, the process of removing blood, and answer any questions you may have." The nurse attempts to overcome resistance behavior by allowing the client to maintain control; this also promotes a trusting relationship with the client.

Use critical thinking to answer the following questions:

1. How would you respond if the client answered, "No thank you. That's not necessary. I can look it up on the internet"?
2. If the client agrees to listen to the nurse, what phase of the relationship will they be in once the nurse begins teaching?
3. What other types of resistance behaviors have you, or might you, encounter and how would you attempt to overcome them?

TABLE 36–4 Tasks and Skills for Each Phase of the Therapeutic Relationship

PHASE	TASKS	SKILLS
Preinteraction Phase	The nurse reviews pertinent assessment data and knowledge, considers potential areas of concern, and develops plans for interaction.	Gathering data, recognizing limitations, and seeking assistance as required.
Introductory Phase		
1. Opening the relationship	Both client and nurse identify each other by name. When the nurse initiates the relationship, it is important to explain the nurse's role to give the client an idea of what to expect. When the client initiates the relationship, the nurse needs to help the client express concerns and reasons for seeking help. Vague, open-ended questions, such as "What's on your mind today?" are helpful at this stage.	A relaxed, attending attitude to put the client at ease. It is not easy for all clients to receive help.
2. Clarifying the problem	Because the client initially may not see the problem clearly, the nurse's major task is to help clarify the problem.	Attentive listening, paraphrasing, clarifying, and other effective communication techniques discussed in this chapter. A common error at this stage is to ask too many questions of the client. Instead focus on priorities.
3. Structuring and formulating the contract (obligations to be met by both the nurse and client)	Nurse and client develop a degree of trust and verbally agree about (a) location, frequency, and length of meetings; (b) overall purpose of the relationship; (c) how confidential material will be handled; (d) tasks to be accomplished; and (e) duration and indications for termination of the relationship.	Communication skills listed previously and ability to overcome resistive behaviors if they occur.
Working Phase	Nurse and client accomplish the tasks outlined in the introductory phase, enhance trust and rapport, and develop caring.	Listening and attending skills, empathy, respect, reflecting, clarifying, paraphrasing, and confrontation. Skills acquired by the client are nondefensive listening and self-understanding.
1. Exploring and understanding thoughts and feelings	The nurse assists the client to explore thoughts and feelings and acquires an understanding of the client. The client explores thoughts and feelings associated with problems, develops the skill of listening, and gains insight into personal behavior.	
2. Facilitating and taking action	The nurse plans programs within the client's capabilities and considers long- and short-term goals. The client needs to learn to take risks (i.e., accept that either failure or success may be the outcome). The nurse needs to reinforce successes and help the client recognize failures realistically.	Decision-making and goal-setting skills. Also, for the nurse: reinforcement skills; for the client: risk taking.
Termination Phase	Nurse and client accept feelings of loss. The client accepts the end of the relationship without feelings of anxiety or dependence.	For the nurse: summarizing skills; for the client: ability to handle problems independently.

WORKING PHASE The working phase has two major stages: exploring and understanding thoughts and feelings, and facilitating and taking action. The nurse helps the client to explore thoughts, feelings, and actions and helps the client plan a program of action to meet preestablished goals.

The nurse requires the following skills for this phase of the therapeutic relationship:

■ *Empathetic listening and responding.* As discussed previously, nurses must listen attentively and communicate (respond) in ways that indicate the nurse acknowledges the client's concerns and feelings as important. Nonverbal behaviors indicating empathy include moderate head nodding, a steady gaze, moderate gesturing, and little activity or body movement.

■ *Respect.* The nurse must show respect for the client's willingness to be available, a desire to work with the client, and a manner that conveys the idea of taking the client's point of view seriously.

- *Genuineness.* Nurses exude a genuine care for the client by maintaining professional behaviors that promote the therapeutic helping relationship. Egan (1998) has outlined five behaviors that are components of genuineness (see Box 36–9).
- *Concreteness.* The nurse must assist the client to be concrete and specific rather than to speak in generalities. When the client says, "My blood pressure has been very unstable," the nurse narrows the topic to the specific by pointing out, "Show me your blood pressure log for the past two weeks."
- *Reflecting, Paraphrasing, Clarifying, and Confronting.* These skills, as described earlier, assist nurses in making sure they understand the client's messages and feelings and help them identify discrepancies that inhibit the client's self-understanding or exploration of specific areas and ideas.

During this first stage of the working phase, the intensity of interaction increases, and feelings such as anger, shame, or self-consciousness may be expressed. If the nurse is skilled in this stage and if the client is willing to pursue self-exploration, the outcome is a beginning understanding on the part of the client about behavior and feelings.

Ultimately the client must make decisions and take action to become more effective. The responsibility for action belongs to the client. The nurse, however, collaborates in these decisions, provides support, and may offer options or information.

PRACTICE ALERT

Clients with dementia or cognitive impairments may not move between phases of the nurse–client relationship the same as those with normal cognitive function. Nurses working with these clients find a need to reintroduce themselves at each meeting.

TERMINATION PHASE The termination phase of the relationship is often expected to be difficult and filled with ambivalence. However, if the previous phases have evolved effectively, the client generally has a positive outlook and feels able to handle problems independently. On the other hand, because caring attitudes have developed, it is natural to expect some feelings of loss, and each person needs to develop a way of saying good-bye.

Many methods can be used to terminate relationships. Summarizing or reviewing the process can produce a sense of

Box 36–9 **Components of Genuineness**

- The genuine helper does not take refuge in or overemphasize the role of counselor.
- The genuine person is spontaneous.
- The genuine person is nondefensive.
- The genuine person displays few discrepancies—that is, the person is consistent and does not think or feel one thing but say another.
- The genuine person is capable of deep self-disclosure (selfsharing) when it is appropriate, although this type of self-disclosure is not appropriate in the context of a therapeutic helping relationship.

accomplishment. This may include sharing reminiscences of how things were at the beginning of the relationship and comparing them to how they are now. It is also helpful for both the nurse and the client to express their feelings about termination openly and honestly. Thus termination discussions need to start in advance of the termination interview. This allows time for the client to adjust to independence. In some situations referrals are necessary, or it may be appropriate to offer an occasional standby meeting to give support as needed. Follow-up phone calls or e-mails are other interventions that ease the client's transition to independence.

CLINICAL EXAMPLE

The nurse may terminate a relationship simply by saying, "I have to leave now but will follow up with you tomorrow," or "It was a pleasure meeting you. Good-bye." How the nurse terminates the relationship is largely determined by how long the nurse–client relationship has existed, the amount the client depends on the nurse, and the client's response to the termination of the relationship. The client who is highly dependent on the nurse or who has worked with the nurse for extended periods of time requires preparation for termination, which can be accomplished by statements made by the nurse such as, "You're doing so well. After next Monday you'll be able to function independently and won't require my constant attention."

Developing Therapeutic Relationships

Whatever the practice setting, the nurse establishes some type of therapeutic relationship in which mutual goals (outcomes) are set with the client or, if the client is unable to participate, with support persons. Although special training in counseling techniques is advantageous, there are many ways of helping clients that do not require special training.

- *Listen actively.*
- *Help to identify what the person is feeling.* Often clients who are troubled are unable to identify or to label their feelings and consequently have difficulty working them out or talking about them. Responses such as "You seem angry about taking orders from your boss" or "You sound as if you've been lonely since your wife died" can help clients recognize what they are feeling and talk about it.
- *Put yourself in the other person's shoes (i.e., empathize).* Communicate to the client in a way that shows an understanding of the client's feelings and the behavior and experience underlying these feelings.
- *Be honest.* In effective relationships nurses honestly recognize any lack of knowledge by saying "I don't know the answer to that right now"; openly discuss their own discomfort by saying, for example, "I feel uncomfortable about this discussion"; and admit tactfully that problems do exist, for instance, when a client says "I'm a mess, aren't I?"
- *Be genuine and credible.* Clients will sense whether the nurse is truly concerned.
- *Use your ingenuity.* There are always many courses of action to consider in handling problems. Whatever course is chosen needs to further the achievement of the client's goals

(outcomes), be compatible with the client's value system, and offer the probability of success.

- *Be aware of cultural differences that may affect meaning and understanding.* To facilitate nurse–client interaction, recognize the language(s) and/or dialect(s) the client uses. Provide a bilingual interpreter as needed for clients limited in the English language.
- *Maintain client confidentiality.* To maintain the client's right to privacy, share information only with other health care professionals as needed for effective care and treatment.
- *Know your role and your limitations.* Every person has unique strengths and problems. When you feel unable to handle some problems, the client should be informed and referred to the appropriate health professional. Clarify functions and roles, specifically what is expected of the client, the nurse, and the primary care provider.

SPECIAL CONSIDERATIONS WHEN WORKING WITH CHILDREN AND FAMILIES

The focus of nursing interventions is facilitation of effective therapeutic communication with the child and family, and the resulting establishment of an effective nurse–child–family relationship (Table 36–5). The techniques the nurse uses to develop a therapeutic relationship with the child and family are not significantly different from those already described: The nurse tailors the techniques to the needs of the child and family (Figure 36–7 ■). See Developmental Considerations: Establishing Rapport With Children. Providing an appropriate environment will foster effective nurse–child–family communication. Remember to provide privacy to ensure confidentiality.

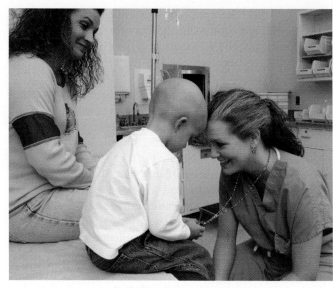

Figure 36–7 ■ Taking time to listen to the family members and child is important to the establishment of trust and developing rapport with the child and family.

Establishing Trust

Trust plays a critical role for an effective nurse–child–family relationship. To establish an atmosphere of trust, the nurse should do the following:

- Follow through with promises to the child and family—this ensures secure feelings for the family.
- Respect confidentiality—this promotes protection of the family.
- Be truthful with the child and family—they will respect the nurse, even if the truth is not what they want to hear.

DEVELOPMENTAL CONSIDERATIONS Establishing Rapport With Children

A child will be more responsive to the nurse when efforts are made to help the child feel like he or she is an important person in the interaction. By following the following guidelines, nurses can help establish rapport with the child and encourage the child to share personal information and feelings:

- Sit or otherwise lower yourself so that you are at the child's eye level. Sitting at eye level suggests that the nurse cares.
- Note what the child is playing with or reading; ask about his or her favorite cartoon character. Interest displayed by the nurse encourages the child's feeling of security.
- Agree with the child when appropriate and share your feelings: "I don't like the taste of that medicine either, but sometimes I have to take it when I am sick—but then I have juice." This statement offers encouragement to the child and family.
- Compliment a physical feature or activity performed by the child: "You are really strong" or "You picked really nice colors for that picture." This observational statement may reduce anxiety and imparts status for the child.
- Use a calm tone of voice, with developmentally appropriate language. Children want to talk and share information on their level of comprehension.

- Pace the discussion or procedure in a nonhurried manner. Trying to rush the child will only add to his or her anxiety.
- Preschoolers have a limited concept of time. Explain concepts in terms they understand: "Your mother will be back after lunch." This type of response provides them with a concrete time frame.
- Include the adolescent in discussion about his or her care. They have the cognitive ability to employ abstract communication and comprehend scientific terminology.
- Listen more than you talk, and avoid distractions. This attentive behavior of the nurse conveys an attitude of interest in the child.
- Be truthful with the child. He or she will respect your honesty.

Source: Data from Boggs, K. U. (2007a). Communicating with children. In E. C. Arnold, & K. U. Boggs, *Interpersonal relationships: Professional communication skills for nurses* (5th ed., pp. 395–416). St. Louis, MO: Saunders; Adubato, S. (2004). Making the communication connection. *Nursing Management, 35*(9), 33–36; Fleitas, J. (2003). The power of words: Examining the linguistic landscape of pediatric nursing. MCN. *The American Journal of Maternal Child Nursing, 28*(6), 384–388.

TABLE 36–5 Using Therapeutic Communication Techniques With Children

COMMUNICATION TECHNIQUE	EXAMPLE	NURSING IMPLICATIONS
Accepting	"It is okay to cry. I know that this hurts."	The nurse should empathize with the child's thoughts and feelings. Conveying acceptance includes respecting the child's emotions by allowing the child to cry when in pain or letting the child know that crying is okay.
Active listening	Pay attention to what the child says, acknowledge the child's feelings, and avoid interruption.	Involve children in the discussion and encourage them to relay their points of view.
		Face the child and parents when talking to let the child and family know that the nurse is listening and understands what is being communicated.
Broad openings	"What do you want to talk about right now?"	Use open-ended questions to allow the child to choose the discussion topic.
Clarifying	*Child*: "Whenever the doctor tells me I have to stay in the hospital longer, I get so mad."	Communicate understanding by asking the child to clarify or elaborate on the thoughts expressed.
	Nurse: "It sounds like you are very angry. What does that feel like?"	
Collaborating	"Perhaps we can work together and figure out the best way to go about handling this."	Assist the child and family through the problem-solving process.
		The nurse first suggests collaboration with the child and/or family, and then assists them to work through each step of the problem-solving process.
Exploring	"Can you tell me more about how you feel after you receive your chemotherapy?"	Exploring helps the child to organize thoughts and focus on particular issues. It also encourages the child to freely discuss issues in more detail.
Focusing	"I do want to hear about your dog in a little while, but right now could you tell me about your stomachache?"	Utilize focusing to guide the direction of the conversation. This is useful for small children who often wish to discuss a variety of topics rather than focus on one topic.
		Focusing allows the nurse to explore the child's concern further.
Giving recognition	"That is a very colorful picture you are drawing."	Identify observed behaviors or cues of the child. This indicates an interest in the child.
Observations	"You tell me you aren't hurting, but your fists are clenched and your mouth is quivering."	Pay close attention to the behavioral aspect of communication.
	"You seem sad today."	The nurse acknowledges behaviors that indicate the child's thoughts and feelings.
Offering self	"I will stay with you while your mother goes to the cafeteria to eat lunch."	The nurse is available to listen and be with the child.
Placing the event in time or sequence	"Which happened first...?"	Assist the child to determine what happened and in what order.
	"When did you first start feeling...?"	The goal is to help the child and nurse understand the progression of events.
Reflection	*Adolescent*: "I keep thinking about what my friends are doing while I am in the hospital, and if they miss me."	Repeat a phrase or sentence the child just said.
	Nurse: "It is hard not being with your friends."	By reflection, the nurse indicates an interest in the discussion and validates the child's concerns.

(continued)

TABLE 36–5 **Using Therapeutic Communication Techniques With Children** (continued)

COMMUNICATION TECHNIQUE	EXAMPLE	NURSING IMPLICATIONS
Restatement or paraphrasing	*Child:* "I think I should tell my mother that I have been smoking."	The nurse repeats what the child has said using different words.
	Nurse: "You want to tell your mother about your smoking?"	By restating, the nurse is acknowledging to the child that he or she is listening. It also provides a means to validate the interpretation of the child's statement.
Summarizing	"The two things that you are most concerned about are...."	Highlight the key facts obtained in the conversation by condensing the information the child related.
		Summarizing provides the child and nurse an opportunity to consider further direction of the discussion or to give the discussion closure.
		The nurse can summarize at various points during the conversation; it is not necessary to wait until the discussion is nearing completion.
Validating perceptions	"It sounds like you are sad about being sick. Is that correct?"	The nurse shares the conclusions drawn from the discussion with the child.
		Validating perceptions provides an opportunity for the child to confirm or deny the nurse's interpretation of the meaning of their communication.

Source: Data from Antai-Otong, D. (2007). *Nurse-client communication.* Sudbury, MA: Jones and Bartlett; Fontaine, K. L. (2003). Relating, communicating, and educating. In *Mental health nursing* (5th ed.). Upper Saddle River, NJ: Prentice Hall; Muñoz, C., & Luckmann, J. (2005). *Transcultural communication in nursing* (2nd ed.). Clifton Park, NY: Delmar Learning.

If a child asks whether a procedure is painful, answer truthfully, but follow with positive words. For example, if a child asks if his "shot" is going to hurt, you might reply, "Yes, most people say that a shot hurts, but it will only hurt for a moment, and then it will be over. Your mother can hold your hand while I give you the medicine, if that will make you feel better." By following difficult information with a positive rationale or comforting statement, the nurse can maintain credibility while still providing compassionate care.

CONCLUSION

The nurse's role, whether teaching, advocating, assessing, planning, documenting, or intervening, requires strong communication skills. The ability to communicate effectively plays a large role in the nurse's ability to deliver the highest quality of care to clients. Whether talking with clients, other members of the health care team, distraught family members, or peers, the nurse needs to be understood and understand the messages he or she receives. Strong verbal and written communication skills are required of the effective nurse who must also monitor nonverbal communication to maintain consistency in the messages sent to others.

REVIEW Therapeutic Communication

RELATE: LINK THE CONCEPTS

Linking the exemplar of Therapeutic Communication with the concept of Advocacy:
1. How do strong therapeutic communication skills contribute to the nurse's role as a client advocate?
2. How do strong therapeutic communication skills contribute to the nurse's ability to work within groups to advocate for clients?

Linking the exemplar of Therapeutic Communication with the concept of Teaching and Learning:
3. The nurse is preparing to teach a newly diagnosed diabetic client about self-care. Describe the three phases of the therapeutic relationship as it applies to the client teaching plan.
4. While teaching the diabetic client the nurse accidentally creates a barrier to the therapeutic relationship by misspeaking. What should the nurse do next?

REFER: GO TO MYNURSINGKIT

REFLECT: CASE STUDY

Kate Swanson is a newly graduated nurse working at the Neighborhood Hospital. She is assigned the care of Mrs. Ocampo, diagnosed with Alzheimer's disease.

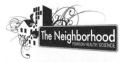

Mrs. Ocampo was admitted with a fractured hip following a fall at home that occurred when she was wandering around her house late

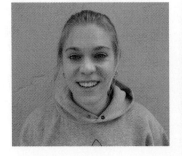 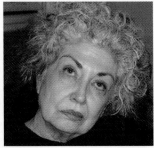

one night. Mrs. Ocampo was assigned a different nurse yesterday but Dr. Ocampo, her husband, complained to the nurse manager when he came to visit and found her restrained and yelling for help with an untouched breakfast tray in front of her. Dr. Ocampo requested a different nurse be assigned to her care from now on; Ms. Swanson is happy to act as her primary nurse. She develops rapport with Dr. Ocampo and gets satisfaction from caring for Mrs. Ocampo and helping her to feel more comfortable.

1. When communicating with a client diagnosed with later-stage Alzeheimer's disease what strategies will Ms. Swanson employ?
2. Why does the development of rapport with Mr. Ocampo improve the client's ability to meet expected outcomes?
3. Dr. Ocampo complains to Ms. Swanson about the poor care provided to his wife by the other nurse, Bobby. How should Ms. Swanson respond to this statement?

36.2 ASSERTIVE COMMUNICATION

KEY TERMS

Aggressive communicators, *2179*
Assertive communicators, *2179*
Passive communicators, *2179*

BASIS FOR SELECTION OF EXEMPLAR

NLN Competencies
National Institute of Mental Health

LEARNING OUTCOMES

After reading about this exemplar, you will be able to:

1. Contrast various styles of communicating including positive and negative results of each style.
2. Explore the characteristics of an assertive communicator.
3. Predict the impact on client care when the nurse communicates assertively.
4. Demonstrate assertive communication techniques.

OVERVIEW

Different people have different ways or styles of communication. Gender, culture, personality type, and degree of confidence can all play a role in how a nurse communicates with others. Communication is complex and requires that the nurse use a thoughtful process to communicate effectively. It is something that is used daily in both the work and home environment and often is not viewed as important until there is a problem with it.

Most people tend to express themselves in one of three ways—aggressively, assertively, or passively. **Aggressive communicators** focus primarily on their own needs and can become impatient when needs are not satisfied. **Passive communicators** focus primarily on the needs of others and often deny themselves power, causing frustration. **Assertive communicators** are able to declare and affirm their opinions while respecting the rights of others to do the same. Assertive behavior strikes a balance between aggression and passivity and promotes the most productive communication. Box 36–10 contrasts the characteristics of these three styles.

People who use assertive communication express themselves effectively and stand up for their beliefs while respecting the rights of others (Mayo Clinic, 2009). Assertive communicators are honest, direct, and appropriate while being open to ideas and showing concern for the needs and of others. Assertive communication promotes client safety by minimizing miscommunication with colleagues. Failure to communicate can result in negative client outcomes.

COMMUNICATION STYLES

An important characteristic of assertive communication includes the use of "I" statements versus "you" statements. The "you" statement places blame and puts the listener in a defensive

position. On the other hand, the "I" statement encourages discussion. For example, a nurse who states "I am concerned about ..." to a physician will gain the attention of the doctor while also giving the message of the importance to work together for the benefit of the client. Once the nurse has the doctor's attention, it is important for the nurse to be clear, concise, organized, and fully informed when presenting the client concern.

Box 36–10 Aggressive, Passive, and Assertive Styles

AGGRESSIVE
- Loud, heated arguing
- Physically violent encounters
- Blaming, name-calling, and verbal insults
- Walking out of arguments before they are resolved
- Being demanding: "Do this"

PASSIVE
- Concealing one's own feelings
- Denying one's own anger
- Feeling that one has no right to express anger
- Avoiding arguments
- Being noncommittal: "You don't have to do this unless you really want to . . . "

ASSERTIVE
- Expressing feelings without being nasty or overbearing
- Acknowledging emotions but staying open to discussion
- Expressing self and giving others the chance to express themselves equally
- Using "I" statements to defuse arguments
- Asking and giving reasons: "I would appreciate it if you would do this, and here's why . . . "

Source: Katz, J. (2001). *Keys to nursing success* (p. 267). Upper Saddle River, NJ: Prentice Hall. Reprinted with permission.

When people use a submissive communication style they allow their rights to be violated by others (Catalano, 2006). They meet the demands and requests of others without regard to their own feelings and needs as they believe their own feelings are not important. Some experts believe that people who use the submissive behaviors or communication styles are insecure and try to maintain their self-esteem by avoiding conflict (e.g., negative criticism and disagreement from others).

There is a fine line between assertive and aggressive communication. Assertive communication is an open expression of ideas and opinions while respecting the rights, opinions, and ideas of others. Aggressive communication strongly asserts the person's legitimate rights and opinions with little regard or respect for the rights and opinions of others (Catalano, 2006, p. 278). Aggressive communication is often perceived as a personal attack by the other person because aggressive communication humiliates, dominates, controls, or embarrasses the other person. By lowering the other person's self-esteem, the person using aggressive communication may feel superior, which helps increase his or her self-esteem. Catalano (2006) states that aggressive communication can take several different forms, including screaming, sarcasm, rudeness, belittling jokes, and even direct personal insults (p. 278).

A nurse's approach to communication can have far-reaching impact on the quality of client care delivered. Consider the following scenario:

CLINICAL EXAMPLE

The client has a standing order for vital signs every 2 hours because on admission to the facility the client's temperature was elevated. Since admission, the client's temperature has normalized and vital signs have consistently been within normal limits. The client tells the nurse assigned to his care that he isn't sleeping well because the nurses keep coming in and waking him every 2 hours and it takes him almost an hour to fall back to sleep. As a result, the client says he is sleeping in 1-hour intervals and feels extremely sleep deprived. The nurse approaches the physician and requests the order be changed to every 4 hours during the day with 6 hours of uninterrupted sleep from midnight to 6:00 a.m. The physician responds by saying, "If he wants to sleep he'll have to wait until he goes home. I want vital signs every 2 hours as ordered."

Depending on the nurse's communication style the response may be one of the following:

- Aggressive: "Well, you're very inconsiderate and obviously don't care at all about your client's well-being!"
- Passive: "Oh, okay. Thank you."
- Assertive: "I'm concerned that if the client fails to obtain adequate rest it will negatively impact his condition and potentially extend his hospital stay. Is there a different schedule we could use at night to allow us to monitor him closely as you requested while not interrupting his sleep so frequently?"

You can clearly see that both the aggressive approach as well as the passive approach will not serve the best interests of the client. Further, the aggressive approach will most likely cause the provider to become defensive, further reducing the chance for compromise in a manner that will best serve the client's needs. In addition to being ineffective, the aggressive approach to communication is also unprofessional and diminishes others' opinions of the nurse.

ASSERTIVE COMMUNICATION

Beliefs about personal boundaries play a role in determining communication style. The passive communicator does not respect his or her own values and as such is often ignored, manipulated, or taken advantage of by more aggressive individuals. Aggressive communicators do not respect the boundaries of others and are willing to say or do anything necessary to get their way. The goal of all professionals is to achieve a mutual respect for boundaries in order to promote the best outcome for everyone involved.

Assertive communication allows the nurse to express all ideas in a direct and non-confrontational manner that promotes both the rights of the nurse (or the client) while respecting the rights of others to have a different outlook. Assertive communication does not use name calling, is not judgmental, and does not blame others. It increases the likelihood of creating a win-win result where both parties walk away feeling like their point of view was heard and understood while reaching a conclusion satisfactory to them both.

Characteristics of assertive communicators include freedom to express oneself, awareness of one's own rights, and self-control over strong emotions such as anger, fear, or frustration. Assertive communicators are professional and serve as the best advocate for the client. Assertive communicators express their opinions but are open to listening to others' points of view. They do not use sarcasm, biting comebacks, or passive-aggressive wounding to promote their superiority.

Much of conversation is nonverbal, so the body language of the assertive communicator should be upright, relaxed, and open to the words of others. The tone of voice should be well modulated with inflection, but avoid raised voices, whispering, or aggressive overtones.

An assertive person receives feedback from others with a willingness to consider both the positive and the negative perspective of the evaluator. While an assertive person may not believe everything that is said, he or she will listen to another person's opinion without becoming defensive, attacking the speaker, or becoming angry. Seeking clarification is appropriate in order to be sure that the perception of the message is the same as what the sender intended.

Some people may have more trouble accepting positive feedback and will dismiss it or negate it when offered. The assertive person simply says "Thank you" and considers the value of the positive feedback for later application to similar situations.

Benefits of Assertive Communication

Assertiveness is an effective and professional communication style because it is based on mutual respect. An assertive style improves communication and reduces stress by de-escalating conflict, improving outcomes, and reducing the likelihood of angry encounters. Passive communicators tend to feel increased stress, resentment, anger, feelings of victimization, and a desire to exact revenge, which is eliminated when assertive communication styles are used (Mayo Clinic, 2009). Aggressive communication often results in a perception by others that the person is a bully and is unprofessional. This can impact future interactions, as those who deal with the aggressor on a regular basis may become defensive before communication even begins, because they anticipate an aggressive encounter.

Techniques for Assertive Communication

Because no one technique works in every situation, it is essential to have an arsenal of strategies to use when faced with a situation requiring assertive communication. These techniques include the following:

- *"I" statements.* An assertive communicator voices his or her own feelings and wishes based on sound evidence without placing blame or raising the defenses of the person to whom he or she is speaking. For example, "I have assessed that Client A is...."
- *Fogging.* Finding some area, no matter how small, on which both parties agree and building from there is a technique that assertive communicators use. In the example of the sleep-deprived client described previously, both the nurse and the physician can agree that they want to maintain client safety through careful monitoring of the client's condition. This gives them a starting point from which to reach consensus where both can feel client care has been optimized.
- *Negative assertion.* An assertive communicator can agree with criticism without becoming upset or angry, thus moving the focus of the communication toward the desired goal. This method can be particularly important to the nurse when receiving feedback related to the quality of the care he or she delivers. For example, when the evaluator says, "While you are very caring, I would like to see you improve your decision-making ability," the nurse may respond, "I could use improvement in my decision-making ability, but I believe the quality of the care I deliver is excellent." This prevents an ongoing debate about something that is agreed upon and allows the communication to move forward regarding the more important topic.
- *Repetition.* Repeating the request every time you meet with resistance is another technique that can be useful. However, each time the request is repeated, the power of the words is diminished. This strategy is effective only if the nurse has power within the relationship. For example, the nurse calls the pharmacy to request a newly ordered medication that is to be given within the hour and is told the pharmacy is very busy and cannot fill the prescription right now and will not

be able to deliver it to the unit for 3–4 hours. The nurse repeats, "I must give this medication within the hour" or "The client needs the medication within the hour." The effectiveness of this approach is improved if differing attempts to reach a compromise are suggested as well. The nurse might say, "I need to administer this medication within the hour" to which the pharmacy responds, "I'm sorry, I can't have it to the floor that quickly." The nurse then responds, "The client needs that medication within the hour. What if I come to the pharmacy so you don't have to deliver it?" This allows for both the nurse and the pharmacy to collaborate to reach a mutually effective solution to the problem.

- *Confidence.* Confidence is essential to assertive communication. A choppy or weak tone of voice implies uncertainty. Nurses should maintain an air of confidence in order to help others see their needs and wants as having merit.
- *Manage nonverbal communication.* Getting too close to the other person, wagging a finger in someone's face, or an angry glare can all counteract assertive words. By maintaining open, assertive body language and keeping a neutral voice, the nurse promotes shared decision making and compromise.
- *Think before speaking.* Consider both your words and your tone of voice before speaking. This helps the nurse avoid saying something he or she will later regret or that will reduce the effectiveness of his or her communication style.
- *Avoid apologizing whenever possible.* This is particularly important for women, who have a tendency to say "I'm sorry" even when there is no call for an apology. A woman may say, "I'm sorry, I didn't hear you," or "I'm sorry to bother you but...." An unnecessary apology immediately places the communicator in a somewhat submissive position. Apologies should be given only when warranted.
- *Perform a post-conversation evaluation.* Assertive communicators can continue to improve their skills by reviewing what was said and how it might have been done differently to improve the final outcome. This should be done even when the communication interaction was successful because evaluation of what went well and what did not go well helps the nurse improve his or her assertive communication skills.

While assertive communication may not be an individual's preferred style, and may not be comfortable for the individual, it is possible for every nurse to become an assertive communicator and reach more positive outcomes through practice, self-evaluation, and ongoing efforts to improve communication approach.

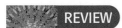 **REVIEW** **Assertive Communication**

RELATE: LINK THE CONCEPTS

Link the exemplar of Assertive Communication with the concept of Professional Behaviors:

1. How does the use of assertive communication promote others' perceptions of you as a professional?
2. How does the lack of assertive communication promote others' perceptions of you as unprofessional?

Linking the exemplar of Assertive Communication with the concept of Safety:

3. How does the nurse's use of assertive communication skills improve client safety?
4. Provide specific examples of how an assertive nurse can improve a client's safety.

REFER: GO TO MYNURSINGKIT

REFLECT: CASE STUDY

Dr. Danilo Ocampo is a 74-year-old retired pathologist. He lives in his home with Lydia, his wife of 51 years. Their only child, a son, was killed at age 22 in an automobile accident. Dr. Ocampo was born and raised in the Philippines and came to the United States when he was 23. He is the last living member of his immediate family. He has a few nephews and nieces in the Philippines, but no relatives live nearby.

Dr. Ocampo's health has been declining for the past few years. He has a medical history that includes hypertension, myocardial infarction, angina, and class 2 heart failure. Because of these cardiovascular disorders, he takes multiple medications, including metoprolol, lisinopril, Aldactone, furosemide (intermittently as needed), K+ when taking furosemide, aspirin, isosorbide dinitrate, and nitroglycerin. He has a good understanding of the pharmaceutical properties of the medications. At times, he is not sure he gets good health care because of all the medications he takes. He often does not believe the medications are helpful because he experiences many side effects and he has required multiple admissions to the hospital. He usually feels better after a few days in the hospital but typically checks himself out of the hospital against medical advice. He has

been known to adjust his own dosages of medications based on his symptoms and how he feels.

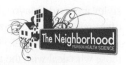

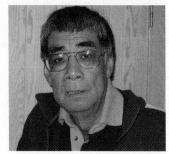

1. With Dr. Ocampo's disdain for his medications, how would the use of assertive communication provide useful when talking to him about safe medication self-administration and the need to consult his doctor before adjusting dosages?

2. If the nurse talks with Dr. Ocampo in an assertive manner but does not achieve the objectives because Dr. Ocampo refuses to comply with the nurse's safe self-medication request, what can the nurse do next?

3. If the nurse relies on a communication style other than assertiveness, how might that impact Dr. Ocampo's perception of the nurse and his response to health teaching?

36.3 DOCUMENTATION

KEY TERMS

Chart, *2183*
Charting, *2182*
Charting by exception (CBE), *2189*
Client record, *2183*
Discussion, *2182*
Documenting, *2182*
Flow sheet, *2187*
Focus charting, *2187*
Kardex, *2193*
Narrative charting, *2184*
Problems, interventions, evaluation (PIE), *2187*
Problem-oriented medical record (POMR), *2185*
Problem-oriented record (POR), *2185*
Record, *2182*
Recording, *2182*
Report, *2182*
SOAP, *2187*
Source-oriented record, *2184*
Variance, *2192*

BASIS FOR SELECTION OF EXEMPLAR

The Joint Commission

LEARNING OUTCOMES

After reading about this exemplar, you will be able to:

1. List the measures used to maintain the confidentiality of client records.

2. Discuss reasons for keeping client records.

3. Compare and contrast different documentation methods: source-oriented and problem-oriented medical records; the problems, interventions, evaluation (PIE) model; focus charting; charting by exception; computerized records; and the case management model.

4. Explain how various forms in the client record (e.g., flow sheets, progress notes, care plans, critical pathways, Kardexes, discharge/transfer forms) are used to document steps of the nursing process (assessment, diagnosis, planning, implementation, and evaluation).

5. Compare and contrast the documentation needed for clients in acute care, home health care, and long-term care settings.

6. Identify and discuss guidelines for effective documentation that meets legal and ethical standards.

7. Identify prohibited abbreviations, acronyms, and symbols that cannot be used in any form of clinical documentation.

OVERVIEW

Effective communication among health care professionals is vital to the quality of client care. Generally, health care personnel communicate through discussion, reports, and records. A **discussion** is an informal oral consideration of a subject by two or more health care personnel to identify a problem or

establish strategies to resolve a problem. A **report** is oral, written, or computer-based communication intended to convey information to others. For instance, nurses always report on clients at the end of a hospital work shift. A **record** is written or computer-based. The process of making an entry on a client record is called **recording**, **charting**, or **documenting**.

A clinical record, also called a **chart** or **client record**, is a formal, legal document that provides evidence of a client's care. Although health care organizations use different systems and forms for documentation, all client records have similar information.

Each health care organization has policies about recording and reporting client data, and each nurse is accountable for practicing according to these standards. Agencies also indicate which nursing assessments and interventions can be recorded by RNs and which can be charted by unlicensed personnel. In addition, the Joint Commission requires client record documentation to be timely, complete, accurate, confidential, and specific to the client.

ETHICAL AND LEGAL CONSIDERATIONS

The American Nurses Association (ANA) code of ethics (2001) states that ". . . the nurse has a duty to maintain confidentiality of all patient information" (p. 12). The client's record is also protected legally as a private record of the client's care. Access to the client's record is restricted to health care professionals involved in giving care to the client. The institution or agency is the rightful owner of the client's record. This does not, however, exclude the client's rights to the same records. Ethics will be covered further in Concept 42 and legal issues are covered in Concept 47.

On April 14, 2003, changes were made regarding HIPAA regulations to maintain privacy and confidentiality of protected health information (PHI). PHI is identifiable health information that is transmitted or maintained in any form or medium, including verbal discussions, electronic communications with or about clients, and written communications (Clark, 2003, p. 7).

PRACTICE ALERT

Take safety measures before faxing confidential information. A fax cover sheet should contain instruction that the faxed material is to be given only to the named recipient. Consent is needed from the client to fax information. Make sure that personally identifiable information has been removed or is not immediately visible on the top sheet. Finally, check that the fax number is correct, check the number on the display of the machine after dialing, and check a third time before pressing the "send" button. Some facilities require the recipient agency to return a signed receipt.

For purposes of education and research, most agencies allow student and graduate health care professionals access to client records. The records are used in client conferences, clinics, rounds, client studies, and written papers. The student or graduate is bound by a strict ethical code and legal responsibility to hold all information in confidence. It is the responsibility of both students and practicing nurses to protect the client's privacy by not using a name or any statements that may identify the client in their worksheets, notes for class, or any notations they make that could potentially leave the facility's premises. Facilities provide shredders or other receptacles for discarding material with client personal information.

Ensuring Confidentiality of Computer Records

Because of the increased use of computerized client records, health care agencies have developed policies and procedures to ensure the privacy and confidentiality of client information stored in computers. In addition, the Security Rule of HIPAA governs the security of electronic protected health information (Gallagher, 2004). Following are some suggestions for ensuring the confidentiality and security of computerized records:

1. A personal password is required to enter and sign off computer files. Do not share this password with anyone, including other health care team members.
2. After logging on, never leave a computer terminal unattended.
3. Do not leave client information displayed on the monitor where others may see it.
4. Shred all unneeded computer-generated worksheets.
5. Know the facility's policy and procedure for correcting an entry error.
6. Follow agency procedures for documenting sensitive material, such as a diagnosis of AIDS.
7. Information technology (IT) personnel must install a firewall to protect the server from unauthorized access.

PURPOSES OF CLIENT RECORDS

Client records are kept for a number of purposes. These include communication among health care professionals who are treating the same client, tracking services provided for reimbursement purposes, and quality assurance purposes, among others:

- *Communication.* The record serves as the vehicle by which different health care professionals who interact with a client communicate with each other. This prevents fragmentation, repetition, and delays in client care.
- *Planning Client Care.* Each health care professional uses data from the client's record to plan care for that client. A primary care provider, for example, may order a specific antibiotic after establishing that the client's temperature is steadily rising and that laboratory tests reveal the presence of a certain microorganism. Nurses use baseline and ongoing data to evaluate the effectiveness of the nursing care plan.
- *Auditing Health Agencies.* An audit is a review of client records for quality-assurance purposes (see Concept 48, Quality Improvement). Accrediting agencies such as the Joint Commission may review client records to determine if a particular health agency is meeting required standards.
- *Research.* The information contained in a record can be a valuable source of data for research. The treatment plans for a number of clients with the same health problems can yield information helpful in treating other clients.
- *Education.* Students in health disciplines often use client records as educational tools. A record can frequently provide a comprehensive view of the client, the illness, effective treatment strategies, and factors that affect the outcome of the illness.
- *Reimbursement.* Documentation helps a facility receive reimbursement from the federal government. For a facility to obtain

payment through Medicare, for example, the client's clinical record must contain the correct diagnosis-related group (DRG) codes and reveal that the appropriate care has been given.

Codable diagnoses, such as DRGs, are supported by accurate, thorough recording by nurses. Accurate coding not only facilitates reimbursement from the federal government, but also facilitates reimbursement from insurance companies and other third-party payers. If additional care, treatment, or length of stay becomes necessary for the client's welfare, thorough charting will help justify these needs.

- *Legal Documentation.*   The client's record is a legal document and usually is admissible in court as evidence. In some jurisdictions, however, the record is considered inadmissible as evidence when the client objects, because information the client gives to the physician is confidential.
- *Health Care Analysis.*   Information from records may assist health care planners to identify agency needs, such as overutilized and underutilized hospital services. Records can be used to establish the costs of various services and to identify those services that cost the agency money and those that generate revenue.

DOCUMENTATION SYSTEMS

A number of documentation systems are in current use: the source-oriented record; the problem-oriented medical record; the problems, interventions, evaluation (PIE) model; focus charting; charting by exception (CBE); and computerized documentation.

Source-Oriented Record

The traditional client record is a **source-oriented record**. Each person or department makes notations in a separate section or sections of the client's chart. For example, the admissions department has an admission sheet; the physician has a physician's order sheet, a physician's history sheet, and progress notes; nurses use the nurses' notes; and other departments or personnel have their own records. In this type of record, information about a particular problem is distributed throughout the record. For example, if a client had left hemiplegia (paralysis of the left side of the body), data about this problem might be found in the physician's history sheet, on the physician's order sheet, in the nurses' notes, in the physical therapist's record, and in the social service record. Box 36–11 lists the components of a source-oriented record.

Narrative charting is a traditional part of the source-oriented record. It consists of written notes that include routine care, normal findings, and client problems. There is no right or wrong order to the information, although chronological order is frequently used. Few institutions use only narrative charting today. Narrative recording is being replaced by other systems, such as charting by exception and focus charting. However, narrative charting is expedient in emergency situations (see Figure 36–8 ■). Many agencies combine narrative charting with another system. For example, an agency using a charting-by-exception system (discussed later) may use narrative charting when describing abnormal findings. When using narrative charting, it is important to organize the information in a clear,

NURSING NOTES		
Date	Time	
6/6/09	1400	Passive ROM exercises provided for R arm and leg.
		Active assistive exercises to L arm and leg. Has scratch
		marks on L and R forearms. States, My skin on my back
		and arms has been itchy for a week. Rash not evident.
		No previous history of pruritus. Is allergic to elastoplast
		but has not been in contact. Dr. J. Wong notified.
		T. Ritchie, RN
	1430	Applied calamine lotion to back and arms. Incontinent
		of urine. Is restless. T. Ritchie, RN

Figure 36–8 ■ An example of narrative notes.

Box 36–11 Components of the Source-Oriented Record

FORM	INFORMATION
Admission (face) sheet	Legal name, birth date, age, gender
	Social Security number
	Address
	Marital status; closest relatives or person to notify in case of emergency
	Date, time, and admitting diagnosis
	Food or drug allergies
	Name of admitting (attending) physician
	Insurance information
	Any assigned DRGs
Initial nursing assessment	Findings from the initial nursing history and physical health assessment
Graphic record	Body temperature, pulse rate, respiratory rate, blood pressure, daily weight, and special measurements such as fluid intake and output and oxygen saturation
Daily care record	Activity, diet, bathing, and elimination records
Special flow sheets	Examples: fluid balance record, skin assessment
Medication record	Name, dosage, route, time, date of regularly administered medications
	Name or initials of person administering the medication
Nurses' notes	Pertinent assessment of client
	Specific nursing care, including teaching and client's responses
	Client's complaints and how client is coping
Medical history and physical examination	Past and family medical history, present medical problems, differential or current diagnoses, findings of physical examination by the primary care provider
Physician's order sheet	Medical orders for medications, treatments, and so on
Physician's progress notes	Medical observations, treatments, client progress, and so on
Consultation records	Reports by medical and clinical specialists
Diagnostic reports	Examples: laboratory reports, x-ray reports, CT scan reports
Consultation reports	Physical therapy, respiratory therapy
Client discharge plan and referral summary	Started on admission and completed on discharge; includes nursing problems, general information, and referral data

coherent manner. Using the nursing process as a framework is one way to do this (see Box 36–12).

Source-oriented records are convenient because (a) care providers from each discipline can easily locate the forms on which to record data and (b) it is easy to trace the information specific to one's discipline. The disadvantage is that information about a particular client problem is scattered throughout the chart, making it difficult to find chronological information on a client's problems and progress. This can lead to decreased communication among the health care team, an incomplete picture of the client's care, and a lack of coordination of care (Lippincott, Williams, & Wilkins, 2003, 2007).

Problem-Oriented Medical Record

The **problem-oriented medical record (POMR)**, or **problem-oriented record (POR)**, was established by Lawrence Weed in the 1960s. In POMR, data are arranged according to the problems the client has rather than the source of the information. Members of the health care team contribute to the problem list,

Box 36–12 Example of Organizing Narrative Charting

Situation: Client is postop day # 2 after abdominal surgery.
  Questions to ask yourself:
- What assessment data are relevant?
- What nursing interventions have I completed?
- What is my evaluation of the result of the interventions and/or what is the client's response to the interventions?

EXAMPLE
1000 Diminished breath sounds in all lung fields with crackles in LLL. Temperature 99.6. Not using incentive spirometer (IS). Stated he's "not sure how to use it." Instructed how to use IS. Discussed the importance of deep breathing and coughing after surgery. Administered analgesic for c/o abdominal pain rating of 5/10. After pain relief (1/10), able to demonstrate correct use of IS. _____
_____ S. Martin, RN
1400 Using IS each hour. Lungs less diminished with fewer LLL crackles. Temp 99. _____S. Martin, RN

plan of care, and progress notes. Plans for each active or potential problem are drawn up, and progress notes are recorded for each problem.

The advantage of POMR is that (a) it encourages collaboration and (b) the problem list in the front of the chart alerts caregivers to the client's needs and makes it easier to track the status of each problem. Its disadvantages are that (a) caregivers differ in their ability to use the required charting format, (b) it takes constant vigilance to maintain an up-to-date problem list, and (c) it is somewhat inefficient because assessments and interventions that apply to more than one problem must be repeated.

The POMR has four basic components:

- Database
- Problem list
- Plan of care
- Progress notes.

In addition, flow sheets and discharge notes are added to the record as needed.

DATABASE The database of a POMR consists of all information known about the client when the client first enters the health care agency. It includes the nursing assessment, the physician's history, social and family data, and the results of the physical examination and baseline diagnostic tests. Data are constantly updated as the client's health status changes.

PROBLEM LIST The problem list (see Figure 36–9 ■) is derived from the database. It is usually kept at the front of the chart and serves as an index to the numbered entries in the progress notes. Problems are listed in the order in which they are identified, and the list is continually updated as new problems are identified and others resolved. All caregivers may contribute to the problem list, which includes the client's

No.	Date Entered	Date Inactive	Client Problem
#1	3/9/09		CVA resulting in Rt hemiplegia and left-sided weakness
#1A	3/9/09		Self-care deficit (hygiene, toileting, grooming, feeding)
#1B	3/9/09		Impaired physical mobility (unable to turn and position self) Redefined 2/7/10
#1C	3/9/09		Total urinary incontinence Redefined 1/17/10
#1D	3/9/09		Progressive dysphasia
#2	3/9/09		Constipation r/t immobility Redefined 6/10/09
#3	3/9/09		History of depression
#4	3/9/09		Essential hypertension
~~#5~~	~~6/6/09~~	~~7/11/09~~	~~Pruritus~~
#2	6/10/09		Risk for constipation r/t insufficient fiber intake
#1C	1/17/10		Urge urinary incontinence at night
#1B	2/7/10		Impaired physical mobility (needs 2-person assistance to transfer and walk)

Figure 36–9 ■ A client's problem list in the POMR. Note that the problems 1B, 1C, and 2 were redefined on the dates indicated and listed subsequently.

physiologic, psychologic, social, cultural, spiritual, developmental, and environmental needs. Primary care providers write problems as medical diagnoses, surgical procedures, or symptoms; nurses write problems as nursing diagnoses.

As the client's condition changes or more data are obtained, it may be necessary to "redefine" problems. Figure 36–9 illustrates how this has been done for Problems 1B, 1C, and 2. When a problem is resolved, a line is drawn through it and the number is not used again for that client.

PLAN OF CARE In the POMR method, the initial list of orders or plan of care is made with reference to the active problems. Care plans are generated by the person who lists the problems. Physicians write physician's orders or medical care plans; nurses write nursing orders or nursing care plans. The written plan in the record is listed under each problem in the progress notes and is not isolated as a separate list of orders.

PROGRESS NOTES A progress note in the POMR is a chart entry made by all health care professionals involved in a client's care, who all use the same type of sheet for notes. Progress notes are numbered to correspond to the problems on the problem list and may be lettered for the type of data. The SOAP format is frequently used. **SOAP** is an acronym for subjective data, objective data, assessment, and planning.

- S—*Subjective data* consist of information obtained from what the client says. Subjective data describe the client's perceptions of and experience with the problem. When possible, the nurse quotes the client's words; otherwise, they are summarized. Subjective data are included only when it is important and relevant to the problem.
- O—*Objective data* consist of information that is measured or observed by use of the senses (e.g., vital signs, laboratory and x-ray results).
- A—*Assessment* is the interpretation or conclusions drawn about the subjective and objective data. During the initial assessment, the problem list is created from the database, so the "A" entry should be a statement of the problem. In all subsequent SOAP notes for that problem, the "A" should describe the client's condition and level of progress rather than merely restating the diagnosis or problem.
- P—The *plan* is the plan of care designed to resolve the stated problem. The initial plan is written by the person who enters the problem into the record. All subsequent plans, including revisions, are entered into the progress notes.

Over the years, the SOAP format has been modified. The acronyms *SOAPIE* and *SOAPIER* refer to formats that add interventions, evaluation, and revision.

- I—*Interventions* refer to the specific interventions that have actually been performed by the caregiver.
- E—*Evaluation* includes client responses to nursing interventions and medical treatments. This is primarily reassessment data.

- R—*Revision* reflects care plan modifications suggested by the evaluation. Changes may be made in desired outcomes, interventions, or target dates.

Newer versions of this format eliminate the subjective and objective data and start with *assessment*, which combines the subjective and objective data. The acronym then becomes *AP*, *APIE*, or *APIER*. See Figure 36–10 ■.

PIE

The **PIE** documentation model groups information into three categories. PIE is an acronym for problems, interventions, and evaluation of nursing care. This system consists of a client care assessment flow sheet and progress notes. The **flow sheet** uses specific assessment criteria in a particular format, such as human needs or functional health patterns. The time parameters for a flow sheet can vary from minutes to months. In a hospital intensive care unit, for example, a client's blood pressure may be monitored by the minute, whereas in an ambulatory clinic a client's blood glucose level may be recorded once a month.

After the assessment, the nurse establishes and records specific problems on the progress notes, often using North American Nursing Diagnosis Association (NANDA) diagnoses to word the problem. If there is no approved nursing diagnosis for a problem, the nurse develops a problem statement using NANDA's three-part format: client's response, contributing or probable causes of the response, and characteristics manifested by the client. The *problem statement* is labeled "P" and referred to by number (e.g., P #5). The *interventions* employed to manage the problem are labeled "I" and numbered according to the problem (e.g., I #5). The *evaluation* of the effectiveness of the interventions is also labeled and numbered according to the problem (e.g., E #5).

The PIE system eliminates the traditional care plan and incorporates an ongoing care plan into the progress notes. Therefore, the nurse does not have to create and update a separate plan. One of the disadvantages to PIE is that the nurse must review all the nursing notes before giving care to determine which problems are current and which interventions were effective.

Focus Charting

Focus charting is intended to make the client and the client's concerns and strengths the focus of care. Three columns for recording are usually used: date and time, focus, and progress notes (see Figure 36–11 ■). The *focus* may be a condition, a nursing diagnosis, a behavior, a sign or symptom, an acute change in the client's condition, or a client strength. The progress notes are organized into (D) data, (A) action, and (R) response, referred to as DAR. The *data* category reflects the assessment phase of the nursing process and consists of observations of client status and behaviors, including data from flow sheets (e.g., vital signs, pupil reactivity). The nurse records both subjective and objective data in this section.

SOAP Format

6/6/09 #5 Generalized pruritus

1400 S— "My skin is itchy on my back and arms, and it's been like this for a week."

O— Skin appears clear—no rash or irritation noted. Marks where client has scratched noted on left and right forearms. Allergic to elastoplast but has not been in contact.
No previous history of pruritus.

A— Altered comfort (pruritus): cause unknown.

P— Instructed not to scratch skin.
— Applied calamine lotion to back and arms at 1430 h.
— Cut fingernails.
— Assess further to determine whether recurrence associated with specific drugs or foods.
— Refer to physician and pharmacist for assessment.
T. Ritchie, RN

SOAPIER Format

6/6/09 #5 Generalized pruritus

1400 S— "My skin is itchy on my back and arms, and it's been like this for a week."

O— Skin appears clear—no rash or irritation noted. Marks where client has scratched noted on left and right forearms. Allergic to elastoplast but has not been in contact.
No previous history of pruritus.

A— Altered comfort (pruritus): cause unknown.

P— Instruct to not scratch skin.
— Apply calamine lotion as necessary.
— Cut nails to avoid scratches.
— Assess further to determine whether recurrence associated with specific drugs or foods.
— Refer to physician and pharmacist for assessment.

I — Instructed not to scratch skin. Applied calamine lotion to back and arms at 1430 h. Assisted to cut fingernails. Notified physician and pharmacist of problem.

1600 E— States, "I'm still itchy. That lotion didn't help."

R— Remove calamine lotion and apply hydrocortisone cream as ordered.
T. Ritchie, RN

APIE Format

6/6/09 A— Generalized pruritus r/t unknown cause

1400 States, "My skin is itchy on my back and arms, and it's been like this for a week." Skin appears clear. No rash or irritations noted. Marks where client has scratched noted on left and right forearms. Allergic to elastoplast but has not been in contact. No previous history of pruritus.

P— Instruct to not scratch skin.
— Apply calamine lotion as necessary.
— Cut nails to avoid scratches.
— Assess further to determine whether recurrence associated with specific drugs or foods.
— Refer to physician and pharmacist for assessment.

I — Instructed not to scratch skin. Applied calamine lotion to back and arms at 1430 h. Assisted to cut fingernails. Notified physician and pharmacist of problem.

E— States, "I'm still itchy. That lotion didn't help."
T. Ritchie, RN

Figure 36–10 ■ Examples of nursing process notes using SOAP, SOAPIER, and APIE formats.

Date/Hour	Focus	Progress Notes
2/11/09 0900	Pain	**D:** Guarding abdominal incision. Facial grimacing. Rates pain at 8 on scale of 0–10.
		A: Administered morphine sulfate 4 mg IV.
0930		**R:** Rates pain at 1. States willing to ambulate.

Figure 36–11 ■ Example of the focus charting system.

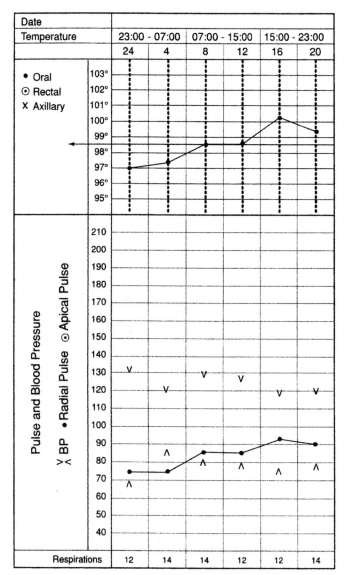

Figure 36–12 ■ Sample vital signs graphic record.

Charting by Exception

Charting by exception (CBE) is a documentation system in which only abnormal or significant findings or exceptions to norms are recorded. CBE incorporates three key elements (Guido, 2005):

1. *Flow sheets.* Examples of flow sheets include a graphic record (Figure 36–12 ■), fluid balance record, daily nursing assessments record (Figure 36–13 ■), client teaching record, client discharge record, and skin assessment record (Figure 36–14 ■).
2. *Standards of nursing care.* Documentation by reference to the agency's printed standards of nursing practice eliminates much of the repetitive charting of routine care. An agency using CBE must develop its own specific standards of nursing practice that identify the minimum criteria for client care regardless of clinical area. Some units may also have unit-specific standards unique to their type of client. For example, "The nurse must ensure that the unconscious client has oral care at least q4h." Documentation of care according to these specified standards involves only a check mark in the routine standards box on the graphic record. If all of the standards are not implemented, an asterisk on the flow sheet is made with reference to the nurses' notes. All exceptions to the standards are fully described in narrative form on the nurses' notes.
3. *Bedside access to chart forms.* In the CBE system, all flow sheets are kept at the client's bedside to allow immediate recording and to eliminate the need to transcribe data from the nurse's worksheet to the permanent record.

The advantages to this system are the elimination of lengthy, repetitive notes and that it makes client changes in condition more obvious. Inherent in CBE is the presumption that the nurse did assess the client and determined what responses were normal and abnormal. Many nurses believe in the saying "not charted, not done" and subsequently may feel uncomfortable with the CBE documentation system. Sullivan (2004) suggests writing N/A on flow sheets where the items are not applicable and to not leave blank spaces. This would then avoid the possible misinterpretation that the assessment or intervention was not done by the nurse.

Computerized Documentation

Computerized clinical record systems are being developed as a way to manage the huge volume of information required in contemporary health care. Nurses use computers to store the client's database, add new data, create and revise care plans, and document client progress (see Figure 36–15 ■). Some institutions have a computer terminal at each client's bedside, or nurses carry a small handheld terminal, enabling the nurse to document care immediately after it is given.

The *action* category reflects planning and implementation and includes immediate and future nursing actions. It may also include any changes to the plan of care. The *response category* reflects the evaluation phase of the nursing process and describes the client's response to any nursing and medical care.

The focus charting system provides a holistic perspective of the client and the client's needs. It also provides a nursing process framework for the progress notes (DAR). The three components do not need to be recorded in order and each note does not need to have all three categories. Flow sheets and checklists are frequently used on the client's chart to record routine nursing tasks and assessment data.

medication order, the expiration date, the medication name and dose, the frequency of administration and route, and the nurse's signature. Some records also include a place to document the client's allergies.

■ *Skin Assessment Record.* A skin or wound assessment is often recorded on a flow sheet such as the one shown in Figure 36–14. These records may include categories related to stage of skin injury, drainage, odor, culture information, and treatments.

Progress Notes

Progress notes made by nurses provide information about the progress a client is making toward achieving desired outcomes. Therefore, in addition to assessment and reassessment data, progress notes include information about client problems and nursing interventions. The format used depends on the documentation system in place in the institution.

Nursing Discharge/Referral Summaries

A discharge note and referral summary are completed when the client is being discharged and transferred to another institution or to a home setting where a visit by a community health nurse is required. Many institutions provide forms for these summaries. Some records combine the discharge plan, including instructions for care, and the final progress note. Many are designed with checklists to facilitate data recording.

If the discharge plan is given directly to the client and family, it is imperative that instructions be written in terms that can be readily understood. For example, medications, treatments, and activities should be written in layman's terms, and use of medical abbreviations (such as t.i.d.) should be avoided.

If a client is transferred within the facility or from a long-term facility to a hospital, a report needs to accompany the client to ensure continuity of care in the new area. It should include all components of the discharge instructions, but also describe the condition of the client prior to transfer. Any teaching or client instruction that has been done should also be described and recorded.

If the client is being transferred to another institution or to a home setting where a visit by a home health nurse is required, the discharge note takes the form of a referral summary. Regardless of format, discharge and referral summaries usually include some or all of the following:

■ Description of client's physical, mental, and emotional status at discharge or transfer
■ Resolved health problems
■ Unresolved continuing health problems and continuing care needs; may include a review-of-systems checklist that considers integumentary, respiratory, cardiovascular, neurological, musculoskeletal, gastrointestinal, elimination, and reproductive problems
■ Treatments that are to be continued (e.g., wound care, oxygen therapy)
■ Current medications
■ Restrictions that relate to (a) activity such as lifting, stair climbing, walking, driving, work; (b) diet; and (c) bathing, such as sponge bath, tub, or shower

■ Functional/self-care abilities in terms of vision, hearing, speech, mobility with or without aids, meal preparation and eating, preparing and administering medications, and so on
■ Comfort level
■ Support networks including family, significant others, religious adviser, community self-help groups, home care and other community agencies available, and so on
■ Client education provided in relation to disease process, activities and exercise, special diet, medications, specialized care or treatments, follow-up appointments, and so on
■ Discharge destination (e.g., home, nursing home) and mode of discharge (e.g., walking, wheelchair, ambulance)
■ Referral services (e.g., social worker, home health nurse).

FACILITY SPECIFIC DOCUMENTATION

Documentation systems and requirements vary by facility. The documentation required in an acute care setting, as discussed in the early part of this exemplar, is different from the documentation required by long-term care, home care, or other care delivery sites.

Long-Term Care Documentation

Long-term facilities usually provide two types of care: skilled or intermediate. Clients needing skilled care require more extensive nursing care and specialized nursing skills. In contrast, an intermediate care focus is needed for clients who usually have chronic illnesses and may only need assistance with activities of daily living (such as bathing and dressing).

Requirements for documentation systems in long-term care settings are based on professional standards, federal and state regulations, and the policies of the health care agency. Laws influencing the kind and frequency of documentation required are found in the Health Care Financing Administration and the Omnibus Budget Reconciliation Act (OBRA) of 1987. The OBRA law, for example, requires that (a) a comprehensive assessment (the Minimum Data Set [MDS] for Resident Assessment and Care Screening) be performed within 4 days of a client's admission to a long-term care facility, (b) a formulated plan of care must be completed within 7 days of admission, and (c) the assessment and care screening process must be reviewed every 3 months.

DEVELOPMENTAL CONSIDERATIONS
Long-Term Care

OLDER ADULTS

Older adults in long-term care facilities tend to have chronic conditions and generally experience subtle small changes in their condition. However, when problems do occur, such as a hip fracture, CVA, or pneumonia, they are serious and require prompt attention. This points out the importance of keeping Kardexes and charting in long-term facilities current and up to date in the event that the client needs to be transferred for more skilled care and further treatment. A thorough transfer summary will facilitate communication and promote continuity of care in these situations.

Documentation must also comply with requirements set by Medicare and Medicaid. These requirements vary with the level of service provided and other factors. For example, Medicare provides little reimbursement for services provided in long-term care facilities except for services that require skilled care such as chemotherapy, tube feedings, ventilators, and so on. For these clients, the nurse must provide daily documentation to verify the need for service and reimbursement.

Nurses need to familiarize themselves with regulations influencing the kind and frequency of documentation required in long-term care facilities. Usually the nurse completes a nursing care *summary* at least once a week for clients requiring skilled care and every 2 weeks for those systems requiring intermediate care. Summaries should address the following:

- Specific problems noted in the care plan
- Mental status
- Activities of daily living
- Hydration and nutrition status
- Safety measures needed
- Medications
- Treatments
- Preventive measures
- Behavioral modification assessments, if pertinent (if client is taking psychotropic medications or demonstrates behavioral problems).

See Box 36–14 for some of the documentation required in long-term care facilities.

Home Care Documentation

In 1985, the Health Care Financing Administration, a branch of the U.S. Department of Health and Human Services, mandated that home health care agencies standardize their documentation methods to meet requirements for Medicare and Medicaid and other third-party disbursements. Two records are required: (a) a home health certification and plan of treatment form and (b) a medical update and client information form. The nurse assigned to the home care client usually completes the forms, which must be signed by both the nurse and

---

Box 36–15 Home Health Care Documentation

- Complete a comprehensive nursing assessment and develop a plan of care to meet Medicare and other third-party payer requirements. Some agencies use the certification and plan of treatment form as the client's official plan of care.
- Write a progress note at each client visit, noting any changes in the client condition, nursing interventions performed (including education and instructional brochures and materials provided to the client and home caregiver), client responses to nursing care, and vital signs as indicated.
- Provide a monthly progress nursing summary to the attending physician and to the reimburser to confirm the systems need to continue services.
- Keep a copy of the care plan in the client's home and update it as the client's condition changes.
- Report changes in the plan of care to the physician and document that these were reported. Medicare and Medicaid will reimburse only for the skilled services provided that are reported to the physician.
- Encourage the client or home caregiver to record data when appropriate.
- Write a discharge summary for the physician to approve the discharge and to notify the reimbursers that services have been discontinued. Include all services provided, the client's health status at discharge, outcomes achieved, and recommendations for further care.

---

the attending physician. See Box 36–15, Home Health Care Documentation.

Some home health agencies provide nurses with laptop or handheld computers to make records available in multiple locations. This allows the nurse to add new client information to records at the agency without systems traveling to the office.

GENERAL GUIDELINES FOR RECORDING

Because the client's record is a legal document and may be used to provide evidence in court, many factors are considered in recording. Health care personnel must not only maintain the confidentiality of the client's record but also meet legal standards in the process of recording.

Date and Time

Document the date and time of each recording. This is essential not only for legal reasons but also for client safety. Record the time in the conventional manner (e.g., 9:00 a.m. or 3:15 p.m.) or according to the 24-hour clock (military clock), which avoids confusion about whether a time was a.m. or p.m. (see Figure 36–18 ▪).

Timing

Follow the agency's policy about the frequency of documenting, and adjust the frequency as a client's condition indicates; for example, a client whose blood pressure is changing requires

---

Box 36–14 Long-Term Care Documentation

- Complete the assessment and screening forms (MDS) and plan of care within the time period specified by regulatory bodies.
- Keep a record of any visits and of phone calls from family, friends, and others regarding the client.
- Write nursing summaries and progress notes that comply with the frequency and standards required by regulatory bodies.
- Review and revise the plan of care every 3 months or whenever the client's health status changes.
- Document and report any systems change in the client's condition to the primary care provider and the client's family within 24 hours.
- Document all measures implemented in response to a change in the client's condition.
- Make sure that progress notes address the client's progress in relation to the goals or outcomes defined in the plan of care.

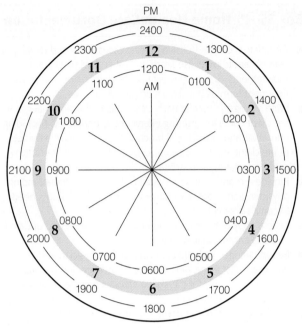

Figure 36–18 ■ The 24-hour clock.

more frequent documentation than a client whose blood pressure is constant. As a rule, documenting should be done as soon as possible after an assessment or intervention. No recording should be done *before* providing nursing care.

Legibility
All entries must be legible and easy to read to prevent interpretation errors. Hand printing or easily understood handwriting is usually permissible. Follow the agency's policies about handwritten recording.

Permanence
All entries on the client's record are made in dark ink so that the record is permanent and changes can be identified. Dark ink reproduces well on microfilm and in duplication processes. Follow the agency's policies about the type of pen and ink used for recording.

Accepted Terminology
Use only commonly accepted abbreviations, symbols, and terms that are specified by the agency. Many abbreviations are standard and used universally; others are used only in certain geographic areas. Many health care facilities supply an approved list of abbreviations and symbols to prevent confusion. When in doubt about whether to use an abbreviation, write the term out in full until certain about the abbreviation. Table 36–7 lists some common abbreviations except those used for medications.

In 2004, the Joint Commission developed National Patient Safety Goals (NPSGs) to reduce communication errors. These goals are required to be implemented by all organizations accredited by the Joint Commission. As a result, the accredited organizations must develop a "Do Not Use" list of

TABLE 36–7 Commonly Used Abbreviations

ABBREVIATION	TERM
Abd	Abdomen
ABO	The main blood group system
ac	Before meals
ADL	Activities of daily living
ad lib	As desired
Adm	Admitted or admission
a.m.	Morning
amb	Ambulatory
amt	Amount
approx	Approximately
bid	Twice daily
BM (bm)	Bowel movement
BP	Blood pressure
BRP	Bathroom privileges
$\bar{c}$	With
C	Celsius (centigrade)
CBC	Complete blood count
c/o	Complains of
DAT	Diet as tolerated
drsg	Dressing
Dx	Diagnosis
ECG (EKG)	Electrocardiogram
F	Fahrenheit
fld	Fluid
GI	Gastrointestinal
gtt	Drop
h (hr)	Hour
H_2O	Water
I&O	Intake and output
IV	Intravenous
LMP	Last menstrual period
(L)	Left
meds	Medications
mL (ml)	Milliliter
mod	Moderate
neg	Negative
Ø	None
#	Number or pounds
NPO (NBM)	Nothing by mouth
NS (N/S)	Normal saline
OD	Right eye or overdose
OOB	Out of bed

TABLE 36–7 Commonly Used Abbreviations (continued)

ABBREVIATION	TERM
OS	Left eye
pc	After meals
PE (PX)	Physical examination
per	By or through
p.m.	Afternoon
po	By mouth
postop	Postoperatively
preop	Preoperatively
prep	Preparation
prn	When necessary
qid	Four times a day
(R)	Right
$\bar{s}$	Without
stat	At once, immediately
tid	Three times a day
TO	Telephone order
TPR	Temperature, pulse, respirations
VO	Verbal order
VS	Vital signs
WNL	Within normal limits
wt	Weight

*Institutions may elect to include some of these abbreviations on their "Do Not Use" list. Check the agency's policy.

abbreviations, acronyms, and symbols. This list must include those banned by the Joint Commission (see Table 36–8).

Correct Spelling

Correct spelling is essential for accuracy in recording. If unsure how to spell a word, look it up in a dictionary or other resource book. Two decidedly different medications may have similar spellings, for example, Fosamax and Flomax.

PRACTICE ALERT
Incorrect spelling gives a negative impression to the reader and, thus, decreases the nurse's credibility.

Signature

Each recording on the nursing notes is signed by the nurse making it. The signature includes the name and title, for example, "Susan J. Green, RN" or "SJ Green, RN." Some agencies have a signature sheet and after signing this signature sheet, nurses can use their initials. With computerized charting, each nurse has his or her own code, which allows the documentation to be identified.

The following title abbreviations are often used, but nurses need to follow agency policy about how to sign their names.

RN	registered nurse
LVN	licensed vocational nurse
LPN	licensed practical nurse
NA	nursing assistant
CNA	certified nursing assistant
MA	medical assistant
NS	nursing student
PCA	patient care associate
SN	student nurse

Accuracy

The client's name and identifying information should be stamped or written on each page of the clinical record. Before making any entry, check that it is the correct chart. Do not identify charts by room number only; check the client's name. Special care is needed when caring for clients with the same last name.

Notations on records must be accurate and correct. Accurate notations consist of facts or observations rather than opinions or interpretations. It is more accurate, for example, to write that the client "refused medication" (fact) than to write that the client "was uncooperative" (opinion); to write that a client "was crying" (observation) is preferable to noting that the client "was depressed" (interpretation). Similarly, when a client expresses worry about the diagnosis or problem, this should be quoted directly on the record: "Stated: 'I'm worried about my leg.'" When describing something, avoid general words, such as *large*, *good*, or *normal*, which can be interpreted differently. For example, chart specific data such as "2 cm × 3 cm bruise" rather than "large bruise."

When a recording mistake is made, draw a line through it and write the words *mistaken entry* above or next to the original entry, with your initials or name (depending on agency policy). Do not erase, blot out, or use correction fluid. The original entry must remain visible. When using computerized charting, the nurse needs to be aware of the agency's policy and process for correcting documentation mistakes. (See Figure 36–19 ■ for an example.)

Write on every line but never between lines. If a blank appears in a notation, draw a line through the blank space so that no additional information can be recorded at any other time or by any other person, and sign the notation.

PRACTICE ALERT
Avoid writing the word *error* when a recording mistake has been made. Some believe that the word error is a "red flag" for juries and can lead to the assumption that a clinical error has caused a client injury.

Sequence

Document events in the order in which they occur; for example, record assessments, then the nursing interventions, and then the client's responses. Update or delete problems as needed.

Appropriateness

Record only information that pertains to the client's health problems and care. Any other personal information that the client conveys is inappropriate for the record. Recording

TABLE 36–8 Official "Do Not Use" List[1]

DO NOT USE	POTENTIAL PROBLEM	USE INSTEAD
U (unit)	Mistaken for "0" (zero), the number "4" (four) or "cc"	Write "unit"
IU (International Unit)	Mistaken as IV (intravenous) or 10 (ten)	Write "International Unit"
Q.D., QD, q.d., qd (daily) Q.O.D., QOD, q.o.d, qod (every other day)	Mistaken for each other Period after the Q mistaken for "I" and the "O" mistaken for "I"	Write "daily" Write "every other day"
Trailing zero (X.0 mg)* Lack of leading zero (.X mg)	Decimal point is missed	Write X mg Write 0.X mg
MS MSO_4 and $MgSO_4$	Can mean morphine sulfate or magnesium sulfate Confused for one another	Write "morphine sulfate" Write "magnesium sulfate"

[1] Applies to all orders and all medication-related documentation that is handwritten (including free-text computer entry) or on pre-printed forms.

*Exception: A "trailing zero" may be used only where required to demonstrate the level of precision of the value being reported, such as for laboratory results, imaging studies that report size of lesions, or catheter/tube sizes. It may not be used in medication orders or other medication-related documentation.

Additional Abbreviations, Acronyms and Symbols
(For possible future inclusion in the Official "Do Not Use" List)

DO NOT USE	POTENTIAL PROBLEM	USE INSTEAD
> (greater than) < (less than)	Misinterpreted as the number "7" (seven) or the letter "L" Confused for one another	Write "greater than" Write "less than"
Abbreviations for drug names	Misinterpreted due to similar abbreviations for multiple drugs	Write drug names in full
Apothecary units	Unfamiliar to many practitioners Confused with metric units	Use metric units
@	Mistaken for the number "2" (two)	Write "at"
cc	Mistaken for U (units) when poorly written	Write "mL" or "ml" or "milliliters" ("mL" is preferred)
μg	Mistaken for mg (milligrams) resulting in one thousand-fold overdose	Write "mcg" or "micrograms"

Note: © Joint Commission Resources. (2010). 2010 National Patient Safety Goals—FAQs. Oakbrook Terrace, IL: Joint Commission on Accreditation of Healthcare Organizations. Reprinted with permission.

irrelevant information may be considered an invasion of the client's privacy and/or libelous. A client's disclosure that she was addicted to heroin 15 years ago, for example, would *not* be recorded on the client's medical record unless it had a direct bearing on the client's health problem.

Completeness
Not all data that a nurse obtains about a client can be recorded. However, the information that is recorded needs to be complete and helpful to the client and health care professionals.

Date	Time	Progress Notes
9/12/2009	0800	~~Breath sounds diminished throughout all lung fields. C/O "shortness of breath".~~ N. Smith, RN.
9/12/2009	0805	Mistaken entry above, wrong client --N. Smith, RN.

Figure 36–19 ■ Correcting a charting error.

Nurses' notes need to reflect the nursing process. Record all assessments, dependent and independent nursing interventions, client problems, client comments and responses to interventions and tests, progress toward goals, and communication with other members of the health team.

Care that is *omitted* because of the client's condition or refusal of treatment must also be recorded. Document what was omitted, why it was omitted, and who was notified.

PRACTICE ALERT
Do not assume that the person reading your charting will know that a common intervention (e.g., turning) has occurred because you believe it to be an "obvious" component of care.

Conciseness
Recordings need to be brief as well as complete to save time in communication. The client's name and the word *client* are omitted. For example, write "Perspiring profusely. Respirations shallow, 28/min." End each thought or sentence with a period.

Legal Prudence
Accurate, complete documentation should give legal protection to the nurse, the client's other caregivers, the health care facility, and the client. Admissible in court as a legal document, the clinical record provides proof of the quality of care given to a client. Documentation is usually viewed by juries and attorneys as the best evidence of what really happened to the client.

PRACTICE ALERT
Complete charting by using the steps of the nursing process as a framework is the best defense against malpractice.

For the best legal protection, the nurse should not only adhere to professional standards of nursing care but also follow agency policy and procedures for intervention and documentation in all situations—especially high-risk situations (see Box 36–16).

Box 36–16 Do's and Don'ts of Documentation

DO
- Chart a change in a client's condition *and* show that follow-up actions were taken.
- Read the nurses' notes prior to care to determine if there has been a change in the client's condition.
- Be timely. A late entry is better than no entry; however, the longer the period of time between actual care and charting, the greater the suspicion.
- Use objective, specific, and factual descriptions.
- Correct charting errors.
- Chart all teaching.
- Record the client's actual words by putting quotes around the words.
- Chart the client's response to interventions.
- Review your notes—are they clear and do they reflect what you want to say?

DON'T
- Leave a blank space for a colleague to chart later.
- Chart in advance of the event (e.g., procedure, medication).
- Use vague terms (e.g., "appears to be comfortable," "had a good night").
- Chart for someone else.
- Use "patient" or "client," as it is his or her chart.
- Alter a record even if requested by a superior or a physician.
- Record assumptions or words reflecting bias (e.g., "complainer," "disagreeable").

CLINICAL EXAMPLE
1100—c/o of feeling dizzy. Raised top two side rails and instructed to stay in bed and ring call bell if requiring assistance. 1130—found lying on floor beside the bed. Stated, "I climbed out of bed all by myself." When asked about pain, replied, "I feel fine but a little dizzy." Helped into bed. BP 100/60 P90 R24. Dr. RJ Naden notified. _____ RS Woo RN

 EVIDENCE-BASED PRACTICE **Does Nursing Documentation Reflect Individualized Client Care?**

Using qualitative metasynthesis, the researchers reviewed and analyzed qualitative research reports focusing on the documentation of nursing care published between 1996 and 2003. The aim of this study was to increase understanding of the content of documenting nursing care and to show how ethical principles relating to individualized care are visible in the documentation. Ethical care includes the value of respecting clients and, therefore, documenting what the clients believe to be important in their care.

Three different themes emerged. One of the themes reflected the demands of the organization. That is, the organizations wanted the documentation to show measurable results of nursing care that could subsequently affect financial implications. The second theme reflected nurses' attitudes and duties. Nurses did not consider documentation to be important and viewed it negatively or with indifference. The third theme reflected clients' involvement in their care. It became clear that the client's views were seldom referred to in the documentation. Nurses mainly documented physical functions of the client.

Implications
This study reflected the small amount of documentation given to clients' wishes and needs. The researchers point out that the more structured the documentation system (i.e., computerized charting), the more the focus will be on nursing tasks rather than individualizing nursing care for the health of the client. Although nurses advocate the need for individualized client care, it is not visible in the nursing documentation. Is it time to clearly define the purpose of documentation? Who is the documentation for—the organization, the nurse, or the client?

Note: From Karkkainen, O., Bondas, T., & Eriksson, K. (2005). Documentation of individualized patient care: A qualitative metasynthesis. *Nursing Ethics, 12*(2), pp. 123–132. Copyright © Sage Publications Ltd, 2005. Reproduced with permission of Sage Publications, London.

REVIEW Documentation

RELATE: LINK THE CONCEPTS

Linking the exemplar of Documentation with the concept of Legal Issues:

1. How does proper documentation reduce the risk of lawsuits?
2. What components of nursing care must be included in the nurse's documentation to meet legal requirements?

Linking the exemplar of Documentation with the concept of Quality Improvement:

3. How is nursing documentation used to assess the quality of nursing care delivered?
4. How can incomplete documentation result in a negative evaluation of the quality of nursing care delivered?

REFER: GO TO MYNURSINGKIT

REFLECT: CASE STUDY

Kate Swanson is a 23-year-old nurse from a small, rural community. Kate graduated from nursing school a few months ago and took a job working on a general medical-surgical inpatient unit at Neighborhood Hospital. At some point, her goal is to work in an adult intensive care unit. She recently received a sign-on bonus and looks forward to buying her first new car.

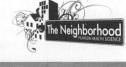
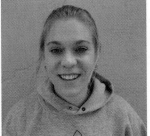

Kate has a busy week because of increased client loads—she has seven to eight clients of her own. She has trouble managing her charting with all the client care she has to do. She ends up staying up to 2 hours after each shift to get it done. Kate's manager, Pat, talks with her about this and reviews the importance of point-of-care charting. The feedback he gives her is generally positive.

1. Why is Kate's manager trying to improve her point-of-care charting?
2. What are potential dangers of waiting until the end of the shift to document care?
3. What strategies might you suggest to Kate to help her improve point-of-care charting during a busy shift?

36.4 REPORTING

KEY TERMS

Change-of-shift report, 2200
Reporting, 2200

BASIS FOR SELECTION OF EXEMPLAR

The Joint Commission

LEARNING OUTCOMES

After reading about this exemplar, you will be able to:

1. Explain the purpose of reporting.
2. Describe various types of reporting used by nurses.
3. Identify essential guidelines for reporting client data.
4. Demonstrate each form of reporting following all of the essential steps.

OVERVIEW

The purpose of **reporting** is to communicate specific information to a person or group of people. A report, whether oral or written, should be concise, including pertinent information but no extraneous detail. In addition to change-of-shift reports and telephone reports, reporting can also include the sharing of information or ideas with colleagues and other health professionals about some aspect of a client's care. Examples include the care plan conference and nursing rounds.

Change-of-Shift Reports

A **change-of-shift report** is given to all nurses on the next shift. Its purpose is to provide continuity of care for clients by providing the new caregivers a quick summary of client needs and details of care to be given.

Change-of-shift reports may be written or given orally, either in a face-to-face exchange or by audiotape recording. The face-to-face report permits the listener to ask questions during the report; written and tape-recorded reports are often briefer and less time consuming. Reports are sometimes given at the bedside, and clients as well as nurses may participate in the exchange of information. Box 36–17 lists key elements of

a change-of-shift report. Figure 36–20 ■ provides a sample change-of-shift report.

PRACTICE ALERT

Be aware of where the shift report takes place in order to maintain client confidentiality. An area that is private and free from interruption is best.

ROOM 201—C.W.
Admitted last night for pneumonia
Allergic to penicillin
DNR
IV of D5/0.45 NS infusing at 100 mL/hour in (L) forearm
Need sputum specimen for C&S
Temp 102.4. Tylenol given at 0600
Lung sounds diminished in lower lobes

ROOM 202—G. H.
Admitted for (L) total knee arthroplasty. POD # 3
Has discharge orders to go to rehab today
Dressing clean, dry, and intact
Regular diet. Taking fluids well.
Had BM yesterday
Pain rating of 4/10—last medicated with Percocet at 0400

Figure 36–20 ■ Sample change-of-shift report.

Box 36–17 **Key Elements of a Change-of-Shift Report**

- Follow a particular order (e.g., follow room numbers in a hospital).
- Provide basic identifying information for each client (e.g., name, room number, bed designation).
- For new clients, provide the reason for admission or medical diagnosis (or diagnoses), surgery (date), diagnostic tests, and therapies in past 24 hours.
- Include significant changes in the client's condition and present information in order (i.e., assessment, nursing diagnoses, interventions, outcomes, and evaluation). For example, "Mr. Ronald Oakes said he had an aching pain in his left calf at 1400 hours. Inspection revealed no other signs. Calf pain is related to altered blood circulation. Rest and elevation of his legs on a footstool for 30 minutes provided relief."
- Provide exact information, such as "Ms. Jessie Jones received morphine 6 mg IV at 1500 hours," not "Ms. Jessie Jones received some morphine during the evening."
- Report clients' need for special emotional support. For example, a client who has just learned that his biopsy results revealed malignancy and who is now scheduled for a laryngectomy needs time to discuss his feelings before preoperative teaching is begun.
- Include current nurse-prescribed and primary care provider–prescribed orders.
- Provide a summary of newly admitted clients, including diagnosis, age, general condition, plan of therapy, and significant information about the client's support people.
- Report on clients who have been transferred or discharged from the unit.
- Clearly state priorities of care and care that is due after the shift begins. For example, in a 7 a.m. report the nurse might say, "Mr. Li's vital signs are due at 0730, and his IV bag will need to be replaced by 0800." Give this information at the end of that client's report because memory is best for the first and last information given.
- Be concise. Don't elaborate on background data or routine care (e.g., do not report "Vital signs at 0800 and 1150" when that is the unit standard). Do not report coming and going of visitors unless there is a problem or concern, or visitors are involved in teaching and care. Social support and visits are the norm.

Telephone Reports

Health care professionals frequently report about a client by telephone. Nurses inform primary care providers about a change in a client's condition, a radiologist reports the results of an x-ray study, or a nurse may report to a nurse on another unit about a transferred client.

The nurse receiving a telephone report should document the date and time, the name of the person giving the information, and the subject of the information received, and sign the notation. For example:

6/6/03 1035 GL Messina, laboratory technician, reported by telephone that Mrs. Sara Ames's hematocrit was 39/100 mL. _____*B. Ireland RN*

The person receiving the information should repeat it back to the sender to ensure accuracy.

When giving a telephone report to a primary care provider, it is important that the nurse be concise and accurate. Begin with name and relationship to the client (e.g., "This is Jana Gomez, RN; I'm calling about your client, Dorothy Mendes. I'm her nurse on the 7 p.m. to 7 a.m. shift").

Telephone reports usually include the client's name and medical diagnosis, changes in nursing assessment, vital signs related to baseline vital signs, significant laboratory data, and related nursing interventions. The nurse should have the client's chart ready to give the primary care provider any further information.

After reporting, the nurse should document the date, time, and content of the call:

> **CLINICAL EXAMPLE**
> 1200-Admitted from ED. c/o burning upper right quadrant abdominal pain. Rates pain at 6/10. BP 115/80, P100, R15. Demerol 100 mg given IM per order. 1300-BP 100/40, P115, R30. Pain unchanged. Color pale and diaphoretic. Reported by telephone to Dr. Burns at 1305.
> _____TS Jones RN

Telephone Orders

Physicians often order a therapy (e.g., a medication) for a client by telephone. Most agencies have specific policies about telephone orders. Many agencies allow only registered nurses to take telephone orders.

While the primary care provider gives the order, *write* the complete order down and *read* it back to the primary care provider to ensure accuracy. Question the primary care provider about any order that is ambiguous, unusual (e.g., an abnormally high dosage of a medication), or contraindicated by the client's condition. Then transcribe the order onto the physician's order sheet, indicating it as a verbal order (VO) or telephone order (TO). See Box 36–18 for selected guidelines.

Once the order is transcribed on the physician's order sheet, the order must be countersigned by the primary care provider within a time period described by agency policy. Many acute care hospitals require that this be done within 24 hours.

Care Plan Conference

Care plan conferences allow for collaborative reporting among the health care professionals who provide care to the client. They are most often used for clients who have complex care needs. During the conference, the client's health care providers discuss possible solutions to certain problems of the client, such as inability to cope with an event or lack of progress toward goal attainment. The care plan conference allows each member of the health care team an opportunity to offer an opinion in order to reach a solution to the problem. The choice of health care professionals who are invited to attend the conference is based on the needs of the client. Family members

Box 36–18 Guidelines for Telephone and Verbal Orders

Taking verbal orders for medications from a primary provider increases the risk for error and should be avoided whenever possible. If a verbal order must be taken, the order should be signed by the provider as soon as possible. Guidelines provided by facility policy vary, so the nurse should become familiar with his or her facility's policy. General guidelines include:

1. Verbal orders should not be used when a written order is possible.
2. Always read the order back to the prescribing provider after writing it in the medical record. Make sure to include client name, drug name and spelling of the drug, dosage (pronounce dosage in single digits), route, and frequency if the order involves a medication. If the order involves something other than a medication, repeat the order verbatim as written to assure the order was written as intended.
3. Ask the provider about the indications for the medication; this helps avoid errors.
4. If there is any uncertainty about the order, ask the provider.
5. Record the order directly into the client's chart or electronic health record while receiving the order. Writing the order down on a scrap of paper and then recording it increases the risk for error.

6. Note the order according to procedure, including date and time, and sign the order. How the order is written will depend on facility policy, but is generally signed with the prescriber's name and title followed by a / and the signature of the person writing the order. For example: Dr. Monica Wilson/T. Johnson R.N. Most facilities require orders be signed within a specific period of time ranging from 4–24 hours. If no policy exists, the prescribing provider should sign the order as soon as possible.
7. Each state has its own regulations regarding the categories of personnel (e.g., registered nurse, pharmacist) who may accept a verbal order for a prescription. Know the regulations for your state.
8. Each facility has policies regarding what type of verbal orders can be accepted. For example, facilities may not allow verbal orders for narcotics, TPN, or chemotherapy and often require these orders be written directly by the provider.

Note: Adapted from: Institute for Safe Medication Practices. (2001). Instilling a measure of safety into those "whispering down the lane" verbal orders. *ISMP Medication Safety Alert.* Retrieved May 17, 2010 from http://www.ismp.org/newsletters/acutecare/articles/20010124.asp; and Vancouver Coastal Health. 2010. *Prescribing policies: telephone/verbal orders.* Retrieved May 17, 2010 from http://www.vhpharmsci.com/VHFormulary/Policies/4.2-TELEPHONE-VERBA-%20ORDERS.htm

are an important part of the care plan conference, especially for clients who are unable to advocate for themselves. Other professionals may be invited. For example, a social worker may be present to discuss support for the family of a burned child or a pharmacist may be present for the conference when the client requires multiple medications.

Care plan conferences are most effective when there is a climate of respect—that is, nonjudgmental acceptance of others even though their values, opinions, and beliefs may seem different. Interdisciplinary collaboration is discussed further in Concept 35, Collaboration. Nurses need to accept and respect each person's contributions, listening with an open mind to what others are saying even when there is disagreement.

Nursing Rounds

Nursing rounds allow two or more nurses to report to each other while visiting selected clients at each client's bedside to

- Obtain information that will help plan nursing care.
- Provide clients the opportunity to discuss their care.
- Evaluate the nursing care the client has received.

During rounds, the nurse assigned to the client provides a brief summary of the client's nursing needs and the interventions being implemented. Nursing rounds offer advantages to both clients and nurses: Clients can participate in the discussions, and nurses can see the client and the equipment being used. To facilitate client participation in nursing rounds, nurses need to use terms that the client can understand. Medical terminology excludes the client from discussion.

REVIEW Reporting

RELATE: LINK THE CONCEPTS

Linking the exemplar of Reporting with the concept of Legal Issues:
1. What legal obligations does the nurse providing change-of-shift reporting to the oncoming nurse have?
2. How can the nurse assure that all legal obligations were met when accepting telephone orders from the primary provider?

Linking the exemplar of Reporting with the concept of Safety:
3. How does change-of-shift reporting contribute to the safety of the client?
4. When providing a telephone report to the primary provider because of a client's sudden change in condition what information should be included to maintain the safe care of the client?

REFER: GO TO MYNURSINGKIT

REFLECT: CASE STUDY

Marjorie Newman, 64 years old, was admitted to the coronary care unit (CCU) with the diagnosis of acute anterior myocardial infarction. Her condition has remained stable; she is to be transferred to the telemetry unit tomorrow or sooner if the CCU bed is required for an acutely ill client. The nurse assigned to her care is called to the monitors by the monitor technician because Ms. Newman has suddenly begun having frequent premature ventricular contractions (PVCs). When the nurse enters Ms. Newman's room, she assesses the client and finds her to be short of breath, experiencing severe left-sided chest pain radiating to the left arm, and very diaphoretic. Vital signs are T 98.6, P 108 and irregular, R 28, BP 92/44. The nurse analyzes Ms. Newman's rhythm strip and finds elevated ST segments, tachycardia, with 10–14 PVCs per minute. A coworker agrees to stay with

Ms. Newman and monitor her condition while the nurse assigned to Ms. Newman's care calls the primary care provider.

1. What information would the nurse report to the primary care provider when calling to notify of the change in the client's condition?

2. Why did the nurse have a coworker stay with the client while calling the primary care provider?

3. If the nurse's shift ended while this event was occurring with Ms. Newman, what should the nurse do before leaving for the day?

PEARSON

EXPLORE **mynursingkit**™

MyNursingKit is your one stop for online chapter review materials and resources. Prepare for success with additional NCLEX®-style practice questions, interactive assignments and activities, web links, animations and videos, and more!

Register your access code from the front of your book at **www.mynursingkit.com**.

REFERENCES

American Association of Critical-Care Nurses (AACN). (2005). *AACN standards for establishing and sustaining healthy work environment: A journey to excellence.* Aliso Viejo, CA: Author.

American Nurses Association. (2001). *Code of ethics for nurses with interpretive statements.* Washington, DC: Author.

Anonymous. (2005). Meeting security regulations for e-mail. *Health Management Technology, 26*(10), 52–54.

Austin, S. (2006). E-mail: So fast, so convenient, so ... risky? *Nursing, 36*(2), 76–77.

Beyea, S. C. (2004). Improving verbal communication in clinical care. *AORN Journal, 79*(5), 1053–1057.

Catalano, J. T. (2006). *Nursing now! Today's issues, tomorrow's trends* (4th ed.). Philadelphia: F. A. Davis.

Clark, A. P. (2003). What's all the HIPAA hype? *Nurse Practitioner Supplement: The 2004 Sourcebook for Advanced Practice Nurses,* 6–11.

Delbanco, T., & Sands, D. Z. (2004). Electrons in flight—E-mail between doctors and patients. *New England Journal of Medicine, 350*(17), 1705–1708.

Dochtermaun, J. M., & Bulachek, G. H. (2004). *Nursing Interventions Classification (NIC),* (4th ed.). St. Louis: Mosby.

Editors of Nursing 2004. (2004). JCAHO says watch your p's and q's. *Nursing, 34*(3), 55.

Egan, G. (1998). *The skilled helper: A problem-management approach to helping* (6th ed.). Pacific Grove, CA: Brooks/Cole.

Fenwick, J., Barclay, L., & Schmeid, V. (2001). Chatting: An important clinical tool in facilitating mothering in neonatal nurseries. *Advances in Nursing Science, 24,* 34–49.

Gallagher, P. M. (2004). Maintain privacy with electronic charting. *Nursing Management, 35*(2), 16–17.

Guido, G. W. (2005). *Legal and ethical issues in nursing* (4th ed). Upper Saddle River, NJ: Prentice Hall.

Haskard, K., DiMatteo, M., & Heritage, J. (2009). Affective and instrumental communication in primary care interactions: Predicting the satisfaction of nursing staff and patients. *Health Communication, 24*(1), 21–32.

Joint Commission on Accreditation of Healthcare Organizations. (2006). *2006 National Patient Safety Goals–FAQs.* Retrieved April 30, 2006, from http://www .jointcommission.org/NR/rdonlyres/7C116D6D-AE82-449E-BA45-1DE49D2A0A34/0/06_npsg_faq.pdf

Kozier, B., Erb, G., Berman, A. J., & Snyder, S. (2004). *Fundamentals of nursing: Concepts, process, and practice* (7th ed.). Upper Saddle River, NJ: Prentice Hall Health.

Lindeke, L. L., & Sieckert, A. M. (2005). Nurse-physician workplace collaboration. *Online Journal of Issues in Nursing, 10*(1), manuscript 4. Retrieved February 2, 2005, from http://www.nursingworld.org/ojin/topic26/tpc26_4.htm

Lippincott Williams & Wilkins. (2003). *Complete guide to documentation.* Philadelphia: Author.

Lippincott Williams & Wilkins. (2007). *Chart smart* (2nd ed.). Philadelphia: Author.

MacDonald, C. M. (2004). A chuckle a day keeps the doctor away: Therapeutic humor & laughter. *Journal of Psychosocial Nursing & Mental Health Services, 42*(3), 18–25.

Maxfield, D., Grenny, J., McMillan, R., Patterson, K., & Switzler, A. (2005). *Silence kills. The seven crucial conversations for healthcare.* VitalSmarts, L.C.

Mayo Clinic (2009). *Being assertive: Reduce stress, communicate better.* Retrieved on December 12, 2009, from http://www.mayoclinic.com/health/assertive/ SR00042

Moorhead, S., Johnson, M., & Maas, M. (2004). *Nursing Outcomes Classification (NOC).* (3rd ed.). St. Louis: Mosby.

NANDA International. (2007). *NANDA nursing diagnosis: Definitions & classification 2007–2008.* Philadelphia: Author.

The Office for Civil Rights. (2010). Effective communication in hospitals. Retrieved March 7, 2010, from http://www.hhs .gov/ocr/civilrights/resources/specialtopics/ hospitalcommunication/index.html

Perry, J., Galloway, S., Bottorff, J. L., & Nixon, S. (2005). Nurse-patient communication in dementia: Improving the odds. *Journal of Gerontological Nursing, 31*(4), 43–52.

Rondeau, K. V. (1992). Effective communication means really listening. *Canadian Journal of Medical Technology, 52*(2), 78–80.

Rosenstein, A. H., & O'Daniel, M. (2005). Disruptive behavior & clinical outcomes: Perceptions of nurses & physicians. *American Journal of Nursing, 105*(1), 54–64.

Smith, C. M., & Dougherty, M. (2001). Practice brief: Requirements for the acute care record. *Journal of AHIMA, 72*(3), 56A–56G.

Sullivan, G. H. (2004). Legally speaking: Does your charting measure up? *RN, 67*(3), 61–65.

Tamparo, C. T., & Lindh, W. Q. (2000). *Therapeutic communications for health professionals* (2nd ed.). Albany, NY: Delmar: Thomson Learning.

Wilkinson, J. M. (2005). *Nursing diagnosis handbook with NIC interventions and NOC outcomes* (8th ed.). Upper Saddle River, NJ: Prentice Hall Health.

Williams, K., Kemper, S., & Hummert, M. L. (2004). Enhancing communication with older adults: Overcoming elderspeak. *Journal of Gerontological Nursing, 30*(10), 17–25.

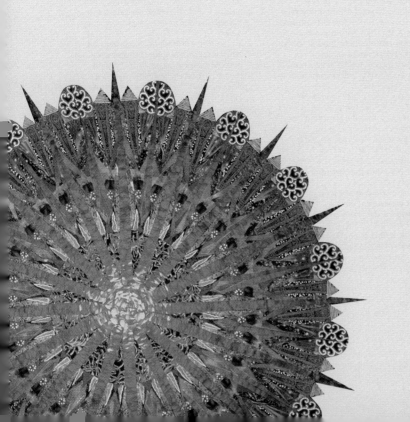

Managing Care

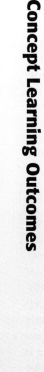

Concept at-a-Glance

About Managing Care, *2205*

37.1   Care Coordination, *2208*

37.2   Cost-Effective Care, *2209*

37.3   Delegation, *2217*

Concept Learning Outcomes

After reading about this concept, you will be able to:

1. Describe the goals and emphasis of managed care.

2. Explain the role of the case manger in a managed care environment.

3. List different frameworks for delivering care, and explain how each differs, including the advantages and disadvantages of each.

Concept Key Terms

Case management, *2206*
Client-focused care, *2206*
Differentiated practice, *2206*
Licensed practical nurses (LPNs), *2206*
Managed care, *2206*

Registered nurses (RNs), *2206*
Team nursing, *2206*
Unlicensed assistive personnel (UAPs), *2206*

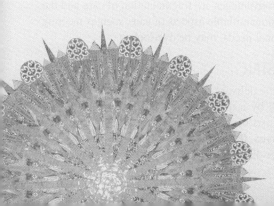

About Managing Care

A number of options for the delivery of nursing care support the continuity of care and cost-effectiveness. These options include managed care, case management, client-focused care, differentiated practice, shared governance, the case method, the functional method, team nursing, and primary nursing (described in Concept 44, Health Care Systems). Each of these systems of care has evolved as organizations attempt to decrease health care costs; maximize limited human and physical resources; meet increasingly complex federal, state, and local regulations; and improve the quality of client care. A particular agency may use more than one configuration—for example, team nursing on the medical surgical units and primary nursing on the cardiac surgery unit. ●

MANAGED CARE

Managed care describes a health care system in which the goals are to provide cost-effective, quality care that focuses on decreased costs and improved outcomes for groups of clients. The care of a client is carefully planned from the initial contact to the conclusion of the specific health problem. In managed care, health care providers and agencies collaborate to render the most appropriate, fiscally responsible care possible. Managed care denotes an emphasis on cost controls, customer satisfaction, health promotion, and preventive services. Health maintenance organizations and preferred provider organizations are examples of provider systems committed to managed care.

Managed care can be used with primary and team nursing, the functional method, and alternative nursing care delivery systems. Although managed care has been embraced as a model for health care reform, many question the application of this business approach to a commodity as precious as health.

CASE MANAGEMENT

Case management describes a range of models for integrating health care services for individuals or groups. Generally, case management involves multidisciplinary teams that assume collaborative responsibility for planning and assessing needs, and for coordinating, implementing, and evaluating care for groups of clients from preadmission to discharge or transfer and recuperation. A case manager may be a nurse, social worker, or other appropriate professional. In some areas of the United States, case managers may be referred to as discharge planners. This topic is discussed in greater detail in Concept 35, Collaboration.

CLIENT-FOCUSED CARE

Client-focused care is a delivery model that brings all services and care providers to the client. The idea is that if activities normally provided by various members of the health care team (e.g., physical therapy, respiratory therapy, electrocardiographic testing, and phlebotomy) are moved closer to the client, then the number of personnel involved and the number of steps needed to get the work done are decreased. To succeed, client-focused care requires cross-training (development of multiskilled workers who can perform tasks or functions in more than one discipline) of health care personnel.

DIFFERENTIATED PRACTICE

Differentiated practice is a system in which the best possible use of nursing staff members is based on their educational preparation and resultant skill sets. Thus, differentiated practice models consist of specific job descriptions for nurses according to their education or training—for example LVN, ADN, BSN RN, MSN RN, or APN. In order to establish a differentiated practice system, each health care agency must first identify the nursing competencies required by the clients that agency serves. This model further requires the delineation of roles between both licensed nursing personnel and unlicensed

assistive personnel (UAPs). This enables nurses to progress and assume roles and responsibilities appropriate to their level of experience, capability, and education. As with managed care and case management, differentiated nursing practice seeks to provide quality care at an affordable cost.

SHARED GOVERNANCE

The shared governance model can be used in concert with other models of nursing delivery. In this organizational model, nursing staff participate with administrative personnel in making, implementing, and evaluating client care policies. The focus of this model is to encourage participation of nurses in decision making at all levels of the organization. Individuals may participate either at their own request or as part of their job role criteria. More commonly, nurses participate through serving in decision-making groups, such as committees and task forces. The decisions made may also address employment conditions, cost-effectiveness, long-range planning, productivity, and wages and benefits. The underlying principle of shared governance is that employees will be more committed to the organizational goals if they have input into planning and decision making.

CASE METHOD

The case method, also referred to as total care, is one of the earliest nursing models developed. In this client-centered method, one nurse is assigned to, and is responsible for, the comprehensive care of a group of clients during an 8- or 12-hour shift. For each client, the nurse assesses needs, makes nursing plans, formulates diagnoses, implements care, and evaluates the effectiveness of care. In this method, a client has consistent contact with one nurse during a shift but may have different nurses on other shifts. Considered to be the precursor of primary nursing, the case method continues to be used in a variety of practice settings, such as intensive care nursing.

FUNCTIONAL METHOD

The functional method focuses on the jobs to be completed (e.g., bed making and temperature measurement). In this task-oriented approach, personnel with less preparation than the professional nurse perform those aspects of care with less complex requirements. The method is based on a production and efficiency model that gives authority and responsibility to the person assigning the work—for example, the head nurse. Clearly defined job descriptions, procedures, policies, and lines of communication are required. The functional approach to nursing is economical and efficient, and it permits centralized direction and control. Its disadvantages are fragmentation of care and the possibility that nonquantifiable aspects of care, such as meeting the client's emotional needs, may be overlooked.

TEAM NURSING

Team nursing is the delivery of individualized nursing care to a group of clients by a team led by a professional nurse. A nursing team consists of the following:

■ **Registered nurses (RNs)**, who are specially licensed and trained to deliver direct client care, including assessment and

EVIDENCE-BASED PRACTICE Do the Types of Nurses and Delivery Models in Hospitals Influence Client Outcomes?

Researchers in one study correlated the number of professional nursing staff on a total of 77 medical, surgical, and obstetrical units in 19 hospitals with costs and quality of care. Quality of care was measured through client outcomes: rates of medication errors, falls, and certain infections. More than 1,000 nurses were surveyed for the care delivery model used on their units. These models included total care, team nursing, and primary care nursing. The nurses were also asked about communication and coordination within the nursing unit.

Quality, coordination, and communication were statistically superior on those units that had all registered nurse staffing as opposed to staff that included unlicensed assistive personnel and practical nurses. Quality was lower on those units that used the total care delivery model.

Implications

In every case, the larger the percentage of registered nurses among the total care staff, the lower the incidence of adverse client outcomes, such as falls, errors, and preventable infections. It is more difficult to compare outcomes with care delivery models because each unit may employ slight variations of the model. However, it is important to continue to examine delivery models and their effectiveness in order to allow optimal deployment of registered nurses in a time of a shortage.

Source: From Hall, L. M., Doran, D., and Pink, G. H. (2004). Nurse staffing models, nursing hours, and patient safety outcomes. *Journal of Nursing Administration, 34*, 41–45.

---

identification of health problems and development and coordination of care.

- **Licensed practical nurses (LPNs)**, who provide direct client care under the direction of an RN, physician, or other licensed practitioner.
- **Unlicensed assistive personnel (UAPs)**, or health care staff, who assume delegated aspects of basic client care such as bathing, assisting with feeding, and collecting specimens. UAPs include certified nurse assistants, hospital attendants, nurse technicians, and orderlies.

The RN retains responsibility and authority for client care but delegates appropriate tasks to the other team members. Proponents of this model believe the team approach increases the efficiency of the RN. Opponents feel that inpatient clients with acute illnesses require greater attention from the professional nurse and allow little room for delegation.

PRIMARY NURSING

Primary nursing is a system in which one nurse is responsible for overseeing the total care of a number of clients 24 hours a day, 7 days a week, even if he or she does not deliver all the care personally. It is a method of providing comprehensive, individualized, and consistent care.

Primary nursing uses the nurse's technical knowledge and management skills. The primary nurse assesses and prioritizes each client's needs, identifies nursing diagnoses, develops a plan of care with the client, and evaluates the effectiveness of care. Associates provide some care, but the primary nurse coordinates it and communicates information about the client's health to other nurses and health professionals. Primary nursing encompasses all aspects of the professional role, including teaching, advocacy, decision making, and continuity of care. The primary nurse is the first-line manager of the client's care, with all its inherent accountabilities and responsibilities.

NURSING PRACTICE

Regardless of the model of care delivery an agency uses, nurses carry a great deal of responsibility for the management of client care. Managing care has implications on direct client care, on coordination of client care, and on cost containment. For example, by scheduling the dietician to come at a different time than the physical therapist, the nurse makes sure that neither professional wastes time (and therefore money) waiting for the other one to finish seeing the same client. This also may prevent the client from becoming overtired by seeing too many providers within a short period of time.

Like everything in nursing, managing care is a learned skill that requires strong communication, assessment, and time-management skills. It also requires, when necessary, appropriate delegation. Nurses who manage these activities successfully will contribute significantly to client well-being and to the cost of care delivery.

REVIEW About Managing Care

RELATE: LINK THE CONCEPTS

Linking the concept of Managing Care with the concept of Communication:

1. How does the nurse's ability to communicate effectively contribute to managing the client's care?
2. Describe a situation in which conflict management may be necessary when managing care for a client who requires the services of several departments within the hospital.

Mr. Montoya is to be discharged from the acute care facility after removal of a metastatic brain tumor. He will receive chemotherapy intrathecally as well as intravenously. The unit clerk has scheduled follow-up appointments with his surgeon, family provider, oncologist, and neurologist as well as with the infusion therapy department. The doctor has provided referrals for consultation with a dietician, social services, and home nursing care.

Linking the concept of Managing Care with the concept of Collaboration:

3. How can the nurse prioritize care to meet the client's needs while assuring that each of these services meets his or her own needs in preparing for the client's discharge (e.g., nutritional screening predischarge, social services interview, and home nursing assessment to determine home care needs)?

4. What is the nurse's role in managing this client's care and collaborating with the other members of the health care team?

REFER: GO TO MYNURSINGKIT

REFLECT: CASE STUDY

Katelyn Donmoyer, 8 years old, was brought to the emergency department following a severe burn to more than 55% of her body. Police accompanied Katelyn to the hospital and explained that her burn was the result of parental abuse and that both parents had been arrested and were facing charges of child abuse, neglect, and attempted murder.

Katelyn was admitted to the pediatric burn unit with an endotracheal tube in place to preserve her airway; she required mechanical ventilation for 3 weeks. At the end of the first week, a tracheotomy was created and, even after the mechanical ventilator was discontinued, was maintained in order to preserve her airway, which was severely burned. She has had numerous surgeries to remove eschar and for skin grafting.

Shortly after Katelyn's admission, authorities located her grandparents, who agreed to assume custody of her. They have obtained the necessary court papers to make them legal guardians and are responsible for making all medical and legal decisions for her.

1. What team members would be important to include in managing Katelyn's care?
2. When it is time to discharge Katelyn, what type of facility may appropriately receive her?
3. What factors would influence Katelyn's care management by the nurse?

 37.1 CARE COORDINATION

KEY TERMS

Collaboration, *2208*
Coordination, *2208*

BASIS FOR SELECTION OF EXEMPLAR

Institute of Medicine
National League for Nursing Competencies
Standards of Nursing Practice

LEARNING OUTCOMES

After reading about this exemplar, you should be able to:

1. Differentiate between coordination and collaboration.
2. Predict potential barriers to effective coordination along with strategies to overcome or avoid these barriers.
3. Relate skills to achieve effective coordination.
4. Expand upon the anticipated benefits when care coordination is effective.

OVERVIEW

In March 2008, researchers presented findings from a study funded by the Robert Wood Johnson Foundation (RWJF) on nursing care coordination. In the presentation, the researchers defined **coordination** as "actions initiated by nurses with patients, families, and/or members of the health care team to manage and correct the sequence, timing, and/or effectiveness of patient care" (RWJF, 2008).

Coordination shares some similarities with **collaboration** (two or more people working toward a common goal) in that it requires the nurse to interact with others on behalf of the client. When considering client care, however, two critical differences emerge between collaboration and coordination:

1. Coordination is an action initiated by the nurse. Collaboration may be initiated by the client, a family member, or any member of the health care team.
2. Collaboration requires direct interaction with the client or other individual with whom one is collaborating. Coordination of care may or may not involve direct client care and, thus, may not require direct interaction with another individual. For example, the nurse may ensure that all plans for the client's discharge are complete or that the various treatment and exam procedures are scheduled appropriately.

BARRIERS TO EFFECTIVE COORDINATION

As health care organizations and services become more complex and use more interdisciplinary teams, team members may not always have the same view of the clients, problems, or priorities. In situations like this, it is critical that the team find a way to work collaboratively in order to provide coordinated client care and prevent errors, disorganized care, and care that does not produce effective outcomes.

Team members need to have a better understanding of individual responsibilities and stress levels in order to appreciate each other and develop more realistic working relationships. Coordination is also more effective when those involved have a better understanding of their respective roles and work stresses. Recognizing this will make coordination less frustrating.

If resources are not available when and in the manner required, this will act as a barrier to coordination. Team members who are not willing to listen and include others will find that coordination may not be as successful as planned. Other barriers include a lack of interdisciplinary understanding, lack of resources, and inadequate communication. Ineffective problem solving is also a critical barrier.

SKILLS THAT PROMOTE EFFECTIVE COORDINATION

To coordinate care effectively, nurses need to solve problems, plan, use the abilities or skills of other staff, identify resources required, communicate, and be willing to collaborate. Because delegation often is required, delegation skills are important. The nurse also must develop evaluation skills to determine if outcomes are met as well as when to change course or make adjustments. The skills required for coordination are the same as those required for collaboration, which shares the primary goal of working together to reach agreed-upon goals. Box 37–1 highlights the skills needed for effective coordination.

Box 37–1 Skills Needed for Effective Coordination

- Problem solving
- Planning
- Ability to use the skills of others
- Identification of needed resources
- Communication
- Collaboration
- Delegation
- Evaluation

APPLICATION OF COORDINATION

Coordination is integral to daily operations, short- and long-range planning, and the daily care process. All of these activities require coordination of clinical and administrative resources. The following strategies are helpful in improving coordination:

- All team members should have a clear understanding of goals.
- All team members should use effective communication.
- All team members should have knowledge of policies and procedures, with an understanding of what has to be done, by whom, and how it will help to facilitate coordination.

- Orientation and staff development programs should emphasize the importance of coordination and how to use it.
- All team members need to accept that different expertise is required to meet complex client needs (Finkelman, 1996, pp. 1–1:17).

Health care agencies use many tools that focus on coordination of care. Some of these are case management, clinical pathways, practice guidelines, and disease management. To be successful and meet expected outcomes, these tools also require collaboration with clients, clients' families and significant others, and other health care providers. Coordination plays a major role in reaching managed care's goals of effective and efficient care. Coordination requires that the nurse understand the client's needs and the resources that are available to meet these needs. This includes understanding the association between costs and services.

In conclusion, coordination is a very important part of care delivery and management within the health care delivery system. Coordination is required to provide client care, get resources, schedule staff, plan work activities, implement quality improvement, and perform all types of functions related to the delivery of health care. As this system becomes more complex, however, communication and coordination also become more complex.

REVIEW   Care Coordination

RELATE: LINK THE CONCEPTS

Linking the exemplar of Care Coordination with the concept of Development:

1. How might care coordination differ with clients who are at differing stages of development?
2. Who might be included when coordinating care for a young child versus care for an older adult?

Linking the exemplar of Care Coordination with the concept of Diversity:

3. How does the diversity of clients impact care coordination?
4. How might the diversity of the health care team impact care coordination?

REFER: GO TO MYNURSINGKIT

REFLECT: CASE STUDY

Michel Goulian, 22 years old, experienced severe head trauma in a motor vehicle accident 2 months ago and has been hospitalized ever since. He has Broca's aphasia and, as a result of damage to his frontal region, has difficulty putting words together to form complete sentences, which has also altered his personality, leaving him moody, temperamental, and prone to outbursts of frustration. His mobility is hampered by weakness in both legs and difficulty controlling movement. He has strong family support, and his parents want him to live with them until he is able to function independently. After discharge he will receive speech therapy, occupational therapy, and physical therapy. Social services has been involved in helping him pay for the cost of health care (he has no medical insurance) as well as in meeting his financial needs after discharge until he can return to his job. Dietary services would like to meet with both the client and his mother, who will be providing his meals, to help Mr. Goulian meet his nutritional needs. Secondary to extended need for mechanical ventilation, respiratory therapy is involved in his care and will facilitate home oxygen administration due to what is expected to be an extended need for maintenance of his tracheostomy.

1. How can the nurse facilitate this client's care, coordinating all of the different departments and team members involved?
2. How can care coordination help to reduce the cost of the client's care?
3. What complications might be anticipated if this client's care is inadequately coordinated?

37.2 COST-EFFECTIVE CARE

KEY TERMS

Coinsurance, 2211
Deductible, 2211
Diagnosis-related groups (DRGS), 2211
Health maintenance organization (HMO), 2212
Integrated delivery system (IDS), 2212
Mandatory health insurance, 2213

Medicaid, 2211
Medicare, 2210
Physician/hospital organization (PHO), 2212
Preferred provider organization (PPO), 2212
Private insurance, 2210
Prospective payment system (PPS), 2211
Public insurance, 2210

State Children's Health Insurance Program (SCHIP), *2211*
Socialized insurance, *2213*
Socialized medicine, *2213*
Supplemental Security Income (SSI) benefits, *2211*
Voluntary insurance, *2213*

BASIS FOR SELECTION OF EXEMPLAR

National League for Nursing Competencies
Standards of Nursing Care

LEARNING OUTCOMES

After reading about this exemplar, you will be able to:

1. Contrast the various types of payment sources available in the United States.

2. Contrast the U.S. system of health care with those of other countries.

3. Expand upon the challenges faced by the U.S. health care system.

4. Describe the nurse's role in creating a cost-conscious nursing practice.

OVERVIEW

Between the years 1980 and 2004, health care spending, despite efforts to control the costs of health care, grew faster than the economy (Stanton, 2005). Employers, legislators, insurers, and health care providers continue to collaborate in efforts to resolve the issues surrounding how to best finance health care costs. Among these efforts, the United States has implemented several cost-containment strategies, including health promotion and illness prevention activities, managed care systems, and alternative insurance delivery systems. The U.S. Center for Outcomes and Effectiveness Research (COER) conducts and supports studies on the outcomes and effectiveness of diagnostic, therapeutic, and preventive health care services and procedures, including cost.

In 1972, Congress directed the Department of Health, Education, and Welfare to create professional standards review organizations in order to monitor the appropriateness of hospital use under the Medicare and Medicaid programs. This opened the door to the establishment of health systems agencies throughout the United States for comprehensive health planning. In 1978, the Rural Health Clinics Act provided for the development of health care in medically underserved rural areas. The government's increasing commitment to provide health care to the medically underserved resulted in the ability of nurse practitioners to provide primary care.

At the time this book is being published, the U.S. federal government is struggling to create a health care reform bill that will help to lower the cost of health care while increasing the number of people who have health care coverage (Box 37–2). The effort is complicated by the fact that many in the United

States feel all persons should have access to health care regardless of their ability to pay for it. Others feel that individuals should be able to pay their own way, either by getting a job that offers health care insurance or by paying directly for whatever care they can afford. The skyrocketing costs of care threaten to cripple the nation's economy and are driving some families into bankruptcy while others are living a much lower quality of life because they cannot access the care they need.

PAYMENT SOURCES IN THE UNITED STATES

Payment for health care services in the United States may be made from one or more of several sources. For example, an older client may have Medicare coverage and supplement the difference with private insurance and, if the combination does not cover all services, his or her own money (Figure 37–1 ■). Insurance is often classified as **public insurance** (insurance financed by the government) or **private insurance** (insurance provided by private or publicly owned companies such as Blue Cross Blue Shield, Kaiser, or Aetna). Many insurance plans, public or private, include a per-visit or per-prescription copayment.

Public Insurance

Public insurance programs exist to support children, older adults, and those with disabilities. Part of the discussion of health care reform revolves around whether these programs should be expanded to serve additional people. While public insurance programs are funded primarily at the federal level, states are

---

Box 37–2 Five Principles for Addressing the Problem of the Underinsured

From 2001 to 2004, the Institute of Medicine (IOM) issued six research reports identifying the scope of the problem of the underinsured in America. The IOM recommended five principles for addressing the problem:

1. Health coverage should be for everyone.
2. Health coverage should be ongoing/uninterruptible.
3. Individuals and families need to have coverage they can afford.
4. A national approach must be cost-effective and able to be maintained by the society.
5. This coverage must ensure care that is "effective, safe, timely, patient centered, and equitable" (Jennings, 2004, p. 101).

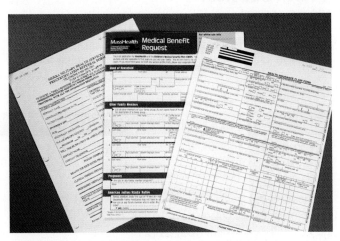

Figure 37–1 ■ Medicare helps defray the costs of health care.

TABLE 37–2 **Trends in Health Care Delivery**

FROM	TO
Illness emphasis	Preventive emphasis
Acute care	Preventive, home care
Hospital/institution-based	Noninstitution-based (clinic/home)
Fee-for-service (cost-based)	Prospective payment and managed care
Physician-directed	Diverse decision makers and managed care
If it helps (at all), use it (regardless of cost)	Outcomes measurement and cost-effectiveness
Independent decisions (practice variation)	Protocols/guidelines (best practice)
Local perspective (practice variation, standards/benchmarking)	Global perspective (protocols/guidelines/practice)
Introduce new technologies (regardless of cost)	Outcomes measurement and cost-effectiveness
Paper records, medical charts	Information systems, computer records
Change in:	
Orientation	
Illness, crisis	Prevention
Specific, specialist	Holistic
Quantity of care	Quality of care
Location of service	
Inpatient	Outpatient, clinic, home
Payment mode	
Retrospective	Prospective
Fee-for-service	Managed care
Outlook	
Just do it	Outcomes measurement
	Quality of care; quality of life

Source: From Cherry, B. and Jacob, S. R. (1999). *Contemporary nursing: Issues, trends, and management* (p. 162). St. Louis, MO: Mosby. Used by permission.

Advances in medical technology also contributed to this move from a traditional hospital to an outpatient setting. Many surgeries, such as cholecystectomies, hernia repairs, and some orthopedic surgeries, that once necessitated several days in the hospital at one time could now be done on an outpatient or ambulatory surgery basis. These outpatient services are less costly.

Within the integrated system, the goal is to create a "seamless" system of client care, in which movement from service to service is coordinated and well organized. Such a plan could improve quality of care and outcomes while increasing client satisfaction and providing better control of costs by more efficient use of resources. If the system is efficient, it can decrease transaction costs and allow greater accountability.

NURSING ECONOMICS

Quality care and cost trade-offs in hospitals have dominated the literature of the past decade. Both consumers and health care professionals express concerns about diminished quality of care resulting from cost constraints, early discharge,

periodic nursing shortages, and increased use of UAPs. Determining the precise cost of nursing services is a major challenge for nursing. What are the exact costs of high-quality nursing care? How many nursing care hours are required for each DRG? What is the best skill mix—that is, ratio of RNs to LPNs and nursing assistants—on each hospital unit? Since 1983, many studies have been undertaken to determine the actual costs of nursing care and the cost-effectiveness of nursing care. Researchers have investigated such topics as the impact of nurse–physician collaboration; new cost-effective interventions; cost benefits of primary nursing, nurse practitioners, and nurse–midwives; cost-effectiveness of home care; and so on. The quality of the nursing care of the future will rely on ongoing research.

Nursing Shortages

One factor that must be considered when discussing the economics of nursing is that at various times, the country experiences a national shortage of nurses. These shortages usually are cyclic in nature, with periods of acute shortage followed by periods in which the problem seems to have been resolved.

The measure commonly used to indicate a shortage of nurses is the *nursing vacancy rate*, the percentage of unfilled positions for which an organization is recruiting.

When shortages occur, employers are forced to increase wages in order to be able to hire and retain staff as other employers increase their wages in their attempts to maintain staffing during a shortage. As employers fill positions or more nurses enter the workforce as a result of other factors, employers begin to decrease the rate at which they increase salaries and wages. Fluctuations in salaries as a result of nursing shortages add another challenge to attempts to determine actual costs of nursing.

The trends of the past 15 years in health care have added to the complexity of the problem. When length of stay decreased, clients were sent home "sicker and quicker," and care shifted to the home, outpatient settings, and skilled-nursing facilities. Cost-containment companies began hiring nurses to do utilization review and case management. For a period of time, hospitals were downsizing nursing departments as a cost-cutting measure and adding UAPs. With these changes, some nurses experienced disillusionment with health care and left the profession, feeling that they could no longer provide quality care.

Ending the cycle of nursing shortages will require some adjustment to the approaches used by employers and nurses. New opportunities and new roles for nurses may attract more people into the profession. To the extent that RNs are able to perform more highly valued functions, their presence will be more valuable to administrators in health care organizations.

Cost-Conscious Nursing Practice

All nurses must be concerned about the cost of health care to ensure a viable health care system in the future (Vere-Jones, 2006). Because the nursing budget can account for as much as half of an organization's total expenses, nurses at all levels face significant pressure to become more cost conscious in the budgeting process, to allocate resources, and to control and monitor expenditures (Finkler & Kovner, 2007). This level of financial accountability is new to the nursing profession and comes at a time when nursing must compete with other departments within the organization for limited resources. Consider the following:

- Compared with other providers, nurses use the most resources, such as supplies and equipment. Nurses increase their awareness of issues related to use of supplies and equipment. Careful use of supplies, for example, reduces waste. Appropriate use and preventive maintenance of equipment prolongs the life span of equipment and reduces the risk of a malfunction that may impact client care.
- Because nursing staff levels have been impacted by the efforts of health care organizations to control costs, nurses have to assess how they deliver care and to search for more efficient methods of care delivery.
- Efforts at cost containment in managed care have increased the focus on health promotion and prevention of illness and disease—important aspects of nursing care. This has resulted in new professional opportunities for nurses in a variety of settings.

Whether nurses work in a hospital, a school, home health care, or another setting, they are increasingly required to participate in strategies to make care more cost effective. While this is an essential component to their ability to compete in the workforce, it does not negate their roles as client advocates and care coordinators. Nurses everywhere must continue to advocate for care that meets the standards of best practice while trying to find new ways to contain costs.

REVIEW Cost-Effective Care

RELATE: LINK THE CONCEPTS

Linking the exemplar of Cost-Effective Care with the concept of Health, Wellness, and Illness:

1. Explain how health promotion activities reduce the cost of care.
2. You are caring for an adolescent client who admits to smoking "a couple" cigarettes per week. What impact would helping this client quit smoking have on the lifetime cost of his health care?

Linking the exemplar of Cost-Effective Care with the concept of Infection:

3. How does the cost of a hospital-acquired infection impact the cost of a client's admission?
4. How does the cost of reducing the risk of hospital-acquired infections compare to the cost of treating a client who contracts a hospital-acquired infection?

REFER: GO TO MYNURSINGKIT

REFLECT: CASE STUDY

The nurse works on an oncology unit with 30 beds, including a six-bed bone-marrow transplant unit. Each nurse is usually assigned four or five clients each, depending on the acuity. Only nurses with advanced training are allowed to administer chemotherapy, so it is not uncommon to have one nurse assigned to be a medication nurse when many others are also working who have not yet attended or completed the chemotherapy certification course.

1. What actions could you, as a staff nurse on this unit, take to reduce the cost of providing care to these clients?
2. An automated medication distribution unit was recently purchased that allows nurses to receive their medications after entering the client information without having to go to the pharmacy. Explain both the positive and the negative impact on costs as a result of using this new equipment.
3. The hospital is considering replacing its 10-year-old x-ray machine with a newer model that uses less radiation and is completely digital, eliminating the need for film cartridges and making it easier for radiologists to read x-rays from computers in their offices or homes. However, the cost of the machine is very high. You are asked to join the committee that will make the decision whether to purchase this equipment. What are the pros and cons of buying this new radiology equipment?

37.3 DELEGATION

KEY TERMS

Assignment, *2218*
Authority, *2218*
Delegate, *2217*
Delegation, *2217*
Delegator, *2217*
Overdelegation, *2222*
Reverse delegation, *2222*

BASIS FOR SELECTION OF EXEMPLAR

National League for Nursing Competencies
Standards of Nursing Care

LEARNING OUTCOMES

After completing this exemplar, you will be able to:

1. Describe the need for responsibility, accountability, and authority when delegating.
2. Contrast the terms *assignment* and *delegation*.
3. Describe how effective delegation benefits the delegator, the delegate, and the organization.
4. Explain the delegation process and key behaviors when delegating tasks.
5. Identify obstacles that can impede effective delegation.
6. Explain the liability of delegation.

OVERVIEW

Delegation is the transference of responsibility and authority for an activity to a competent individual. The **delegate** is the individual who assumes responsibility for the actual performance of the task or procedure. The **delegator** is the individual who assigns the task and retains accountability for the outcome.

Delegation is a tool that allows the delegator to devote more time to tasks that cannot be delegated. It also enhances the skills and abilities of the delegate, which builds self-esteem, promotes morale, and enhances teamwork and attainment of the organization's goals. In nursing, delegation refers to indirect care—the intended outcome is achieved through the work of someone supervised by the nurse—and involves defining the task, determining who can perform the task, describing the expectation, seeking agreement, monitoring performance, and providing feedback to the delegate regarding performance.

Delegation is a difficult leadership skill for nurses to learn, because nurses have a tendency to feel that no one can do things as well as they can. Given the confusion over what tasks UAPs can perform and those that are the unique purview of RNs (Kleinman & Saccomano, 2006), nurses may be reluctant to delegate. Never before, however, has delegation been as critical a skill for nurses to perfect as it is today, with the emphasis on doing more with less. Once nurses learn how to delegate, they will extend their ability to accomplish more by using others' help. No nurse working in health care today can afford not to delegate. Tools for successful delegation are listed in Box 37–3.

PRINCIPLES OF DELEGATION

Registered nurses increasingly delegate components of nursing care to other health care workers, especially UAPs. An RN who delegates a task to another health care worker is accountable for selecting an appropriately skilled caregiver and for continued evaluation of the client's care. These "nurse extenders" may be identified by a variety of titles, including certified nursing aides/assistants, home health aides, client care

---

Box 37–3 Tools for Delegating Successfully

1. Delegate only tasks for which you have responsibility.
2. Transfer authority when you delegate responsibility.
3. Be sure you follow state regulations, job descriptions, and agency policies when delegating.
4. Follow the delegation process and key behaviors for delegating.
5. Accept delegation when you are clear about the task, time frame, reporting, and other expectations.
6. Confront your fears about delegation; recognize those that are realistic and those that are not.

---

technicians, orderlies, or surgical technicians, and they have diverse levels of training and experience. They are employees and do not include family members or friends who provide some client care.

It is not possible to generate an exhaustive list of exactly which actions may or may not be delegated to UAPs. Examples of tasks that may and may not be delegated are given in Box 37–4. A statement regarding delegation is included with the steps for each procedure in this book.

Principles guiding the nurse's decision to delegate ensure the safety and quality of outcomes. These principles are listed in Box 37–5. Even if the task is one that may legally be delegated, the individual nurse must still determine if the task can be delegated to a particular UAP for a specific client. (The unlicensed person may not delegate tasks to another person.) Once the decision has been made to delegate, the nurse must communicate clearly to the UAP and verify that the UAP understands the following:

■ The specific tasks to be done for each client.
■ When each task is to be done.
■ The expected outcomes for each task, including parameters outside of which the unlicensed person must immediately report to the nurse (and any action that must urgently be taken).
■ Who is available to serve as a resource if needed.
■ When and in what format (written or verbal) a report on the tasks is expected.

Box 37–4 Examples of Tasks That May and May Not Be Delegated to Unlicensed Assistive Personnel

TASKS THAT MAY BE DELEGATED TO UNLICENSED ASSISTIVE PERSONNEL

- Taking of vital signs
- Measuring and recording intake and output
- Client transfers and ambulation
- Postmortem care
- Bathing
- Feeding
- Gastrostomy feedings in established systems
- Attending to safety
- Weighing
- Performing simple dressing changes
- Suctioning of chronic tracheostomies
- Performing basic life support (e.g., cardiopulmonary resuscitation)

TASKS THAT MAY NOT BE DELEGATED TO UNLICENSED ASSISTIVE PERSONNEL

- Assessment
- Interpretation of data
- Making a nursing diagnosis
- Creation of a nursing care plan
- Evaluation of care effectiveness
- Care of invasive lines
- Administering parenteral medications
- Insertion of nasogastric tubes
- Client education
- Performing triage
- Giving telephone advice

Box 37–5 Principles Used by the Nurse to Determine Delegation to Unlicensed Assistive Personnel

1. The nurse must assess the individual client before delegating tasks.
2. The client must be medically stable or in a chronic condition and not fragile.
3. The task must be considered as routine for this client.
4. The task must not require a substantial amount of scientific knowledge or technical skill.
5. The task must be considered as safe for this client.
6. The task must have a predictable outcome.
7. The nurse must learn the agency's procedures and policies about delegation.
8. The nurse must know the scope of practice and the customary knowledge, skills, and job description for each health care discipline represented on the team.

9. The nurse must be aware of individual variations in work abilities. Along with different categories of caregivers are individual variations. Each individual has different experiences and may not be capable of performing every task cited in the job description.
10. The nurse, when unsure about an assistant's abilities to perform a task, must observe while the person performs it or must demonstrate it to the person and get a return demonstration before allowing the person to perform it independently.
11. The nurse must clarify reporting expectations to ensure the task is accomplished.
12. The nurse must create an atmosphere that fosters communication, teaching, and learning. For example, the nurse should encourage the unlicensed assistive personnel (UAP) to ask questions, listen carefully to concerns, and make use of every opportunity to teach.

A specific task that can be delegated to one UAP may not be appropriate for a different UAP, depending on each UAP's experience and individual skill sets. Also, a task that is appropriate for the UAP to perform with one client may not be appropriate with a different client, or with the same client under altered circumstances. For example, the taking of routine vital signs may be delegated to the UAP for a client who is in stable condition, but it would not be delegated for the same client who has become unstable.

PRACTICE ALERT

Each nurse or other licensed or unlicensed health care provider is responsible for his or her own actions. Anyone who feels unqualified to perform a delegated task must decline to perform it.

Differentiating Delegation From Assignment

Delegation is often confused with work allocation or assignment. Delegation transfers both responsibility and **authority** (the right to act or to accomplish the task). In **assignment**, no transfer of authority occurs. Instead, assignments are a bureaucratic function that reflect job descriptions and client or organizational needs.

Too often, the principle of authority is neglected, and delegators hamper delegates from accomplishing tasks successfully, setting them up for failure.

Delegation Versus Dumping

Nurses delegate because it is the best use of time, not in order to dump an undesirable task or to reward a productive employee with even more work. Delegation should be practiced in a way that provides the greatest benefit to the client, makes the best use of the time of all staff members, and provides delegates with opportunities for growth. Delegation also requires that the delegate provide a clear, precise description of the task to be performed, including its objective, limits, and expectations.

BENEFITS OF DELEGATION

The proper delegation of duties can benefit the nurse, the delegate, the client, and the organization.

Benefits to the Nurse

When nurses are able to delegate some tasks to UAPs, more time can be devoted to those tasks that cannot be delegated, especially complex client care. Thus, delegation enhances client care, increases nurses' job satisfaction, and improves retention within the organization.

CLINICAL EXAMPLE

Nancy, RN, has three central line dressing changes to complete as well as two client transfers to another unit before the end of shift in 1 hour. Nancy delegates the transfer duties to Shelley, LPN, and completes the central line dressing changes.

Benefits to the Delegate

Delegation allows delegates to gain new skills and abilities that can help them advance within a given organization or in their overall careers. In addition, delegation often brings with it trust and support, thereby helping build the self-esteem and confidence of the delegate. Subsequently, job satisfaction and motivation are enhanced as individuals feel stimulated by new challenges, morale improves, and a sense of pride and belonging develops, as does as greater awareness of responsibility. Individuals feel more appreciated and learn to appreciate the roles and responsibilities of others, increasing cooperation and enhancing teamwork.

Benefits to the Manager

Delegation also yields benefits for the manager. First, if nurses are delegating appropriately to UAPs, the manager will have a better-functioning unit. Also, the manager may be able to delegate some tasks to staff members and devote more time to management tasks that cannot be delegated. With more time available, the manager can develop new skills and abilities, facilitating the opportunity for career advancement.

Benefits to the Organization

As teamwork improves, the organization benefits by achieving its goals more efficiently. Overtime and absences decrease. Subsequently, productivity increases, and the organization's financial position may improve. As delegation increases efficiency, the quality of care improves, and as quality improves, client satisfaction increases.

THE DELEGATION PROCESS

Nurses delegate only work for which they have responsibility and authority. These tasks include the following:
- Routine tasks
- Tasks for which the nurse does not have time
- Tasks that have moved down in priority.

The delegation process has five steps:

1. Define the task.
2. Decide on the delegate.
3. Determine the task.
4. Reach agreement.
5. Monitor performance and provide feedback.

Determine the Task

In order to define the task, the nurse must consider some critical questions, including the following:
- Does the task involve technical skills or cognitive abilities?
- Are specific qualifications necessary?
- Is performance restricted by practice acts, standards, or job descriptions?
- How complex is the task?
- Is training or education required?

Certain tasks should never be delegated. Discipline of other employees, highly technical tasks, and complex client care tasks that require specific levels of licensure, certification, or training should not be delegated. Also, any situation that involves confidentiality or controversy should not be delegated to others.

Decide on the Delegate

The nurse delegating a task should match the task to the individual. This requires analyzing individuals' skill levels and abilities to evaluate their capability to perform the task. It also requires that the nurse consider what characteristics might prevent a delegate from accepting responsibility for the task. A rule of thumb is to delegate to the lowest person in the hierarchy who has the requisite capabilities and is allowed to do the task both legally and by organizational policy.

The nurse who needs to delegate a task must also determine availability. For example, Su Ling might be the best candidate, but if she is leaving early or is not available, the nurse will need to consider other possible delegates.

Describe the Task

The next step in delegation is to clearly describe the expectations for the delegate and decide when to delegate the task. Attempting to delegate in the middle of a crisis is not delegation; that is directing. The delegator must provide for enough time to describe the task and its expectations and to entertain questions from the delegate.

Key behaviors that nurses should use when delegating tasks include effective communication, motivation, and validation. Box 37–6 discusses these key behaviors in more detail.

Reach Agreement

After describing the task and its expectations, the delegator must be sure that the delegate agrees to accept responsibility and authority for the task. The delegator must also be prepared to equip the delegate to complete the task successfully. This might mean providing additional information or resources or informing others about the arrangement as needed to empower the delegate. Before meeting with the delegate, the delegator anticipates areas of negotiation and identifies what he or she must be prepared and able to provide.

Box 37–6 Key Behaviors When Delegating Tasks

Nurses who are delegating should:
- Describe the task using "I" statements (e.g., "I would like . . .") and appropriate nonverbal behaviors (e.g., open body language, face-to-face positioning, and eye contact). The delegate needs to know what is expected, when the task should be completed, and also where and how (if appropriate). The more experienced delegates may be able to define for themselves the where and how. The nurse must decide whether written reports are necessary or if brief oral reports are sufficient. If written reports are required, indicate whether tables, charts, or other graphics are necessary. Be specific about reporting times. In client care tasks, it is also important to determine who has responsibility and authority to chart certain tasks: UAPs can enter vital signs, but if they observe changes in client status, the RN must investigate and chart his or her assessment.

- Describe the importance of the task to the organization, the delegator, the client, and the delegate. Provide the delegate with an incentive for accepting both the responsibility and the authority to do the task.
- Clearly describe the expected outcome and the timeline for completion. Establish how closely the assignment will be supervised. Monitoring is important because the nurse remains accountable for the task. However, controls should never limit an individual's opportunity to grow.
- Identify any constraints on completing the task or any conditions that could change. For example, the nurse may ask an assistant to feed a client as long as the client is coherent and awake, but the nurse will feed the client if he or she is confused.
- Validate the assistant's understanding of the task and its expectations by eliciting questions and providing feedback.

CLINICAL EXAMPLE
Nancy, RN, delegates the measurement of vital signs to Pat, CNA. When asking Pat to complete this task Nancy explains by saying, "Mrs. Campbell has hypertension and has been stable, but if her systolic blood pressure is greater than 140 or less than 110, or her diastolic is higher than 90 or less than 60 please let me know immediately. Can you measure these vital signs within the next 10 minutes?"

Monitor Performance and Provide Feedback

Monitoring performance provides a mechanism for feedback and control that ensures delegated tasks are carried out as agreed. The nurse who is delegating a task must give careful thought to monitoring efforts when objectives are established. When defining the task and expectations, clearly establish the where, when, and how. Remain accessible. Support builds confidence, reassures the delegate of your interest, and negates any concerns about dumping undesirable tasks.

Monitoring the delegate too closely, however, conveys distrust. If problem areas are identified, the nurse should privately investigate and explain the problem, provide an opportunity for feedback, and inform the individual how to correct the mistake in the future. Equally important is giving praise and recognition for a job well done.

The following Clinical Example shows how a school nurse handled delegating medication administration.

CLINICAL EXAMPLE
Lisa Ford is a school nurse for a suburban school district. She has responsibility for three school buildings, including a middle school, a high school, and a vocational rehabilitation workshop for mentally and physically handicapped secondary students. Her management responsibilities include providing health services for 1,000 students, 60 faculty members, and 25 staff members and supervising two unlicensed school health aides and three special education health aides. The logistics of managing multiple school sites results in the delegation of many daily health room tasks, including medication administration to the school-based health aides.

Nancy Andrews is an unlicensed health aide at the middle school. This is her first year as a health aide, and she has a limited background in health care. The nurse practice act in her state allows delegation of medication administration in the school setting. Lisa is responsible for training Nancy to safely administer medication to students, documenting the training, evaluating Nancy's performance, and providing ongoing supervision. Part of Nancy's training will also include a discussion of those medication-related decisions that must be made by a registered nurse. To delegate medication administration to Nancy, Lisa must do the following:
- Understand the state nurse practice act and its applicability to the school setting.
- Implement school district policies related to health services and medication administration.
- Develop and implement an appropriate training program.
- Limit opportunities for error and decrease liability by ensuring that unlicensed health aides are appropriately trained to handle delegated tasks.
- Maintain documentation related to training and observation of medication administration by unlicensed staff.
- Audit medication administration records to ensure accuracy and completeness.
- Conduct several "drop-in" visits during the school year in order to track the competency of health aides.
- If necessary, report any medication errors to administration, and follow up with focused training and closer supervision.

FACTORS AFFECTING DELEGATION

A number of factors may affect delegation, including organizational culture and the personal qualities of the participants. Resource availability, such as having sufficient staff to whom the nurse may delegate tasks, also impacts delegation.

Accepting Delegation

Before accepting a task, the delegate is responsible for making sure he or she understands what is being asked. This includes examining whether he or she has the skills and abilities for the task and the time to do it. If the delegate does not have the necessary skills, he or she must inform the delegator. However, this does not mean the delegate cannot accept the responsibility provided the delegator is willing to train or otherwise equip the delegate to do the task. A delegate who does not have time should not be afraid to say no. When that is necessary, the delegate should thank the delegator for the offer and clearly explain why he or she must decline the task.

Accepting delegation means accepting full responsibility for the outcome and its benefits or liabilities. Just as the delegator has the option to delegate parts of a task, the delegate also has the option to negotiate for those aspects of a task the delegate feels he or she can accomplish. A delegate who is not qualified to do the task or does not have time should not be afraid to say no, and should explain why he or she must decline the task.

Once the delegate agrees on the role and responsibilities, the delegate should clarify the time frame, feedback mechanisms, and other expectations. Delegates should not assume anything. At a minimum, they should repeat to the delegator their understanding of the task and all the related requirements and expectations. Outlining the task in writing may be helpful.

Throughout the project, the delegate should keep the delegator informed, reporting any concerns that may arise. Most important, the delegate should complete the task as agreed. This fosters trust with the delegator and indicates the delegate is dependable, improving the chances for increased responsibility and opportunity in the future.

Obstacles to Delegation

Although delegation can yield many benefits, there are potential barriers to delegation. Some barriers are environmental; others are the result of the delegator's or delegate's beliefs or inexperience (Table 37–3).

A NONSUPPORTIVE ENVIRONMENT Some environments do not support delegation. For example, the culture of an organization may restrict delegation through rigid chains of command and autocratic leadership styles. In this type of organizational culture, the norm is to do the work oneself because others are not capable or skilled. These types of environments promote an atmosphere of distrust as well as a poor tolerance for mistakes.

Lack of resources also inhibits delegation. For example, there may not be adequate staff to whom the nurse can delegate certain responsibilities. Consider the sole RN in a skilled nursing facility. If practice acts define a task as one that only an RN can perform, there is no one else to whom that nurse can delegate that task.

Financial constraints also can interfere with delegation. For instance, if someone from the department must attend the annual conference in your nursing specialty area but the organization will only pay the manager's travel and conference expenses, then no one else will be able to attend.

Educational resources may be another limiting factor. Perhaps others could learn how to do a task if they could practice with the equipment, but the equipment or a trainer is not available.

Time resources can limit the ability to delegate as well. For example, it is Friday and the schedule needs to be posted on Monday. The nurse manager in charge of scheduling needs to go out of town for a family emergency, however, no one on staff has experience in developing schedules, so there is no one else to do the schedule.

DELEGATOR INSECURITY Delegators often feel insecure about delegation, because they remain accountable for the tasks involved. Fears that are common among delegators include the following:

■ *Fear of competition or criticism.* Delegators fear losing respect and being outdone at their job. The delegator who selects the right task and matches it to the right individual has no need to fear either competition or criticism. In fact, the delegate's success provides evidence of the delegator's leadership and decision-making abilities.

■ *Fear of liability.* Some liability risks are inherent in delegation, and related to the fear of liability is the fear of being blamed for the delegate's mistakes. If the delegator follows the steps of delegation in selecting the task and the delegate, however, then the risks of liability can be minized and the responsibility for any mistakes is solely that of the delegate.

TABLE 37–3 **Potential Obstacles to Delegation**

ENVIRONMENTAL	DELEGATOR	DELEGATE
Practice acts	Lack of trust and confidence	Inexperience
Standards	Believe others incapable	Fear of failure and reprisal
Job descriptions	Believe self indispensable	Lack of confidence
Policies	Fear of competition	Overdependence on others
Organizational structure	Fear of criticism	Avoidance of responsibility
Management styles	Fear of liability	
Norms	Fear of blame for others' mistakes	
Resources	Fear of loss of control	
	Fear or overburdening	
	Fear of decreased job satisfaction	
	Insecurity	
	Inexperience in delegation	
	Inadequate organizational skills	

Source: Reprinted with permission from Hansten, R. and Washburn, M. (1992). Delegation: How to deliver care through others. *American Journal of Nursing, 92*(3), 87–88.

- *Fear of loss of control.* This is a typical concern of inexperienced or insecure delegators, but also a frequent concern in individuals who tend toward perfectionism and autocratic styles of leadership. The key to retaining control is to clearly identify the task and expectations and then to monitor the delegate's progress and provide feedback.
- *Fear of overburdening others.* Delegators should not fear overburdening others, because delegation is a voluntary, contractual agreement. Acceptance of a delegated task indicates the availability and willingness of the delegate to perform the task. Often, the delegate welcomes the diversion and stimulation, and what the delegator perceives as a burden is actually a blessing.
- *Fear of decreased personal job satisfaction.* Because the type of tasks recommended to delegate are those that are familiar and routine, the delegator's job satisfaction should actually increase with the opportunity to explore new challenges and obtain other skills and abilities.

Additional barriers to delegation include inadequate organizational skills, such as poor time management, and inexperience in delegation.

AN UNWILLING DELEGATE Inexperience and fear of failure can motivate a potential delegate to refuse a delegated task. This delegate needs much reassurance and support. In addition, the delegator needs to equip this delegate to be able to handle the task. If the delegator follows the proper selection criteria and the steps of delegation, then the delegate should not fail.

The delegator can boost the delegate's lack of confidence by building on simple tasks. The delegate needs to be reminded that everyone was inexperienced at one time. Another common concern is how mistakes will be handled. When describing the task, the delegator should provide clear guidelines for handling problems—guidelines that adhere to organizational policies.

Another barrier is the individual who avoids responsibility or is overdependent on others. Success breeds success; therefore, it is important to use an enticing incentive to engage the individual in a simple task that guarantees success.

Ineffective Delegation
When the steps of delegation are not followed or barriers remain unresolved, delegation is often ineffective. Ineffective delegation can also result from unnecessary duplication, underdelegation, reverse delegation, and overdelegation.

UNNECESSARY DUPLICATION If staff are duplicating the work of others, related tasks may have been given to too many people (Barter, 2002). To avoid unnecessary duplication, try delegating associated tasks to as few people as possible. This allows the person to complete the assignment without spending time negotiating with others about which task should be done by which person. This also simplifies reporting for both the delegate and the delegator.

To prevent work duplication, Barter (2002, p. 57) suggests that nurses ask the following:

- How often does staff duplicate an activity that someone else has recently performed?
- Why does this duplication occur, and is it necessary?
- What needs to done to prevent duplication?

UNDERDELEGATION Underdelegation occurs in the following situations:
- The delegator fails to transfer full authority to the delegate.
- The delegator takes back responsibility for aspects of the task.
- The delegator fails to equip and direct the delegate.

As a result, the delegate is unable to complete the task, and the delegator must resume responsibility for its completion.

CLINICAL EXAMPLE
After completing Lisa's training (see prior Clinical Example) Nancy gives her the authority to begin administering medications to the students in the school. During the first week of school, Lisa tries to "speed up" the medication administration process and sets out all of the noon medications in individual, unlabeled cups for the students. The cups are rearranged by students trying to find their medications, and Lisa cannot identify what meds belong to which students. Nancy is called back to the school to administer the correct medications, students are late to class, and Lisa is frustrated that she couldn't handle the task.
1. Which of the five steps of delegation did Nancy fail to follow?
2. Which step or steps did Lisa fail to follow?
3. What should Nancy do to prevent this situation from happening again?

REVERSE DELEGATION In **reverse delegation**, someone with a lower rank delegates to someone with more authority.

CLINICAL EXAMPLE
Thomas is a nurse practitioner for the burn unit. He recently arrived on the unit to find several clients whose dressing changes have not been completed due to a code situation earlier in the morning. Dawn, LPN, asks Thomas to complete a few dressing changes to help the staff before physician rounds begin.

OVERDELEGATION **Overdelegation** occurs when the delegator loses control over a situation by providing the delegate with too much authority or too much responsibility. This places the delegator in a risky position, increasing the potential for liability.

CLINICAL EXAMPLE
Ellen, GN, is in her 6th week of orientation in the trauma ICU. Her mentor, Dolores, RN, notes that Mr. Anderson is scheduled for an MRI off the unit. Dolores delegates to Ellen the task of escorting Mr. Anderson to the MRI unit. Ellen is not ACLS certified. During the MRI, Mr. Anderson is accidentally extubated and suffers respiratory and cardiac arrest. A code is called in the MRI suite and ER nurses must respond since an ACLS certified nurse is not with the client.

LIABILITY AND DELEGATION
Fear of liability often keeps nurses from delegating. State nurse practice acts determine the legal parameters for practice, professional associations set practice standards, and organizational policy and job descriptions define delegation appropriate to the specific work setting.

Several guidelines can help. The American Nurses Association and the National Council of State Boards of Nursing (2006) identified the five rights of delegation:

1. **Right task** (task is one that can be delegated for specific client)
2. **Right circumstances** (setting is appropriate and resources are available)
3. **Right person** (give the right task to the right delegate for the right client)
4. **Right direction and communication** (describe objectives, limits, and expectations)

5. **Right supervision** (monitor, evaluate, give feedback, and intervene if necessary) (ANA & NCSBN, 2006).

In addition, the American Nurses Association and the National Council of State Boards of Nursing have issued a joint statement on delegation to explain both the profession's practice guidelines and the legal requirements for delegation (ANA & NCSBN, 2006). Figure 37–2 ■ shows a decision tree for delegation from the joint statement.

One situation that may present a challenge is when the staff receives written or verbal orders from a physician's office nurse (Austin, 2004). The same legal guidelines for the

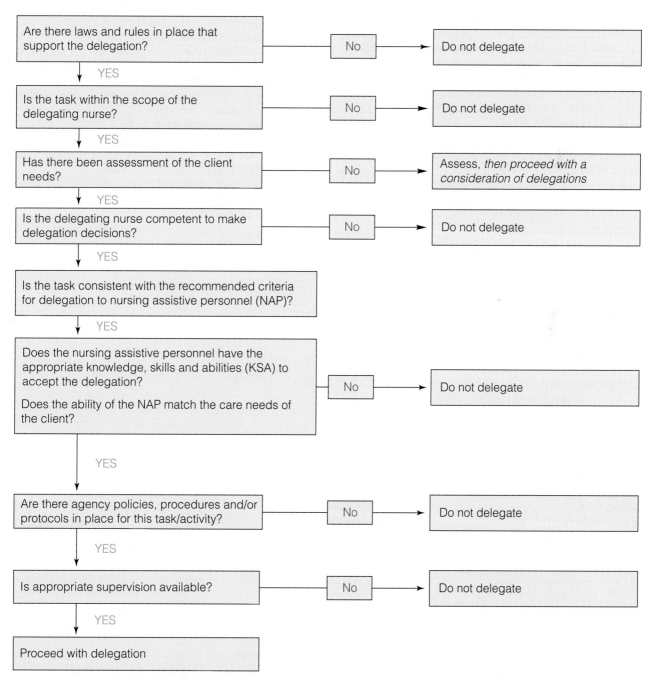

Figure 37–2 ■ Decision tree for delegation to unlicensed assistive personnel.

Source: Adapted from National Council of State Boards of Nursing. (2006). *Joint statement on delegation.* Retrieved December, 2007, from http://www.ncsbn.org/Joint_statement.pdf

nurse giving the orders apply to the staff receiving them. If the nurse calling from the physician's office has a license that allows prescribing privileges, such as a nurse practitioner, the staff can accept appropriate orders from the physician's nurse.

Otherwise, the orders must also be verified by the prescribing physician. The staff members put their own licenses in jeopardy if they do not obtain verification from the physician when necessary.

REVIEW Delegation

RELATE: LINK THE CONCEPTS

You are an RN working on a medical unit with two other RNs, a LPN, and two UAPs, and you receive a call informing you that two clients (both of whom are assigned to your care) must be transferred to another unit in order to make room for two clients who are to be admitted as soon as the rooms are ready.

Linking the exemplar of Delegation with the concept of Collaboration:

1. You delegate collection of a client's possessions in preparation for transfer to the UAP who says, "Why are you dumping this work on me? You do it." How would you manage this conflict?
2. The LPN working on the unit is a new graduate and has only been employed for 4 weeks. How would you collaborate with this nurse when delegating tasks for completion?

Linking the exemplar of Delegation with the concept of Teaching and Learning:

3. How can you facilitate the new LPN's education in performing tasks that are commonly delegated?
4. How would you evaluate the LPN's learning related to delegated tasks?

REFER: GO TO MYNURSINGKIT

REFLECT: CASE STUDY

You are working the night shift on a medical unit and have been assigned charge nurse responsibilities. You are working with four RNs, one LPN, and two UAPs. A client becomes pulseless and is not breathing, and the nurse assigned to the client's care calls a code. The nurse is occupied at this client's bedside for 1½ hours until the resuscitation effort is completed and the client is transferred to the intensive care unit. This nurse also has four other assigned clients. In addition to the nurse assigned to care for the client requiring resuscitation, two of the other nurses working on your unit are assisting in the code.

1. What tasks could you delegate to the UAP?
2. How will you maintain the safety of the clients on your unit while three nurses are occupied with the client requiring resuscitation?
3. How might effective delegation to other team members contribute to care of the clients on the unit?

PEARSON

EXPLORE 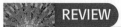 ™

MyNursingKit is your one stop for online chapter review materials and resources. Prepare for success with additional NCLEX®-style practice questions, interactive assignments and activities, web links, animations and videos, and more!

Register your access code from the front of your book at
www.mynursingkit.com.

REFERENCES

Abood, S., & Franklin, P. (2002). Billing for nursing services. *Nevada Reformation, 11*(2), 12.

American Nurses Association (ANA) & National Council of State Boards of Nursing (NCSBN). (2006). *Joint statement on delegation.* Retrieved March 2, 2010, from https://www.ncsbn.org/Joint_statement.pdf

Austin, S. (2004). Respect the scope of your license and practice. *Nursing Management, 35*(12): 18, 20.

Barter, M. (2002). Follow the team leader. *Nursing Management, 33*(10), 54–57.

Centers for Disease Control and Prevention. (2009). *Uninsured Americans: Newly released health insurance statistics.* Retrieved March 2, 2010, from http://www.cdc.gov/Features/Uninsured/

Feldstein, P. J. (2003). *Health policy issues: An economic perspective on health reform* (3rd ed.). Chicago: Health Administration Press.

Finkelman, A. (1996). *Psychiatric nursing administration manual.* Gaithersburg, MD: Aspen Publishers, Inc.

Finkler, S. A., & Kovner, C. T. (2007). *Financial Management for nurse managers and executives* (3rd ed.). St. Louis, MO: Saunders.

Finkler, S. A., & McHugh, M. (2007). *Budgeting concepts for nurse managers* (4th ed.). St. Louis, MO: Saunders.

Gordon, J. A., Emond, J. A., & Camargo, C. A. (2005). The State Children's Health Insurance Program: A multicenter trial of outreach through the emergency department. *American Journal of Public Health, 95,* 250–253.

Hall, L. M., Doran, D., & Pink, G. H. (2004). Nurse staffing models, nursing hours, and patient safety outcomes. *Journal of Nursing Administration, 34,* 41–45.

Jennings, C. P. (2004). Insuring America's health: Principles and recommendations: IOM report. *Policy, Politics, and Nursing Practice, 5,* 100–101.

Kerr, P. (2000). Comparing two nursing outcome reporting initiatives. *Outcomes Management for Nursing Practice, 4*(3), 144.

Kleinman, C. S., & Saccomano, S. J. (2006). Registered nurses and unlicensed assistive personnel: An uneasy alliance. *The Journal of Continuing Education in Nursing, 37*(4), 162–170.

Milstead, J. A. (2004). *Health policy in the new millennium: Vision, values, and leadership.* Boston, MA: Jones and Bartlett Publishers.

Morrison, I. (2000). *Health care in the new millennium: Vision, values, and leadership.* San Francisco: Jossey-Bass.

National Center for Health Statistics. (2005). *Health: United States, 2005.* Hyattsville, MD: Author.

Peters, R. M. (2000). Using NOC outcome of risk control in prevention, early detection, and control of hypertension. *Outcomes Management for Nursing Practice, 4*(1), 39–45.

Robert Wood Johnson Foundation (2008). *Measuring the work nurses do in coordinating care.* Retrieved February 21, 2010, from http://www.rwjf.org/qualityequality/product.jsp?id=27811

Stanton, M. W. (2005).*The high concentration of U.S. health care expenditures.* Rockville, MD: Agency for Healthcare Research and Quality.

Vere-Jones, E. (2006). The business of nursing. *Nursing Times, 102*(23), 14–17.

Professional Behaviors

38

Concept at-a-Glance

About Professional Behaviors, *2225*

38.1   Commitment to Profession, *2230*

38.2   Leadership Principles, *2233*

38.3   Work Ethic, *2236*

Concept Learning Outcomes

After reading about this concept, you will be able to:

1. Connect professional behaviors to the development of trust in the nurse.
2. Provide examples of how the nurse uses professional behaviors to meet the primary responsibility of nursing.
3. Explore nursing behaviors that demonstrate professionalism.
4. Create strategies for avoiding unprofessional behaviors.
5. Provide examples of behaviors that may be interpreted as sexual harassment and strategies to avoid them.

Concept Key Terms

Abuse of power, *2228*

Compassion, *2228*

Integrity, *2227*

Professional behaviors, *2226*

Socialization, *2226*

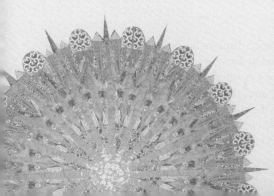

About Professional Behaviors

Nurses hold the public's trust. In Gallup's annual survey of professions released in December of 2009, 83% of Americans call nurses' honesty and ethical standards either high or very high. Nurses have topped Gallup's honesty and ethics ranking survey every year but one since being added to the list in 1999 (ANA, 2009), continuing to be the most well-respected of 21 professions. In a society where image is everything, consistently holding the public's trust is a remarkable accomplishment.

How does nursing earn and keep this trust? Clients know that nurses are there 24 hours a day, 7 days a week during some of the most difficult times of clients' lives. When a client has a problem or concern, he or she asks to see the nurse. When family members have difficulty navigating the health care system, they ask to see their nurse. When a physician has an issue with order implementation, he or she asks to see the nurse. Clients, physicians, family members, and interdisciplinary health team members may not know a name, but they all know to ask for the nurse. **Professional behaviors** are those actions by the nurse that invite trust and inspire confidence. Learning to exemplify those behaviors requires an understanding of leadership principles, a commitment to the profession, and an acceptance of a work ethic. ●

COMPONENTS OF PROFESSIONALISM IN NURSING

Part of the process of nursing education is the acculturation, or socialization, of the student into the nursing profession. **Socialization** is the process by which people (a) learn to become members of groups and society and (b) learn the social rules defining relationships into which they will enter. Through socialization, the nursing student becomes immersed into the culture, behaviors, and expectations of the profession. Clinical experiences, nursing labs, classroom time, individual study, and student work all help the nursing student assume the responsibilities inherent in the nursing profession.

The nurse's primary professional responsibility, task, or behavior is always to maintain the client at the center of every nursing action. The nurse should not wear artificial fingernails, excessive jewelry, or long flowing hair styles because of the increased risk of infection to the client. The nurse should not chew gum while caring for clients because it is disrespectful and can be annoying rather than calming or supportive, as well as serving as a reservoir for pathogens. No matter where a nurse practices, whether in a facility, in the community, or in a privately owned business, the nurse's behaviors should be governed by concern for the client. Further, the nurse acts as a role model when not on duty and must always consider the impact he or she has on others' perception of the nursing profession. A nurse is always a nurse, even when off duty, and is always being observed and judged.

How does a nurse begin to acquire the behaviors that invite trust and inspire confidence? In 2003, Via Christi Health System conducted a survey of 300 nurses and asked them to name three characteristics they felt best expressed the behaviors that demonstrated professionalism. The top seven responses were knowledge, competence, appearance, teamwork, respect for integrity, a positive attitude, and compassion (Via Christi Regional Medical Center, 2003).

Knowledge

Knowledge is central to maintaining client safety and meeting expected outcomes. Students are required to learn the information that is essential for the entry-level practicing nurse to know in order to meet the minimal competency required for nursing practice. Learning all of the information essential to the practice of nursing is a daunting challenge: Nursing students must acquire knowledge of anatomy and physiology, biology, psychology, technology, group processes, and many other disciplines. Once licensed, nurses are expected to continue to update and maintain their knowledge base throughout their careers. Health care is changing constantly with new drugs entering the market every year, new treatments and technology being introduced, and research demonstrating the effectiveness of existing or past information. If nurses do not participate in continuing education, their knowledge base quickly becomes obsolete and their practice may even endanger the client.

Competence

The expectation of competency begins when the student enrolls in a nursing program and it continues throughout nursing practice, whether the nurse is caring for clients, managing a department, or acting in an advanced practice role. The nurse must learn how to operate new equipment before it is put into general use; maintain an evidenced-based practice that is current on the latest findings; and seek help from peers, mentors, and instructors to learn new skills and techniques. Each nurse is accountable for determining his or her own areas of weakness. Once the nurse identifies an area of practice in which he or she is not competent, the nurse should take responsibility to seek opportunities to gain competency.

Components of competency include the nurse's awareness of factors, both positive and negative, that affect client care. Competency is required in many areas, including the following:

- Understanding the culture of the client and the facility
- The ethics of the nursing profession
- The many responsibilities of the nurse including legal, professional, ethical, and client centered roles
- The procedures to follow when performing skills
- Recognizing the client's needs for individualized care
- Proper documentation
- The ability to show compassion for the needs of others.

Each state's nurse practice act defines professional competence and outlines those behaviors or actions that indicate incompetence or that may result in loss of licensure. It is important for nurses to know the requirements set forth in the nurse practice acts in their home states. For example, the North Carolina nurse practice act defines competence as "the ongoing application of knowledge and the decision-making, psychomotor, and interpersonal skills expected of the licensed nurse within a specific practice setting resulting in nursing care that contributes to the health and welfare of clients served" (North Carolina Board of Nursing, 2008).

Appearance

The nurse's appearance displays his or her commitment to professionalism. Not only does this include a clean, pressed uniform and clean shoes, but it also includes how the nurse walks, speaks, gestures, and the tone of voice the nurse uses. Appearance affects the client's first impression of the nurse, and this can make a difference in the client's level of trust and respect toward the nurse. Consider the clinical example that follows.

CLINICAL EXAMPLE

Mark views himself as one of the smartest nurses on the unit because he belongs to several nursing organizations and works hard to maintain knowledge and competence by attending in-services, seminars, and regularly reading several nursing journals. However, when he enters clients' rooms wearing a wrinkled uniform and chewing gum, and then fails to answer clients' questions about their plan of care, the clients often discount what he is saying.

Appearance also affects how others within the medical community see the nurse. It is a form of nonverbal communication that evokes a response from others. Imagine a nurse approaching a doctor to question the validity of an order while talking on her cell phone. Will the doctor have enough confidence in the nurse to accept her concern and change the decision regarding the client's plan of care?

While simple rules of dress may seem obvious, some beginning nurses underestimate their importance. Nurses should take care to do the following:

■ Wear a clean uniform every day.
■ Keep hair contained and pulled back from the face to avoid it falling on a client or contaminating a sterile field.
■ Keep nails trimmed and filed to avoid scratching the client.
■ Shower daily and use deodorant or antiperspirant.
■ Avoid wearing jewelry that could injure the client (rings, bracelets, dangling earrings).
■ Avoid using perfumes or highly scented products (e.g., laundry detergent) that might irritate the allergic client or nauseate a client.
■ Avoid artificial fingernails, which harbor bacteria and increase the client's risk of infection.

Maintaining a professional appearance supports the nurse's credibility and increases the likelihood of gaining the trust of clients and colleagues (Figure 38–1 ■).

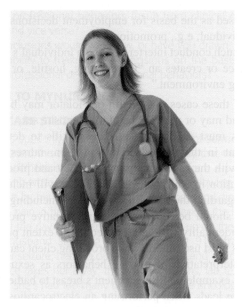

Figure 38–1 ■ A professional appearance supports the nurse's credibility.

Teamwork

How to work as a member of the team is discussed in detail in Concept 35, Collaboration. The nurse's skill in working as a team member contributes to others' opinions of the nurse as a professional and improves the quality of care delivered to the client. Consider the clinical example that follows.

CLINICAL EXAMPLE

Jose Guarez, 63 years old, is admitted to the unit with a medical diagnosis of angina, congestive heart failure, and left lower lobe pneumonia. Initially when Mr. Guarez is admitted, his condition is very unstable, with rapid respirations, hypoxia, and a weak productive cough. He requires endotracheal intubation and mechanical ventilation while receiving antibiotics and other medications. As his condition improves, Mr. Guarez is extubated and placed on oxygen, first by face mask and then by nasal cannula.

1. What members of the team would the nurse work with to provide care for Mr. Guarez?
2. How would nurse-to-nurse collaboration be important to the care of this client?
3. How would this client's care potentially suffer if the nurse preferred to function independently instead of as a member of the team?

Integrity

Integrity is the adherence to a strict moral or ethical code. Nurses adhere to the ANA Code of Ethics for Nurses (discussed in Concept 42, Ethics). Nurses demonstrate integrity by accepting feedback (positive or negative) as a tool for improving delivery of client care, by maintaining accountability for their actions and freely admitting when they make mistakes, and by following the nurse practice act and never working outside their scope of practice. Consider the clinical example that follows.

CLINICAL EXAMPLE

The nurse is caring for Julie Ong, a 36-year-old woman and the mother of three children. Ms. Ong was admitted to the hospital for surgery after discovering that her breast cancer had metastasized to her brain. She underwent a lengthy procedure to remove the brain tumor and is now experiencing a great deal of pain. The nurse calls the physician, explaining that current analgesic dosages are inadequate and that the client is not achieving adequate comfort levels after administration. The physician declines to increase the dose and gives no explanation. The nurse, who is the same age as Ms. Ong and also has three children, identifies strongly with this client and feels that the most important intervention for Ms. Ong is to help her obtain pain relief. Since the doctor will not increase the dosage, the nurse decides to administer the dosage more frequently and forge the documentation to make it look as though it was given as ordered. Mrs. Ong is so grateful for the pain relief and praises the nurse's action, thanking her repeatedly for "taking such good care of me." The nurse is convinced that the actions taken were justified and in the best interest of the client.

1. Is this nurse demonstrating integrity? Why or why not?
2. Did the nurse maintain a practice within the nurse's scope of practice?
3. What could the nurse have done to maintain a respect for integrity?

daughters through their teenage years, be the mother of the bride at their weddings, or hold her first grandchild. Lori will even sit down on her bed and hold her hand, providing a shoulder to cry on, or just sit quietly in silence while Sally gathers the thoughts she so desperately needs to express.

The wait to see which nurse opens the door is interminable. Yes, they will all provide her with the medication to relieve her physical pain. But tonight, this night, Sally needs so much more.

1. Of the three nurses discussed, are any of them unprofessional? Which one(s) and why do you see their behavior as lacking professionalism? What could they do differently to be perceived as more professional?
2. What professional roles or characteristics does this client require from the nurse providing her care?
3. If you were the nurse who responded to this client's call bell, what would you do when you entered the client's room?

38.1 COMMITMENT TO PROFESSION

KEY TERMS
Affective commitment, *2231*
Burnout, *2232*
Commitment, *2230*
Continuance commitment, *2231*
Normative commitment, *2231*
Organizational commitment, *2230*

BASIS FOR SELECTION OF EXEMPLAR
Standards of Nursing Practice
NLN Competencies

LEARNING OUTCOMES
After reading about this exemplar, you will be able to:

1. Discuss concepts of organizational commitment as applied to the profession of nursing.
2. Apply factors of professional commitment to the role of nursing student.
3. Analyze your personal level of commitment to the nursing profession.

OVERVIEW

Many experienced nurses say that nursing is not what they *do*, it's who they *are*. They have made a commitment to their profession, incorporating the ethics and expectations of nursing into every aspect of their lives, whether at home or at work.

The Merriam-Webster Dictionary (2009) defines **commitment** as the state or an instance of being obligated or emotionally impelled (motivated). To understand commitment as it is applied to the profession of nursing, one must first look at the concept of organizational commitment. The most widely accepted definition of **organizational commitment** is the relative strength of an individual's relationship and sense of belonging to an organization. Originally, this definition was used by researchers exploring commitment to a specific place of employment. It is more helpful for the nursing student to view organizational commitment as applying to the profession of nursing regardless of the specific job location. Thus, the concept of organizational commitment will be synonymous with professional commitment.

FACTORS OF PROFESSIONAL COMMITMENT

There are three factors associated with professional commitment:

1. A strong belief in and acceptance of the profession's goals and values
2. A willingness to exert considerable personal effort on behalf of the profession
3. A strong desire to maintain membership in the profession.

As was discussed earlier, nursing education not only is concerned with teaching students how to think like a nurse, but also is charged with the acculturation or socialization of students into the profession. This process begins when the student enters the first nursing class. Many of the policies and rules associated with a nursing program may seem harsh or "old-fashioned," but their purpose is to prepare the student for entry into the profession of nursing. For example, tardiness to clinical may not be tolerated and may result in significant consequences for the offender. The student may ask, "So, what's the big deal with being a few minutes late?" The big deal is that time and attendance are critical in nursing. Even during a nursing shortage, the nurse who is chronically late for or excessively absent from work will be subject to disciplinary action that could include suspension and termination. With frequent staff shortages, it is even more important for managers to be able to rely on staff to be on the job when scheduled. Chronic lateness and frequent absenteeism place a greater burden on colleagues, compromise client care, and lead to conflict among staff. The student who violates or ignores school policy is in danger of becoming the nurse who ignores agency policy.

The values and goals of professional nursing are clearly delineated through standards of nursing practice, codes of ethics, nurse practice acts, national client safety goals, and many other such resources. Students must always remember that they are entering a profession, not just a job.

Most students can easily identify with the willingness to exert considerable effort on behalf of the profession. Nursing programs have high standards of admission, and many receive more applications than they have openings available. In times of economic recession, this is even more prevalent as displaced workers seek job security in health professions with staff shortages. Nursing education is a rigorous program of study requiring considerable time and effort, which prepares students for entry into a demanding, yet rewarding, profession.

Students also can identify with the strong desire to maintain membership in the profession. Most students have already made sacrifices while taking related general education and science courses in preparation for the nursing major. The sacrifices required during nursing courses are even greater, as the number of credit hours per course increases when hours spent in lab and clinical are added. Most students accepted into a nursing program have a strong desire to complete the program, especially as their time in the program increases.

After graduation, the commitment to maintain membership in the nursing profession is demonstrated by membership in professional organizations and various committees and by contributing to community organizations seeking to establish laws related to health care and health promotion. Nurses must always maintain current knowledge related to changes in health care and the profession of nursing in order to keep nursing practice and, therefore, clients safe.

TYPES OF COMMITMENT

Three types of commitment have been identified to describe the psychological link between an individual and the decision to continue in a profession: affective, normative, and continuance. **Affective commitment** is defined as an attachment to a profession and includes identification with and involvement in the profession. Affective commitment develops when involvement in a profession produces a satisfying experience. The student or nurse who is affectively committed has a strong desire to continue in the profession, is more involved in keeping up with current information, and becomes involved with profession-specific organizations and service activities (Figure 38–3 ■). This individual is in school or working as a nurse because he or she wants to be a nurse.

Normative commitment is defined as a feeling of obligation to continue in the profession. Normative commitment develops as a result of having received benefits or having had positive experiences through engagement in the profession. The nurse who enters the field or remains in it because personal or family experiences with illness have created a desire to work in the health care field exemplifies normative commitment.

Continuance commitment, or the awareness of costs associated with leaving the profession, develops when negative consequences of leaving, such as loss of income, are seen as reasons to remain. Individuals who experience this type of commitment do not manifest the same ties to the profession as do those who are motivated by affective or normative commitment. In general, such individuals are not inclined to promote their profession. These students and nurses are in the field for the money and job security.

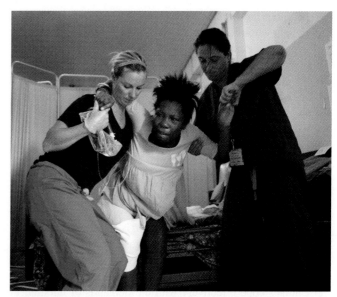

Figure 38–3 ■ Affective commitment leads nurses and other health care professionals to volunteer their services to help those in disasters, such as the January 2010 earthquake in Haiti. Here, Michele Shiel, an ER nurse from the U.S. Virgin Islands (left), helps to carry a woman from the hallway into a delivery room at the Haitian Community Hospital in Petionville, Haiti.

STAGES OF COMMITMENT DEVELOPMENT

Commitment to a profession is a process that develops in stages. The first stage is the *exploratory stage*, in which individuals explore the positive aspects of the profession. Commitment begins to occur as exploration leads to a positive orientation toward the profession. Examples of this stage may be seen in the excitement felt by nursing students during the first weeks of their program as they model their new uniforms and ransack their lab kits.

The second stage is the *testing stage* of commitment, during which individuals discover negative elements of the profession. In this stage, individuals start to assess their willingness and ability to deal with those negative elements. Some nursing students never get beyond this stage and drop out of school or change majors, deciding that the sacrifices are not worth the effort or that they are not suited to the nursing profession.

The third stage is the *passionate stage* of commitment, which begins as the individual synthesizes the positive and negative elements from stages one and two. Students in this stage not only are willing to commit to the profession but also are willing to contribute to its well-being. These students are the ones who become involved in student nursing associations, serve as class officers, or volunteer for activities not associated with a grade.

The fourth stage is the *quiet-and-bored stage* of commitment, in which students settle into the humdrum routines of the nursing program. This often occurs during the middle or late middle of the nursing program, as students begin to become more comfortable in their role and feel less anxiety about their performance.

The *integrated stage* is the final stage of commitment. Individuals who reach this stage have integrated both positive and negative elements of the profession into a more flexible, complex, and enduring form of commitment. They act out their commitment as a matter of habit. These students are in the final stages of their nursing program and are beginning to see themselves as nurses, eager to take the NCLEX-RN® and begin employment. As new graduates, they will once again proceed through the stages of commitment while transitioning from nursing student to registered nurse.

MANAGING STRESS

Part of a commitment to any profession is learning how to manage the stress associated with that profession. Nursing can be a particularly stressful profession, with clients and work situations bringing both physical and emotional demands. Although most nurses cope effectively with the demands of nursing, in some situations nurses become overwhelmed and develop **burnout**, a complex syndrome of behaviors that can be likened to the exhaustion stage of the general adaptation syndrome (see Concept 28, Stress and Coping). The nurse with burnout manifests physical and emotional depletion, a negative attitude and self-concept, and feelings of helplessness and hopelessness.

Nurses can prevent burnout by using healthy techniques to manage stress. To do so, nurses must first recognize their stress and become attuned to responses such as feelings of being overwhelmed, fatigue, angry outbursts, physical illness, and increases in coffee drinking, smoking, or substance abuse. Once attuned to stress and their own personal reactions, nurses must identify which situations produce the most pronounced reactions. This will help them take steps to reduce the stress. Suggestions include the following:

- Plan a daily relaxation program with meaningful quiet times to reduce tension (e.g., read, listen to music, soak in a tub, or meditate).
- Establish a regular exercise program to direct energy outward.
- Study assertiveness techniques to overcome feelings of powerlessness in relationships with others. Learn to say no.
- Learn to accept failures and turn them into constructive learning experiences. Recognize that most people do the best they can. Learn to ask for help, to show feelings with colleagues, and to support colleagues in times of need.
- Accept what cannot be changed. There are certain limitations in every situation.
- Get involved in efforts toward constructive change if organizational policies and procedures cause stress.
- Develop collegial support groups to deal with feelings and anxieties generated in the work setting.
- Participate in professional organizations to address workplace issues.
- Seek counseling if indicated to help clarify concerns.

Nursing is a profession like few others. Nurses work odd hours and carry great responsibility. They face the knowledge that the choices they make and actions they take often involve life and death decisions. While most nurses feel their work is highly satisfying and that they make a difference in their clients' lives, they also know they need to maintain their commitment to their profession or face the potential for burnout and movement away from nursing into another career.

REVIEW   Commitment to Profession

RELATE: LINK THE CONCEPTS

Linking the exemplar of Commitment to Profession with the concept of Development:

1. How might nurses in different life stages commit to the profession of nursing in different ways?
2. Describe the impact of the nurse's moral development, according to Kohlberg, on commitment to the profession of nursing.

Linking the exemplar of Commitment to Profession with the concept of Collaboration:

3. How is the nurse's commitment to profession demonstrated by his or her ability and willingness to collaborate with others?
4. The nurse, working on a medical unit, is approached by a newly graduated licensed practical nurse who asks for help in improving her skill when initiating an IV catheter. How would nurses with different levels of commitment to the profession respond to this request?

REFER: GO TO MYNURSINGKIT

REFLECT: CASE STUDY

Hakeem Kamara is a nurse working on a very busy and often understaffed oncology unit. Two clients have died within the past week. They were both well known to the staff because they had been admitted several times with complications of their disease and treatment. The staff members who were working all cried, first for one client and then, a few days later, for the other client. Today, one of Hakeem's assigned clients required cardiopulmonary resuscitation and was sent to the ICU, another developed septicemia and required many diagnostic tests and procedures, and a third client was given bad news regarding her prognosis and was tearful and frightened. At the end of the day, Hakeem felt that he hadn't done his best job because he was so busy and wished he could spend more time with each of his assigned clients caring more for their emotional needs.

1. How will Hakeem's commitment to the profession of nursing affect how he responds to his feelings of inadequacy and grief?
2. If Hakeem is fully committed to nursing, how will he resolve his feelings about the quality of the care he delivers?
3. If Hakeem has a continuance commitment to nursing, how will he respond to the shift he worked and his feelings?

38.2 LEADERSHIP PRINCIPLES

KEY TERMS

Autocratic (authoritarian) leader, 2233
Bureaucratic leader, 2234
Charismatic leader, 2234
Democratic leader, 2234
Formal leader, 2233
Informal leader, 2233
Laissez-faire leader, 2234
Leader, 2233
Shared governance, 2235
Shared leadership, 2235
Situational leader, 2234
Transactional leader, 2234
Transformational leader, 2235

LEARNING OUTCOMES

After reading about this exemplar, you will be able to:

1. Differentiate between formal and informal leaders.
2. Contrast different leadership theories and styles.
3. Explore strategies and characteristics of a successful leader.

BASIS FOR SELECTION OF EXEMPLAR

Standards of Nursing Practice
NLN Competencies

OVERVIEW

It is important not to confuse leadership with management. A manager has an official position offered by the facility to run a unit, department, or facility depending on the level of management. A leader does not require an official position to lead. **Leaders** are people with the ability to rule, guide, or inspire others to think or act as they recommend. A leader influences others to work together to accomplish a specific goal. Leadership may be formal or informal. The **formal leader**, or appointed leader, is selected by an organization and given official authority to make decisions and act. An **informal leader** is not officially appointed to direct the activities of others but, because of seniority, age, or special abilities, is recognized by the group as a leader and plays an important role in influencing colleagues, coworkers, or other group members to achieve the group's goals. Leaders can be negative or positive in their appeal and approach. While they may not always be liked by others, leaders are able to create trends, instigate actions, and influence behaviors.

Leaders tend to be very productive and persuasive people. They are often highly competent, efficient, charismatic, and powerful. Leaders can be visionary. Leaders tend to be informed, articulate, confident, and self-aware. Many leaders also have outstanding interpersonal skills and are excellent listeners and communicators. They have initiative and the ability and confidence to innovate change, and to motivate, facilitate, and mentor others.

Within their organizations, nurse leaders participate in and guide teams that assess the effectiveness of care, implement evidence-based practice, and construct process improvement strategies. They may be employed in a variety of positions—from shift team leader to institutional president. Leaders may also hold volunteer positions such as chairperson of a professional organization or a community board of directors.

LEADERSHIP THEORIES

Early leadership theories focused on what leaders are (trait theories), what leaders do (behavioral theories), and how leaders adapt their leadership style according to the situation (contingency theories). Theories about leadership style describe traits, behaviors, motivations, and choices used by individuals to influence others.

Classic Leadership Theories

Trait theories of leadership hold that leaders often possess specific traits and abilities, including good judgment, decisiveness, knowledge, adaptability, integrity, tact, self-confidence, and cooperativeness. Behavioral theorists believe that through education, training, and life experiences, leaders develop a particular leadership style. These styles have been characterized as autocratic, democratic, laissez-faire, and bureaucratic.

An **autocratic (authoritarian) leader** makes decisions for the group based on the belief that individuals are externally motivated (their driving force is extrinsic, they desire rewards from others) and are incapable of independent decision making. Likened to a dictator, the autocratic leader determines policies, giving orders and directions to the group. Under this leadership style, the group may feel secure because procedures are well defined and activities are predictable. Productivity may also be high. Under the autocratic leader, however, the group's needs for creativity, autonomy, and self-motivation are not met, and the degree of openness and trust between the leader and the group members is minimal or absent. Although group members are often dissatisfied with this leadership style, at times an autocratic style is the most effective. When urgent decisions must be made (e.g., a cardiac arrest, a unit fire, or a terrorist attack), one person must assume the responsibility without being challenged by other team members. When group members are unable or do not wish to participate in making a decision, the authoritarian style solves the problem and enables the individual or group to move on. This style can also be effective when a project must be completed quickly and efficiently.

A **democratic** (participative, consultative) **leader** encourages group discussion and decision making. This type of leader acts as a catalyst or facilitator, actively guiding the group toward achieving the group goals. Group productivity and satisfaction are high as group members contribute to the work effort. The democratic leader assumes that individuals are internally motivated (their driving force is intrinsic, they desire self-satisfaction), are capable of making decisions, and value independence. Democratic leaders typically provide constructive feedback, offer information, make suggestions, and ask questions to gain information or to help group members grow in their ability to make decisions. This leadership style demands that the leader have faith in the group members to accomplish the goals. Although democratic leadership has been shown to be less efficient and more cumbersome than authoritarian leadership, it allows more self-motivation and more creativity among group members. It also calls for a great deal of cooperation and coordination. This leadership style can be extremely effective in the health care setting.

The **laissez-faire leader** recognizes the group's need for autonomy and self-regulation. The leader assumes a "hands-off" approach, being less directive and more permissive than other types of leaders. The laissez-faire leader presupposes that the group is internally motivated. However, a laissez-faire style can result in group members working at cross-purposes due to a lack of cooperation and coordination. A laissez-faire style is most effective for groups whose members have both personal and professional maturity, so that once the group has made a decision, the members become committed to it and have the required expertise to implement it. Individual group members then perform tasks in their area of expertise while the leader acts as resource person.

Table 38–1 compares the authoritarian, democratic, and laissez-faire leadership styles.

The **bureaucratic leader** does not trust him- or herself or others to make decisions and instead relies on the organization's rules, policies, and procedures to direct the group's work efforts. Group members are usually dissatisfied with the leader's inflexibility and impersonal relations with them.

Contingency theory proposes yet another type of leader. According to contingency theorists, effective leaders adapt their leadership style to the situation. The **situational leader** (a) is flexible in task and relationship behaviors, (b) considers the staff members' abilities, (c) knows the nature of the task to be done, and (d) is sensitive to the context or environment in which the task takes place. The task orientation focuses the leader on activities that encourage group productivity to get the work done. The relationship orientation style is concerned with interpersonal relationships and focuses on activities that meet group members' needs.

Situational leaders adapt their leadership style to the readiness and willingness of the individual or group to perform the assigned task. When employees are insecure, unable, or unwilling to perform the task, the leader uses a highly directive style, providing specific instructions and close supervision. If the group is motivated and willing but unable to perform the task, the leader again uses a highly directive style but, in this case, explains decisions and provides the opportunity for clarification. When the group is able but unwilling or lacking in confidence, the leader shares ideas and facilitates decision making. For a group that is willing, able, and confident to perform the task, the leader delegates, turning the responsibility for decision making and implementation over to the group.

Contemporary Leadership Theories

Contemporary theorists have described charismatic leaders, transactional leaders, transformational leaders, and shared leadership.

A **charismatic leader** is rare and is characterized by an emotional relationship between the leader and the group members. The charming personality of the leader evokes strong feelings of commitment to both the leader and the leader's cause and beliefs. The followers of a charismatic leader often overcome extreme hardship to achieve the group's goals because of faith in the leader.

The **transactional leader** has a relationship with followers based on an exchange for some resource valued by the follower. These incentives are used to promote loyalty and performance. For example, in order to ensure adequate staffing on the night shift, the nurse manager might entice a staff nurse to work the night shift in exchange for a weekend shift off. The transactional leader has a traditional

TABLE 38–1 Comparison of Authoritarian, Democratic, and Laissez-Faire Leadership Styles

	AUTHORITARIAN (AUTOCRATIC)	DEMOCRATIC (PARTICIPATIVE)	LAISSEZ-FAIRE (PERMISSIVE)
Degree of control	Makes decisions alone	Collaborative	No control
Leader activity level	High	High	Minimal
Assumption of responsibility	Primarily the leader	Shared	Relinquished
Output of the group	High quantity, good quality	Creative, high quality	Variable, may be of poor quality
Efficiency	Very efficient	Less efficient than authoritarian	Inefficient

---

Box 38–1 Characteristics of Effective Leaders

Effective leaders do the following:
- Use a leadership style that is natural to them.
- Use a leadership style appropriate to the task and the members.
- Assess the effects of their behavior on others and the effects of others' behavior on themselves.
- Are sensitive to forces acting for and against change.
- Express an optimistic view about human nature.
- Are energetic.
- Are open and encourage openness, so that real issues are confronted.

- Facilitate personal relationships.
- Plan and organize activities of the group.
- Are consistent in behavior toward group members.
- Delegate tasks and responsibilities to develop members' abilities, not merely to get tasks performed.
- Involve members in all decisions.
- Value and use group members' contributions.
- Encourage creativity.
- Encourage feedback about their leadership style.
- Assess for and promote use of current technology.

---

managerial style, focused on the day-to-day tasks of achieving organizational goals and understanding and meeting the needs of the group.

In contrast, a **transformational leader** fosters creativity, risk taking, commitment, and collaboration by empowering the group to share in the organization's vision. The leader inspires others with a clear, attractive, and attainable goal and enlists them to participate in attaining the goal. Through shared values, honesty, trust, and continual learning the transformational leader empowers the group. This facilitates independence, individual growth, and change.

Shared leadership recognizes that a professional workforce is made up of many leaders. No one person is considered to have knowledge or ability beyond that of other members of the work group. Appropriate leadership is thought to emerge in relation to the challenges that confront the work group. Examples of shared leadership in nursing are self-directed work teams, co-leadership, and shared governance. **Shared governance** is a method that aims to distribute decision making among a group of people.

Effective Leadership

Much has been written about effective leadership and style; some descriptive statements about effective leaders are listed in Box 38–1.

Stephen Covey's bestselling book, *Seven Habits of Highly Effective People*, presents a framework for personal effectiveness (see Box 38–2 for Covey's list of the seven habits) that has been adopted by leaders and managers throughout the world. Covey's philosophy emphasizes an approach to effectiveness that is centered on principles and character. This character ethic assumes that there are some absolute principles that exist in all humans, such as fairness, honesty, integrity, human dignity, quality, potential, and growth. Character is a collection of habits that have a powerful role in life. Effective leadership results from interdependence. Covey's philosophy has many parallels to the nursing profession. For example, the fifth habit, "Seek first to understand, then to be understood," exemplifies active, effective listening. Covey asserts that empathic listening (discussed in Concept 36, Communication) is necessary to be an effective

leader (Covey, 1989). Nursing is a profession that demands interdependence—between the client and the nurse, among all members of the nursing team, and in collaboration with other health care professionals.

Leadership is a learned process. To be an effective leader requires an understanding of factors such as needs, goals, and rewards that motivate people; knowledge of leadership skills and of the group's activities; and possession of the interpersonal skills to influence others. Principles of effective leadership include vision, influence, and acting as a role model.

Vision is a mental image of a possible and desirable future state. Leaders transform visions into realistic goals and communicate their visions to others, who accept the visions as their own.

Influence is an informal strategy used to gain the cooperation of others without exercising formal authority. Influence is exercised through persuasion and excellent communication skills; it is based on a trusting relationship with the followers.

An effective leader needs to show sensitivity to being a *positive role model*, demonstrating caring toward coworkers and clients. As is appropriate for any health and caring profession, leadership can also be humanistic, that is, acting in a way that stresses individuals' dignity and worth. Being a good leader takes thought, care, insight, commitment, and energy. In this way, the leader sets the example for others to follow.

Box 38–2 Covey's Seven Habits of Highly Effective People

1. Be proactive.
2. Begin with the end in mind.
3. Put first things first.
4. Think win–win.
5. Seek first to understand, then to be understood.
6. Synergize.
7. Sharpen the saw.

REVIEW Leadership Principles

RELATE: LINK THE CONCEPTS

Linking the exemplar of Leadership Principles with the concept of Communication:

1. How important are communication skills to effectiveness as a leader?
2. Can a person with poor communication skills act as a competent leader? Why or why not?

Linking the exemplar of Leadership Principles with the concept of Advocacy:

3. Are all nursing advocates leaders? Explain your answer.
4. How do leadership principles increase the effectiveness of advocacy?

REFER: GO TO MYNURSINGKIT

REFLECT: CASE STUDY

Martha Rivaldo is a staff nurse who has worked in the neonatal ICU for 7 years. She is not well liked. She tends to be very critical of the performance of new nurses on the unit and can frequently be heard talking with her friends and complaining about how the unit is managed. Several nurses have complained to the nurse manager, but nothing ever seems to be done about her behavior. Martha is a very skilled and competent NICU nurse and is always the first person the staff members call on when they have difficulty initiating an IV line on one of the babies. Martha is also a good resource for people she likes, as she is knowledgeable about responding to emergency situations. However, once she decides someone is lacking in competence, she has no use for them.

1. Is Martha a leader? Explain your answer.
2. If you were Martha's nurse manager and several people came to you, one at a time, to complain about Martha's cruel comments about newly hired nurses, how would you respond?
3. Why do you think Martha reacts the way she does to newly hired NICU nurses?

38.3 WORK ETHIC

KEY TERMS

Arrogance, *2238*
Corrective action, *2237*
Dismissal, *2237*
Generational cohort, *2238*
Insubordination, *2237*
Optimism, *2238*
Pessimism, *2238*
Punctual, *2236*
Work ethic, *2236*

BASIS FOR SELECTION OF EXEMPLAR

Standards of Nursing Practice
NLN Competencies

LEARNING OUTCOMES

After reading about this exemplar, you will be able to:

1. Apply the concept of work ethic to the behavior of the professional nurse.
2. Differentiate between work ethics commonly seen in the four generations of nurses in today's workplace.
3. Predict the impact of generational differences in work ethic as it relates to learning to work as a cohesive nursing team.

OVERVIEW

Ask any employer what characteristic is most important in a good employee and the majority will respond, "A strong **work ethic**." An individual with a strong work ethic places high value on hard work and diligence. Employees with a strong work ethic stay focused and leave their personal problems at home. They apply themselves to the task at hand and take a thorough approach to getting the work done right the first time. If they do make any mistakes, they take responsibility for them and repair any damage, or willingly accept the consequences. They exercise self-discipline and self-control. They know what management expects of them, and they measure up. They don't wait to be told what to do, and they demonstrate a positive attitude and enthusiasm for their work.

By examining some of the factors involved in developing a strong work ethic and demonstrating a commitment to their job and to their employer, nursing students can better understand some of the expectations of the nursing profession.

ATTENDANCE AND PUNCTUALITY

It's nearly impossible to demonstrate a commitment to a job without being there. Performing the duties of a job requires showing up for work every day and being **punctual** (on time) (Figure 38–4 ■).

When an employee has poor attendance, others are required to cover for that individual. Even when the employee has a good reason for being absent, frequent absences increase the stress of other employees and decrease productivity. Many health care agencies are forced to employ as few people as required due to funding shortages. Each nurse (and nursing student) is counted on to be at work and to arrive on time.

The employee who is late for work holds things up and inconveniences other people. When a nurse is late, a client's procedure might have to be rescheduled, possibly delaying that client (or another's) diagnosis, treatment, surgery, or discharge from the hospital. Needed supplies might not get

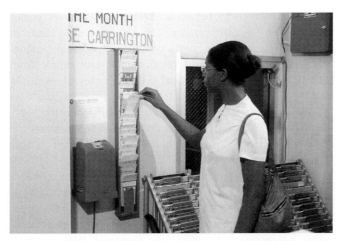

Figure 38–4 ■ It is essential for nurses to arrive at work on time.

delivered on time, paperwork might be filed too late to meet a deadline, or other people might have to work beyond their shifts. Because the roles of health care professionals are interconnected, it is essential that the nurse reports to work on time. "On time" does not mean arriving at the parking lot at the time one is supposed to report for work; "on time" means being at work and in place, ready to begin work at the start of the shift.

Almost everyone must miss work or arrive late on occasion. But when poor attendance or lack of punctuality becomes a habit, it also becomes a performance issue and possible grounds for **corrective action** (steps taken to overcome a job performance problem) or **dismissal** (termination of employment).

As part of his or her professional commitment, each nursing student must make the commitment to show up for work every day, arrive on time, and be ready to work when the shift starts. Those who have set up contingency plans to cover possible situations such as a child being sick or a car being in the shop will be most successful.

For nurses, a good work ethic includes protecting their own health and safety by making sure to get enough rest, avoid unnecessary risks, and considering preventive measures, such as flu shots.

Individuals who possess a good work ethic do not take excessively long or unscheduled breaks. They try to allow some extra time at the end of the shift in case they are held over. Above all, nurses never leave a client, coworker, visitor, or guest hanging by rushing out the door the minute the shift ends. It is the nurse's responsibility (and the nursing student's) to stay long enough to complete work or to hand it off to the person who follows. The nurse makes sure there is a smooth transition between shifts and does not leave any work for other people to finish.

RELIABILITY AND ACCOUNTABILITY

Being reliable and being accountable are key factors in professionalism. From a systems perspective, each nurse is responsible for completing the duties of his or her job appropriately so

that other people can complete their work, too. This responsibility extends to following through on commitments, such as agreeing to trade shifts or taking on additional work when someone is absent. Following through on commitments is a big part of the team effort (Figure 38–5 ■).

Accepting responsibility and the consequences of one's actions is also important. Professionals hold themselves personally accountable and avoid shifting the blame to others. When the nurse makes a mistake (and everyone does occasionally), he or she should admit it and accept full responsibility. The next step is to apologize to those who have been inconvenienced. Although it is important to apologize for a mistake, the apology does not erase the fact that a mistake was made. Learn from the experience and avoid making the same mistake twice. Supervisor, coworkers, and other people appreciate a "the buck stops here" attitude.

Professional nurses accept all work assignments for which they are qualified and that they are prepared to perform. If a nurse is given a work assignment that he or she is not qualified for or prepared to perform, the nurse should discuss the situation with his or her supervisor immediately. Refusal to complete a task as assigned may be construed as **insubordination** and grounds for dismissal.

However, a responsible person would never perform a task that he or she is not capable of performing appropriately. When serving the needs of clients, it's important to avoid passing judgment or projecting one's own personal beliefs on others. If a nurse objects to an assignment because it conflicts with his or her religious beliefs, morals, or values, the nurse must discuss these concerns with his or her supervisor.

It's best to resolve issues like these when the nurse first considers a job offer. If a nurse wishes not to participate in abortions, sex change operations, end-of-life procedures, or other activities that conflict with his or her beliefs or morals, many employers will allow that nurse to opt out. However, this must be discussed ahead of time so that client care is not delayed or jeopardized.

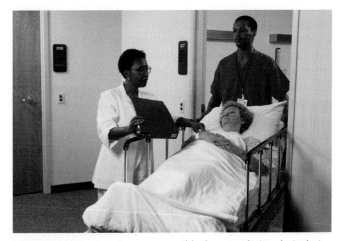

Figure 38–5 ■ Nurses are responsible for completing their duties so that other people can complete their work too.

ATTITUDE AND ENTHUSIASM

As was mentioned earlier, nurses view having a positive attitude as an essential professional characteristic. This sense of **optimism**, a feeling that things will turn out for the best, is common among professional nurses. Unfortunately, for some people a negative attitude is a way of life. Those with a sense of **pessimism** see the glass as half empty. From their perspective, the situation is always bad and may become worse. They complain about everything, and nothing seems to satisfy them. Pessimists rarely smile, appear happy, or convey enthusiasm about their work. They may try to spread negativity to everyone around them and undermine morale, teamwork, and a spirit of cooperation. Pessimism is a dangerous attitude that does not invite trust or inspire confidence. Nurses must convey a sense of optimism and convey enthusiasm about their work to clients and their families. Nurses who maintain a positive attitude among their colleagues contribute to a more pleasant and, ultimately, more productive work environment.

Pessimism is not the only negative attitude that can endanger the nurse's professionalism. **Arrogance**, defined as excessive pride and a feeling of superiority, can be an extremely dangerous characteristic in the nurse, as it can lead to a false belief that the nurse is always right and does not need input from others in guiding his or her actions. For example, when the unit begins using a new IV infusion pump, the arrogant nurse doesn't bother attending the in-service and believes that it is possible to "figure things out" independently. The nurse's ability to accurately assess both strengths and weakness, as well as to accept feedback from others, is a professional characteristic that promotes both safety and growth.

GENERATIONAL DIFFERENCES IN WORK ETHIC

For the first time in American history, four generations of people work shoulder to shoulder. Typically, discussions about diversity focus on multiracial or multiethnic perspectives (see Concept 6, Culture, and Concept 8, Diversity). Diversity can also occur when nurses and other health care workers from different generations work together. Research has clearly shown that generational membership is a key variable in the determination of behavior. Different generations hold different ideals, values, traits, goals, and characteristics. These generational differences play a significant role in how employees of one group relate to the others and include communication styles, expectations, work styles, values and norms, attitudes about work and life, comfort with technology, views regarding loyalty and authority, and acceptance of change.

The term **generational cohort** refers to people born in the same general time span who share key life experiences, including historical events, public heroes, pastimes, and early work experiences. These common life experiences create cohesiveness in perspectives and attitudes. As a result, generational cohorts develop distinct values and workforce patterns. Differences between generations (what is sometimes called a *generation gap*) can have negative effects in the workplace, causing conflicts and interpersonal tension. Learning to create collegial relationships with people from different generations is a critical skill for nurses who work in multigenerational teams.

While the literature sometimes disagrees on specific years or generational names, there is consistent agreement on the characteristics of each generational cohort. Members of the oldest generation were born between 1925 and 1944. They have been called veterans, survivors, traditionalist, or the silent generation and are between about 66 and 85 years of age. The baby boomers were born during the post–World War II population surge from approximately 1945 to 1960, a time of economic prosperity and opportunity. Currently, baby boomers are between about 50 and 65 years of age and represent the largest cohort in the nursing workforce. Generation X was born between 1961 and 1980, and its members are currently 30–49 years of age. The generation after generation X, known as the millennial generation, has nearly as many members as the baby boomer generation and was born between 1981 and 2000. The millennials are currently 10–29 years of age and have also been called generation Y, generation next, and the net generation. An understanding of each generation's historical influences, life experiences, and the workforce the members entered when first employed is necessary to understand their attitudes and values related to work (see Table 38–2).

Different generational styles can lead to workplace conflict. Older nurses may experience considerable conflict over younger nurses' behaviors and may describe younger nurses as arrogant, lacking in commitment, and having a "slacker" attitude. Younger nurses, however, see themselves as self-reliant rather than arrogant. Older nurses may be dismayed and struggle with a perceived lack of professionalism among their younger colleagues evidenced by younger nurses' dress, hair styles, piercings, and tattoos. Younger nurses may be disillusioned by older nurses' perceived unwillingness to become technologically competent.

While differences between generations are not new, two significant changes over the past 60 years have forced the current generations in the workforce into more intense interaction. First, the nature of the work itself has shifted. In traditional bureaucratic structures, interactions between generations followed hierarchical lines. People from younger generations traditionally held entry-level positions and reported to people of the older generation in more senior positions. As a result, younger employees took direction from and followed the rules of people who were older. With the advent of continuous quality improvement and shared governance structures, today individuals from various "levels" of the organization are placed as equal members of a team. This has increased the interaction of employees from different generations.

Second, the transformation from the industrial age to the information age has altered the interactions between people of differing generations. Historically, the most senior members of

TABLE 38–2 Description of Four Generations in the American Workforce

GENERATIONAL COHORT	LIFE EXPERIENCES	WORKFORCE ENTERED	WORK ETHIC
Veterans (born 1925–1944) Great Depression World War II	News came from newspapers and radio Long-distance phone calls were rare and expensive Shopping was mostly done at locally owned stores Movies were only seen in theaters Attitude toward children to be "seen and not heard"	End of depression and war Economic prosperity Emergence of middle class Able to thrive in a nice home on a single income Large, bureaucratic organizations Rules, policies, and procedures plainly outlined	Sacrifice and hard work are rewarded Seniority is important to advance career Value loyalty Respect authority Like working in teams with designated leaders Prefer personal forms of communication
Baby Boomers (born 1945–1960) Introduction of television Man landed on the moon Assassination of President Kennedy Vietnam War Civil Rights Movement Summer of Love Woodstock Watergate	Grew up in a healthy, flourishing economy Watched variety shows, movies, and sitcoms within their own home News became more visual and dramatic Raised in two-parent households in which father worked and mother was home caretaker Member of smaller families	Emphasis on freedom to be yourself—the "me" generation Heroes were those who questioned status quo People in positions of power were not to be trusted Raised to be independent, critical thinkers Many female college graduates went on to become secretaries, nurses, or teachers due to perception these were "primarily female professions"	Workaholics Embrace sense of professionalism Self-worth closely tied to work ethic Question authority Status quo can be transformed by working together Desire financial prosperity but long to make a significant contribution with their experience and expertise
Generation X (born 1961–1980) Rising divorce rates Microwaves Video games Computers Spaceship *Challenger* disaster Numerous scandals involving high-profile public figures	Lived in two-career households Many raised in single parent homes Watched parents work extremely long hours and sacrifice leisure time for success at work "Latch key" generation; learned to manage on their own; becoming adept, clever, and resourceful Allowed to be equal participants in family discussions, learned at an early age to participate in conversations, advocate for their point of view, and expect to have their opinions considered	Dramatic downsizing, reengineering, and layoffs seen with more senior colleagues, parents, and grandparents Hierarchical structures had begun to flatten, eliminating promotional opportunities for younger workers Large cohort of baby boomers remained in workforce filling limited managerial positions Assumed responsibility to keep themselves employable by constantly updating their skills	Seek challenges Self-directed Comfortable with technology Expect instant access to information Desire employment where they can create balance in work and personal life Prefer managers to be mentors and coaches Limited motivation to stay with same employer but loyal to their profession Desire more control over their own schedule Pragmatic focus on outcomes rather than process
Millennial Generation (born 1981–2000) Established infrastructure (childcare, preschool, after-school care) to assist dual-career parents Global generation Internet Bombing of federal building in Oklahoma City Columbine High School shootings Terrorist attack of September 11, 2001	Mostly children of baby boomers born to older mothers; "baby on board" signs in automobiles Live highly structured and scheduled with everything from soccer camp to piano lessons Parents heavily involved in their upbringing, often chaperoning or coaching extracurricular activities Accept multiculturalism Grew up using e-mail or the Internet more often than the telephone Raised enmeshed in digital technology with computer games at nursery school "Extreme sports" generation Mass consumption of television and pop culture	Economic downturn Job opportunities in many industries dried up Wall Street and banking industry crisis Believe education is the key to success Resurgence of heroism and patriotism Diversity a given Renewed sense of interest in contributing to collective good Volunteer for community service Joining organizations in record numbers	Social, confident, optimistic, talented, well-educated, collaborative, open-minded, achievement-oriented Expect daily feedback, high maintenance Potential to become the highest-producing workforce in history Thrive on the adrenaline rush of new challenges and new opportunities Consider personal cell phones a necessity for daily life and interpersonal communication

an organization offered the most reliable information and knowledge (Figure 38–6 ■). Young nurses relied on their more senior colleagues for instruction and advice when confronted with an unusual diagnosis or a complex client situation. With the advent of the information age, young nurses are not as reliant on their older peers, since they can easily access information from around the world on their computers and smartphones. Computerization has not only broken the dependence of younger generations on more senior generations for information, it has also resulted in the unprecedented situation of having the youngest in the workforce be the most expert at a critical skill. Instead of younger nurses turning to their older colleagues for advice, older nurses are often dependent upon their younger peers for guidance in using the computer and other new technologies (Figure 38–7 ■).

Members of each generation operate as if their own values and expectations are universal. For example, veteran nurses who entered the workforce when success occurred through long-term employment with one organization assume that the same approach will ensure achievement today. They see their younger colleagues' frequent job changes or working as independent agents as unreliability or a lack of commitment. Younger nurses may assume that their older peers who have remained in one place of employment have done so because of failure to take advantage of opportunities. Also, having grown up in a world where their voice and contributions are expected, younger nurses are often misunderstood when they advise their more senior colleagues who were taught to respect and listen to their elders. An older nurse may see the voiced criticisms of a novice nurse at a staff meeting as disrespectful and therefore discount him or her. From the younger nurse's perspective, speaking up even with limited experience is seen as contributing to the unit.

Learning to develop collegial relationships with people from different generations is a critical skill for nurses who work in multigenerational teams. Working with nurses from different generations offers the opportunity to explore new and different ways of thinking. Rather than focusing on what's "wrong" with another generation, nurses should capitalize on

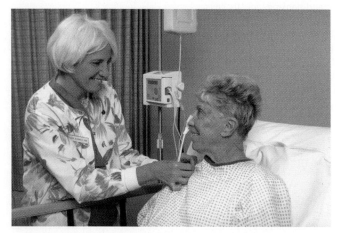

Figure 38–6 ■ Experienced nurses should be valued for their clinical experience.

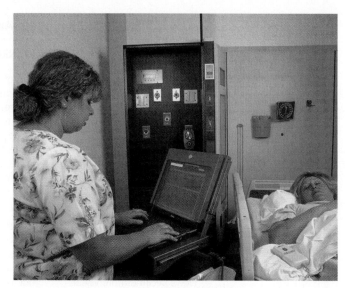

Figure 38–7 ■ Younger nurses should be valued for their understanding of technology.

each generation's strengths. Veteran nurses value hard work and respect authority, whereas baby boomers value teamwork. Generation X nurses value self-reliance, and millennial nurses value achievement. In the workplace, a veteran nurse might say, "Do it because I say so," and a baby boomer nurse might say, "Let's get together and reach a consensus about how to do it." The generation X staff nurses might say they will do it themselves, and the millennial nurses might not care who does it as long as the work gets done.

Veteran nurses should be valued for the wisdom and organizational history they bring to nursing teams. When technology fails, veteran nurses can assist a unit to quickly shift back to the traditional ways of assessing and caring for clients. Baby boomers should be valued for their clinical and organizational experience and be utilized to coach and mentor younger nurses. Generation X nurses should be valued for their innovative ideas and creative approaches to unit issues and problems. They can be important in helping organizations design new approaches to nursing care delivery. Millennial nurses should be valued for their understanding of technology and insights into how it can be used in practice. They can also serve as technology coaches to members of older generational cohorts.

Negative, nonsupportive, unpleasant, and uncooperative peers and coworkers are key impediments to nurses' ability to find joy in their work. Teams that work together, support one another, value one another's strengths and abilities, and resolve conflicts are critical factors in staff nurse retention. Box 38–3 gives examples of questions to be considered about each generational cohort to assist in capitalizing on the strengths of each.

Learning from the unique strengths of each generation can decrease interpersonal tension and facilitate personal growth. Nurses who learn to acknowledge and appreciate their colleagues from different backgrounds, including generational backgrounds, have a distinct advantage. Successful teamwork

Box 38–3 Questions to Highlight the Strengths of Each Generation of Nurses

VETERAN GENERATION
- Where does the unit have a need for resource conservation?
- Which tasks require close attention to timeliness and detail?
- Where are skills in listening and problem solving most needed?

BABY BOOMERS
- Where are nurses who can "roll with the punches" most needed?
- Which tasks require independent thinking?
- Where are skills in coaching and mentoring most needed?

GENERATION X
- Where are new approaches to nursing care delivery needed?
- Which tasks call for an entrepreneurial spirit?
- Where can troubleshooting skills best be utilized?

MILLENNIAL GENERATION
- Where are culturally sensitive viewpoints most needed?
- What tasks require an outspoken nature?
- Where can advanced computer or other technological skills best be utilized?

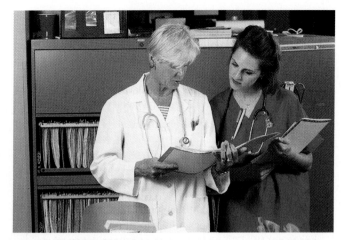

Figure 38–8 ■ The best nursing teams utilize the contributions of each generation's strengths.

is increasingly required for job satisfaction and the ability to positively affect client outcomes. This is reflected in the recent introduction of relationship-based nursing care delivery systems. All too frequently, intergenerational interactions lead to conflicts due to lack of appreciation, understanding, or just misinterpretation of other perspectives.

Particular attention should be paid to engaging the perspective of younger nurses, as this generation is always at a distinct disadvantage. It's not unusual to hear the phrase "Nurses eat their young." The existing organizational structure is based upon strategies that were used successfully in the past rather than designed for the future. Because of their longevity, older generations often dominate in leadership positions of power and are more influential when changes are

made. These nurses update processes and rewards in a way that makes sense from their generational perspective, not recognizing that younger nurses might not hold this perspective. Incorporating younger nurses' values of participation, access to information, and balance into nursing operations is important. Older nurses need to learn to welcome input from their younger colleagues, encouraging them to use their fresh viewpoints to identify where opportunities exist. Younger nurses need to be taught and learn to value the experience and expertise of more senior nurses who have a wealth of lived experiences to share.

The best teams utilize the contributions of each generation's skill set and strength. The hardworking, loyal veterans; the idealist, passionate baby boomers; the techno-literate, adaptable generation Xers; and the young, optimistic millennials can come together into a powerful network of nurses with a remarkable ability to support each other and maximize their contribution to client care (Figure 38–8 ■).

REVIEW Work Ethic

RELATE: LINK THE CONCEPTS

Linking the exemplar of Work Ethic with the concept of Collaboration:
1. How does the work ethic of the individual nurse affect collaboration?
2. How might nurses from different generations respond to a rude and confrontational physician?

Linking the exemplar of Work Ethic with the concept of Teaching and Learning:
3. How does the nurse's generational work ethic affect how the nurse teaches clients?
4. How does the nurse's generational work ethic affect learning style?

REFER: GO TO MYNURSINGKIT

REFLECT: CASE STUDIES

How would you respond to each of the following situations?
1. You were out with friends until very late last night and had to report for work this morning at 7:00 a.m. You know that your coworkers won't arrive for another half an hour. You've got just enough time for a quick run to the corner coffee shop before your coworkers arrive.
2. You promised your coworkers that you would work the day shift on Thanksgiving so they could be home with their families. Two days before the holiday, an old friend from out of town calls to say that he would like you to be his guest for lunch on Thanksgiving Day.
3. You have an appointment with your supervisor next week to review the results of your annual performance evaluation. You overhear one of your teammates telling another person that she gave you a low score on your 360-degree feedback evaluation because you refused to trade shifts with her over the Easter weekend.
4. Your shift ends in 30 minutes, and you've got about 30 minutes of work left to do, but you haven't been able to take your afternoon break yet.

5. One of your neighbors is admitted to the unit where you work. A relative of yours calls to tell you he's heard a rumor that the neighbor has a communicable disease. Because you work on the unit and have access to records, your relative asks you to find out whether the rumor is true.

6. A new piece of equipment gets installed in your department, but you miss the in-service session when everyone gets trained on how to operate it. The next day there's a procedure to be done using this equipment, and it's your responsibility to use it.

7. A coworker invites you to a party. When you arrive, you notice three other people that you work with complaining about low wages and telling a group of strangers that one of the surgeons at your hospital made a mistake in surgery last week and lied to the client's family to try to cover it up.

PEARSON

EXPLORE mynursingkit™

MyNursingKit is your one stop for online chapter review materials and resources. Prepare for success with additional NCLEX®-style practice questions, interactive assignments and activities, web links, animations and videos, and more!

Register your access code from the front of your book at
www.mynursingkit.com.

REFERENCES

American Nurses Association. (2009). *Gallup poll votes nurses most trusting profession* (News Release December 9, 2009). Silver Spring, MD: Author. Retrieved March 22, 2010 from http://www.nursingworld.org/FunctionalMenuCategories/MediaResources/PressReleases/2009-PR/Gallup-Votes-Nurses-Most-Trusted-Profession.aspx

Battell, C. (2006). *Effective listening.* Alexandria, VA: American Society for Training and Development.

Brody, M., & Alati, D. (2004), Learn to listen. *Incentive, 178*(5), 57–59.

Carver, L & Candela, L. (2008). Attaining organizational commitment across different generations of nurses. *Journal of Nursing Management, 16*, 984–992.

Covey, S. R. (1989). *The 7 habits of highly successful people.* New York: Simon & Schuster.

Dunn, D., & Goodnight, L.J. (2008). *Communication: embracing differences.* Boston: Pearson Education/Allyn and Bacon.

Hill, J. (2004). Listen.... it will change your life: a practical guide to effective listening. *Presentations, 18*(4), 41.

Hill, K. S. (2004). Defy the decades with multigenerational teams. *Nursing Management, January 2004*, 33–35.

Hu, J., Herrick, C., & Hodgin, K. A. (2004). Managing the multigenerational nursing team. *The Health Care Manager, 23*(4), 334–340.

Kupperschmidt, B. (2006). Addressing multigenerational conflict: Mutual respect and carefronting as a strategy. *Online Journal of Issues in Nursing, 11*(2), 19p.

Lavoie-Tremblay, M., O'Brien-Pallas, L., Gelinas, C., Desforges, N., & Marhchionni, C. (2008). Addressing the turnover issue among new nurses from a generational viewpoint. *Journal of Nursing Administration, 16*, 724–734.

Merriam-Webster Online Dictionary (2010). *Commitment.* Retrieved February 22, 2010, from www.merriam-webster.com/dictionary/commitment

Merriam-Webster Online Dictionary (2009). *Commitment and work ethic.* Retrieved March 1, 2009, from www.merriam-webster.com

Nogueras, D. J. (2006). Occupational commitment, education, and experience as a predictor of intent to leave the nursing profession. *Nursing Economics, 24*(2), 86–93

North Carolina Board of Nursing (2008). *Continuing competence.* Retrieved February 6, 2010, from www.ncbon.com/content.aspx?id=1078&terms=definition+of+competent

Parry, J. (2008). Intention to leave the profession: Antecedents and role in nurse turnover. *Journal of Advanced Nursing, 64* (2), 157–168.

Saad, L. (2008, November 24). *Nurses shine, bankers slump in ethics poll.* U.S.A. Today/Gallup Poll, p12.

Sherman, R. O. (2006). Nursing generations in the contemporary workforce. *Online Journal of Issues in Nursing, 11*(2), 5p.

Sherman, R. O. (2006). Leading a multigenerational nursing workforce: Issues, challenges, and strategies. *Online Journal of Issues in Nursing, 11*(2).

Shwu-Ru, L. (2008). An analysis of the concept of organizational commitment. *Nursing Forum, 43*(3), 116–125.

University of Kansas School of Medicine (2010). *Professionalism initiative.* Retrieved February 6, 2010, from www.kumc.edu/som/professionalism.html

Via Christi Regional Medical Center (2003). Survey on professionalism. Retrieved on February 6, 2010, from www.via-christi.org/workfiles/Professionalism%20in%20Nursing.ppt

Wagner, C. M. (2007). Organizational commitment as a predictor variable in nursing turnover research: Literature review. *JAN Review Paper*, Blackwell Publishing, 235–247.

Ward, K. S. & Parsons, L. C. (2006). A look at generational diversity: Managing the differences. *SCI Nursing, 23*(4), 14p.

Weston, M. J. (2006). Integrating generational perspectives in nursing. *Online Journal of Issues in Nursing 11*(2), 11p.

Young, S. (2007). Speak easy: The power of quality questions and the art of listening. *Public Relations Tactics, 14*(3), 23.

Teaching and Learning

39

Concept at-a-Glance

About Teaching and Learning, *2243*

39.1   Client Education, *2253*

39.2   Mentoring, *2269*

39.3   Staff Education, *2272*

Concept Learning Outcomes

After reading about this concept, you will be able to:

1. Discuss the importance of the teaching role of the nurse.
2. Describe the attributes of learning.
3. Compare and contrast andragogy, pedagogy, and geragogy.
4. Discuss the characteristics of adult learners.
5. Describe the three domains of learning.
6. Identify factors that affect learning.
7. Discuss the implications of using the Internet as a source of health information.

Concept Key Terms

Adherence, *2245*
Affective domain, *2247*
Andragogy, *2245*
Behaviorist theory, *2246*
Cognitive domain, *2247*
Cognitive theory, *2246*
Compliance, *2245*
Constructivism, *2248*
e-health, *2251*
Geragogy, *2245*
Humanistic learning
    theory, *2248*

Imitation, *2247*
Learning, *2243*
Learning need, *2245*
Modeling, *2247*
Motivation to learn, *2249*
Observational learning, *2247*
Pedagogy, *2245*
Positive reinforcement, *2246*
Psychomotor domain, *2247*
Readiness to learn, *2249*
Teaching, *2243*

About Teaching and Learning

Teaching is a system of activities designed to produce learning. **Learning** is a change in human disposition or capability that persists and that cannot be solely accounted for by growth. Learning is represented by a change in behavior; in other words, the learner is able to apply or demonstrate what has been learned. (See Box 39–1 for attributes of learning.)

The teaching–learning process involves dynamic interaction between teacher and learner. Each participant in the process communicates information, emotions, perceptions, and attitudes to the other. This concept discusses the teaching–learning process, the

> ### Box 39–1 **Attributes of Learning**
>
> Learning is
> - An experience that occurs inside the learner
> - The discovery of the personal meaning and relevance of ideas
> - A consequence of experience
> - A collaborative and cooperative process
> - An evolutionary process that builds on past learning and experiences
> - A process that is both intellectual and emotional.

A number of factors affect teaching clients and others in the health care system. Federal and state regulations influence the content to be taught and the documentation required of nursing schools, certifying agencies, and agencies employing and training nurses and other health care professionals. Nurses providing client education do so for clients who vary in age, cultural and socioeconomic background, primary language, and previous knowledge and experience. Information is constantly changing as new research becomes available. Today's resources are numerous and readily available through the Internet. These factors combine to make providing clients with accurate, current information a challenge for nurses.

nurse's responsibility as a client and family educator, the domains and theories of learning, the factors that affect an individual's ability to learn, and how nurses can use this information to design more successful client and family education activities.

Nurses as Teachers

The ANA Standards of Practice for Registered Nurses identifies teaching as one of the many roles of the professional nurse. Although nurses teach a variety of learners in various settings, nurses primarily teach clients and their families. Such instruction includes discharge teaching about how to perform self-care; about taking medications, including side effects; and about how to perform prescribed treatments. Although most teaching is done directly with clients, family members or caregivers also may be instructed in care of the client. This is especially important for those clients who have difficulty performing self-care. For example, parents who need to give medication to their children must be instructed in the proper administration of that medication. A client with diabetes who has visual impairment may need assistance in administering insulin or in assessing his or her feet and lower extremities for skin breakdown. The caregiver or family member must be included in the client's instruction. When teaching clients about diet, it is important to include the person who purchases and prepares the food.

Nurses also teach professional colleagues and other health care personnel in academic institutions such as vocational schools, colleges, and universities, and in health care facilities such as hospitals or nursing homes. Nurses teach each other through a variety of experiences, including mentoring, continuing education classes, and clinical experiences for nursing students.

Nurses as Learners

Nursing education programs prepare the new practitioner with effective beginning nursing skills. However, because changes occur quickly and often in nursing and health care, nurses must continue learning to keep current. The ANA Standards of Professional Performance recognize this (see Box 39–2). Each state's Board of Nursing outlines requirements for nurses to participate in continuing education programs designed to increase their knowledge and skill. To assist nurses in maintaining their licenses and ensuring quality of care, many employers provide continuing education programs at the work site. Sometimes nurses need to travel to specialized centers to gain advanced specialized skills. Many nurses return to school to obtain advanced degrees in nursing and other health-related disciplines. ●

THE ART OF TEACHING

Teaching is a system of activities intentionally designed to produce specific learning. It is a goal-directed activity that results in improved learning for the learner. Teaching is more than giving information; the art of teaching lies in creating a learning environment conducive for the learner to gain knowledge, skills, and a desire within the learner to change some aspect of his or her life. Effective teaching requires knowledge of the subject matter, understanding of the learning process, judgment, and intuition (Box 39–3).

The relationship between the teacher and the learner is essentially one of trust and respect. The learner trusts that the teacher has the knowledge and skill to teach, and the teacher

---

Box 39–2 **American Nurses Association Standards of Professional Performance Related to Teaching and Learning**

- *Standard 8. Education:* The nurse attains knowledge and competency that reflects current nursing practice. Measurement criteria include participating in educational activities related to appropriate knowledge bases and professional issues; demonstrating a commitment to lifelong learning through self-reflection and inquiry to identify personal learning needs; seeking experiences that reflect current practice in order to maintain skills and competence in clinical practice or role performance; acquiring knowledge and skills appropriate to the specialty area, practice setting, role, or situation; maintaining professional records that provide evidence of competency and lifelong learning; and seeking experiences and formal and independent

learning activities to maintain and develop clinical and professional skills and knowledge.
- *Standard 10. Collegiality:* The nurse interacts with and contributes to the professional development of peers and other health providers as colleagues. Measurement criteria for this standard include sharing knowledge and skills with peers and colleagues; providing peers with feedback regarding their practice and/or role performance, and contributing to an environment that is conducive to the education of health care professionals.

Source: Adapted from American Nurses Association. (2004). *Nursing: Scope and standards of practice* (pp. 35, 37). Washington, DC: ANA.

Box 39-3 **Characteristics of Effective Teaching**

- Holds the learner's interest.
- Involves the learner in the learning process, and creates a partnership between the learner and the teacher.
- Fosters a positive self-concept in the learner; learner believes learning is possible and probable.
- Sets realistic goals.
- Is directed at helping learners meet their objectives.
- Supports the learner with positive reinforcement.
- Is accurate and current.
- Is appropriate for the learner's age, condition, and abilities.
- Is optimistic, positive, and nonthreatening.
- Uses several methods of teaching to accommodate a variety of learning styles, and provides learning opportunities through hearing, seeing, and doing.
- Gathers information from reliable sources.
- Is cost-effective (i.e., cost of nurse's time spent teaching is less than the cost of treating health problems occurring when clients do not follow recommended treatments, fail to take medications correctly, or do not adapt lifestyle to changing health needs).

respects the learner's ability to attain the recognized goals. Once a nurse starts to instruct a client and/or other learner, it is important that the teaching process continues until the participants achieve the mutually agreed upon learning goals, change the goals, or decide that the goals cannot be met.

As teachers, nurses must understand a number of learning theories. By understanding how people learn and the factors that impact learning, nurses can develop more successful client teaching plans for both individual clients and their families, as well as for various types of groups of learners.

LEARNING

All people have a variety of learning needs. A **learning need** is a desire or a requirement to know something that is presently unknown to the learner. Learning needs may include new knowledge or information, a new or different skill or physical ability, a new behavior, or a need to change an old behavior.

An important aspect of learning is the individual's desire to learn and to act on learning, which is referred to as compliance. In the health care context, **compliance** is the extent to which an individual's behavior coincides with medical or health advice. Compliance is best illustrated when the individual recognizes and accepts the need to learn, then follows through with the appropriate behaviors that reflect the learning. For example, a client diagnosed as having diabetes willingly learns about the recommended special diet and then plans and follows the diet. Many people, however, view the term *compliance* in a negative light because it implies the learner is submissive, and this is in conflict with the learner's right to determine his or her own health care decisions rather than be told what to do by a health care professional. Conversely, some professionals can be too quick to label a

client as noncompliant. It is important to determine why a client is not following a recommended course of action before applying this label. For example, the client may have intended to comply but was unable to do so because he could not afford the cost of the medications.

Another term seen in health care literature is **adherence**, which is commitment or attachment to a regimen. Bastable (2003) explains that both compliance and adherence refer to the "ability to maintain health-promoting regimens, which are determined largely by a health care provider" (p. 169).

Although **pedagogy** has historically been defined as the study or science of teaching, the term has increasingly been used to specifically refer to teaching children and adolescents. **Andragogy** is the art and science of teaching adults, while **geragogy** refers to the process of stimulating and helping older adults to learn (Hayes, 2005; John, 1988). The different learning needs of adults, versus children or older adults, has led to the science of developing specific approaches to teaching and learning, requiring the differentiation of terms. For example, when teaching a young child about what will happen in surgery a doll may be used. This approach would be far less successful with a cognizant adult, but could work with a client who has a cognition deficit.

Learning Theories

A number of different learning theories help nurses understand how people learn. Adult learning theory, behaviorist theory, cognitive theory, and humanistic learning theory are among the theories most commonly used by nurses to teach individuals and groups of learners. Other theories that may be used include social learning theory, informational processing theory, categorization, constructivism, and multiple intelligence.

ADULT LEARNING THEORY Knowles, Holton, and Swanson (2005) proposed the adult education theory, which described differences in the learning styles of adults and children. Prior to their work, it was assumed that the same teaching principles could be used for both children and adults. Knowles et al. suggested four basic conceptual differences between adult and child education:

1. Self-concept
2. Experience
3. Readiness to learn
4. Time perspective.

These characteristics are described in Table 39–1.

Further research in andragogy has determined a number of factors about adult learners that nurses can use as guides for client teaching (Hayes, 2005; Knowles, 1984):

- As people mature, they move from dependence to independence.
- An adult's previous experiences can be used as a resource for learning.
- An adult's readiness to learn is often related to a developmental task or social role (i.e., perceive a need in his or her life situation).
- An adult is more oriented to learning when the material is useful immediately, not sometime in the future.

TABLE 39–1 **Characteristics of Adult Learners and Educational Implications**

ADULT LEARNER CHARACTERISTICS	IMPLICATIONS FOR ADULT LEARNING
1. The need to know	Adults need to know why they need to learn something before undertaking to learn it. The first task of the facilitator of learning is to help the learners become aware of the "need to know." At the very least, facilitators can make an intellectual case for the value of the learning in improving the effectiveness of the learners' performance or the quality of their lives. Even more potent tools for raising the level of awareness of the need to know are real or simulated experiences in which the learners discover for themselves the gaps between where they are now and where they want to be. Personnel appraisal systems, job rotation, exposure to role models, and diagnostic performance assessments are examples of such tools.
2. The learners' self-concept	Adults have a self-concept of being responsible for their own decisions, for their own lives. Once they have arrived at that self-concept, they develop a deep psychological need to be seen and treated by others as being capable of self-direction. They resent and resist situations in which they feel others are imposing their wills on them. This presents a serious problem in adult education: The minute adults walk into an activity labeled "education," "training," or anything synonymous, they hark back to their conditioning in their previous school experience, put on their dunce hats of dependency, fold their arms, sit back, and say, "Teach me."
3. The role of the learners' experiences	Adults come into an educational activity with both a greater volume and a different quality of experience from youths. The emphasis in adult education is on experiential techniques—techniques that tap into the experience of the learners, such as group discussion, simulation exercises, problem-solving activities, case method, and laboratory methods instead of transmittal techniques. Also, greater emphasis is placed on peer-helping activities.
4. Readiness to learn	Adults become ready to learn those things they need to know and be able to do in order to cope effectively with their real-life situations. An especially rich source of "readiness to learn" is the developmental tasks associated with moving from one developmental stage to the next. The critical implication of this assumption is the importance of timing learning experiences to coincide with those developmental tasks.
5. Orientation to learning	There are ways to induce readiness through exposure to models of superior performance, career counseling, simulation exercises, and other techniques. In contrast to children's and youths' subject-centered orientation to learning (at least in school), adults are life-centered (or task- or problem-centered) in their orientation to learning. Adults are motivated to learn to the extent that they perceive that learning will help them perform tasks or deal with problems that they confront in their life situations. Furthermore, they learn new knowledge, understandings, skills, values, and attitudes most effectively when they are presented in the context of application to real-life situations.
6. Motivation	While adults are responsive to some external motivators (better jobs, promotions, higher salaries, and the like), the most potent motivators are internal pressures (the desire for increased job satisfaction, self-esteem, quality of life, and the like), but this motivation is frequently blocked by such barriers as negative self-concept as a student, inaccessibility of opportunities or resources, time constraints, and programs that violate principles of adult learning.

Source: From Knowles, M. S., Holton, E. F., Swanson, R. A.(1998). *The adult learner* (6th ed). Houston: Butterworth-Heinemann. Reprinted with permission from Elsevier.

BEHAVIORIST THEORY   According to **behaviorist theory**, learning takes place when an individual's reaction (called a *response)* to a stimulus is either positively or negatively reinforced. Thus, to modify a person's attitude and response, a behaviorist would either alter the stimulus condition in the environment or change what happens after a response occurs (Bastable, 2003, p. 45). Major contributors to behaviorist theory include Thorndike, Skinner, Pavlov, and Bandura.

Skinner's and Pavlov's work focused on conditioning behavioral responses to a stimulus that causes the response or behavior. To increase the probability of a response, Skinner introduced the importance of **positive reinforcement** (e.g., a pleasant experience such as praise and encouragement) in fostering repetition of an action.

Nurses applying behavioristic theory will

- Provide sufficient practice time and both immediate and repeat testing and redemonstration.
- Provide opportunities for learners to solve problems by trial and error.

- Select teaching strategies that avoid distracting information and that evoke the desired response.
- Praise the learner for correct behavior and provide positive feedback at intervals throughout the learning experience.
- Provide role models of desired behavior.

COGNITIVE THEORY   **Cognitive theory**, or *cognitivism*, recognizes the developmental level of learners and acknowledges the learner's motivation and environment. It depicts learning as primarily a mental, intellectual, or thinking process. The learner structures and processes information (see Box 39–4). Perceptions are selectively chosen by the learner, and personal characteristics have an impact on how a cue is perceived. Cognitive theorists also emphasize the importance of social, emotional, and physical contexts in which learning occurs, such as the teacher–learner relationship and the environment. Developmental readiness and individual readiness (expressed as motivation) are other key factors associated with cognitive approaches.

Major cognitive theorists include Piaget and Bloom. Piaget's five major phases of cognitive development include:

1. The sensorimotor phase
2. The preconceptual phase
3. The intuitive phase
4. The concrete operations phase
5. The formal operations phase.

These are discussed in detail in Concept 7, Development.

Bloom (1956) identified three domains or areas of learning. The **cognitive domain**, of the "thinking" domain, includes six intellectual abilities and thinking processes, beginning with knowing, comprehending, and applying to analysis, synthesis, and evaluation. The **affective domain**, also known as the "feeling" domain, is divided into categories that specify the degree of a "person's depth of emotional response to tasks"

Box 39–4 Cognitive Learning Processes

Cognitive theory proposes that learning involves three cognitive (mental) processes: acquiring information, processing the information, and using the information. These three processes can occur sequentially or simultaneously.

ACQUIRING INFORMATION

Acquiring information involves two processes: sensory reception and discrimination. Sensory reception is made possible by the neurosensory system. Stimuli in the environment signal the appropriate sense, such as sight, hearing, or smell. Impulses then travel by the nervous system to the brain. Sensory reception generally is continuous, but it is not always a conscious process.

The second aspect of acquiring information is discrimination. Discrimination is the ability to determine which stimuli are relevant in a particular situation. Stimuli can be objects, ideas, actions, or facts. They may be internal (i.e., inside the body) or external. Discrimination is the most difficult when there are multiple, complex stimuli.

PROCESSING INFORMATION

Processing provides meaning to the information. Information is processed in three steps:

1. *Association,* which is the joining of two or more ideas. For example, a person may associate an object such as a needle with the word *needle* and/or with the experience of pain.
2. *Generalization,* which is the perceiving of similarities among various stimuli, for example, the similarities between three different syringes.
3. *Concept formation,* which is the organization of stimuli that have some attributes in common. For example, a nurse who understands the concept of caring appreciates the characteristics associated with caring. The nurse can then help others to convey caring in the health care setting.

USING INFORMATION

Using information is the application of information in the cognitive, affective, and psychomotor areas. The ability to formulate and relate concepts is an essential critical thinking skill. In addition, relating concepts is essential for creative thinking and problem solving.

(Bastable, 2003, p. 330). It includes feelings, emotions, interests, attitudes, and appreciations. The **psychomotor domain**, or the "skill" domain, includes motor skills, such as the fine motor skills required to give an injection.

Nurses should include each of Bloom's three domains in client teaching plans. For example, teaching a client with diabetes how to self-administer insulin is in the psychomotor domain. Teaching the client why insulin is needed and what to do when not feeling well is in the cognitive domain. Helping the client accept the chronic implications of diabetes and maintain self-esteem is in the affective domain.

Nurses applying cognitive theory will

- Provide a social, emotional, and physical environment conducive to learning.
- Encourage a positive teacher–learner relationship.
- Select multisensory teaching strategies since perception is influenced by the senses.
- Recognize that personal characteristics have an impact on how cues are perceived and develop appropriate teaching approaches to target different learning styles.
- Assess a person's developmental and individual readiness to learn and adapt teaching strategies to the learner's developmental level.
- Select behavioral objectives and teaching strategies that encompass the cognitive, affective, and psychomotor domains of learning.

SOCIAL LEARNING THEORY Social learning theorists, such as Bandura, agree with Skinner that the environment exerts a great deal of control over overt behavior. However, they believe that the entire learning process involves three highly interdependent factors:

1. The characteristics of the person
2. The person's behavior
3. The environment.

Bandura claims that most learning comes from observational learning and instruction rather than from overt trial-and-error behavior. **Observational learning** is the acquisition of new skills or the alteration of old behaviors simply by watching other children and adults. It is especially important for acquiring behavior in situations when mistakes can be life-threatening or costly—for example, driving a car or administering medication.

Bandura's research focuses on **imitation** (the process by which individuals copy or reproduce what they have observed) and on **modeling** (the process by which a person learns by observing the behavior of others). Imitation is regarded as one of the most powerful socialization forces. Various imitative behaviors are reinforced by a process of operant conditioning. For example, a boy may be praised for being "just like his father." The child may even self-reinforce the imitations by repeating an adult's words of praise. According to Bandura, models influence others mainly by providing information rather than by eliciting matching behavior, so that learning can occur without even once performing the model's behavior.

In recent years, Bandura's theory has become more cognitive, and he now calls his theory a "social cognitive theory." Learning is defined as "knowledge acquisition through cognitive processing information" (Bandura, 1971, p. xii). For example, the effects of television on children depend on both cognitive and imitative processes. Whether the child can comprehend the story affects the child's perceptions of the model and the tendency to imitate the model. (It is interesting to note that Bandura's research explored the concerns regarding the influence of televised violence.)

Social learning theory often is applied when nurses teach clients new skills necessary for their self-care by providing information and, when necessary, modeling how to perform the new skill. For example, nurses may apply social learning theory when teaching clients how to

- Administer an injection
- Change a wound dressing
- Change a suprapubic catheter
- Use assistive technology devices.

HUMANISTIC LEARNING THEORY **Humanistic learning theory** focuses on both cognitive and affective qualities of the learner. According to humanistic theory, learning is believed to be self-motivated, self-initiated, and self-evaluated. Each individual is viewed as a unique composite of biologic, psychologic, social, cultural, and spiritual factors. Learning focuses on self-development and achieving full potential; it is most likely to occur when the information or skill being learned is relevant to the learner. Autonomy and self-determination are important; the learner identifies the learning needs and takes the initiative to meet these needs. The learner is an active participant and takes responsibility for meeting individual learning needs.

Prominent members of this school of thought include Maslow and Rogers. Maslow's hierarchy of needs suggests a way of prioritizing nursing interventions so that physiologic needs are met first, followed by safety and security needs, love and belonging needs, esteem and self-esteem needs, and ultimately, growth needs (see Concept 28, Stress and Coping). Rogers was particularly concerned with personalized approaches. He emphasized that independence, creativity, and self-reliance are all facilitated when self-criticism and self-evaluation are of primary importance; evaluation by others is of secondary importance.

The major attributes of humanistic learning theory are its focus on the feelings and attitudes of learners, on the importance of the individual in identifying learning needs and taking responsibility for them, and on the self-motivation of the learners to work toward self-reliance and independence. Nurses applying humanistic theory will

- Convey empathy in the nurse–client relationship.
- Encourage the learner to establish goals and promote self-directed learning.
- Encourage active learning by serving as a facilitator, mentor, or resource for the learner.
- Use active learning strategies to assist the client's adoption of new behavior.
- Expose the learner to new relevant information and ask appropriate questions to encourage the learner to seek answers.

GAGNE'S INFORMATION PROCESSING THEORY Gagne (1974) postulates eight levels of intellectual skills: (1) signal; (2) stimulus-response; (3) chaining, which involves at least two stimulus-response connections; (4) verbal association, which involves assembling verbal chains from previous learning; (5) multiple discrimination involving differentiated responses to variable stimuli; (6) concept formation, which involves identifying and responding to a class of objects that serve as stimuli; (7) principle formation, which involves applying a principle that is made up of at least one chain of two or more concepts; and (8) problem solving, which involves processing at least two or more principles to produce a higher-level principle.

CATEGORIZATION According to Bruner (1966), perception, conceptualizing, learning, and decision making all depend on categorizing information. People interpret information in terms of the similarities and differences detected, and they arrange the information in related categories. For example, the human body contains hundreds of bones. By categorizing them into major bone types (e.g., long bones and flat bones) or areas of the body (e.g., bones of the head, bones of the hand, and vertebrae), it is easier to learn them. This theory of cognitive learning emphasizes the formation of a coding system. These systems serve to facilitate transfer, enhance retention, and increase problem-solving motivation. Bruner advocates discovery-oriented learning to help students discover relationships between categories. Bruner's work is sometimes considered to be among the theories of the constructivists.

CONSTRUCTIVISM **Constructivism** is a relatively recent term. It represents a collection of theories with the common thread of individuals actively constructing knowledge in order to solve realistic problems, often in collaboration with others. The constructivist described learning as a change in meaning constructed from experience. Knowledge becomes an individual interpretation of experience; learning is the construction of new interpretations. Constructivists encourage learning inquiry, acknowledge the critical role of experience in learning, and encourage cooperative learning. Constructivist theory is applicable to learning with technology.

The ideas of constructivism emerged with Dewey and continued with Bruner (learning as discovery). Gagne, Bruner, and Ausubel, as well as the social development theorist Vygotsky and the social learning theorist Bandura, are associated with the constructivists; however, their focus is more on the learning, not the teaching, with language as a process.

MULTIPLE INTELLIGENCE Early psychologists gauged intelligence by use of the intelligence quotient, or IQ. They felt that intelligence at too low a level inhibited individuals from participating in intellectually demanding learning situations and that intelligence at a higher level indicated a genius. Those in between were considered to be normal. Many individuals were incorrectly labeled and, as a result, were never encouraged to reach higher potential.

Today, new theories have emerged disputing IQ as the only indicator of intelligence, arguing that intelligence has a number of dimensions and, contrary to previous thinking, is not fixed and unchangeable by training. Howard Gardner, head of the Project of Human Potential at Harvard, has presented a theory of multiple intelligence. This is based on observations of how brain damage from a stroke might affect one area, such as language, while other areas of mental functioning remain intact. Gardner (1983) first cited seven intelligences:

1. Linguistic
2. Musical/rhythmic (music)
3. Logical/mathematical
4. Spatial (visual)
5. Body/kinesthetic/movement (body)
6. Personal
7. Symbols as intellectual strengths or ways of knowing.

Gardner has since added an eighth intelligence: naturalist. Gardner offers a fresh perspective to learning.

Factors Affecting Learning

Many factors can facilitate or inhibit a client's ability to learn, such as stress level, effects of medication, fatigue, or pain. The nurse should be aware of these factors, particularly when available teaching time is limited.

FACTORS FACILITATING LEARNING A number of factors promote learning. While these factors are common to all people, how they promote learning in the individual learner will vary. What motivates one individual to learn, for example, may not motivate another individual at all.

Motivation **Motivation to learn** is the desire to learn. It greatly influences how quickly, and how much, a person learns. Motivation is generally greatest when a person recognizes a need and believes the need will be met through learning. It is not enough for the need to be identified and verbalized by the nurse; it must be experienced by the client. Often the nurse's task is to help the client work through the problem and identify the need. Sometimes clients or support people need help identifying information relevant to their situation before they can see a need. For instance, clients with heart disease may need to know the effects of smoking before they recognize the need to stop smoking. Similarly, adolescents may need to know the consequences of an untreated sexually transmitted disease before they see the need for treatment.

Readiness **Readiness to learn** is the demonstration of behaviors or cues that reflect the learner's motivation to learn at a specific time. Readiness reflects not only the desire or willingness to learn but also the ability to learn at a specific time. The nurse's role is often to encourage the development of readiness. For example, a client may want to learn self-care during a dressing change, but if the client is experiencing pain or discomfort, he or she may not be able to learn. In this case, the nurse can provide pain medication to make the client more comfortable and more able to learn.

Active Involvement When the learner is actively involved in the process of learning, learning becomes more meaningful. If the learner actively participates in planning and discussion, the learner will learn more quickly and retain more information (Figure 39–1 ■). Active learning promotes critical thinking, enabling learners to solve problems more effectively. Clients who are actively involved in learning about their health care may be more able to apply the learning to their own situation. For example, clients who are actively involved in learning about their therapeutic diets may be more able to apply the principles being taught to their cultural food preferences and usual eating habits. Passive learning, such as listening to a lecture or watching a film, does not foster optimal learning.

Relevance Clients learn more quickly, and retain what they learn better, when what they are learning is personally relevant to them. It also helps when they can connect the new knowledge to that which they already know or have experienced. For example, if a client is diagnosed with hypertension, is overweight, and has symptoms of headaches and fatigue, he is more likely to understand the need to lose weight if he remembers having more energy when he weighed less. The nurse needs to validate the relevance of learning with the client throughout the learning process.

Feedback Feedback is information regarding a person's performance in relation to a desired goal. It has to be meaningful to the learner. Feedback that accompanies the practice of psychomotor skills helps the person to learn those skills. Nurses provide positive feedback regarding desired behavior through praise, positively worded corrections, and suggestions of alternative methods. Negative feedback, such as ridicule, anger, or sarcasm, can lead people to withdraw from learning. Such feedback, viewed as a type of punishment, may cause the client to avoid the teacher in order to avoid punishment.

Nonjudgmental Support People learn best when they believe they are accepted and will not be judged. The person who expects to be judged as a "poor" or "good" client will not learn as well as the person who feels no such threat. Once learners have succeeded in accomplishing a task or understanding a concept, they gain self-confidence in their ability to learn. This reduces their anxiety about failure and can motivate greater learning. For

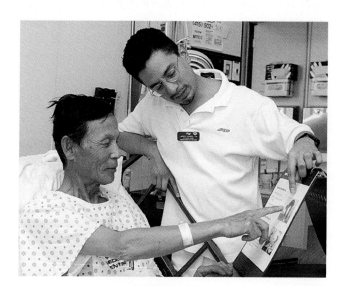

Figure 39–1 ■ Learning is facilitated when the client is interested and actively involved.

example, when the nurse cares for a client who did not graduate from high school, it is important that the nurse independently assess the client's ability to learn, and not make a judgment about the client's ability based on education level. Completing high school is an indication of the client's level of formal education, but not an indication of the client's intellect or ability to learn. The client may be highly intelligent and self-taught, so the nurse must begin by assessing the client's ability to learn.

Simple to Complex Learning is facilitated by material that is logically organized and proceeds from the simple to the complex. Such organization enables the learner to comprehend new information, assimilate it with previous learning, and form new understandings. Of course, *simple* and *complex* are relative terms, depending on the level at which the person is learning. What is simple for one person may be complex for another.

Repetition Repetition of key concepts and facts facilitates retention of newly learned material. Practice of psychomotor skills (particularly with feedback from the nurse) improves performance of those skills and facilitates their transfer to another setting.

Timing People retain information and psychomotor skills best when there is a short time interval between learning and using what they learn; the longer the time interval, the easier it is for people to forget what they have learned. For example,

a client who is only shown literature and videotapes about administering insulin but is not permitted to administer his or her own insulin until discharge from the hospital is unlikely to remember what was learned. However, giving his or her own injections while in the hospital (and with feedback from the nurse) enhances the client's learning.

Environment An optimal learning environment facilitates learning by reducing distraction and providing physical and psychologic comfort. It has adequate lighting that is free from glare, a comfortable room temperature, and good ventilation. Most students know what it is like to try to learn in a hot, stuffy room; the consequent drowsiness interferes with concentration. Noise can also distract the student and interfere with listening and thinking. To facilitate learning in a hospital setting, nurses should choose a time when no visitors are present and interruptions are unlikely.

In some situations, privacy during the learning process is essential. For example, when a client is learning to change a colostomy bag, the presence of others can be embarrassing and thus interfere with learning. However, when a client is particularly anxious, having a support person present may give the client confidence.

FACTORS INHIBITING LEARNING Many factors inhibit learning. Some of the most common barriers to learning are described next and in Table 39–2.

TABLE 39–2 Barriers to Learning

BARRIER	EXPLANATION	NURSING IMPLICATIONS
Acute illness	Client requires all resources and energy to cope with illness.	Defer teaching until client is less ill.
Pain	Pain decreases ability to concentrate.	Conduct pain assessment before teaching.
Prognosis	Client can be preoccupied with illness and unable to concentrate on new information.	Defer teaching to a better time.
Biorhythms	Mental and physical performances have a circadian rhythm.	Adapt time of teaching to suit client.
Emotion (e.g., anxiety, denial, depression, or grief)	Emotions require energy and distract from learning.	Deal with emotions and possible misinformation first.
Language	Client may not be fluent in the nurse's language.	Obtain services of an interpreter or nurse with appropriate language skills.
Age		
Older adults	Vision, hearing, and motor control can be impaired in older adults.	Consider sensory and motor deficits, and adapt in teaching plan.
Children	Children have a shorter attention span and vocabulary differences.	Plan shorter and more active learning episodes.
Culture/religion	There may be cultural or religious restrictions on certain types of knowledge (e.g., birth control information).	Assess the client's cultural/religious needs when planning learning activities.
Physical disability	Visual, hearing, sensory, or motor impairments may interfere with a client's ability to learn.	Plan teaching activities appropriate to the learner's physical abilities. For example, provide audio learning tools for the client who is blind or large-print materials for the client whose vision is impaired.
Mental disability	Impaired cognitive ability may affect the client's capacity for learning.	Assess client's capacity for learning, and plan teaching activities to complement the client's ability while planning more complex learning for the client's caregivers.

Emotions   Emotions such as fear, anger, and depression can impede learning. A high level of anxiety resulting in agitation and the inability to focus or concentrate can also inhibit learning. Clients or families who are experiencing extreme emotional states may not hear spoken words or may retain only part of the communication. Emotional responses such as fear and anxiety decrease with information that relieves uncertainty. Medications may be prescribed for clients, or even families, who are extremely distraught in order to reduce their anxiety and put them in an emotional state in which understanding or learning can occur.

Physiologic Events   Physiologic events such as a critical illness, pain, or sensory deficits inhibit learning. Because the client cannot concentrate and apply energy to learning, the learning itself is impaired. The nurse should try to reduce the physiologic barriers to learning as much as possible before teaching. For clients experiencing a physiologic event, analgesics and rest before teaching is often helpful.

Cultural Aspects   Cultural barriers to learning arise when the client's language, beliefs, or values are different from those of the health care team. The most obvious barrier is that of language: The client who does not understand the nurse's language may learn very little. Another impediment to learning is differing values held by the client and the health care team. For example, if a client comes from a culture that views being overweight or "plump" as positive, the nurse negotiates with the client to determine an acceptable weight, and they develop a plan together (Purnell & Paulanka, 2005). Western medicine also may conflict with a client's cultural healing beliefs and practices. To be effective, nurses must be culturally sensitive and competent; otherwise, the client may be partially or totally noncompliant with recommended treatments.

Psychomotor Ability   It is important that the nurse be aware of a client's psychomotor ability when planning teaching. Psychomotor skills can be affected by health. For example, an older client who has severe osteoarthritis of the hands may not be able to wrap a bandage. The following physical abilities are important for learning psychomotor skills:

■ *Muscle strength.*   For example, an older client who cannot rise from a chair because of insufficient leg and muscle strength cannot be expected to learn to lift him- or herself out of a bathtub.

■ *Motor coordination.*   Gross motor coordination is required for movements such as walking, and fine motor coordination is needed to eat with utensils. For example, a client who has advanced amyotrophic lateral sclerosis involving the lower limbs will probably be unable to use a walker.

■ *Energy.*   Energy is required for most psychomotor skills, and learning these skills uses more energy. People who are ill or older often have limited energy resources; learning and carrying out these skills must be timed for when the client's energy sources are at their peak.

■ *Sensory acuity.*   Sight is used for most learning (e.g., walking with crutches, changing a dressing, or drawing a medication into a syringe). Clients who have a visual impairment often need the assistance of a support person to carry out such tasks.

CLINICAL EXAMPLE

Angela Simpson is a new mother who believes a fat baby is a healthy baby. She has grown up with this value and is being told this repeatedly by her mother (the baby's grandmother). When developing a plan for teaching infant nutrition to this mother:

1. What essential information would you want Ms. Simpson to learn?
2. How could you increase Ms. Simpson's motivation to apply the information?
3. In what setting would Ms. Simpson be most likely to learn and retain the information?

THE INTERNET AND HEALTH INFORMATION

The Internet has become a part of the lives of many Americans, allowing them to communicate and obtain information quickly. Internet technology has dramatically changed the activities of business, including health care. The term **e-health** is defined as "the application of Internet and other related technologies in the health care industry to improve the access, efficiency, effectiveness, and quality of clinical and business processes utilized by health care organizations, practitioners, clients, and consumers in an effort to improve the health status of clients" (Healthcare Information and Management Systems Society E-Health Special Interest Group, 2003, p. 4). E-health includes many aspects, such as online appointment access, billing review, e-mail access between the client and health care provider, and online health information.

Online Health Information

Using the Internet to locate health information is common. Health care online usage is growing twice as fast as any other online type of usage (Curran & Curran, 2005, p. 496). Fox and Jones (2009) report 74% of American adults go online, 57% have broadband connections, and 61% adults look online for health information. Two thirds of those looking at online health information talk with someone, usually a friend or spouse, about their findings. In addition, 41% have read someone else's commentary or experience related to their own health issue, and 19% have signed up to receive updates about health or medical issues. More telling, 60% say the information they found online affected a health decision about how to treat an illness or condition, while only 53% say it led them to talk to a health care provider and 38% said it affected a decision about whether to see a doctor. Three percent report they or someone they know was harmed by following health information found on the Internet, which has been a stable figure since 2006 (Fox & Jones, 2009).

EVIDENCE-BASED PRACTICE Do College Students Use the Internet to Obtain Health Information?

Previous studies have found that a majority of college students use the Internet, with the most frequent activities being e-mail and instant messaging. Little research data was found, however, about college students' use of the Internet for locating health information. This study examined college students' Internet use, health-seeking behaviors on the Internet, and attitudes toward use of the Internet for health information.

The researchers used an anonymous, cross-sectional survey that was completed by college students from two universities over a two-semester time frame. The questionnaire was administered either by paper survey or online. The 743 students who completed the survey were primarily women (58%), first-year (49%) or sophomore (25%), and white (78%).

The findings indicated the following:

- More than 98% of the college students in the study used the Internet, and 68% reported being very experienced with the Internet.
- Fifty-three percent reported that they would like to get health information on the Internet.
- Seventy-three percent reported getting health information from the Internet for themselves. Of this group, the majority (91%)

reported retrieving from "some" to "a little" information. About 37% of this group seeking health information felt the information improved the way they took care of their health.

- The majority of the students used a variety of search engines to locate health information. However, 89% of the students did not always find the desired information.
- The top topics researched included fitness/exercise, diet and nutrition, and prescription drugs or medications.

Implications

The research suggests that there is great potential for using the Internet for health education at colleges and universities. Campus health centers could use the Internet as a tool for health education. The results also suggest a need for training students how to search for and evaluate the health information.

Source: From *Journal of American College Health, 53*(4), pp. 183–188. Reprinted with permission of Helen Dwight Reid Educational Foundation. Published by Heldref Publications, 1319 Eighteenth St., NW, Washington, DC 20036-1802. Copyright © 2005.

Older Adults and Use of the Internet

The American Association of Retired Persons (Keenan, 2009, pp. 6–7) conducted a survey that updated statistics on Internet usage for health information by midlife and older adults. Key findings of the report included the following:

- Twenty-two percent of adults between ages 50 and 65 do not use a computer. This number increases to 51% in adults 65 and older.

- Of those who do not use a computer, 71% have no interest in learning how to use it (78% over age 65 and 63% between ages 50 and 65).
- Fifty-seven percent used the computer to research information (Table 39–3).
- Those respondents with incomes of $25,000 or higher are more likely to use a computer, and those with incomes above $50,000 are even more likely to use computers.

Table 39–4 demonstrates locations of computer use by age, gender, and income.

TABLE 39–3 Reasons for Using the Internet by Age and Gender

REASON	AGE		GENDER	
	50–64 (n = 655)	>65 (n = 358)	MALE (n = 472)	FEMALE (n = 541)
Send and receive e-mail or instant messages	64%	41%	60%	53%
Use it for work	46%	14%	37%	33%
Take online courses	16%	3%	11%	12%
Read newspapers, magazines, and books	37%	18%	36%	26%
Join "affinity" groups to participate in political, health, or social discussions	10%	5%	9%	7%
Buy a product online, such as books, music, toys, or clothing	53%	27%	43%	45%
Research information about a topic or issue of interest	68%	38%	62%	53%
Watch a video on a video-sharing site (e.g., YouTube or Google Video)	30%	12%	25%	23%
Use an online social or professional networking site (e.g., MySpace, Facebook, or LinkedIn)	26%	10%	18%	23%
Play online games	26%	13%	15%	28%
Search for a job	22%	3%	21%	11%
Do your banking online	43%	17%	34%	33%
Make travel reservations	50%	25%	46%	37%

Source: From Keenan, T. (2009). *Internet use among midlife and older adults: An AARP Bulletin poll.* Retrieved March 10, 2010, from http://assets.aarp.org/rgcenter/general/bulletin_internet_09.pdf

TABLE 39–4 Locations of Computer Use by Age, Gender, and Income

LOCATION	AGE		GENDER		INCOME			
	50–64 (*n* = 655)	>65 (*n* = 358)	MALE (*n* = 472)	FEMALE (*n* = 541)	<$25K (*n* = 242)	$25K–$49,999 (*n* = 214)	$50K–$74,999 (*n* = 123)	>$75K (*n* = 214)
Anywhere (net)	78%	48%	71%	65%	41%	65%	84%	92%
At home	68%	45%	64%	57%	35%	57%	78%	84%
At work	37%	8%	25%	28%	9%	20%	31%	54%
At a library	5%	2%	4%	4%	3%	6%	5%	4%
At a computer store	3%	—	1%	3%	—	—	—	1%
Remotely	1%	—	1%	—	—	—	—	1%
At a friend or family member's house	6%	2%	2%	7%	1%	3%	5%	5%
I don't use a computer	22%	51%	29%	34%	58%	34%	16%	8%

Source: From Keenan, T. (2009). *Internet use among midlife and older adults: An AARP Bulletin poll.* Retrieved March 10, 2010, from http://assets.aarp.org/rgcenter/general/bulletin_internet_09.pdf

REVIEW About Teaching and Learning

RELATE: LINK THE CONCEPTS

Linking the concept of Teaching and Learning with the concept of Communication:

1. How does the quality of the nurse's communication skills impact the ability to teach?
2. How does the ability to communicate with those who speak a different language impact the teaching process?

Linking the concept of Teaching and Learning with the concept of Advocacy:

3. How does the role of the nurse as teacher combine with the role of the nurse as advocate?
4. The nurse teaches a client newly diagnosed with diabetes how to provide self-care to reduce the risk of complications. How does teaching this client serve the nurse's advocacy role?

REFER: GO TO MYNURSINGKIT

REFLECT: CASE STUDY

The nurse, Martin Dalcone, has worked on the medical unit of a local acute care facility for the past 4 years. He has 9 years of nursing experience, having worked at another facility for 5 years before accepting this position. The unit is usually staffed with registered nurses (RNs), nursing assistants, and licensed practical nurses, along with a clinical secretary who transcribes orders, answers the phone, and obtains supplies. Throughout the course of an average day, Martin interacts with many different members of the health care team.

1. What teaching opportunities is Martin likely to encounter on a normal workday?
2. What teaching opportunities might Martin encounter on his days off?
3. How does teaching impact Martin's self-evaluation of his work performance?

39.1 CLIENT EDUCATION

KEY TERM

Health literacy, *2257*

BASIS FOR SELECTION OF EXEMPLAR

Healthy People 2010

NLN Competencies

Standards of Nursing Practice

LEARNING OUTCOMES

After reading about this exemplar, you will be able to:

1. Assess learning needs of learners and the learning environment.
2. Identify nursing diagnoses that reflect the learning needs of clients.
3. Describe the essential aspects of a teaching plan.
4. Discuss guidelines for effective teaching.
5. Suggest effective strategies for teaching clients from different cultures across the life span.
6. Identify methods to evaluate learning.
7. Demonstrate effective documentation of teaching–learning activities.

OVERVIEW

Client education is a major aspect of nursing practice and an important independent nursing function. In 1992, the American Hospital Association passed *A Patient's Bill of Rights*, mandating client education as a right of all clients. State nurse practice acts include client teaching as a function of nursing, thereby making teaching a legal and professional responsibility. In addition, The Joint Commission has expanded its standards of client education by nurses to include "evidence that patients and their significant others understand what they have been taught. This requirement means that providers must consider the literacy level, educational background, language skills, and culture of every client during the education process" (Bastable, 2003, p. 5).

Client education involves promoting, protecting, and maintaining health, which in turn involves teaching about reducing health risk factors, increasing a person's level of wellness, and taking specific protective health measures. Box 39–5 lists specific areas of health teaching.

TEACHING CLIENTS AND THEIR FAMILIES

Nurses may teach individual clients in one-on-one sessions. For example, the nurse may teach about wound care while changing a client's dressing or may teach about diet, exercise, and other lifestyle behaviors that minimize the risk of a heart attack for a client who has a cardiac problem. Nurses may also be involved in teaching family members or other support people who are caring for the client. Nurses working in obstetric and pediatric areas teach parents, and sometimes grandparents, how to care for children.

Because of decreased length of hospital stays, time constraints on client education may occur. Nurses need to provide client education that will ensure his or her safe transition from one level of care to the next and make appropriate plans for follow-up education in the home. Discharge plans must include information about what the client has been taught before transfer or discharge and what remains for the client to learn in order to perform self-care in the home or other residence.

NURSING PROCESS

Clients and families have the right to health education in order to make informed decisions about their health. The nurse is in a position to promote healthy lifestyles through the application of health knowledge, the change process, learning theories, and the nursing and teaching process. The teaching process shares many similarities with the nursing process (Table 39–5), including assessment of needs, planning, implementation, and evaluation.

Assessment

A comprehensive assessment of client learning needs incorporates data from the nursing history and physical assessment and includes information about the client's support system. It also considers client characteristics that may influence the learning process: readiness to learn, motivation to learn, and reading and comprehension level.

The nurse's knowledge of common learning needs required by clients experiencing similar health problems is another source of information. Nurses must constantly reassess client learning needs as the client's needs change with changes in the client's health status.

Nursing History

Several elements in the nursing history provide clues to the client's learning needs. These elements include the following:

- Age
- Understanding and perceptions of the health problem
- Health beliefs and practices
- Cultural factors

Box 39–5 Areas for Client Education

PROMOTION OF HEALTH
- Increasing a person's level of wellness
- Growth and development topics
- Fertility control
- Hygiene
- Nutrition
- Exercise
- Stress management
- Lifestyle modification
- Resources within the community

PREVENTION OF ILLNESS/INJURY
- Health screening (e.g., blood glucose levels, blood pressure, blood cholesterol, Pap test, mammogram, testicular examination, vision, hearing, and routine physical examinations)
- Reducing health risk factors (e.g., lowering cholesterol level)
- Specific protective health measures (e.g., immunizations, use of condoms, use of sunscreen, use of medication, and umbilical cord care)

- First aid
- Safety (e.g., using seat belts, helmets, and walkers)

RESTORATION OF HEALTH
- Information about tests, diagnosis, treatment, and medications
- Self-care skills or skills needed to care for a family member
- Resources within the health care setting and community

ADAPTING TO ALTERED HEALTH AND FUNCTION
- Adaptations in lifestyle
- Problem-solving skills
- Adaptation to changing health status
- Strategies to deal with current problems (e.g., receiving home IV therapy, medications, diet, activity limits, and prostheses)
- Strategies to deal with future problems (e.g., fear of pain with terminal cancer, future surgeries, or treatments)
- Information about treatments and likely outcomes
- Referrals to other health care facilities or services
- Facilitation of strong self-image
- Grief and bereavement counseling

TABLE 39–5 Comparison of the Teaching Process and the Nursing Process

STEP	TEACHING PROCESS	NURSING PROCESS
1	Collect data; analyze client's learning strengths and deficits.	Collect data; analyze client's strengths and deficits.
2	Make educational diagnoses.	Determine appropriate nursing diagnoses.
3	Prepare teaching plan: ■ Write learning outcomes. ■ Select content and time frame. ■ Select teaching strategies.	Plan nursing goals/desired outcomes, prioritize needs, and select interventions.
4	Implement teaching plan.	Implement nursing strategies.
5	Evaluate client learning based on achievement of learning outcomes.	Evaluate client outcomes based on achievement of goal criteria.

■ Economic factors
■ Learning style
■ Support systems.

Examples of interview questions to elicit this information are shown in the accompanying Assessment Interview feature. Note the number of open-ended questions in that feature.

Age

The client's age provides information on the person's developmental status that may indicate distinctive health teaching content and teaching approaches. Simple questions to school-age children and adolescents will elicit information on what they know. Observing children at play provides information about their motor and intellectual development as well as their relationships with other children. For older people, conversation and questioning may reveal slow recall or limited psychomotor skills, sensory deficits, and learning difficulties (see the Developmental Considerations feature that follows).

CLIENT PERCEPTIONS AND CONCERNS The client's perceptions of his or her current health problems and concerns may indicate deficient knowledge or misinformation. For example, the client with benign prostatic hypertrophy may be anxious about the outcome of surgery and its long-term effects on his sexuality. The parent of a child with asthma may misunderstand the need to administer a preventive medication on a daily basis, not just when the child is symptomatic.

The effects of the problem on the client's usual activities can alert the nurse to other areas requiring instruction. For example, clients who cannot manage self-care at home often need information about community resources and services.

HEALTH BELIEFS AND PRACTICES The client's health beliefs and practices are important to consider in any teaching plan. Because so many factors impact a person's health beliefs and practices, it may be unreasonable to expect a client to change his or her beliefs completely.

CULTURAL FACTORS Many cultural groups have their own folk beliefs and practices, many of which relate to diet, health, illness, and lifestyle. It is therefore important to discuss the client's cultural perspective on illness and therapy. The cultural practices and values held by clients will affect their learning needs. For example, the client may understand the health care information being taught, but the client may not act son that information if he or she primarily believes in folk medical practices.

ECONOMIC FACTORS Economic factors can also affect a client's learning. For example, a client who cannot afford to obtain a new sterile syringe for each injection of insulin may find it difficult to learn to administer insulin when the nurse teaches that a new syringe should be used each time.

LEARNING STYLE Considerable research has been done on people's learning styles. The best way to learn varies with the individual. Some people are visual learners and learn best by watching. Other people do not visualize an activity well; they learn best by actually manipulating equipment and discovering how it works. Other people can learn well from reading things presented in an orderly fashion. Still others learn best in groups where they can relate to other people. For some, emphasizing the thinking part of a skill and its logic will promote learning. For others, stressing the feeling part or interpersonal aspect motivates and promotes learning.

A client's learning style may be based in his or her cultural background. For example, clients from cultures that have a strong oral tradition may prefer educational videos presented in their native language (Munoz & Luckmann, 2005).

The nurse seldom has the time or skills to assess each learner, identify the person's particular learning style, and then adapt his or her teaching accordingly. What the nurse can do, however, is ask clients how they have learned things best in the past or how they like to learn. Many people know what helps them learn, and the nurse can use this information in planning the teaching. Using a variety of teaching techniques and varying activities during teaching are good ways to match learners with learning styles. One technique will be most effective for some clients, whereas other techniques will be suited to clients with different learning styles.

CLIENT SUPPORT SYSTEM The nurse explores the client's support system to determine the extent to which others may enhance learning and offer support. Family members or a close friend may help the client perform required skills at home and maintain required lifestyle changes.

Physical Examination

The general survey part of the physical examination provides useful clues to the client's learning needs, such as mental status, energy level, and nutritional status. Other parts of the physical examination reveal data about the

DEVELOPMENTAL CONSIDERATIONS **Special Teaching Considerations**

OLDER ADULTS

Older adults often have chronic illnesses that require multiple treatments and/or medications. Health teaching with older adults will focus on the same areas as with other ages—health and wellness promotion and prevention of illness and accidents—but older adults often need help learning how to manage their lives in relation to managing their chronic health condition and maintaining optimal health and functioning.

Older adults possess a lifetime of experiences and learned knowledge of their own. Respect this, and always have them use their strengths to work with any problems. Positive reinforcement and ongoing evaluation of what has been taught are important factors in effective health teaching with older adults. For older adults to be motivated to learn, however, the material must be practical and have meaning for them individually, especially if the information is new. Special considerations in teaching older adults include the following:

- Promote healthy habits, including in these areas:
  a. Exercise
  b. Nutrition
  c. Safety habits
  d. Having regular health checkups
  e. Understanding medications.
- Set achievable goals; involve the client and family in doing this.
- If developing written materials:
  a. Use large print (e.g., at least 14-point font) in bulleted format.
  b. Use buff-colored paper (avoids the glare of white paper).
  c. Present the information at a fifth- to sixth-grade reading level.
- Increase time for teaching, and allow rest periods because processing of information may be slower.
  a. Verbal presentation of material should be well organized.
  b. Ensure that there is minimal distraction.
- Repeat information if necessary.
- Use return demonstrations with psychomotor skills, such as teaching someone to perform insulin injections.
- Determine where clients obtain most of their health information (e.g., newspapers, magazines, or television).
- Use examples that clients can relate to in their daily lives.

- Be aware of sensory deficits, such as hearing and vision.
- Use the setting with which the individual is most comfortable (i.e., a group or one-on-one setting).
- Investigate the cause of noncompliance if it occurs. Noncompliance can result from a number of factors, including financial difficulties, transportation problems, and poor access to medical care.

CHILDREN

The parent is a child's first and most important teacher. Every interaction between a child and parent (or between other adults and children) is a moment when teaching and learning occur, often unconsciously. Sometimes the results are ones that parents desire and strive for; sometimes they are not what the parents would have wished.

In order to make parents more aware of the teaching they are doing, nurses can discuss how the parent is using the concept of a "teaching loop" and how "formal" teaching strategy may be applied more consciously to many parent–child interactions. The teaching loop consists of four specific teaching behaviors that give children verbal instruction, role modeling, and positive feedback:

1. *Alerting:* Get children's attention by calling their name, touching them, or making a noise.
2. *Instructing:* Give the child a short, specific instruction about what is to be done; modeling or demonstrating behavior can also be done (e.g., "Try it like this...").
3. *Performing:* Give the child an opportunity to practice the task, play with the toy, and explore the materials being used. Provide "enough" time, but with some structure or direction.
4. *Reinforcing:* Give the child feedback; a positive or negative comment (e.g., "You poured the milk very well" or "No, that's not quite right; try turning it this way") that is specific to the task lets children know how they have done and encourages them to continue to learn.

Source: From Stanley, M., Blair, K., & Beare, P. G. (2005). *Gerontological nursing: Promoting successful aging with older adults* (3rd ed., pp. 67–75). Philadelphia: F. A. Davis; Hayes (2005), adapted with permission; and Steward D., & Steward M. (1973). The observation of Anglo-Mexican and Chinese-American mothers teaching their young sons. *Child Development, 44,* 329–337.

---

client's physical capacity to learn and to perform self-care activities. For example, visual ability, hearing ability, and muscle coordination affect the selection of content and approaches to teaching.

READINESS TO LEARN Clients who are ready to learn often behave differently from those who are not. A client who is ready may search out information by asking questions, reading books or articles, talking to others, and generally showing interest. The person who is not ready to learn is more likely to avoid the subject or situation. In addition, the client who is not ready may change the subject when it is brought up by the nurse. For example, the nurse might say, "I was wondering about a good time to show you how to change your dressing," and the client responds, "Oh, my wife will take care of everything."

The nurse assesses for the following readiness characteristics:

- *Physical readiness.* Is the client able to focus on things other than physical status, or are pain, fatigue, and immobility using up all of the client's time and energy?

- *Emotional readiness.* Is the client emotionally ready to learn self-care activities? Clients who are extremely anxious, depressed, or grieving over their health status are not ready.
- *Cognitive readiness.* Is the client able to think clearly at this point? Are the effects of anesthesia and analgesia altering the client's level of consciousness?

Nurses can promote readiness to learn by providing physical and emotional support during the critical stage of recovery. As the client stabilizes physically and emotionally, the nurse can provide opportunities to learn.

MOTIVATION TO LEARN Motivation to learn relates to whether the client wants to learn and is usually greatest when the client is ready and the information being offered is meaningful to the client. Assessment of motivation, however, may be difficult. Sometimes, through conversation, the nurse can elicit helpful information indicating a readiness for change, such as "I'm really ready to lose weight this time." On the other hand, nonverbal behaviors such as disinterest, lack of attention, and missed appointments can indicate a decreased motivation to learn.

Assessment Interview   Learning Needs and Characteristics

PRIMARY HEALTH PROBLEM
- Tell me what you know about your current health problem. What do you think caused it?
- What concerns do you have about it?
- How has the problem affected what you can or cannot do during your usual activities (e.g., work, recreation, shopping, or housework)?
- What do you or did you do at home to relieve the problem? How helpful was it?
- Tell me about the tests (surgery, treatments) you are going to have.

HEALTH BELIEFS
- How would you describe your health generally?
- What things do you usually do to keep healthy?
- What health problems do you think you may be at risk for because of family history, age, diet, occupation, inadequate exercise, or other habits, such as smoking?
- What changes would you be willing to make to decrease your risk for these problems or to improve your health?

CULTURAL FACTORS
- What language do you use most often when speaking and writing?
- Do you seek the advice of another health practitioner?
- Do you use herbs or other medications or treatments commonly used in your cultural group?
- If you use herbs or other medications or treatments, does your current primary care provider know about these?

- What advice or treatments given previously by your primary care provider conflicted with values or beliefs you consider to be important?
- If a conflict arose, what did you do?

LEARNING STYLE
- Note the client's age and developmental level.
- What level of education have you received?
- Do you like to read?
- Where do you obtain health information (e.g., primary care provider, nurse, magazines, books, or pharmacist)?
- How do you best learn new things?
  a. By reading about them
  b. By talking about them
  c. By watching a movie or demonstration
  d. By using a computer
  e. By listening to the teacher
  f. By first being shown how something works and then doing it
  g. On your own
  h. In a group

CLIENT SUPPORT SYSTEM
- Would you like a family member or friend to help you learn about things you need to do to take care of yourself?
- Who do you think would be interested in learning with you?

Nurses can increase a client's motivation in several ways:
- By relating the learning to something the client values and helping the client see the relevance of the learning
- By making the learning environment pleasant and non-threatening
- By encouraging self-direction and independence
- By demonstrating a positive attitude about the client's ability to learn
- By offering continuing support and encouragement as the client attempts to learn (i.e., positive reinforcement)
- By creating a learning situation in which the client is likely to succeed (e.g., succeeding in small tasks motivates the client to continue learning)
- By assisting the client to identify the benefits of changing behavior.

HEALTH LITERACY **Health literacy** is the ability to read, understand, and act on health information, including such tasks as comprehending prescription labels, interpreting appointment slips, completing health insurance forms, and following instructions for diagnostic tests (Redman, 2004, pp. 30–31). Limited health literacy skills are often greater among certain groups: older adults, people with limited education, poor people, minority populations, and people with limited English proficiency.

Low health literacy skills are associated with poor health outcomes and higher health care costs (Institute of Medicine, 2004). For example, a client may not be able to read a prescription to know how many pills to take or may misread a prescription and take the wrong number of pills (e.g., "once" means eleven in Spanish). Clients with low literacy skills have less information about health promotion and/or management of a

disease process for themselves and their families because they are unable to read the educational materials. As a result, they have higher rates of hospitalization than people with adequate health literacy.

It is a challenge for the nurse to teach clients with low or no reading and writing skills. However, such teaching is vitally important, because clients with low literacy skills need learning opportunities to improve their health practices.

PRACTICE ALERT
The majority of people at the lowest reading levels will report that they "read well."

It is difficult, however, to assess a client's literacy skills because the shame and stigma associated with limited health literacy skills are major barriers. Clients may be too embarrassed to admit they cannot read. The following client behaviors may cause a nurse to suspect a literacy problem:
- Pattern of noncompliance
- Insisting that they already know the information
- Having a friend or family member read the document for them
- Pattern of excuses for not reading the instructions (e.g., glasses broken, stating they will read later or when they get home).

Many formulas for assessing the reading level of written material are available. Most word-processing programs have a feature that will automatically calculate the readability (Box 39–6). Nurses involved in developing written health teaching materials

Box 39–6 Determining Readability Using the FOG Index

The FOG index was created by Robert Gunning. It is a simple method to determine the readability level of text.

- Choose a sample of at least 100 words.

DETERMINE THE AVERAGE NUMBER OF WORDS IN YOUR SENTENCES

- Count the words in your sample (or check the word count in your word processing program). Count the number of sentences in your sample.
- Divide the number of words by the number of sentences to determine the average number of words per sentence in your sample.

COUNT THE NUMBER OF THREE-SYLLABLE WORDS IN YOUR SAMPLE

- Then count the number of words in your sample that are three syllables or more.

- Do not count proper names. Do not count words that become three syllables because –es or –ed was added.
- Divide the number of three syllable words by the total words in your sample to determine the percentage of hard words in your sample.

DETERMINE THE FOG INDEX

- Add the average words per sentence to the percentage of three-syllable words.
- Multiply the total by .04.
- The resulting number corresponds to the number of years of education the reader needs in order to successfully read the text.

Source: Adapted from "The Gunning's Fog Index (or FOG) Readability Formula." Retrieved May 20, 2010, from http://www.readabilityformulas.com/gunning-fog-readability-formula.php

should write for lower reading levels (see Client Teaching: Developing Written Teaching Aids). The goal is to have the education materials at a fifth- or sixth-grade reading level (Aldridge, 2004). People with good reading skills are not offended by simple reading material and prefer easy-to-read information. Even the simplest written directions, however, won't be helpful for the client with low or no reading skills (see Client Teaching: Teaching Clients With Low Literacy Levels).

Diagnosis

Nursing diagnoses for clients with learning needs can be designated in two ways: as the client's primary concern or problem or as the etiology of a nursing diagnosis associated with the client's response to health alterations or dysfunction.

Learning Need as the Diagnostic Label

The North American Nursing Diagnosis Association (NANDA) includes the following diagnostic labels appropriate to a client's learning needs when the learning need is the primary concern:

- Deficient Knowledge: absence or deficiency of cognitive information related to a specific topic (NANDA International, 2005, p. 109).
- Health-Seeking Behavior: active seeking (by a person in stable health) of ways to alter personal health habits and/or the environment in order to move toward a higher level of health (NANDA International, 2005, p. 88).
- Noncompliance: behavior of person and/or caregiver that fails to coincide with a health-promoting or therapeutic plan agreed on by the person (and/or family and/or community) and health-care professional. In the presence of an agreed-on, health-promoting or therapeutic plan, the person's or caregiver's behavior is fully or partially nonadherent and may lead to clinically ineffective or partially ineffective outcomes (NANDA International, 2005, p. 120).

DEFICIENT KNOWLEDGE Whenever the diagnostic label deficient knowledge is used, either the client is seeking health information or the nurse has identified a learning need. The area of deficiency should always be included in the diagnosis.

Following are examples using the NANDA label deficient knowledge as the primary concern:

- Deficient Knowledge (Low-Calorie Diet) related to inexperience with newly ordered therapy
- Deficient Knowledge (Home Safety Hazards) related to denial of declining health and living alone.

Wilkinson (2009) stresses that if deficient knowledge is used as the primary concern, one client goal must be "client will acquire knowledge about." The nurse needs to provide information that has the potential to change the client's behavior rather than focus on the behaviors caused by the client's lack of knowledge.

HEALTH-SEEKING BEHAVIOR When the diagnostic label health-seeking behavior is used, the client is seeking health information; the client may or may not have an altered response or dysfunction at the time but may be seeking information to improve health or prevent illness. This diagnosis is especially appropriate for clients attending community health education

CLIENT TEACHING Developing Written Teaching Aids

- Keep language level at or below the fifth-grade reading level.
- Use active, not passive, voice.
- Use easy, common words of one or two syllables (e.g., *use* instead of *utilize*, or *give* instead of *administer*).
- Use the second person (*you*) rather than the third person (*the client*).
- Use a large type size (14–16 point).
- Write short sentences.
- Avoid using all capital letters.
- Place priority information first, and repeat this information more than once.
- Use bold for emphasis.
- Use simple pictures, drawings, or cartoons, if appropriate.
- Leave plenty of white space.
- Obtain feedback from nurses and clients.

CLIENT TEACHING Teaching Clients With Low Literacy Levels

■ Use multiple teaching methods: Show pictures. Read important information. Lead a small group discussion. Role-play. Demonstrate a skill. Provide hands-on practice.
■ Emphasize key points in simple terms, and provide examples.
■ Limit the amount of information presented in a single teaching session. Instead of one long session with a great deal of information, have more frequent sessions with one major point at each session.
■ Associate new information with something the client already knows and/or associates with his or her job or lifestyle.
■ Reinforce information through repetition.
■ Involve the client in the teaching.
■ Obtain feedback: Ask the client specific questions about the information presented, or ask the client to repeat it in his or her own words.
■ Avoid handouts with many pages and classroom lecture format with a large group.

programs. The following are examples using the NANDA label health-seeking behavior as the primary concern:

■ Health-Seeking Behavior (Exercise and Activity) related to desire to improve health behaviors and decrease risk of heart disease. This diagnosis may be appropriate for the client who has identified a personal health risk for a cardiac condition and wants to minimize that risk through exercise.
■ Health-Seeking Behavior (Home Safety Hazards) related to desire to minimize risk of injury. This diagnosis may be appropriate for parents of a toddler who are seeking information to ensure that their home is safe for their child. The diagnosis might also be used when an adult child seeks information to ensure that the home of an older parent is free of risk factors for falls or other injuries common to older adults.

NONCOMPLIANCE The diagnostic label noncompliance should be used with caution. In general, this diagnosis is associated with the *intent* to comply, but situational factors make it difficult (Wilkinson, 2009, p. 323). Factors that influence a client's compliance with health teaching include understanding or comprehension of the teaching, the experienced negative side effects of the treatment, financial inability to carry out the treatment plan, language barriers, or poor teaching on the part of the health care team. The diagnostic label noncompliance should *not* be used for a client who is unable to follow instructions (e.g., cognitive disability) or for a client who makes an informed decision to refuse or not follow the medical treatment (Wilkinson, 2009, p. 323).

PRACTICE ALERT
The term *noncompliance* is often perceived as a negative label. Be sure to state the etiology in neutral, nonjudgmental words.

Deficient Knowledge as the Etiology
Another way to deal with identified learning needs of clients is to write *deficient knowledge* as the etiology, or second part, of the diagnosis statement. Such nursing diagnoses are written in the following format: *Risk for (Specify) related to deficient knowledge (specify)*. Examples include the following:

■ Risk for Impaired Parenting related to deficient knowledge of skills in infant care and feeding
■ Risk for Infection related to deficient knowledge of sexually transmitted diseases and their prevention
■ Anxiety related to deficient knowledge of bone marrow aspiration.

Other nursing diagnoses in which a knowledge deficit can be the etiology include the following:

■ Risk for Injury
■ Ineffective Breast-feeding
■ Impaired Adjustment
■ Ineffective Coping
■ Ineffective Health Maintenance.

EVIDENCE-BASED PRACTICE Can Animated Cartoons Increase Knowledge of Educational Information?

Printed client information may not be helpful because of low English-language literacy levels. The researchers in this study compared the gain of knowledge about polio vaccination from information presented in two formats: printed pamphlet and videotape of animated cartoons. Both formats contained the same information. The participants were parents/caretakers of pediatric clinic clients. The treatment group consisted of 96 participants who watched the videotape in the clinic waiting room in the midst of intense client traffic. The comparison group consisted of 96 participants who were given a written pamphlet to read. Both groups completed a pretest that included demographics and five questions related to understanding polio vaccine. After the two groups completed either reading the pamphlet or viewing the videotape, the participants completed a posttest that included the five pretest questions and three additional questions.

No statistical difference was found between the two groups regarding demographic information or pretreatment knowledge. A significant statistical difference was found between the two groups in posttest knowledge. Both groups scored higher on the posttest in comparison to the pretest. However, 30% of the participants in the videotape group answered all of the posttest questions correctly, while none of the participants in the pamphlet group responded correctly to all the questions.

Implications
This study shows that animated cartoons can improve client knowledge independent of the level of literacy. The production cost of the videotape used in this study was $6,000, with a production time of 6 weeks. Printed material is less costly and can be developed quickly; however, if the client does not or cannot read the material, what is the ultimate cost to the client and the health care system?

Source: From Leiner, M., Handal, G., & Williams, D. (2004). *Health Education Research.* Copyright 2004 by Oxford University Press Journals. Reproduced with permission of Oxford University Press Journals in the format Textbook via Copyright Clearance Center.

Note also that most NANDA-approved nursing diagnoses imply a teaching–learning need. For example, the nursing diagnosis constipation suggests the need for a review of bowel hygiene practices, including diet, hydration, and exercise/activity.

Plan

Developing a teaching plan is accomplished in a series of steps. Involving the client at this time promotes the formation of a meaningful plan and stimulates client motivation. The client who helps develop the teaching plan is more likely to achieve the desired outcomes (see Client Teaching: Sample Teaching Plan for Wound Care).

PRACTICE ALERT
Knowing the client's stage of change helps determine which interventions will be useful to help the client change.

Determining Teaching Priorities

The client's learning needs must be ranked according to priority. The client and the nurse should do this together, with the client's priorities always being considered. Once a client's priorities have been addressed, he or she is generally more motivated to concentrate on other identified learning needs. For example, a man who wants to know all about coronary artery disease may not be ready to learn how to change his lifestyle until he meets his own need to learn more about the disease. Nurses can also use theoretical frameworks, such as Maslow's hierarchy of needs, to establish priorities.

Setting Learning Outcomes

Learning outcomes can be considered to be the same as desired outcomes for other nursing diagnoses. They are also written in the same way. Like client outcomes, learning outcomes:

- State the client (learner) behavior or performance, not the nurse behavior. For example, "Identify personal risk factors for heart disease" (client behavior), *not* "Teach the client about cardiac risk factors" (nurse behavior).
- Reflect an observable, measurable activity. The performance may be visible (e.g., walking) or invisible (e.g., adding a column of figures). It is necessary, however, to be able to evaluate whether an unobservable activity has been mastered based on some performance that represents the activity. For example, the performance of an outcome might be written: "Selects low-fat foods from a menu" (observable), *not* "Understands low-fat diet" (unobservable). Examples of measurable verbs used for learning outcomes are shown in Box 39–7. Avoid using words such as *knows*, *understands*, *believes*, and *appreciates*, because they are neither observable nor measurable.
- May add conditions or modifiers as required to clarify what, where, when, or how the behavior will be performed. Examples are "Demonstrates four-point crutch gait *correctly*" (condition), "Administers own insulin *independently* as taught" (condition), or "States *three* factors that affect blood sugar level" (condition).

Box 39–7 Examples of Verbs for Writing Learning Outcomes

COGNITIVE DOMAIN	AFFECTIVE DOMAIN	PSYCHOMOTOR DOMAIN
Compares	Accepts	Assembles
Describes	Attends	Calculates
Evaluates	Chooses	Changes
Explains	Discusses	Demonstrates
Identifies	Displays	Measures
Labels	Initiates	Moves
Lists	Joins	Organizes
Names	Participates	Shows
Plans	Shares	
Selects	Uses	
States		
Writes		

- Include criteria specifying the time by which learning should have occurred. For example, "The client will state three things that affect blood sugar level *by end of second diabetic class*."

Learning outcomes can reflect the learner's command of simple to complex concepts. For example, the learning outcome "The client will list cardiac risk factors" is a low-level knowledge outcome that simply requires the learner to identify all cardiac risk factors; it does not suggest application of the knowledge to the learner's own behaviors. The learning outcome "The client will list personal cardiac risk factors" requires that the learner not only know cardiac risk factors in general but also know the personal behaviors that place him or her at risk for cardiac disease.

In writing learning outcomes, the nurse must be specific about what behaviors and knowledge (cognitive, psychomotor, and affective) learners must have in order to positively influence their health state. In most cases, the learning needs are more complex than simple acquisition of knowledge and include the application of that knowledge to oneself.

Choosing Content

The content, or what is to be taught, is determined by the learning outcomes desired. For instance, "Identify appropriate sites for insulin injection" means the nurse must include content about the body sites suitable for insulin injections. Nurses can select among many sources of information, including books, nursing journals, Internet, and other nurses and primary care providers. Whatever sources the nurse chooses, content should be

- Accurate
- Current
- Based on learning outcomes
- Adjusted for the learner's age, culture, and ability

CLIENT TEACHING   Sample Teaching Plan for Wound Care

Assessment of Learner: A 24-year-old male college student suffered a 7-cm (2.5-inch) laceration on the left lower anterior leg during a hockey game. The laceration was cleaned, sutured, and bandaged. The client was given an appointment to return to the health clinic in 10 days for suture removal. Client states that he lives in the college dormitory and is able to do wound care if given instructions. Client is able to understand and read English. He is assessed to be in the "preparation" and "action" stages of change.

Nursing Diagnosis: Deficient Knowledge (Care of Sutured Wound) related to no prior experience.
Long-Term Goal: Client's wound will heal completely without infection or other complications.
Intermediate Goal: At clinic appointment, client's wound will be without signs of infection, loss of function, or other complication.
Short-Term Goals: Client will (a) correctly list three signs and symptoms of wound infection and (b) correctly perform a return demonstration of wound cleansing and bandaging.

LEARNING OUTCOMES	CONTENT OUTLINE	TEACHING METHODS
Upon completion of the instructional session, the client will		
1. Describe normal wound healing.	I. Characteristics of normal wound healing	Describe normal wound healing with the use of audiovisuals.
2. Describe signs and symptoms of wound infection.	II. Infection Signs and symptoms include wound warm to touch, misalignment of wound edges, and purulent wound drainage. Signs of systemic infection include fever and malaise.	Discuss the mechanism of wound infection. Use audiovisuals to demonstrate appearance of an infected wound. Provide handout describing signs and symptoms of wound infection.
3. Identify equipment needed for wound care.	III. Wound care equipment a. Cleansing solution as prescribed by physician (e.g., clear water, mild soap and water, or antimicrobial solution) b. Bandaging material: Telfa, gauze wrap, or tape	Demonstrate equipment needed for cleansing and bandaging wound. Provide handout listing equipment needed.
4. Demonstrate wound cleansing and bandaging.	IV. Demonstration of wound cleansing and bandaging on the client's wound or a mannequin	Demonstrate wound cleansing and bandaging on the client's wound or a mannequin. Provide handout describing procedure for cleansing and bandaging wound.
5. Describe appropriate action if questions or complications arise.	V. Resources available for client questions include health clinic and emergency department	Discuss available resources. Provide handout listing available resources and follow-up treatment plan.
6. Identify date, time, and location of follow-up appointment for suture removal.	VI. Follow-up treatment plan: where and when	Provide written instructions.

Evaluation: The client will
1. Respond to questions regarding self-care of wound.
2. Return demonstration of wound cleansing and bandaging.
3. State contact person and telephone number to obtain assistance.
4. State date, time, and location of follow-up appointment.

- Consistent with information the nurse is teaching
- Selected with consideration of how much time and what resources are available for teaching.

Selecting Teaching Strategies
The method of teaching that the nurse chooses should be suited to the individual and to the material to be learned (Figure 39–2 ■). For example:

- The individual who cannot read will not benefit from written material, but may need to review a video or receive a demonstration.
- A discussion is usually not the best strategy for teaching how to give an injection.
- A nurse using group discussion for teaching should be a competent group leader.

As stated earlier, some people are visually oriented and learn best through seeing; others learn best through hearing and having the skill explained. Table 39–6 lists selected teaching strategies.

Organizing Learning Experiences
To save nurses time in constructing their own teaching guides, some health agencies have developed guides for teaching sessions that nurses commonly give to clients. These guides standardize content and teaching methods and make it easier for the nurse to plan and implement client teaching. Standardized teaching plans also ensure consistency of content, thereby decreasing the risk of confusion if different practices are taught. For example, when teaching infant bathing, the nurse on the unit should be consistent about which soaps are appropriate

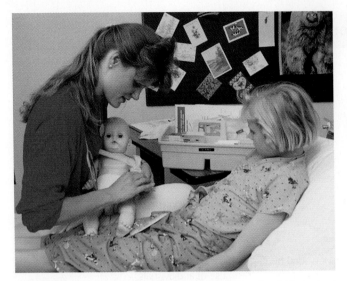

Figure 39–2 ■ Teaching materials and strategies should be suited to the client's age and learning abilities.

for the infant's bath and distinguish those that are not. Whether the nurse is implementing a plan devised by another or developing an individualized teaching plan, some guidelines can help the nurse sequence the learning experience:

- Start with something the learner is concerned about (e.g., before learning how to administer insulin to himself, an adolescent wants to know how to adjust his lifestyle and yet still play football).
- Discover what the learner knows, and then proceed to the unknown. This gives the learner confidence. Sometimes you will not know the client's knowledge or skill base and will need to elicit this information either by asking questions or by having the client fill out a form (e.g., a pretest).
- Address early any area that is causing the client anxiety. A high level of anxiety can impair concentration in other areas. For example, a woman who is highly anxious about her fear of the needle breaking off into the skin may not be able to learn how to self-administer an insulin injection until her fear is resolved.
- Teach the basics before proceeding to the variations or adjustments (e.g., simple to complex). It is confusing to have to consider possible adjustments and variations before learners master the basic concepts. For example, when teaching a female client how to insert a retention catheter, it is best to teach the basic procedure before teaching any adjustments that might be needed if the catheter stops draining after insertion.
- Schedule time for review of content and questions the client(s) may have in order to clarify information.

PRACTICE ALERT
If the client has no questions, you can help introduce questions by saying, "A few frequently asked questions are...."

Implementation

The nurse needs to be flexible in implementing any teaching plan, because the plan may need revising. The client may tire sooner than anticipated or be faced with too much information too quickly. Or the client's needs may change, or external factors may intervene. For instance, the nurse and the client may have planned to change his dressing at 10 a.m., but the client wants to observe the nurse once more before actually doing it himself. In this case, the nurse alters the teaching plan and discusses any desired information, provides another demonstration, and defers teaching the psychomotor skill until the next day. It is also important for nurses to use teaching techniques that enhance learning and reduce or eliminate any barrier to learning, such as pain or fatigue.

PRACTICE ALERT
Many nurses find that they teach while performing nursing care (e.g., giving medication). Remember to document this informal teaching.

Guidelines for Teaching

Knowledge alone is not enough to motivate a person to change a behavior. Do not assume that providing information will automatically result in clients changing their behavior. Learning what needs to be done in order to change behavior and acting on that knowledge are two different processes (Saarmann, Daugherty, & Riegel, 2000, p. 281). The stages of change, the person's willingness and perceived need to change, and barriers to change are important elements to reflect on when implementing a teaching plan. When a client is ready to change a health behavior and when implementing a teaching plan, the nurse may find the following guidelines helpful:

- Rapport between teacher and learner is essential. A relationship that is both accepting and constructive will best assist learning. Knowledge of the learner and the previously described factors that may affect his or her learning should be established before planning the teaching.
- The teacher who uses the client's previous learning in the present situation encourages the client and facilitates learning new skills. For instance, a person who already knows how to cook can use this knowledge when learning to prepare food for a special diet.
- The optimal time for each session depends largely on the learner. Whenever possible, ask the client to help in choosing the best time—for example, when the client feels most rested or when no other activities are scheduled. Look for "teachable moments" that may occur during normal routine care (Hohler, 2004). For example, if a client asks you why he or she needs a certain medication (e.g., Coumadin), it is an opportunity to explain the reason for the medication, signs to watch for, and if follow-up laboratory work is needed.
- The nurse teacher must be able to communicate clearly and concisely. The words used need to have the same meaning to the client as to the teacher. For example, a client who is taught not to put water on an area of skin

TABLE 39–6 Selected Teaching Strategies

STRATEGY	MAJOR TYPE OF LEARNING	CHARACTERISTICS
Explanation or description (e.g., lecture)	Cognitive	Teacher controls content and pace. Learner is passive; therefore, learner retains less information than when actively participating. Feedback is determined by teacher. May be given to individual or group.
One-on-one discussion	Affective, cognitive	Encourages participation by learner. Permits reinforcement and repetition at learner's level. Permits introduction of sensitive subjects.
Encourage and answer client questions	Cognitive	Teacher controls most of content and pace. Learner may need to overcome cultural perception that asking questions is impolite and may embarrass the teacher. Can be used with individuals and groups. Teacher sometimes needs to confirm whether question has been answered by asking learner (e.g., "Does that answer your question?").
Demonstration	Psychomotor	Often used with explanation. Can be used with individuals and with small or large groups. Does not permit use of equipment by learner; learner is passive.
Discovery	Cognitive, affective	Teacher guides problem-solving situation. Learner is active participant; therefore, retention of information is high.
Group discussions	Affective, cognitive	Learner can obtain assistance from supportive group. Group members learn from one another. Teacher needs to keep discussion focused and prevent monopolization by one or two learners.
Practice	Psychomotor	Allows repetition and immediate feedback. Permits hands-on experience.
Printed and audiovisual materials	Cognitive	Forms include books, pamphlets, films, programmed instruction, and computer learning. Learners can proceed at their own speed. Nurse can act as resource person and need not be present during learning. Potentially ineffective if reading level of the material is too high for the client. Teacher needs to select language of materials that meets learner needs (e.g., Spanish) if English is a second language.
Role playing	Affective, cognitive	Permits expression of attitudes, values, and emotions. Can assist in development of communication skills. Involves active participation by learner. Teacher must create supportive, safe environment for learners in order to minimize anxiety.
Modeling	Affective, psychomotor	Nurse sets example by attitude and psychomotor skill.
Computer-assisted learning programs	All types of learning	Learner is active. Learner controls pace. Provides immediate reinforcement and review. Use with individuals or groups.

may think a wet washcloth is permissible for washing the area. In effect, the nurse needs to explain that no water or moisture should touch the area.

- Using a layperson's vocabulary enhances communication. Often nurses use terms and abbreviations that have meaning to other health professionals but make little sense to clients. Even words such as *urine* or *feces* may be unfamiliar to clients, and abbreviations such as ICU (intensive care unit) or PACU (postanesthesia care unit) are often misunderstood.

- The pace of each teaching session also affects learning. Nurses should be sensitive to any signs that the pace is too fast or too slow. A client who appears confused or who does not comprehend material when questioned may be finding the pace too fast. When the client appears bored and loses interest, the pace may be too slow, the learning period may be too long, or the client may be tired.

- The environment can detract from or assist learning. For example, noise or interruptions usually interfere with concentration, as does a chair that is the wrong size or a room that is too hot or too cold. A quiet, comfortable environment promotes learning. If possible, the client should be out of bed for learning activities. Most people associate their bed with rest and sleep, not with learning. Placing the client in a position and location associated with activity or learning may influence the amount of learning that takes place. For instance, a client who is shown a videotape while in bed may be more likely to become drowsy during instruction than a client who is watching from a bedside chair.

- Teaching aids can foster learning and help focus a learner's attention. To ensure the transfer of learning, the nurse should use the type of supplies or equipment the client will eventually use. Before the teaching session, the nurse needs to assemble all equipment and visual aids and ensure that all audiovisual equipment is functioning effectively.
- Teaching that involves a number of the learner's senses often enhances learning, for instance, when teaching about changing a surgical dressing, the nurse can tell the client about the procedure (hearing), show how to change the dressing (sight), and show how to manipulate the equipment (touch).
- Learning is more effective when the learners discover the content for themselves. Ways to increase learning include stimulating motivation and self-direction by providing specific, realistic, achievable outcomes; by giving feedback; and by helping the learner derive satisfaction from learning. The nurse may also encourage self-directed independent learning by encouraging the client to explore sources of information required. If certain activities do not assist the learner to attain outcomes, these need to be reassessed; perhaps other activities can replace them. For example, explanation alone may not be able to teach a client how to handle a syringe; actually handling the syringe may be more effective (Figure 39–3 ■).
- Repetition reinforces learning. Summarizing content, rephrasing (using other words), and approaching the material from another point of view are ways of repeating

and clarifying content. For instance, after discussing the kinds of foods that can be included in a diet, the nurse describes the foods again, but in the context of the three meals eaten during one day.

- It is helpful to employ "organizers" to introduce material to be learned. Advanced organizers provide a means of connecting unknown material to known material and generating logical relationships. The following statement can be an advanced organizer: "You understand how urine (this term may need to be replaced with "pee," "tinkle," or other term depending on client's development and ability to understand this terminology) flows down a catheter from the bladder. Now I will show you how to inject fluid so that it flows up the catheter into the bladder." The details that follow are then seen within a framework that adds meaning.
- The anticipated behavioral changes that indicate learning has taken place must always be within the context of the client's lifestyle and resources. It would be unreasonable to expect a woman to soak in a tub of hot water two times a day if she did not have a bathtub or had to heat water on a stove.

Special Teaching Strategies

One-on-one discussion is the most common method of teaching used by nurses. However, nurses can choose from a number of special teaching strategies: client contracting, group teaching, computer-assisted instruction, discovery/problem solving, and behavior modification. Transcultural teaching also requires different teaching strategies. Whatever strategy the nurse selects must be appropriate for the learner and the learning objectives.

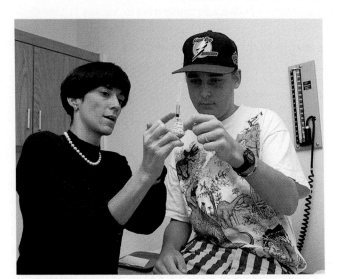

Figure 39–3 ■ Teaching activities may need to include hands-on client participation.

CLIENT TEACHING Teaching Tools for Children

- *Visits.* Visiting the hospital and treatment rooms; seeing people dressed in uniforms, scrub suits, protective gear.
- *Dress-up.* Touching and dressing up in the clothing they will see and wear.
- *Coloring books.* Using coloring books to prepare for treatments, surgery, or hospitalization; shows what rooms, people, and equipment will look like.
- *Storybooks.* Storybooks describe how the child will feel, what will be done, and what the place will look like. Parents can read these stories to children several times before the experience. Younger children like this repetition.
- *Dolls.* Practicing procedures on dolls or teddy bears that they will later experience; gives a sense of mastery of the situation. Custom dolls are often available for inserting tubes, giving injections, and so on.
- *Puppet play.* Puppets can be used in role-play situations to provide information and show the child what the experience will be like; they help the child express emotions.
- *Health fairs.* Health fairs can educate children about their bodies and ways to stay healthy. Fairs can focus on high-risk problems children face, such as accident prevention, poison control, and other topics identified in the community as a concern.

CLIENT CONTRACTING Client contracting involves establishing a learning contract, drawn up and signed by the client and the nurse, that specifies certain learning outcomes and when they are to be met. The contract may also specify the responsibilities of the client and the nurse as well as the methods of follow-up and evaluation. Here is an example of such a contract:

I, Amy Martin, will exercise strenuously for 20 minutes three times per week for a period of 2 weeks and will then buy myself six yellow roses.

Amy Martin   A. Ward, RN

July 30, 2009

The contract can be changed in two ways: first, if the client meets the contract outcomes and wants to negotiate new learning outcomes, and second, if the client decides that he or she is unable to meet the existing learning outcomes and wants to revise them (Rankin, Stallings, & London, 2005, pp. 207–209). The learning contract allows for freedom, mutual respect, and mutual responsibility.

GROUP TEACHING Group instruction is economical, and it provides members with an opportunity to share with and learn from others. A small group allows for discussion in which everyone can participate. A large group often necessitates a lecture technique or use of films, videos, slides, or role playing by teachers.

It is important that all members involved in group instruction have a common need (e.g., prenatal health or preoperative instruction). It is also important that sociocultural factors be considered in the formation of a group. Women from certain cultures, for example, may be uncomfortable participating in group teaching in which men are present. Single working parents may be unable to attend a class or discussion that occurs during working hours or may need child care to be provided in conjunction with the class.

COMPUTER-ASSISTED INSTRUCTION Initially, the primary use of computer educational methods was to help people learn factual information. Now, however, computer-assisted instruction can also be used to teach the following:

- Application of information (e.g., answering questions after reading the information about a health subject)
- Psychomotor skills (e.g., filling a syringe on the computer screen to the correct dosage line on the syringe)
- Complex problem-solving skills (e.g., responding to questions based on a client situation).

Individuals using a computer are able to set the pace that meets their particular learning needs, but a single computer can be used in other ways as well. Families or small groups of three to five clients may gather around one computer, take turns running the program, and answer questions together. A teacher or one learner may use the keyboard while the computer display is projected onto an overhead screen for a large group to see. Small groups are less able to set pace that meets everyone's individual learning needs, however, and large groups will progress through the program at a pace that may be too slow

for some learners and too fast for others. It is therefore helpful to group learners of similar needs and abilities together.

Whether using the computer alone or in large groups, learners read and view informational material, answer questions, and receive immediate feedback. The correct answer is usually indicated by the use of colors, flashing signs, or written praise. When the learner selects an incorrect answer, the computer may respond with an explanation of why that was not the best answer and encouragement to try again. Many programs ask learners whether they want to review material on which the question and answer were based. Some programs feature simulated situations that allow learners to manipulate objects on the screen in order to learn psychomotor skills. When used to teach such skills, computer-assisted instruction must be followed up with practice on actual equipment supervised by the teacher.

Some clients may have a negative attitude about computers that could act as a barrier to learning. The nurse helps these clients by explaining how the computer can help meet their needs. Matching a computer program or website to the client's individual health circumstances may encourage computer use. Providing a resource list of free available community sites for training and access may also help. For clients who use the Internet, it is important for the nurse to teach the client how to evaluate if the site is a relevant and credible source for health information.

Most media catalogs, professional journals, and health care libraries contain information about computer software programs available to the nurse for client education. The media specialist or librarian in a health care facility or college is an excellent resource to help the nurse locate appropriate computer programs. Computer educational material is also available for clients with different language needs, for clients with special visual needs, and for clients at different growth and development levels.

DISCOVERY/PROBLEM SOLVING In using the discovery/problem-solving technique, the nurse presents some initial information, then asks the learners a question or presents a situation related to the information. The learner applies the new information to the situation and decides what to do. Learners can work alone or in groups. This technique is well suited to family learning. The teacher guides the learners through the thinking process necessary to reach the best solution to the question or the best action to take in the situation. This may also be referred to as anticipatory problem solving. For example, the nurse educator might present information on diabetes and glucose management. Then, the nurse might ask the learners how they think their insulin and/or diet should be adjusted if their morning glucose was too low. In this way, clients learn what critical components they need to consider in order to reach the best solution to the problem.

BEHAVIOR MODIFICATION Behavior modification is a method that is used to prompt individuals to change behavior. It has as its basic assumptions, first, that human behaviors are learned and can be selectively strengthened, weakened, eliminated, or replaced and, second, that a person's behavior is under conscious control. Under this system, desirable behavior is rewarded and undesirable behavior is ignored. The client's response is the key to behavior change. For example, clients trying to quit smoking are not criticized when they smoke, but they are praised or rewarded when they go without a cigarette for a certain period of time. For some people, a learning contract is combined with behavior modification and includes the following pertinent features:

- Positive reinforcement (e.g., praise) is used.
- The client participates in development of the learning plan.
- Undesirable behavior is ignored, not criticized.
- The expectation of the client and the nurse is that the task will be mastered (i.e., the behavior will change).

TRANSCULTURAL TEACHING Nurses and clients with different cultural and ethnic backgrounds have additional barriers to overcome in the teaching–learning process. These barriers include language and communication problems, differing concepts of time, conflicting cultural healing practices, beliefs that may positively or negatively influence compliance with health teaching, and unique high-risk or high-frequency health problems that can be addressed with health promotion instruction. Nurses should consider the following guidelines when teaching clients from various ethnic backgrounds:

- *Obtain teaching materials, pamphlets, and instructions in languages used by clients.* Nurses who are unable to read the foreign language material for themselves can have the translator read the material to them. The nurse can then evaluate the quality of the information and update it with the translator's help as needed.
- *Use visual aids, such as pictures, charts, or diagrams, to communicate meaning.* Audiovisual material may be helpful if the English is spoken clearly and slowly. Even if understanding the verbal message is a problem for the client, seeing a skill or procedure may be helpful. In some instances, a translator can be asked to clarify the video. Alternatively, the video may be available in several languages, and the nurse can request the necessary version from the company.
- *Use concrete rather than abstract words.* Use simple language (short sentences and short words), and present only one idea at a time.
- *Allow time for questions.* This helps the client mentally separate one idea or skill from another.
- *Avoid the use of medical terminology or health care language.* For example, avoid phrases such as "taking your vital signs" or "apical pulse." Rather, nurses should say they are going to take a blood pressure or listen to the client's heart.
- *If understanding another's pronunciation is a problem, validate brief information in writing.* For example, during assessments, write down numbers, words, or phrases, and have the client read them to verify accuracy.
- *Use humor very cautiously.* Meaning can change in the translation process.
- *Do not use slang words or colloquialisms.* These may be interpreted literally.
- *Do not assume that a client who nods, uses eye contact, or smiles is indicating an understanding of what is being taught.* These responses may simply be the client's way of indicating respect. The client may feel that asking the nurse questions or stating a lack of understanding is inappropriate because it might embarrass the nurse or cause the nurse to "lose face."
- *Invite and encourage questions during teaching.* Let clients know they are urged to ask questions and be involved in making information clearer. When asking questions to evaluate client understanding avoid asking negative questions. These can be interpreted differently by people for whom English is a second language. For example, "Do you understand how far you can bend your hip after surgery?" is better than the negative question "You don't understand how far you can bend your hip after surgery, do you?" With particularly difficult information or skills teaching, the nurse might say, "Most people have some trouble with this. May I please help you go through this one more time?" In some cultures, expressing a need is not appropriate, and expressing confusion or asking to be shown something again is considered to be rude.
- *When explaining procedures or functioning related to personal areas of the body, it may be appropriate to have a nurse of the same sex do the teaching.* Because of modesty concerns in many cultures and beliefs about what is considered to be appropriate and inappropriate male–female interaction, it is wise to have a female nurse teach a female client about personal care, birth control, sexually transmitted diseases, and other potentially sensitive areas. If a translator is needed during explanation of procedures or teaching, the translator should also be female.
- *Include the family in planning and teaching.* This promotes trust and mutual respect. Identify the authoritative family member, and incorporate that person into the planning and teaching in order to promote compliance and support of health teaching. In some cultures, the male head of household is the critical family member to include in health teaching; in other cultures, it is the eldest female member. (See the Focus on Diversity and Culture feature that follows.)
- *Consider the client's time orientation.* The client may be more oriented to the present than the nurse. Cultures with a predominant orientation to the present include the Mexican American, Navajo Native American, Appalachian, Eskimo, and Filipino American cultures. Preventing future problems may be less significant for these clients than for others, so teaching prevention may be more difficult. For example, teaching a client why and when to take medications may be more difficult if the client is oriented to the present. In such instances, the nurse can emphasize preventing short-term problems rather than long-term problems. Failure to keep clinic appointments or to arrive on time is common in clients who have a present-time orientation. The nurse can help by accommodating these clients when they arrive for their appointment.

Schedules may be very flexible in present-oriented societies, with sleeping and eating patterns varying greatly. Teaching clients to take medications at bedtime

FOCUS ON DIVERSITY AND CULTURE Examples of Cultures That Value Family Inclusion in Client Teaching

HISPANIC AMERICANS

- Because of the value of family, it is important for the nurse to direct teaching to include all interested family members. Hispanic families provide support to each other, and decision making is usually made by the male and older adult figures in the family.
- Ensure adequate space when teaching to allow all family members who may accompany the client seeking health information and care.

BLACK AMERICANS

- The family structure has traditionally been matriarchal.
- It is important to recognize the dominant role that black women have in decision making and to share health information with them.
- Grandmothers play a central role in the Black American family and are often involved in support and care of their grandchildren.

ASIAN/PACIFIC ISLANDERS

- Decision making is often a family matter. Therefore, it is important to include the family, especially the male authority figure, in the process of decision making for a situation.
- Respect is automatically given to health care professionals, because they are viewed as knowledgeable.
- Asians often want to "save face" for themselves and others. As a result, they may agree to what is being said or nod their heads in agreement in order to avoid being considered offensive or disruptive by disagreeing with the nurse or doctor. They may need to be given permission to ask questions.

Source: Adapted from Bastable, S. (2003). *Nurse as educator: Principles of teaching and learning for nursing practice* (2nd ed.). Boston: Jones & Bartlett.

---

or with a meal does not necessarily mean that these activities will occur at the same time each day. For this reason, the nurse should assess the client's daily routine before teaching the client to pair a treatment or medication with an event the nurse assumes occurs at the same time every day. When teaching a client when to take medication, the nurse should determine whether a clock or watch is available to the client and whether the client can tell time.

- *Identify cultural health practices and beliefs.* Noncompliance with health teaching may be related to conflict with folk medicine beliefs. Noncompliance may also be related to lack of understanding or fatalism, a belief system in which life events are held to be predestined or fixed in advance and the individual is powerless to change them. To encourage compliance, the nurse needs to learn the client's explanation of why the illness developed and how it might be treated (Munoz & Luckmann, 2005).

The nurse should treat the client's cultural healing beliefs with respect and try to identify whether any are in agreement or in conflict with what is being taught. The nurse can then focus on the ones in agreement in order to promote the integration of new learning with the familiar health practices. The goal is to arrive at a mutually agreeable plan: Decide which instructions must be followed for client safety, and negotiate less crucial folk healing practices.

Evaluation

Evaluation is both an ongoing and a final process in which the client, the nurse, and often the support people determine what has been learned. The process of evaluating learning is the same as evaluating client achievement of desired outcomes for other nursing diagnoses. Learning is measured against the predetermined learning outcomes selected in the planning phase of the teaching process. Thus, the outcomes serve not only to direct the teaching plan but also to provide outcome criteria for evaluation. For example, the outcome "Selects foods that are low in carbohydrates" can be evaluated by asking the client to name such foods or to select low-carbohydrate foods from a list.

Evaluating Learning

The best method for evaluating learning depends on the type of learning. In cognitive learning, the client demonstrates acquisition of knowledge. Examples of the evaluation tools for cognitive learning include the following:

- Direct observation of behavior (e.g., observing the client selecting the solution to a problem using the new knowledge)
- Written measurements (e.g., tests)
- Oral questioning (e.g., asking the client to restate information or correct verbal responses to questions)
- Self-reports and self-monitoring. These can be useful during follow-up phone calls and home visits. Evaluating individual self-paced learning, as might occur with computer-assisted instruction, often incorporates self-monitoring.

The acquisition of psychomotor skills is best evaluated by observing how well the client carries out a procedure, such as self-administration of insulin. However, affective learning is more difficult to evaluate. Whether attitudes or values have been learned may be inferred by listening to the client's responses to questions, noting how the client speaks about relevant subjects, and observing the client's behavior that expresses feelings and values. For example, have parents learned to value health sufficiently to have their children immunized? Do clients who state that they value health actually use condoms every time they have sex with a new partner?

Following evaluation, the nurse may find it necessary to modify or repeat the teaching plan if the objectives have not been met or have been met only partially. Follow-up teaching in the home or by phone may be needed for the client discharged from a health facility.

Behavior change does not always take place immediately after learning. Often individuals accept change intellectually first and then change their behavior only periodically (for example, a client who knows that she must lose weight diets and exercises off and on). If the new behavior is to replace the old behavior, it must emerge gradually; otherwise, the old behavior may prevail. The nurse can assist clients with behavior change by allowing for client vacillation and by providing encouragement.

Evaluating Teaching

It is important for nurses to evaluate their own teaching and the content of the teaching program, just as they evaluate the effectiveness of nursing interventions for other nursing diagnoses. Evaluation should include a consideration of all factors—the timing of the program, the teaching strategies used, the amount of information provided, whether the teaching was helpful to the learner, and so on. The nurse may find, for example, that the client was overwhelmed with too much information, was bored, or was motivated to learn more.

Both the client and the nurse should evaluate the learning experience. The client may tell the nurse what was helpful, interesting, and so on. Feedback questionnaires and videotapes of the learning sessions can also be helpful.

The nurse should not feel ineffective as a teacher if the client forgets some of the information provided. Forgetting is normal and should be anticipated. Strategies that help clients retain information include the following:

- Having clients write down information
- Repeating information during teaching
- Giving handouts on the information
- Having clients be active in the learning process.

Documenting the Teaching Process

Documentation of the teaching process is essential because it provides a legal record that the teaching took place and communicates the teaching to other health professionals. If teaching is not documented, then legally, it did not occur.

It is also important to document the responses of the client and support people to teaching activities. What did the client or support person say or do to indicate that learning occurred? Has the client demonstrated mastery of a skill or the acquisition of knowledge? The nurse records this in the client's chart as evidence of learning. A sample documentation of charting follows:

6/8/2007 1130 Demonstrated correct technique using glucometer. Stated that she is "feeling more comfortable" each time she does it but still "needs to stop and think about the process." Will continue to monitor client's progress

S. Brown, RN

Many agencies have multiple-copy client teaching forms that include the medical and nursing diagnoses, the treatment plan, and the client education. After the teaching session is completed, the client and the nurse sign the form, and a copy of the form is given to the client as a record of teaching and as reinforcement of the content taught. A second copy of the completed and signed form is placed in the client's chart. The parts of the teaching process that should be documented in the client's chart include the following:

- Diagnosed learning needs
- Learning outcomes
- Topics included in the session
- Client outcomes
- Need for additional learning opportunities or sessions
- Resources provided.

For additional documentation, the written teaching plan that the nurse uses as a resource to guide future teaching sessions might also include the following elements:

- Information and skills included in the session
- Teaching strategies used
- Time framework and content for each class
- Teaching outcomes and methods of evaluation.

CLINICAL EXAMPLE

Mrs. Yorty is a 59-year-old African American bank vice president who is heavily relied on by her boss and co-workers. Three days ago she was admitted to the hospital with complaints of shortness of breath and mild chest pain. A diagnostic evaluation indicates that she has significant coronary artery disease but has not yet suffered a heart attack. Her primary care provider has indicated that Mrs. Yorty will need to make significant lifestyle changes in order to reduce her heart attack risk.

As her nurse, you have been requested to inform Mrs. Yorty about her disease process, diet, exercise, and stress reduction. As you begin the information session with Mrs. Yorty, you note that she is very pleasant and frequently nods her head, but she also seems preoccupied and is readily distracted.

1. How would you evaluate Mrs. Yorty's readiness to learn?
2. What benefit would a learning needs assessment be since Mrs. Yorty is obviously a well-educated client?
3. You recognize that you have a great deal of information to deliver to Mrs. Yorty and you are concerned that you will not be able to present it all in the given timeframe. What can you do to help Mrs. Yorty and still accomplish the learning outcomes?
4. How will you evaluate client learning?
5. How might your teaching differ if you were teaching Mrs. Yorty at home rather than in a hospital or acute care setting?

REVIEW Client Education

RELATE: LINK THE CONCEPTS

Linking the exemplar of Client Teaching with the concept of Infection:
1. You are required to teach a class on hand hygiene to a group of preschoolers. Discuss the teaching plan for this class.
2. How would you evaluate the effectiveness of your presentation after it is completed?

Linking the exemplar of Client Teaching with the concept of Perfusion:
3. The nurse wishes to reduce the rate of coronary artery disease in the community. Describe a teaching program you would design to address this issue, including the topics to be covered, the method of presenting material, and the group you would likely target.
4. How would the information to be presented differ if the class were being offered in the acute care facility for those with existing coronary artery disease?

REFER: GO TO MYNURSINGKIT

REFLECT: CASE STUDY

Mathew Derambasko, 76 years old, has been experiencing chronic constipation and is seen in the emergency room with abdominal pain secondary to a fecal impaction. He is married and has three children who live close by. He is retired from an upper-level management position and gets little exercise, preferring to watch sports on TV or putter around his garage. After removal of the impaction the nurse is preparing him for discharge.

1. What information would you consider important to teach this client?

2. What nursing diagnosis would you select related to his learning needs?
3. Would you include anyone else from Mr. Derambasko's family in the teaching session?
4. How would you evaluate the client's learning?

39.2 MENTORING

KEY TERMS

Coaching, *2270*
Mentors, *2269*
Networking, *2271*
Preceptor, *2270*

BASIS FOR SELECTION OF EXEMPLAR

Healthy People 2010
NLN Competencies
Standards of Nursing Practice

LEARNING OUTCOMES

After reading about this exemplar, you will be able to:

1. Differentiate between mentoring, precepting, coaching, and networking, including indications for the use of each.
2. Differentiate between actions in each stage of the mentoring process.
3. List the advantages of networking to the nurse.

OVERVIEW

Mentoring is an important career development tool that can be used by nurses in any type of setting or speciality. It has been identified in nursing literature as particularly important for career development in nursing administration and nursing education. **Mentors** are "competent, experienced professionals who develop a relationship with a novice for the purpose of providing advice, support, information, and feedback in order to encourage development of the individual" (Schutzenhofer, 1995, p. 487).

Both beginning and more experienced nurses can benefit from mentoring and from other career development strategies that involve repeated contact with other professional nurses. These include precepting, coaching, and networking.

MENTORING

Mentoring is an essential tool for the professional nurse who seeks to improve both practice and leadership skills. "All successful leaders have had mentors and are mentors. They had someone they could confide in, seek advice from, and get help from, and they do the same for others. Being influential and making a difference often are the result of learning leadership skills from others. The skill of gaining recognition and power and the ability to influence others often are learned from those who have recognition, power, and influence" (Bower, 2000, p. 255).

Seeking out a mentor is not a sign of inadequacy, but rather a sign of a professional who knows the value of support and positive criticism. "Mentors awaken our confidence in our capacity and work with us on how we view ourselves" (Klein & Dickenson-Hazard, 2000, p. 20). Mentors act as teachers by sharing knowledge and expertise; as counselors by providing psychological support; as intervenors by providing access to resources and protection; and as sponsors by promoting the protégé as he or she facilitates development of independence, self-confidence,

job satisfaction, upward mobility, decision-making skills, and problem-solving skills (Gordon, 2000). Mentoring does not just occur with new graduates; it may be sought at various points in a nurse's career (Domrose, 2002). "The conclusions drawn from the literature indicate that mentorship has some bearing on career advancement, social and political skill development, and work satisfaction" (Carey & Campbell, 1994, p. 40).

In most circumstances, mentoring has a positive impact on the mentor, the protégé, and the profession as the experienced nurse fosters the professional growth of the new graduate, who may choose to mentor those who follow. Mentoring, however, may have negative effects, particularly if there is not a good match between mentor and protégé. As this may lead to intimidation, overmanipulation, and demands for loyalty (Gordon, 2000), it is important to explore the relationship aspect of mentoring.

There are three steps in the mentoring relationship (Bower, 2000).

1. *The first phase is the selection process.* Does the mentor select the protégé or does the protégé select the mentor? Typically, the mentor selects the protégé; however, a protégé may approach someone and suggest a mentorship. Mentoring is not new to nurses, although when stress increases (such as during times of high staff shortage) there can be less interest in mentoring and less energy available to reach out to others. The mentoring process is a socializing relationship as the mentor guides the protégé. Even though it may be more common for the mentor to select the protégé, it is perfectly acceptable for a nurse who wants career guidance to select a mentor to help guide the process. Mentoring should be a win–win experience for the protégé and the mentor (Shaffer, Tallarica, & Walsh, 2000). Compatibility is important for a successful mentoring experience. Critical questions to consider are (a) Does the mentor have time for the relationship? (b) Does the mentor have the skills that can assist the

protégé? (c) Is the mentor willing to include the protégé in his or her professional activities? Vance (2003) identifies some of the important characteristics of the mentor and the protégé. The mentor should demonstrate generosity, competence, self-confidence, and openness to mutuality. The protégé should demonstrate initiative, career commitment, self-identity, and openness to mutuality. A mentor is not a friend or supervisor and should be well-respected. Protégés should expect mentors to challenge them and stimulate new considerations.

2. *The second phase is goal-setting.* The protégé develops goals detailing what he or she hopes to accomplish by having a mentor. Mentors also have goals for the relationship. They work together to ensure that goals do not conflict and are reasonable, given time and skills. Goals need to be periodically evaluated.

3. *The third phase is the working phase.* The relationship develops as boundaries are established and both decide how and what type of contact they will have with one another. Then they begin to exchange feedback and resources. Transition during the working phase happens subtly as the protégé gradually becomes a colleague, although it is possible to be a colleague and be mentored.

Nurses who wish to improve and advance their professional practice, whether in education, administration, or clinical practice, should seek mentors to assist them. Mentors usually are of the same sex, 8–14 years older, and have a position of authority in the organization. Most are knowledgeable individuals who are willing to share their knowledge and experience. Mentors often choose protégés because of their leadership or managerial qualities.

One assumes that a mentor and protégé must be in the same location in order to interact; however, e-mail may be used as well as the telephone to exchange information and resources. These methods may actually provide more accessibility even when the mentor and protégé live in the same location.

PRECEPTING

A **preceptor** is "an experienced nurse who provides emotional support and is a strong clinical role model for the new nurse" (Marquis & Huston, 2003, p. 265). Preceptors are usually assigned to nurses who are new to the nursing unit to assist them in learning routines, policies, and procedures and in improving clinical nursing skill and judgment necessary for effective practice in their environment. They also serve as role models by demonstrating how to set priorities, solve problems and make decisions, manage time, complete or delegate tasks, and interact with others. Preceptors must be patient and willing to teach new nurses, and they must be willing to answer questions and clarify the expectations of the nurse's role within the practice environment. If new nurses experience discrepancies between their educational preparation or their expectations and the realities of working as a professional nurse, the preceptor can prove invaluable by helping them cope with "reality shock." In addition to providing training, modeling, and counseling, the preceptor also evaluates the new nurse's performance and provides both verbal and written feedback to encourage development.

Preceptors are usually assigned to assist in the growth process of the new nurse; preceptors may have duties defined as part of their job description within the organization. Mentors serve in a voluntary capacity, and the mentorship process is one of mutual growth. Mentors and preceptors are important for the successful development of a nurse from a beginning care provider to an expert practitioner and professional.

COACHING

Coaching is "a personal performance-focused conversation of discovery. Not only to help nurses improve performance, it can renew their commitment to self-sufficiency, organizational goals and values, continuous learning, and improved achievement" (Kinlaw, 1999; as cited in Lachman, 2000, p. 19). Coaching provides nurses the opportunity to improve performance through four strategies:

1. Helping the nurse master challenges, remembering that success breeds success.
2. Using vicarious experience to encourage action. The coach is a role model for providing customer service, portraying confidence with peers, and dealing with difficult families.
3. Using social persuasion, as self-confidence can improve with others who have confidence, such as the coach.
4. Promoting self-care, as taking care of oneself improves self-sufficiency (Lachman, 2000, p. 15).

When nurses have performance problems, coaching may be used to help these nurses develop solutions. Other strategies that can be used in the coaching process include:

■ *Create a positive mind-set.* Shifting the focus to performance improvement rather than the problem and negative consequences.

■ *Get the facts straight.* Arriving at a clear and complete assessment of the problem.

■ *Start on an up note.* When the coaching process begins it should focus on the qualities of the staff member rather than jumping right into the problem.

■ *Present the problem concisely.* From the perspective of its effect on the team, unit, division, and organization.

■ *Ask about the nurse's perspective of the problem.* Using open-ended questions to involve the staff member, summarizing and repeating to get to the issues, avoiding blame placing and overemphasis on resentments that may come out, then agreeing on major causes.

■ *Search for solutions.* Involve the nurse by asking what the nurse would do to solve the problem; avoid the temptation to set a strict direction for the solution even when the nurse cannot seem to identify one.

Preceptors and coaches may sound very similar to mentors, but they are different. Gordon (2000) compares these three roles (see Box 39–8).

Box 39–8 Comparing Preceptors, Mentors, and Coaches

A preceptor is a formalized role with a definite time period and a focus on task accomplishment. Typically, preceptors are assigned. An example of a preceptorship is what may occur in a health care setting when a new nurse is assigned to an experienced nurse for a specific time period for assistance with orientation. Characteristics of an effective preceptor include:

- Sufficient experience with confidence and competence, typically at least 2 years
- Excellent communication skills exercised with peers, medical staff, and clients
- The ability to successfully use mechanisms for coping with stress and conflicting priorities
- Excellent teaching and mentoring skills
- The ability to identify and assess alternatives for problem solving

- The willingness to share knowledge and experience
- Experience in evaluating job performance objectively
- The ability to recognize bad habits in self and others and the willingness to make efforts to correct them promptly (Jackson, 2001, p. 24C).

In comparing preceptorship with mentoring, the mentor–protégé relationship usually occurs more naturally with no designated beginning and ending time, and each agrees to enter the relationship. There is also less focus on tasks. The mentor and protégé may not even be employed by the same employer. As described earlier, a mentorship continues over a period of time, allowing the development of a close relationship with the mentor in the role of guide over a long period of time. A coach focuses on a specific event, and there is less emphasis on the development of an interpersonal relationship.

NETWORKING

Networking is a process by which people develop linkages throughout the profession to communicate, share ideas and information, and offer support and direction to each other.

It allows for informal communication with others—exchanging information, ideas, and other contacts to meet professional goals. Nurses develop networks through contacts they make in school, work, professional organizations, professional meetings, and even from the nurse's personal life, as there may be someone who is met in a personal encounter who may be helpful later. When attending meetings, nurses should make an effort to meet other nurses and exchange contact information. The Internet and e-mail offer additional methods for networking, from making initial contact with someone who might be helpful to continuing networking with long-term colleagues. Many people feel more comfortable contacting someone they do not know by e-mail than calling him or her on the telephone.

The advantages of building a network include the following:

- Build support systems
- Foster self-help
- Improve productivity and work life

- Foster a sense of belonging
- Expedite the exchange of information
- Encourage the development of new ideas
- Generate other connections and develop the network
- Enhance both personal and professional development
- Liberate creativity and innovation
- Emphasize cooperation (Henderson & McGettigan, 1994, p. 286).

Networking is not a "one-way street": All members in a network help one another. Sharing information is one way to begin to initiate a networking relationship. This sets a positive tone. Competition does not lead to effective networking.

Networking can be useful to student nurses in a number of ways. After graduation, peers who have already found employment become an excellent source of information about potential jobs and employers. Student nurses should also take advantage of networking opportunities that may result from their participation in clinical settings. The likelihood of employment increases when a former classmate or contact from a clinical experience can provide a character reference for the beginning nurse seeking employment.

REVIEW Mentoring

RELATE: LINK THE CONCEPTS

Linking the exemplar of Mentoring with the concept of Collaboration:
1. Can the nurse mentor members of the health care team other than nurses? Explain your answer.
2. How might the RN serve as a mentor for a physician?

Linking the exemplar of Mentoring with the concept of Professional Behaviors:
3. How can a nurse serve to improve the professionalism of others in a mentoring capacity?
4. Is it possible for the professional nurse to mentor others without entering into a formal agreement, or even being aware of other's views of the nurse as a mentor? Explain your answer.

REFER: GO TO MYNURSINGKIT

REFLECT: CASE STUDY

Frankie Meningio is a new graduate and has recently passed the NCLEX-RN®. He has accepted a position in an acute care facility and attends hospital orientation followed by nursing orientation. He is scheduled to begin working on his assigned unit tomorrow and meets his preceptor on the last day of hospital-wide orientation.
1. What purpose does the preceptor serve as Frankie begins working on his assigned unit?
2. Why is a preceptor necessary?
3. What actions can Frankie take to increase his likelihood of success as a new RN on the unit?

39.3 STAFF EDUCATION

KEY TERMS

On-the-job instruction, *2274*
Orientation, *2272*
Peer coaching, *2275*
Staff development, *2272*

BASIS FOR SELECTION OF EXEMPLAR

National League for Nursing Competencies
Standards of Nursing Practice

LEARNING OUTCOMES

After reading about this exemplar, you will be able to:

1. Explain the contribution of staff development to improving job performance.
2. Demonstrate how educational programs enhance the effectiveness of an organization.

OVERVIEW

As discussed earlier in this concept, nurses must seek opportunities to maintain currency in their practice. Many educational opportunities are provided in the workplace. Nurses participate in staff education through continuing education, in-service programs, and staff development. More experienced nurses participate in staff education for their own benefit as well as for the benefit of others. For example, experienced nurses may function as preceptors for new graduate nurses or for newly employed nurses. Nurses with specialized knowledge and experience may share that knowledge and experience with nurses who are new to that practice area, either in the clinical setting or through continuing education and certification programs. Courses offered in specialty areas include critical-care nursing, perioperative nursing, and quality improvement/quality assurance. In addition, nurses in nursing practice settings are often involved in the clinical instruction of nursing students.

Nurses are also involved in teaching other health professionals. Nurses may participate in the education of medical students or allied health students. In this capacity, the nurse educator clarifies the role of the nurse for other health professionals and discusses how nurses can assist them in their care of the client.

Because each person is unique, nurses vary in education, skills, and ability. There are a few common denominators; for example, all new staff nurses will have passed state board examinations. Because educational preparation and clinical opportunities for nurses vary, all nurses do not graduate with identical skills and knowledge. Furthermore, new developments in nursing practice and technology call for ongoing staff education. One of the nurse manager's major responsibilities is to enhance staff performance through a planned series of activities usually referred to as **staff development**. In most organizations, the cornerstone of staff development is the orientation process.

ORIENTATION

Helping new employees start their jobs successfully is important to every organization. Among other things, a well-planned **orientation** (a series of planned activities designed to acclimate new employees to the workplace) helps provide new employees with important information they need to begin working. It also contributes to workplace efficiency by reducing employee dissatisfaction, absenteeism, and turnover.

Orientation is typically the responsibility of the organization's staff development manager and the nursing manager. In larger organizations, the staff member in charge of development may be the human resource officer; in smaller organizations, it may be an office manager or finance director. The development staff provides information involving matters that are relevant to all new employees, such as benefits, mission, governance, general policies and procedures, safety, quality improvement, infection control, and common equipment. The nurse manager typically concentrates on those items unique to the nurse's specific job.

Because nurse managers are an extremely important part of the orientation process, they should be specific when discussing what they expect of new members of the nursing staff. Nurse managers should address everything from standards of performance, attendance, and treatment of clients to the feedback the employee should expect in performance appraisals. Nurse managers should also correct any unrealistic expectations or misconceptions that new nurses may have regarding their employment. A thorough orientation helps prevent job dissatisfaction, low productivity, and early departures from the organization and, possibly, the nursing profession.

New employees sometimes experience difficulty integrating all the information provided during the orientation process. Managers may need to repeat information during the first few days or weeks following orientation, and new employees should not hesitate to ask questions to clarify information or expectations.

The preceptor model is one method that may be used to help new employees adapt to their work environment. (see Exemplar 39.2, Mentoring). Preceptors offer new nurses the advantage of an on-the-job instruction program tailored specifically to their needs. Preceptors also benefit from the experience, which gives them an opportunity to sharpen their skills and increase their personal and professional satisfaction.

Residency programs, usually 12 or 18 months in length, are also designed to orient new graduates to the work environment and have been shown to be effective in reducing turnover (McPeck, 2006; Williams et al., 2007).

STAFF DEVELOPMENT PROCESS

In most organizations, staff development includes orientation for new employees as well as ongoing education and training activities for all employees. Ongoing activities usually are provided to meet local, state, or federal requirements or to improve employee performance in areas identified by supervisors and managers.

The staff development process may proceed along lines similar to that of the nursing process: needs assessment, planning, implementation, and evaluation. Three main questions should be considered in assessment and planning:

1. Can the learner do what is required?
2. How should the staff development program be arranged to facilitate learning?
3. What can be done to ensure that what is learned will be transferred to the job?

Needs Assessment

The first step in planning staff development opportunities is to perform a needs assessment.. Too often, staff development programs are used simply because they have been done in the past, or because other organizations have offered them. Sometimes a program is chosen because it has been advertised and marketed by an organization specializing in staff development, and comes with pre-developed materials for ease of use. Because staff development programs can be expensive, managers must justify how an educational activity can achieve an organizational goal, such as improving client care, reducing operating costs, or producing more efficient or satisfied personnel.

Successful educational programs
- Teach more effective and efficient behaviors (e.g., a streamlined dressing technique).
- Help employees maintain currency in techniques (e.g., cardiopulmonary resuscitation [CPR] or infection control).
- Teach essential information (e.g., required documentation).
- Provide information that employees who are transferred or promoted need to learn (e.g., a nurse who transfers to intensive care and needs education about thermodilution catheters).
- Provide new evidence for practice or information about new technology (e.g., a new chemotherapeutic agent).

Managers can assess and identify employee learning needs through a variety of strategies. These strategies include the following:
- Checklists and surveys
- Advisory groups
- Quality improvement data
- Professional standards
- Group brainstorming.

Some educational programs are dictated by federal, state, or local regulations. Mandatory programs may include:
- Infection control
- Employee fire and client safety
- Quality assurance/quality improvement

- CPR
- Handling of hazardous materials (including bloodborne pathogens).

Additional requirements may be established through professional organization standards. For example, The Joint Commission (2002) requires organizations to provide education and training necessary to maintain a knowledgeable and skilled staff.

Planning

Once a manager determines employee learning needs through some type of assessment, the next step is to plan staff development programs. The planning process involves identifying learner objectives and matching them with educational methods.

Learner objectives, like client outcomes, should be specific, measurable statements about desired behaviors, skills, or knowledge to be acquired within a specific time frame. Box 39–9 illustrates learning objectives for an infection control class on handwashing.

When choosing educational methods, nurse managers have a variety of media at their disposal, including closed-circuit television, online Web-based instruction, satellite programs, competency-based programs, self-study, and traditional didactic programs. Other alternatives include using experienced staff members as teachers, preceptors, or mentors; unit-based educators; or off-site continuing education programs.

For effective adult education, the student needs:
- Material to be presented
- Opportunities to practice using the new knowledge and/or skill
- Feedback about performance.

For instance, if an individual is shown how to perform CPR correctly, practices it under instructor supervision, and receives feedback on his or her success, the individual could be expected to be able to perform CPR. Reading about or listening to a lecture about how to do CPR provides no assurance that the learner actually could resuscitate an individual in an emergency.

Implementation

Implementation involves bringing together educators, learners, and the materials and methods needed for education. Implementation of staff development can be divided into internal (on the unit) and external (off the unit). Internal sources of

---

Box 39–9 Staff Development Learning Objectives

INFECTION CONTROL – HAND WASHING UNIT
Following completion of the handwashing unit, the employee will be able to
1. Explain to the instructor why correct handwashing is important.
2. Correctly identify situations when the employee should wash his or her hands.
3. Identify handwashing and hand sanitizing products used in the facility.
4. Demonstrate correct handwashing technique.

implementation include on-the-job instruction, workshops for staff, and in-service programs. External sources are formal workshops and educational activities provided outside the organization, such as college courses, conferences, Web-based learning, and continuing education workshops.

ON-THE-JOB INSTRUCTION **On-the-job instruction** is widely used among organizations to provide staff development opportunities. On-the-job instruction often involves assigning new employees to experienced nurse peers, preceptors, or the nurse manager. The learner is expected to learn the job by observing the experienced employee and by performing the actual tasks under supervision.

On-the-job instruction has several positive features, one of which is cost-effectiveness. Nurses learn as they provide nursing services. Moreover, this method reduces the need to use outside facilities or rely on professional instructors. Transfer of learning becomes less of an issue, because the learning occurs while performing the actual job. However, on-the-job instruction often fails, because there is no assurance that accurate and complete information is presented. If the employee providing the on-the-job instruction has no understanding of the principles involved in adult learning, he or she may unknowingly omit an important teaching strategy, such as providing feedback. Another drawback to on-the-job instruction is that the staff members involved may not view it as having equal value to more standardized and formal classroom instruction.

Strategies for implementing successful on-the-job instruction include the following:

1. Ensuring that experienced employees who are providing instruction understand that doing so will in no way jeopardize their own job security, pay level, seniority, or status.
2. Pairing teachers and learners to minimize any differences in background, language, personality, attitudes, or age that may inhibit communication and understanding.
3. Selecting employees to provide instruction based on their ability to teach and their desire to take on this added responsibility.
4. Ensuring that staff nurses chosen to provide instruction are educated in the proper methods of instruction including assessing needs, planning interventions, and evaluating learning.
5. Formalizing assignments so that those participating do not view on-the-job instruction as less valuable than formal training opportunities.
6. Rotating learners so that each is exposed to the experience of a number of staff nurses or education department teachers.
7. Ensuring that employees serving as teachers understand that their new assignment is in addition to their regular workload.
8. Ensuring that on-the-job instruction is one of several types of staff development opportunities provided to all employees.
9. Ensuring close supervision of learners in order to prevent errors.

OTHER EDUCATIONAL TECHNIQUES As technology continues to advance and the number of people requiring instruction increases, teaching is becoming more efficient, and the learning process is accelerating. Many organizations are using self-learning modules, such as online classes, closed-circuit television, computerized clinical simulations, interactive video instruction, satellite broadcasts (some of which are interactive), CDs, DVDs, and long-distance learning via cable television. These methods allow an instructor to convey information in a uniform manner on several occasions or at several locations at one time.

Evaluation

Few issues in education create as much controversy or discussion as evaluation. Evaluation helps managers determine whether a staff development activity was cost-effective, its objectives were met, and whether those who participated applied what they learned in their jobs. Educators usually agree on the need for evaluating staff development programs, but they seldom agree on the best method of evaluation and rarely perform empirical evaluation. Typically, a program is reviewed at the corporate level before its implementation and then used over and over until someone in authority decides the program is no longer useful or no longer effective or, more commonly, until attendance decreases.

The purpose of evaluation is to determine whether the staff development program has a positive effect on day-to-day operating problems and to identify elements of the program that need improvement. Although designing sound evaluation tools is difficult and costly, it is necessary. Four evaluation criteria should be used:

1. *Learner reaction.* Learning reaction can be evaluated by distributing a questionnaire or survey at the end of a program. The questionnaire may ask about the program's content, the educator, the program's objectives, the teaching methods used, physical facilities, and meals. Only required questions should be asked; irrelevant data should not be gathered. Learner reactions are important because
   a. Positive reactions ensure organizational support for a program.
   b. Reactions can be used to assess the program.
   c. Reactions indicate whether the learners liked the program.
2. *Learning acquired.* Learning criteria assess the knowledge—the facts and figures—learned in the educational program. Paper-and-pencil tests are just one way to assess knowledge, whether through multiple-choice items, true/false questions, or essay questions.
3. *Behavior change.* Just because the learner acquires knowledge does not mean that the learner will apply that knowledge in the workplace. One of the biggest problems in staff education is that instruction does not necessarily transfer from the classroom to the job—often because learners are taught the theory and the technique but never learn how to translate these into behavior in the workplace. There is a big difference between learning and

doing; if behavior is not measured after the program (or on the job), it cannot be determined whether the instructional program has affected behavior or helped the employee transfer the new behavior to the job.

One technique to ensure transfer of learning to clinical practice is **peer coaching** (Waddell & Dunn, 2005). Peer coaching uses partners who have both participated in the same educational program. Each partner observes the other practicing the skill, asks appropriate questions during the demonstration, and offers feedback about the performance.

4. *Organizational impact.* The objective of many staff development programs can be expressed in terms of organizational impact, such as reduced turnover, fewer employee grievances or client complaints, reduced absenteeism, improved quality of care, fewer accidents, and, ultimately cost savings for the organization.

REVIEW **Staff Education**

RELATE: LINK THE CONCEPTS

Linking the exemplar of Staff Education with the concept of Accountability:

1. What responsibility does the nurse have toward attending staff education opportunities in order to maintain competence?
2. How does the nurse, teaching a course for staff members, contribute to the staff's ability to maintain competence?

Linking the exemplar of Staff Education with the concept of Safety:

3. How does staff development contribute to safe practice?
4. Can a nurse maintain a safe practice without participating in staff education?

REFER: GO TO MYNURSINGKIT

REFLECT: CASE STUDY

Bobby Wester is an experienced nurse working in the operating room as a circulating nurse; he also works occasionally in the postanesthesia recovery unit. The facility has purchased new cardiorespiratory monitors that it hopes to put into use within the next 2 months. The manufacturer has offered to provide a class on the new monitors. The hospital has decided to select a few nurses to attend the class; these nurses will then use the knowledge they gain to educate the remaining staff members. Bobby has been selected to be one of the nurses attending the class.

1. In addition to attending the manufacturer's class, what other actions should Bobby take in order to assure accurate information is taught to staff members at the completion of the class?
2. What things might Bobby do when teaching the staff about the monitors to improve the comfort and safety of the first clients to use the new equipment?
3. How can Bobby determine the effectiveness of the staff classes before the monitors are used for client care?

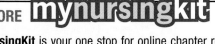

PEARSON
EXPLORE mynursingkit™

MyNursingKit is your one stop for online chapter review materials and resources. Prepare for success with additional NCLEX®-style practice questions, interactive assignments and activities, web links, animations and videos, and more!

Register your access code from the front of your book at
www.mynursingkit.com.

REFERENCES

Aldridge, M. D. (2004). Writing and designing readable patient education materials. *Nephrology Nursing Journal, 31*(4), 373–377.

American Nurses Association. (2004). *Nursing: Scope and standards of practice.* Washington, DC: Author.

Bandura, A. (Ed.). (1971). Analysis of modeling processes. In *Psychological modeling.* Chicago: Aldine.

Bastable, S. (2003). *Nurse as educator: Principles of teaching and learning for nursing practice* (2nd ed.). Boston: Jones & Bartlett.

Bloom, B. S. (Ed.). (1956). *Taxonomy of education objectives. Book 1, Cognitive domain.* New York: Longman.

Bower, F. (2000). Mentoring others. In F. Bower (Ed.), *Nurses taking the lead* (pp. 255–276). Philadelphia: W. B. Saunders Company.

Bruner, J. (1966). *Toward a theory of instruction.* Cambridge, MA: Harvard University Press.

Carey, S., & Campbell, S. (1994). Preceptor, mentor, and sponsor roles. *Journal of Nursing Administration, 24*(12), 39–48.

Curran, M. A., & Curran, K. E. (2005). The e-health revolution: Competitive options for nurse practitioners as local providers. *Journal of the American Academy of Nurse Practitioners, 17*(12), 495–498.

Domrose, C. (2002). A guiding hand. *Nurse Week Great Lakes, 2*(3), 9–10.

Edmunds, M. (2005). Health literacy a barrier to patient education. *Nurse Practitioner, 30*(3), 54.

Internet use for health information among college students. *Journal of American College Health, 53*(4), 183–188.

Fox, S., & Jones, S. (2009). *The social life of health information.* Pew Internet/California HealthCare Foundation. Retrieved January 21, 2010, from http://www.pewinternet.org/Reports/2009/8-The-Social-Life-of-Health-Information.aspx

Gagne, R. M. (1974). *Essentials of learning of instruction.* Hinsdale, IL: Dryden Press.

Gardner, H. (1983). *Frames of mind: The theory of multiple intelligences.* New York: Basic Books.

Gordon, P. (2000, March). The road to success with a mentor. *Journal of Vascular Nursing,* 30–33.

Hayes, K. (2005). Designing written medication instructions: Effective ways to help older adults self-medicate. *Journal of Gerontological Nursing, 31*(5), 5–10.

Box 40-1 National Student Nurses' Association, Inc., Code of Academic and Clinical Conduct

PREAMBLE

Students of nursing have a responsibility to society in learning the academic theory and clinical skills needed to provide nursing care. The clinical setting presents unique challenges and responsibilities while caring for human beings in a variety of health care environments.

The Code of Academic and Clinical Conduct is based on an understanding that to practice nursing as a student is an agreement to uphold the trust with which society has placed in us. The statements of the code provide guidance for the nursing student in the personal development of an ethical foundation and need not be limited strictly to the academic or clinical environment but can assist in the holistic development of the person.

A CODE FOR NURSING STUDENTS

As students are involved in the clinical and academic environments we believe that ethical principles are a necessary guide to professional development. Therefore within these environments we:

1. Advocate for the rights of all clients.
2. Maintain client confidentiality.
3. Take appropriate action to ensure the safety of clients, self, and others.
4. Provide care for the client in a timely, compassionate and professional manner.
5. Communicate client care in a truthful, timely and accurate manner.
6. Actively promote the highest level of moral and ethical principles and accept responsibility for our actions.
7. Promote excellence in nursing by encouraging lifelong learning and professional development.
8. Treat others with respect and promote an environment that respects human rights, values and choice of cultural and spiritual beliefs.

9. Collaborate in every reasonable manner with the academic faculty and clinical staff to ensure the highest quality of client care.
10. Use every opportunity to improve faculty and clinical staff understanding of the learning needs of nursing students.
11. Encourage faculty, clinical staff, and peers to mentor nursing students.
12. Refrain from performing any technique or procedure for which the student has not been adequately trained.
13. Refrain from any deliberate action or omission of care in the academic or clinical setting that creates unnecessary risk of injury to the client, self, or others.
14. Assist the staff nurse or preceptor in ensuring that there is full disclosure and that proper authorization is obtained from clients regarding any form of treatment or research.
15. Abstain from the use of alcoholic beverages or any substances in the academic and clinical setting that impair judgment.
16. Strive to achieve and maintain an optimal level of personal health.
17. Support access to treatment and rehabilitation for students who are experiencing impairments related to substance abuse and mental or physical health issues.
18. Uphold school policies and regulations related to academic and clinical performance, reserving the right to challenge and critique rules and regulations as per school grievance policy.

Note: Adopted by the NSNA House of Delegates, Nashville, TN, on April 6, 2001. Reprinted with permission.

---

of nursing practice (see Exemplar 40.2, Professional Development), and in the legal system itself (see Concept 47, Legal Issues). Additionally, in 2001 the National Student Nurses' Association (NSNA) adopted a code of academic and clinical conduct (see Box 40–1).

FACTORS INFLUENCING NURSING PRACTICE AND ACCOUNTABILITY

A number of social factors influence nursing as a profession. These forces usually affect the entire health care system, and nursing, as a major component of that system, cannot avoid the effects.

Economics

Greater financial support provided through public and private health insurance programs has increased the demand for nursing care. As a result, people who could not afford health care in the past are increasingly using such health services as emergency department care, mental health counseling, and preventive physical examinations.

Costs of health care have also increased during the past two decades. In 1982, the Medicare payment system to hospitals and physicians was revised to establish reimbursement fees

according to the client's medical diagnosis. This classification system is known as *diagnostic-related groups (DRGs)*. The system has categories that establish pretreatment diagnosis billing categories. With the implementation of this legislation, clients in hospitals are more acutely ill than before and clients once considered sufficiently ill to be hospitalized are now treated at home; however, health care costs continue to rise.

These changes present challenges to nurses. Currently, the health care industry is shifting its emphasis from inpatient to outpatient care with preadmission testing, increased outpatient same-day surgery, post-hospitalization rehabilitation, home health care, health maintenance, physical fitness programs, and community health education programs. As a result, more nurses are being employed in community-based health settings, such as home health agencies, hospices, and community clinics. These changes in employment for nurses have implications for nursing education, nursing research, and nursing practice, particularly in relationship to the nurse's competence in being able to practice within these various settings.

Consumer Demands

A **consumer** is an individual, a group of people, or a community that uses a service or commodity. Consumers of nursing services (e.g., the public) have become an increasingly effective force in changing nursing practice. On the whole, people are better educated and have more knowledge about health and illness than in the past. Through the Internet, more people have more access to a great amount of information. Consumers also have become more aware of others' needs for care. The ethical and moral issues raised by poverty and neglect have made people more vocal about the needs of minority groups and the poor.

The public's concepts of health and nursing have also changed. Many now believe that health is a right of all people, not just a privilege of the rich. The media emphasize the message that individuals must assume responsibility for their own health by obtaining a physical examination regularly, knowing risks factors for diseases such as cancer, and maintaining their mental well-being by balancing work and recreation. Interest in health and nursing services is therefore greater than ever. Furthermore, many people now want more than freedom from disease—they want energy, vitality, and a feeling of wellness.

Increasingly, the consumer has become an active participant in making decisions about health and nursing care. Planning committees concerned with providing nursing services to a community usually have active consumer membership, meaning that clients are having an increasing influence on the accountability of the nursing profession. Recognizing the legitimacy of public input, many state nursing associations and regulatory agencies have consumer representatives on their governing boards.

Science and Technology

Advances in science and technology affect nursing practice, competence, and accountability. For example, people with AIDS are receiving new drug therapies to prolong life and delay the onset of AIDS-associated diseases. Nurses must be knowledgeable about the action of such drugs and the needs of clients receiving them. Biotechnology also is affecting health care. For example, nurses are exposed to emerging genetic technology such as the field of cancer gene therapy (Cashion, Driscoll, & Sabek, 2004; Liu, 2003). Nurses will need to expand their knowledge base and technical skills as they adapt to meet the new needs of clients.

In some settings, technological advances have required that nurses learn how to use sophisticated computerized equipment to monitor or treat clients. As technologies change, nursing education changes, and nurses require increasing education to provide effective, safe nursing practice.

The space program has developed advanced technologies for space travel based on the need for long-distance monitoring of astronauts and spacecraft, lighter materials, and miniaturization of equipment. Health care has benefited as this new technology has been adapted in such health care aids as Viewstar (an aid for the visually impaired), the insulin infusion pump, the voice-controlled wheelchair, magnetic resonance imaging, laser surgery, filtering devices for intravenous fluid control devices, and monitoring systems for intensive care.

Information and Telecommunications

The Internet has already affected health care, with more and more clients becoming well informed about their health concerns. People with chronic health conditions or battling life-threatening disease are the hungriest information seekers (DeLenardo, 2004). As a result, nurses may need to help clients and families interpret information that they find on the Internet. Because not all of the Internet-based information is accurate, nurses need to know how to help people to access high-quality, valid websites; interpret the information; and then help clients evaluate the information and determine if it is useful to them.

Telecommunications is the transmission of information from one site to another, using equipment to send information in the form of signs, signals, words, or pictures by cable, radio, or other systems (Chaffee, 1999, p. 27). Greenberg (2000) explains that terms with the prefix *tele-*, meaning distance, are used to describe the many health care services provided via telecommunications. The common denominators of teleservices are distance and technology (p. 220).

Telehealth uses telecommunication technology to provide long-distance health care. It can include using videoconferencing, computers, or telephones. *Telenursing* occurs when the nurse delivers care through a telecommunication system. Examples of telenursing include the nurse who telephones clients at home to assess their progress or to answer questions, the nurse who participates in a video teleconference where consultants or experts at various sites discuss a client's health care plan, and the nurse who uses videophone technology to assess a client living in a rural area.

Telehealth does not recognize state boundaries and, subsequently, licensure issues have been raised. For example, if a nurse licensed in one state provides health information to a client in another state, does the nurse need to maintain licensure in both states? The National Council of State Boards of Nursing endorses a change from single-state licensure to a mutual recognition model. Many state legislatures have adopted mutual recognition language into statute and are currently implementing it. See Concept 47, Legal Issues for more information.

Legislation

Legislation about nursing practice and health matters affects both the consumer and the nursing profession. Changes in legislation relating to health also affect nursing. For example, the **Patient Self-Determination Act (PSDA)** requires that every competent adult be informed in writing on admission to a health care institution about his or her rights to accept or refuse medical care and to use advance directives. This law, which in many institutions is implemented by nurses, affects the nurse's role in supporting clients and their families.

Demography

Demography is the study of population, including statistics about distribution by age and place of residence, mortality (death), and morbidity (incidence of disease). From demographic data, needs of the population for nursing services can be assessed. For example:

- The total population in North America is increasing. The proportion of elderly people has also increased, creating an increased need for nursing services for this group.

- The population is shifting from rural to urban settings. This shift signals an increased need for nursing related to problems caused by pollution and by the effects on the environment of concentrations of people. Thus, most nursing services are now provided in urban settings.
- Mortality and morbidity studies reveal the presence of risk factors. Many of these risk factors (e.g., smoking) are major causes of death and disease that can be prevented through changes in lifestyle.

The Current Nursing Shortage

The multiple factors influencing the current nursing shortage (see Box 40–2) are different from previous nursing shortages. Registered nurses make up the largest group of health care providers. Fewer nurses, however, are entering the workforce, and certain geographic areas are experiencing acute nursing shortages. The supply is inadequate to meet the demand, especially for specialized nurses (e.g., critical care), and it is expected to worsen during the next 20 years (National League for Nursing, 2005).

Addressing the nursing shortage requires collaborative activities among health care systems, policy makers, nursing educators, and professional organizations. Recommendations include but are not limited to the following:

- Develop mechanisms for nursing students to progress to and through educational programs more efficiently and quickly.
- Recruit young people to nursing early (e.g., grade school).
- Improve the nurse's work environment: Provide greater flexibility in work hours, reward experienced nurses who serve as mentors, ensure adequate staffing, and increase salaries.
- Increase nursing education funding.

NURSING PRACTICE

Accountability is one of the single most important components of nursing practice. It is influenced by a variety of factors, including the individual's own values and beliefs, the values and ethics inherent to the profession as a whole, and many

---

Box 40–2 Factors Affecting the Nursing Shortage

AGING NURSE WORKFORCE
- Number of nurses under 30 decreasing
- Between 2010 and 2020, over 40% of the RN workforce will be over 50 years of age, and many RNs are expected to retire and withdraw from the workforce (Norman, et al., 2005)
- New graduates entering workforce at an older age and will have fewer years to work

AGING OF NURSING FACULTY
- As nursing faculty retire, nursing programs may have fewer faculty to educate future nurses

AGING POPULATION
- Individuals 65 and older to double between 2000 and 2030
- Increasing health care needs of aging population

INCREASED DEMAND FOR NURSES
- Increased acuity of hospital clients requiring skilled and specialized nurses
- Shorter hospital stays, resulting in transfer of clients to long-term care and community settings, creating increased demand for nurses in the community

WORKPLACE ISSUES
- Inadequate staffing
- Heavy workloads
- Increased use of overtime
- Lack of sufficient support staff
- Inadequate wages
- Difficulty recruiting and retaining nurses

---

social factors that affect, either directly or indirectly, nursing practice and accountability.

Accountability is either supported or undermined by the competency of the individual nurse, the professional development of nurses as individuals, and the development of the nursing profession itself. Competence and professional development are discussed in the exemplars that follow.

REVIEW Accountability

RELATE: LINK THE CONCEPTS

Linking the concept of Accountability with the concept of Legal Issues:
1. What is the nurse's legal obligation to the client related to accountability, and how is it regulated?
2. The nurse makes a medication error that results in harm to the client. The nurse demonstrates accountability by immediately informing the physician and nursing supervisor when the error is recognized. How does the nurse's proper accountability impact the nurse's legal responsibility?

Linking the concept of Accountability with the concept of Ethics:
3. How does the nurse's code of ethics reflect the expectation that the nurse is accountable when providing client care?
4. The nurse believes that the physician has written orders that may endanger the client. After consulting the physician, who refuses to alter the orders, what is the nurse's ethical obligation to the client in order to demonstrate accountability?

REFER: GO TO MYNURSINGKIT

REFLECT: CASE STUDY

Carol Ramsey is a 51-year-old certified nurse-midwife at Neighborhood Women's Health Specialists (NWHS). She has been a midwife for 21 years; before that she worked for 8 years as a labor and delivery room nurse. Four physicians and three midwives (including Ms. Ramsey) work at NWHS. Ms. Ramsey works 4 ½ days a week at NWHS and one afternoon a week at the Neighborhood Community Health Department.

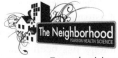

At her job at NWHS, Ms. Ramsey sees her own clients; the large majority require prenatal care, delivery, and postpartum care, although she also provides routine gynecologic care for many of her clients as well. At the Community Health Department, Ms. Ramsey sees a variety of clients, many of whom are seen for sexually transmitted infection and pregnancy testing.

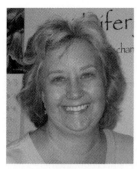

Ms. Ramsey is not feeling well this week. She has been trying to recover from a mild cold, but it has really zapped her energy. She has a full caseload this week because one of the midwives in the practice is out on medical leave for the next couple of months. Ms. Ramsey and the other two midwives at NWHS clinic have to work extra clients into their day; which is a bit tough, and Ms. Ramsey feels she is already working at full capacity. She finds it hard to do this in addition to her once-a-week position at the Community Health Department.

1. How does the nurse respond to understaffing in order to maintain accountability?
2. Is Ms. Ramsey demonstrating accountability when she comes to work with a mild cold? Explain your answer.
3. How might Ms. Ramsey's situation impact her ability to function at optimal levels? How does Ms. Ramsey demonstrate accountability for her action in this situation?

40.1 COMPETENCE

KEY TERM
Competence, *2285*

BASIS FOR SELECTION OF EXEMPLAR
Standards of Nursing Practice
NLN Competencies

LEARNING OUTCOMES
After reading about this exemplar, you will be able to:

1. Discuss Benner's levels of nursing proficiency.
2. Identify four major areas of competency within the scope of nursing practice.
3. Describe ways to promote lifelong competence in nursing.

OVERVIEW

Competence is defined as possessing the knowledge and skills necessary to perform one's job appropriately and safely on a daily basis (Makely, S., 2009, p. 9). In the past, nurses were considered able to do their job simply if they could provide care and comfort. Today nurses are held to a higher standard of competency. Each nurse is expected to achieve and maintain competency within four main areas: health promotion, illness prevention, health restoration, and caring for the dying.

AREAS OF COMPETENCY

The four areas described here encompass a variety of knowledge bases, professional skills, and expertise. Within each area, the nurse is expected to achieve competency in application of the nursing process as well as in those skills necessary to provide safe and appropriate client care.

Health and Wellness Promotion

Wellness is a process in which an individual engages in activities and behaviors that enhance quality of life and maximize personal potential (Anspaugh, Hamrick, & Rosata, 2003, p. 490). Nurses promote wellness in clients who are both healthy and ill. This may involve individual and community activities to enhance healthy lifestyles, such as improving nutrition and physical fitness, preventing drug and alcohol misuse, restricting smoking, and preventing accidents and injury in the home and workplace. Client teaching and other strategies to promote health and wellness are discussed throughout Volume 1 of this text.

Illness Prevention

Nurses engage in illness prevention in every setting in which they work. In community settings, illness prevention programs are designed to maintain optimal health by preventing disease.

Most communities offer illness prevention programs in areas such as immunizations, prenatal and infant care, and prevention of sexually transmitted disease. These are frequently taught by nurses working in school settings, hospital outreach programs, and local health departments.

Within clinical settings, nurses engage in illness prevention in a variety of ways. Many of these, such as sterile precautions and client teaching, are discussed throughout Volume 1 of this text.

Health Restoration

Restoring health focuses on the ill client, and it extends from early detection of disease through helping the client during the recovery period. Nursing competencies include the following:

- Providing direct care to the ill person, such as administering medications, baths, and specific procedures and treatments
- Performing diagnostic and assessment procedures, such as measuring blood pressure and examining feces for occult blood
- Consulting with other health care professionals about client problems
- Teaching clients about recovery activities, such as exercises that will accelerate recovery after a stroke
- Rehabilitating clients to their optimal functional level following physical or mental illness, injury, or chemical addiction.

Caring for the Dying

This area of nursing practice involves comforting and caring for people of all ages who are dying. End-of-life care includes helping clients live as comfortably as possible until death and helping support persons cope with death. Nurses carrying out these activities work in homes, hospitals, and extended care facilities. End-of-life care is one of the exemplars in Concept 5, Comfort.

PROMOTING LIFELONG COMPETENCE

Nothing contributes more to the client's safety than the competence of the nurses caring for him or her. Nurses gain competency gradually throughout nursing school until they reach an entry level when they are judged safe enough to function as a newly graduated nurse. The nurse continues to build competence throughout his or her career, with expertise coming from experience, gaining new knowledge, and improving the performance of skills.

Growth and maintaining competence in nursing requires the nurse to continue learning. Professional development and continuing education opportunities come in a variety of forms: seminars offered by colleges and professional organizations, professional and peer-reviewed journals, hospital- or employer-sponsored classes on new equipment or procedures, and formal and informal discussions with peers and other members of the health care team.

With the expanding body of knowledge surrounding health care, it is unlikely that any one nurse can maintain competency in all areas. The nurse generalist knows something about many things, while the nurse specialist knows a great deal about his or her specific area of expertise. Each nurse must assess his or her own level of knowledge and be able to identify the need to gain additional knowledge to provide appropriate client care.

Even the most competent nurses encounter situations that make them question how best to respond. Luckily, nurses are able to collaborate with each other and with others on the interdisciplinary team, sharing opinions, ideas, and information. While collaboration is helpful, and even critical, each nurse is accountable for the choices he or she makes, and must weigh all information and choose the best course of action. The nurse who recognizes that there will always be a need to collaborate with others maintains a safe practice.

Various models of the competency process have been developed. Benner's model (2001) describes five levels of proficiency in nursing based on the Dreyfus general model of skill acquisition. The five stages, which have implications for teaching and learning, are novice, advanced beginner, competent, proficient, and expert. Benner writes that experience is essential for the development of professional expertise (see Box 40–3).

Box 40–3 **Benner's Stages of Nursing Expertise**

STAGE I, NOVICE

No experience (e.g., nursing student). Performance is limited, inflexible, and governed by context-free rules and regulations rather than experience.

STAGE II, ADVANCED BEGINNER

Demonstrates marginally acceptable performance.
Recognizes the meaningful "aspects" of a real situation. Has experienced enough real situations to make judgments about them.

STAGE III, COMPETENT

Has 2 or 3 years of experience. Demonstrates organizational and planning abilities. Differentiates important factors from less important aspects of care. Coordinates multiple complex care demands.

STAGE IV, PROFICIENT

Has 3 to 5 years of experience. Perceives situations as wholes rather than in terms of parts, as in Stage II. Uses maxims as guides for what to consider in a situation. Has holistic understanding of the client, which improves decision making. Focuses on long-term goals.

STAGE V, EXPERT

Performance is fluid, flexible, and highly proficient; no longer requires rules, guidelines, or maxims to connect an understanding of the situation to appropriate action. Demonstrates highly skilled intuitive and analytic ability in new situations. Is inclined to take a certain action because "it felt right."

Source: Benner, P., (2001). *Novice to expert: Excellence and power in clinical nursing practice, commemorative edition* (1st ed.). Upper Saddle River, NJ: Pearson Education, Inc. Reproduced with permission.

NURSING PRACTICE

Nurses hold themselves accountable by weighing and assessing their own competence frequently. Nurses know that it is honorable to say "I don't know" or ask "Would you help me?" as opposed to taking the attitude that "I'm not sure but I think this is right" or "I'll figure it out as I go along." Rule one of competence when providing client care is to ask for help when the certainty of safety in any given action is missing. By doing so, nurses (1) invite opportunities to increase their own levels of competence and (2) hold themselves accountable for providing the highest quality of client care.

REVIEW Competence

RELATE: LINK THE CONCEPTS

Linking the exemplar of Competence with the concept of Legal Issues:
1. What is the nurse's legal obligation to society and the profession to maintain competency?
2. How can a nurse who lacks competence in one area of nursing strengthen his or her knowledge and skills?

Linking the exemplar of Competence with the concept of Ethics:
3. What is the nurse's ethical obligation related to competence?
4. How does the nursing code of ethics address the issue of competence?

REFER: GO TO MYNURSINGKIT

REFLECT: CASE STUDY

Tyree Campbell has worked in the labor and delivery unit of a large metropolitan hospital since graduating from nursing school 8 years ago. A new private hospital recently opened in town and the census on Ms. Campbell's unit has been significantly lower. Tonight, Ms. Campbell reports to work and learns there are more nurses scheduled to work than clients. The decision has been made to float the excess staff to other units and Ms. Campbell is asked to float to the neonatal intensive care unit (NICU). When she hears the request, her heart sinks and she begins to feel the early signs of panic as she thinks to herself, "How can I work in the NICU? I don't have any experience working there!"

1. What is Ms. Campbell's responsibility in this situation?

2. Can Ms. Campbell agree to float to the NICU if she is not competent to care for the clients on this unit?

3. What should Ms. Campbell say to her nursing supervisor who has given her this assignment?

40.2 PROFESSIONAL DEVELOPMENT

KEY TERMS

Clara Barton, *2290*
Client, *2292*
Consumer, *2292*
Florence Nightingale, *2290*
Harriet Tubman, *2288*
Mary Mahoney, *2290*
Patient, *2292*
Sojourner Truth, *2288*
Standards of Practice, *2293*
Standards of Professional Performance, *2293*

BASIS FOR SELECTION OF EXEMPLAR

NLN Competencies
Standards of Nursing Practice

LEARNING OUTCOMES

After reading about this exemplar, you will be able to:

1. Discuss historical and contemporary factors influencing the development of nursing.

2. Describe the roles of nurses.

3. Describe the expanded career roles available to nurses and their functions.

OVERVIEW

Professional development takes on different meanings in the many different areas of nursing. Some associate the term with advanced education, some think it refers to increase in experience or seniority, some view it as involvement or membership in an organization that governs the profession, and others associate it primarily with continuing education classes or offerings. Professional development encompasses all of these activities.

Nursing today is far different from nursing as it was practiced years ago, and it is expected to continue changing during the twenty-first century. To comprehend present-day nursing and at the same time prepare for the future, one must understand not only past events but also contemporary nursing practice and the sociological and historical factors that affect it.

HISTORICAL PERSPECTIVES

Nursing has undergone dramatic changes in response to societal needs and influences. A look at nursing's beginnings reveals its continuing struggle for autonomy and professionalization. In recent decades, a renewed interest in nursing history has produced a growing amount of related literature. This section highlights only selected aspects of events that have influenced nursing practice. Recurring themes of women's roles and status, religious (Christian) values, war, societal attitudes, and visionary nursing leadership have influenced nursing practice in the past. Many of these factors still exert their influence today.

Women's Roles

Traditional female roles of wife, mother, daughter, and sister have always included the care and nurturing of other family members. From the beginning of time, women have cared for infants and children; thus, nursing could be said to have its roots in "the home." Additionally, women, who in general occupied a subservient and dependent role, were called on to care for others in the community who were ill.

Generally the care provided was related to physical maintenance and comfort. Thus, the traditional nursing role has always entailed humanistic caring, nurturing, comforting, and supporting.

Religion

Religion has also played a significant role in the development of nursing. Although many of the world's religions encourage benevolence, it was the Christian value of "love thy neighbor as thyself" and Christ's parable of the Good Samaritan that had a significant impact on the development of Western nursing. During the third and fourth centuries, several wealthy matrons of the Roman Empire, such as *Fabiola*, converted to Christianity and used their wealth to provide houses of care and healing (the forerunner of hospitals) for the poor, the sick, and the homeless. Women were not, however, the sole providers of nursing services.

The Crusades saw the formation of several orders of knights, including the Knights of Saint John of Jerusalem (also known as the Knights Hospitalers), the Teutonic Knights, and the Knights of Saint Lazarus (Figure 40–1 ■). These brothers in arms provided nursing care to their sick and injured comrades. These orders also built hospitals, the organization and management of which set a standard for the administration of hospitals throughout Europe at that time. The *Knights of Saint Lazarus* dedicated themselves to the care of people with leprosy, syphilis, and chronic skin conditions.

The deaconess groups, which had their origins in the Roman Empire of the third and fourth centuries, were groups of nursing providers that surfaced occasionally throughout the centuries, most notably in 1836 when Theodore Fliedner reinstituted the Order of Deaconesses and opened a small hospital and training school in Kaiserswerth, Germany. Florence Nightingale received her "training" in nursing at the Kaiserswerth School.

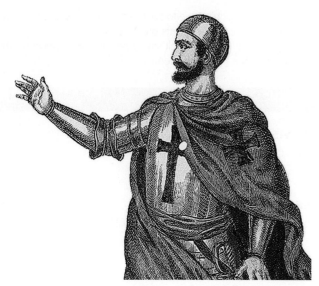

Figure 40–1 ■ The Knights of Saint Lazarus (established circa 1200) dedicated themselves to the care of people with leprosy, syphilis, and chronic skin conditions. From the time of Christ to the mid-thirteenth century, leprosy was viewed as an incurable and terminal disease.
CORBIS Images.

Early religious values, such as self-denial, spiritual calling, and devotion to duty and hard work, have dominated nursing throughout its history. Nurses' commitment to these values often resulted in exploitation and few monetary rewards. For some time, nurses themselves believed it was inappropriate to expect economic gain from their "calling."

War

Throughout history, wars have accentuated the need for nurses. During the Crimean War (1854–1856), the inadequacy of care given to soldiers led to a public outcry in Great Britain. The role Florence Nightingale (Figure 40–2 ■) played in addressing this problem is well known. She was asked by Sir Sidney Herbert of the British War Department to recruit a contingent of female nurses to provide care to the sick and injured in the Crimea.

Nightingale and her nurses transformed the military hospitals by setting up sanitation practices, such as hand washing and washing clothing. Nightingale is credited with performing miracles: The mortality rate in the Barrack Hospital in Turkey, for example, was reduced from 42% to 2% (Donahue, 1996, p. 197).

During the American Civil War (1861–1865), several nurses emerged who were notable for their contributions to a country torn by internal strife. **Harriet Tubman** and **Sojourner Truth** (Figures 40–3 ■ and 40–4 ■) provided care and safety to slaves fleeing to the North on the Underground Railroad. Mother Biekerdyke and Clara Barton searched the battlefields and gave care to injured and dying soldiers. Noted authors Walt Whitman and Louisa May Alcott volunteered as nurses to give care to injured soldiers in military hospitals. Another woman leader who provided nursing care during the Civil War was *Dorothea Dix*. She became the Union's superintendent of female nurses responsible for recruiting nurses and supervising the nursing care of all women nurses working in the army hospitals.

The arrival of World War I resulted in American, British, and French women rushing to volunteer their nursing services. These nurses endured harsh environments and treated injuries never seen before. A monument, entitled "The Spirit of Nursing," stands in Arlington National Cemetery (Figure 40–5 ■). It honors the nurses who served in the U.S. Armed Services in World War I, many of whom are buried in Section 21, the "Nurses Section" (Military District of Washington, n.d.). Progress in health care occurred during World War I, particularly in the field of surgery. For example, there were advancements in the use of anesthetic agents, infection control, blood typing, and prosthetics (Holder, 2004, p. 915).

World War II casualties created an acute shortage of caregivers, and the Cadet Nurse Corps was established in response to a marked shortage of nurses. Also at that time, auxiliary health care workers became prominent. "Practical" nurses, aides, and technicians provided much of the actual nursing care under the instruction and supervision of better prepared nurses. Medical specialties also arose at that time to meet the needs of hospitalized clients.

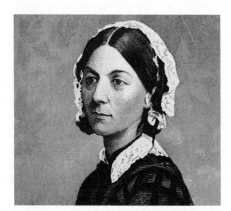

Figure 40–2 ■ Considered the founder of modern nursing, Florence Nightingale (1820–1910) was influential in developing nursing education, practice, and administration. Her publication, *Notes on Nursing: What It Is, and What It Is Not*, first published in England in 1859 and in the United States in 1860, was intended for all women.
© Bettman/CORBIS.

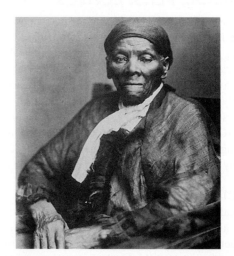

Figure 40–3 ■ Harriet Tubman (1820–1913) was known as "The Moses of Her People" for her work with the Underground Railroad. During the Civil War, she nursed the sick and suffering of her own race.
© CORBIS.

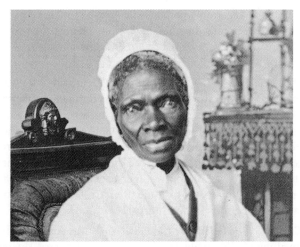

Figure 40–4 ■ Sojourner Truth (1797–1883), abolitionist, Underground Railroad agent, preacher, and women's rights advocate, was a nurse for over 4 years during the Civil War and worked as a nurse and counselor for the Freedmen's Relief Association after the war.

Randall Studio (1805–1875) Sojourner Truth (c. 1797–1883–), abolitionist. © 1870. Photograph, Albumen Silver Print. Copyright National Portrait Gallery, Smithsonian Institution/Art Resources, NY.

During the Vietnam War, approximately 90% of the 11,000 American military women stationed in Vietnam were nurses. Most of them volunteered to go to Vietnam right after they graduated from nursing school. This made them the youngest group of medical personnel ever to serve in wartime (Vietnam Women's Memorial Foundation, n.d.). Near the Vietnam Veterans Memorial ("The Wall") stands the Vietnam Women's Memorial (Figure 40–6 ■). This monument was established to "honor the women who served and also for the families who lost loved ones during the war ... to let them know about the women who provided comfort, care and a human touch for those who were suffering and dying" (Vietnam Women's Memorial Foundation, n.d.).

Societal Attitudes

Society's attitudes about nurses and nursing have significantly influenced professional nursing.

Before the mid-1800s, nursing was without organization, education, or social status; the prevailing attitude was that a woman's place was in the home and that no respectable woman should have a career. The role for the Victorian middle-class woman was that of wife and mother, and any education she obtained was for the purpose of making her a pleasant companion to her husband and a responsible mother to her children. Nurses in hospitals during this period were poorly educated; some were even incarcerated criminals. Society's attitudes about nursing during this period are reflected in the writings of Charles Dickens. In his book *Martin Chuzzlewit* (1896), Dickens reflected his attitude toward nurses through his character Sairy Gamp. She "cared" for the sick by neglecting them, stealing from them, and physically abusing them (Donahue, 1996, p. 192). This literary portrayal of nurses greatly influenced the negative image and attitude toward nurses up to contemporary times.

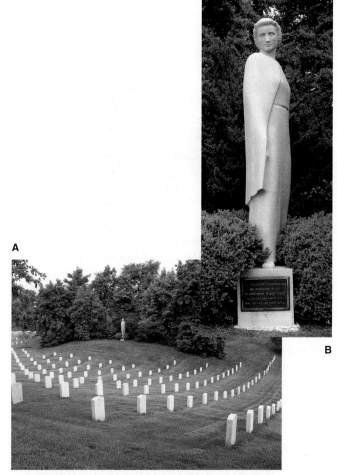

Figure 40–5 ■ *A,* Section 21 in Arlington National Cemetery honors the nurses who served in the Armed Services in World War I. *B,* The "Spirit of Nursing" monument that stands in Section 21. The plaque at the base of the monument reads *THIS MONUMENT WAS ERECTED IN 1938 AND REDEDICATED IN 1971 TO COMMEMORATE DEVOTED SERVICE TO COUNTRY AND HUMANITY BY ARMY, NAVY, AND AIR FORCE NURSES.*

Photo by Sherrilyn Coffman, PhD, RN.

In contrast, the *guardian angel* or *angel of mercy* image arose in the latter part of the nineteenth century, largely because of the work of Florence Nightingale during the Crimean War. After Nightingale brought respectability to the nursing profession, nurses were viewed as noble, compassionate, moral, religious, dedicated, and self-sacrificing.

Another image arising in the early nineteenth century that has affected subsequent generations of nurses and the public and other professionals working with nurses is the image of *doctor's handmaiden*. This image evolved when women had yet to obtain the right to vote, when family structures were largely paternalistic, and when the medical profession portrayed increasing use of scientific knowledge that, at that time, was viewed as a male domain. Since that time, several images of nursing have been portrayed. The *heroine* portrayal evolved from nurses' acts of bravery in World War II and their contributions in fighting poliomyelitis—in particular, the work of

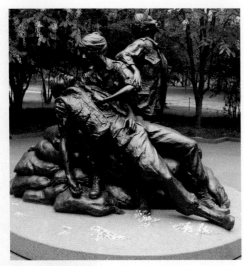

Figure 40–6 ■ Vietnam Women's Memorial. Four figures include a nurse tending to the chest wound of a soldier, another woman looking for a helicopter for assistance, and a third woman (behind the other figures) kneeling while staring at an empty helmet in grief.

Photo by Sherrilyn Coffman, PhD, RN.

the Australian nurse Elizabeth Kenney. Other images in the late 1900s include the nurse as sex object, surrogate mother, and tyrannical mother.

During the past few decades, the nursing profession has taken steps to improve the image of the nurse. In the early 1990s, the Tri-Council for Nursing (the American Association of Colleges of Nursing, the ANA, the American Organization of Nurse Executives, and the NLN) initiated a national effort (titled "Nurses of America") to improve the image of nursing. More recently, the Johnson & Johnson corporation contributed $20 million in 2002 to launch a "Campaign for Nursing's Future" to promote nursing as a positive career choice (Anonymous, 2003; Fitzpatrick, 2002). In addition, nursing schools and hospitals are targeting men in their recruitment efforts (Meyers, 2003).

Nursing Leaders

Florence Nightingale, Clara Barton, Lillian Wald, Lavinia Dock, Margaret Sanger, and Mary Breckinridge are among the leaders who have made notable contributions both to nursing's history and to women's history. These women were all politically astute pioneers. Their skills at influencing others and bringing about change remain models for political nurse activists today. Contemporary nursing leaders Virginia Henderson, who created a modern worldwide definition of nursing, and Martha Rogers, a catalyst for theory, played important roles in nursing.

NIGHTINGALE (1820–1910) **Florence Nightingale**'s contributions to nursing are well documented. Her achievements in improving the standards for the care of war casualties in the Crimea earned her the title "Lady with the Lamp." Her efforts in reforming hospitals and in producing and implementing public health policies also made her an accomplished political nurse: She was the first nurse to exert political pressure on government. Through her contributions

to nursing education—perhaps her greatest achievement—she is also recognized as nursing's first scientist-theorist for her work *Notes on Nursing: What It Is, and What It Is Not* (1860/1969).

BARTON (1812–1912) **Clara Barton** (Figure 40–7 ■) was a schoolteacher who volunteered as a nurse during the American Civil War. Her responsibility was to organize the nursing services. Barton is noted for her role in establishing the American Red Cross, which linked with the International Red Cross when the U.S. Congress ratified the Treaty of Geneva (Geneva Convention). It was Barton who persuaded Congress in 1882 to ratify this treaty so that the Red Cross could perform humanitarian efforts in times of peace.

RICHARDS (1841–1930) Linda Richards was America's first trained nurse. She graduated from the New England Hospital for Women and Children in 1873. Richards is known for introducing nurse's notes and doctor's orders. She also initiated the practice of nurses wearing uniforms (American Nurses Association, 2006a). She is credited for her pioneer work in psychiatric and industrial nursing.

MAHONEY (1845–1926) **Mary Mahoney** (Figure 40–8 ■) was the first African American professional nurse. She graduated from the New England Hospital for Women and Children in 1879. She constantly worked for the acceptance of African Americans in nursing and for the promotion of equal opportunities (Donahue, 1996, p. 271). The ANA (2006b) gives a Mary Mahoney Award biennially in recognition of significant contributions in interracial relationships.

WALD (1867–1940) Lillian Wald is considered the founder of public health nursing. Wald and Mary Brewster were the first to offer trained nursing services to the poor in the New York slums. Their home among the poor on the upper floor of a tenement, called the Henry Street Settlement and Visiting Nurse Service, provided nursing services, social services, and organized educational and cultural activities. Soon after the founding of the Henry Street Settlement, school nursing was established as an adjunct to visiting nursing.

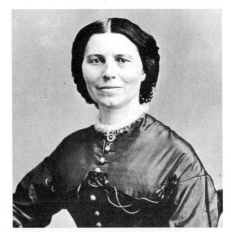

Figure 40–7 ■ Clara Barton (1821–1912) organized the American Red Cross, which linked with the International Red Cross when the U.S. Congress ratified the Geneva Convention in 1882.

© Bettman/CORBIS.

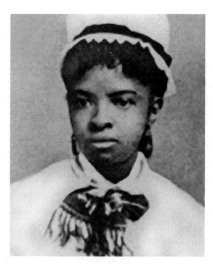

Figure 40–8 ■ Mary Mahoney (1845–1926) was the first African American trained nurse.
Schomburg Center for Research in Black Culture, New York Public Library.

DOCK (1858–1956) Lavinia L. Dock was a feminist, prolific writer, political activist, suffragette, and friend of Wald. She participated in protest movements for women's rights that resulted in the 1920 passage of the 19th Amendment to the U.S. Constitution, which granted women the right to vote. In addition, Dock campaigned for legislation to allow nurses rather than physicians to control their profession. In 1893, Dock, with the assistance of Mary Adelaide Nutting and Isabel Hampton Robb, founded the American Society of Superintendents of Training Schools for Nurses of the United States and Canada, a precursor to the current National League for Nursing.

SANGER (1879–1966) Margaret Higgins Sanger, a public health nurse in New York, has had a lasting impact on women's health care. Imprisoned for opening the first birth control information clinic in America, she is considered the founder of Planned Parenthood. Her experience with the large number of unwanted pregnancies among the working poor was instrumental in addressing this problem.

BRECKINRIDGE (1881–1965) After World War I, Mary Breckinridge, a notable pioneer nurse, established the Frontier Nursing Service (FNS). In 1918, she worked with the American Committee for Devastated France, distributing food, clothing, and supplies to rural villages and taking care of sick children. In 1921, Breckinridge returned to the United States with plans to provide health care to the people of rural America. In 1925, Breckinridge and two other nurses began the FNS in Leslie County, Kentucky. Within this organization, Breckinridge started one of the first midwifery training schools in the United States.

CONTEMPORARY NURSING PRACTICE

An understanding of contemporary nursing practice includes a look at definitions of nursing, recipients of nursing, settings for nursing practice, nurse practice acts, and current standards of clinical nursing practice.

Definitions of Nursing

Florence Nightingale defined nursing nearly 150 years ago as "the act of utilizing the environment of the patient to assist him in his recovery" (Nightingale, 1860–1969). Nightingale considered a clean, well-ventilated, and quiet environment essential for recovery. Often considered the first nurse theorist, Nightingale raised the status of nursing through education. Nurses were no longer untrained housekeepers but people educated in the care of the sick.

Virginia Henderson was one of the first modern nurses to define nursing. She wrote, "The unique function of the nurse is to assist the individual, sick or well, in the performance of those activities contributing to health or its recovery (or to peaceful death) that he would perform unaided if he had the necessary strength, will, or knowledge, and to do this in such a way as to help him gain independence as rapidly as possible" (Henderson, 1966, p. 3). Like Nightingale, Henderson described nursing in relation to the client and the client's environment. Unlike Nightingale, Henderson saw the nurse as concerned with both healthy and ill individuals, acknowledged that nurses interact with clients even when recovery may not be feasible, and mentioned the teaching and advocacy roles of the nurse.

In the latter half of the twentieth century, a number of nurse theorists developed their own theoretical definitions of nursing. Theoretical definitions are important because they go beyond simplistic common definitions. They describe what nursing is and the interrelationship among nurses, nursing, the client, the environment, and the intended client outcome.

Certain themes are common to many of these definitions:

- Nursing is caring.
- Nursing is an art.
- Nursing is a science.
- Nursing is client centered.
- Nursing is holistic.
- Nursing is adaptive.
- Nursing is concerned with health promotion, health maintenance, and health restoration.
- Nursing is a helping profession.

Professional nursing associations have also examined nursing and developed their definitions of it. In 1973, the ANA described nursing practice as "direct, goal oriented, and adaptable to the needs of the individual, the family, and community during health and illness" (ANA, 1973, p. 2). In 1980, the ANA changed its definition of nursing to this: "Nursing is the diagnosis and treatment of human responses to actual or potential health problems" (ANA, 1980, p. 9). In 1995, the ANA recognized the influence and contribution of the science of caring to nursing philosophy and practice. Its most recent definition of professional nursing is much broader and states, "Nursing is the protection, promotion, and optimization of health and abilities, prevents of illness and injury, alleviation of suffering through the diagnosis and treatment of human response, and advocacy in the care of individuals, families, communities, and populations" (ANA, 2003, p. 6).

Research to explore the meaning of caring in nursing has been increasing. For example, Coffman (2004) conducted a metasynthesis of qualitative studies describing cultural caring in nursing practice. Likewise, Graber and Mitcham (2004) sought to identify actions, interventions, and interpersonal relationships that demonstrated caring and compassion.

Recipients of Nursing

The recipients of nursing are sometimes called consumers, sometimes patients, and sometimes clients. A **consumer** is an individual, a group of people, or a community that uses a service or commodity. People who use health care products or services are consumers of health care.

A **patient** is a person who is waiting for or undergoing medical treatment and care. The word *patient* comes from a Latin word meaning "to suffer" or "to bear." Traditionally, the person receiving health care has been called a patient. Usually people become patients when they seek assistance because of illness or for surgery. Some nurses believe that the word *patient* implies passive acceptance of the decisions and care of health professionals. Additionally, with the emphasis on health promotion and prevention of illness, many recipients of nursing care are not ill. Moreover, nurses interact with family members and significant others to provide support, information, and comfort in addition to caring for the patient.

For these reasons, nurses increasingly refer to recipients of health care as *clients*. A **client** is a person who engages the advice or services of another who is qualified to provide this service. The term *client* presents the receivers of health care as collaborators in the care, that is, as people who are also responsible for their own health. Thus, the health status of a client is the responsibility of the individual in collaboration with health professionals. In this book, *client* is the preferred term, although *consumer* and *patient* are used in some instances.

Settings for Nursing

In the past, the acute care hospital was the main practice setting open to most nurses. Today many nurses work in hospitals, but increasingly they work in clients' homes, community agencies, ambulatory clinics, long-term care facilities, health maintenance organizations (HMOs), and nursing practice centers (see Figure 40–9 ■).

Nurses have different degrees of nursing autonomy and nursing responsibility in the various settings. They may provide direct care, teach clients and support persons, serve as nursing advocates and agents of change, and help determine health policies affecting consumers in the community and in hospitals.

Nurse Practice Acts

Nurse practice acts, or legal acts for professional nursing practice, regulate the practice of nursing in the United States and Canada. Each state in the United States and each province in Canada has its own act. Although nurse practice acts differ in various jurisdictions, they all have a common purpose: to

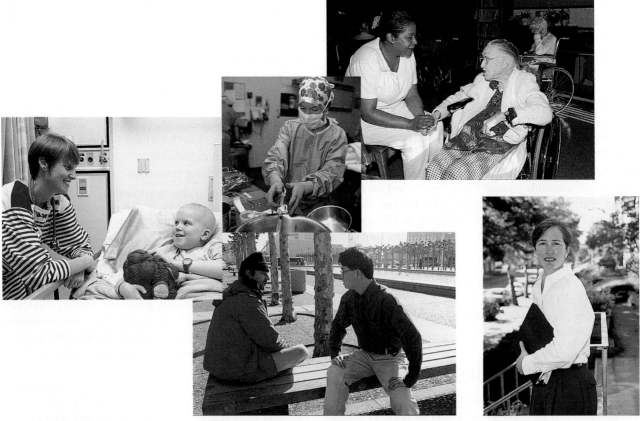

Figure 40–9 ■ Nurses practice in a variety of settings. Clockwise from top left: pediatric nursing, operating room nursing, geriatric nursing, home nursing, and community nursing.

protect the public. Nurses are responsible for knowing their state's nurse practice act as it governs their practice. These are discussed in detail in Concept 47, Legal Issues.

Standards of Nursing Practice

Establishing and implementing standards of practice are major functions of a professional organization. The purpose of the ANA's **Standards of Practice** is to describe the responsibilities for which nurses are accountable (see Box 40–4). By using the nursing process as a foundation, the ANA developed standards of nursing practice that are generic in nature, and provide for the practice of nursing regardless of area of specialization. Various specialty nursing organizations have further developed specific standards of nursing practice for their area. For nurses in Canada, each province or territory establishes its own standards of practice. The ANA's **Standards of Professional Performance** (see Box 40–4) describe behaviors expected in the professional nursing role.

ROLES AND FUNCTIONS OF THE NURSE

Nurses assume a number of roles when they provide care to clients. Nurses often perform multiple roles simultaneously. For example, the nurse may act as a counselor while providing physical care and teaching aspects of that care. The roles required at a specific time depend on the needs of the client and aspects of the particular environment. These roles are discussed throughout this text and are briefly outlined in Table 40–1.

As the nursing profession has grown in autonomy through professional organizations, nursing leaders and managers have seen a need for a number of expanded roles in the nursing profession. Some of these roles, such as that of the nurse midwife, have also come about, in part, as a response to needs expressed by clients themselves. Other expanded roles, such as that of the nurse educator, result primarily from the profession's recognition to continue to improve, educate, and renew its own members.

Expanded Career Roles for Nurses

Nurses are fulfilling expanded career roles, such as those of nurse practitioner, clinical nurse specialist, nurse midwife, nurse educator, and nurse anesthetist, all of which allow greater independence and autonomy.

NURSE PRACTIONER Nurse practioners have advanced education and are graduates of a nurse practitioner program. These nurses are certified by the American Nurses Credentialing Center in areas such as adult nurse practitioner, family nurse

---

Box 40–4 ANA Standards

The ANA's Standards of Practice for the Registered Nurse describe a competent level of nursing care as demonstrated by the nursing process:

1. *Assessment*
   Collects comprehensive data pertinent to the client's health or the situation.
2. *Diagnosis*
   Analyzes the assessment data to determine the diagnoses or issues.
3. *Outcomes identification*
   Identifies expected outcomes for a plan individualized to the client or the situation.
4. *Planning*
   Develops a plan that prescribes strategies and alternatives to attain expected outcomes.
5. *Implementation*
   Implements the identified plan.
   5A. *Coordination of care*
   5B. *Health teaching and health promotion*
   5C. *Consultation*
       The advanced practice registered nurse and the nursing role specialist provide consultation to influence the identified plan, enhance the abilities of others, and effect change.
   5D. *Prescriptive authority and treatment*
       The advanced practice registered nurse uses prescriptive authority, procedures, referrals, treatments, and therapies in accordance with state and federal laws and regulations.
   5E. *Treatment and evaluation*
6. *Evaluation*
   Evaluates progress toward attainment of outcomes.

The ANA's Standards of Professional Performance describe a competent level of behavior in the professional role:

7. *Quality of practice*
   Systematically enhances the quality and effectiveness of nursing practice.
8. *Education*
   Attains knowledge and competency that reflects current nursing practice.
9. *Professional practice evaluation*
   Evaluates one's own nursing practice in relation to professional practice standards and guidelines as well as relevant statutes, rules, and regulations.
10. *Collegiality*
    Interacts with and contributes to the professional development of peers and colleagues.
11. *Collaboration*
    Collaborates with client, family, and others in the conduct of nursing practice.
12. *Ethics*
    Integrates ethical provisions in all areas of practice.
13. *Research*
    Integrates research findings into practice.
14. *Resource utilization*
    Considers factors related to safety, effectiveness, cost, and impact on practice in the planning and delivery of nursing services.
15. *Leadership*
    Provides leadership in the professional practice setting and the profession.

Source: American Nurses Association. (2004). *Nursing: Scope and standards of practice.* Silver Spring, MD: Nursebooks.org. Reprinted with permission.

TABLE 40–1 Roles and Functions of the Nurse

NURSING ROLE	FUNCTIONS
Caregiver	As a caregiver, the nurse engages in activities that assist the client physically and psychologically while preserving the client's dignity.
Communicator	As a communicator, the nurse identifies client problems and then communicates these to other members of the health care team. See Concept 36, Communication.
Teacher	Nurses help clients learn about their health and health care procedures in order to restore or maintain their health. Nurses also teach unlicensed assistive personnel (UAP) to whom they delegate care, and they share their expertise with other nurses and health care professionals. See Concept 39, Teaching and Learning, and the many examples provided in Volume 1 of this text.
Client advocate	In this role the nurse may represent the client's needs and wishes to other health professionals, such as relaying the client's wishes for information to the physician. He or she also assists clients in exercising their rights and helps them speak up for themselves.
Counselor	Nurses counsel primarily healthy individuals with normal adjustment difficulties and focus on helping these persons develop new attitudes, feelings, and behaviors by encouraging them to look at alternative behaviors, recognize the choices, and develop a sense of control. Nurses counsel ill clients in how to develop more healthy and protective behaviors and how to recognize and respond to triggers, signs, and symptoms in a timely manner.
Change agent	The nurse acts as a change agent when assisting clients to make modifications in their behavior. Nurses also often act to make changes in a system, such as clinical care, if it is not helping a client return to health. Nurses are continually dealing with change in the health care system. Technological change, change in the age of the client population, and changes in medications are just a few of the changes nurses deal with daily.
Leader	A leader influences others to work together to accomplish a specific goal. The leader role can be employed at different levels: individual client, family, groups of clients, colleagues, or the community. Effective leadership is a learned process requiring an understanding of the needs and goals that motivate people, the knowledge to apply the leadership skills, and the interpersonal skills to influence others. Leadership is discussed further in Concept 38, Professional Behaviors.
Manager	The nurse manages the nursing care of individuals, families, and communities. The nurse manager also delegates nursing activities to ancillary workers and other nurses, and supervises and evaluates their performance. Managing requires knowledge about organizational structure and dynamics, authority and accountability, leadership, change theory, advocacy, delegation, and supervision and evaluation. See Concept 35, Collaboration, for more information.
Case manager	Nurse case managers work with the multidisciplinary health care team to measure the effectiveness of the case management plan and to monitor outcomes. Each agency or unit specifies the role of the nurse case manager. In some institutions, the case manager works with primary or staff nurses to oversee the care of a specific caseload. In other agencies, the case manager is the primary nurse or provides some level of direct care to the client and family. Insurance companies have also developed a number of roles for nurse case managers, and responsibilities may vary from managing acute hospitalizations to managing high-cost clients or case types. Regardless of the setting, case managers help ensure that care is oriented to the client, while controlling costs. See Concept 37, Managing Care, for more information.
Research consumer	Nurses often use research to improve client care. In a clinical area, nurses need to (a) have some awareness of the process and language of research, (b) be sensitive to issues related to protecting the rights of human subjects, (c) participate in the identification of significant researchable problems, and (d) be a discriminating consumer of research findings.

practitioner, school nurse practitioner, pediatric nurse practitioner, or gerontology nurse practitioner. They are employed in health care agencies or community-based settings. They usually deal with nonemergency acute or chronic illness and provide primary ambulatory care.

CLINICAL NURSE SPECIALIST A clinical nurse specialist is a nurse who has an advanced degree or expertise and is considered to be an expert in a specialized area of practice (e.g., gerontology, oncology). The nurse provides direct client care, educates others, consults, conducts research, and manages care. The American Nurses Credentialing Center provides national certification of clinical specialists.

NURSE ANESTHETIST A nurse who has completed advanced education in an accredited program in anesthesiology may qualify to be a nurse anesthetist. The nurse anesthetist carries out preoperative visits and assessments, and administers general anesthetics for surgery under the supervision of a physician prepared in anesthesiology. The nurse anesthetist also assesses the postoperative status of clients.

NURSE-MIDWIFE A nurse-midwife is a registered nurse who has completed a program in midwifery and is certified by the American College of Nurse Midwives. The nurse gives prenatal and postnatal care and manages deliveries in normal pregnancies. The midwife practices in association with a health care agency and can obtain medical services if complications occur. The nurse-midwife may also conduct routine Papanicolaou smears, family planning, and routine breast examinations.

NURSE RESEARCHER   Nurse researchers investigate nursing problems to improve nursing care and to refine and expand nursing knowledge. They are employed in academic institutions, teaching hospitals, and research centers such as the National Institute for Nursing Research in Bethesda, Maryland. Nurse researchers usually have advanced education at the doctoral level.

NURSE ADMINISTRATOR   The nurse administrator manages client care, including the delivery of nursing services. The administrator may have a middle management position, such as head nurse or supervisor, or a more senior management position, such as director of nursing services. The functions of nurse administrators include budgeting, staffing, and planning programs. The educational preparation for nurse administrator positions is at least a baccalaureate degree in nursing and frequently a master's or doctoral degree.

NURSE EDUCATOR   Nurse educators are employed in nursing programs, at educational institutions, and in hospital staff education. The nurse educator usually has a baccalaureate degree or more advanced preparation and frequently has expertise in a particular area of practice. The nurse educator is responsible for classroom and often clinical teaching.

NURSE ENTREPRENEUR   The nurse entrepreneur usually has an advanced degree and manages a health-related business. The nurse may be involved in education, consultation, or research, for example.

CONCLUSION

Nurses fulfill a variety of roles and functions within the profession of nursing. They work in various organizations providing care to clients and their families in various forms. All nurses, regardless of where they work or their level of degree, experience, or practice, are required to maintain competency and to seek professional development as necessary to provide appropriate and safe client care.

REVIEW Professional Development

RELATE: LINK THE CONCEPTS

Linking the exemplar of Professional Development with the concept of Legal Issues:

1. What role does the nurse's continued professional development play in meeting the legal requirements for the profession?
2. What nursing regulations require continued professional development?

Linking the exemplar of Professional Development with the concept of Ethics:

3. Can the nurse meet the ethical responsibilities of the profession without belonging to a professional organization?
4. How does the nursing code of ethics address the issue of professional development?

REFER: GO TO MYNURSINGKIT

REFLECT: CASE STUDY

Francois Guardiene graduated from nursing school 4 years ago and accepted a position working in the coronary care unit of a large metropolitan hospital. He was required to attend 6 weeks of hospital orientation, a 3-month class for CCU nurses, and worked under the supervision of a preceptor for an additional 3 months. During his first year of practice he checked with more experienced nurses frequently, but with time he began to have more confidence in his competence and established a more autonomous practice. Over the past 2 years he has noticed that some people actually collaborate with him and he considers himself a good CCU nurse.

1. Has Mr. Guardiene satisfied the need for professional development? Explain your answer.
2. What obligations does Mr. Guardiene have going forward to developing his professional practice?
3. How would a nurse's hospital orientation differ if the position accepted involved an area less specialized that the CCU?

PEARSON
EXPLORE mynursingkit™

MyNursingKit is your one stop for online chapter review materials and resources. Prepare for success with additional NCLEX®-style practice questions, interactive assignments and activities, web links, animations and videos, and more!

Register your access code from the front of your book at **www.mynursingkit.com**.

or by assisting clients in exercising their rights and helping them to speak up for themselves.

Successful advocacy is a positive experience for nurses as well as for clients. Clients derive a benefit, and nurses feel good about their ability to be agents of change. Not all advocating, however, will be successful. Unsuccessful advocating can be hard for the nurse to cope with and has the potential to lead to frustration, anger, and burnout. ●

THE ADVOCATE'S ROLE

The complexities of the health care system are challenging even to the most educated of clients. Those at lower levels of literacy, those who do not speak English, and those who are very ill or very poor face great difficulty navigating the system, and as a result many of them "fall through the cracks." These clients need an advocate to penetrate the layers of bureaucracy and help them access the resources they require (Figure 41–1 ■). Some values basic to client advocacy are shown in Box 41–1.

The overall goal of the client advocate is to protect clients' rights. Clients must understand their rights in order to be able to defend them. The nurse serves as both a teacher and an advocate by informing clients about their rights. To help clients and health care providers understand clients' rights, a number of professional and consumer organizations have developed Bills of Rights for patients. Patient rights are discussed in detail in Exemplar 42.2, Patient Rights.

As an advocate, the nurse provides clients with the information they need to make informed decisions and supports the clients' rights to make their own health care decisions. In some cases, the decision making may be shared by the client and the provider. When the client makes decisions about his or her treatment other than what is recommended, it is the nurse's role to ensure the client is making an informed decision and, if so, then the nurse must advocate for the client's right to make autonomous choices, even when those choices run counter to the nurse's own beliefs. The advocate must be careful to

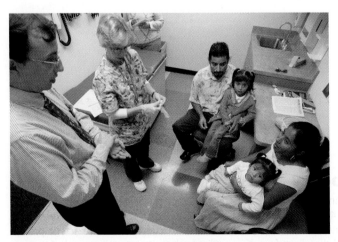

Figure 41–1 ■ At this clinic in Pittsburgh, Pennsylvania, clients not only receive health care, but also are helped to find English lessons, the closest Hispanic grocery store, and anything else they might need.

Box 41–1 Values Basic to Client Advocacy

■ The client is a holistic, autonomous being who has the right to make choices and decisions.
■ The client has the right to expect a nurse–client relationship that is based on shared respect, trust, collaboration in solving problems related to health and health care needs, and consideration of his or her thoughts and feelings.
■ The nurse has the responsibility to ensure the client has access to health care services that meet health needs.

remain objective and should not convey approval or disapproval of the client's choices. Advocacy requires accepting and respecting the client's right to decide, even if the nurse believes the decision to be wrong.

If a client lacks decision-making capacity, is legally incompetent, or is a minor, these rights can be exercised on the client's behalf by a designated health care surrogate or legal guardian. It is important, however, for the nurse to remember that client control over health decisions is a Western view, and is not necessarily accepted in other cultures. In other societies, such decisions may normally be made by the head of the family or a member of the community. The nurse must respect the client's and family's views and honor their traditions regarding health care decision making.

To be an effective advocate, the nurse must
■ Be assertive.
■ Recognize that the rights and values of clients and families must take precedence when they conflict with those of health care providers.
■ Be aware that conflicts may arise over issues that require consultation, confrontation, or negotiation between the nurse and administrative personnel or between the nurse and primary care provider.

DEVELOPMENTAL CONSIDERATIONS
Advocating for Safety

The nurse's role as an advocate includes assessing and protecting vulnerable clients from abuse. Children who are being abuse by a family member or caregiver are often powerless to speak. Older adults may be abused by their primary caregiver, who may be a spouse or one of their adult children. The risk for abuse of the older adult is greater when the adult is dependent on others for help with activities of daily living. Women may seek care for injuries resulting from abuse by a spouse or significant other.

The nurse must be alert for signs of abuse during the initial assessment and recognize that the abuse victim will often deny abuse for fear of retribution from the abuser. The nurse advocates for these clients by keeping them safe, educating them in regards to other options, and by identifying and helping them access additional resources to ensure their safety once they leave the health care system. Maintaining an awareness of resources in the community and advocating for victims of abuse through political and legislative initiatives are components of the advocacy role.

CARE SETTINGS · Advocacy in Home Care

The goals of advocacy in the home care setting pose unique concerns for the nurse advocate. For example, while in the hospital, people often operate from the values of the nurses and primary care providers by following instructions and complying with provider requests. Once they return home, however, people tend to operate from their own personal values and may revert to old habits that may not be beneficial to their health. Although the

nurse may view this as noncompliance, the nurse must respect client autonomy.

In home care, limited resources and a lack of client care services may shift the focus from client welfare to concerns about resource availability and allocation. Financial considerations can limit a client's access to services and materials, making it difficult to ensure that the client's needs are met.

- Work with community agencies and lay practitioners.
- Understand that advocacy may require political action—communicating a client's health care needs to government and other officials who have the authority to do something about these needs.

Empowering the Client

Because of the special nurse–client relationship, nurses support and advocate for clients and families facing difficult choices and for those living with the results of their choices. Through knowing the client and engaging in a mutual relationship, the nurse is able to identify and build upon client/family strengths. This empowering relationship includes mutual respect, trust, and confidence in the other's abilities and motives.

Rather than viewing the nurse as *empowering* the client, Swanson (1993), describes a caring behavior of *enabling* that is defined as "facilitating the other's passage through life transitions and unfamiliar events" (p. 356). Enabling also includes coaching, informing, explaining, supporting, assisting, guiding, focusing, and validating. There are times when enabling involves the nurse providing substitutive care (i.e., doing for the client who is unable to do for oneself), but never more than is needed at the time. At other times, enabling involves providing an environment in which the client is able to function safely and effectively, or mediating on the client's behalf. For example, the nurse may ask the primary care provider to review the reasons for a recommended therapy with the client, because the client says he or she always forgets to ask the primary care provider. The nurse should remain mindful of professional boundaries and responsibilities to avoid enabling pathological choices by the client. The goal is always to facilitate growth and development.

Nurses both *advocate* (verb) for and are *advocates* (noun) for clients and families. Knowlden (1998) explored the meaning of caring in nursing and identified four dimensions of advocacy:

1. Being a client advocate
2. Following through or following up
3. Providing resources
4. Going above and beyond.

A client in Knowlden's study described how his nurse served as an advocate for him: "She keeps in touch with [my practitioner] to find out what's to be done. She gets through right away. They give us the run-around and get back 5 days later... She has been instrumental in getting the tube changed"

(p. 37). Through advocacy, nurses are champions for their clients. They empower clients and families through activities that enhance well-being, understanding, and self-care.

Educating Providers and Others

Sometimes the gap between the rights that clients have in theory and the rights that clients have in practice results from a knowledge deficit on the part of treatment providers. If so, the remedy is simple: Educate the treatment providers so that they in turn can educate and provide appropriate care to their clients.

Another, more complicated possibility that may not be so easily solved is that direct care providers sometimes feel threatened by the expansion of client rights. Health care providers have been known to express concern that some new regulations not only hamper treatment but also make their job both more difficult and more dangerous. For example, a mother brings her adolescent to the provider's office and requests a drug screen be performed because of suspected substance abuse. Federal regulations require confidentiality of test results, which prevents the provider from sharing test results with anyone other than the adolescent. The nurse, advocating for the client, is required to maintain confidentiality as well and may need to find a means of either convincing the adolescent to allow information be shared with the parent so appropriate drug treatment may be initiated or explaining to the parent why the information cannot be shared if the adolescent refuses.

Local, state, and national advocacy programs exist to protect and advocate for those with mental illness or disability (see Box 41–2).

Box 41–2 Advocacy Programs

The federal government has encouraged states to develop advocacy programs to provide information about and serve as a resource regarding the rights of those with mental illness or disability. Each state designates an agency or group to advocate for the rights of those with mental illness or a disability and to investigate reported incidents involving neglect and abuse of these vulnerable clients in public or private mental health treatment settings, research facilities, and nursing homes. Disability Rights California is an example of a state agency designated to protect and advocate for those with disabilities. Independent organizations, such as the Legal Center for People with Disabilities and Older People of Colorado, also operate at local, state, and national levels to advocate for clients who cannot advocate for themselves.

Professional and Public Advocacy

The role of advocacy in nursing extends to professional organizations, who advocate at the state and national levels for the profession of nursing, its members, and from those who benefit from the services that nurses provide. Professional organizations include the American Nurses Association and are discussed in Exemplar 45.2, Professional Organizations.

Individual nurses and professional nursing organizations have great opportunities to speak publicly for the health, welfare, and safety of their clients; to take steps to protect client rights; to inform the public about issues and concerns by writing articles for the popular press; to lobby their congressional representatives on behalf of better health care for all people; and to run for political office. Gains that nursing makes in developing and improving health policy at the institutional and governmental levels help to achieve better health care for the public.

Nurses who function responsibly as professional and public advocates are in a position to effect change. They need an understanding of the ethical issues in nursing and health care as well as knowledge of the laws and regulations that affect nursing practice and the health of society.

ADVOCATING FOR CHILDREN AND FAMILIES Advocacy for children and their families is directed at helping the child and family to adjust to the changes in the child's health in their own way. To be an effective advocate, the nurse must be aware of the child's and the family's needs, the family's resources, and the health care options available to them. The nurse can then assist the family and the child to make informed decisions and to act in the child's best interests. For example, the nurse works to make sure the family member and child (to his or her level of understanding) have adequate information about treatment options to make an informed decision. The nurse must also protect the child and family by taking appropriate actions related to any potential or actual incidents of incompetent, unethical, or illegal practices by any member of the health care team.

As advocates, nurses also ensure that the policies and resources of health care agencies meet the psychosocial needs of children and their families. This sometimes requires nurses to become active participants on committees that develop policies or guidelines for nursing and medical care or for modernizing the health care facility design. In each case, the knowledge that the nurse contributes about the developmental and psychosocial needs of children is important in ensuring that the needs of children are appropriately addressed in their health care facility (Figure 41–2 ■).

Table 41–1 lists some examples of how nurses can advocate for children and families in their community.

Advocating for Vulnerable Populations

Throughout history, nurses have been strong advocates for vulnerable populations such as the poor, those who have a disability or mental illness, and any client who is unable to advocate for him- or herself. In the twenty-first century, there is a need for new energy and political activism. In this era of health care reform, nurses must be particularly concerned

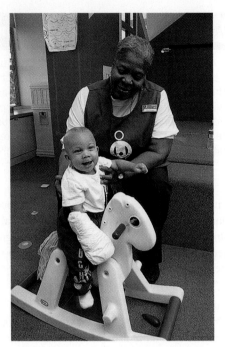

Figure 41–2 ■ Play is a significant component of childhood: It provides opportunities for learning as well as relaxation. The stress of illness and hospitalization increases the value of play. Sometimes, however, the importance of play can be overlooked in the day-to-day activities of providing care for acutely ill children. Nurses must be aware of the needs of pediatric clients for play time and advocate for children to have play time as well as rest time and appropriate nutrition. In this photo, a volunteer grandmother plays with a young boy to provide stimulation and nurturing during his lengthy hospitalization.

with ensuring that the needs and the rights of those within vulnerable populations are not overlooked or ignored. As the explosion of knowledge in science and technology revolutionizes how nurses practice (Figure 41–3 ■), nurses must continue to advocate for fair and equitable access to high quality care for all clients. Nurses advocate for these clients in a variety of settings, including hospitals, free clinics, and primary care and specialty practices.

CLINICAL EXAMPLE

Mrs. Potter is a 68-year-old woman with a number of medical conditions, including Parkinson's disease, which causes frequent tremors in her hands. One of her medications is a weekly injection. Mrs. Potter's insurance company refuses to pay for her to receive the injection at her primary care provider's office, but will pay if she gives the injection to herself at home. Mrs. Potter is on a very limited income and cannot afford to pay a weekly injection fee. The nurse working with Mrs. Potter at her primary care provider's office realizes that Mrs. Potter is not able to self-inject.

1. What options does the nurse have for advocating that Mrs. Potter receive the injection at her primary care provider's office?
2. How can the nurse advocate for the client without removing her need for dignity?
3. What goal would you advocate for this client?

TABLE 41-1 Advocating for Children and Families

HEALTH NEED EXAMPLE	NURSE ADVOCACY ACTIONS
Members of the community who need information about places to obtain immunizations.	■ Make a list of agencies that provide immunizations. ■ Check on cost and special programs. ■ Obtain financial assistance from a local foundation to print your findings. ■ Make copies available in childcare centers and other community agencies.
A local homeless shelter has little in the way of self-care amenities for the clients.	■ Obtain donations of hotel lotions, soaps, and shampoos from classmates and faculty that can be given to the shelter. ■ Visit several local hotels and ask if they will each donate a box of small toiletries for the residents. ■ Encourage volunteers to provide haircuts and styling, or obtain donations to provide this service.
Your state has a law protecting the rights of any woman to bring her unwanted newborn baby to certain sites for the purpose of giving up her baby without legal recriminations. Because many women do not know about the law, babies are abandoned in unsafe locations.	■ Find a local newspaper reporter who is willing to write an article about the law. ■ Print copies of the article to distribute. ■ Make posters with necessary information for several community sites.

CLIENTS WITH DISABILITIES Two pieces of federal legislation have implications for the rights of clients. In 1990, the Americans with Disabilities Act (ADA) extended federal protection to individuals with physical and/or mental health disabilities for access to public services, employment, and benefits. In an effort to increase the involvement of individuals in directing their own medical care, Congress enacted the Patient Self-Determination Act (PSDA) in 1991 to protect the rights of clients to accept or reject aspects of their medical care (see Concept 47, Legal Issues, for more information about the PSDA).

Figure 41-3 ■ Clients with late-stage dementia often are unable to advocate for themselves. Nurses in long-term care should be experts in assessing for pain and providing effective pain control in this population.

Although laws may protect certain aspects of human rights, they cannot prevent errors and misunderstandings. Even when the letter of the law is followed, the spirit of the law may not be satisfied. For example, even if a client is read his rights, the client may not understand the information, may not remember it, or may be so distracted by worry that the client fails to grasp the information completely. Nurses are often in a position to ensure that both the letter of the law and the spirit of the law are followed. It is the spirit of the law that many health care providers overlook when working with clients with disabilities. Nurses are in the unique position to advocate for clients with disabilities as they navigate the health care system.

CLINICAL EXAMPLE

Marina Commodore is an RN with 20 years of clinical experience and advanced degrees. While caring for a client, Marina injures her back and is no longer able to work as a clinical nurse. During a visit to her primary care provider the nurse finds Marina crying and asks what caused her tears. Marina says she is no longer able to perform clinical work and doesn't know how she'll pay her monthly bills. Marina reports that she applied for a position as a telephone advice nurse, but says she did not even get an interview when the agency discovered she had physical limitations.

1. If you were Marina's nurse, how would you advocate on Marina's behalf?
2. What would you say to Marina at this time?
3. Would you best advocate for this client professionally or publicly? Explain your answer.

ISSUES IN MENTAL HEALTH SETTINGS Clients with mental health disorders are particularly vulnerable to both physical and psychological abuse and often do not have the ability to defend themselves. When these clients enter treatment, they may exhibit some of the same inappropriate behaviors and unrealistic expectations in which they engage outside of treatment. As a result, they are also vulnerable to abuse within the treatment facility.

Although little actual data is available regarding how much client abuse exists in treatment settings. One advocacy group ranked client abuse as the most frequent rights-violation complaint, while another ranked it third. The types of abuse that reportedly occur with some frequency include the following:

- Supplying clients with drugs or alcohol in return for favors
- Making privileges contingent on favors from clients
- Slapping and kicking clients when staff members feel frustrated
- Using restraints when other, less intrusive alternatives are available
- Verbal harassment, including threats, sarcasm, and other "put-downs"
- General threats of harm if clients do not behave "appropriately" or as they are told
- Inhumane physical facilities
- Sexual misconduct.

Some identified causes that that may lead to client abuse include the following:

- Unsuitability of certain staff members who do not have the patience or understanding to work with clients having trouble with self-control
- A buildup of stresses that have reduced the staff's patience and ability to problem solve (burnout)
- An actual lack of knowledge regarding other means of interacting with clients in a high-stress situation.

ADVOCACY INTERVENTIONS

When designing and conducting advocacy interventions, it is important to:

- Assess the client for his or her ability to cooperate and to make decisions.
- Assess the reliability of information provided by the client, especially if he or she exhibits impairment of cognitive function or mental instability.
- Assess the client's medical history and family situation.

Additionally, when nurses not only partner with family members but also teach family members to be advocates, clients experience greater improvement in their health outcomes.

Specific areas of advocacy interventions include the following:

- Educating clients and their families about their legal rights
- Monitoring treatment planning and delivery of service for the abuse of client rights
- Evaluating policies and procedures regarding infringement of client rights
- Ensuring that clients have the necessary information to make an informed decision or give informed consent
- Questioning other health care professionals when they provide care that is based on stereotypic ideas rather than on an assessment of the individual client's needs
- Speaking out for safe practice conditions when threatened by budget cutbacks.

Responsibility to Communicate and Collaborate

The nurse's duty to intervene and advocate on behalf of the client requires the nurse to communicate clearly with others, particularly the client and family members or other health care professionals participating in the decision-making process. Clear communication by all members of the client's health care team ensures client safety, enhances client care, and increases the likelihood of positive outcomes for the client.

Formulating a Plan to Intervene

Nurses often complain of not having "think time" (time to consider all options before acting). It is essential that nurses formulate a plan of care prior to implementing interventions. Many nurses report that time constraints prevent them from considering options for care and that they often respond based on past experience or intuition (Negarandeh, Oskouie, Ahmadi, Nikravesh & Hallberg, 2006). While this may work for many expert nurses, beginning nurses need to carefully think through options and learn to assess the clinical and legal implications of their actions before providing care for their clients.

ILLEGAL, IMMORAL, OR UNETHICAL ACTIVITIES OF PROFESSIONALS

Nurses are advocates for all clients, not just those in their care. As such, they have a legal responsibility to report any professional whom they suspect of engaging in illegal, immoral, or unethical activities. Normally, nurses making such a report will do so following established procedures at the facility at which they are employed. Nurses suspecting another nurse of impairment should also follow guidelines set forth by the board of nursing for the state in which they work. At other times, nurses may need to seek the guidance of the state board of nursing or the American Nurses Association. A nurse who fails to act when he or she suspects a colleague of engaging in illegal, immoral, or unethical conduct is in direct violation of the ANA Code of Ethics for Nurses (ANA, 2005).

Impairment of a coworker or team member is the most common situation encountered by health care professionals. Impairment may result from use of alcohol or drugs or from emotional overload as a result of a stressful personal experience (e.g., a nurse who returns to work too soon following the death of a close family member). Impairment from drugs or alcohol may be linked with other illegal acts, such as theft of drugs or a client's personal property. Impairment has the potential to interfere with job performance and may result in unsafe clinical practice. Nurses who observe or suspect impairment in another professional are obligated to immediately report it to a supervisor (ANA, 2001, p 15). Although an impaired health care provider may view this intervention as an invasion of privacy, this prompt action will safeguard the client from harm, while at the same time offer the impaired health care provider a chance at recovery. Many hospitals have programs to help impaired employees recover.

NURSING PRACTICE

Nurses are morally obligated to act as advocates for all clients, but particularly those who cannot advocate for themselves. This obligation extends to time off duty as well including time at work.

Clients from vulnerable population particularly benefit from nursing advocacy. Advocacy by nurses can greatly impact clients' well-being by helping eliminate barriers to accessing to health care services. Learning the role of a client advocate begins in nursing school and, with experience, is incorporated into daily professional practice.

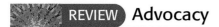 **REVIEW Advocacy**

RELATE: LINK THE CONCEPTS

Linking the concept of Advocacy with the concept of Diversity:

1. Consider each of the different groups generally included within the description of vulnerable people, and provide examples of how the nurse can advocate for each.
2. Why might clients with more diverse characteristics from the general population require greater advocacy?

Linking the concept of Advocacy with the concept of Ethics:

3. How does the nursing code of ethics address advocacy?
4. Differentiate between the nurse's role of advocate for those who are unable to speak for themselves versus the role of advocate for those who are competent to speak for themselves but, for whatever reason, do not.

REFER: GO TO MYNURSINGKIT

REFLECT: CASE STUDY

Heather Adams is a neighbor in your apartment building. On weekends, the two of you sometimes get together for morning coffee. Last weekend, Heather shared a concern that has been troubling her for a few weeks. She is 31 years old, unmarried, and lives alone. Her father is deceased, and her mother, who was diagnosed with Alzheimer's disease several years ago, is now a resident in a long-term care facility for the cognitively impaired. Heather is estranged from her only brother and next of kin. When she was in her early 20s, Heather was hospitalized and treated for depression. Her fear is that, should she become incapacitated again with depression, the brother whom she actively dislikes and with whom she does not get along will make treatment decisions as her next of kin.

You have decided to invite Heather for coffee. Because Heather seems to be a person who would benefit from a health care power of attorney, you intend to educate her about her choices.

1. On what basis do you act as an advocate for Heather?
2. Would it be ethical for you to serve as the surrogate decision maker?
3. In your discussion with Heather, should you encourage her to see an attorney?

EXPLORE PEARSON **mynursingkit™**

MyNursingKit is your one stop for online chapter review materials and resources. Prepare for success with additional NCLEX®-style practice questions, interactive assignments and activities, web links, animations and videos, and more!

Register your access code from the front of your book at **www.mynursingkit.com**.

REFERENCES

American Nurses Association. (2005). *Code of Ethics for Nurses with Interpretive Statements.* Retrieved May 2, 2010, from http://nursingworld.org/ethics/code/protected_nwcoe813.htm

Knowlden, V. (1998). *The communication of caring in nursing.* Indianapolis, IN: Center Nursing Press.

Negarandeh, R., Oskouie, F., Ahmadi, F., Nikravesh, M., & Hallberg, I.R. (2006). Patient advocacy: barriers and facilitators. *BMC Nursing,* Mar 1;5:3.

Swanson, K. (1993). Nursing as informed caring for the well-being of others. *IMAGE: Journal of Nursing Scholarship,* 25(4), 352–357.

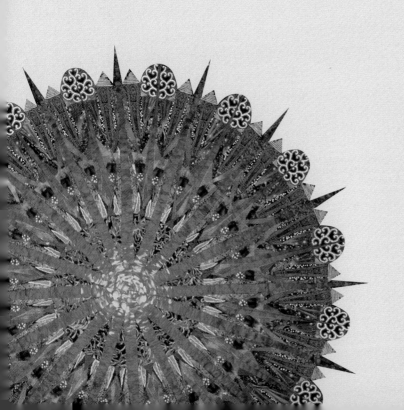

Ethics

42

Concept at-a-Glance

About Ethics, *2305*

42.1   Ethical Dilemmas, *2312*

42.2   Patient Rights, *2318*

BASIS FOR SELECTION OF CONCEPT
American Hospital Association

NLN Competencies

Nursing Practice

Standards of Nursing Practice

Concept Learning Outcomes

After reading about this concept, you will be able to:

1. Summarize the relationship between values and ethics in the nursing profession.
2. Identify principles of ethical decision making.
3. Explain the ANA Code of Ethics.
4. Apply the ANA Code of Ethics in providing individual client care.
5. Discuss how personal values influence individual care.
6. Apply a model to processing an ethical dilemma.
7. Apply ethical principles in situations involving ethical dilemmas.
8. Demonstrate appropriate steps to approaching ethical dilemmas.
9. Analyze ethical principles used to make decisions in providing individual client care.
10. Propose solutions to ethical dilemmas based on an individual's problem and ethical principles.
11. Discuss the rights of clients in the health care system.
12. Describe support systems that exist for clients who feel that their rights have been violated by a health care agency or provider.
13. Compare the contents of different documents or laws that address patient rights.

Concept Key Terms

Active euthanasia, *2314*

Advocate, *2306*

Altruism, *2306*

Assisted suicide, *2314*

Autonomy, *2306*

Beliefs, *2306*

Beneficence, *2308*

Bioethics, *2313*

Code of ethics, *2308*

Ethics, *2305*

Euthanasia, *2314*

Human dignity, *2306*

Integrity, *2306*

Justice, *2308*

Morality, *2306*

Nonmaleficence, *2308*

Social justice, *2307*

Values, *2306*

Veracity, *2308*

Withdrawing or withholding life-sustaining therapy (WWLST), *2314*

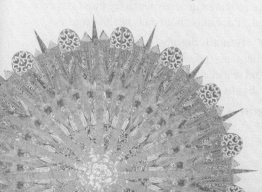

About Ethics

Ethics, as applied in professional nursing, is defined as a system of moral principles or standards governing behaviors and relationships that is based on professional nursing beliefs and values. More broadly defined, "ethics is concerned with motives and attitudes and the relationship of these attitudes to the individual" (Guido, 2010, p. 3). Ethics refers to the standards of right and wrong that influence human behavior, usually in terms of rights, obligations, benefits to society, fairness, or specific virtues. Ethical standards are based on the values of the group that holds to those standards, whether the group comprises individuals of the same religion, people from the same community, or those who share the same profession. Ethical standards of nursing include standards relating to the rights of clients and their families, such as the right to privacy.

The term *ethics* also refers to the study and development of the ethical standards of an individual, a community, or a profession. It is necessary for nurses to constantly examine their personal ethical standards and understand how their personal ethics and morals compare to the ethical standards of the nursing profession.

Morality (or morals) is similar to ethics, and many use the terms interchangeably. **Morality** usually refers to private, personal standards of what is right and wrong in conduct, character, and attitude. Sometimes the first clue to the moral nature of a situation is the awareness of feelings such as guilt, hope, or shame. Another indicator is the tendency to respond to the situation with words such as *ought*, *should*, *right*, *wrong*, *good*, and *bad*. Moral issues are concerned with important social values and norms; they are not about trivial things.

Nurses should be able to distinguish between morality and law. Laws reflect the moral values of a society, and they offer guidance in determining what is moral. However, an action can be legal but not moral. For example, an order for full resuscitation of a dying client is legal, but one could still question whether the act is moral. On the other hand, an action can be moral but illegal. For example, if a child at home stops breathing, it is moral but not legal to exceed the speed limit when driving to the hospital. Legal aspects of nursing practice are covered in Concept 47.

When people are ill, they frequently are unable to assert their rights as they would if they were healthy. When this happens, nurses have an ethical responsibility to advocate on behalf of the client based on what the client would want. An **advocate** is one who expresses and defends the cause of another. Therefore, the nurse advocates for the client's best interest based on the client's values, not based on the nurse's own ethical or moral values. Nursing advocacy takes many forms and is discussed in detail in Concept 41. In order to function successfully in this capacity, each nurse needs an understanding of the ethical issues in nursing and health care. ●

VALUES

Guido defines **values** as "personal beliefs about the truth and the worth of thoughts, objects, or behaviors" (Guido, 2010, p. 3). A **belief** is an interpretation or conclusion that one accepts as true. Values can reflect both beliefs that are based on a particular tenet (doctrine) or a body of tenets accepted by a group of persons and beliefs that are based on a pattern of mental views established by cumulative prior experience. For example, many of the traditional Jewish beliefs are based on the tenets found in the Jewish Torah, but individual Jews may hold other or additional beliefs based on their experiences within their own communities. Personal values are developed through individual observation and experience and may be heavily influenced by social traditions and the cultural, ethnic, and religious norms experienced within the family and associated groups.

Nurses acquire professional values through socialization into the nursing profession by established professional codes of ethics, faculty, and other nurses and through clinical and life experiences. As part of this socialization, nurses develop insight into their own values and how their values influence their actions. One of the most helpful ways for nurses to develop such insight is through values clarification. Through the process of consciously identifying, examining, and developing individual values, nurses become able to choose actions on the basis of deliberately adopted values. Values clarification is important to both nurses and clients in supporting the provision of client-centered care, because it helps nurses learn how to identify client values and distinguish client values from their own. Values clarification is not a once in a lifetime activity but an ongoing process of examining what one values and how one's values inform or affect one's decisions and actions. Nursing students and professional nurses need to have a clear sense of their values specific to life, death, health, and illness. Values clarification exercises and real-life experience in carrying out treatment plans that contradict or challenge their beliefs about the best interest of the client will assist nurses at all levels in developing expertise in responding to ethical issues.

One model of values clarification is the unit-based discussion. This has been utilized by Lucia Wocial, a nurse ethicist at the Fairbanks Center for Medical Ethics, as a developmental strategy to address particular client situations happening on the unit or typical to that unit. Unit-based discussions provide real-time opportunities for nurses to speak openly about ethics concerns and develop effective strategies for managing their distress or resolving the ethical issues. Wocial speaks to the need to utilize the interdisciplinary team, including the nurse's unique relationship with the client, in addressing the development of an ethical treatment plan (Nurses, 2008).

Values Essential for the Professional Nurse

The American Association of Colleges of Nursing (AACN, 2008) has identified five values that are essential for the professional nurse: altruism, autonomy, human dignity, integrity, and social justice.

ALTRUISM **Altruism** is a concern for the welfare and well-being of others. In practice, altruism is reflected by the nurse's concern for the welfare of clients, other nurses, and other health care providers.

AUTONOMY **Autonomy** is the right to self-determination. Professional practice reflects autonomy when the nurse respects clients' rights to make decisions about their health care.

HUMAN DIGNITY **Human dignity** refers to the inherent worth and uniqueness of individuals and populations. The nurse who values and respects all clients and colleagues shows respect for human dignity.

INTEGRITY **Integrity** is acting in accordance with an appropriate code of ethics and accepted standards of practice. Integrity is reflected in professional practice when the nurse is

Box 42–1 Professional Behaviors Associated With Ethical Nursing Values

- Demonstrate the professional standards of moral, ethical, and legal conduct.
- Assume accountability for personal and professional behaviors.
- Promote the image of nursing by modeling the values and articulating the knowledge, skills, and attitudes of the nursing profession.
- Demonstrate professionalism, including attention to appearance, demeanor, respect for self and others, and attention to professional boundaries with patients and families as well as among caregivers.
- Demonstrate an appreciation of the history of and contemporary issues in nursing and their impact on current nursing practice.
- Reflect on one's own beliefs and values as they relate to professional practice.
- Identify personal, professional, and environmental risks that impact personal and professional choices and behaviors.
- Communicate to the health care team one's personal bias on difficult health care decisions that impact one's ability to provide care.

- Recognize the impact of attitudes, values, and expectations on the care of the very young, frail older adults, and other vulnerable populations.
- Protect client privacy and confidentiality of client records and other privileged communications.
- Access interprofessional and intraprofessional resources to resolve ethical and other practice dilemmas.
- Act to prevent unsafe, illegal, or unethical care practices.
- Articulate the value of pursuing practice excellence, lifelong learning, and professional engagement to foster professional growth and development.
- Recognize the relationship between personal health, self renewal, and the ability to deliver sustained quality care.

Note: From American Association of Colleges of Nursing. (2008). *The essentials of baccalaureate education for professional nursing practice* (p. 29). Washington, DC. Reprinted with permission.

honest and provides care based on an ethical framework that is accepted within the profession (e.g., the ANA Code of Ethics).

SOCIAL JUSTICE **Social justice** refers to the upholding of justice, or what is fair, on a social scale. Nurses act in accordance with social justice by treating all clients equally without regard to economic status, ethnicity, age, citizenship, disability or sexual orientation.

Professional behaviors associated with these ethical values are outlined in Box 42–1.

Clarifying Client Values

To plan effective care, nurses need to identify clients' values as those values influence and relate to a particular health problem. For example, a client with failing eyesight will probably place a high value on the ability to see, and a client with

chronic pain will value comfort. Normally, people take such things for granted. When clients hold unclear or conflicting values that are detrimental to their health, the nurse should use values clarification as an intervention. Examples of behaviors that may indicate the need for clarification of health values are listed in Table 42–1.

The following process may help clients clarify their values:

1. *List alternatives.* Make sure that the client is aware of all alternative actions. Ask, "Are you considering other courses of action? Tell me about them."
2. *Examine possible consequences of choices.* Make sure the client has thought about possible results of each action. Ask, "What do you think you will gain from doing that?" "What benefits do you foresee from doing that?"
3. *Choose freely.* To determine whether the client chose freely, ask, "Did you have any say in that decision?" "Do you have a choice?"
4. *Feel good about the choice.* To determine how the client feels, ask, "How do you feel about that decision (or action)?" Because some clients may not feel satisfied with their decision, a more sensitive question might be "Some people feel good after a decision is made; others feel bad. How do you feel?"
5. *Affirm the choice.* Ask, "How will you discuss this with others (family, friends)?"
6. *Act on the choice.* To determine whether the client is prepared to act on the decision, ask, for example, "Tell me how you plan to start doing this."
7. *Act with a pattern.* To determine whether the client consistently behaves in a certain way, ask, "How many times have you done that before?" or "Would you act that way again?"

When implementing these seven steps to clarify values, the nurse assists the client to think each question through but does

TABLE 42–1 Behaviors That May Indicate Unclear Values

BEHAVIOR	EXAMPLE
Ignoring a health professional's advice	A client with heart disease who values hard work ignores advice to exercise regularly.
Inconsistent communication or behavior	A pregnant woman says she wants a healthy baby but continues to drink alcohol and smoke tobacco.
Numerous admissions to a health agency for the same problem	A middle-aged, obese woman repeatedly seeks help for back pain but does not lose weight.
Confusion or uncertainty about which course of action to take	A woman wants to obtain a job to meet financial obligations but also wants to stay at home to care for an ailing husband.

not impose personal values. The nurse rarely, if ever, offers an opinion when the client asks for it—and then only with great care or when the nurse is an expert in the content area. Since each situation is different, what the nurse would choose in his or her own life might not be relevant to the client's circumstances. Thus, if the client asks the nurse "What would you have done in my situation?" it is best to redirect the question back to the client rather than answering from the nurse's personal view.

PRINCIPLES OF ETHICAL DECISION MAKING

An individual's personal, community, and professional values inform his or her decision-making processes. Behind those values, a framework of four primary principles has been used to guide ethical decision making among professional nurses (Chally & Loritz, 1998).

As was mentioned previously, autonomy is defined as the right to self-determination (Guido, 2010, p. 8). Clients have the right to determine their own care. The nurse honors this principle by respecting the client's decision even if it is in conflict with what the nurse believes is in the client's best interest.

Beneficence requires that "the actions one takes should promote good" (Guido, 2010, p. 8). The nurse's ethical duty goes beyond beneficence to include **nonmaleficence**, which requires that the nurse do no harm and safeguard the client. Intentional harm is clearly not in keeping with this principle, but there can be also risk of harm in performing nursing interventions that are intended for good. Nonmaleficence does not mean that the nurse performs only actions that carry no risk to the client. Many actions, such as administering medications, carry some degree of risk. In most cases, the risk of harm is weighed against the potential for benefit. Prior to the action, the client is given information regarding the potential benefits and risks, and the client decides whether or not to accept the treatment. Take the example of administering pain medication to a client following an operation. The risk of discomfort from the injection or side effects from the medication is outweighed by the need to relieve the client's suffering.

Nurses treat clients fairly and with **justice**, the upholding of what is just, especially fair treatment and due reward in accordance with honor, standards, or law. This principle is challenging when decisions related to allocation of scarce resources must be made.

Individuals who always tell the truth reflect the principle of **veracity** (Guido, 2010, p. 8). Veracity can be a particularly challenging principle for the nurse, who may be faced with providing a client with complete information regarding the client's illness when family members or significant others want the information withheld. Veracity is the principle behind giving complete information before obtaining a client's informed consent for any procedure. Veracity is one of several principles behind timely and accurate documentation of nursing interventions.

NURSING CODES OF ETHICS

Ethical standards and behaviors are at the core of nursing practice. As a result, the nursing profession has developed codes of ethics to guide nurses in their work with clients and other health care professionals. A **code of ethics** is a general guide for a profession's membership and a social contract with the public that it serves. The Nightingale Pledge is considered the first code of nursing ethics in the United States. Written in 1893 by Lystra Gretter, the principal of the Farrand Training School for Nurses in Detroit, and patterned after the Hippocratic Oath for medicine, the Nightingale Pledge was named for Florence Nightingale. It is still used at many nursing schools' graduation ceremonies. The Nightingale Pledge reads as follows:

> I solemnly pledge myself before God and in the presence of this assembly: To pass my life in purity and to practice my profession faithfully. I will abstain from whatever is deleterious and mischievous, and will not take or knowingly administer any harmful drug. I will do all in my power to elevate the standard of my profession, and will hold in confidence all personal matters committed to my keeping, and all family affairs coming to my knowledge in the practice of my profession. With loyalty will I endeavor to aid the physician in his work and devote myself to the welfare of those committed to my care (Gretter, 1910).

There are two major national and international codes of ethics for the nursing profession: the American Nurses Association Code of Ethics for Nurses and the International Council of Nurses Code of Ethics. Both codes were initially formally adopted in the early 1950s and have undergone changes to reflect social and technological change. The current versions are presented in Box 42–2 and Box 42–3.

The ANA Code of Ethics for Nurses (2001) serves as a statement of ethical obligations and duties of the nurse, as the profession's nonnegotiable ethical standard, and as the nursing profession's statement of commitment to society.

The terms "ethical" and "moral" are used throughout the ANA Code. The Code is not simply a reference tool; nurses should use it to direct how they perform their duties in their daily life. The Code needs to be read and reread as the nurse develops ethical decision-making ability through his or her professional career. Provision 1 of the Code addresses the valuing of humans without modifiers (such as color, race, gender, or religious preferences). Nurses are expected to move beyond feelings and recognize the humanity of the client and respond with compassion and respect. A brief discussion of the provisions of the Code is provided here.

1. Interpretive statement 1.4, the right to self-determination, requires that the nurse be knowledgeable about the client's moral and legal rights (see Concept 47, Legal Issues). The ethical standard is that the nurse supports the client's decisions about care regardless of the nurse's own values.

Box 42–2 **International Council of Nurses Code of Ethics**

PREAMBLE

Nurses have four fundamental responsibilities: to promote health, to prevent illness, to restore health and to alleviate suffering. The need for nursing is universal.

Inherent in nursing is respect for human rights, including cultural rights, the right to life and choice, to dignity and to be treated with respect. Nursing care is respectful of and unrestricted by considerations of age, colour, creed, culture, disability or illness, gender, sexual orientation, nationality, politics, race or social status.

Nurses render health services to the individual, the family and the community and coordinate their services with those of related groups.

THE ICN CODE

The *ICN Code of Ethics for Nurses* has four principal elements that outline the standards of ethical conduct.

Elements of the Code

1. Nurses and People

   The nurse's primary professional responsibility is to people requiring nursing care.

   In providing care, the nurse promotes an environment in which the human rights, values, customs and spiritual beliefs of the individual, family and community are respected.

   The nurse ensures that the individual receives sufficient information on which to base consent for care and related treatment.

   The nurse holds in confidence personal information and uses judgement in sharing this information.

   The nurse shares with society the responsibility for initiating and supporting action to meet the health and social needs of the public, in particular those of vulnerable populations.

   The nurse also shares responsibility to sustain and protect the natural environment from depletion, pollution, degradation and destruction.

2. Nurses and Practice

   The nurse carries personal responsibility and accountability for nursing practice, and for maintaining competence by continual learning.

   The nurse maintains a standard of personal health such that the ability to provide care is not compromised.

   The nurse uses judgment regarding individual competence when accepting and delegating responsibility.

   The nurse at all times maintains standards of personal conduct which reflect well on the profession and enhance public confidence.

   The nurse, in providing care, ensures that use of technology and scientific advances are compatible with the safety, dignity and rights of people.

3. Nurses and the Profession

   The nurse assumes the major role in determining and implementing acceptable standards of clinical nursing practice, management, research and education.

   The nurse is active in developing a core of research-based professional knowledge.

   The nurse, acting through the professional organization, participates in creating and maintaining safe, equitable social and economic working conditions in nursing.

4. Nurses and Co-workers

   The nurse sustains a co-operative relationship with co-workers in nursing and other fields.

   The nurse takes appropriate action to safeguard individuals, families and communities when their health is endangered by a co-worker or any other person.

Note: From International Council of Nurses. (2006). *The ICN code of ethics for nurses.* Geneva: Imprimeries Populaires. Reprinted with permission.

2. Provision 2 mandates that the nurse's primary commitment be to the client. Davis (ANA, 2008) states that ethical problems often arise from tensions among responsibilities as well as from differing value and belief systems. She suggests that in applying Provision 2 to an ethical problem, the nurse needs to ask the following questions:

■ What do I know about this client's situation?

■ What do I know about the client's values and moral preferences?

■ What assumptions am I making that require more data to clarify?

■ What are my own feelings (and values) about the situation? How might they be influencing how I view and respond to the situation?

■ Are my own values in conflict with those of the client?

■ What else do I need to know about this case and where can I obtain this information?

■ What can I never know about this case?

■ Given my primary obligation to the client, what should I do to be ethical?

CLINICAL EXAMPLE

Carolyn Jetty, a 35-year-old woman diagnosed with cancer of the breast that has metastasized to the lung, has refused all chemotherapy and radiation treatment. Her husband, George, wants everything possible done to save his wife's life. They have three children ages 3, 7, and 9. The physician tends to go along with the husband for the sake of the children. Using the questions identified by Davis, determine what else you, as Ms. Jetty's nurse, would need to do to provide competent, ethical care for Ms. Jetty.

3. Provision 3 reflects the need to apply the principle of autonomy to specific bioethical issues, including the use of humans in research. In the current revision of the Code, privacy and confidentiality are separate interpretive statements. Privacy involves the aspects of information that the client can control. Confidentiality is how the information is handled once it is shared by the client (see Exemplar 47.2, HIPAA). The nurse's responsibility to the client involved in research is addressed in statement 3-3. Continuing competency in providing client-centered care is addressed in the interpretive statement 3-4. All nurses, regardless of position

Box 42–3 American Nurses Association Code of Ethics for Nurses (Approved July 2001)

1. The nurse, in all professional relationships, practices with compassion and respect for the inherent dignity, worth, and uniqueness of every individual, unrestricted by considerations of social or economic status, personal attributes, or the nature of health problems.
   - 1.1 Respect for human dignity
   - 1.2 Relationships to patients
   - 1.3 The nature of health problems
   - 1.4 The right to self-determination
   - 1.5 Relationships with colleagues and others
2. The nurse's primary commitment is to the patient, whether an individual, family, group, or community.
   - 2.1 Primacy of patient's interests
   - 2.2 Conflict of interest for nurses
   - 2.3 Collaboration
   - 2.4 Professional boundaries
3. The nurse promotes, advocates for, and strives to protect the health, safety, and rights of the patient.
   - 3.1 Privacy
   - 3.2 Confidentiality
   - 3.3 Protection of participants in research
   - 3.4 Standards and review mechanisms
   - 3.5 Acting on questionable practice
   - 3.6 Addressing impaired practice
4. The nurse is responsible and accountable for individual nursing practice and determines the appropriate delegation of tasks consistent with the nurse's obligation to provide optimum patient care.
   - 4.1 Acceptance of accountability and responsibility
   - 4.2 Accountability for nursing judgment and action
   - 4.3 Responsibility for nursing judgment and action
   - 4.4 Delegation of nursing activities
5. The nurse owes the same duties to self as to others, including the responsibility to preserve integrity and safety, to maintain competence, and to continue personal and professional growth.
   - 5.1 Moral self-respect
   - 5.2 Professional growth and maintenance of competence
   - 5.3 Wholeness of character
   - 5.4 Preservation of integrity
6. The nurse participates in establishing, maintaining, and improving health care environments and conditions of employment conducive to the provision of quality health care and consistent with the values of the profession through individual and collective action.
   - 6.1 Influence of the environment on moral virtues and values
   - 6.2 Influence of the environment on ethical obligations
   - 6.3 Responsibility for the health care environment
7. The nurse participates in the advancement of the profession through contributions to practice, education, administration, and knowledge development.
   - 7.1 Advancing the profession through active involvement in nursing and health care policy
   - 7.2 Advancing the profession by developing, maintaining, and implementing professional standards in clinical, administrative, and educational practice
   - 7.3 Advancing the profession through knowledge development, dissemination, and application to practice
8. The nurse collaborates with other health professionals and the public in promoting community, national, and international efforts to meet health needs.
   - 8.1 Health needs and concerns
   - 8.2 Responsibilities to the public
9. The profession of nursing, as represented by associations and their members, is responsible for articulating nursing values, for maintaining the integrity of the profession and its practice, and for shaping social policy.
   - 9.1 Assertion of values
   - 9.2 The profession carries out its collective responsibility through professional associations
   - 9.3 Intraprofessional integrity
   - 9.4 Social reform

Note: Reprinted with permission from American Nurses Association. (2001). *Code of ethics for nurses with interpretive statements.* Silver Spring, MD: Nursesbooks.org.

and setting, are accountable for ensuring that all nursing care is provided to clients by nurses who meet the profession's standards.

Statements 3-5 and 3-6 address the responsibility to identify any practice of an individual that is questionable, to recognize the need to do something about it, and to determine possible appropriate actions. This is consistent with mandatory reporting laws (see Exemplar 47.3) and the ethical responsibility that nurses have to address colleagues who may be impaired (refer to Concept 2, Addiction Behaviors).

4. Provision 4 identifies that, at all times, the responsibility and accountability for each nurse's actions and judgments belong to the individual nurse. Accountability is the professional implied contract with the public (see Concept 40, Accountability).

5. Provision 5 identifies the nurse's duty to self in seeking professional growth and maintaining competence, wholeness of character, and integrity. Fowler defines integrity as a lived conformity with the values one holds dear, both personal and professional (ANA, 2008, p. 66).

6. Provision 6 focuses on the role of the nurse in creating, promoting, and maintaining an ethical environment. A healthy, supportive workplace environment is essential to meet the needs of both the nurse and the clients. Many professional organizations have focused on the importance of developing a healthy workplace which provides for an environment that promotes ethical treatment of both the employees and the clients. The ANA (2001) developed the Bill of Rights for Registered Nurses as a policy statement with specific attention to the workplace environment. The American Nurses Credentialing Center Magnet Recognition Program recognizes organizations that demonstrate excellence in nursing practice and provide a culture of excellence.

7. Provision 7 encourages individual nurses to use their own talents and interests in contributing to the advancement of the profession through engagement in refining

professional standards or through the development, adaptation, and communication of knowledge.

8. Provisions 8 and 9 address the responsibility of the nurse in shaping public health policy and participating in social reform and the nurse's obligation to society to eliminate social inequity, prejudice, and oppression.

MODELS OF ETHICAL DECISION MAKING

Responsible ethical reasoning is rational and systematic. It should be based on ethical principles and codes rather than on emotions, intuition, fixed policies, or precedent (i.e., an earlier similar occurrence). Two decision-making models are shown in Box 42–4.

A good decision is one that is in the client's best interest and at the same time preserves the integrity of all the people involved. Nurses have ethical obligations to their clients, to the agency that employs them, and to primary care providers. Therefore, nurses must weigh competing factors when making ethical decisions. See Box 42–5 for examples.

Although ethical reasoning is principle-based and has the client's well-being at the center, being involved in ethical problems and dilemmas is stressful for the nurse. The nurse may feel torn among obligations to the client, the family, and the employer. What is in the client's best interest might be contrary to the nurse's personal belief system. In settings in which ethical issues arise frequently, nurses should establish support

---

Box 42–4 **Ethical Decision-Making Models**

THOMPSON AND THOMPSON MODEL (1985)
- Review the situation to determine health problems, decision needs, ethical components, and key individuals.
- Gather additional information to clarify the situation.
- Identify the ethical issues in the situation.
- Define personal and professional moral positions.
- Identify moral positions of key individuals involved.
- Identify value conflicts, if any.
- Determine who should make the decision.
- Identify range of actions with anticipated outcomes.
- Decide on a course of action and carry it out.
- Evaluate/review results of decision/action.

CASSELLS AND REDMAN MODEL (1989)
- Identify the moral aspects of nursing care.
- Gather relevant facts related to a moral issue.
- Clarify and apply personal values.
- Understand ethical theories and principles.
- Utilize competent interdisciplinary resources.
- Propose alternative actions.
- Apply nursing codes of ethics to help guide actions.
- Choose and implement resolutive action.
- Participate actively in resolving the issue.
- Apply state and federal laws governing nursing practice.
- Evaluate the resolutive action taken.

Note: From Thompson, J. B., & Thompson, H. O. (1985). *Bioethical decision-making for nurses* (p. 99). Norwalk, CT: Appleton-Century-Croft and Cassells, J., & Redman, B. (1989). Preparing students to be moral agents in clinical nursing practice. *Nursing clinics of North America, 24*(2), pp. 463–473. Reprinted with permission.

Box 42–5 **Examples of Nurses' Obligations in Ethical Decisions**

- Maximize the client's well-being.
- Balance the client's need for autonomy with family members' responsibilities for the client's well-being.
- Support each family member and enhance the family support system.
- Carry out hospital policies.
- Protect other clients' well-being.
- Protect the nurse's own standards of care.

---

systems such as team conferences and use of counseling professionals to allow expression of their feelings.

Many nursing problems are not moral problems at all, but simply questions of good nursing practice. An important first step in ethical decision making is to determine whether a moral dilemma exists. The following criteria may be used:

- A difficult choice exists between actions that conflict with the needs of one or more persons.
- Moral principles or frameworks exist that can be used to provide some justification for the action.
- The choice is guided by a process of weighing reasons.
- The decision is freely and consciously chosen.
- The choice is affected by personal feelings and by the particular context of the situation.

Although the nurse's input is important, in reality several people are usually involved in making an ethical decision. The client, family, spiritual support persons, and other members of the health care team work together in reaching ethical decisions (see Figure 42–1 ■). Therefore, collaboration, communication, and compromise are important skills for health professionals.

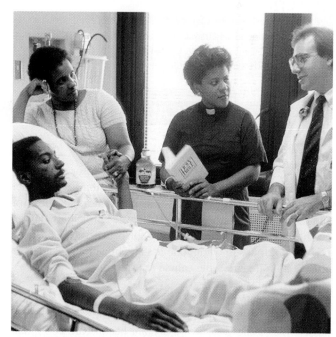

Figure 42–1 ■ When there is a need for ethical decisions of client advocacy, many different people contribute to the final outcome.
A. Ramsey/PhotoEdit

STRATEGIES TO ENHANCE ETHICAL DECISIONS AND PRACTICE

Several strategies help nurses overcome possible organizational and social constraints that can hinder the ethical practice of nursing and create moral distress for nurses. Nurses should do the following:

■ Become aware of their own values and the ethical aspects of nursing.

■ Be familiar with nursing codes of ethics.

■ Seek continuing education opportunities to stay knowledgeable about ethical issues in nursing.

■ Respect the values, opinions, and responsibilities of other health care professionals that may be different from your own.

■ Participate in or establish ethics rounds. Ethics rounds use hypothetical or real cases that focus on the ethical dimensions of client care rather than the client's clinical diagnosis and treatment.

■ Serve on institutional ethics committees.

■ Strive for collaborative practice in which nurses function effectively in cooperation with other health care professionals.

One resource that is available to help nurses maintain a current, evidence-based ethical practice is the National Guideline Clearinghouse (www.guideline.gov). The clearinghouse provides an index to more than 2,000 guidelines for evidence-based practice on a number of health issues, including ethical issues. For example, the Hartford Institute of Geriatric Nursing has developed a number of evidence-based nursing protocols for working with geriatric clients. These protocols address topics such as advance directives and health care decision making, working with older adults with dementia, and discussing sexual health with the older adult (NGC, 2010).

PRACTICE ALERT
When an ethical dilemma arises in a clinical practice, nurses should begin an ethical analysis and communicate with colleagues to seek a solution. The process is a way to seek balance, address issues, and understand the needs of all involved.

One strategy that hospitals and other organizations can use to enhance ethical decision making is to implement a multidisciplinary ethics committee. Ethical standards of The Joint Commission mandate that health care institutions provide ethics committees or a similar structure to write guidelines and policies and to provide education, counseling, and support on ethical issues (Joint Commission, 2006). These multidisciplinary committees, which include nurses, physicians, and hospital administrators, can be asked to review a case and provide guidance to a competent client, an incompetent client's family, or to a health care provider. These committees provide a forum in which diverse views can be expressed, support is provided for caregivers, and the institution's legal risks can be reduced (see Exemplar 47.5, Risk Management).

CONCLUSION

The ANA Code of Ethics outlines the ethical standards that nurses are expected to use to inform their behavior towards clients and their families, other nurses and health care professionals, and the larger community. Ethical standards do not fall solely within the realm of the nursing profession. No one profession is responsible for ethical decisions, nor does expertise in one discipline, such as nursing, necessarily make a person an expert in ethics.

As discussed, determining whether or not a moral problem exists is the first step in ethical decision making. The nursing profession has identified a number of ethical dilemmas that nurses face in a variety of settings. Nursing students as well as professional nurses should examine their values related to these identified dilemmas and understand how their values may impact their own professional nursing practice. Several of the dilemmas are discussed in Exemplar 42.1.

42.1 ETHICAL DILEMMAS

OVERVIEW

An ethical dilemma exists when there are two or more conflicting rights, values, obligations, or responsibilities. Conflict may arise between the nurse's personal values and those of another person or the organization, between principles and the need to achieve a desired outcome, or between two or more persons or groups to whom one has an obligation, such as the client, a colleague, the nurse's profession, the nurse's employer, and society.

Rapidly changing technology, conflicting societal and cultural values, conflicting loyalties and obligations among nurses, increasing pressure to contain health care costs, and reduced staffing are some of the factors that contribute to the development of ethical dilemmas in nursing.

Social and Technological Changes

Technology creates new issues that did not exist in earlier times. Before monitors, respirators, and intravenous (IV) or artificial tube feedings, there was no question about whether to "allow" an 800-gram premature infant to die. Before organ transplantation, death did not require a legal definition that might still permit viable tissues to be removed and given to other living persons. Advances in the ability to decode and control the growth of tissues through gene manipulation present new potential ethical dilemmas related to cloning organisms and altering the course of hereditary diseases and biological characteristics. Today, with treatments that can prolong and enhance biologic life, these questions arise: Should we do what we know we can? Who should be treated—everyone, only those who can pay, only those who have a chance to improve?

Conflicting Loyalties and Obligations

Because of their unique position in the health care system, nurses experience conflicts among their loyalties and obligations to clients, families, primary care providers, employing institutions, and licensing bodies. Client needs may conflict with institutional policies, primary care provider preferences, needs of the client's family, or even state or federal laws. According to the ANA Code of Ethics for Nurses (2001), the nurse's first loyalty is to the client. However, it is not always easy to determine which action best serves the client's needs. For instance, the nurse may be aware that marijuana has been shown to be effective for a condition a client has that has not responded to mainstream therapies. Although legal issues are involved, the nurse must determine whether, ethically, the client should be made aware of a potentially effective alternative. Another example is individual nurses' decisions regarding whether to honor picket lines during employee strikes. The nurse may experience conflict among feeling the need to support co-workers in their efforts to improve working conditions, feeling the need to ensure that clients receive care and are not abandoned, and feeling loyalty to his or her employer.

BIOETHICAL ISSUES

Bioethics refers to ethics as applied to human life or health. Bioethical dilemmas may arise during the care of clients and families dealing with HIV/AIDS, abortion, organ transplantation, and end-of-life decisions.

Acquired Immune Deficiency Syndrome (AIDS)

Because of its association with sexual behavior and illicit drug use, AIDS bears a social stigma. According to an ANA position statement, the moral obligation to care for the client infected with HIV cannot be set aside unless the risk exceeds the responsibility (ANA, 1994).

Other ethical issues center on testing for HIV status and for the presence of AIDS in health care professionals and clients. Questions arise as to whether testing of all providers and clients should be mandatory or voluntary and whether test results should be released to insurance companies, sexual partners, or caregivers. As with all ethical dilemmas, each possibility has both positive and negative implications for specific individuals.

Abortion

Abortion is a highly publicized issue about which many people feel very strongly. Debate continues, pitting the principle of sanctity of life against the principle of autonomy and the woman's right to control her own body. This is an especially volatile issue because no public consensus has yet been reached.

Most state laws have provisions known as conscience clauses that permit individual physicians and nurses, as well as institutions, to refuse to assist with an abortion if doing so violates their religious or moral principles. However, nurses have no right to impose their values on a client. Nursing codes of ethics support clients' rights to information and counseling in making decisions.

PRACTICE ALERT
Working with a teenager who is seeking information about abortion can be a particularly difficult ethical challenge for the nurse. Nurses working in emergency rooms and in clinics that serve teenagers should examine their beliefs and values about teens having abortions. They should also know the legal requirements of their state: Some states require parental consent for a minor to have an abortion, though the age at which consent is required may vary by state; some states require only notification of the minor's parents; some require neither consent nor notification.

Organ Transplantation

Organs for transplantation may come from living donors or from donors who have just died. Many living people choose to become donors by giving consent under the Uniform Anatomical Gift Act. Ethical issues related to organ transplantation include allocation of organs, selling of body parts, involvement of children as potential donors, consent, clear definition of death, and conflicts of interest between potential donors and recipients. In some situations, a person's religious belief may also present conflict. For example, certain religions forbid the mutilation of the body, even for the benefit of another person.

End-of-Life Issues

Advances in technology and the growing number of older adults have expanded the ethical dilemmas faced by older adults and the health care professionals who work with them. Providing these clients with information and professional assistance, as well as the highest quality of care and caring, is of the utmost importance. Some of the most frequent disturbing ethical problems for nurses involve issues that arise around death and dying. These include euthanasia, assisted suicide, termination of life-sustaining treatment, and withdrawing or withholding of food and fluids. For more information on end-of-life issues, see Exemplar 5.2.

PRACTICE ALERT
Nurses working with clients who are terminally ill and their families need special preparations to meet the needs of these individuals and to manage their own personal stress, particularly when the client's decisions regarding end-of-life care conflict with the nurses' personal values. Nurses working with these clients should seek support from their peers or from group sessions with mental health professionals. Participating in team decisions regarding a dying client's palliative plan of care helps many nurses manage their distress.

EVIDENCE-BASED PRACTICE How Do Nurses Feel About Abortion Based on the Reasons for Aborting?

There are many reasons why women decide to terminate a pregnancy. Some of these reasons include physiological impairment in the fetus, conditions life-threatening to the mother, the mother's desire not to have the child, and preference for a specific gender of the child. The researchers found few existing studies of nurses' attitudes about abortion. The ANA Code of Ethics supports the nurse's choice to avoid participation in an abortion under ethical opposition reasons. The purpose of this study was to determine how often nurses refused to care for clients choosing an abortion and for what reasons. Seventy-five labor and delivery nurses working in California participated in the study. The majority of respondents said they would care for a woman having an abortion for fetal death (95%) and when fetal defects were incompatible with life (77%). Between 20% and 37% would care for a client with fetal birth defects compatible with life, and between 8% and 29% for clients choosing to reduce the number of fetuses in multifetal pregnancies, depending on how far along was the pregnancy. Although 32% of nurses would care for a client terminating the pregnancy in the first trimester for personal reasons, only 4% would do so during the third trimester.

Less than 5% of the nurses would participate in an abortion being done for gender selection at any time in the pregnancy. Nurses listed a variety of influences on their decisions to care or not care for these clients, including ethical beliefs (57%), spiritual beliefs (48%), and previous work experiences with termination and grief/loss (28%).

Implications

Although ethical guidelines permit nurses to refuse care in nonemergency situations for ethical reasons, little is known about when, why, and how this occurs. Nurses face ethical challenges when there is no other provider available who can provide competent care for the client. Nurses must consider their ethical beliefs when accepting assignments to work in areas known to commonly experience particular ethical issues and, very importantly, must communicate their willingness or refusal to provide care to the team so that safe client care can be assured.

Note: From Marek, M. J. (2004). Nurses' attitudes toward pregnancy termination in the labor and delivery setting. *Journal of Obstetric, Gynecologic, and Neonatal Nursing, 33*, pp. 472–479.

ADVANCE DIRECTIVES Many moral problems surrounding the end of life can be resolved if clients complete advance directives. Currently, all 50 states have enacted advance directive legislation. Advance directives instruct caregivers as to the client's wishes about treatments, providing an ongoing voice for clients when they have lost the capacity to make or communicate their decisions. See Concept 47, Legal Issues, and Exemplar 5.2, End-of-Life Care, for more information about advance directives. An advanced directive may provide instructions regarding Do-Not-Resuscitate (DNR) orders, the withholding of emergency measures to sustain life, the termination of life sustaining measures, or any combination thereof. Nurses working with clients who are experiencing life-threatening events or who are approaching the end of life should make sure they understand both the client's advance directive as well as the policies and procedures regarding advance directives at their place of employment.

EUTHANASIA AND ASSISTED SUICIDE Euthanasia, a Greek word meaning "good death," is popularly known as "mercy killing." **Active euthanasia** involves actions to bring about the client's death directly, with or without client consent. An example of this would be the administration of a lethal dose of medication to end the client's suffering. Regardless of the caregiver's intent, active euthanasia is forbidden by law and can result in criminal charges against the individual who brings about the client's death.

A variation of active euthanasia is **assisted suicide**, or giving clients the means to kill themselves if they request it (e.g., providing pills or a weapon). Some countries and some states have laws permitting assisted suicide for clients who are severely ill, who are near death, and who wish to commit suicide. Although some people may disagree with the concept, in January 2006, the U.S. Supreme Court ruled to uphold the assisted suicide regulations in the state of Oregon. In any case, the nurse should recall that legality and morality are not the same thing. Determining whether an action is legal is only one aspect of deciding whether it is ethical. The questions of suicide and assisted suicide are still controversial in our society. The American Nurses Association's position statement on assisted suicide (ANA, 1995) states that active euthanasia and assisted suicide are in violation of the Code of Ethics for Nurses.

WITHDRAWING, WITHHOLDING, OR TERMINATING LIFE-SUSTAINING TREATMENT Withdrawing or withholding life-sustaining therapy (WWLST) involves the withdrawal of extraordinary means of life support, such as removing a ventilator or withholding special attempts to revive a client, and allowing the client to die of the underlying medical condition (e.g., aspiration pneumonia). WWLST is both legally and ethically more acceptable to most people than assisted suicide (Ersek, 2005).

Antibiotics, organ transplants, and technological advances (e.g., ventilators) help to prolong life but do not necessarily restore health. Clients may specify that they wish to have life-sustaining measures terminated, they may have advance directives on this matter, or they may appoint a health care surrogate to make the decision on their behalf. Regardless, it is usually more troubling for health care professionals to withdraw a treatment than to decide initially not to begin it. Nurses must understand that a decision to withdraw treatment is not a decision to withdraw care. As the primary caregivers, nurses must ensure that sensitive care and comfort measures (palliative care) are given as the client's illness progresses after withdrawal of treatment. When the client is at home, nurses often provide this type of education and support through hospice services (see Concept 5 for more information regarding hospice and end-of-life care).

Because it is difficult for families to withdraw treatment, it is very important that they fully understand the client's treatment. Families often misunderstand which treatments are life sustaining. Keeping clients and families well informed is an ongoing process, as they need time to ask questions and discuss the situation. It is also essential that clients and families understand that they can reevaluate and change their decision if they wish.

PRACTICE ALERT

Nurses provide ethical care to dying clients and their families by respecting client autonomy; by providing competent, culturally sensitive care; and by providing nursing presence.

WITHDRAWING OR WITHHOLDING FOOD AND FLUIDS It is generally accepted that providing food and fluids is part of ordinary nursing practice and, therefore, a moral duty. However, some people consider it an extraordinary measure to administer food and fluids by tube to a dying client or to administer them over a long period to an unconscious client who is not expected to improve. A nurse is morally obligated to withhold food and fluids (or any treatment) if it is determined to be more harmful to administer them than to withhold them. The nurse must also honor competent and informed clients' refusal of food and fluids. The ANA Code of Ethics for Nurses (2001) supports this position through the nurse's role as a client advocate and through the moral principle of autonomy.

ETHICAL ISSUES IN NURSING PRACTICE

Nursing is the undisputed leader in the list of professions viewed as honest and ethical. Nursing has been ranked first among all professions in all but one year since they were added to the list in 1999 (Saad, 2009). While nurses are perceived as being honest and ethical, their identity as moral agents is shaped by contextual and organizational forces. Patricia Benner (2000) describes how shifts in governmental

and corporate health care values profoundly influence nurses' ablility to exercise their moral agency at the level of practice. While biomedical ethicists have tended to focus on high profile medical cases, the nursing profession has identified the need for more models of practice that deal with situations that nurses confront on a daily basis.

Ethical behavior is the day-by-day expression of one's commitment to other persons and the ways in which human beings relate to one another in their daily interaction (Levine, 1977). Some everyday ethical challenges identified by nurses are categorized by Varcoe and colleagues (2004) as working the "in-betweens." Nurses identify being caught in between various players including health care providers and the client, and between the client and the family. Nurses are also caught between family members, between staff members, and between managers and various other colleagues. Within these relationships there are conflicting loyalties. Nurses balance loyalties to the client, family, employer, profession, and community. Nurses also identify conflicts arising from traditional power structures in health care such as the focus on providing curative treatment and the emphasis on the role of the physician. For example, nurses have expressed concerns about being intimidated or dismissed by physicians when reporting observations incongruent with proposed medical treatment plan or being ignored by senior medical staff when reporting concerns related to physician behavior. Additional conflict arises when operating under staffing shortages or other situations in which organizational efficiency is at issue. Nurses who must balance limited time available with care that needs to be provided operate in such a conflict. Frequently the activities that suffer the most include client teaching, counseling, and support as the nurse's focus moves to the performance of physical tasks and functions. Nurses reporting conflict with corporate values have experienced being threatened by administrators and fear of job and license loss. Important resources for ethical practice that have been identified are supportive colleagues, educators, and

FOCUS ON CULTURE AND DIVERSITY   Variations in Applying Moral Principles

Although a moral principle may exist and be valued in different cultures, the degree to which it is valued and the manner by which it is used in health care may be quite variable. Nurses must become familiar with how moral principles are viewed within the cultural groups with which they practice.

PRINCIPLE	EXAMPLES OF ETHNIC/CULTURAL VARIATIONS
Autonomy	Family members, rather than the client, receive information on the client's condition and take primary responsibility for decision making. The family and community are viewed as affected by the client's condition and decisions as much as the individual is affected: Chinese, Koreans, Mexican Americans, Bosnian Americans.
Veracity	Prefer client not to be told directly of a life-threatening condition: Hispanics, Asians, Pakistanis, Bosnian Americans, Italian Americans, Canadian Aboriginals.
Nonmaleficence	Discussion of advance directives and issues such as cardiopulmonary resuscitation are viewed as physically and emotionally harmful to the client: Filipino, Native American, Chinese.
Beneficence	Health care providers should promote client well-being and hope: Asian cultures, Native Americans, Russians.

Note: From Ellerby, J. H., McKenzie, McKay, J.S., Gariepy, G. J., & Kaufert, J. M. (2000). Bioethics for clinicians: 18 aboriginal cultures. *Canadian Medical Association Journal*, 163, 845–850; Searight, H. R., & Gafford, J. (2005). Cultural diversity at the end of life: Issues and guidelines for family physicians. *American Family Physician*, 71, 515–522; Searight, H. R. & Gafford, J. (2005). It's like playing with your destiny: Bosnian immigrants' views of advance directives and end-of-life decision-making. *Journal of Immigrant Health*, 7, 195–203.

approachable responsible managers. Nurses have reported that having the opportunity to discuss ethical concerns is both personally and professionally sustaining (Varcoe, et al., 2004).

Dr. Patricia Benner has identified that the behavior of nurses is shaped by their organizational and professional roles and the settings in which they work and that their responses to ethical problems are inseparable from the settings in which they arise. The Carnegie study of nursing education (Benner, 2010) demonstrated that clinical experiences (including pre and post clinical conferences) of nursing students were strong in developing six essential ethical behaviors when compared to the clinical experiences of other professions. The ethical behaviors examined included meeting the client as a person, preserving the dignity and personhood of clients, how to respond to substandard practice related to client advocacy, learning to do "good" nursing practice, and how to be present with client and family suffering. Dr Benner identified the need for nursing students to learn social ethics and for greater emphasis on the role of the nurse as advocate, as traditional classroom teaching emphasizes bioethics and has been critical of the effects of developing technology and the ethics of its use.

Academic Dishonesty

Through reading, class time, and clinical experiences, nursing students can begin to imagine some aspects of ethical decision making in the clinical context. With increased experience and exposure, each student can identify increasing conflicting values and variables that affect the practicing nurse. The development of professional ethical behavior, social roles, and responsibilities builds on the individual's personal ethics. Ethical decision-making is a situational or contextual process. Academic dishonesty presents an ethical situation which nursing students may confront early in their ethical development. Examples of academic dishonesty include cheating, plagiarism, and failure to follow academic policies, such as the requirement to return examinations following a test review session. See the Clinical Example that follows and Box 42–6, An Exercise in Ethical Decision Making.

CLINICAL EXAMPLE

Elizabeth, a first year nursing student, has obtained a copy of the first examination given last year in Nursing 110 from Jasmine, her assigned "Big Sister" from the second year class. Jasmine emphasized that questions on nursing examinations are much harder to answer because they require application of information, not just recall. Elizabeth informs her selected study group that she has the exam and she is willing to share to help them focus their study time. You are a member of Elizabeth's study group.

1. Will you participate? Why or why not?
2. Will you report Elizabeth to your instructor?
3. What ethical principle is involved in your decision process?
4. What conflicting values are involved in this scenario?
5. What additional information might help you make your decision? What difference does it make if you learn that Jasmine did not turn in the exam following a test review session?
6. What school policies are involved? What aspects of the ANA Code of Ethics apply?

Box 42–6 An Exercise in Ethical Decision Making

Referring to the clinical example of Elizabeth and Jasmine:
1. **Identify a range of actions with potential outcomes**
   What are the pros? What are the cons?
   If you choose to participate in the study group *and* then inform the instructor?
   If you choose to participate and not tell the instructor?
   If you choose not to participate and not tell the instructor?
   If you choose not to participate and to tell the instructor?
2. **Decide on a course of action and carry it out**
   So what are you going to decide?
   On what do you base your decision?
   What does your decision tell others about you and your values?
   Does your decision predict future decisions/actions?
3. **Evaluate/revaluate the consequences of your decision/action**
   What tools would you use to evaluate your decision/action after the fact?
   How would you determine what effect your decision/action had on others?

In a personal ethical dilemma, the decision is made by the individual based on the individual's values and best interests. The individual will be primarily accountable for the consequences of that action, including those affecting others. This is in direct contrast to a professional ethical dilemma in which the decision should reflect the autonomy of the client and in which the nurse is accountable to the client's values, and best interests.

Workplace Issues

Financial restraints, personnel issues, and other organizational challenges can contribute to ethical conflicts in the work place. Limited resources and short staffing are two ethical challenges which nurses frequently experience in the workplace.

ALLOCATION OF LIMITED HEALTH RESOURCES Allocation of limited supplies of health care goods and services, including organ transplants, artificial joints, and the services of specialists, has become an especially urgent issue as health care costs continue to rise and more stringent cost-containment measures are implemented. The moral principle of autonomy cannot be applied if it is not possible to give each client what he or she chooses. In these situations, health care providers may use the principle of justice by attempting to choose what is most fair to all. Nurses, other health care professionals, legislators, and clients must continue to look for ways to balance economics and care in the allocation of health resources. For more information on resource allocation in health care, see Concept 37, Managing Care, and Concept 44, Health Care Systems.

SHORT STAFFING With a nationwide shortage of nurses, nursing care is becoming a limited health resource. Short staffing is a critical concern as a number of studies link staffing levels to safe client care (AACN, 2010). Unfortunately, some facilities continue to staff nursing units with fewer registered nurses and more unlicensed caregivers. When this occurs, nurses become concerned that staffing in their institutions is not adequate to ensure client safety, much less to allow them to provide the level of care that they value. California is the first state to enact legislation mandating specific nurse-to-client ratios in hospitals and other health-care settings. This is not the simple solution that it seems: Another ethical dilemma arises when organizations begin to turn away clients in need in order to ensure adequate staffing levels.

CLINICAL EXAMPLE

The director of nursing is having difficulty staffing all the units adequately. Two units have already been closed. The director can either spread the available staff around the facility and keep the remaining units open, but with fewer nurses than is really safe, or close additional units. The director needs to consider the welfare of the institution, the nursing staff, and the clients.

1. How would you assess the ethical aspects of this issue?
2. What actions would you take? Why?
3. How does the Code of Ethics inform the possible actions?

Working With Clients and Families

Working with clients and families can be both rewarding and challenging. Clear communication and good clinical decision making skills help the nurse develop a positive relationship with clients and their families. Ethical challenges which may arise include maintaining client privacy and confidentiality and ensuring client autonomy.

CLIENT PRIVACY AND CONFIDENTIALITY In keeping with the principle of autonomy, nurses are obligated to respect clients' privacy and confidentiality. Privacy is both a legal and an ethical mandate. The Health Insurance Portability and Accountability Act of 1996 (HIPAA) includes standards protecting the confidentiality, integrity, and availability of data and standards defining appropriate disclosures of identifiable health information and client rights protection (see Concept 47, Legal Issues). Clients must be able to trust that nurses will reveal details of the clients' situations only as appropriate and will communicate only the information necessary to provide for their health care. Computerized client records make sensitive data accessible to more people and accent issues of confidentiality. Nurses should help develop and follow security measures and policies to ensure appropriate use of client data (see Concept 46, Informatics).

CLIENT AUTONOMY Nurses have an ethical obligation as well as a legal mandate to respect the right of each client to make his or her own decisions regarding health care treatment. It is not uncommon for nurses to come across situations in which the client's autonomy is at risk. In these situations, the nurse has an ethical obligation to advocate for the client's right to make his or her own health care decisions, whether or not the risk comes in the form of a well-meaning family member who disagrees with the client's decision or a physician or other health care provider who either fails to hear the client's concerns or who disagrees with the client's request or decision. See the Clinical Example that follows.

CLINICAL EXAMPLE

David Lewis is a 50-year-old African American male who is recovering from a stroke at a rehabilitation facility. He is medically stable and able to participate fully in his therapies. However, he has requested DNR (do not resuscitate) status. He reasons that if he has another stroke or cardiac arrest, he could lose much more cognitive and motor function and that if he were resuscitated, it would place too heavy a burden of care on his family. Day after day he and his family ask about the DNR order. The nurses working with Mr. Lewis repeatedly ask the attending physician for an order, and the physician continues to respond that Mr. Lewis does not need a DNR order—he is stable. Finally, the primary nurse goes to the facility's ethics committee to discuss the problem. This results in another physician reviewing the chart, speaking with the client and family, and entering the DNR order.

1. What ethical dilemma did the primary nurse working with Mr. Lewis face?
2. What principles did the primary nurse follow in going to the ethics council?
3. How do you feel about DNR orders? Why?
4. In what ways did the nurses working with Mr. Lewis advocate on his behalf? How is the nurse's role as an advocate related to nursing ethics?

CONCLUSION

Coping with ethical dilemmas can be a challenge for even the most experienced nurse. Changes as a result of developments in research and technology make it essential for nurses to maintain a current, evidence-based, ethical practice. Thorough knowledge of the ANA Code of Ethics, assessment and understanding of the client's personal values and beliefs, and recognizing one's own personal values and beliefs will help each nurse address ethical dilemmas in a professional, responsible manner that ensures the nurse's credibility while respecting client autonomy.

Box 42–7 Nurses Coping With Ethical Dilemmas

Nurses maintain ethical practice through maintaining knowledge of the ANA Code of Ethics, ANA standards of practice, recognition of personal values, understanding ethical decision-making processes, and recognizing and understanding the importance of legal issues. As nurses confront ethical dilemmas, they should take care to avoid these decision-making traps:

- Reaching a decision prematurely
- Overconfidence in their own judgment
- Failing to follow systems and policies of their workplace
- Inability to recognize the effect of their own personal values
- Inability to recognize when a conflict arises between what is best for the client and what is best for the organization (Wocial, 1996, p. 155).

42.2 PATIENT RIGHTS

OVERVIEW

All clients have certain rights. Some of these are guaranteed by federal law, such as the right to informed consent mandated in the Patient Self-Determination Act (see Concept 47, Legal Issues). Many states have additional laws protecting clients, and health care facilities often have a patient bill of rights. The importance of patient rights are evident in the American Nurses Association's Standards of Practice and Code of Ethics as well as in the standards set for accreditation of various types of health care agencies by The Joint Commission. The Joint Commission offers a wealth of information on patients' rights, including brochures for clients (see www.jointcommission.org).

Nurses should be aware of national and state laws pertaining to patient rights, as well as the policies and procedures that their own employers establish in an effort to protect patient rights and ensure employee compliance with applicable laws and standards. For example, in a procedure that describes preoperative care, a hospital or surgical facility would include patient rights by identifying how informed consent should be obtained, by whom, when, and how it is to be documented.

PROTECTING PATIENT RIGHTS

Despite the many assurances that patients' rights will be protected, many people encounter what they view as mistreatment or violations of their rights during the course of their experiences in the health care system. Individual clients who feel their rights have been violated or are endangered have a number of options available to them. Many hospitals and large provider agencies have patient advocates who can help clients navigate their system and intervene to ensure that their rights are maintained. Many states have an office designated by the governor or secretary of health to assist clients with issues related to patient rights in long term care. The state's department of health may also be able to

help. Nursing homes, homes for the aged, and licensed facilities for the disabled are regulated at the state level, and violations committed by these agencies may be reported for investigation. Legislatures in many states have legislated declarations of patient rights that must be followed by nursing homes and other agencies who provide medical care and housing for clients at various points in the health care system. Box 42–8 provides North Carolina's Declaration of Patient Rights as an example.

In addition to the bills of rights provided in this exemplar, there are many others. Among them are bills of rights for hospice clients and for mental health clients and patient bills of rights legislated in certain states. Insurance plans sometimes have lists of rights for subscribers.

Most of these documents give information regarding where to go if a client has problems with his or her care. The American Hospital Association has a list of rights that is accompanied by a list of patient responsibilities to help clients be more active partners in their own health care (see Box 42–10). The AHA's list of patient rights includes those required under the Patient Self-Determination Act, but goes beyond that to include additional rights, such as the patient's right to considerate and respectful care and the patient's right to ask and be informed of the any business relationships that the hospital may have that may influence the patient's treatment and care (AHA, 1998).

CONCLUSION

Ethical issues impact nursing practice on a daily basis. Nurses who engage in ethical practice follow the ANA Code of Ethics, their own employers' policies and procedures regarding the rights of clients and their families, employ values clarification exercises as necessary, and make use of additional resources, such as peers and multidisciplinary ethics committees, to ensure clients are provided the best possible nursing care.

Box 42–8 **Patient Rights in North Carolina**

In the state of North Carolina, General Statute chapter 131E addresses Health Care Facilities and Services. N.C.G.S. §131E-117 addresses patients' rights:

DECLARATION OF PATIENTS' RIGHTS
All facilities shall treat their patients in accordance with the provisions of this Part.
   Every patient shall have the following rights:
1. To be treated with consideration, respect, and full recognition of personal dignity and individuality;
2. To receive care, treatment and services which are adequate, appropriate, and in compliance with relevant federal and State statutes and rules;
3. To receive at the time of admission and during the stay, a written statement of the services provided by the facility, including those required to be offered on an as needed basis, and of related charges. Charges for services not covered under Medicare or Medicaid shall be specified. Upon receiving this

statement, the patient shall sign a written receipt which must be on file in the facility and available for inspection;
4. To have on file in the patient's record a written or verbal order of the attending physician containing any information as the attending physician deems appropriate or necessary, together with the proposed schedule of medical treatment. The patient shall give prior informed consent to participation in experimental research. Written evidence of compliance with this subdivision, including signed acknowledgments by the patient, shall be retained by the facility in the patient's file;
5. To receive respect and privacy in the patient's medical care program. Case discussion consultation, examination, and treatment shall remain confidential and shall be conducted discreetly. Personal and medical records shall be confidential and the written consent of the patient shall be obtained for their release to any individual, other than family members, except as needed in case of the patient's transfer to another health care institution or as required by law or third party payment contract;

Box 42–8 Patient Rights in North Carolina (continued)

6. To be free from mental and physical abuse and, except in emergencies, to be free from chemical and physical restraints unless authorized for a specified period of time by a physician according to clear and indicated medical need;

7. To receive from the administrator or staff of the facility a reasonable response to all requests;

8. To associate and communicate privately and without restriction with persons and groups of the patient's choice on the patient's initiative or that of the persons or groups at any reasonable hour; to send and receive mail promptly and unopened, unless the patient is unable to open and read personal mail; to have access at any reasonable hour to a telephone where the patient may speak privately; and to have access to writing instruments, stationery, and postage;

9. To mange the patient's financial affairs unless authority has been delegated to another pursuant to a power of attorney, or written agreement, or some other person or agency has been appointed for this purpose pursuant to law. Nothing shall prevent the patient and facility from entering a written agreement for the facility to manage the patient's financial affairs. In the event that the facility manages the patient's financial affairs, it shall have an accounting available for inspection and shall furnish the patient with a quarterly statement of the patient's account. The patient shall have reasonable access to this account at reasonable hours; the patient or facility may terminate the agreement for the facility to manage the patient's financial affairs at any time upon five days' notice.

10. To enjoy privacy in visits by the patient's spouse, and, if both are inpatients of the facility, they shall be afforded the opportunity where feasible to share a room;

11. To enjoy privacy in the patient's room;

12. To present grievances and recommend changes in policies and services, personally or through other persons or in combination with others, on the patient's personal behalf or that of others to the facility's staff, the community advisory committee, the administrator, the Department, or other persons or groups without fear of reprisal, restraint, interference, coercion, or discrimination;

13. To not be required to perform services for the facility without personal consent and the written approval of the attending physician;

14. To retain, to secure storage for, and to use personal clothing and possessions, where reasonable;

15. To not be transferred or discharged from a facility except for medical reason, the patient's own or other patients' welfare, nonpayment for the stay, or when the transfer or discharge is mandated under Title XVIII (Medicare) or Title XIX (Medicaid) of the Social Security Act. The patient shall be given at least five days advance notice to ensure orderly transfer or discharge, unless the attending physician orders immediate transfer, and these actions, and the reasons for them, shall be documented in the patient's medical record.

16. To be notified within 10 days after the facility has been issued a provisional license because of violation of licensure regulations or received notice of revocation of license by the North Carolina Department of Human Resources and the basis on which the provisional license or notice of revocation of license was issued. The patient's responsible family member or guardian shall also be notified. (1977, c.)

Source: North Carolina, General Statute chapter 131E (N.C.G.S. §131E-117). The U. S. Advisory Commission on Consumer Protection and Quality in the Health Care Industry adopted a Bill of Rights in 1998. This Bill of Rights now applies to the insurance plans offered to federal employees. A summary of this Bill of Rights is provided in Box 42–9.

Box 42–9 A Summary of the Bill of Rights of the U. S. Advisory Commission on Consumer Protection and Quality in the Health Care Industry

- *Information Disclosure:* You have the right to accurate and easily understood information about your health plan, health care professionals, and health care facilities. If you speak another language, have a physical or mental disability, or just don't understand something, help should be provided so you can make informed health care decisions.

- *Choice of Providers and Plans:* You have the right to a choice of health care providers who can give you high-quality health care when you need it.

- *Access to Emergency Services:* If you have severe pain, an injury, or sudden illness that makes you believe that your health is in serious danger, you have the right to be screened and stabilized using emergency services. These services should be provided whenever and wherever you need them, without the need to wait for authorization and without any financial penalty.

- *Participation in Treatment Decisions:* You have the right to know your treatment options and to take part in decisions about your care. Parents, guardians, family members, or others that you select can represent you if you cannot make your own decisions.

- *Respect and Nondiscrimination:* You have a right to considerate, respectful care from your doctors, health plan representatives, and other health care providers that does not discriminate against you.

- *Confidentiality of Health Information:* You have the right to talk privately with health care providers and to have your health care information protected. You also have the right to read and copy your own medical records. You have the right to ask that your doctor change your record if it is not accurate, relevant, or complete.

- *Complaints and Appeals:* You have the right to a fair, fast, and objective review of any complaint you have against your health plan, doctors, hospitals, or other health care personnel. This includes complaints about waiting times, operating hours, the actions of health care personnel, and the adequacy of health care facilities.

Source: Adapted from *Consumer bill of rights and responsibilities.* Retrieved March 18, 2010, from http://www.hcqualitycommission.gov/press/cbor.html#head1

Box 42–10 Patient Responsibilities

The partnership nature of health care requires that patients, or their families/surrogates, take part in their care. The effectiveness of care and patient satisfaction with the treatment depends, in part, on the patient fulfilling certain responsibilities. The following are patient responsibilities:

- Patients are responsible for providing information about past illnesses, hospitalizations, medications, and other matters related to health status. To participate effectively in decision making, patients are take responsible for asking for additional information or explanation about their health status or treatment when they do not fully understand information and instructions.
- Patients are also responsible for ensuring that the health care institution has a copy of their written advance directive if they have one.
- Patients are responsible for telling their doctors and other caregivers if they expect problems in following prescribed treatment.

- Patients should be aware of the hospital's duty to be reasonably efficient and fair in providing care to other patients and the community. The hospital's rules and regulations are intended to help the hospital meet this responsibility. Patients and their families are responsible for making reasonable accommodations to the needs of the hospital, other patients, medical staff, and hospital employees.
- Patients are responsible for giving necessary information for insurance claims and for working with the hospital to make payment arrangements, when necessary.
- A person's health depends on much more than health care services. Patients are responsible for recognizing the impact of their lifestyle on their personal health.

Source: Maryland Hospital Performance Evaluation Guide. Patient guide. Retrieved March 29, 2010, from http://mhcc.maryland.gov/consumerinfo/hospitalguide/patients/consumer_help/bill_of_rights.htm

REVIEW Ethics

RELATE: LINK THE CONCEPTS

Linking the concept of Ethics with the concept of Addiction Behavior:
1. How does substance abuse affect an individual's ability to make ethical decisions based on his or her personal values and beliefs?
2. What parts of the ANA Code of Ethics for Nurses address impaired nurses?

Linking the concept of Ethics with the concept of Reproduction:
3. What are your personal beliefs about fertility treatments? How would you feel towards a client who has conceived multiple fetuses through fertility treatments and now wants to have selective reduction to reduce the number of children she will carry to term?
4. As a nurse, what are your responsibilities to the teenager seeking information on birth control methods?

REFER: GO TO MYNURSINGKIT

REFLECT: CASE STUDY

Keith Morgan, a 46-year-old male, had a fall and broke his leg several weeks ago. He is now receiving home health care. You are a home health nurse case manager, and you arrive at Mr. Morgan's home to assess his ability to ambulate. He is alert and oriented but continues to report a high pain level. During your assessment, Mr. Morgan tells you that the Tylenol just isn't effective in controlling his pain. When you ask him about the effect of the narcotic that has been prescribed and documented as given by the primary nurse, Mr. Morgan tells you that the nurse told him all he needed was the Tylenol and that he has not taken any other pain medication.
1. How do you respond?
2. What is your legal responsibility? What is your ethical responsibility? What actions do you need to take?

REFERENCES

American Association of Colleges of Nursing. (2010). Nursing shortage fact sheet. Retrieved May 3, 2010, from http://www.aacn.nche.edu/media/FactSheets/NursingShortage.htm

American Association of Colleges of Nursing. (2008). *The essentials of baccalaureate education for professional nursing practice.* Washington, DC.

American Cancer Society. (1998). *Patient bill of rights.* Retrieved September 27, 2008, from http://www.cancer.org/docroot/mit/content/mit_3_2_patients_bill_of_rights.asp

American Hospital Association. (1998). *A patient's bill of rights.* Retrieved March 29, 2010, from http://www.patienttalk.info/AHA-Patient_Bill_of_Rights.htm

American Nurses Association. (2001). Code of ethics for nurses with interpretive statements. Silver Springs, MD.

American Nurses Association. (2002). Nursing's agenda for the future. A call to the nation. Washington, DC: American Nurses Publishing.

American Nurses Association. (2008). Guide to the code of ethics for nurses. Silver Springs, MD.

Baum, N., Gollust, S., Goold, S., & Jacobson, P. (2007, December). Looking ahead: Addressing ethical challenges in public health practice. *Journal of Law, Medicine & Ethics, 35*(4), 657–667. Retrieved September 14, 2008, from CINAHL with Full Text database.

Benner, P., Sutphen, M., Leonard-Kahn, V., & Day, L. (2008). Formation and everyday ethical comportment. *American Journal of Critical Care, 17*(5), 473–476. Retrieved May 2, 2010, from CINAHL with Full Text database.

Benner, P., Sutphen, M., Leonard, V., & Day, L. (2010). *Educating nurses: A call for radical transformation. San Francisco: Jossey-Bass.*

Blacksher, E. (2008, July). Children's health inequalities: Ethical and political challenges to seeking social justice. *Hastings Center Report, 38*(4), 28–35. Retrieved September 14, 2008, from CINAHL with Full Text database.

Buchanan, D. (2008). Autonomy, paternalism, and justice: Ethical priorities in public health. *American Journal of Public Health, 98*(1), 15–21. Retrieved September 14, 2008, from CINAHL with Full Text database.

Chally, P., & Loriz, L. (1998). Decision making in practice: A practical model for resolving the types of ethical dilemmas you face daily. *American Journal of Nursing, 98*(6), 17–20.

Corley, M. (2002). Nurse moral distress: a proposed theory and research agenda. *Nursing Ethics, 9*(6), 636–650. doi:10.1191/0969733002ne557oa

Corley, M., Minick, P., Elswick, R., & Jacobs, M. (2005). Nurse moral distress and ethical work environment. *Nursing Ethics, 12*(4), 381–390. doi:10.1191/0969733005ne809oa.

Gretter, L. (1910). Florence Nightingale pledge: Autograph manuscript dated 1893. *American Journal of Nursing 10*(4), 271.

Guido, G. W. (2010). *Legal and ethical issues in nursing* (5th ed.).Upper Saddle River, NJ: Prentice Hall.

Ham, K. (2004). Principled thinking: a comparison of nursing students and experienced nurses. *Journal of Continuing Education in Nursing, 35*(2), 66–73. Retrieved May 2, 2010, from CINAHL with Full Text database.

International Council of Nurses. (2006). The ICN Code of Ethics for Nurses. Geneva Switzerland.

Kirsch, R. (2008). Ethical issues and students: Case two. *PT: Magazine of Physical Therapy, 16*(4), 48–51. Retrieved September 13, 2008, from Academic Search Premier database.

Kirsch, R. (2008). Ethical issues and students: Case two. *PT: Magazine of Physical Therapy, 16*(5), 48–50. Retrieved September 13, 2008, from Academic Search Premier database.

Levine, M. (1977). Nursing ethics and the ethical nurse. *American Journal of Nursing, 77*, 845–849.

Manthey, M. (2008, April). Social justice and nursing: The key is respect. *Creative Nursing, 14*(2), 62–65. Retrieved September 14, 2008, from CINAHL with Full Text database.

Meulenbergs, T., Verpeet, E., Schotsmans, P., & Gastmans, C. (2004, May). Professional codes in a changing nursing context: literature review. *Journal of Advanced Nursing, 46*(3), 331–336. Retrieved September 13, 2008, from CINAHL with Full Text database.

National Guideline Clearinghouse. (2010). Guideline index. Retrieved April 15, 2010, from http://www.guideline.gov/browse/guideline_index.aspx

Noone, J. (2009). Teaching to the three apprenticeships: Designing learning activities for professional practice in an undergraduate curriculum. *Journal of Nursing Education, 48*(8), 468–471. Retrieved from CINAHL with Full Text database.

North Carolina General Statute §131E-117, Retrieved March 8, 2010, from http://www.ncga.state.nc.us/EnactedLegislation/Statutes/HTML/ByChapter/Chapter_131E.html

Nurses learn to 'speak the language of ethics': Program helps nurses add to ethics discussions. (2008, June). *Hospital Home Health*. Retrieved September 14, 2008, from CINAHL with Full Text database.

Pauly, B., Varcoe, C., Storch, J., & Newton, L. (2009). Registered nurses' perceptions of moral distress and ethical climate. *Nursing Ethics, 16*(5), 561–573. Retrieved May 2, 2010, from, Health Source: Nursing/Academic Edition database.

Rodriguez, L. (2007). Confronting life and death responsibility: The lived experiences of nursing students and nursing faculty response to practice breakdown and errors in nursing school. Retrieved May 2, 2010, from CINAHL with Full Text database.

Saad, L. (2009). Gallop honesty and ethics poll. Retrieved May 2, 2010, from http://www.gallup.com/poll/124625/honesty-ethics-poll-finds-congress-image-tarnished.aspx

Varcoe, C., Doane, G., Pauly, B., Rodney, P., Storch, J. L., Mahoney, K., Mcpherson, G., Brown, H., & Starsomski, R. (2004). Ethical practice in nursing: Working the in-betweens. *Journal of Advanced Nursing, 45*(3), 316–325.

White, J. (1999). Ethical comportment in organizations: A synthesis of the feminist ethic of care and the Buddhist ethic of compassion. *International Journal of Value-Based Management, 12*, 109–128.

Wocial, L. (1996). Achieving collaboration in ethical decision making: Strategies for nurses in clinical practice. *Dimensions of Critical Care Nursing, 15*(3), 150–158.

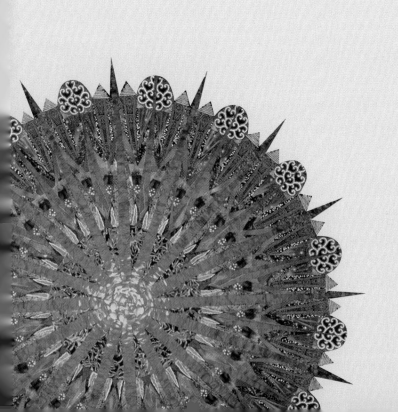

Evidence-Based Practice

43

Concept at-a-Glance

About Evidence-Based Practice, *2323*

BASIS FOR SELECTION OF CONCEPT
Institute of Medicine
NLN Competencies
Standards of Nursing Practice

Concept Learning Outcomes

After reading about this concept, you will be able to:

1. Describe the goals and purpose of evidence-based practice.
2. List the benefits of evidence-based practice.
3. Suggest strategies for overcoming barriers to evidenced-based practice.
4. Discuss the four goals of nursing research.
5. Contrast definitions of nursing research.
6. Identity sources of nursing knowledge.
7. Identify the significance of the American Nurses Association's standards of professional performance pertaining to research.
8. Analyze the impact of education on the different roles of nurses in nursing research.
9. Predict priority areas for nursing research in the future.
10. Explain the significance of the National Institute of Nursing Research.
11. Suggest nursing strategies for maintaining ethics in nursing research.
12. Recommend strategies for developing an evidence-based nursing practice.

Concept Key Terms

Applied research, *2329*
Basic research, *2329*
Clinical nursing research, *2326*
Empirical data, *2327*
Evidence-based practice, *2323*
Nursing research, *2326*
Population, *2327*
Replication studies, *2332*
Research utilization, *2331*
Sample, *2329*

About Evidence-Based Practice

Evidence-based practice (EBP) means that nurses make clinical decisions based on the best research evidence, their clinical expertise, and the health care preferences of their clients. Although EBP may be based on factors other than research findings, such as available resources and the expertise of clinicians, the aim of EBP is to provide the best possible care based on the best available research. The best evidence-based research for nurses to use comes from the body of research that has been developed to answer clinical questions specifically about nursing practice and its impact on client care and outcomes. Nursing students and

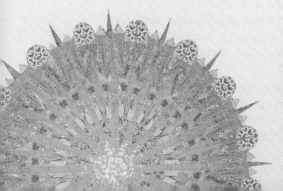

professional nurses must know how to find evidence-based research, determine its suitability for practice, form clinical questions, and implement research into their daily practice.

Although the evidence-based practice movement was started in the early 1970s by Dr. Archie Cochrane, a British epidemiologist, the push for the integration of more evidence-based research in nursing did not come until the Institute of Medicine's (IOM) publication of *To Err Is Human* in 2000. In this document, the IOM discussed medical errors and their costs, both in terms of dollars and human life, and recommended strategies for improvement. The IOM's 2001 publication *Crossing the Quality Chasm*: *A New Health System for the 21st Century* addressed the failure of the health care delivery system to provide consistent, high quality health care to all people and included discussions of issues such as organizational problems and complexity in health care and how they are contributing to the gap in the provision of health care services. The IOM identified 10 strategies for improving the health care delivery system:

1. Care is based on continuous healing relationships.
2. Care is customized according to client needs and values.
3. The client is the source of control.
4. Knowledge is shared and information flows freely.
5. Decision making is evidence-based.
6. Safety is a system property.
7. Transparency is necessary.
8. Needs are anticipated.
9. Waste is continuously decreased.
10. Cooperation among clinicians is a priority.

It is important that nurses be knowledgeable about the health care environment. They must also recognize that they will be expected to make informed decisions about the best care to provide to the public they serve. Additionally, nurses need to be aware that neither the health care environment nor the evidence they use to build their practice is static. On the contrary, it is dynamic, constantly building and sometimes changing. Nursing, according to the American Nurses Association Scope and Standards of Practice (2004) "is a dynamic profession, blending evidence-based practice with intuition, caring, and compassion to provide quality care." Nurses have a responsibility to maintain professional creditability. This is accomplished in part through participation in continuing education activities, which may include reading professional journals. Keeping abreast of this new information is no easy task. For example, there are approximately 7,000 articles published monthly in just five primary care journals (Alper, 2004). To keep up with the information in those journals would mean that a nurse wanting to stay up-to-date with the most current evidence in primary care would need to spend more than 600 hours a month just reading articles. Obviously it is impossible to spend 25 days a month just reading, however, this example is helpful to show just how much information is available in one journal and why users of information need to be able to make critical judgments about the information they read to ensure that changes in their practice are effective and efficient.

Sigma Theta Tau International Honor Society of Nursing supports the development and implementation of evidence-based nursing and has adopted a position statement in which it defined evidence-based nursing as "an integration of the best evidence available, nursing expertise, and the values and preferences of the individuals, families and communities who are served. This approach to nursing care serves to bridge the gap between the best evidence available and the most appropriate nursing care for individuals, groups, and populations with varied needs" (Sigma Theta Tau, 2005). ●

THE BENEFITS OF EVIDENCE-BASED PRACTICE

Nurses play a critical part in the chain of client care. They help clients navigate the health care environment. They assume many roles such as provider of care, advocate, teacher, and researcher. Nurses help to ensure that there is open and effective communication and continuity between all members of the health care team and clients and their families. When nurses are actively involved in evidence-based practice, they are able to access and use evidence from a variety of sources and disciplines that will help to guide their clinical practice and improve client care. By using evidence-based practice, nurses also ensure the credibility of their profession and provide accountability for nursing care.

RESEARCH EXAMPLE

Nurses are instrumental in providing and analyzing health care in a variety of settings. In one project, a school nurse and physical education teacher partnered to establish an evidence-based guideline to provide strategies to increase physical activity in kindergarten through eighth grade. The extensive guideline provides tools for monitoring children, observing play, evaluating student knowledge, and structuring physical education (Bagby & Adams, 2007). Another example of nurse activity is the construction of an evaluation tool for use with teens at a nurse-managed health center (Benkert, George, Tanner, et al., 2007). Adolescent ratings of care can influence their acceptance of care provided, so ratings of student perception are important to consider when evaluating outcomes of health centers.

BARRIERS TO EVIDENCE-BASED PRACTICE

Despite the benefits of EBP to the profession of nursing, some common barriers to EBP prevent nurses from participating in research and implementing it in their daily practice. These include the following:

- Lack of knowledge
- Negative attitudes
- Lack of institutional support
- Limited research findings applicable to nursing
- Lack of time to access and review the data
- Lack of access to information technology
- Problems accessing journals
- Lack of confidence in their ability to understand research based articles and apply them to practice
- Lack of support from colleagues and employers
- Resistance to changing current methods of practice (Hodge, Kochie, and Santiago, 2003; Vratny, 2007, Bertulis, 2008).

Nurses must be aware of these barriers in order to be able to combat them. For example, the nurse who has difficulty accessing electronic databases from work or home should make use of local reference librarians and other resources that may be available. Many libraries, particularly at colleges and universities, have access to nursing journals both online and in print (see Box 43–1). The nurse who fails to get support from employers and colleagues may want to do more networking with local chapters of professional organizations such as the ANA.

NURSING RESEARCH

In order to implement an evidence-based practice, every nurse must understand a number of aspects of nursing research, including its goals, sources, history, and the roles of nurses in research. Each nurse must also have a thorough understanding of terms frequently used in research and an understanding of the types and methods of research, including protections available to individuals who participate as research subjects.

Goals of Nursing Research

The importance of nursing research cannot be stressed enough. Four goals for conducting research are to (a) promote evidence-based nursing practice, (b) ensure credibility of the nursing profession, (c) provide accountability for nursing practice, and (d) document the cost effectiveness of nursing care.

PROMOTE EVIDENCE-BASED NURSING PRACTICE As stated earlier, nursing research helps nursing students and professional nurses improve their daily practice. By asking themselves a series of questions about interventions they

---

Box 43–1 Nursing Research Journals

EXAMPLES OF RESEARCH JOURNALS IN NURSING
Advances in Nursing
Science
Applied Nursing Research
Evidence-Based Nursing
International Journal of Nursing Studies
Journal of Nursing Scholarship
Nursing Research
Research in Nursing and Health
Scholarly Inquiry for Nursing Practice
Western Journal of Nursing Research

EXAMPLES OF CLINICAL AND SPECIALTY NURSING JOURNALS THAT PUBLISH RESEARCH
American Journal of Critical Care
American Journal of Nursing
Heart and Lung
Journal of Gerontologic Nursing
Journal of Neuroscience Nursing
Journal of Nursing Administration
Journal of Nursing Education
Journal of Obstetric, Gynecologic & Neonatal Nursing
Journal of Pediatric Nursing
Journal of Professional Nursing
MedSurg Nursing
Nursing Administration Quarterly
Nursing Outlook
Oncology Nursing Forum

---

perform or see performed, both nursing students and professional nurses can increase their ability to incorporate research into practice.

- Am I performing this intervention because someone told me to or because this is the intervention that has *always* been used?
- What evidence exists that this is the most effective intervention for the problem?

If an intervention is not based on research evidence, there is no way to determine that this intervention is the optimum one.

PRACTICE ALERT

Each facility dictates its own procedures for performing nursing skills. Following these procedures as written protects the nurse from liability. The nurse should never take it upon him- or herself to change the way a procedure is performed. The nurse who discovers evidence that indicates there may be a better way to perform a skill or procedure must follow the appropriate chain of command and share the evidence. In many facilities, this may involve talking with the nurse manager or the Standards and Practice Committee members for the unit.

ENSURE THE CREDIBILITY OF THE NURSING PROFESSION
In the past, nursing was frequently thought of as a vocation rather than a profession. In fact, the struggle to gain professional status has been long and difficult. One of the criterion for a profession is the existence of a body of knowledge that is distinct from that of other disciplines. Nursing has traditionally borrowed knowledge from the natural and social sciences, and only in recent years have nurses concentrated on establishing a unique body of knowledge that would allow nursing to be clearly identified as a distinct profession. The most valid means of developing this knowledge base is scientific research. Through research, nurses can determine what it is that they do and how they do it that distinguishes them from other groups in the health care field. Nurses must demonstrate to the general public that nursing makes a difference in the health status of people. Americans have ranked nurses highest in honesty and ethical standards when comparing them to other professionals, except for 2001, when firefighters scored higher following the terrorist attacks of 9/11 (ANA, 2009). By using research to build an evidence-based practice, nurses ensure the continued credibility of the nursing profession in both the eyes of the general public and in the eyes of members of the other health care professions.

PRACTICE ALERT

Balas (2001) stated there is an approximate 17-year lag between the discovery of more effective forms of treatment and their incorporation into routine client care. Nurses can decrease that lag time by searching for the best evidence-based research and incorporating it into their practice.

Box 43–2 American Nurses Association's Standards of Professional Performance Pertaining to Research

STANDARD 13: RESEARCH
The registered nurse integrates research findings into practice.

Measurement Criteria
The registered nurse:

Utilizes best available evidence, including research findings, to guide practice decisions.

Actively participates in research activities at various levels appropriate to the nurse's level of education and position. Such activities may include:

■ Identifying clinical problems specific to nursing research (patient care and nursing practice).

■ Participating in data collection (surveys, pilot projects, and formal studies).

■ Participating in a formal committee or program.

■ Sharing research activities and/or findings with peers and others.

■ Conducting research.

■ Critically analyzing and interpreting research for application to practice.

■ Using research findings in the development of policies, procedures, and standards of practice in patient care.

■ Incorporating research as a basis for learning.

Note: Reprinted with permission from American Nurses Association. (2004). *Nursing: Scope and standards of practice.* Silver Spring, MD:.Nursebooks.org.

Box 43–3 Clinical Research at a Glance

Clinical research seeks to answer questions that ultimately will improve client care. For example:

■ What are the links between diet and the development of diabetes and cardiovascular disease?

■ Is a new drug or medical device more effective than one already on the market?

■ Do clients who undergo surgery at one medical center have a higher complication rate than those who are treated at another?

■ Are clients satisfied with their care during hospitalization?

These sorts of questions are answered by research. A familiarity with research methodology is becoming increasingly important in nursing practice. Nurses may be involved in a variety of types of clinical research during the course of their work. When implementing evidence-based practice, weighing the scientific merit of a research study is key to considering its interpretation and implications.

Not all research is created equal. A number of different methodologies are used in clinical research. Which methodology used is determined by the researcher based on the resources that are available and the issues being investigated. Practical and ethical issues also factor in to decisions about research methodology.

Quantitative Research
Quantitative research uses precise measurement for data collection and analyzes numerical data. Quantitative research uses a rigorously controlled design and employs statistical analysis to summarize and describe findings or to test relationships among variables. Two examples of research questions that lend themselves to the quantitative approach are:

■ Is the use of therapeutic touch effective in reducing pain perception postoperatively?

■ Are there differences in skin breakdown between premature infants who are bathed with plain water and those who are bathed with bacteriostatic soap?

Qualitative Research
Qualitative research investigates a question through narrative data that describe events or occurrences in an in-depth and holistic fashion. The research design is typically more flexible and less controlled than quantitative designs. For example, the researcher may gather data from the transcripts of interviews. Qualitative research often is used to explore the subjective experiences of human beings and can provide nursing with a better understanding of the client's perspective. Two examples of research questions which lend themselves to qualitative research are:

■ What is the nature of coping and adjustment after a radical masectomy?

■ What is the nature of the bereavement process in spouses of clients who have terminal cancer?

Observational Study
An *observational study* seeks to capture a picture of the real world, such as the incidence of birth defects in a population of people. Surveys and focus groups are types of observational studies. An *interventional* or *experimental design* involves testing a hypothesis by manipulating conditions, usually in a controlled environment.

One of the tasks facing the scientist is to determine whether an observed relationship—for example, a change in a client's condition after taking a medication—is cause-and-effect or just a random coincidence. Several strategies are employed to reduce the risk that an observation is due to chance:

■ A *control group* is a set of people who are very similar to those being studied, typically matched for age, weight, sex, illness severity, and other relevant factors. The experimental group will be given an experimental treatment while the control group receives the existing therapy or a *placebo* with no therapeutic effect.

■ To reduce the chance that a client may be influenced by the appearance of medication, he or she is not told whether a tablet contains active ingredient or is a placebo—a strategy known as *blinding.* In a *double-blind* research design, neither the client nor the researchers know which tablet contains a therapeutic agent until the study is concluded.

diagnosis of moderate or severe persistent asthma ages 21–55). The **sample** is the segment of the population from whom the data will actually be collected (those who volunteer to participate in the study). Sample size may be an important indicator of whether or not a research study should be considered for incorporation into daily nursing practice. A sample of 15 may indicate that further research is needed. A carefully designed study with a sample size of 5,000 may be more likely to generate meaningful information.

There are many similarities between scientific research and the problem-solving approach that is familiar to all nurses. Both processes involve identifying a problem area, establishing a plan, collecting data, and evaluating the data. The purposes of these two activities are, however, quite different. Problem solving attempts to seek a solution to a problem that exists for a person or persons in a given setting. The purpose of scientific research is much broader. It seeks to obtain knowledge that can be generalized to other people and to other settings. For example, the nursing staff might be concerned about the best approach to teaching Mrs. Smith, a blind client, how to operate an insulin pump. This would be an example of an immediate problem that needs a solution. Scientific research, in contrast, would be concerned with the best approach to use in teaching blind people, in general, how to operate insulin pumps. Scientific research is concerned with the ability to generalize research results.

RESEARCH EXAMPLE

The Children's Health Study is a large longitudinal study of children across the United States designed to identify long-term effects of exposure to a variety of environmental factors. The study began in 1992 with a focus on air pollution effects on California children. Reduced lung development in children exposed to high amounts of particulate contaminants was observed, although children improved if they moved to other communities. A wide range of natural and human-caused environmental conditions, social factors, genetics, and other issues will be considered in the coming years (Children's Health Study, 2005, 2006). Nurses should understand the environmental hazards in the areas where they work and tailor teaching during health care visits to minimize them.

1. Are there days with unsafe air in your community? What resources are available to help you determine air quality in your community?
2. What are the rates of radon, lead, or other hazardous substances in homes in your area?

Purposes of Nursing Research

The overall purpose of nursing research is to develop a body of knowledge specific to the nursing profession and to provide research that supports evidence-based practice. Research may be classified, according to the general purpose of the study, as basic or applied research. The purpose of **basic research** is to generate new knowledge; **applied research** is concerned with using knowledge to solve immediate problems. Basic research is also referred to as pure research.

Basic research is conducted to develop, test, and refine theories and generate new knowledge (Kerlinger, 1986; Oman, Krugman, & Fink, 2003; Polit & Beck, 2004). Sometimes it is said that basic research seeks "knowledge for knowledge's

sake." Whether basic research seeks to generate or develop theories, immediate application of the results usually does not occur. In fact, it may take years before the usefulness of the results of the research is determined or acknowledged. Basic research often uses laboratory animals as subjects. The following example of a basic research study was conducted with peripheral catheters. The object was to determine a way to keep these catheters from becoming occluded.

RESEARCH EXAMPLE

Nurses must intervene when peripherally inserted central catheters (PICCs) become occluded. Fetzer and Manning (2004) maintained that pharmacological interventions are costly and involve risks. They explored the use of a mechanical percussive technique. A 5- to 10-mL syringe was filled with 1 mL of normal saline and then attached to the hub of the occluded catheter. The plunger was pulled back and released at 2-second intervals until patency was restored. When the plunger was released, a "pop" sound was heard, thus, the technique was named POP. Thirty PICC catheters were clotted with human blood and incubated for 8 hours in a 35°F saline bath. Using the POP technique, patency was restored in 86% of the occluded catheters.

Applied research is directed toward generating knowledge that can be used in the near future. It is often conducted to seek solutions to existing problems (Burns & Grove, 2005; Kerlinger, 1986; Polit & Beck, 2004). The majority of nursing studies have been examples of applied research as many of these studies focus on nursing interventions for clients and their families.

The distinction between basic and applied research is really not as clear cut as it may seem. Sometimes the findings of basic research are applied rather quickly in the clinical setting, whereas the findings of applied research may actually lead to basic studies. Studies contain elements of both basic and applied research when testing theory that will have immediate implications for nursing. The distinction between basic and applied research may have more to do with financial support for the project than with the purpose of the study. In this sense, basic research may imply that the researcher has financial support to work on a particular project without having to indicate the immediate practical usefulness of the findings.

Although nursing research is generally of the applied type, which is more likely to receive funding than basic research, nurses must search for funding for both types of research. The federal government has the most money available for research (Colling, 2004). Nurses receive the largest amount of government funding through the National Institute for Nursing Research. The budget for this institute was over $138 million for 2005 (Grady, 2005). Other sources for nursing research include private foundations, corporations, and professional organizations, such as Sigma Theta Tau International, Honor Society of Nursing. This organization, in conjunction with its chapters and grant partners (corporations, associations, and foundations), provides more that $650,000 annually for nursing research through grants, scholarships, and monetary awards (Sigma Theta Tau International, Honor Society of Nursing, 2005). Johnson & Johnson is an excellent example of a corporation that has long supported the profession of nursing. The

Robert Wood Johnson foundation is a private foundation that contributes financially to nursing research.

Roles of Nurses in Research

In 1981, the ANA Council of Nurse Researchers developed guidelines for the roles of nurses in research according to level of educational preparation. The guidelines were revised in 1993 and 1994. Expectations are presented for nurses prepared at the following educational levels: associate's degree in nursing, baccalaureate degree in nursing, master's degree in nursing, doctoral education, and postdoctoral education. Nurses with associate's degrees should be prepared to participate in research activities in order to assist in identifying clinical problems in nursing practice; assist with the collection of data; and, alongside nurses with more advanced credentials, use research findings to develop evidence-based practice. Nurses prepared at the baccalaureate level should be able to read research critically and determine if research results are ready for use in clinical practice. They should be able to identify clinical problems that need to be investigated. Baccalaureate-prepared nurses should also assist experienced investigators to gain access to clinical sites. They should help select appropriate data collection methods and collect data. Finally, they should implement research findings in their practice (ANA, 1994). The American Association of College of Nursing (AACN) published a position statement on nursing research in 1999. This statement lists research expectations and outcomes for graduates of baccalaureate, master's, doctoral, and postdoctoral programs. These expectations are similar to those of the American Nurses Association (Box 43–4).

The latest revision of the American Nurses Association guidelines and the AACN guidelines include expectations of those with postdoctoral preparation. Postdoctoral study involves agreements between novice researchers, usually with recent doctorates, and established investigators. These seasoned investigators agree to mentor the novices for a period of 2 or 3 years. Private and federal funding is available for postdoctoral preparation.

Overall, there are many roles that nurses can assume in association with research projects. Some of these include the following:

1. Principal investigator
2. Member of a research team
3. Identifier of researchable problems
4. Evaluator of research findings
5. User of research findings
6. Patient/client advocate during studies
7. Subject/participant in studies.

PRINCIPAL INVESTIGATOR Nurses can and should serve as principal investigators in scientific investigations. To be a principal investigator, special research preparation is necessary. It might be possible for a beginning researcher to conduct a small-scale survey study, but preparation beyond the baccalaureate level is necessary for independent investigator status in most nursing research studies.

MEMBER OF A RESEARCH TEAM Nurses can serve as members of a research team. They may act as data collectors or administer the experimental intervention of the study (Figure 43–1 ■). Many nurses who participate in research gain interest and enthusiasm in conducting their own investigations. In 1982, Rittenmeyer wrote that research would become a higher priority as knowledge of the benefits of research increases. She predicted that by 1990 research would be part of the nurse's normal workload. Unfortunately, this has not yet become true.

Myers and Kosinski (2005) have proposed that nursing research is slowly gathering momentum because bedside nurses and health care leaders are trying to validate the impact of nursing on client outcomes and the health care system in general. Hopefully, as this trend continues, evidence-based practice will become the standard for nursing care.

IDENTIFIER OF RESEARCHABLE PROBLEMS All nurses from associate's degree to doctoral-level preparation have the responsibility of trying to identify areas of needed research.

Box 43–4 Research Roles at Various Levels of Nursing Education According to the ANA Position Statement on *Education for Participation in Nursing Research*

ASSOCIATE'S DEGREE IN NURSING
- Help to identify clinical problems in nursing practice
- Assist in the collection of data within a structured format
- In conjunction with nurses holding more advanced credentials, appropriately use research findings in clinical practice

BACCALAUREATE DEGREE IN NURSING
- Identify clinical problems requiring investigation
- Assist experienced investigators gain access to clinical sites
- Influence the selection of appropriate methods of data collection
- Collect data and implement nursing research findings

MASTER'S DEGREE IN NURSING
- Be active members of research teams
- Assume the role of clinical expert collaborating with experienced investigators in proposal development, data collection, data analysis, and interpretation
- Appraise the clinical relevance of research findings

- Help create a climate that supports scholarly inquiry, scientific integrity, and scientific investigation of clinical nursing problems
- Provide leadership for integrating findings in clinical practice

DOCTORAL EDUCATION
- Conduct research aimed at theory generation or theory testing
- Design studies independently as well as collaborate with other clinicians and researchers
- Acquire funding for research
- Disseminate research findings

POSTDOCTORAL EDUCATION
- Develop a systematic program of research
- Become a sustaining member of the scientific community

Source: Based on the ANA Position Statement: *Education for Participation in Nursing Research,* originated by the Council of Nurse Researchers and Council of Nursing Practice and adopted by the ANA Board of Directors, April, 1994.

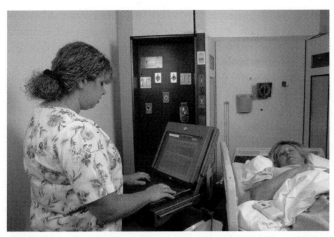

Figure 43–1 ■ Collecting data at the client's bedside is an important component of research.

Nurses at the bedside are particularly well situated to identify client-related researchable problems.

EVALUATOR OF RESEARCH FINDINGS   Every nurse should be involved in the evaluation of research findings. As research consumers, nurses have the obligation to become familiar with research findings and determine the usefulness of these findings in the practice area. Beginning researchers should critique research articles, first with the help of an experienced researcher and eventually on their own, through the use of knowledge gained in a structured research course (either in their basic nursing education program or in a continuing education course).

As evidence of the expectation that all nurses know how to evaluate research articles, *AJN* published an article in December 1996 on critiquing research (Rankin & Esteves, 1996). The article began by stating that many nurses do not feel confident that they can evaluate research articles. However, the authors cautioned against nurses relying on the mass media report and interpret research findings. Media discussions of research frequently lack the objectivity needed by nurses to determine if findings are appropriate for use in nursing practice.

USER OF RESEARCH FINDINGS   Through the years, nurses have tended to carry out nursing procedures and provide nursing care "the way we've always done it." Change is difficult, both to accomplish and to accept, but research findings have no value if they are not put into use. After evaluating research findings, nurses should use relevant findings in their practice. The primary goal of nursing research is to improve care for clients. To ensure client safety and quality of care, nurses must be judicious in their use of research findings. The results of one small study conducted with a sample of 15 volunteers would not provide sufficient evidence for a change in nursing practice.

Research utilization and evidence-based nursing practice are related because both processes place emphasis on research findings. The term research utilization is one which may be confused with evidence-based practice. **Research utilization** is knowledge that is based upon evidence generated from research alone or the implementation of findings based solely on one or more research studies and is dependent upon the availability of published research (Newhouse, et al, 2007). Research utilization is not interested in the implementation of research specifically to impact nursing care or in conjunction with critical review or client preferences. Evidence-based practice, which has evolved from research utilization, is much more involved. Evidence-based practice focuses on the question of how can nurses provide the best nursing care and results from a critical review of information. It is a systematic search to find the best answer to a clinical question. Evidence-based practice is influenced by the clinical expertise of the health care provider within a specific health care environment and is strongly focused upon the individual preferences and values of the client. It is important for nurses, therefore, to strive to keep up with current evidence and technology, adapt to those changes, and carefully integrate those changes into their clinical practice. See Box 43–5 for strategies to implement EBP in clinical practice.

PATIENT/CLIENT ADVOCATE DURING STUDIES   All nurses have the responsibility to act as patient/client advocates when their patient/clients are involved in research. This advocacy involves making sure that the ethical aspects of research are

---

Box 43–5 Strategies for Implementing Evidence-Based Practice

1. Assess the extent to which your practice is evidenced based.
2. Review literature that provides evidence to strengthen your belief that EBP results in better client outcomes.
3. Ask questions about your current practice strategies (e.g., Is use of distraction really effective in reducing children's distress during intrusive procedures? Does nonnutritive sucking alleviate pain in infants?).
4. Determine whether other colleagues at your practice site have an interest in the same clinical question so that you can form a collaboration to search for and review the evidence.
5. Conduct a search for studies or systematic reviews in the specific area of your clinical question. (Remember that randomized clinical trials are typically the gold standard for producing the best evidence.)
6. Critique the studies from your search to determine whether you have the "best evidence" to guide your practice.
7. Develop a practice guideline using the "best evidence."
8. Establish measurable outcomes that you can use to determine the effectiveness of your guideline.
9. Implement the practice guideline.
10. Measure the established outcomes.
11. Evaluate the effectiveness of the practice guideline and determine whether you should continue the practice guideline as established or whether there is a need for revision.
12. Develop a mechanism for routinely disseminating and discussing evidence-based literature upon which decisions can be made to improve practice at your clinical site (e.g., EBP rounds).

Source: From Melnyk, B.M., Stone, P., Fineout-Overhold, E., & Ackerman, M. (2000). Evidence-based practice: The past, the present, and recommendations for the millennium. *Pediatric Nursing, 26*(1), 77–80. Used by permission.

upheld. Nurses should help answer questions and explain a study to potential participants before the study begins. They also may need to be available during the study to answer questions or provide support to study participants. Habel published an article in the March 15, 2005, edition of *NurseWeek*, "Can You Answer Patients' Questions about Clinical Trials?" The purpose of the article was to help nurses answer questions about participation in research that might be posed by clients, friends, and neighbors. Some of the questions that research subjects should have answered include why is the study being done? Who is conducting the study? Who is going to be in the study? What kind of tests and treatments are involved? How long will the study last? What are alternatives to participation (p. 24)? Habel wrote that nurses can serve as valuable resources for information about clinical trials whether they are in the health care setting or in the community.

SUBJECT/PARTICIPANT IN STUDIES Nurses may act as subjects or participants in research. Many nurses are involved in a long-term survey study, the Nurses' Health Study that is being conducted by researchers at Harvard Medical School. The study was designed to examine some of the health risks that pose special threats to women. Women nurses were chosen as subjects, according to Frank Speizer, the principal investigator, because the study called for "a sophisticated group of individuals who could report exposure and diseases more accurately than the general population" (Massive Nurses' Health Study, 1983, p. 998). The study was begun in 1976 and was originally intended to last for 4 years, but additional funding was received and the study has continued for approximately 30 years. In 1989, a new cohort of younger nurses was added to the study in what is called Nurses' Health Study II. Approximately 650 publications (as of summer 2005) have resulted from the data obtained in these studies.

Research Priorities for the Future

Professional nursing organizations and individual nurse leaders are united in identifying the need for research that will help build a scientific knowledge base for nursing practice.

In 1985 the ANA Cabinet on Nursing Research identified 10 priority areas. These included (a) promoting health, well-being, and the ability to care for oneself among all age, social, and cultural groups; (b) minimizing or preventing behaviorally and environmentally induced health problems that compromise the quality of life and reduce productivity; and (c) minimizing the negative effects of new health technologies on the adaptive abilities of individuals and families experiencing acute or chronic health problems.

In November 1987, Dr. Ada Sue Hinshaw, then the director of the National Center for Nursing Research (NCNR), invited nursing organizations to identify their research priorities. Since that time, many nursing organizations have conducted surveys of their membership to determine research priorities. Replication studies should be a high priority for nursing research. **Replication studies** involve repeating a study with all the essential elements of the original study held intact. Different samples and settings may be used. Replication studies in nursing have not been numerous, and the lack of these studies has hindered the development of a cumulative body of nursing knowledge. This type of study is of particular importance in

clinical nursing research. Because of the small nonrandom samples used in many studies, nurses need to conduct many similar studies on the same topic to allow for generalization of findings. Nursing studies have generally been one of a kind. It is rare that the results of a single study provide enough evidence for making decisions about nursing practice.

The National Institute of Nursing Research (NINR) was officially established within the National Institutes of Health (NIH) on June 10, 1993. It replaced the National Center for Nursing Research (NCNR), which had been established in 1986. With the creation of the NINR, nursing research received a big boost in respectability. Funding for nursing research has increased a great deal. In 1986 the NCNR had a budget of $16 million. In 1995 the NINR received an appropriation of close to $50 million from Congress. By 2001 funding had been increased to almost $90 million. In 2005 the budget for the NINR was over $138 million.

The mission statement of the NINR (National Institute of Nursing Research, 2005) indicates support for "clinical and basic research to establish a scientific basis for the care of individuals across the life span—from management of patients during illness and recovery to the reduction of risks for disease and disability, the promotion of healthy lifestyles, promoting quality of life in those with chronic illness, and care for individuals at the end of life" (¶ 1). The entire mission statement and strategic plans for the twenty-first century are found at http://www.ninr.nih.gov/AboutNINR/NINRMissionandStrategicPlan/. The areas of research emphasis identified in NINR's 2006–2010 Mission and Strategic Plan are

■ Promoting Health and Preventing Disease
■ Improving Quality of Life
■ Eliminating Health Disparities
■ Setting Directions for End of Life Research.

In 2000 the NINR joined with more than 50 societies that represent the behavioral and social sciences to usher in the Decade of Behavior: 2000–2010. This broad-based research and public policy initiative focuses on improving health, education, and safety. For more information on the Decade of Behavior, visit www.decadeofbehavior.org.

ETHICAL CONSIDERATIONS IN NURSING RESEARCH

How long does it take for body parts to freeze when people are kept naked outdoors in subfreezing temperatures? What signs and symptoms are seen when people are kept in tanks of ice water for 3 hours? These questions were asked by so-called researchers in Germany in the early 1940s. They were trying to determine the most effective means of treating German Air Force pilots who had been exposed to cold conditions. The so-called subjects for these experiments were prisoners in the German concentration camps.

Because the United States is a country with a strong Judeo-Christian background, it may seem unlikely that such heinous research could ever be conducted in this country. But the following examples of research were, in fact, carried out in the United States.

One of the most widely known unethical studies was started in Macon County, Alabama, in 1932 by the U.S. Public Health

Service. The study was titled "Tuskegee Study of Untreated Syphilis in the Negro Male." Of the 600 black male subjects, 399 had syphilis, and 201 did not have the disease. Those subjects with active cases were given *no* treatment. All subjects were given free medical exams, free meals, and burial expenses (Centers for Disease Control and Prevention, 2006). Even after penicillin was accepted as the treatment of choice for syphilis in 1945, subjects were still given no treatment. This unethical study became common knowledge 40 years after it was begun. On May 16, 1997, President Bill Clinton made a public apology on behalf of the nation.

Development of Ethical Codes and Guidelines

The need for ethical guidelines becomes clear after reading these accounts of unethical research projects. The development of appropriate guidelines is not simple. Ethics is concerned with rules and principles of human behavior. Because human behavior is a very complex phenomenon, rules to govern the actions of human beings are difficult to formulate. Studies of recorded history show that people have always been interested in this topic. The biblical Ten Commandments are an example of a code of conduct that has endured through the centuries. Ethical principles frequently change with time and the development of new knowledge. The present ethical standards used in nursing research, and in research conducted by other disciplines, are based on the guidelines developed after World War II. The atrocities committed in the German prison camps led to the Nuremberg Trials after the war. The 1947 Nuremberg Code resulted from the revelations of unethical human behavior that occurred during the war. This code is concerned with several criteria for research including the following:

1. Researcher must inform subjects about the study.
2. Research must be for the good of society.
3. Research must be based on animal experiments, if possible.
4. Researcher must try to avoid injury to research subjects.
5. Researcher must be qualified to conduct research.
6. Subjects or the researcher can stop the study if problems occur.

In 1978 The National Commission for the Protection of Human Subjects of Biomedical and Behavioral Research was formed. The goals of this commission were to (a) identify basic ethical principles that should guide the conduct of research involving human subjects and (b) develop guidelines based on principles that had been identified. The report published by this commission in 1979 was titled *The Belmont Report*. The report identified three basic principles related to research subjects:

1. Respect for Persons—research subjects should have autonomy and self-determination
2. Beneficence—research subjects should be protected from harm
3. Justice—research subjects should receive fair treatment.

The U.S. Department of Health, Education and Welfare (HEW) (now the Department of Health and Human Services,

DHHS) published general guidelines for research in 1981. These have been revised several times. Also, special guidelines exist for research with vulnerable groups such as children, the mentally retarded, and prisoners. Any institution that receives federal money for research must abide by the DHHS guidelines or risk losing federal money.

The federal government guidelines resulted in the creation of institutional review boards (IRBs). These review boards are given various names, such as Human Research Committee, Human Subjects Committee, and Committee for the Protection of Human Subjects. Every agency or institution that receives federal money for research must have an IRB to review research proposals. The federal government, through the Office of Protection from Research Risk (OPRR), oversees IRBs.

Agencies may also have internal research committees that review research proposals. Some institutions have nursing research committees specifically concerned with nursing research in that particular institution. Because research policies and procedures vary from agency to agency, the researcher should become informed about the requirements of specific institutions that will be used for data collection.

Researchers must also be aware of the Health Insurance Portability and Accountability Act (HIPAA), which was implemented on April 14, 2003. Known as the HIPAA Privacy Rule, this act protects an individual's health information. It was designed to protect the unauthorized use and disclosure of a person's medical and health information. Authorization for use and disclosure must be obtained in writing from the person. This requirement pertains not only to health care but also to research conducted in a health care setting. Researchers may be required to obtain the person's signature on a separate document or integrate the information into the research informed consent document that is signed by potential research subjects (Arford, 2004).

Research Guidelines for Nurses

In 1968 the American Nurses Association Research and Studies Commission published a set of guidelines for nursing research. These guidelines were revised in 1975 and 1985 and are titled *Human Rights Guidelines for Nurses in Clinical and Other Research*. These guidelines address the rights of research subjects and nurses involved in research. Subjects must be protected from harm, their privacy should be ensured, and their dignity preserved. Nurses who are asked to participate in research should be fully informed about the research, and nurses should be included on the IRBs that review research proposals. The American Nurses Association published another set of guidelines in 1995. This document is titled *Ethical Guidelines in the Conduct, Dissemination, and Implementation of Nursing Research* (Silva, 1995). Although much of this document covers the same material as the earlier sets of guidelines, there is more emphasis in this document on research integrity and the reporting of suspected, alleged, or known incidents of scientific misconduct in research.

ELEMENTS OF INFORMED CONSENT The principal means for ensuring that the rights of research subjects are protected is through informed consent. Informed consent concerns subjects' participation in research in which they have full understanding of the study before the study begins (Figure 43–2 ■). These are the major elements of informed consent:

1. Researcher is identified and credentials presented.
2. Subject selection process is described.
3. Purpose of study is described.
4. Study procedures are discussed.
5. Potential risks are described.
6. Potential benefits are described.
7. Compensation, if any, is discussed.
8. Alternative procedures, if any, are disclosed.
9. Anonymity or confidentiality is assured.
10. Right to refuse to participate or to withdraw from study without penalty is assured.
11. Offer to answer all questions is made.
12. Means of obtaining study results is presented.

PEDIATRIC RESEARCH ISSUES Children are vulnerable subjects who cannot provide truly informed consent, and as such require additional protections. Because of the ethical principles of beneficence and nonmaleficence, it is imperative that there be a risk–benefit ratio that is favorable to the individual child or to children in general. Risk needs to be minimized as much as possible while maintaining a sound research design. Harm must be considered from the perspective of the child, such as pain, distress related to procedures, or any psychological harm, and minimized as much as possible (Diekema, 2006).

PRACTICE ALERT
Subpart D of the HHS regulations at 45 CFR part 46 provides protections for children participating in human subject research that must be followed, usually in addition to the protections outlined for adults. Some of the additional requirements in Subpart D are that an Institutional Review Board review may be required for some research activities involving children that would be exempt if the research subjects were adults and the use of parental permission and child assent instead of the procedures for obtaining informed consent used for research involving adults (OHRP, 2008).

DEVELOPING EVIDENCE-BASED PRACTICE

Two factors in the move towards evidence-based practice in nursing have been the report from the Institute of Medicine regarding clinical errors and the increasing complexity of client care related to increasing numbers of clients who suffer from multiple health problems and experience more frequent and more severe episodes of acute illness. In order to assure that the nurse is using best practices when delivering client care, the nurse must be able to find the evidence to support each client action.

Evidence-based practice is a combination of the knowledge that is generated from the experience of the clinician, the research evidence, and the preferences of the client. For nurses to develop an evidence-based practice, they need to first be able to identify information that is relevant and accurate. The sheer volume of information that may be published on a certain topic can make this a daunting task.

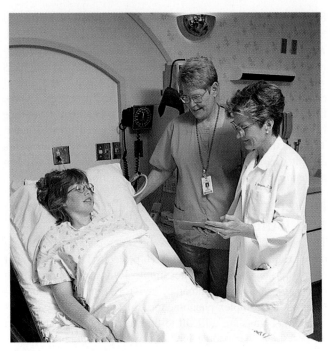

Figure 43–2 ■ It is important for clients to be fully informed before they participate in a research study.

There are several steps in the evidence-based process. The first step involves developing a question. This question will probably be developed from the clinical problems or needs of the client. This may include information like their diagnosis, prognosis, and treatment needs. The second step requires the nurse to begin searching the literature for relevant research to answer the question. There are many sources that can be searched. The third step is to engage in a critical appraisal of the evidence, determining the validity (truthfulness) of the evidence and its implications for the needs, values, and preferences of the client. The fourth step is to formulate a plan and apply the intervention based upon what the evidence points to the best intervention, in combination with the nurse's clinical experience, and with consideration for the client's values and preferences. The final step is to evaluate the intervention: Was it done correctly? Did it yield the intended results? Were the results unexpected? What are the areas in need of improvement?

If this process sounds familiar, it should because they are very similar to the components of the nursing process in which the nurse engages in assessment, planning, implementing, and evaluation. It has been written that the process of evidence-based practice is very similar to the nursing process with one additional step of searching for, finding, and evaluating pertinent evidence to answer defined clinical questions. This searching for the evidence would be done between the assessment and planning phases (Hoss, 2008).

Developing a Question
Major clinical questions can be generated in many ways but usually occur because of a question or problem encountered during client care. These questions should be asked in the

PICO format, which helps to construct the problem in a clear and concise way by identifying key words.

Patient Population attributes such as race, gender, age, etc.

Intervention of Interest Interventions such as treatments, education plan, etc.

Comparison Intervention A comparison group may not always exist.

Outcome May include issues such as quality of life, cost, etc.

Finding and Reviewing the Evidence

Finding the evidence in EBP will lead the nurse on a journey into some familiar places such as existing policies and standards of practice within the institution in which they practice or it may take them into a new territory of computerized bibliographic databases.

The best way to become proficient with literature searches is to frequently just go out and visit the different databases. Many databases have a tutorial available. Some databases will offer only abstracts, which is a synopsis of the article, while others will offer the reader the full text article. All sources and sites should be judged on their degree of credibility.

To obtain the most relevant information and narrow the search, the nurse should choose the best terms to define. The results obtained from the search depend upon whether the abstract, a synopsis of the study, or a full text of the article is available. Reference librarians at local libraries are good sources of information for nursing students and nurses who are confused about how to start searching for relevant articles.

In addition to formal databases, there are several national and international nursing organizations which develop and disseminate evidence-based resources (see Box 43–6). Some of these organizations include The Johanna Briggs Institute, Arizona State University Center for the Advancement of Evidence-Based Practice, University of Texas Academic Center for Evidence-Based Practice (ACE), Sigma Theta Tau International, Honor Society for Nursing, Canadian Center for Evidence-Based Practice, Case Western Reserve University Sarah Cole Hirsch Institute, The Indiana Center for Evidence-Based Nursing Practice, Agency for Healthcare Research and Quality (AHRQ), and Substance Abuse and Mental Health Services Administration.

In 1997 the Agency for Healthcare Research and Quality (AHRQ) established 12 Evidence-based Practice Centers (EPCs). The number of these centers is now up to 14 and includes Blue Cross and Blue Shield Association, Duke University, ECRI Institute, Johns Hopkins University, McMaster University, Oregon Evidence-Based Practice Center, RTI International–University of North Carolina at Chapel Hill, Southern California Evidence-Based Practice Center–RAND Corporation, Tufts New England Medical Center, University of Alberta, University of Connecticut, Minnesota Evidence-Based Practice Center, University of Ottawa, and Vanderbilt University. Through their efforts, these centers improve the quality and effectiveness of health care by reviewing all relevant scientific literature, synthesizing the evidence, and helping to translate the evidence-based research findings so that they are more readily available to those clinicians who are at the bedside providing care.

A significant source of evidence-based practice data is the Cochrane Database of Systematic Reviews. The data found in this resource often combine research to increase the power of the findings of numerous studies, each too small to produce reliable results individually. The Cochrane Collection is an international not-for-profit organization dedicated to making up-to-date, accurate information about the effects of health care readily available worldwide. Other major resources for information on evidence-based practice are the Healthlinks search engine at the University of Washington, the Academic Center for Evidence-Based Nursing at the University of Texas Health Science Center at San Antonio, and the National Guideline Clearinghouse, a public resource for evidence-based clinical practice guidelines.

Integrating Information

How can the average staff nurse integrate information gained from research studies into an evidence-based practice centered on client care? By following these steps: formulate the clinical question; search relevant databases for research evidence; critically judge the quality of the evidence; develop a plan that takes into consideration the evidence, your clinical expertise, and the preferences and values of your client; implement the plan; and evaluate the practice change (Melnyk and Fineout-Overholt, 2005). Having the knowledge to search the literature by using current technology will facilitate the process. Access to the Internet and databases on the clinical unit (where the questions arise), and knowledge of medical information technology and a willingness to learn technology increase the nurse's ability to access research findings that may have implications for client care. Today technology goes beyond the Internet. New technologies create a better work environment for nurses by improving quality of care, safety, and efficiency. Such advances include electronic client care records, electronic medication administration with bar coding, electronic clinical documentation, wireless communication, delivery robots, and more. The integration of these and other types of technology add quality to nursing care and ultimately save client lives.

Evidence-based research on medication safety has implemented the need for safe delivery of medications. Medication errors account for a high percentage of errors related to client care and increased health care costs. Electronic medication administration with bar coding is one strategy that many facilities have implemented to decrease the amount of medication

---

Box 43–6 Selected Internet Sites for Evidence-Based Resources

- Cochrane Database of Systemic Reviews
  www.cochrane.org/reviews/
- Agency for Healthcare Research and Quality
  www.ahrq.gov
- National Guideline Clearinghouse
  http://guideline.gov

errors. Some facilities have instituted the use of handheld devices for nursing and medical staff. These devices provide the users with large amounts of electronic data that can be upgraded at frequent intervals. Meeting the need for current information and practice standards requires institutional support to ensure that nurses and other care providers have access to the resources and a computer or handheld device to use.

Nurses need to communicate their findings with their work colleagues and then incorporate changes into their practice. Implementation of these practice changes will hopefully make a positive change in the care of the client, decrease the length of stay, and become more cost effective. Additionally, unit-based policies and procedures, and protocols must reflect current research based information.

Sharing Information

When positive practice changes are realized, it is important that the nurse "close the EBP loop" by sharing the findings with other colleagues. This dissemination of results can be done in a variety of ways both informally at the agency level and, more importantly, formally through presentations at national conferences and by submission of articles for publication in professional journals.

The explosion of informatics in health care has also generated a need for a common language that can be used by individuals to access information and to share information. This common language allows nurses to code information to track nursing care processes and revise as necessary. Information technology is not simply improving access to information, but is developing new ways for nurses to share information on best practice. Listservs, blogs, and videoconferencing are just a few of the ways that information may be shared through technology.

Because of the importance of research to improving client care and to nursing as a profession, each nurse must make a personal commitment to engage in efforts to further expand the implementation of research to the profession. It is through these efforts that nurses will continue their quest for the provision of safe, effective, quality client care.

REVIEW | ## Evidence-Based Practice

RELATE: LINK THE CONCEPTS

Linking the concept of Evidence-Based Practice with the concept of Cellular Regulation:

1. While caring for a pediatric client with severe stomatitis secondary to chemotherapy, the nurse is concerned because the mouth ulcers are not responding to current treatment. How can the nurse assure the practice used is evidence based?
2. The nurse learns of a new treatment that has had great results with treatment-resistant stomatitis. What should the nurse do next?

Linking the concept of Evidence-Based Practice with the concept of Advocacy:

3. How can the nurse best advocate for a client considering becoming a participant in a research study?
4. The nurse is caring for a client who is involved in a clinical research study. The client says to the nurse, "I don't want to be a part of this study any longer. How do I get out of it?" How can the nurse best advocate for this client?

REFER: GO TO MYNURSINGKIT

REFLECT: CASE STUDY

The nurse is caring for a client diagnosed with recurrent metastatic testicular cancer. The client has been invited to join a research study to determine the effects of a new medication showing some success at treating this particular form of cancer. The lead researcher has provided the client with the necessary information for informed consent. The client has asked for time to think about it and discuss it with his spouse. When the nurse enters the room, the client asks, "What if I agree to participate and receive the placebo? Doesn't that mean I'm receiving no treatment for my cancer?" Later, the client says, "How do I know this new medication isn't more dangerous than the cancer?"

1. How can the nurse best respond to each of the client's questions?
2. How can the nurse best advocate for this client?
3. What are the nurse's ethical obligations to help this client?
4. Would the client actually get a placebo if not selected for the study?

REFERENCES

Abdellah, F. G., & Levine, E. (1965). *Better patient care through nursing research*. New York: Macmillan.

Abdellah, F. G., & Levine, E. (1994). *Preparing nursing research for the 21st century*. New York: Springer.

Alper, B.S., Hand, J.A., Elliott, S.G., Kinkade, S., Hauan, M. Onion, D.K., Sklar, B.M. (2004). How much effort is needed to keep up with the literature relevant for primary care? *Journal of the Medical Library Association 92*(4), 429–437.

American Nurses Association *Nursing scope and standards of practice* (2004) Silver Srping, MD: Author

The American Nurses Association. (2001). *Code of ethics for nurses*. Kansas City, MO: Author. Retrieved April 26, 2010, from http://www.nursingworld.org/MainMenuCategories/EthicsStandards/CodeofEthicsforNurses.aspx

American Nurses Association. (1994). *Archived position statement: Education for participation in nursing research*. Retrieved March 24, 2010, from http://www.nursingworld.org/MainMenuCategories/HealthcareandPolicyIssues/ANAPositionStatements/Archives.aspx

Balas, E. A. (2001). Information systems can prevent errors and improve quality. *Journal of the American Medical Informatics Association 8*(4): 398–399.

Bagby, K., & Adams, S. (2007). Evidence-based practice guideline: Increasing physical activity in schools—Kindergarten through 8th grade. *Journal of School Nursing, 23*, 137–143.

Bayley, E. W., MacLean, S. L., Desy, P., & McMahon, M. (2004). ENA's Delphi study on national research priorities for emergency nurses in the United States. *Journal of Emergency Nursing, 30*, 12–21.

Benkert, R., George, N., Tanner, C., Barkauskas, V. H., Pohl, J. M., & Marszalek, A. (2007). Satisfaction with a school-based teen health center: A report card on care. *Pediatric Nursing, 33*, 103–109.

Berger, A. M., Berry, D. L., Christopher, K. A., Greene A. L., Maliski, S., Swenson, K. K., et al. (2005). Oncology Nursing Society year 2004 research priorities survey. *Oncology Nursing Forum, 32*, 281–290.

Bertulis, R. (2008). Barriers to accessing evidence-based information. *Nursing Standard, 22*(36), 35–39.

Bourdeaux, L., Matthews, L., Richards, N. L., SanAgustin, G., Thomas, P., & Veltigian, S. (2005). Comparative study of case management program for patients with syncope. *Journal of Nursing Care Quality, 20*, 140–144.

Brooten, D., Kumar, S., Brown, L. P., Butts, P., Finkler, S. A., Bakewell-Sachs, S., et al. (1986). A randomized clinical trial of early hospital discharge and home follow-up of very-low-birth-weight infants. *New England Journal of Medicine, 315*, 934–939.

Brown, J., Tanner, C., & Padrick, K. (1984). Nursing's search for scientific knowledge. *Nursing Research, 33*, 26–32.

Burns, N., & Grove, S. K. (2005). *The practice of nursing research: Conduct, critique and utilization* (5th ed.). St. Louis, MO: Elsevier Saunders.

Children's Health Study. (2005). *Fact sheet*. Retrieved July 20, 2007, from http://www.arb.ca.gov/research/chs/chs.htm

Children's Health Study. (2006). *What is the National Children's Study?* Retrieved April 26, 2010, from http://www.nationalchildrensstudy.gov/Pages/default.aspx

Colling, J. (2004). Procedures, ethics, and funding sources. *Urologic Nursing, 24*, 130–133.

Diekema, D. S. (2006). Conducting ethical research in pediatrics: A brief historical overview and review of pediatric regulations. *Journal of Pediatrics, 149*, S3–S11.

Domrose, C. (2005, August 15). Nursing's new frontier. *NurseWeek—South Central Edition*, 10–11.

Downs, F. S. (1994). Hitching the research wagon to theory [Editorial]. *Nursing Research, 45*, 195.

Duffey, L., Hepburn, K., Christensen, R., & Brugge-Wiger, P. (1989). A research agenda in care for patients with Alzheimer's disease. *Image: Journal of Nursing Scholarship, 21*, 254–257.

Evidence-based Practice Centers Overview. (November 2007). Agency for healthcare research and quality, Rockville, MD. Retrieved from http://www.ahrq.gov/clinic/epc/

Ferguson, L. A. (1996). Enhancing health care to underserved populations. *AAOHN Journal, 44*, 332–335.

Fitzpatrick, J. (2007). Finding the research for evidence-based practice-part one-the development of EBP. *Nursing Times.net 103* (17), 32–33.

Fitzpatrick, J. J. (1999). Lateness is not greatness. *Nursing and Health Care Perspectives, 20*, 231.

Fitzpatrick, J. J. (2004). Making a commitment to go public [Editorial]. *Applied Nursing Research, 17*, 223.

Grady, P. A. (2005). Minutes of the National Advisory Council for Nursing Research—May 17–18, 2005. Retrieved August 28, 2005, from http://www.ninr.nih.gov/AboutNINR/NACNR/CouncilMinutesArchive/

Greenberg, M. E. (2000). Telephone nursing: Evidence of client and organizational benefits. *Nursing Economics, 18*, 117–123.

Grier, M. (1982). Editorial. *Research in Nursing and Health, 5*, 111.

Habel, M. (2005, March 14). Can you answer patients' questions about clinical trials? *NurseWeek—South Central Edition*, 23–25.

Henderson, V. (1956). Research in nursing practice—when? *Nursing Research, 4*, 99.

Hlipala, S. I., Meyer, K. A., Wallace, T. O., & Zaremba, J. A. (2005). Profile of an admission nurse. *Nursing Management, 36*, 44–47.

Hodge, M., Kochie, L., & Santiago, M. (2003). Clinician-implemented research utilization in critical care. *American Journal of Critical Care, 12*(4), 361–366.

Hoss, B., Hanson, D. (2008). Evaluating the evidence: Web sites. *AORN Journal, 87*(1), 125–141.

Johnson, J. (2008). Impact of the professional environment on knowledge. *Create the Future, 5*(6). Retrieved April 26, 2010, from http://www.nursingsociety.org/Publications/Newsletter/Pages/June08_CTF_ImpactoftheProfessionalEnvironmentonKnowledge.aspx

Kennedy, M. S. (2004). Not your grandma's nursing research [Editorial]. *American Journal of Nursing, 104*, 11.

Kerlinger, F. (1986). *Foundations of behavioral research* (3rd ed.). New York: Holt, Rinehart & Winston.

Lake, E. T. (2006). Multilevel models in health outcomes research: Part I. Theory, design, and measurement. *Applied Nursing Research, 19*, 51–55.

Leininger, M. M. (Ed.). (1985). *Qualitative research methods in nursing*. Orlando, FL: Grune & Stratton.

Marvin, M. (1927). Research in nursing. *American Journal of Nursing, 27*, 331–335.

Massive nurses' health study in seventh year, reports first findings on disease links in women. (1983). *American Journal of Nursing, 83*, 998–999.

Melnyk and Fineout-Overholt. (2005). *Evidence-based practice in nursing and healthcare*. Philadelphia: Lippincott Williams and Wilkins.

Myers, G., & Kosinski, M. (2005). Research in the perianesthesia setting: The basics of getting started. *Journal of PeriAnesthesia Nursing, 20*, 35–41.

National Institute of Nursing Research. (2005). *Mission statement*. Retrieved April 26, 2010, from http://www.ninr.nih.gov/NR/rdonlyres/E54A777C-FAAA-474A-BDFF-5B85EC8B9E7E/0/StrategicMission.pdf

Newhouse, R., Dearholt, S., Poe, S., Pugh, L., White, K. (2007). Johns Hopkins Nursing evidence-based practice model and guidelines. Sigma Theta Tau International: Indianapolis, IN.

Nightingale, F. (1859). Notes on nursing, What it is and what it is not (p. 59). Facsimile of the first edition printed in London, 1859, and reproduced by Edward Stern and Company, Inc., Philadelphia.

Nuremberg Military Tribunals. (1949). *Trials of war criminals before the Nuremberg Military Tribunals under Control Council Law No. 10* (Publication No. 1949–841584, Vol. 2). Washington, DC: U.S. Government Printing Office.

Office for Human Research Protection. (2008). *OHRP research involving children frequently asked questions*. Retrieved March 26, 2010, from http://www.hhs.gov/ohrp/researchfaq.html#q1

Oman, K. S., Krugman, M. E., & Fink, R. M. (2003). *Nursing research secrets*. Philadelphia: Hanley & Belfus.

Paul, I. M., Phillips, T. A., Widome, M. D., & Hollenbeak, C. S. (2004). Cost-effectiveness of postnatal home nursing visits for prevention of hospital care for jaundice and dehydration. *Pediatrics, 114*, 1015–1022.

Polit, D. F., & Beck, C. T. (2004). *Nursing research: Principles and methods* (7th ed.). Philadelphia: Lippincott Williams & Wilkins.

Pullen, L., Tuck, I., & Wallace, D. C. (1999). Research priorities in mental health nursing. *Issues in Mental Health Nursing, 20*, 217–227.

Rankin, M., & Esteves, M. D. (1996). How to assess a research study. *American Journal of Nursing, 96*, 33–36.

Rittenmeyer, P. (1982). The evolution of nursing research. *Western Journal of Nursing Research, 4*, 223–225.

Sackett, D.L., Rosenberg, W. M., Gray, J. A., Haynes, R. B., and Richardson, W. S. (1996). Evidence based medicine: What it is and what it isn't [Editorial]. *BMJ, 312*, 71–72.

Salmond, S.W. (2007). Advancing evidence-based practice: A primer. *Orthopaedic Nursing, 26*(2).

Salmond, S. W. (1994). Orthopaedic nursing research priorities: A Delphi study. *Orthopaedic Nursing, 13*, 31–45.

Sedlak, C., Ross, D., Arslanian, C., & Taggart, H. (1998). Orthopaedic nursing research priorities: A replication and extension. *Orthopaedic Nursing, 17*(2), 51–58.

Sigma Theta Tau International, Honor Society for Nursing. (2005). The society's vision and mission. Retrieved April 26, 2010, from http://www.nursingsociety.org/aboutus/mission/Pages/factsheet.aspx

Silva, M. C. (1995). *Ethical guidelines in the conduct, dissemination, and implementation of nursing research*. Washington, DC: American Nurses Association.

Simmons, L. W., & Henderson, V. (1964). *Nursing research—a survey and assessment*. New York: Appleton-Century-Crofts.

Strumpf, L., & Evans, L. (2008). *Individualized restraint free care*. University of Pennsylvania, Hartford Center for Geriatric Nursing Excellence. Retrieved February 11, 2008, from http://www.nursing.upenn.edu/centers/hcgne/restraints.htm

Tucker-Allen, S. (2003). Nursing education as a respected area of research [Editorial]. *The Association of Black Nursing Faculty Journal, 14*, 115.

Ulrich, B. (2005, August 15). Intersecting worlds: Nursing and NASA. *NurseWeek—South Central Edition*, 3.

Vratney, A. (2007). A conceptual model for growing evidence based practice. *Nursing Administration Quarterly, 31*(2). 162–170.

Williams, S. (2005, January 31). The science of care. *NurseWeek—South Central Edition*, 10.

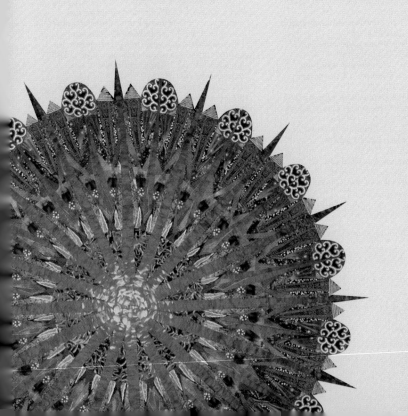

Health Care Systems

44

Concept at-a-Glance

About Health Care Systems, *2339*

44.1   Access to Health Care, *2345*

44.2   Allocation of Resources, *2349*

44.3   Emergency Preparedness, *2351*

Concept Learning Outcomes

After reading about this concept, you will be able to:

1. Discuss the three levels of prevention and give examples of each level.

2. Differentiate different types of health care agencies and describe the type of health care service provided at each.

3. List factors that influence the delivery of health care and explain how each factor affects the delivery of care.

4. List different frameworks for delivering care and explain how they differ, including the advantages and disadvantages of each.

Concept Key Terms

Case management, *2343*
Client-focused care, *2344*
Diagnosis-related groups (DRG), *2343*
Functional nursing, *2344*
Health literacy, *2342*
Managed care, *2343*

Primary nursing, *2344*
Primary prevention, *2340*
Secondary prevention, *2340*
Team nursing, *2344*
Tertiary prevention, *2340*
Unlicensed assistive personnel (UAP), *2344*

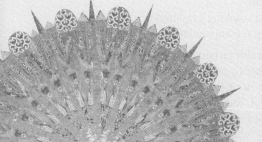

About Health Care Systems

The concept of health care systems relates to the methods of health care delivery and management, including financing and coordination of services. Particularly in the last two decades, new cost-containment strategies and advances in technology—both informatics and medical technology—have combined to bring about significant changes to health care systems in the United States. Table 44–1 demonstrates the impact of those changes. ●

TABLE 44–1 Comparison of Old Health Care Paradigm With New Paradigm

OLD PARADIGM	NEW HEALTH CARE PARADIGM
Hospital-based, acute care	Short-term hospital: same-day surgery, 23-hour stays; prehospital testing and precertification; telehealth/telemedicine; home health; mobile vans; school and mall clinics
Specialty units	Cross-training (multiskilled workers): LDRP, OR/PACU, CCU/telemetry
Hierarchical management	Decentralization (unit budget, scheduling, variance); shared governance; strategic plan
Physician "captain of ship"; others are followers	Inter/multidisciplinary team, collaboration; case management (registered nurse/broker)
Nurse as employee: job-focused, limited responsibilities and opportunities	Nurse as professional: career focused; clinical ladder; continuing credentials; tuition reimbursement, paid certification exam
Medical condition, focus on segment	Holistic person in family/community; pastoral care, parish nurse
"Sick care," focus on cure	Health care, health promotion, prevention programs; care and continuity of care; complementary health alternatives
Cost containment, focus on billing	Focus on patient and accountability of caregivers/agency; electronic patient record, continuous quality improvement, care maps
Written medical record	Integrated electronic records: smart card, bedside computers
Fee for service	Managed competition (HMO, PPO, IPA)
Physician as employer	Physician as employee; capitation system
One insurance plan	Variety of insurance options ("covered lives"): basic plan plus dental, eye, long-term care, cancer, disability
80–100% covered by insurance	Greater deductible, lower percentage coverage, or copayment

Source: From J. A. Milstead. (2004). Health policy and politics: A nurse's guide (2nd ed., p. 14). Sudbury, MA: Jones and Bartlett Reprinted by permission.

TYPES OF HEALTH CARE SERVICES

Health care delivery can be classified by the type of services offered. A **primary prevention** service focuses on health promotion and illness prevention. **Secondary prevention** services include the diagnosis and treatment of disease. **Tertiary prevention** consists of the restoration of health following an illness or accident and includes rehabilitation and palliative services.

Primary Prevention

Primary prevention avoids development of disease as much as possible and promotes healthy living. Until the 1980s, health care was actually illness/disease care. Individuals typically accessed the health care system only when confronted with an illness or accident. The 1979 Surgeon General's Report from *Healthy People* laid the foundation for a national prevention agenda. Since 1979, *Healthy People* has set and monitored national health objectives to meet a broad range of health needs, encourage collaborations across sectors, guide individuals toward making informed health decisions, and measure the impact of prevention activity. *Healthy People* identifies a number of leading health indicators (discussed in Concept 13, Health, Wellness, and Illness), which, if addressed, should result in an increase in the quality and length of life and the elimination of health disparities. Every 10 years, the U.S. Department of Health and Human Services (DHHS) updates the *Healthy People* with scientific insights and lessons learned from the past decade, along with new knowledge of current data, trends, and innovations. *Healthy People 2020*, due to be launched in 2010, will reflect assessments of major risks to

health and wellness, changing public health priorities, and emerging issues related to our nation's health preparedness and prevention (U.S. DHSS, 2008).

Programs for health promotion are developed to address the need to control the rising cost of health care and the idea that prevention of disease is more cost effective than treatment of disease. The nurse has an integral role in health promotion. Some examples of how nurses participate in health promotion include the following:

- Facilitating client involvement in the assessment, implementation, and evaluation of health goals
- Educating clients to be effective health care consumers
- Guiding clients' development in effective problem solving and decision making
- Advocating in the community for changes that promote a healthy environment.

Specific health promotion topics that have been identified both by *Healthy People* and by individual states and communities include the following:

- Childhood obesity and nutrition
- Physical activity across the lifespan
- Dental/oral health
- Tobacco use and smoking cessation
- Health screening recommendations.

In designing health promotion strategies, it is important to remember that health promotion can be offered to all clients regardless of their health and illness status or age. For example, weight-control measures can benefit both overweight clients without disease and clients with cardiac or joint disease.

Secondary Prevention

Secondary prevention activities are aimed at early disease detection and treatment to prevent the progression of the disease and development of more symptoms. Traditionally, secondary prevention has been the largest segment of health care services and has occurred primarily in hospitals and physicians' offices. Independent community-based diagnostic and treatment centers have grown in popularity. Examples of these include outpatient surgery and diagnostic imaging centers. Early detection of diseases is provided through screening. Different types of screening, such as screening for high blood pressure or vision problems, may be provided by primary health providers or through health fairs. Screenings can be offered to the general population or focused on groups at high risk.

Tertiary Prevention

Tertiary prevention involves restoring function and decreasing disease-related complications of an already established disease. When restoration to the previous level of functioning is not possible, care is focused on controlling symptoms and promoting the highest quality of life. Rehabilitation and palliative care are included in tertiary prevention.

Table 44–2 outlines the three levels of prevention.

TYPES OF HEALTH CARE SETTINGS

Primary care is delivered in a variety of settings, including physicians' offices, hospital-based clinics, community health centers, and public health service organizations (Figure 44–1 ■). Community health centers and public health organizations frequently offer health promotion activities at locations throughout their communities, such as churches, shopping malls, and cultural events.

In the context of managed care, the primary care setting is often the point of entry and the gatekeeper for all other care. Primary care involves health maintenance services such as routine physicals, immunizations, treatment of common acute illnesses, and support for psychosocial needs.

Secondary care may be delivered in a hospital, outpatient surgical center, or specialist's office. For example, an adult with a basal cell carcinoma may have it removed at the dermatologist's office. As it is an outpatient treatment that involves only local anesthesia, the office setting can provide the most appropriate, cost-effective point of care for removing the basal cell.

Tertiary care that involves complicated diagnostic or therapeutic procedures may be provided in a hospital, an acute care facility, a rehabilitation center, or an extended care facility. Regardless of the type of facility in which the client is receiving tertiary care, nurses will coordinate the client's activities and ensure the client's compliance with treatment during the course of the client's stay.

FACTORS AFFECTING DELIVERY OF HEALTH CARE

A number of factors affect the ability of nurses to deliver client care, regardless of the level of care or the setting in which care is being delivered. These include changing demographics, advances in technology, and levels of health literacy of clients in the community.

TABLE 44–2 Levels of Prevention

LEVEL AND DESCRIPTION	EXAMPLES
Primary prevention: Provides generalized health promotion and specific protection against disease. It precedes disease or dysfunction and is applied to generally healthy individuals or groups.	■ Health education about injury and poisoning prevention, standards of nutrition and of growth and development for each stage of life, exercise requirements, stress management, protection against occupational hazards, and so on ■ Immunizations ■ Risk assessments for specific disease ■ Family planning services ■ Environmental sanitation and provision of adequate housing, recreation, and work conditions
Secondary prevention: Emphasizes early detection of disease, prompt intervention, and health maintenance for individuals experiencing health problems. Includes prevention of complications and disabilities.	■ Screening surveys and procedures of any type (e.g., Denver Developmental Screening Test, hypertension screening) ■ Encouraging regular medical and dental checkups ■ Teaching self-examination for breast and testicular cancer ■ Assessing the growth and development of children ■ Nursing assessments and care provided in home, hospital, or other agency to prevent complications (e.g., maintaining skin integrity; turning, positioning, and exercising clients; ensuring adequate rest, food, and fluid intake; promoting fecal and urinary elimination; administering medical therapies such as medications; and so on)
Tertiary prevention: Begins after an illness, when a defect or disability is fixed, stabilized, or determined to be irreversible. Its focus is to help rehabilitate individuals and restore them to an optimum level of functioning within the constraints of the disability.	■ Referring a client who has had a colostomy to a support group ■ Teaching a client who has diabetes to identify and prevent complications ■ Referring a client with a spinal cord injury to a rehabilitation center to receive training that will maximize use of remaining abilities

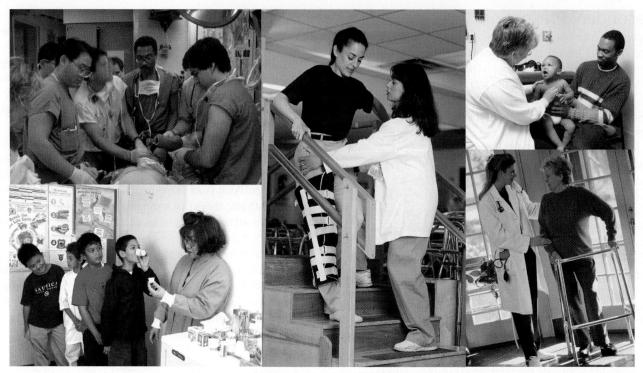

Figure 44–1 ■ Various health care settings.

Changing Demographics

The nation will be more racially and ethnically diverse, as well as much older, by midcentury, according to projections released by the U.S. Census Bureau (2008):

- Minorities, now roughly one-third of the U.S. population, are expected to become the majority in 2042 with the nation projected to be 54% minority in 2050. By 2023, minorities will comprise more than half of all children.
- In 2030, when all of the baby boomers will be 65 and older, nearly one in five U.S. residents is expected to be 65 and older. This age group is projected to increase to 88.5 million people in 2050, more than doubling the number in 2008 (38.7 million).
- Similarly, the 85 and older population is expected to more than triple from 5.4 million to 19 million people between 2008 and 2050.

Effects of aging, long-term illnesses, and lack of primary care of these three groups will increase the need for management of health care and support systems to assist those living in the community.

Advances in Technology

Scientific knowledge and technology related to health care are rapidly increasing. Information management systems are being created and refined that utilize bedside charting, laboratory testing, and the availability of online evidenced-based guidelines to provide care. New strategies for early identification and prevention of disease, new drugs, and new less invasive surgical techniques are being developed that change where and how care may be provided. For example, the use of laparoscopic surgical techniques has decreased length of stay and requirements for hospitalization. Many advances in technology require specialized personnel, creating new opportunities for individuals seeking employment in the health care sector.

Health Literacy

Health literacy is defined as the degree to which individuals can obtain, act on, and understand basic health information and services needed to make appropriate health care decisions (IOM, 2004). In 2003, the National Center for Educational Statistics conducted the National Assessment of Adult Literacy (NAAL). The study assessed health literacy in more than 19,000 adults (ages 16 and older) in households or prisons through the measurement of tasks completed. This study identified the following:

- A slight majority of adults had an intermediate level of health literacy.
- Thirty-six percent of respondents had a basic or below basic level of health literacy.
- Lower health literacy was seen in the elderly, those with lower socioeconomic status, and those with lower education attainment.
- Caucasian and Asian/Pacific Islander adults had higher average health literacy than African Americans, Hispanic, American Indian/Alaska Native, and multiracial adults.
- Hispanic adults had lower average health literacy than adults in any of the other racial/ethnic groups.

Health care illiteracy and ineffective communication place clients at risk for poor health outcomes. According to the National Institutes of Health (2006), African Americans, Hispanics, Native Americans, and Asian Pacific Islanders, representing about 25% of the U.S. population, continue to experience heath disparities including shorter life expectancy and higher rates of diabetes, cancer, heart disease, stroke, substance abuse, infant mortality, and low birth weight. One of the strategies for overcoming this health disparity is health education programs for these populations. Unless health literacy is addressed, this strategy is likely to be unsuccessful. Strategies for working with clients who have low levels of health literacy are discussed in Exemplar 13.6, Consumer Education, in Volume 1.

FRAMEWORKS FOR PROVIDING CARE

In the United States, most health care providers work within a specific framework for providing care. Managed care, case management, and client-focused care are just three of the models used. Sometimes frameworks overlap: services may be coordinated through a case management model to clients whose health insurance plan uses a managed care model.

Managed Care

Managed care, discussed in detail in Concept 37, Managing Care, is a method of organizing care delivery that emphasizes cost-effective, quality care that focuses on decreased costs and improved outcomes for groups of clients. It became an extended responsibility of the registered nurse following the introduction of prospective payment systems in 1983. The function of managed care can be adapted across all health care settings. As discussed in Concept 37, **diagnosis-related groups (DRGs)** establish fees according to a diagnosis to simplify billing and limit reimbursement for services by Medicare. One advantage of managed care is that care of the client is carefully planned from the initial contact to the conclusion of the specific health problem. In managed care, costs for services are predetermined,

allowing clients to know ahead of time what their copayment for a service will be. However, some benefits, such as the number of days in the hospital, may be limited under managed care, as may be the circumstances under which the client may access specialty care and be covered for those services. For example, many managed care insurance plans cover services provided by health care providers who are "in network," or who have agreed to operate within the cost structure of the plan, and will not cover services by health care providers who are under no such agreement (called "out of network").

Case Management

Case management is a framework for care in which multidisciplinary teams assist clients and their families access necessary resources in a timely manner while managing and allocating available resources. The overall goal of case management is to provide a service delivery approach that ensures cost-effective care, provides alternatives to institutionalization, provides access to care, coordinates services, and improves the client's functional ability (Lyon, 1993). Case managers may be nurses, social workers, or other health care team members. The case manager may or may not provide direct care depending on the model used. Case management may be limited to a hospitalization or may occur across settings for clients receiving care in the community and/or at home. This enables clients to experience continuity of care, regardless of the location at which the care is provided. See Figure 44–2 ■. Advantages of case management include support for the client by a variety of health care providers (e.g., nurses, physicians, speech and occupational therapists, and social workers), increased access to care, and collaborative responsibility for cost-effective care. Disadvantages may include poor communication among

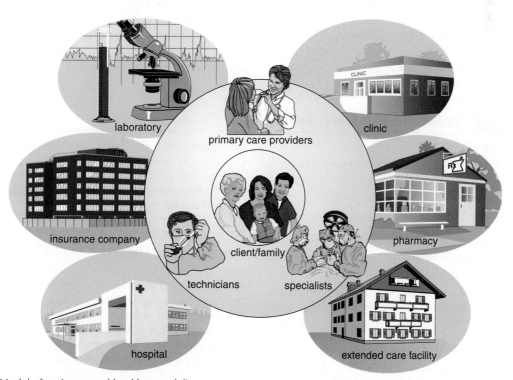

Figure 44–2 ■ Model of an integrated health care delivery system.

members of the health care team, which can result in the client "slipping through the cracks," or in less cohesive provision of services.

Client-Focused Care

Client-focused care is a delivery model that brings all services and care providers to the client. The idea is that if activities normally provided by various members of the health care team (e.g., physical therapy, respiratory therapy, electrocardiographic testing, and phlebotomy) are moved closer to the client, then the number of personnel involved and the number of steps needed to get the work done are decreased. To succeed, client-focused care requires cross-training (development of multiskilled workers who can perform tasks or functions in more than one discipline) of health care personnel. An advantage of client-focused care is that the services are closer to the client. A disadvantage is that the decreased focus on cost considerations may result in increasing costs to the client or the client's insurance plan.

Nursing Care Delivery Systems

Three models of nursing care delivery may be used regardless of the framework in which health care is delivered to the client.

Functional nursing arose at the end of World War II, as large numbers of unskilled workers entered the health care workforce. This system divides health care along functional lines, so that the task requiring the least skill is done by the least skilled worker. The head nurse delegates tasks to the staff members as available; clients are not assigned to a specific nurse. The RN remains accountable for performing tasks accurately and competently (Zander, 1980). Functional nursing is one model being proposed to address the nursing shortage. The goal would be to increase the number of tasks that unlicensed assistive personnel (UAP) are trained to accomplish and free the RN for activities requiring professional judgment and decision making or a higher degree of skill level. **Unlicensed assistive personnel (UAP)** are those health care

staff members who assume delegated aspects of basic client care, such as bathing, assisting with feeding, and collecting specimens. Advantages of functional nursing include cost efficiency and centralization of control. A primary disadvantage is that it overlooks nursing care that cannot be quantified easily, such as care of the client's emotional needs.

Under the **team nursing** model, a professional nurse leads a team that provides individualized care to clients. The registered nurse leading each team retains responsibility and authority but delegates tasks to a nursing assistant, who spends the most time giving direct care to the client. The work is identified by the tasks to be completed during each shift. While this model frees the professional nurse to attend to more complex client care tasks, frequent changes in assignments may lead to a lack of continuity of care for clients.

Primary nursing means that the registered nurse plans and oversees client care directly. Each client is assigned to a primary nurse, who assesses and prioritizes client needs, develops a plan of care, and provides direct care. While less skilled personnel may provide some care, especially in the absence of the primary nurse, the primary nurse coordinates all care and retains authority and responsibility for the care provided (Zander, 1980).

NURSING PRACTICE

Nurses need to have a solid understanding of the different types of health care settings and frameworks for providing care. Some agencies use a combination of models, and each agency has its own specific policies and procedures. Nurses must know the requirements of the agency in which they practice. In addition, nurses must understand the barriers to accessing health care that their clients face, the issues they themselves face when resources are insufficient to meet client needs, and their agency's and community's procedures for how they are to respond in the event of a disaster.

 REVIEW About Health Care Systems

RELATE: LINK THE CONCEPTS

You are a registered nurse leading a team that includes LPNs and UAPs on a critical care unit of a hospital. You are planning care for a client on a mechanical ventilator.

Linking the concept of Health Care Systems with the concept of Oxygenation:

1. What aspects of this client's care may be delegated to UAPs?
2. What factors that affect the delivery of health care may impact your ability to provide care for this client, and how?

You are a registered nurse working in the emergency department (ED) of a rural hospital. Harvesting season has brought large numbers of Spanish-speaking families to the community. Almost all of the men and many of the women work as migrant workers. A mother who speaks limited English brings her 5-year-old son to the ED saying that he has been vomiting for 2 days. He has a fever of 102 degrees. She says he does not have a regular physician; he is not enrolled in any type of health insurance plan.

Linking the concept of Health Care Systems with the concept of Clinical Decision Making:

3. What factors will impact your ability to plan care for the child?
4. Which model of nursing care delivery would most benefit the child and his mother? Why?

REFER: GO TO MYNURSING KIT

REFLECT: CASE STUDY

Juan Santiago, 41 years old, makes an appointment with a provider he's never seen before for an annual physical examination. When he arrives for his appointment, the nurse escorts him back to the examination room and begins the assessment process. The client explains that he has never had a complete physical before because he has always been healthy and never had health insurance. He has recently graduated from college and accepted a new job that offered full benefits so he decided it was time he take care of his health. His wife, two daughters, and one son have all had their physical examination and he realized he needed to do this too. He is obviously anxious about what will happen, but does not ask any questions and avoids making eye contact with the nurse.

During the nurse's collection of Mr. Santiago's health history he reveals he smokes approximately 20 cigarettes per day, drinks 2–3 alcoholic beverages per week, and up until recently has worked as a landscaper in a very physically demanding job. He describes his new job as involving "a little bit of walking but mostly desk work."

During the physical examination the nurse notes a wound the size of a quarter on the anterior aspect of his left foot, which is erythematous, warm to the touch, and has a small amount of purulent drainage seeping from the side of the wound. Mr. Santiago reports the wound has been there for more than 6 weeks and won't heal

despite over-the-counter antibiotic cream he has been applying daily. The nurse questions the client about his weight and Mr. Santiago admits he has lost approximately 10 pounds in the past month but denies any change in his diet.

1. Describe primary, secondary, and tertiary care requirements for this client.
2. What referrals to other health care providers might be appropriate to assist in the treatment plan for this client?
3. What type of assessment of health literacy would the nurse conduct with this client before providing written information?
4. What factors will influence care delivery to this client and how will that alter the nurse's approach to providing care for this client?

44.1 ACCESS TO HEALTH CARE

KEY TERMS
Underinsured, 2345
Uninsured, 2345

BASIS FOR SELECTION OF EXEMPLAR
Agency for Healthcare Research and Quality
Healthy People 2010
U.S. Department of Health and Human Services
World Health Organization

LEARNING OBJECTIVES
After reading about this exemplar, you will be able to:
1. Describe barriers to access to health care services.
2. Explain what it means to be uninsured or underinsured.
3. Discuss ways to increase access to health care for uninsured and underinsured people.

OVERVIEW

For most Americans who have health care coverage through an employer, high-quality health care is available without a long wait and at a reasonable cost. However, high-quality health care is often beyond the reach of the many Americans who work for small employers, the unemployed and underemployed, the self-employed, the poor, and underserved minorities. These groups face many challenges to accessing health care and, as a result, often have poorer health outcomes—in some cases worse than those of residents of developing countries. As was demonstrated by previous National Healthcare Disparities Reports (2007), racial and ethnic minorities and people of low socioeconomic status are disproportionately represented among those with access problems. Inadequate access to care has a larger impact on society. For example, a failure to receive immunizations or early treatment of a contagious disease can result in community outbreaks. The health care reform act signed into law by President Obama in early 2010 is an attempt to remedy some of the disparities in access to health insurance coverage and to remedy other, related problems (see Box 44–1 for more information on the health care reform act).

Uninsured individuals are those without any type of health care coverage. Uninsured individuals do not qualify for public insurance programs, such as Medicaid, and cannot buy health insurance usually because they work for employers who do not offer health insurance coverage. Uninsured clients also include those who cannot afford to purchase insurance through their employer because the insurance premiums are too expensive.

Increasingly, individuals who are self-employed are unable to purchase health insurance privately, either because the premiums are unaffordable or because they are denied coverage due to a pre-existing condition or chronic illness (Alboher, 2008). It is expected that the Health Care and Education Reconciliation Act of 2010 will significantly reduce the number of individuals in the United States who are currently uninsured, but the outcome of this act is yet to be measured.

Underinsured individuals have health care coverage that is insufficient to meet their needs. Examples include the child who is covered under a parent's company policy but the policy does not include immunizations and the client with a chronic illness whose insurance does not include coverage for medications. Recent health care reform will attempt to resolve these gaps in coverage.

BARRIERS TO ACCESS

According to the Institute of Medicine (1993), access to health care means having "the timely use of personal health services to achieve the best health outcomes." Accessing health care requires three discrete steps:

1. Gaining entry into the health care system.
2. Getting access to sites of care where clients can receive needed services.
3. Finding providers with whom the client can communicate, develop a trusting relationship, and have their individual needs met.

Box 44-1 2010 Health Care and Education Reconciliation Act

In 2010 Congress passed the Health Care and Education Reconciliation Act. The new law is intended to:

- Curb medical costs that are growing much faster than the rate of inflation
- Return insurance premiums to less costly rates so that more individuals and companies, especially small businesses, can afford to purchase insurance
- Remedy many unpopular insurance industry practices, such as denying coverage for clients with preexisting conditions or dropping coverage for clients who become ill
- Extend coverage to 32 million Americans, many of whom are working poor who do not qualify for public insurance programs and who work for employers who do not offer health insurance benefits.

Some of the provisions of the health care reform take effect immediately, while others will be implemented over several years.

Among provisions of the new law that take effect immediately:

- Children can no longer be denied health insurance coverage for preexisting conditions.
- Insurance companies can no longer drop clients when they become ill.
- Lifetime caps on coverage are eliminated. Annual caps on benefits are limited and will be eliminated in 2014. These measures help those who experience catastrophic illness or who live with costly chronic conditions such as hemophilia.
- Children will be allowed to remain on their parents' insurance plan until the age of 26.
- New health insurance plans must offer preventive care with no co-payment or deductible.
- Small employers that offer health insurance benefits to employees will receive a 35% tax credit for their share of premiums.
- Retirees aged 55-64 will be offered access to a re-insurance program.
- Medicare Part D recipients will receive a $250 credit.

BY 2011:

- Medicare must provide plans for preventive care with no copayment or deductible.
- Medicare Part D recipients in the "doughnut hole" of coverage will receive a 50% discount off prescription drugs.
- Health insurance companies will have to justify any premium increases or risk being taken out of state insurance exchange pools.

BY 2014:

- The uninsured and self-employed will be able to purchase insurance through state-based exchanges. Separate exchanges will be established for small companies.
- The IRS will impose a penalty of $750 per individual or 2% of income—whichever is greater—for those that choose not to purchase health insurance.
- Individuals and families who make between 100% to 400% of the Federal Poverty Level (FPL) and want to purchase their own health insurance on an exchange will be eligible for federal subsidies. In order to be eligible, these people cannot qualify for Medicare or Medicaid and cannot be covered by an employer. Eligible buyers will receive premium credits and there will be a limit to how much they have to contribute to their premiums.
- Private insurers will be required to accept all applicants without varying premiums on the basis of a person's health status. Insurance companies will not be able to deny coverage on the basis of preexisting conditions.
- Annual limits on benefits will be eliminated.
- The temporary high-risk pools for those unable to receive coverage prior to the law will be eliminated as people enroll in state insurance exchanges.

BY 2018:

- All insurance plans will be required to offer preventive care with no copayment or deductible.
- Insurance companies will pay a 40% excise tax on high-end benefit plans worth over $27,500 for families ($10,200 for individuals). Dental and vision plans will be exempt and will not be counted in the total cost of a family's plan.

Sources: Binckes J, Wing N. Health reform bill summary: The top 18 immediate effects. *Huffington Post*. Retrieved March 23, 2010, from http://www.huffingtonpost.com/2010/03/22/health-reform-bill-summary_n_508315.html#s75159. Jackson J, & Nolen J. Health care reform bill summary: A look at what's in the bill. *CBS News*, Retrieved March 23, 2010, from http://www.cbsnews.com/8301-503544_162-20000846-503544.html. Health care reform. *New York Times*, Retrieved March 26, 2010, from http://topics.nytimes.com/top/news/health/diseasesconditionsandhealthtopics/health_insurance_and_managed_care/health_care_reform/index.html. Health Care and Education Reconciliation Act of 2010. *Wikipedia*. Retrieved from http://en.wikipedia.org/wiki/Health_Care_and_Education_Reconciliation_Act_of_2010

Lack of Health Insurance

Some reports estimate that 46 million Americans are uninsured in the United States. More than 8.3 million of the uninsured are children. More than 8 out of 10 uninsured people are in working families that cannot afford health insurance, and most of them are not eligible for public programs. Following are more facts about uninsured Americans:

- 83% of the uninsured are in working families
- 62.1% live in households with a full-time worker, and 21.3 percent live in households with a part-time worker
- 17.8% of non-elderly Americans are uninsured
- 21.2% of African Americans are uninsured
- 34.3% of Hispanics are uninsured (U.S. Census Bureau, August 2008).

The financial implications for a large population of uninsured individuals and families are many. In the United States, for example, the costs of early death and poor health among the uninsured range from $65 billion to $130 billion per year. Nearly 50% of those filing bankruptcy each year are forced to do so because of medical expenses. Uninsured individuals are diagnosed at later stages of disease and typically get less therapeutic treatment, increasing their mortality rates (AHRQ, 2007).

Insurance is even more critical for children. In the publication *Why Health Insurance Matters to Children*, the Campaign for Children's Health Care gives six reasons why children should have health insurance:

1. Children with insurance are more likely to have a usual source of care.

2. Children with insurance are more likely to have access to preventive care.
3. Children with insurance get the health care services they need.
4. Insured children will help close the racial disparities gap.
5. Health insurance helps improve social and emotional development.
6. Insured children are better equipped to do well in school.

The document details how children who have insurance, regardless of the funding source of that insurance, experience better health outcomes, and, over time, have better attendance rates in school and experience better social and emotional development (Families USA, 2006). There are two provisions of the Health Care and Education Reconciliation Act that are expected to increase the access of children to health care insurance within 6 months of the law's passing. First, insurance companies will no longer be able to deny coverage to children based on preexisting conditions. Second, insurance companies will be prevented from dropping clients who become ill. This second provision means that families who already have insurance but who experience the serious illness of a family member will no longer have to worry about losing their health insurance coverage (Appleby, 2010).

PRACTICE ALERT
Emergency departments have the only legal mandate to provide health care, as dictated by the Emergency Medical Treatment and Labor Act (EMTALA, 1986). This law ensures that anyone who comes to an emergency department, regardless of insurance status or ability to pay, must receive a medical screening exam and be stabilized.

Lack of a Usual Source of Care

According to the Agency for Healthcare Research and Quality (AHRQ), individuals with a *usual source of care*, defined as a facility where one regularly receives care, experience improved health outcomes and reduced disparities (smaller differences between groups) and costs. A usual source of care is sometimes referred to as a *medical home* or *health care home*.

Having a usual primary care provider, defined as a doctor or nurse from whom one regularly receives care, is associated with clients' greater trust in their provider and with good client-provider communication, which, in turn, increases the likelihood that clients will receive appropriate care, according to AHRQ (2007). By learning about the client's diverse health care needs over time, the primary care provider can coordinate care to better meet these needs. Having a usual primary care provider correlates with receipt of higher-quality care, yet over 40 million Americans do not receive regular care.

Children in particular need a usual source of health care. When a family has an established partnership with a care provider, comprehensive, family-centered health services can be provided on the basis of the family's risks and protective factors. The U.S. Department of Health and Human Services (DHHS), the American Academy of Pediatrics (AAP), and the American Medical Association have developed national guidelines for preventive health services for infants, children, and adolescents

(Box 44–2). The National Association of Pediatric Nurse Associates and Practitioners (NAPNAP) supports the list of comprehensive services identified by the AAP (Box 44–3).

Perceptions of Need

Perceptions of need often affect individuals' ability to access the health care system. These include perceived difficulties or delays in obtaining care and problems getting care as soon as it is wanted. Although clients may not always be able to assess their own need for care, problems getting care when people perceive that they are ill or injured can increase their perception that care is difficult to access.

CLINICAL EXAMPLE
A nurse working for a large insurance company as a telephone triage nurse receives a call from a member reporting that her 4-year-old daughter woke with ear pain that has not responded to acetaminophen administered by mouth 15 minutes ago. The mother reports the child is crying in pain and requests authorization to go to the hospital emergency room. The nurse provides strategies to treat the child's pain and explains that oral analgesics require 45–60 minutes to begin taking effect. The nurse offers to make an appointment with the primary care provider in the morning. When the mother states the child must be seen immediately, the nurse suggests that the mother take the child to a 24-hour urgent care center. The mother declines, insisting that the child be treated immediately at the emergency room.

1. Does this nurse have the right to inform parents they cannot take the child to the emergency room because this is not an emergency?
2. How does the mother's perception of need impact her response?
3. What else might the nurse do help the parent more accurately perceive the child's health care needs?

Uneven Distribution of Services

Serious problems in the distribution of health care services exist in the United States, primarily in terms of uneven distribution and increased specialization. In some areas, particularly remote and rural locations, not enough health care professionals and services are available to meet the needs of the people who live there. Rural clients may need to drive large distances to obtain the services they require. Uneven distribution is evidenced by the relatively higher number of nurses per capita in the New England states and the lowest number in the

Box 44–2 National Guidelines for Health Promotion

- *Bright Futures*, American Academy of Pediatrics (original editions by Maternal and Child Health Bureau, Health Resources and Services Administration, DHHS)
- *Put Prevention into Practice*, Agency for Healthcare Quality and Research
- *The Guide to Clinical Preventive Services*, U.S. Preventive Services Task Force
- *Guidelines for Adolescent Preventive Services*, American Medical Association

Box 44-3 Elements of a Pediatric Health Care Home

The AAP and NAPNAP concur that a pediatric health care home should offer:

- Family-centered care and trusting partnership
- Sharing of unbiased and clear information
- Provision of primary care to include acute and chronic care; breastfeeding promotion; immunizations; growth and development screenings; healthcare supervision; and counseling about health, nutrition, safety, parenting, and psychosocial issues
- Continuously accessible care
- Continuity of care
- Provision of compassionate, developmentally appropriate, and culturally competent care
- Referral to early intervention and child care
- Coordination of services and collaboration of professionals
- Maintenance of a comprehensive central record
- Referral to specialists as needed.

Sources: Data from American Academy of Pediatrics. (2002). The medical home. Policy statement. *Pediatrics*, 110, 184–186; Pan, R.J. (2006). A Jacobian future: Can everyone have a medical home? *Pediatrics*, 118, 1254–1256; National Association of Pediatric Nurse Associates and Practitioners (2002). *NAPNAP position statement on the pediatric health care home.* Retrieved May 26, 2007, from http://www.napnap.org/practice/positions/healthcarehome.html

Southwest. Physicians are also unevenly distributed: In 2006, Mississippi, Idaho, Wyoming, and Nevada had the fewest physicians per 100,000 people, whereas the District of Columbia, Massachusetts, New York, and Maryland had the most (National Center for Health Statistics, 2009).

An increasing number of health care personnel provide specialized services. Specialization can lead to fragmentation of care and, often, increased cost of care. To clients, it may mean receiving care from 5 to 30 people during their hospital experience. This seemingly endless stream of personnel and the paperwork required is often confusing and frightening to the client.

SOLUTIONS

Communities across the country are seeking ways to increase access to health care services for their uninsured and underinsured citizens. Local health departments, for example, use federal and state funding as well as grants from private foundations to meet the needs of their communities, including hiring translators and maternal–child care nurses and purchasing vans to provide dental services in remote areas. In some communities, federally qualified community health centers and free clinics serve those who do not have access to regular health care.

Community Health Centers

In 1991, the Federally Qualified Health Center benefit was added under Medicare. These centers specialize in treating the medically underserved in communities, public housing projects, and Native American reservations across the United States. Because most of community health centers operate as nonprofit entities, they are able to rely on federal, state, and private funding. Community health centers serve people who are on Medicaid and Medicare and see other clients who are charged sliding-scale fees. Services offered include health promotion and prevention, primary care, dental, and mental health services. For example, on a given morning in a community health center, one might see a class of Head Start students coming for dental examinations, older clients coming for a physical exam or blood pressure screening, and an array of other clients coming for diagnostic screenings.

Although some services vary by agency and by state, community health centers typically offer services provided by physicians, nurse practitioners, certified nurse midwives, physician assistants, clinical psychologists, and clinical social workers (DHHS, 2009).

Free Clinics

Many communities have free clinics, which are nonprofit organizations established by health care professionals to serve the uninsured and underinsured. Free clinics typically maintain limited hours and see a limited number of individuals. Staffed by volunteer physicians, nurses, and pharmacists, free clinics provide a critical service in their community. Clients must participate in an intake process and prove that they qualify for services. Services vary but typically include primary care, acute care, dental and mental health services, and prescription services.

REVIEW Access to Health Care

RELATE: LINK THE CONCEPTS

Linking the exemplar of Access to Health Care with the concept of Ethics:

1. What are the ethical issues involved when individuals are uninsured?
2. What aspects of the ANA Code of Ethics address clients who are uninsured or underinsured?

Linking the exemplar of Access to Health Care with the concept of Reproduction:

3. What resources in your community are available to uninsured pregnant women?
4. Are the risk factors to the fetus any greater or any different when the pregnant mother is uninsured? Explain.

REFER: GO TO MYNURSINGKIT

REFLECT: CASE STUDY

Helena Alvarez is a pregnant, 19-year-old Hispanic woman, who arrives at the emergency department of a small rural hospital with severe cramping pains and bleeding. She has no health insurance. There are no maternity services available at this hospital and no obstetricians available in the community. There is a tertiary care facility about 100 miles away.

1. How would you determine what options are available for providing care for this young mother?
2. As a nurse, what are your obligations to Helena Alvarez?

44.2 ALLOCATION OF RESOURCES

KEY TERMS
Resource allocation, *2349*

BASIS FOR SELECTION OF EXEMPLAR
U.S. Department of Health and Human Services

LEARNING OUTCOMES
After reading about this exemplar, you will be able to:
1. Discuss the reasons for allocating health care resources.
2. Describe examples of resource allocation.
3. Examine the role of the nurse in allocation of resources at the local and national levels.

OVERVIEW

The escalating cost of health care in the United States has been a concern for at least the last two decades, and both the government and private entities have attempted to gain control over health care expenditures. Furthermore, the move toward prospective payment and managed care, fears surrounding the potential for malpractice litigation, and resultant defensive medicine have increased the demand on the available resources. As discussed in Concept 37, Managing Care, employment-negotiated insurance plans, while providing a positive benefit of insurance for employees, created a sense of indifference to the cost because individuals did not pay directly for any health care services. This led to overspending on duplicative services of marginal utility. Because of increasing costs and the resulting efforts at cost containment allocation of health care goods and services, including such things as organ transplants, the services of medical specialists, and care involving expensive technology, has become an especially urgent issue. For example, decisions about the number of office visits and the length of hospital stay are increasingly being influenced not by medical considerations, but by administrative policies of health care facilities and funding entities such as insurance companies, HMOs, and Medicare. Third-party coverage of some expensive and/or experimental treatments is being denied. The term **resource allocation** is used to describe how a resource is allocated, or provided, to clients or communities when there are not enough of the resource for every one who needs it.

Critics dispute the idea that health care is a scarce resource in North America. Instead, they contend that access to health care is limited for certain segments of the population. Increasing people's access to health care is costly, however, and makes decisions about providing and financing health care difficult, as shown in the following example.

No single answer exists to the problem of how to allocate increasingly overstretched health care resources. Debate continues at all levels: in Congress, in state legislatures, within health care organizations, even between and among health care professionals themselves. Some argue for more efforts at prevention, but these efforts are not guaranteed to provide cost savings or reduce use of the health care system (Arvantes, 2009).

EXAMPLES OF RESOURCE ALLOCATION

One method of allocating resources is through rationing. The rationing of health care resources occurs in a variety of ways. For example, on an individual level, many older adults on fixed incomes ration their own medications by taking half of the amount prescribed or by taking a medication every other day instead of every day because they cannot afford their copayments for prescriptions every month. Insurance companies ration health care in a number of ways, most notably through clauses that prevent new insurance plan members from using the plan for health care services related to a pre-existing condition for up to 1 year. Some insurance programs, such as the Oregon Health Plan, have developed specific criteria under which certain services may be administered in order to keep costs at a minimum (Oregon Health Plan, 2009). This results in individuals insured by those programs having access to what is essentially a basic level of care. Advocates of such programs argue that more people benefit when coverage is basic and costs are minimized. Opponents argue that offering only basic care is just another form of rationing that results in further disparities in access to high-quality health care.

The Organ Procurement and Transplantation Network

One of the best-known systems of allocating health care resources is the Organ Procurement and Transplantation Network (OPTN). In the United States, approximately 77 people receive a donated organ each day. Unfortunately, another 19 people die each day waiting for an organ transplant. There simply is not enough supply to meet the demand for organ donations. The OPTN, a contracted service of the U.S. Department of Health and Human Services, maintains the only national client waiting list for organ transplantation.

CLINICAL EXAMPLE
An 8-year-old boy with a chronic blood disorder requires weekly blood transfusions. The hospital struggles to maintain enough of the rare blood type. The 8-year-old arrives at the emergency department at the same time as another client with the same blood type who is bleeding profusely. There is enough blood for only one of these clients.
1. Which client should receive the blood?
2. What models or methods should be used to make the decision? Who should be responsible for making the decision?

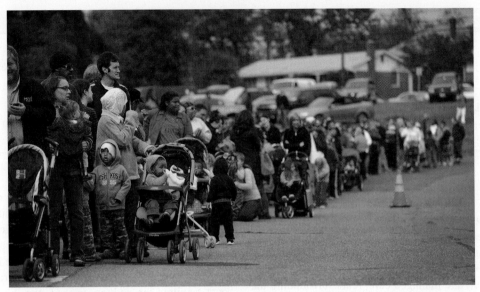

Figure 44–3 ■ Hundreds of county residents wait in a long line for the H1N1 vaccination shot at a clinic held by the Montgomery County Health and Human Services on October 14, 2009, at the Dennis Avenue County Health Center in Silver Spring, Maryland.

Blood and tissue type, medical urgency, organ size, and the geographic distance between the donor and the recipient are just a few of the factors that determine who receives a donor organ (OPTN, 2010). More information on organ donation, including how to register as a donor, can be found at http://optn.transplant.hrsa.gov/.

H1N1 Vaccine Distribution

In 2009, the Centers for Disease Control and Prevention (CDC) developed a protocol for the distribution of H1N1 vaccine across the United States. The protocol was necessitated by an initial lack of available vaccine as the course of H1N1 progressed across the country. Factors that the CDC used in determining how vaccine was allocated as it became available included the amount of vaccine being requested by local health departments and the speed at which the vaccine became available, among others. For example, in addition to allocations for local areas, the vaccine also had to be allocated for active duty military personnel (Centers for Disease Control, 2009).

Once the vaccine arrived in local communities, further decisions were made regarding who could receive the vaccine if the supply was insufficient to meet the demand. Many local health departments screened potential recipients and initially administered the vaccine only to those with risk factors for H1N1, such as small children and adults with diagnosed

respiratory disease (Figure 44–3 ■). Later, when sufficient quantities of the vaccine became available, health care providers were able to administer the vaccine to anyone who asked for it.

NURSES AND ALLOCATION OF RESOURCES

The role of the profession of nursing in the allocation of resources is a collaborative one. Nurses are the largest group of health professionals and, as part of the interdisciplinary health care team, play an integral role in making decisions about how health care resources are allocated. Nurses are also the health care professionals that use and distribute the most direct resources, from adhesive bandages to immunizations. Therefore, nurses must participate in discussions of health care resources in the workplace, in their immediate communities, and at the federal level. As client advocates, nurses are uniquely placed to discuss issues in client care at various levels of their communities. This includes talking with local legislators, writing to politicians, and engaging in discussions in their neighborhoods and social groups. As working professionals, nurses have the opportunity to participate in discussions through a number of professional organizations, such as the American Nurses Association.

REVIEW Allocation of Resources

RELATE: LINK THE CONCEPTS

Linking the exemplar of Allocation of Resources with the concept of Ethics:

1. What provisions of the ANA Code of Ethics address resource allocation?
2. What ethical considerations do you as an individual value that might impact how you would determine resource allocation?

Linking the exemplar of Allocation of Resources with the concept of Safety:

3. What aspects of resource allocation may affect client safety in the operating room? How?
4. What aspects of resource allocation may affect client safety in a long-term care facility, where three people may be required to transfer a client from a bed to a chair?

REFER: GO TO MYNURSINGKIT

REFLECT: CASE STUDY

The general medical–surgical unit of a neighborhood hospital is experiencing a nursing shortage. For the moment, some of the nurses are working extra shifts as a means of helping out the hospital and its clients and of making extra money. When a forest fire breaks out, the unit is forced to accept clients that the emergency department cannot accommodate. That same week, the administration announces that a new mandatory overtime policy is being implemented until more nursing staff can be hired.

1. What aspects of resource allocation are impacting the medical-surgical unit at the hospital?
2. How might these impact nursing staff performance? How might they impact morale?

44.3 EMERGENCY PREPAREDNESS

KEY TERMS

Bioterrorism, *2357*
Cold zone, *2356*
Community Emergency Response Team (CERT) Program, *2355*
Disaster, *2351*
Emergency, *2351*
Emergency preparedness, *2351*
Emergency response, *2353*
Hot zone, *2356*
Local emergency management agency (LEMA), *2355*
Mitigation, *2351*
Pandemic, *2351*
Preparedness, *2351*
Recovery, *2354*
Reverse triage, *2356*
Surge capacity, *2351*
Triage, *2356*
Warm zone, *2356*

BASIS FOR SELECTION OF EXEMPLAR

NLN Competencies
Standards of Nursing Practice
World Health Organization

LEARNING OUTCOMES

After reading about this exemplar, you will be able to:

1. Discuss the four phases of emergency response.
2. Summarize the responsibilities of nurses during each phase of emergency response.
3. Outline the educational competencies required of nurses responding to a mass casualty event.
4. Develop your own individual emergency plan.
5. Describe various biotoxins and how they are disseminated among a population.
6. Propose plans of care based on the emergency and the community resources available.

OVERVIEW

An **emergency** is a sudden, often unforeseen, event that threatens health or safety. A public emergency necessitating assistance from outside the affected community is a **disaster**. Disasters have three things in common: little or no warning before the event; available personnel and emergency services that are overwhelmed initially by the demand; and a combined threat to life, public health, and the environment. Some common types of disasters and resulting injuries are listed in Table 44–3. Infectious diseases may accompany disasters or can become disasters themselves. A **pandemic** is an infection that spreads rapidly around the world.

Surge capacity refers to a community's ability to rapidly meet the increased demand for qualified personnel and resources, including health care resources, in the event of a disaster. **Emergency preparedness** is the act of making plans to prevent, respond to, and recover from emergencies. The Centers for Disease Control and Prevention (CDC) recommend an *all-hazards* approach to emergency preparedness. This approach provides for general preparation, including training that can be applied in a wide variety of emergency situations. The impact on health and the health care system is similar regardless of the nature of the disaster.

THE FOUR PHASES OF EMERGENCY RESPONSE

Four phases have been identified in handling an emergency: preparedness, mitigation, response, and recovery.

Preparedness means having a comprehensive disaster plan in place that coordinates efforts among many people, agencies, and levels of government. Most communities have a number of plans based on their likelihood of experiencing certain natural disasters, such as hurricanes, and the need to respond to potential threats identified by federal organizations like the Federal Emergency Management Agency, the Department of Homeland Security, and the Centers for Disease Control and Prevention. Agencies involved in disaster preparedness activities are typically those that will be involved in any type of emergency response. In developing a disaster plan representatives from each agency are able to share information, offer their respective resources and expertise, and determine any deficiencies in the plan. Planning committees exist on all levels—federal, regional, state, local, and individual agency. Nurses participate in disaster preparedness by having a nurse representative on the planning committee at least at the agency level.

In **mitigation**, agencies and communities identify potential hazards and take measures to prevent or minimize the

TABLE 44–3 Types of Disasters and Common Injuries

TYPE OF DISASTER	COMMON INJURIES	NURSING IMPLICATIONS
Hurricane-related injuries	Drowning; clean-up injuries; aggravation of chronic illnesses; stress-related symptoms; upper respiratory infections; gastrointestinal illnesses; animal, snake, and insect bites; obstetrical complications; contaminated water supplies and insect-breeding grounds; heat-related illnesses; lack of sanitation and safe housing	Asphyxia can occur along with wounds; bone, joint, and muscle injuries; and infections. Also possible are skin irritations and infections, waterborne and insect-borne diseases, dehydration, starvation or malnutrition, and diseases and injuries.
Tsunami-related injuries	"Tsunami lung," a severe infection caused by swallowing muddy, bacteria-laden water. Other water related injuries, such as submersion injuries, and fatalities may also occur.	Requires aggressive respiratory and ventilator management, blood transfusions, antibiotics, and other medical support. Individuals with submersion related injuries may require wound care and infection control.
Thunderstorm-related injuries	Resistance of body tissues to electrical current. *Least resistance:* nerves, blood, mucous membranes, muscle. *Intermediate resistance:* dry skin. *Most resistance:* tendon, fat, bone.	Potential for tissue destruction with longer duration of contact with high-voltage current; if energy current is dissipated at the skin surface, significant surface burns result, especially in calloused areas.
Tornado-related injuries	Flying debris; injuries similar to hurricane-related injuries	Injuries and fatalities can occur.
Earthquake-related injuries	High incidence of mortality and morbidity; explosions	May result in stress-related symptoms; wounds; bone, joint, and muscle injuries; clean-up injuries; gastrointestinal and respiratory problems; aggravation of chronic illnesses; obstetrical complications; burns.
Snowstorm-related injuries	Overexertion and exhaustion; hypothermia	Myocardial infarction can occur. Treatment for hypothermia may be necessary.
Disaster-related eye injuries	"Specks" of dust or debris; cuts, punctures, or stuck objects; blows to the eye	Administer eyewash or flushing versus rubbing; stabilize eye with rigid shield. Apply cold compress, no pressure; client should visit health care professional to rule out serious injury or internal eye damage.
Blast injuries	Auditory	Tympanic membrane rupture, ossicular disruption, and cochlear damage occur; damage from foreign body can occur.
	Eye, orbit, face	Perforated globe, air embolisms, and fractures are common; damage from foreign body can occur.
	Respiratory	May result in blast lung, hemothorax, pneumothorax, pulmonary contusion and hemorrhage, atrioventricular fistulas (source of air embolism), airway epithelial damage, aspiration pneumonitis, or sepsis.
	Digestive	May result in bowel perforation, hemorrhage, ruptured liver or spleen, sepsis, or mesenteric ischemia from air embolism.
	Circulatory	Cardiac contusion, myocardial infarction from air embolism, shock, vasovagal hypotension, peripheral vascular injury, and air embolism-induced injury can occur.
	Central nervous system injury	Concussion, closed and open brain injury, stroke, spinal cord injury, and air embolism-induced injury can occur.
	Renal injury	May result in renal contusion, laceration, acute renal failure due to rhabdomyolysis, hypotension, and hypovolemia.
	Extremity injury	Traumatic amputation, fractures, crush injuries, compartment syndrome, burns, cuts, lacerations, acute arterial occlusion, and air embolism-induced injury can occur.
Blunt trauma	Head and torso blunt trauma, penetrating trauma	Fractured limbs and spinal injury can occur.

TABLE 44–3 Types of Disasters and Common Injuries (continued)

TYPE OF DISASTER	COMMON INJURIES	NURSING IMPLICATIONS
Pressure trauma	Lungs	Tearing of the alveoli cause swelling, fluid accumulation, possible pulmonary emboli, and eventual hypoxia.
	Ear and bowel injury: ear pain, hearing loss	Keep auditory canal clean; make the client comfortable.
Radiological dispersion bomb (dirty bomb) blast	Radiation sickness	Get rid of contaminated clothes, shower, and evacuate the area within a day of a small or medium blast. Those close to the blast could suffer radiation sickness and require hospital care.
Nuclear detonation	Thermal burns	May involve only the epidermis and upper layers of dermis with short duration of heat exposure.
Bright light flash of nuclear detonation	Eye burn injuries	May blind the client momentarily; effects will disappear with time, but can impair a client's ability to perform self-care and other activities of daily living (ADLs).
Radiation exposure injury	Bone marrow and blood cell damage	A reduction in the blood's oxygen-carrying capacity results in nausea, fatigue, and a general feeling of malaise. Reduced platelet production causes clotting disorders and possibly hemorrhage. When the body's white blood cells are destroyed, it is important to reduce the client's exposure to infection. Infection at the time of reduced WBC production can be severe and even fatal.
	Bowel	Cells that reproduce the bowel lining are damaged, resulting in nausea, loss of appetite, vomiting, diarrhea, fluid loss, and malaise in the acute stage; later, dehydration, malnutrition, bowel hemorrhage, and perforation may occur; if radiation exposure is not exacerbated by other injury or pathology, clients will generally survive.
	Integument	Erythema or generalized reddening of the skin occurs when skin cells are damaged, with the appearance of a sunburn; more serious burns may occur with persistent exposure or extremely high radiation doses.
	Nervous and cardiovascular systems	With acute radiation exposure, blood vessel and nerve cells are damaged and the client is incapacitated and experiences cardiovascular collapse, confusion, and even an "on fire" sensation throughout the body; symptoms this severe generally do not permit survival.
Chemical burns	Range from minor to life-threatening injuries	Remove clothing from injury site as well as any jewelry; flush chemical from skin with thorough decontamination; cover wounds loosely with a dry, sterile, or clean cloth.

Source: Adapted from *Centers for Disease Control and Prevention* (2003a), Cooper (1995), DeLorenzo & Porter (2000), and Harris (2005).

emergency. During this phase, communities implement their emergency operations plans including organizing and training personnel and stockpiling equipment and supplies. During mitigation, communities implement communication and warning systems, establish emergency operations centers, and implement response and evacuation plans. A key nursing activity related to mitigation is the anticipation of needed resources and policies to assist nurses and other professionals in implementing an effective disaster response.

When agencies and their communication are well-coordinated and they implement preparedness continually over time,

mitigation efforts will be more effective and result in better outcomes for the community. However, in some instances a variety of factors may result in mitigation efforts that are insufficient to meet community needs. The evacuation of New Orleans in advance of hurricane Katrina and the efforts to provide shelter immediately following Katrina are stunning examples of how mitigation efforts can fail (see Figure 44–4 ■).

The third phase, **emergency response**, is the coordinated response to meet the needs of the individuals in the community affected by the emergency. This may include opening shelters, repairing utility infrastructures, and establishing critical care

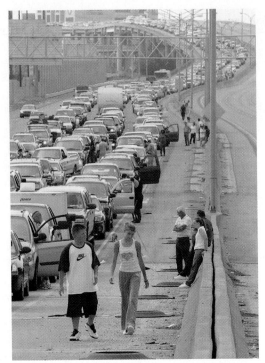

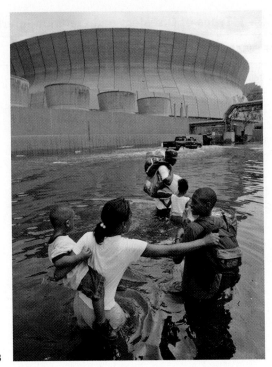

Figure 44–4 ■ *A*, Authorities in New Orleans ordered hundreds of thousands of residents to flee on Sunday, August 28, 2005, as Hurricane Katrina strengthened into a rare top-ranked storm and barreled toward the vulnerable U.S. Gulf Coast city. Those who had vehicles were caught in traffic jams for hours. *B*, Many who had no means to leave the city made their way to the Superdome (pictured here), which eventually housed approximately 30,000 people, and the Convention Center, where another 10,000–20,000 found shelter.

services. The response phase occurs during and immediately after the emergency, simultaneously with the community's assessment of the immediate effects of the disaster. This level of response is carried out by community agencies such as local law enforcement, paramedics and emergency department personnel, and local county or city staff employed in the disaster response unit. State, federal, and other outside resources come in after any initial danger has passed and may bring with them any of the following: first aid, emergency medical assistance, establishment or restoration of communication and transportation, and assessment of infectious diseases and mental health problems.

Nurses should follow the disaster plan of their agencies, communities, and the local emergency management agency. They should also be sure to have a disaster plan for themselves and their immediate family. In this way, the nurse will feel secure about the safety of his or her own family and will be able to respond to the staging area to await instructions without delay.

During the response phase, nurses use their expertise in infectious disease control and in assessing physical as well as psychosocial needs. In a disaster, mental health issues are extremely significant for victims, families, friends, first responders, and all health care workers. Nurses will ensure that clients receive follow-up care for both physical wounds and mental health concerns. Advanced practice nurses may take on significantly greater responsibilities, especially if the nurses are competent and prepared in emergency and trauma

care. Protocols and standards of care are in place to guide the practice of all nurses. It is imperative that nurses determine the boundaries of their practice in times of emergency when mass numbers of victims must be treated without the luxury of an on-site physician.

The **recovery**, or restoration, phase consists of activities and programs aimed at returning the community to normal. During the recovery stage, restoration, reconstitution, and mitigation take place. Restoration may include rebuilding, replacing lost or damaged property, returning to school and work, and continuing life without those who were killed in the disaster. Reconstitution occurs when the life of the community returns to a new "normal."

The work is never complete. Future-oriented activities take place to prevent subsequent disasters or to minimize their effects. Some of these activities may include increased security and surveillance measures. Nurses may suggest ideas for responding to the victims of disasters more effectively and efficiently. For example, nurses may communicate the need for carts stocked with specific items that will assist them in treating clients faster. They may also suggest a more efficient method of tracking clients as they enter the health care system and move from area to area based on the clients' acuity and condition. Nurses participate in mock disasters, read updated protocols, and practice their skills continually to maintain competence. Mock disasters or disaster drills can take the form of tabletop exercises/discussions or simulated drills in which people pretend to be victims. Mock disaster drills allow the participants to become familiar with the plan. During the drill, areas of the plan that need strengthening will become evident (Langan, 2005b).

RESPONSIBILITY FOR EMERGENCY MANAGEMENT AND RESPONSE

Local governments have the primary responsibility for emergency management and response. The U.S. Department of Homeland Security mandates that the federal guidelines called the National Incident Management System (NIMS) be followed. State divisions of emergency management act as the **local emergency management agency (LEMA)** for each state. This is a governmental agency with expertise in public safety, emergency medical services, and management. Training is available for interested individuals through the **Community Emergency Response Team (CERT) Program**. The CERT Program has four major objectives: Present citizens the facts about what to expect following a major disaster in terms of immediate services; give the message about citizens' responsibility for mitigation and preparedness; train citizens in needed life saving skills with emphasis on decision making skills, rescuer safety, and doing the greatest good for the greatest number; and organize teams so that they are an extension of first responder services, offering immediate help to victims until professional help is available.

Nursing Competencies for Emergency Response

Nurses represent the largest number of health care professionals, and emergency preparedness is a necessity, regardless of the nurse's educational preparation, area of expertise, or practice setting. The International Nursing Coalition for Mass Casualty Education (INCMCE) published educational competencies for registered nurses to facilitate their response to mass casualties with a strong recommendation that these core competencies be included in initial nursing education program (see Box 44–4).

Box 44–4 Categories of Educational Competencies for Registered Nurses Responding to Mass Casualty Incidents (MCI)

CORE COMPETENCIES
1. Critical thinking
2. Assessment
3. Technical skills
4. Communication

CORE KNOWLEDGE AREAS
1. Health promotion, risk reduction, and disease prevention
2. Health care systems and policy
3. Illness and disease management
4. Information and health care technologies
5. Ethics
6. Human diversity

PROFESSIONAL ROLE DEVELOPMENT
1. A description of nursing roles in MCIs
2. Identification of the most appropriate or most likely health care role for oneself during an MCI

Source: International Nursing Coalition for Mass Casualty Education. (2003, August). *Educational competencies for registered nurses related to mass casualty incidents.* Retrieved May 1, 2005, from http://www.aacn.nche.edu/Education/pdf/INCMCECompetencies.pdf

---

The ANA (2008) has summarized recommendations for individual registered nurses or other health care professionals that specifies their roles before, during, and after an event. (See Box 44–5.)

Emergency Plans

Individuals and agencies with responsibilities during a disaster or emergency have a series of plans that they must follow. As discussed earlier, each individual nurse needs to have a personal emergency plan. Individual health care agencies, from hospitals to health departments to residential facilities for seniors or the disabled, should have emergency plans that address

---

Box 44–5 Recommendations for Emergency Event Care

PRE-EVENT
- Prepare self and family/significant others for potential emergencies, including the potential for the professional to be away for extended periods during an emergency.
- Participate in continuing education on emergency preparedness.
- Participate in emergency drills and exercises at your practice site.
- Know the legal basis for professional care, and the legal structure of your state regarding health professionals in emergencies.
- Provide clear information to any employer or any volunteer organization where you are enrolled about any limitations or availability or any special skills (e.g., experience with emergency or community triage) applicable to emergency conditions.

DURING AN EVENT
- Use your professional competence to provide the best care possible given the resources and physical conditions under which you are working.

- Use assigned or announced information resources to clarify any changes in protocols or staff roles.
- Use available rapid training to update readiness to respond to the specific event.
- Communicate difficulties responding as expected through the assigned chain of command as quickly as possible.

POST-EVENT
- Participate in post-event evaluation processes.
- Do a psychosocial assessment of self and family, and seek assistance if needed.
- Participate in activities to return to pre-event status.

Source: Adapting standards of care under extreme conditions: Guidance for professionals during disasters, pandemics, and other extreme emergencies (p. 18). American Nurses Association, 2008. Retrieved March 30, 2010, from http://www.nursingworld.org/MainMenuCategories/HealthcareandPolicyIssues/DPR/TheLawEthicsofDisasterResponse/AdaptingStandardsofCare.aspx the roles and responsibilities of all employees in an emergency. In fact, most agencies are mandated by law to develop and implement these types of emergency plans. Every nurse should know the policies and procedures of the agency in which he or she is employed.

TRIAGE

Nurses perform triage every day in emergency departments. The process of **triage** involves prioritizing victims for treatment based on severity of illness or injury and in light of the supplies and resources available. The objective of triage is to ensure early assessment of clients and prioritize clients for care based on severity of symptoms. In a mass casualty (more than 100 victims), **reverse triage** is implemented, with the most severely injured or ill victims who require the greatest resources treated last to allow the greatest number of victims to receive medical attention. A simple color classification system (START) is used to prioritize the clients (see Table 44–4 and Figure 44–5 ■). It is recommended that emergency medical personnel be assigned to triage. This frees physicians and nurses to provide needed care.

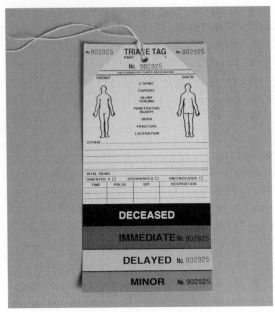

Figure 44–5 ■ On this numbered triage tag, the priority categories are labeled Minor, Delayed, Immediate, and Deceased.

SITE-SPECIFIC DISASTER ZONES

In a disaster in which a weapon is released, such as a bomb, or a site-specific event has occurred, such as a train derailment with tanker cars leaking toxic chemicals, access to the site of contamination is limited, and zones of safety are identified. The initial site of the incident is considered the hot zone. Only personnel with appropriate protective equipment are allowed in the hot zone. See Box 44–6 for more information on zone breakdown.

TABLE 44–4 Simple Triage and Rapid Transport (START) System

PRIORITY	DESCRIPTION
Red (Immediate)	Critically injured, with problems that will require immediate intervention to correct. (Clients with a respiratory rate above 30 are tagged "red." If their respirations are below 30, assess their circulatory status. If capillary refill takes more than 2 seconds, tag them "red." If it is below 2 seconds, assess mental status.)
Yellow (Delayed)	Injured and will require some medical attention, but they will not die if care is delayed while you care for other clients; not ambulatory and will require a stretcher for transportation. (Clients who can follow simple commands such as hand grips are tagged as "yellow." Clients who cannot follow simple commands are tagged "red.")
Green (Ambulatory or Minor)	Not critically injured and can walk and care for themselves. (Have them walk to a safe place, but do not lose track of them; every client triaged at an incident is tracked to the best of the responder's ability.)
Black (Deceased)	Deceased or have such catastrophic injuries that they are not expected to survive to be transported. (If the client is not breathing, open the airway manually. If they remain apneic, tag them "black"; if they begin breathing, they are tagged "red.")

Source: Adapted from Streger (n.d.). *Prehospital Triage.* Retrieved from http://www.emsmagazine.com/articles/emsarts/triage.html

Box 44–6 Hot, Warm, and Cold Zones

HOT ZONE
The site of the disaster where a weapon was released or where the contamination occurred is called the **hot zone**. It is considered contaminated, and only those persons in the appropriate personal protective equipment (PPE) may enter this zone. PPE is equipment used for the protection of personnel and includes gloves, masks, goggles, gowns, and biologic disposal bags (Maniscalco & Christen, 2002). Typically, fire, police, and military personnel will collect evidence and begin their investigation in the hot zone.

WARM ZONE
The **warm zone** is adjacent to the hot zone. Another name for this area is the *control zone*. This area is where decontamination of victims or initial triage and emergency treatment take place. The level of PPE required for the warm zone depends on the dynamic risk assessment of the threat and the agent involved.

COLD ZONE
The **cold zone** is considered to be the safe zone. It is adjacent to the warm zone and is the area where a more comprehensive triage of victims occurs. Survivors may find shelter in this area, and the command and control vehicles are found here, as are the emergency transport vehicles.

BIOTERRORISM

Bioterrorism is the deliberate release of a virus, bacteria, or other microbes used to cause illness or death in people, animals, or plants. One purpose of terrorism is to cause fear and panic. Strategies must be implemented to minimize the threat of bioterrorism and to respond to a potential bioterrorist attack. Because biologic agents are transmitted in a variety of ways (e.g., airborne, food-borne, etc.), local emergency management agencies must have complex, multisystem response plans.

The primary agents identified by the U.S. Army Medical Research Institute of Infectious Diseases as potential bioterrorist threats are *Bacillus anthracis* (anthrax), variola virus (smallpox), *Yersinia pestis* (plague), *Francisella tularensis* (tularemia), botulinum toxin (botulism), and hemorrhagic fever virus (Marburg, Ebola). It is important for the nurse to be aware of the early signs and symptoms as well as the methods of transmission of biological agents. See Table 44–5.

Immediate treatment for the primary biologic agents used in terrorism is limited. Inhalation of anthrax has been effectively

TABLE 44–5 Biological Pathogens of Highest Concern for Bioterrorism Attacks

PATHOGEN	CAUSE	TRANSMISSION	SYMPTOMS
Anthrax	Spore-forming bacterium—*Bacillus anthracis*	■ Not known to spread from one person to another ■ Cutaneous/skin: direct skin contact with spores (most common) ■ Respiratory: inhalation of aerosolized spores (rare) ■ Gastrointestinal: consumption of under-cooked or raw meat products or dairy products from infected animals (rare)	Cutaneous anthrax: ■ Localized itching followed by a lesion that turns vesicular and subsequent development of black eschar (scab) within 7–10 days of initial lesion ■ Fever, flu-like symptoms, nonproductive cough, sore throat
Botulism	Toxin made by a bacterium called *Clostridium botulinum*	■ Not spread from one person to another ■ Food-borne: person ingests preformed toxin ■ Infant: occurs in small number of infants who harbor *C. botulinum* in their intestinal tract ■ Wound: occurs when wounds are infected with *C. botulinum*	Food-borne botulism: ■ Between 12 and 36 hours after eating toxin-containing food: double and blurred vision, slurred speech, difficulty swallowing, and muscle weakness that always descends through the body
Plague	A bacterium found in rodents and their fleas—*Yersinia pestis*	■ Bubonic plague is transmitted through the bite of an infected flea or exposure to infected material through a break in the skin. Bubonic plague is not transmitted person to person. ■ Pneumonic plague would be caused by an aerosol attack (bioweapon). Pneumonic plague can be transmitted person to person.	Pneumonic plague: ■ Fever, weakness, rapidly developing pneumonia with dyspnea, chest pain, cough, and sometimes bloody or watery sputum
Viral hemorrhagic fevers (VHF)	Viruses of most VHFs reside in an animal reservoir host or arthropod host (e.g., rodents are hosts and ticks and mosquitoes can be vectors). However, the hosts of some VHF (e.g., Ebola and Marburg) are unknown.	■ Humans are not natural reservoirs for VHFs. People are infected when they come in contact with infected hosts. However, with some VHFs, after the accidental transmission from the host, humans can transmit the virus to one another.	■ After an incubation period of 5–10 days: abrupt onset of fever, myalgia, headache, nausea and vomiting, abdominal pain, diarrhea, and chest pain ■ A rash on the trunk develops approximately 5 days after onset. ■ Bleeding (e.g., petechiae, bruises, and hemorrhages) occur as disease progresses.
Smallpox	Variola virus	■ Droplet nuclei expelled from the mouth of an infected person or by aerosol. ■ Contaminated clothing or bed linen could also spread the disease. ■ Humans are the only natural host of variola.	■ Incubation period can range from 7 to 17 days where the person has no symptoms and is not contagious. ■ Initial symptoms include high fever, head and body aches, and possibly vomiting. These symptoms last 2–4 days and the person may be contagious. ■ A rash then appears—first on the tongue and in the mouth. These red spots develop into sores that break open and spread large amounts of the virus into the mouth and throat. The person is highly contagious at this point.

(continued)

TABLE 44–5 Biological Pathogens of Highest Concern for Bioterrorism Attacks (continued)

PATHOGEN	CAUSE	TRANSMISSION	SYMPTOMS
			■ The rash then spreads to the entire body. By the third day of the rash, the rash becomes raised bumps, which fill with thick, opaque fluid and have a depression in the center. The bumps become pustules, which begin to form a crust and then scab. ■ The scabs fall off, leaving pitted scars. The person is contagious until all the scabs have fallen off.
Tularemia	The bacterium *Francisella tularensis* found in animals (especially rodents, rabbits, and hares)	■ Not known to be spread from person to person. It is spread in different ways: ■ Being bitten by an infected tick, deer-fly, or other insect ■ Handling infected animal carcasses ■ Eating or drinking contaminated food or water ■ Breathing in/inhaling the *F. tularensis*	■ Sudden fever, chills, headache, diarrhea, muscle aches, joint pain, dry cough, and progressive weakness ■ If *F. tularensis* was used as a biologic weapon and made airborne for exposure by inhalation, the infected people would experience severe respiratory illness, including life-threatening pneumonia and systemic infection.

treated with ciprofloxacin 400 mg administered intravenously every 12 hours. There are no effective therapies for treating clients infected by most of the other viruses that could be used in a bioterrorist attack. For some viruses, a vaccine could be created to stimulate the body's immune system such that the person may be protected from infection if exposed to the virus at a later date.

The Strategic National Stockpile is a program designed to ensure the immediate availability of essential medical materials to a community in the event of a large-scale chemical or biological attack. Managed jointly by the CDC and the Department of Homeland Security, it consists of large quantities of antibiotics; vaccines; and medical, surgical, and client support supplies such as bandages, IV equipment, and airway supplies. The first component of the stockpile is a preassembled "push package" designed to meet the community's needs in case of an undetermined biological or chemical threat. The push packages are stored in locations to enable delivery within 12 hours after an attack. The second component is a vendor-managed inventory package that will be shipped once the threat has been clearly identified. These packages are designed to arrive within 24–36 hours.

COLLABORATION

Emergency preparedness and disaster response are dependent on collaboration of the interdisciplinary health care team with local, state, and federal governmental agencies. Interdisciplinary training and participation in tabletop exercises, simulations, and mock incidents not only prepare the team to assume their roles in case of disaster but also provide an opportunity for evaluation of the plan. This evaluation leads to a more effective emergency plan and facilitates communications in the development, implementation, and evaluation of emergency response.

Nurses often will have contact with members of emergency medical services (EMS) in both emergency departments and disaster situations. A brief overview of the EMS system is presented in Box 44–7.

NURSING PRACTICE

The role of the nurse in a disaster depends greatly on a number of variables including the nature of the disaster; the number of victims and severity of injuries; the location of the disaster as well as the location of the nurse; and the availability of supplies, rescue and command personnel, and other necessary resources. The nurse must be able to perform under stressful conditions but will not be expected to endanger self, other nurses, or other rescuers. Nurses will be expected to follow the emergency preparedness plans outlined in their communities

Box 44–7 The Emergency Medical Services System

The emergency medical services (EMS) system is a network of resources that provides emergency care and transportation, called prehospital care, to victims of illness, injury, or disaster. EMS personnel must be trained and licensed, and they work under the auspices of a medical director, usually a hospital-based physician who is consulted as needed. There are four levels of EMS professionals:

■ *Emergency medical responders (EMRs)* were formerly called *first responders*. EMRs provide initial emergency care including assessment, opening an airway, ventilating, controlling bleeding, performing CPR, stabilizing the spine and injured limbs, assisting with childbirth, and assisting other EMS personnel.

■ *Emergency medical technicians (EMTs)* can do everything EMRs do, and in addition they help clients with prescribed medications and give aspirins, NSAIDs, oral glucose, and other medications when indicated.

EMRs and EMTs provide basic life support.

■ *Advanced emergency medical technicians (AEMTs)* can start IVs and provide IV fluids and medications and have more training in assessment and advanced airway procedures.

■ *Paramedics* have the most training. They can do in-depth assessments, assess abnormal heart rhythms, and perform some invasive procedures.

AEMTs and paramedics provide advanced life support.

and in their agencies of employment. When a disaster occurs, it is not a time for individual creativity.

If it is safe to do so, the nurse may be assigned the responsibility of triaging and assessing the victims for the best care and best use of available resources. Very quick, direct treatment may be given, or the nurse may be involved for extended periods of time with a mobile surgical unit. Local authorities such as the police, fire, and emergency medical services will guide the nurse in securing the area and determining the safe zone for the nurse and others to work. Victim assistance may be offered in the field in mobile shelters, in local clinics, in hospitals, or in makeshift buildings.

Clients who have experienced disasters will present with a variety of individualized needs. Nursing diagnoses that may apply include the following:

- Anxiety
- Impaired Verbal Communication
- Ineffective Coping
- Fear
- Risk for Post-Trauma Syndrome
- Powerlessness
- Risk for Injury
- Risk for Trauma.

Certain disasters tend to cause particular types of injuries. For example, nurses working in a setting where an earthquake has occurred can expect to see a lot of crush injuries. Individuals in an area where there has been an explosion, such as the area in and around the World Trade Center on September 11, 2001, will be more likely to experience eye injuries and blast-related injuries such as hearing impairment and respiratory trauma. Refer to Table 44–3 for different types of disasters and the injuries most commonly associated with them.

Besides providing care in the event of a disaster, nurses should also be leaders in their communities in discussing emergency preparedness and contingency plans before potential disasters strike.

REVIEW Emergency Preparedness

RELATE: LINK THE CONCEPTS

Linking the exemplar of Emergency Preparedness with the concept of Professional Behavior:

1. What is the nurse's professional duty in a time of disaster?

Linking the exemplar of Emergency Preparedness with the concept of Managing Care:

2. Uninsured Americans are the most vulnerable in the event of a pandemic event. How is early recognition related to access to care?

Linking the exemplar of Emergency Preparedness with the concept of Ethics:

3. What are the ethical considerations in allocating scarce resources, such as medication, equipment, and health care personnel, during a disaster?

REFER: GO TO MYNURSINGKIT

REFLECT: CASE STUDY

Mr. Ed Jones, a 75-year-old widower, is a retired cabinet maker who makes small toys in the basement of his home, located on the banks of the Deep River. He is independent and sees his primary care physician for monitoring of his blood pressure, which is controlled with antihypertensive medications. Following a week of heavy rainstorms, flooding occurred in Mr. Jones' neighborhood. His basement sustained much water damage and ruined most of his equipment and wood. He waded through the waist-deep water to get to the rescue boat rather than wait for the boat to get to him. The EMTs who triage him at a fire station subsequently transport him to the nearest emergency department.

You are the nurse assessing Mr. Jones. You observe that he has numerous cuts to his hands from woodworking and an ulcer on his right foot. Mr. Jones report the ulcer resulted from a tool falling on his foot and that he has not sought medical treatment for it. His physical assessment findings include T 100.7F PO, P 96, R 20, and BP 178/100; and his skin is cool and dry with multiple lesions on both hands and a Stage II ulcer on his right dorsal foot with yellow-green exudate. His pain rated at a 2 on a 10 scale with 10 being the worst pain there could be. Lungs are clear, and his heart rate is regular. No edema is noted.

1. What actions did Mr. Jones take that probably exacerbated his skin lesions?
2. What additional information is needed to form nursing diagnoses for Mr. Jones?
3. What nursing diagnoses do you believe would be appropriate?

REFERENCES

Adams, M. P., Holland, L. N., Jr., & Bostwick, P. M. (2008). *Pharmacology for nurses* (2nd ed.). Upper Saddle River, NJ: Prentice Hall.

AHRQ (2007). *National healthcare disparities report.* Retrieved January 9, 2009, from http://www.ahrq.gov/qual/nhdr07/chap3a.htm#Ch3-Edn4

Alboher, M. (2008, March 27). Finding health insurance if you are self-employed. *New York Times.* Retrieved February 23, 2010, from http://www.nytimes.com/2008/03/27/business/smallbusiness/27sbiz.html

Appleby, Julie. (2010, April 6). Changes coming to health insurance plans. *Kaiser Health News.* Retrieved April 9, 2010, from http://www.kaiserhealthnews.org/Stories/2010/April/06/Changes-Coming-To-Insurance-Plans.aspx

Arvantes, James. (2009, January 14). Health experts clash over "cost savings" from prevention measures. *AAFP News Now.* Retrieved February 20, 2010, from http://www.aafp.org/online/en/home/publications/news/news-now/health-of-the-public/20090114hlth-aff-prev.html

Atlas, R., Clover, R., Carrico, R., Wesley, G., Thompson, M., & McKinney, W. (2005, November 2). Recognizing biothreat diseases: Realistic training using standardized patients and patient simulators. *Journal of Public Health Management & Practice.* Retrieved September 14, 2008, from CINAHL with Full Text database.

Berman, A., Snyder, S. J., Kozier, B., & Erb, G. (2008). *Kozier and Erb's fundamentals of nursing* (8th ed.). Upper Saddle River, NJ: Prentice Hall.

Blais, K. K., Hayes, J. S., Kozer, B., & Erb, G. (2006). *Professional nursing practice: Concepts and perspectives* (5th ed.) Upper Saddle River, NJ: Prentice Hall.

Caskey, C. (2006, October). The rule of law and bioterrorism. *Clinical Laboratory Science, 19*(4), 196–202. Retrieved September 14, 2008, from CINAHL with Full Text database.

Centers for Disease Control and Prevention. (2009). *H1N1 flu allocation and distribution Q&A.* Retrieved February 22, 2010, from http://www.cdc.gov/H1N1flu/vaccination/statelocal/centralized_distribution_qa.htm

DeNavas-Walt, C.B. Proctor, and J. Smith. (2008) *Income, poverty, and health insurance coverage in the United States: 2007.* U.S. Census Bureau. August.

Doran, A., & Mulhall, M. (2007, June). Syllabus selection: Innovative learning activity. Bioterrorism in the simulation laboratory: Preparing students for the unexpected. *Journal of Nursing Education, 46*(6), 292–292. Retrieved September 14, 2008, from CINAHL with Full Text database.

Evans, R., & Lawrence, S. (2006, October). Preparing for and responding to bioterrorist attacks: The role of disease management initiatives. *Disease Management & Health Outcomes, 14*(5), 265–274. Retrieved September 14, 2008, from CINAHL with Full Text database.

Families USA. 2006. *Why health insurance matters for children.* Retrieved February 22, 2010, from http://www.familiesusa.org/assets/pdfs/campaign-for-childrens-health-care/kids-why-insurance-matters.pdf

Futterman, L., & Lemberg, L. (2007, November). Inequalities in the healthcare system: A problem, worldwide. *American Journal of Critical Care, 16*(6), 617–620. Retrieved September 14, 2008, from CINAHL with Full Text database.

Garbutt, S., Peltier, J., & Fitzpatrick, J. (2008, November). Evaluation of an instrument to measure nurses' familiarity with emergency preparedness. *Military Medicine, 173*(11), 1073–1077. Retrieved January 17, 2009, from Health Source: Nursing/Academic Edition database.

Horney, J., Sollecito, W., & Alexander, L. (2005, November 2). Competency-based preparedness training for public health practitioners. *Journal of Public Health Management & Practice.* Retrieved September 14, 2008, from CINAHL with Full Text database.

Institute of Medicine (IOM). (2004). *Health literacy: A prescription to end confusion.* Retrieved October 3, 2009, from www.iom.edu/CMS/3775/3827/19723.aspx

Jones, R., & VanGilder, A. (2008, June 26). Bioterrorism agents: What the anesthesiologist needs to know. *Internet Journal of Anesthesiology, 16*(2), 1-1. Retrieved September 14, 2008, from CINAHL with Full Text database.

Kane-Urrabazo, C. (2007, April). Duty in a time of disaster: A concept analysis. *Nursing Forum, 42*(2), 56–64. Retrieved September 14, 2008, from CINAHL with Full Text database.

Katz, R., & Levi, J. (2008, Winter). Should a reformed system be prepared for public health emergencies, and what does that mean anyway? *Journal of Law, Medicine & Ethics, 36*(4), 716–721. Retrieved January 17, 2009, doi:10.1111/j.1748-720X.2008.00327.x

Katz, A., Staiti, A., & McKenzie, K. (2006, July). Preparing for the unknown, responding to the known: Communities and public health preparedness. *Health Affairs, 25*(4), 946–957. Retrieved September 14, 2008, from CINAHL with Full Text database.

LeMone, P., & Burke, K. (2008). Medical-surgical nursing: Critical thinking in client care, 4th edition. Upper Saddle River, NJ: Prentice Hall.

Lookinland, S., Tiedeman, M., & Crosson, A. (2005, February). Nontraditional models of care delivery: Have they solved the problems? *Journal of Nursing Administration, 35*(2), 74–80. Retrieved September 3, 2008, from CINAHL with Full Text database.

Lyon, J. (1993, May). Models of nursing care delivery and case management: Clarification of terms. *Nursing Economic$, 11*(3), 163–169. Retrieved October 3, 2008, from CINAHL with Full Text database.

MacIntyre, C., Seccull, A, Lane, J., & Plant, A. (2006, July). Development of a risk-priority score for category A bioterrorism agents as an aid for public health policy. *Military Medicine, 171*(7), 589–594. Retrieved September 14, 2008, from CINAHL with Full Text database.

Mosca, N., Sweeney, P., Hazy, J., & Brenner, P. (2005, November 2). Assessing bioterrorism and disaster preparedness training needs for school nurses. *Journal of Public Health Management & Practice.* Retrieved September 14, 2008, from CINAHL with Full Text database.

National Center for Health Statistics. (2009). *Health, United States, 2008.* Hyattsville, MD: National Center for Health Statistics.

New videos give advice, tips for emergency preparedness. (2008, February). *Nation's Health.* Retrieved January 17, 2009, from Health Source: Nursing/Academic Edition database.

N.C. Office of Minority Health and Health Disparities and State Center for Health Statistics North Carolina Department of Health and Human Services (2006). *Racial and ethnic health Carolina report card 2006 disparities in north.* Retrieved January 9, 2009, from http://www.schs.state.nc.us/SCHS/pdf/ReportCard2006.pdf

North Carolina Department of Health and Human Services (2006). *Racial and ethnic health Carolina report card 2006 disparities in north.* Retrieved January 9, 2009, from http://www.schs.state.nc.us/SCHS/pdf/ReportCard2006.pdf

O'Boyle, C., Robertson, C., & Secor-Turner, M. (2006, August). Public health emergencies: nurses' recommendations for effective actions. *AAOHN Journal, 54*(8), 427–353. Retrieved September 14, 2008, from CINAHL with Full Text database.

Oregon Health Plan (2009). *The prioritized list.* Retrieved February 22, 2010, from http://www.oregon.gov/DHS/healthplan/priorlist/main.shtml

Organ and Transplantation Network (2010). The matching process – Waiting list. Retrieved February 20, 2010, from http://organdonor.gov/transplantation/matching_process.htm

Richard, J., & Grimes, D. (2008, April). Bioterrorism: Class A agents and their potential presentations in immunocompromised patients. *Clinical Journal of Oncology Nursing, 12*(2), 295–302. Retrieved September 14, 2008, from CINAHL with Full Text database.

Sage, W. (2007, November). Legislating delivery system reform: A 30,000-foot view of the 800-pound gorilla. *Health Affairs, 26*(6), 1553–1556. Retrieved September 14, 2008, from CINAHL with Full Text database.

Shih, A. Davis, K. Schoenbaum, S. Gauthier, A. Nuzum, R. & McCarthy, D. (2008, August). *Organizing the U.S. health care delivery system for high performance.* The Commonwealth Fund.

Silenas, R., Akins, R., Parrish, A., & Edwards, J. (2008, January). Developing disaster preparedness competence: An experiential learning exercise for multiprofessional education. *Teaching & Learning in Medicine, 20*(1), 62–68. Retrieved January 17, 2009, doi:10.1080/10401330701798311

Tiedeman, M., & Lookinland, S. (2004, June). Traditional models of care delivery: What have we learned? *Journal of Nursing Administration, 34*(6), 291–297. Retrieved September 3, 2008, from CINAHL with Full Text database.

The fire next time: Pandemic flu, bioterrorism, and ghost of SARS: Whether from man or nature, one calamity informs the next. (2007, March). *Bioterrorism Watch.* Retrieved September 14, 2008, from CINAHL with Full Text database.

Thomas, J. (2008, May). Self-study: An effective method for bioterrorism training in the OR. *AORN Journal, 87*(5), 915. Retrieved September 14, 2008, from CINAHL with Full Text database.

U.S. Census Bureau (2008) *Press release for 2008 national projections.* Retrieved January 9, 2009, from http://www.census.gov/Press-Release/www/releases/archives/population/012496.html

U.S. Department of Health and Human Services (2003). *3M.* Retrieved October 3, 2008, from http://www.hcup-us.ahrq.gov/db/nation/nis/APR-DRGsV20MethodologyOverviewandBibliography.pdf

U. S. Department of Health and Human Services. (2009). *Federally qualified health center fact sheet.* Retrieved February 23, 2010, from http://www.cms.hhs.gov/MLNProducts/downloads/fqhcfactsheet.pdf

U.S. Department of Health and Human Services (2007). *National healthcare disparities report, 2007.* Retrieved December 30, 2008, from http://www.ahrq.gov/qual/nhdr07/Chap3.htm#barriers

U.S. Department of Health and Human Services (2008). *Healthy people 2020: The road ahead.* Retrieved October 3, 2008, from http://www.healthypeople.gov/hp2020/

Walker-Cillo, G. (2006, April). Bioterrorism! We put our plan to the test. *RN, 69*(4), 36–42. Retrieved September 14, 2008, from CINAHL with Full Text database.

Weiner, E., Irwin, M., Trangenstein, P., & Gordon, J. (2005, November). Emergency preparedness curriculum in nursing schools in the United States. *Nursing Education Perspectives, 26*(6), 342–339. Retrieved September 14, 2008, from CINAHL with Full Text database.

Weiss, M., Weiss, P., & Weiss, J. (2007, November). Anthrax vaccine and public health policy. *American Journal of Public Health, 97*(11), 1945–1951. Retrieved September 14, 2008, from CINAHL with Full Text database.

Westra, B. (1993). Critical pathways in home care. *The Quality Messenger, 1*(1), 1, 6, 8.

Wikler, B. & Bailey, K. (2008, April). Dying for coverage in North Carolina. *Families USA, April.* Retrieved September 14, 2008, from www.familiesusa.org

Wynd, C. (2006). A proposed model for military disaster nursing. *Online Journal of Issues in Nursing, 11*(3). Retrieved September 14, 2008, from CINAHL with Full Text database.

Health Policy

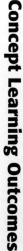

45

Concept at-a-Glance

About Health Policy, *2361*

45.1   Regulatory Agencies, *2363*

45.2   Accrediting Bodies, *2366*

45.3   Professional Organizations, *2366*

45.4   Types of Reimbursement, *2367*

BASIS FOR SELECTION OF CONCEPT

NLN Competencies

OSHA

Standards of Nursing Practice

The Joint Commission

U.S. Department of Health and Human Services

Concept Learning Outcomes

After reading about this concept, you will be able to:

1. Identify factors that influence the development of health policy in the United States.

2. Describe processes by which health policies are developed, implemented, evaluated, changed, and maintained.

3. Identify regulatory agencies and accrediting bodies that develop, administer, or implement health policy.

4. Compare the scope and purpose of specific regulatory agencies and accrediting bodies.

5. Discuss professional organizations that support nurses and the nursing profession.

6. Summarize the types of health care reimbursement.

Concept Key Terms

Accreditation, *2366*

Coinsurance, *2368*

Consumer-driven health care plan (CDHP), *2369*

Copayment, *2368*

Domestic partner, *2369*

Health maintenance organization (HMO), *2369*

Health policy, *2361*

Medicaid, *2368*

Medicare, *2368*

Medigap policy, *2369*

Point of service (POS) plan, *2369*

Preferred provider organization (PPO), *2369*

Primary care provider (PCP), *2369*

State Child Health Insurance Program (SCHIP), *2368*

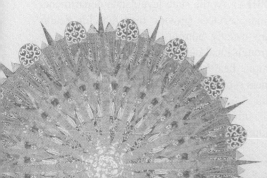

About Health Policy

Public policy and health care delivery systems influence the health and well-being of society. They also have great impact on professional nursing (see Figure 45–1 ■), affecting everything from nursing practice to staffing and education (American Nurses Association, 2003).

The term **health policy** refers to actions and decisions by government bodies or professional organizations that influence the actions and decisions of organizations and individuals within the health care system. Health care policy focuses on how organizations

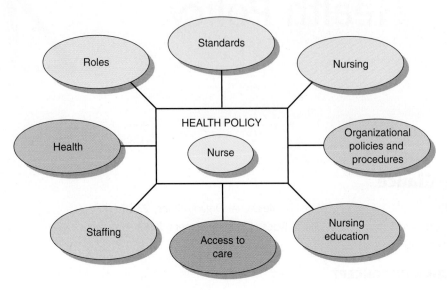

Figure 45–1 ■ Why is health policy relevant to nurses?

function within the socioeconomic and political environment of the United States. These policies affect the provision of services at every level. Every day, nurses identify client problems that are not just clinical, but also relate to the larger health policy environment. For example, the self-employed client whose obesity disqualifies him from being eligible for health insurance has both a clinical problem and a problem related to health policy.

Because of their roles as caregivers, communicators, teachers, advocates, counselors, change agents, leaders, managers, case managers, and research consumers, nurses are in a unique position to help put health policy issues in context and shape policy planning. Policy planning happens in a variety of contexts: within individual organizations, at the local or community level, at the state level, and at the national level. At the national level, the American Nurses Association (ANA) serves as an important voice in policy planning by representing professional nurses and the clients whom they serve. Health care reform is the single most visible national effort in changing health care policy, and ANA has worked tirelessly to promote an agenda in favor of basic health care for all citizens that focuses on primary care, prevention, and chronic disease management:

> ANA believes that health care is a basic human right, and supports the World Health Organization's challenge – originally articulated in 1978, and reaffirmed as late as 2007 – for all nations to provide a basic level of health care to their citizens. The current US system fails in this regard at multiple levels. In fact, it is the only industrialized Western country that does not provide this guarantee to its citizens. It also fails to make the best use of its skilled nursing professionals to provide care throughout all settings and in the varied capacities in which nurses can contribute to significantly patient welfare (ANA, 2009). ●

DEVELOPING HEALTH POLICIES

The process for the development of health policies is a problem-solving framework that is similar to the nursing process. Typical factors that affect the development of health care policy include cost-benefit ratios, client care issues

such as safety, efficiency of service, and equity of access to services. The legislative process required in developing health care policies is outlined in Table 45–1.

Policy making involves three basic phases: the formulation phase, the implementation phase, and the evaluation phase. The *formulation phase* is similar to the assessment and planning phase of the nursing process. During this phase, data are collected through input from key individuals, ideas, interest groups, and research. The data are used to define problems and identify desired outcomes to resolve those problems, as well as the resources necessary to achieve success. The *implementation phase* involves communication of the adopted policies and putting those policies into action. During the *evaluation phase*, additional data are collected and analyzed to determine the degree to which the policy change achieved success.

When public policy is enacted by a governmental entity, it is usually implemented through a specific agency, which is given responsibility for translating the policy into written rules. Once the rules are approved, the agency has responsibility for administering the policy under the rules. As existing policies are evaluated, there may be modifications to adjust to changing circumstances. Typically, these changes are made in an incremental fashion that is less controversial than new policies or massive overhaul. Federal government agencies that develop and administer health policies at the national level include the Department of Health and Human Services (DHHS) and the Occupational Safety and Health Administration (OSHA). At the state level, state departments of health and human services provide oversight for health policies, which are usually administered at the county or municipal level through local departments of health or social services. For example, health policies that affect pet owners and restaurant owners typically are administered through local health departments. Local departments of social services administer public health insurance programs such as Medicare and the State Children's Health Insurance Program.

TABLE 45–1 Applying the Policy Development Process

POLICY PROCESS	APPLIED TO LEGISLATIVE PROCESS	EXAMPLE
Policy issue develops	Senator learns about consumer concern about a health issue and has staff work on the issue.	Staffing levels in acute care hospitals are affecting the quality and safety of care. Examples of errors and poor quality are provided from various hospitals that have led to client deaths and to complications that have extended the need for treatment.
Gather data about issue	Legislative staff gathers data about the issue; some data may come from federal departments or agencies, which act as resources for legislative activity. Criteria are developed to evaluate the data (e.g., cost, efficiency, equity, and political feasibility).	Testimony may be provided by experts, clients, insurers, hospitals, nurses, physicians, and so on. Data related to errors, quality, and access will be used to further understand the problem. Data about enrollment and graduation rates in nursing schools would be important to obtain. Costs would be critical to obtain related to lack of staff: costs for the hospitals, insurers, employers, and clients (consumers).
Coalition building	Senator will form coalitions with other Senators, members of Congress, and stakeholders to back the legislation.	Stakeholders that would be interested in this problem and solution would be health care professionals and their organizations (nurses, physicians), American Hospital Association, insurers, employers, consumer groups, nurse educators, and others. Building a coalition from these groups would help to get the bill passed.
Identify possible solutions	Cost-benefit analysis of data to determine possible solutions; testimony from experts, lobbyists' input and pressure; arrive at list of possible solutions.	Cost data would be used to help assess cost-benefit for each of the possible solutions. Some examples of solutions might be do nothing, require every hospital to have a specific number of staff members, require hospitals to use a client classification system or require that every hospital use the same system, require minimum ratios, and many others.
Select a solution	Federal (or state) written law will probably repeat some of the activities described as part of "identify possible solutions" to gather more data or clarify. Coalition building also continues throughout the process.	For this example, requiring a minimum ratio is selected as the solution. (This does not indicate that it is the best solution but is just used for an example in this scenario.) A law is drafted by the Senator based on information gathered during the first phases of the process. The Senator will need to gain additional support in the Senate and then in the House of Representatives to get the law supported by a Representative(s). The law will wind its way through the legislative process.
Implement policy	Rules and regulations are developed; staff receives feedback on rules and regulations; rules and regulations are revised; rules and regulations become law.	DHHS develops draft of rules and regulations that will be used to implement the law. Professional organizations respond to them by providing feedback. The American Hospital Association submits criticisms. Rules and regulations are revised and may be posted for additional comments. By a specific date, rules and regulations are effective and required by law. Hospitals will have to get this information and make appropriate changes to meet requirements (e.g., increase staffing or alter ratios, recruit more staff, and so on).
Monitor outcomes: evaluation	Federal department or agency responsible for implementation develops evaluation plan and monitors outcomes. The department may have to report to Congress at specific times and may recommend and implement changes as long as within framework of the law. Otherwise, the department will need to recommend legislative changes (new law or amendments to law).	Outcomes analysis is ongoing. What are the outcomes of the plan to establish a minimum staffing ratio? Are hospitals able to meet the requirement deadlines? If not, what are the barriers? Can the barriers be addressed? If so, how?

The most recent change in health policy is the Health Care and Education Reconciliation Act of 2010. Despite the controversy surrounding its passage, this new law is expected to increase access to health insurance for the working poor and self-employed. The Act is discussed in detail in Concept 44, Health Care Systems.

45.1 REGULATORY AGENCIES

OVERVIEW

A number of regulatory agencies function to help health care providers and agencies operate safely, legally, honestly, and effectively. These agencies have a substantial effect on health care by enforcing laws and rules established by legislation. Regulatory agencies typically enforce laws and rules that must be followed at the organizational level; individual health care professionals are regulated by licensure boards (See Concept 47, Legal Issues).

FEDERAL AGENCIES

Changes in health care policy made at the federal level are administered through the U.S. Department of Health and Human Services and the agencies it oversees. The Department of Labor is not without responsibility in this area, however, as it oversees policies that affect worker safety. These policies are administered through the Occupational Safety and Health Administration.

The Department of Health and Human Services

The Department of Health and Human Services (DHHS) is the federal government's principal agency for the protection of the health of all Americans and the provision of essential human services for those least able to care for themselves. The more than 300 divisions and programs within this department range from research and information at the National Institutes of Health (NIH) to health care financing through the Centers for Medicare and Medicaid Services (CMS). Through the Administration for Children and Families and the Administration

---

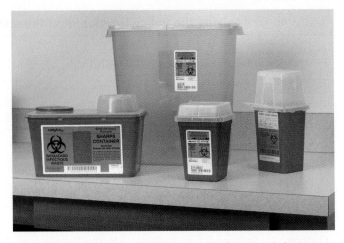

Figure 45–3 ■ OSHA regulations require the use of sharps containers to discard used needles.

---

on Aging, DHHS oversees services for individuals at all stages of life (Box 45–1). With an annual budget of more than 707 billion dollars, the Food and Drug Administration (FDA), Centers for Disease Control and Prevention (CDC), and Agency for Healthcare Research and Quality (AHRQ) all operate out of DHHS. DHHS administers more grant dollars than all other federal agencies combined and represents almost one quarter of all federal outlays (DHHS, 2008).

Occupational Safety and Health Administration

The Occupational Safety and Health Administration (OSHA) works to ensure the health and safety of Americans in the workplace. Employers are responsible for ensuring the health and safety of their employees in the workplace. OSHA provides guidelines and monitors employers' compliance with them by setting and enforcing standards; providing training, outreach, and education; establishing partnerships; and encouraging improvement in workplace safety and health (Figure 45–3 ■). OSHA also establishes and enforces protective standards and reaches out to employers and employees through technical assistance and consultation programs.

Most employees in the nation come under OSHA's jurisdiction. Specific professions that use OSHA services include occupational safety and health professionals, the academic community, lawyers, journalists, personnel of other government entities, and both skilled and unskilled workers who work with or near chemicals or mechanical equipment. Part of OSHA's mission is to provide assistance to employers to reduce or eliminate workplace hazards. OSHA provides a vast array of informational and training materials focusing on numerous safety and health hazards in the workplace. In general, OSHA standards require that employers maintain conditions or adopt practices that are reasonably necessary and appropriate to protect workers on the job; be familiar with and comply with standards applicable to their establishments; and ensure that employees have and use personal protective equipment when

---

Box 45–1 **Let's Move**

The Department of Health and Human Services does more than oversee the implementation of health policies in the United States. It also oversees a number of national health promotion and disease prevention efforts designed to help communities address or prevent health concerns. Let's Move, an initiative to address the issue of childhood obesity, was launched in February 2010 by DHHS with First Lady Michelle Obama at the forefront of the launch efforts (Figure 45–2 ■). Let's Move has donated $230 million to 30 communities across the United States to support programs that promote healthy eating and physical activity among children to expand access to fresh, healthy foods in communities and schools (DHHS, 2010). Nurses can participate in this initiative by joining online, by encouraging parents to make healthier choices for their children, and by lobbying local school boards to provide healthier meals in schools.

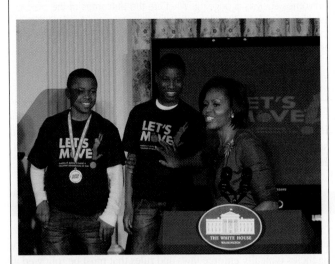

Figure 45–2 ■ Michelle Obama announces the formation of Let's Move.

required for safety and health. OSHA issues standards for a wide variety of workplace hazards including toxic substances, harmful physical agents, electrical hazards, trenching hazards, hazardous waste, and infectious diseases (OSHA, 2008). Many of these standards apply in both industrial and health care settings. Two examples include OSHA standards for Personal Protective Equipment (PPE) and standards related to the availability of emergency eye wash stations (OSHA, n.d.).

STATE AND LOCAL AGENCIES

Each state has its own health policies and regulations that it mandates in conjunction with federal policies and regulations. The majority of these are administered through state divisions of health and human services. At the county or municipal level, local departments of health administer a wide variety of health policies and offer a number of critical services to their communities. Local departments of social services typically have responsibility for administering Medicare, Medicaid, and the State Child Health Insurance Program.

State Divisions of Heath and Health Services

Every state has its own division or department of health and human services, although titles for these agencies may vary from state to state. These departments oversee regulation of county health departments, health care settings such as hospitals and long-term care facilities, child care centers, clinical laboratories, and other service providers such as portable

x-ray suppliers. Additional responsibilities include overseeing planning and construction of medical facilities and receiving complaints regarding facilities that they regulate. State offices of Emergency Medical Services (OEMS) ensure that citizens have access to high-quality emergency medical care through the regulatory oversight of local EMS systems. State divisions of health also oversee environmental health regulations, including those related to animal control and food safety.

Local Health Departments

Local health departments oversee a variety of health policies and their respective regulations. For example, local health departments are responsible for disease monitoring and surveillance in their communities. This includes reporting incidents of disease to state and federal authorities as well as implementing disease prevention efforts, such as offering immunizations. Local departments of health typically oversee child care center sanitation and food safety. They also offer a variety of community-wide prevention programs, whether those are provided through federal efforts or designed in response to local issues. Examples of these efforts include injury prevention campaigns, lead poisoning prevention efforts, and, in some agencies, making smoke detectors, children's bicycle helmets, and infant car seats available to families at no cost. Local departments of health typically administer the Women's, Infants and Children's supplemental nutrition program which provides food assistance to pregnant women and children under five who are at risk for malnutrition (Figure 45–4 ■).

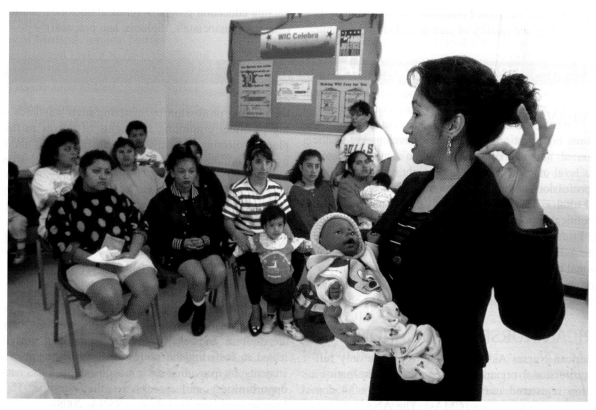

Figure 45–4 ■ An instructor uses a doll to demonstrate breastfeeding techniques to a group of women in a WIC program.

REVIEW Health Policy

RELATE: LINK THE CONCEPTS

Linking the concept of Health Policy with the concept of Ethics:

1. What values or beliefs do those who are for health care reform express as the motivation for their efforts on behalf of health care reform?
2. What values or beliefs do those who are against health care reform express as the motivation for their efforts on behalf of health care reform?
3. What nursing ethics support health care coverage for all people?

Linking the concept of Health Policy with the concept of Diversity:

4. What health policies in your area or in the nation promote discrimination?
5. What health policies address or prevent discrimination?

REFER: GO TO MYNURSINGKIT

REFLECT: CASE STUDY

Mrs. Helen Whitehead is a 70-year-old widow who recently retired from a job as a checkout clerk for a large supermarket chain. Before her retirement, she had group health insurance coverage through her employer. She no longer has her own coverage. She needs cataract surgery and has just been diagnosed with type II diabetes. She has no savings, but she does collect Social Security benefits. Her two children live several hundred miles away from her, and she sees them only about twice a year. She owns her own house and drives her own car. She is an active member of her church, which is also the source of her social group.

1. What options do you think Mrs. Whitehead might have for health care?
2. What resources in your area are available to assist Mrs. Whitehead?

EXPLORE PEARSON mynursingkit

MyNursingKit is your one stop for online chapter review materials and resources. Prepare for success with additional NCLEX®-style practice questions, interactive assignments and activities, web links, animations and videos, and more!

Register your access code from the front of your book at **www.mynursingkit.com**.

REFERENCES

American Association of Colleges of Nursing. (2009). *About us.* Retrieved January 16, 2009, from http://www.aacn.nche.edu/ContactUs/about.htm

Abood, S. (2007, January). Influencing health care in the legislative arena. *Online Journal of Issues in Nursing,* 12(1), 5-5. Retrieved August 16, 2008, from Health Source: Nursing/Academic Edition database.

Agency for Healthcare Research and Quality. (2006). The high concentration of U.S. health care expenditures. *Research in Action, 16,* 1-6. Retrieved April 28, 2010 from http://www.ahrq.gov/research/ria19/expendria.pdf

American Heart Association. (2007). *Managed health care plans.* Retrieved September 3, 2008, from http://www.americanheart.org/presenter.jhtml?identifier=4663

American Nurses Association. (2001). *Hearing on ergonomics safety in the workplace.* Retrieved January 16, 2009, from http://www.nursingworld.org/MainMenuCategories/OccupationalandEnvironmental/occupationalhealth/handlewithcare/Resources/HearingonErgonomicsSafety.aspx

American Nurses Association. (2003). *Nursing's Social Policy Statement* Washington, D.C.: Nursesbooks.org.

American Nurses Association. (2008). *About ANA.* Retrieved January 16, 2008, from http://www.nursingworld.org/FunctionalMenuCategories/AboutANA.aspx

American Nurses Association. (2009). *Frequently asked questions ANA's positions and advocacy on health care reform August 7, 2009.* Retrieved March 28, 2010, from http://www.nursingworld.org/MainMenuCategories/HealthcareandPolicyIssues/HealthSystemReform/FAQ-on-Health-Care-Reform.aspx

Clark, J. (2004, April). An aging population with chronic disease compels new delivery systems focused on new structures and practices. *Nursing Administration Quarterly, 28*(2), 105–115. Retrieved September 3, 2008, from CINAHL with Full Text database.

CMS. (2009).A guide for people with medicare choosing a medicare health plan. Retrieved January 11, 2009, from http://www.medicare.gov/Publications/Pubs/pdf/02219.pdf

CMS. (2009). Choosing a medigap policy: A guide to health insurance for people with medicare. Retrieved January 11, 2009, from http://www.medicare.gov/Publications/Pubs/pdf/02110.pdf

CCNE. (2008). Mission statement and goals. Retrieved January 16, 2009, from http://www.aacn.nche.edu/Accreditation/mission.htm

Department of Health and Human Services. (2010). *Let's move: America's move to raise a healthier generation of children.* Retrieved March 28, 2010, from http://www.letsmove.gov/

Fell-Carlson, D. (2004, October). OSHA 101: An introduction to OSHA for the occupational health nurse. *AAOHN Journal,* 52(10), 442–451. Retrieved August 16, 2008, from CINAHL with Full Text database.

Foley, M., & Leyden, A. (2005, February). Needlestick safety and prevention. *Nevada RNformation, 14*(1), 25–33. Retrieved August 21, 2008, from CINAHL with Full Text database.

Glass, D., Rebstock, J., & Handberg, E. (2004, April). Emergency treatment and labor act (EMTALA): Avoiding the pitfalls. *Journal of Perinatal & Neonatal Nursing, 18*(2), 103–116. Retrieved August 16, 2008, from CINAHL with Full Text database.

Human Rights Campaign. (2010). Domestic partner benefits: cost and utilization. Retrieved March 27, 2010, from http://www.hrc.org/issues/workplace/benefits/domestic_partner_benefit_costs.htm

Keepnews, D. (2008, May). In this issue. *Policy, Politics, & Nursing Practice, 9*(2), 67-67. Retrieved August 16, 2008, from Health Source: Nursing/Academic Edition database.

Lachman, V. (2007, August). Ethics, law, and policy. Moral courage in action: Case studies. *MEDSURG Nursing, 16*(4), 275–277. Retrieved August 16, 2008, from CINAHL with Full Text database.

Lachman, V. (2007, December). Ethics, law, and policy. Patient safety: The ethical imperative. *MEDSURG Nursing, 16*(6), 401–403. Retrieved August 16, 2008, from CINAHL with Full Text database.

Mathes, M. (2005, December). Ethics, law, and policy. On nursing, moral autonomy, and moral responsibility. *MEDSURG Nursing, 14*(6), 395–398. Retrieved August 16, 2008, from CINAHL with Full Text database.

Mayo Clinic. (2010). Health savings accounts: is an HSA right for you? Retrieved April 28, 2010, from http://www.mayoclinic.com/health/health-savings-accounts/GA00053

Miller, T. (2007, September). Making a difference in differences for the health inequalities of individuals. *Health Affairs, 26*(5), 1235–1237. Retrieved September 14, 2008, from CINAHL with Full Text database.

Moore, S, Hutchinson, S, (2007, December) *Developing leaders at every level*. JONA, 37(12), 564–568.

NLN. (2009). About NLN. Retrieved January 16, 2009, from www.nln.org/aboutnln/index.htm

National League for Nursing Accrediting Commission. (2008). About NLNAC. Retrieved January 16, 2009, from http://www.nlnac.org/About%20NLNAC/whatsnew.htm

National Student Nurses Association. (2008). About us. Retrieved January 16, 2009, from http://www.nsna.org/AboutUs.aspx

Nordin, J., Kasimow, S., Levitt, M., & Goodman, M. (2008, May). Bioterrorism surveillance and privacy: Intersection of HIPAA, the Common Rule, and public health law. *American Journal of Public Health, 98*(5), 802–807. Retrieved August 27, 2008, from CINAHL with Full Text database.

North Carolina Division of Health Service Regulation. (2008). Retrieved September 4, 2008, from http://www.ncdhhs.gov/dhsr/whatwedo.htm

Occupational Safety and Health Administration. (n.d.) *OSHA regulations*. Retrieved April 9, 2010, from http://www.osha.gov/SLTC/etools/eyeandface/employer/requirements.html#OSHAStandards

Physicians for a National Health Care Program. (2010). *Pro-single-payer doctors: Health bill leaves 23 million uninsured*. Retrieved March 27, 2010, from http://www.pnhp.org/news/2010/march/pro-single-payer-doctors-health-bill-leaves-23-million-uninsured

Reynolds, B., Fife, P., & Sharp, N. (2008, May). Nurses and policymaking. *American Journal of Nursing, 108*(5), 13–14. Retrieved August 16, 2008, from Health Source: Nursing/Academic Edition database.

Sigma Theta Tau. (2008). Mission and vision. Retrieved January 16, 2009, from http://www.nursingsociety.org/aboutus/mission/Pages/factsheet.aspx

TJC. (2008). Fact sheet. Retrieved January 11, 2009, from http://www.jointcommission.org/AboutUs/Fact_Sheets/joint_commission_facts.htm09

U.S. Department of Health and Human Services. (2008). HHS: What we do. Retrieved September 4, 2008, from http://www.hhs.gov/about/whatwedo.html/

Ward, C. (2005, December). Ethics, law, and policy. Registered Nurse nurse Safe safe Staffing staffing Act of 2005: Part II. *MEDSURG Nursing, 14*(6), 399–401. Retrieved August 16, 2008, from CINAHL with Full Text database.

Ward, C. (2005, October). Ethics, law, and policy. Registered Nurse Safe Staffing Act of 2005: part I. *MEDSURG Nursing, 14*(5), 338–340. Retrieved August 16, 2008, from CINAHL with Full Text database.

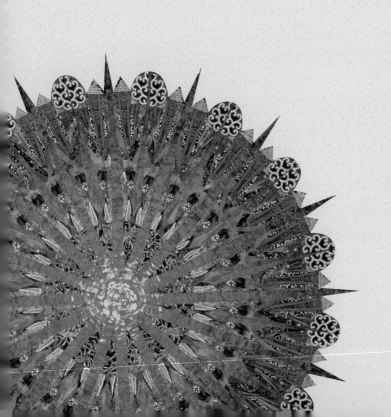

Informatics

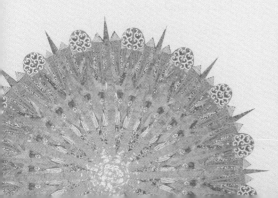

46

Concept at-a-Glance

About Informatics, *2373*

46.1 Clinical Decision Support Systems, *2385*

46.2 Individual Information at Point of Care, *2389*

Concept Learning Outcomes

After reading about this concept, you will be able to:

1. Define informatics and nursing informatics.
2. Describe the common components of a computer system.
3. Contrast the two types of health care information systems and their components.
4. Explain the goals of a nursing information system.
5. Describe current trends in nursing informatics.
6. Distinguish between the electronic medical record and the electronic health record.
7. Describe the advantages, applications, and legal implications of telehealth.
8. List the elements of an ergonomically sound workplace.

Concept Key Terms

Administrative information system, *2375*

Clinical information system, *2375*

Computer vision syndrome (CVS), *2383*

Critical pathways, *2376*

E-health, *2383*

Electronic health record, *2378*

Electronic medical record, *2379*

Ergonomics, *2383*

Hardware, *2374*

Health care information system, *2375*

Informatics, *2373*

Intranet, *2379*

Nursing informatics, *2373*

Repetitive motion disorders, *2383*

Software, *2374*

Telehealth, *2380*

About Informatics

Informatics refers to the science of computer information systems. **Nursing informatics** is the science of using computer information systems in the practice of nursing. During the course of any day, nurses handle large amounts of data and information. This is true for all nurses whether they provide direct care or serve as administrators, educators, researchers, or in some other capacity. Informatics provides tools to help process, manage, and analyze information collected for the purposes of documenting and improving client care, as well as to support knowledge that adds to the scientific foundation for nursing, provides value to nursing knowledge and work, and improves the public image for nursing by building a knowledge-based identity for nurses (American Nurses Association, 2007).

All nurses must have a basic level of computer literacy in order to meet current standards of practice and care. Computers are used to educate nursing students and clients; assess, document, and test client health conditions; manage medical records; communicate among health care providers and clients; and conduct research. Competencies associated with informatics may be categorized as computer skills, information literacy skills, or overall informatics competencies. Basic computer skills include the ability to use a word processing software program, to communicate by e-mail, and to document client care electronically. Information literacy skills include the ability to retrieve research and the ability to evaluate research and incorporate it appropriately into evidence-based practice. Overall informatics competencies include implementing policies to protect the privacy, confidentiality, and security of client information, and recording data relevant to the nursing care of clients. These skills are basic to the entry-level nursing role. Experienced nurses should have even greater competency in using informatics in their daily practice. ●

COMPUTER TERMINOLOGY

A computer is an electronic device that collects, stores, processes, and retrieves data. Information output is provided under the direction of stored sequences of instructions known as computer programs. The physical parts of a computer are frequently referred to as **hardware**, and the instructions, or programs, are collectively known as **software**. A computer system consists of the following components:

■ Hardware
■ Software
■ Data that will be transformed into information
■ Procedures or rules for the use of the system
■ Users.

Rapid advances in technology frequently reshape computer capabilities and user expectations. Many changes have occurred since the introduction of the first computers in the 1940s. In general, computers have become smaller but more powerful and increasingly affordable. This is particularly evident with current notebook, tablet, personal digital assistants (PDAs), and hybrid devices (such as smart phones).

Hardware

Computer hardware is the physical part of the computer and its associated equipment. Computer hardware consists of many different parts, but the main elements are input devices, the central processing unit, primary and secondary storage devices, and output devices. These devices may be contained within one shell or may be separate but connected via cables, infrared, or wireless technology. Figure 46–1 ■ describes the relationship among these components.

INPUT DEVICES   Input devices allow the user to feed data into the computer. Common input devices include the keyboard, mouse or trackball, touch sensitive screen, stylus, microphone, bar code reader, ethernet (network interface) card, joystick, image scanner, fingerprint scanner, digital camera, and Webcam.

CENTRAL PROCESSING UNIT   The central processing unit (CPU) is the "brain" of the computer. It has the electronic circuitry that actually executes computer instructions. The CPU can be divided into the following three components:

■ The arithmetic logic unit (ALU) executes instructions for the manipulation of numeric symbols.
■ Memory is the storage area where programs reside during execution. Memory is subdivided into two categories: read-only memory and random access memory. Read-only memory (ROM) is permanent; it remains when the power is off. It typically cannot be changed by the user unless additional memory is installed. ROM contains start-up instructions that are executed each time the computer is turned on. Random access memory (RAM) is a temporary storage area that is active only while the computer is turned on. It provides storage for the program that is running, as well as for the data that are being processed.
■ The control unit manages instructions to other parts of the computer, including input and output devices. It reads stored programs one instruction at a time and directs other computer parts to perform required tasks.

The CPU is located inside the system cabinet, which is the box that many people think of as "the computer." The CPU and memory are found on the main circuit board, or motherboard, of the personal or desktop computer. The cabinet contains other components as well.

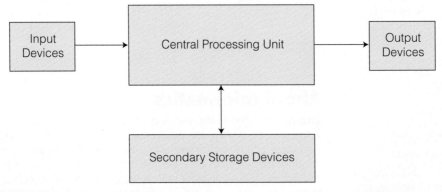

Figure 46–1 ■ Basic components of a computer.

SECONDARY STORAGE Secondary storage provides space to retain data in an area separate from the computer's memory after the computer is turned off. Common mechanisms for secondary storage include hard disk drives, USB flash drives, digital versatile or video discs (DVDs), and high density optical disc format (HD-DVD), which is the successor to DVD. Hard disk drives store digitally encoded data and rotating platters with magnetic surfaces. USB flash drives are portable, fairly inexpensive devices. Slightly smaller than a cigarette lighter, USB flash drives plug into a USB port and can easily be transported from one computer to another. DVDs resemble the CDs that are used to record and play music but offer a larger amount of storage. Blu-ray is a high density optical disc format rival to HD-DVD. Some older machines may still have compact discs (CDs), floppy drives and diskettes, and Zip drive disks, but these are not found on current computers. Floppy diskettes and Zip diskettes come in a square plastic cases. Magnetic tape drives are still used for some large computers.

OUTPUT DEVICES Output devices allow the user to view and possibly hear processed data. Terminals or video monitor screens, projectors, printers, speakers, and fax modem boards are examples of output devices.

COMPUTER INFORMATION SYSTEMS

An *information system* can be defined as the use of computer hardware and software to process data into information to solve a problem. The terms **health care information system** and hospital information system (HIS) both refer to a group of computer systems used by a hospital or organization to support and enhance health care. The HIS comprises two major types of information systems: clinical information systems and administrative information systems. **Clinical information systems** (CISs) are large, computerized database management systems that support several types of activities that may include provider order entry, result retrieval, documentation, and decision support across distributed locations. Health care providers use these systems to access client data in order to plan, implement, and evaluate care. CISs may also be referred to as *client care information systems.* Some examples of CISs include nursing, laboratory, pharmacy, radiology, medical information systems, emergency department systems, physician practice management systems, and long-term and home care information systems. **Administrative information systems** support client care by managing financial and demographic information and providing reporting capabilities. This category includes client management, financial, payroll, and human resources, and quality assurance systems. Coding systems use clinical information to generate charges for care. Figure 46–2 ■ shows the relationships between various components of a hospital information system.

Clinical and administrative information systems may be designed to meet the needs of one or more departments or functions within an organization. In recent years the trend has been to adopt vendor-based solutions with little, if any, customization. This allows system implementation to occur more quickly (Conn, 2007a). Either clinical or administrative systems can be implemented as stand-alone systems, or they may work with other systems to provide information sharing and seamless functionality for the users. Any one health care agency may use one or several clinical and administrative systems. Increasingly, organizations are looking to improve productivity, improve safety, increase the quality of care, and reduce costs throughout the organization. Information technology is seen as the means to achieve these ends through the application of evidenced-based care, improved work flow, and better management of resources. Information technology, however, can only help improve client safety. Organizations must first establish a culture of safety in which all employees work to identify problem areas, seek evidence-based solutions, and solicit feedback for change (Smetzer & Navarra, 2007).

Clinical Information Systems

Although many CISs are designed for use within one hospital department, health care providers and researchers from several areas may use the data collected by each system. For example, the nurse documents client allergies in the initial assessment. The physician, the pharmacist, the dietician, and the radiologist can then use this data during the client's hospital stay. The goal of CISs is to allow health care providers to access information quickly and safely, order appropriate medications and treatments, and implement cost-effective, evidence-based care while avoiding duplicate services. Several tools help health care professionals achieve these goals. These include electronic health records, clinical decision support systems, bedside medication administration using positive client identification, computerized provider order entry (CPOE), client surveillance, and the clinical data warehouse (CDW) (Harrison and Palacio, 2006; Hastings, 2006; Mangalampalli, Chakravarthy, Raja, Jain & Parinam, 2006; Solovy, 2005). Large teaching hospitals are generally better able to afford the investment in information technology. This investment requires other cost containment efforts and a demonstrated return on investment. All health care providers are looking for information technology solutions (Kelley, 2007).

NURSING INFORMATION SYSTEMS A nursing information system supports the use and documentation of nursing processes and interventions, and provides tools for managing the delivery of nursing care (Hendrickson, 1993). An effective nursing information system must accomplish two goals. The first goal is that the system should support the way that nurses function, allowing them the flexibility to use the system to view data and collect necessary information, provide quality client care, and document the client's condition and the care provided to the client. Necessary information includes past health medical history, allergies, test results, and progress notes, among other things. The second goal of an effective nursing information system is that it should support and enhance nursing practice through improved access to information and tools. These include online literature searches such as the Cumulative Index of Nursing and Allied Health Literature (CINAHL) and MEDLINE, and automated drug information and hospital policy/procedure guidelines. Consideration of these two goals in the selection and implementation of a nursing system will ensure that the system benefits nursing.

In general, there are two approaches to nursing care and documentation using automated information systems. These are the *traditional nursing process* approach and the *critical*

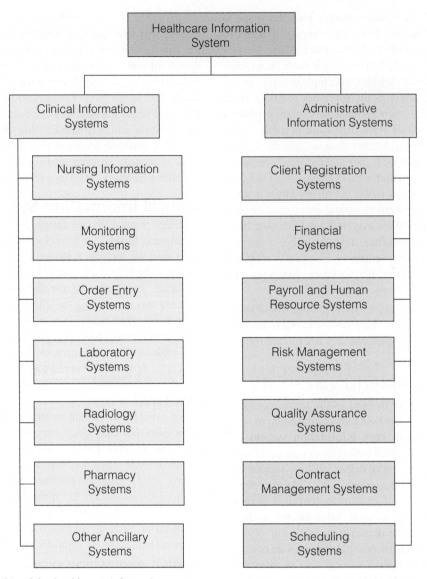

Figure 46–2 ■ Relationship of the health care information system components.

---

pathway, or *protocols*, approach. The traditional nursing process approach allows documentation of nursing care using well-established formats such as admission assessments, problem lists, and care plans. A more organized version of this approach incorporates standardized nursing languages (SNLs) accepted by the American Nurses Association (Prophet, Dorr, Gibbs, & Porcella, 1997). These include nursing diagnoses defined by the North American Nursing Diagnosis Association (NANDA), Nursing Interventions Classification (NIC), and Nursing Outcomes Classification (NOC), and several other languages. SNLs provide a common language across the discipline of nursing that allows all nurses to describe nursing problems, treatments, and outcomes in a consistent manner that is understood by all nurses. Despite progress in representing nursing language in automated systems, the use of interdisciplinary protocols (**critical pathways**) that can be used among multiple types of providers remains popular. These protocols suggest specific treatments related to the client's diagnosis and outline the anticipated outcomes for typical clients with that

diagnosis. The advantages of using a nursing information system are listed in Box 46–1.

The nursing process approach to automated documentation is based on the paper forms traditionally used by nurses. The nursing diagnosis often serves as the organizational framework. Many current information systems follow this format.

■ *Documentation of nursing admission assessment and discharge instructions.* A menu-driven approach to the admission assessment ensures capture of essential information. A menu lists related commands that can be selected from a computer screen to accomplish a task. For example, the menu may include selections such as past medical history, advanced directives, organ donation status, psychosocial history, medications, and review of body systems. This approach can also be used to ensure that all necessary information is covered in the client's discharge instructions, including follow-up appointments and diagnostic studies; diet and activity restrictions; wound care; and medication information such as drug names, instructions for administration,

Box 46–1 Advantages of Using a Nursing Information System

- Better access to information
- Enhanced quality of documentation through prompts
- Improved quality of care
- Increased productivity
- Improved communications
- Reduced errors of omissions
- Reduced hospital costs
- Increased employee satisfaction
- Compliance with agency regulations
- Use of a common clinical database
- Improved client perception of care
- Enhanced ability to track records
- Improved hospital image

NURSING PRACTICE
- Worklists to remind staff of planned nursing interventions
- Computer-generated client documentation including discharge instructions and medication information
- Monitoring devices that record vital signs and other measurements directly into the client record
- Computer-generated nursing care plans and critical pathways
- Automatic billing for supplies or procedures with nursing documentation
- Reminders and prompts that appear during documentation to ensure comprehensive charting
- Quick access to computer-archived patient data from previous encounters
- Online drug information

NURSING ADMINISTRATION
- Automated staff scheduling
- Online bidding for unfilled shifts

- Electronic mail for improved communication
- Cost analysis and finding trends for budget purposes
- Quality assurance and outcomes analysis
- Patient tracking and placement for case management

NURSING EDUCATION
- Online completion of mandatory education requirements
- Online course registration and scheduling
- Computerized student tracking, testing, and grade management
- Course delivery and support for Web-based education
- Remote access to library and Internet resources
- Teleconferencing and Webcast capability
- Presentation software for preparing slides and handouts
- Online test administration
- Communication with students

NURSING RESEARCH
- Computerized literature searching
- The adoption of standardized language related to nursing terms
- The ability to find trends in aggregate data, which is data derived from large population groups
- Use of the Internet for obtaining data collection tools and conducting research
- Collaborate with other nurse researchers

CONSUMER APPLICATIONS
- Communication with health care providers via e-mail and instant messaging
- Remote monitoring and other telehealth services
- Support groups
- Online scheduling

and common side effects that the client should report. The system should generate printed copies of these instructions for clients to review on discharge and for their use at home, as well as for use by the home health staff.

- *Generation of a nursing work list that indicates routine scheduled activities related to the care of each client.* These activities can be grouped according to scheduled time or skill level.
- *Documentation of discrete data or activities such as vital signs, weight, and intake and output measurements.* The automation of this type of data promotes accuracy and allows the data to be readily available to all care providers at any time.
- *Documentation of routine aspects of client care, such as bathing, positioning, blood glucose measurements, notation of dietary intake, and/or wound care in a flow sheet format.*
- *Standardized care plans that the nurse can individualize for clients as needed.* This feature saves time yet allows flexibility to address the client's needs while promoting quality care.
- *Documentation of nursing care in a progress note format.* The nurse may accomplish this through narrative charting, charting by exception, or flow sheet charting. Regardless of the method, automated documentation can improve the overall quality of charting by prompting the nurse with pre-defined selections.

- *Documentation of medication administration.* This multistep task may be performed through the nursing information system, but increasingly it is performed instead through a separate software application. Medication administration applications provide worksheets that list administration times and medications for each client. The nurse uses the worksheets when preparing and administering medications, and the system documents the activity.

The critical pathway or protocol approach to documentation is a popular information system, primarily due to the requirements of managed care. The critical pathway approach may be used by many types of care providers working in the same organization. Nurses, nursing or client care assistants, dietitians, social workers, respiratory therapists, physical and occupational therapists, case managers, and physicians are then able to use the same system to document care and share information. Critical pathway systems include the following features:

- *The nurse, or other care provider, can select one or more appropriate critical pathways for the client.* If more than one path is selected, the system should merge the paths to create one "master" path or protocol.
- *Interaction with physician orders.* Standard physician order sets can be included with each critical pathway and may be automatically processed by the system.

Box 46–2 Administrative Information Systems Used in the Health Care Setting

- *Financial systems* provide the facility with accounting functions. Accurate tracking of financial data is critical for enabling the organization to receive reimbursement for services. Accurate accounting of financial data is essential for preventing fraud.
- *Payroll and human resource systems* track employee time and attendance, credentials, performance evaluations, and payroll compensation information.
- *Contract management systems* manage contracts with third-party payers, such as private insurance plans.
- *Risk management systems* track and plan prevention of unusual occurrences or incidents.

- *Quality assurance systems* monitor outcomes and produce reports that are used to guide quality improvement initiatives.
- *Physician management systems* support client registration, scheduling, coding, and billing in the physician's office and may support results retrieval. These systems also provide better protection of client privacy than paper records.
- *Executive information systems* provide administrators with easy access to summarized information related to the financial and clinical operations of the organization.
- *Materials management systems* facilitate inventory control and charging of supplies.

- *Tracking of protocol variances.* The system should identify variances to the anticipated outcomes as they are charted and provide aggregate variance data for analysis by the providers. This information can be used to fine tune and improve the critical pathways, thereby contributing to improved client outcomes.

Despite the many reasons to establish a nursing information system and the fact that nurses constitute the majority of workers in health care, most systems are designed for use by all health care providers.

Administrative Systems

Various administrative systems may be used in health care organizations to support the process of providing client care. Box 46–2 provides a brief review of some of these systems.

TRENDS IN INFORMATICS

New technologies will impact the practice of nursing informatics in ways that cannot be forecast at present. Nanotechnology, genomics, robotics, wearable monitoring devices, and new developments in educational technology represent some of these trends. The drive for client safety, transparency in healthcare, error reduction, increased efficiency, and additional requirements on the part of regulatory agencies will continue to shape health care delivery and informatics practice for many years to come. Trends shaping nursing care in the twenty-first century are discussed in the section that follows.

Handheld Devices

Personal digital assistants (PDAs) are a well-known type of handheld computer. These small devices were once used to keep appointment calendars, addresses, and telephone numbers. Advances in processing capability, memory, and design make PDAs attractive for a wide variety of functions, including many common software applications and data collection. PDAs can access information from the Internet, store extensive reference materials, and access and exchange client information.

Hybrid or combination devices comprise another category of handheld devices. Hybrids may combine PDA capability with cell phones, MP3 players, or other functions. The BlackBerry, iPhone, and Droid are examples of hybrid devices, or "smart phones." Smart phones are multimedia, Internet-enabled devices. Functions include a camera phone, text messaging, visual voicemail, and a portable media player. Smart phones also support the following Internet services: e-mail, Web-browsing, and local Wi-Fi connectivity. Some have touch screens with a virtual keyboard.

An MP3 player is a small handheld digital music player. MP3 players often support other file types as well. The iPod is a portable music player that supports MP3 and other file types. Its large capacity allows it to download, store, and play music, videos, games, and photo slideshows from a computer or wireless connection. The iPod supports games, can function as a portable hard drive, and offers contact and calendar functions that can synchronize with personal computers.

Computerized Medical Records

Requirements for the management of health care information are evolving—transforming the ways that health care providers store, access, and use information. The traditional paper medical record that reports client status and test results no longer meets the needs of today's health care industry. Paper records are episode-oriented with a separate record for each client visit. Key information, such as allergies or client reports of side effects of medications, may be lost from one episode to the next, threatening client safety. Another drawback to paper records is that only one person can access the record at any given time. As a result, health care providers waste time looking for paper records, and treatment may be delayed (Figure 46–3 ■). Paper records cannot incorporate diagnostic studies that include images and sound, nor do they make use of decision support systems. The **electronic health record** (EHR) has the potential to integrate all pertinent client information into one record as well as to improve the quality of health information. The EHR may also improve client safety and provider productivity, contain costs, support research, decrease wait time for treatment, and contribute to the body of health care knowledge (Gearing et al., 2006; IOM, 2003; Puffer et al., 2007).

While there is no standard term to refer to a client's electronic medical file, EHR has been used as a generic term for all electronic health care systems (NCQHC, 2006). EHR has become the preferred term when referring to the client's lifetime computerized record. Some of the other frequently used terms include electronic medical record (EMR), electronic patient record (EPR), computer-based patient record (CPR) and CPR system, and Shared Electronic Health Record (SEHR).

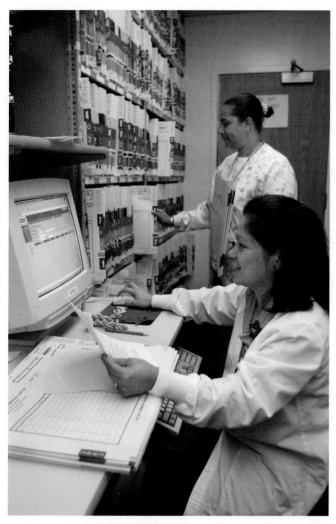

Figure 46–3 ■ Paper records do not meet the needs of today's health care industry. Only one person at a time can use a paper record, paper records can be lost, they don't include images or sounds, and they don't include decision support systems.

The Healthcare Information and Management Systems Society (HIMSS, 2007) outlined the differences between the terms electronic medical record and electronic health record. HIMSS defined the **electronic medical record** (EMR) as the "legal record created in hospitals and ambulatory environments that is the source of data for the EHR." For many years the EMR applied to a single encounter with no, or very limited, ability to carry information from one visit to another within a care delivery system. That situation has changed; it is now possible to bring information forward from prior visits within the organization or delivery system. The basic components of the EMR system are

■ Clinical messaging and e-mail
■ Results reporting
■ Data repository
■ Decision support
■ Clinical documentation
■ Order entry.

The EMR includes unstructured data that may be provided as a text report. Such a report may be produced by transcription

services and may include history and physical assessments, consultation findings, operative reports, and discharge summaries. The EMR also includes structured data, which may be presented in a predefined format. Structured data are often obtained from automated ancillary reporting systems; a primary example is laboratory results from an automated laboratory information system. Electronic imaging produced by diagnostic studies, such as magnetic resonance imaging, is another type of data that may be included in the EMR. The data in the EMR is the legal record of client care during an encounter at the health care organization and is owned by the organization (Garets & Davis, 2006).

Client safety and the need to restructure the health care delivery system to improve the quality of care provided while containing costs are the driving forces behind the development of the EHR (NCQHC, 2006). A well-developed EHR facilitates the provision of quality care and management of costs. The benefits of the EHR can be best understood when considering the needs of various groups of users. Some of the benefits are general, but others relate to nurses, physicians, and other care providers, as well as the health care agency. Benefits of the EHR are listed in Box 46–3.

Information system vendors as well as health care providers are, for the most part, aware of the pressing need to develop the EHR and are continuously working toward its evolvement. Development and cost of an electronic infrastructure are the two major impediments to the creation of a fully functioning EHR. The principal requirement is that the major participants in the health care arena, including health care facilities, payers, and physicians, must be linked electronically. This is a costly undertaking. Other impediments include the lack of a common vocabulary, security and confidentiality issues, resistance among caregivers, and a lack of IT staff to create and support the necessary infrastructure (Rowland, 2007).

Intranets

Intranets are private computer networks that use Internet protocols and technologies, including Web browsers, servers, and languages, to facilitate collaborative data sharing. They were first developed in response to concerns over slowdowns, security breaches, and fears of Internet collapse. Intranets sit behind firewalls or other barriers and may not normally be available to people outside of the organization. In some cases authorized users may be able to access content from remote sites. Intranets permit use of several different information systems within the same organization. Intranets can save money by providing an easy-to-use, familiar interface that is intuitive and therefore requires little training. Most organizations initially use the intranet to share internal documents and information. This cuts down on paper and distribution costs, and makes materials available more quickly and widely. It also provides a mechanism to ensure that everybody has the most recent version of a document, which isn't always possible with hard copies. This type of intranet application may be used to distribute policy and procedure manuals or other reference materials. It also acclimates employees to using the intranet as the single source of information. Additional features may include the ability for employees to view and enroll in benefits, request

Box 46–3 Benefits of the EHR

GENERAL BENEFITS

- *Improved data integrity.* Information is more readable, better organized, and more accurate and complete.
- *Increased productivity.* Caregivers are able to access client information at multiple locations whenever it is needed. This can result in improved client care due to the ability to make timely decisions based on appropriate data.
- *Improved quality of care.* The EHR supports clinical decision-making processes for physicians and nurses. For example, the nurse can tailor a view of client information that shows the most recent labs, vital signs, and current medications on one screen or can select another view that graphs lab values and vital signs over time. This can be especially helpful to show renal response to ordered medications, for example.
- *Increased satisfaction for providers.* Health care providers are able to take advantage of easy access to client data as well as other services, including drug information sources, rules-based decision support, and literature searches.

NURSING BENEFITS

- Facilitates comparisons of current data with data from previous events.
- Supports an ongoing record of the client's education and learning response across multiple encounters or visits.
- Eliminates the need to repeat collection of baseline demographic data with each encounter.
- Provides universal data access to all who have access to the EHR.
- Improves data access and quality for research.
- Provides prompts to ensure administration and documentation of medications and treatments.
- Improves documentation and quality of care (Nelson, 2007).
- Facilitates automation of critical pathways.
- Supports the development of a database that facilitates research, provides information useful to health care providers and administrators, and allows recognition of nursing work in measurable units when used with a common unified structure for nursing language (Simpson, 2007).

BENEFITS FOR HEALTH CARE PROVIDERS

- Simultaneous record access by multiple users.
- Previous encounters may be accessed easily.
- Faster chart access as EHR eliminates the need to wait for old records to be delivered from the medical records department.
- More comprehensive information is available.
- Fewer lost records.
- Improved efficiency of billing.
- Better reporting tools. Trends and clinical graphics are available on demand.

- Reduced liability through better decision making and documentation.
- Improved reimbursement rates.
- Enhanced compliance through system generated prompts with preventive care protocols (Martin, 2007; Mitchell 2007).
- Supports pay-for-performance bonuses (NCQHC, 2006).
- Early warnings of changes in client status.
- Supports benchmarking for how well providers manage clients with chronic disease conditions (Novogoratz, 2007).

HEALTH CARE FACILITY BENEFITS

- Improved client record security.
- Instant notice of authorization for procedures with integration with payer-based health records.
- Strengthened communications.
- Fewer lost records.
- Decreased need for record storage.
- Reduced medical record department costs because pulling, filing, and copying of charts is decreased.
- Improved verification of client eligibility for coverage in managed care settings.
- Faster turnaround for outstanding accounts with electronic coding and claim submission.
- Decreased need for x-ray film and physical filing, storage, and transport of films.
- Improved cost evaluation based on clinical outcomes and resource utilization data.
- Decreased length of stay (NCQHC, 2006).
- Enhanced compliance with regulatory requirements.

CONSUMER BENEFITS

- Decreased wait time for treatment.
- Improved access and control over health information.
- Increased use of best practices with incorporation of decision support.
- Improved ability to ask informed questions.
- Greater responsibility for one's own care.
- Alerts and reminders for upcoming appointments and scheduled tests.
- Increased satisfaction (NCQHC, 2006).
- Improved understanding of treatment choices (Martin, 2007; Mitchell, 2007).

PAYER BENEFITS

- Supports pay for performance as quality measures are gathered (Martin, 2007).
- Supports disease management lowering costs for expensive diagnoses.

vacation days, and apply for internal jobs. Intranets are also an effective tool for marketing and advertising. Intranets in health care facilities may also be used for mail and messaging, conferencing, and access to clinical data. The ability to access clinical data requires that the intranet have a system in place to authenticate authorized users. In some cases, clients may be able to view their own health information, schedule appointments, and register for the hospital online. The concerns associated with intranet use mirror those discussed earlier: issues of data security, the need to develop and implement strong

organizational policies on appropriate intranet use, and the development of the infrastructure to support an intranet.

Telehealth

Telehealth is the use of telecommunication technologies and computers to exchange health care information and to provide services to clients at remote locations. This was once known as telemedicine, but applications are now widely used by other members of the health care community. The American Nurses Association (1996) prefers the term *telehealth* as a more inclusive and accurate description of the services provided. Telehealth services include health promotion, disease prevention, diagnosis, consultation, education, and therapy. Teleconferences and videoconferences are tools used to deliver these services. Electronic, visual, and audio signals sent during these conferences provide information to consultants from remote sites. Many common medical devices have been adapted for use with telemedicine technology. Distant practitioners and clients benefit from the skills and knowledge of the consultants without the need to travel to regional referral centers. Telehealth is a tool that allows health care professionals to do the following (Coyle, Duffy, & Martin, 2007; Cross, 2007; Demiris, Edison, & Vijaykumar, 2005; Liaw & Humphreys, 2006; Merrill, 2007; Yun & Park, 2007):

- Consult with colleagues
- Conduct interviews
- Assess and monitor clients
- View diagnostic images
- Review slides and laboratory reports
- Extend scarce health care resources
- Decrease the number of hospital visits for patients with chronic conditions
- Decrease health care costs
- Tackle isolation and loneliness
- Provide health education
- Improve the coordination of care
- Improve the equity of access to services
- Improve the quality of client care
- Improve the overall quality of the client's record

Box 46–4 lists additional benefits associated with telehealth.

Box 46–4 **Telehealth Benefits**

- *Continuity of care.* Clients can stay in the community and use their regular health care providers.
- *Centralized health records.* Clients remain in the same health care system.
- *Incorporation of the health care consumer as an active member of the health team.* The client is an active participant in videoconferences.
- *Collaboration among health care professionals.* Cooperation is fostered among interdisciplinary members of the health care team.
- *Improved decision making.* Experts are readily available.
- *Education of health care consumers and professionals.* Offerings are readily available.
- *Higher quality of care.* Access to care and access to specialists is improved.
- *Removes geographic barriers to care.* Clients living away from major population centers or in economically disadvantaged areas can access care more readily.
- *May lower costs for health care.* Eliminates travel costs. Clients are seen earlier when they are not as ill. Treatment may take place in local hospitals, which are less costly.
- *Improved quality of health record.* The record contains digitalized records of diagnostic tests, biometric measures, photographs, and communication.

Box 46–5 **Global Telehealth**

Telehealth's ability to support remote monitoring and teleconferencing is of particular importance during large scale disasters when local medical infrastructures are destroyed. In the weeks following the January 2010 earthquake in Haiti, the United States military and other organizations worked diligently to establish sufficient satellite access to enable medical providers on the ground to begin using telehealth to consult with specialists in the United States. Until that was established, health care providers working in Haiti relied on donated Internet access and even ham radio operators to communicate with health care providers working outside the beleaguered nation (Freudenheim, 2010).

TELEHEALTH APPLICATIONS Telehealth applications vary greatly. Examples include monitoring activities, diagnostic evaluations, decision-support systems, storage and dissemination of records for diagnostic purposes, image compression for efficient storage and retrieval, research, electronic prescriptions, voice recognition for dictation, education of health care professionals and consumers, and support of caregivers. Sophisticated equipment is not always necessary (Box 46–5). Some applications are "high tech," whereas others are relatively "low tech."

Real-time videoconferencing between physicians or health care professionals and clients and the transmission of diagnostic images and biometric data are examples of high-tech applications. An example of a low-tech application is a home glucose-monitoring program that uses a touch-tone telephone to report glucose results. Computers with webcams can provide telehealth opportunities for applications that do not require high resolution. Current telehealth technologies can be grouped into at least nine broad categories, although for general discussion purposes there are two types: store-and-forward and interactive conferencing. Store-and-forward is used to transfer digital images and data from one location to another. It is appropriate for nonemergent situations. It is commonly used for teleradiology and telepathology. Interactive conferencing primarily refers to video conferencing and is used in place of face-to-face consultation. Box 46–6 lists some other actual and proposed applications.

BARRIERS TO IMPLEMENTATION OF TELEHEALTH SERVICES Reimbursement and licensure issues remain two of the major barriers to the growth and practice of telehealth (Cwiek, Rafiq, Qamar, Tobey, & Merrell, 2007; Dickens & Cook, 2006; Kennedy, 2005; Starren et al., 2005). The Centers for Medicare & Medicaid Services (CMS) have not formally defined telemedicine for the Medicaid program and Medicaid does not recognize telemedicine as a distinct service. Medicaid reimbursement for telehealth services is available at the discretion of individual states as a cost-effective alternative to traditional services or as a means to improve access for rural residents (CMS, 2007; Cross, 2007; Gray, Stamm, Toevs, Reischl, & Yarrington, 2006).

There are also concerns about the impact of telehealth on record privacy, particularly with the implementation of the Health Insurance Portability and Accountability Act (HIPAA). Who has responsibility for the client when a teleconsult is used? Does the care provider need to be licensed in the state or

Box 46–6 Current and Proposed Telehealth Applications

- *Cardiology.* ECG strips can be transmitted for interpretation by experts at a regional referral center, and pacemakers can be reset from a remote location.
- *Counselling.* Clients may be seen at home or in outpatient settings by a counselor at another site.
- *Data mining.* Research may be conducted on large databases for educational, diagnostic, and cost/benefit analysis.
- *Dermatology.* Primary physicians may ask specialists to see a client without the client waiting for an appointment with the specialist and traveling to a distant site.
- *Diabetes management.* Clients may report blood glucose readings by using the touch-tone telephone.
- *Mobile unit postdisaster care.* Emergency medical technicians (EMTs) and nurses at the site of a disaster can consult with physicians about the health needs of victims.
- *Education.* Health care professionals in geographically remote areas can attend seminars to update their knowledge without extensive travel, expense, or time away from home.
- *Emergency care.* Community hospitals can share information with trauma centers so that the centers can better care for clients and prepare them for transport.
- *Fetal monitoring.* Some high-risk antepartum clients can be monitored from home with greater comfort and decreased expense.
- *Geriatrics.* Videoconference equipment in the home permits home monitoring of medication administration for the client with memory deficits who is otherwise able to stay at home.
- *Home care.* Once equipment is in the client's home, nurses and physicians may evaluate the client at home without leaving their offices.

- *Hospice.* Palliative and end-of-life services via technology can increase access to services in remote areas or supplement traditional care.
- *Military.* Physicians at remote sites can evaluate injured soldiers in the field via the medic's equipment.
- *Pharmacy.* Data can be accessed at a centralized location.
- *Pathology.* The transmission of slide and tissue samples to other sites makes it easier to obtain a second opinion on biopsy findings.
- *Psychiatry.* Specialists at major medical centers can evaluate clients in outlying emergency departments, hospitals, and clinics via teleconferences.
- *Radiology.* Radiologists can take calls from home that receive images from the hospital on equipment they have in place. Rural hospitals do not need to have a radiologist on site.
- *School clinics.* School nurses, particularly in remote areas, can quickly consult with other professionals about problems observed.
- *Social work.* Social workers can augment services with telehealth home visits.
- *Speech–language pathology.* More efficient use can be made of scarce speech–language pathologists.
- *Virtual intensive care units.* Remote monitoring capabilities and teleconferencing allow experts at medical centers to monitor clients in distant, rural hospitals, particularly when weather conditions or other factors do not allow transport.
- *Extended emergency services.* Remote monitoring and teleconferencing support allow emergency care physicians to view and monitor ambulance clients, supervise emergency medical technicians, and initiate treatments early and re-direct clients to the most appropriate facilities such as burn centers or trauma units without being seen first in the emergency department.

province where the client's primary care is given? The National Council of State Boards of Nursing has declared that the applicable regulations are those for where the client resides and not where the provider is located. How is the client's privacy protected? For example, if a provider in state A was tele-consulting with providers in states B, C, and D, which state privacy laws should take precedence over others? What if they conflict? HIPAA and several other projects are under way to answer these questions and to determine the most effective designs for telehealth programs.

BARRIERS TO CLIENT PARTICIPATION IN TELEHEALTH SERVICES Clients expected to participate in home monitoring and other telehealth programs must also have the necessary equipment. This may present more of a challenge than providers imagine. In a recent poll conducted by the American Association of Retired Persons, one-third of those over the age of 50 and 51% of those over the age of 65 reported that they do not use a computer (AARP, 2009). Annie E. Casey Foundation's Kids Count Data Center reports that approximately 41% of families with children in the United States do not have Internet access at home. Kids Count lists five states in which more than 50% of families with children do not have Internet access at home: Mississippi, New Mexico, Arkansas, Louisiana, and Texas (Annie E. Casey Foundation, 2009).

Providers seeking to help clients with chronic diseases through technology may have difficulty. The Pew Internet and American Life Project reports that adults in the United States who live with chronic disease are significantly less likely than healthy adults to have access to the Internet. The project partly attributes this to the fact that chronic disease is associated with being older, African American, less educated, and living on a lower income, all factors associated with lower Internet usage. However, the project reports that those clients with chronic diseases who do have Internet access use it widely to access e-health information and services and to network with others who suffer from the same disease (PIALP, 2010a).

Internet use among Latinos increased from 54% to 64% from 2006 to 2008, and the likelihood of Hispanic users accessing the Internet from home hovers at around 80% (Pew Hispanic Center, 2010). However, Hispanic families with children may be less likely to have Internet access at home. A 2008 study by the Harvard Family Research Project cited that Hispanic families are less likely to have access to the Internet at home than families whose native language is English. The study also found that income was a stronger predictor of Internet access at home among African American families than among other families (Harvard Family Research Project, 2010).

Just as nurses should not make an assumption about a client's beliefs or values based on the client's cultural background or ethnicity, nurses should not make assumptions about Internet access and the client's ability to participate in telehealth experiences. Considering the fact that the Internet café is now the second most popular place to access the Internet in China, and is gaining in popularity in rural areas, it is certainly possible for the client who does not speak English have access to computer equipment (PIALP, 2010b).

CLINICAL EXAMPLE

You are a nurse at St. Theresa's emergency department. A client is brought in with obvious psychiatric problems. You have no psychiatrist available and the nearest psychiatric facility is a 1-hour drive away in another state. St. Theresa is a Tri-State Health Care Alliance Member. Tri-State has telehealth links with the regional hospital, where a psychiatrist is in the emergency department. What steps would you take to initiate a productive teleconference?

E-Health

The term **e-health** has been commonly used to refer to health information, services, and products provided via the Internet (Oh, Rizo, Enkin, & Jadad, 2005). The definition has been expanded to encompass the technology used for education, research and administration, marketing, and customer service (Harrison & Lee, 2006). The Internet is already used for business transactions, electronic prescriptions, online hospital registration, consumer education and support via websites, information about clinical trials, and communication among professionals. It offers the potential to increase access to health care information, empower consumers, educate practitioners, and transmit information quickly, efficiently, and safely. The eHealth Initiative (Foundation for eHealth Initiative, 2007) is an effort to drive improvement in the quality, safety, and efficiency of health care through information and information technology. This initiative represents multiple stakeholders including health care organizations, providers, consumers, and various vendors. As consumers become empowered to select and impact their own care, e-health is changing the ways the health care industry conducts business as well as the relationships between health care professionals and consumers (Saranto et al., 2006). Internet browsers provide a user-friendly environment that allows users to focus on their needs rather than the technology. The Web provides the framework to expedite the delivery of services and revolutionize the way that care is delivered. Web portals help to create virtual communities both for professionals and consumers. Educated consumers come for treatment armed with knowledge that empowers them and may lead them to question treatment modalities. Full realization of the benefits of e-health requires good strategic planning, financial commitment, redesign of processes, and consideration of regulatory demands, physician acceptance, and adequate data protection. E-health affords the opportunity for providers and insurers to offer new services as well as to use their strengths and bargaining powers to lower costs and increase the efficiency of services delivered. E-care is another term used to refer to the automation of all parts of the care delivery process across administrative, clinical, and departmental boundaries. Examples of e-health include wellness tips found on websites, e-mail reminders of appointments,

follow-up e-mail from health care practitioners to consumer questions, electronic prescriptions, centralized storage of health records on the Web, regional telemedicine networks on the Web, consults, and long-term management of chronically ill clients.

Another major application is electronic submission of claims and payment. Electronic claims submission reduces time and costs for claims submission and results in fewer rejections. The use of electronic prescriptions is another e-health service that ultimately benefits the consumer. Electronic prescriptions eliminate the problem of lost or unreadable prescriptions while providing access to Web-based personal health information, drug interaction warnings, formularies, and verifications that reduce the incidence of medication errors. Handheld prescribing devices facilitate the electronic prescription process. The use of the Web to store health care information makes it available from different locations and to practitioners with different computer systems.

The single largest concern related to the Internet is the quality of online information followed by security of client data, collection of personal information, worries over slowdown, collapse, and the ability to transact business smoothly. Lesser concerns include viral contamination and a lack of adherence to Internet standards among some products.

Ergonomic Considerations

Human factors should be considered in every work environment. **Ergonomics** involves the study and design of a work environment that maximizes productivity by reducing operator fatigue and discomfort. Ergonomics considers physical stresses placed on joints, muscles, nerves, and tendons as well as environmental factors that can affect hearing and vision. Poor arrangement of computer equipment leads to somatic complaints that include headaches, eye strain, irritation, stress, fatigue, and neck and back pain. Two health problems associated with poor ergonomics include computer vision syndrome and repetitive motion disorders.

Computer vision syndrome (CVS) is a term the American Optometric Association (AOA) uses to describe eye and vision problems that result from work done in close proximity such as occurs when using a computer for long periods of time (Anshel, 2006). Eye and vision problems comprise the most frequently reported health problems and do impact productivity. However, they receive less attention than do the musculoskeletal disorders primarily because vision problems are largely symptomatic and are often temporary. CVS symptoms include eyestrain, headaches, blurred distance or near vision, dry or red eyes, neck and/or backache, double vision, and light sensitivity. Poor lighting conditions, poor posture, and existing refractive errors contribute to the development of CVS in up to 90% of all computer workers.

Repetitive motion disorders or *repetitive stress injuries* (RSIs) result from using the same muscle groups over and over again without rest (National Institute of Neurological Disorders and Stroke, 2007). One well-known example of a repetitive motion injury is carpal tunnel syndrome. Carpal tunnel syndrome occurs when the median nerve is compressed as it passes through the wrist along the pathway to the hand. This compression results in sensory and motor changes to the thumb, index finger, third finger, and radial aspect of the ring finger. Other

---

Box 46–7 Measures to Ensure Good Ergonomics When Using a Computer-Work Station

- *Determine how a workstation will be used.* Choose optimal settings for the chair, desk, keyboard, and monitor for the person who will use the area or choose equipment that can easily be adjusted for each user. Adjustments are appropriate when wrists are flat and elbow angle is 90 degrees or more to prevent nerve compression.
- *Determine the length of time the user will be at the workstation.* Individual adjustments are less critical if use is occasional or for very brief periods.
- *Configure work areas for specific types of equipment.* Most workstation desks are designed for PCs rather than notebooks. Notebooks may require a docking station or plug in keyboard and stand to ensure proper monitor and keyboard height.
- *Select sturdy surfaces or furniture with sufficient workspace.* Desks should have room to write and use a mouse.
- *Provide chairs with good lumbar support.* Relaxed sitting requires chairs that allow a reclined posture of 100 to 110 degrees.
- *Educate all workers on the need for good body mechanics when working with computers.* Good posture is essential to reduce physical strain whether the individual works from a standing or sitting position.
- *Position monitors just below eye level approximately one arm's length away.* The monitor should be about 30 inches from eye to screen and 20–40 degrees below the line of sight. This will help to prevent neck strain, especially for bifocal wearers.
- *Adjust screen resolution, font size, and brightness as needed.* Sharp screen images help to reduce eye strain.
- *Periodically look away from the monitor to distant objects.* This helps to avoid eye-focusing problems.
- *Minimize screen glare.* Purchase nonglare monitors or place monitors at right angles to windows. Provide blinds or draperies, or adjust area lighting as needed.
- *Take frequent breaks.* Intersperse computer work with other activities to avoid repetitive stress injuries.
- *Avoid noisy locations.* Noise is distracting and stressful.
- *Place the workstation in a well-ventilated area.* Fresh air and a comfortable temperature enhance working conditions.
- *Use ergonomic devices with caution.* Select items that have been researched. Do not continue use an item if it remains uncomfortable after a trial period. Just because an item carries the label "ergonomic" does not mean that it is beneficial.
- *Use optical prescriptions designed for computer work.* Everyday visual correction does not always work well for extended periods of computer work.
- *Provide lighting that can be adjusted to the needs of the individual.* Older individuals need more light than younger persons to clearly view a task. Too little light contributes to eye fatigue and decreased productivity.

---

repetitive motion injuries may involve the neck and shoulders. Good ergonomics helps to avoid occupational injuries and helps employees maintain productivity. Box 46–7 provides a checklist to ensure good ergonomic design when designing and working at computer workstations; Table 46–1 lists several examples of commercially available ergonomic devices. Some controversy exists regarding the degree to which these devices benefit the user and prevent injury. Young (2006) suggests that organizations provide an area where employees can test ergonomic devices before bulk purchases are made. This would also be helpful for employees who need assistance to adapt to new types of devices (Armbrüster et al., 2007).

TABLE 46–1 Examples of Ergonomic Devices

DEVICE	PURPOSE
Glare filter	Reduces eyestrain related to glare or light reflected from a monitor and may help make images appear sharper and text easier to read
Negative tilt keyboard	Tilts away from the user with the keyboard below elbow height to allow the user to rest arms, shoulders, neck, and back during pauses in typing
Document holder	Keeps documents at the same height and distance from the user as the monitor, limiting head and neck movement and tension
Ergonomic mouse	Various designs which aim to reduce wrist and hand pain
	No consistent research findings to support its use
Lumbar support	Maintains the natural curves of the back, minimizing back pain
Wrist rests	May actually increase carpal tunnel pressure unless a broad, flat, firm surface provides a place to rest the palm, not the wrist
Support braces/gloves	May relieve carpal tunnel symptoms when worn at night
	There are no consistent research findings to support use while typing
Ergonomic keyboards	Split keyboard designed to improve posture
	Research fails to support the benefit of this device
Foot rest	Encourages proper posture and supports the lower back to keep the pelvis properly tilted

REVIEW Informatics

RELATE: LINK THE CONCEPTS

As a nurse working for a home care agency in a small, rural town, you would like your clients to receive up-to-date and accurate health information and care. High-speed computer access is available in your office, and many of the residents have computers in their homes since it provides a low-cost way of communicating with friends and relatives who are far away (for example, using e-mail and sending digitized photos). You have a difficult clinical case and want to investigate possible interventions. You decide that sending photos of the client would be useful to your colleagues in providing input. Since time is an issue, you determine that sending them electronically would be most expeditious. The client agrees to the photos but is worried about privacy in sending them through the computer.

Linking the concept of Informatics with the concept of Legal issues:
1. How would you address your client's concerns?
2. Are there any legal considerations?

REFER: GO TO MYNURSINGKIT

REFLECT: CASE STUDY

Agnes Gibbons was admitted through the hospital's emergency department in congestive heart failure. During her admission she was asked to verbally acknowledge whether her demographic data were correct. Ms. Gibbons did so. Extensive diagnostic tests were done, including radiology studies. It was later discovered that all of Ms. Gibbons' information had been entered into another client's file.

1. How would you correct this situation?
2. What departments or other agencies would need to be informed of this situation?
3. How can informatics keep an incident like this from occurring again?

46.1 CLINICAL DECISION SUPPORT SYSTEMS

KEY TERMS

Clinical decision support (CDS), *2385*
Evidence-based practice, *2386*
Expert systems, *2385*

BASIS FOR SELECTION OF EXEMPLAR

Agency for Health Care Research and Quality

Institute for Healthcare Improvement

Institute of Medicine

NLN Competencies

LEARNING OUTCOMES

After reading about this exemplar, you will be able to:

1. Explain the purpose of clinical decision support and expert systems.
2. Describe the importance of a uniform nursing language.
3. List ways that computers and informatics support evidence-based practice and the research process.
4. Discuss advantages of computerized literature searches over manual methods.
5. Identify the role of computers in each step of the research process.
6. Summarize ways computers may be used by nurse administrators in the areas of human resources, facilities management, finance, quality assurance, and accreditation.
7. Evaluate the quality of a health information website.

OVERVIEW

Clinical decision support (CDS) describes a system that provides health care providers with knowledge or specific information that is intelligently filtered, presented at appropriate times, and that enhances health and health care (Kawamioto & Lobch, 2007; Mangalampalli et al., 2006; Osheroff et al., 2007). Decision support systems aid in and strengthen the selection of viable options for care using the information of an organization. Decision support software organizes information to provide analysis and advice to support a choice; the final decision rests with the practitioner. Tools may include clinical practice guidelines, alerts and reminders, order sets, client data reports and dashboards, diagnostic support, workflow tools, and financial applications. Computerized provider order entry (CPOE) with CDS has been show to decrease medication errors by as much as 80 percent (Knowles, Cornish, & Etchells, 2006).

An example of a decision support application is a program that assists nurses performing a skin assessment. The program provides a review available alternatives, from which the best option for maintaining skin integrity may be selected. CDS is best used when available at the point of care. Access is facilitated through the use of wireless devices such as PDAs, tablet computers, and iPhones. These devices may be easily transported by the health care provider to the point of care. While CDS has been proven effective in improving outcomes at many sites, it is not universally available or available at the same level at all locations (Simon, Rundall, & Shortell, 2007). The American Medical Informatics Association has presented a roadmap for national action that calls for improved CDS capabilities and increased used throughout the U.S. health care industry. The financial benefits that result from improved client outcomes are expected to motivate health care organizations to increase adoption of order entry with CDS.

Expert systems use artificial intelligence to model a decision that experts in the field would make. Unlike decision support systems that provide several options from which the user may choose, expert systems provide the best decision based on criteria that experts would use. For example, a nurse enters data and is provided a list of nursing diagnoses. The nurse then selects which diagnoses to accept or reject, and is given a list of associated signs and symptoms. If the nurse accepts the diagnoses based on comparison to actual client data, the next screen will show potential etiologies and so on.

THE ROLE OF UNIFORM LANGUAGES

A standardized nursing language facilitates data collection and allows accurate communication among nurses. This improves decision making, aids research, and subsequently adds to the body of nursing knowledge. The American Nurses' Association (ANA) (2007) has recognized several standardized languages and terminologies to support nursing practice. These include:

- NANDA
- The Nursing Interventions Classification (NIC)
- The Nursing Outcomes Classification (NOC)
- The Clinical Care Classification (CCC), an interface terminology that contains diagnoses, interventions, and outcomes for use in home care
- The Home Health Care Classification (HHCC)
- The Omaha System for capturing community health information
- The Nursing Minimum Data Set (NMDS), which contains clinical data elements
- Nursing Management Minimum Data Set (NMMDS), which contains nursing administrative data elements
- The Patient Care Data Set (PCDS), which has since been retired from use
- The PeriOperative Nursing Data Set (PNDS), a set of diagnoses, interventions, and outcomes for the perioperative area
- ABC codes (Alternative Billing Concept codes) for use of interventions in nursing and other areas
- Logical Observation Identifiers Names and Codes (LOINC®) for use of outcome and assessments
- The Systematic Nomenclature of Medicine Clinical Terms (SNOMED CT®)
- The International Classification for Nursing Practice (ICNP®), which addresses diagnoses, interventions, and outcomes for all of nursing.

In addition to facilitating data collection, uniform languages set the definition of key terms, ensuring that studies can be replicated. Implementation of uniform languages first requires the following:

- Education of staff who are unfamiliar with standardized terms
- Elimination of computer restraints, such as limited characters and lines per field, a common problem among some computer systems
- Database coordination among various health care providers and departments that use terms differently but require access to shared data repositories. This is also known as mapping terms.

UTILIZING RESEARCH

At present there is a gap between theory and practice that results in diminished client care, inefficient practice, and an excessive time lag between the discovery of knowledge and its incorporation into clinical practice (Salmond, 2007). The landmark Institute of Medicine (IOM) (2001) report, *Crossing the Quality Chasm*, called for the implementation of evidence-based practice as a means to improve the quality of care. Evidence-based practice is applicable to all health care disciplines and it contributes to the evolution of nursing as a profession (Courey, Benson-Soros, Deemer, & Zeller, 2006). There is widespread recognition that evidence-based practice is essential to transform health care by providing proven effective treatments.

Evidence-based practice (EBP) is an approach to providing care that integrates nursing experience and intuition with valid and current clinical research to achieve best client outcomes (Dracup & Bryan-Brown, 2006; Drenning, 2006; Hanberg & Brown, 2006; Salmond, 2007). Sigma Theta Tau International (STTI), the Honor Society of Nursing, defines evidence-based practice as "an integration of the best evidence available, nursing expertise, and the values and preferences of the individuals, families and communities who are served" (STTI, 2005). EBP entails development of best practices based on outcomes and the ability of nurses to access and evaluate current professional literature found both in print and online sources. For information on the process of evidence-based practice, see Concept 43.

EBP advances client health and safety by ensuring the provision of quality care based on systematic examination of the scientific literature. EBP is reported to contribute to increased job satisfaction and vitality because it increases the confidence and self-esteem of nurses and other health care providers (Hockenberry, Wilson, & Barrera, 2006). Evidence-based practice provides a mechanism for hospitals and other health care delivery systems to meet research and excellence requirements inherent in the American Association of Colleges of Nursing (AACN) Magnet designation (Shirey, 2006).

COMPUTERS IN NURSING RESEARCH

Computers are invaluable assistants in the conduct of both quantitative and qualitative nursing research. In each step of the research process, computers facilitate generation, refinement, analysis, and output of data. Computer resources are an important component of the planning phase of any research project: The size of the computer and its storage capacity must be adequate for the amount of data that will be collected, and the proper software programs must be in place to manage and analyze the data. Computerized word processing is also an integral component in the publication and dissemination of research. Common computer applications that support evidence-based practice and research can be found in Box 46–8.

Problem Identification

The first step of the research process is to identify and describe the problem of interest. The computer can be useful in locating current literature about the problem and related concepts. Perhaps, unknown to the researcher, a solution to the problem has already been found and reported. A search of existing documents, and e-mail to colleagues, may help define the problem.

Box 46–8 Common Computer Applications Supporting Evidenced-Based Practice and Research

- *Topic identification or searchable questions.* Online literature searches, research reports, e-mail, online communities, and discussion groups can be used to identify areas in need of research.
- *Online literature and database searches.* Electronic searches enable the researcher to identify systematic reviews, prior research in an area as well as articles pertaining to the theoretical framework for proposed studies.
- *Full text retrieval of articles.* This eliminates the need to physically locate journals and photocopy them.
- *Development of resource files.* Computer files replace handwritten and may be searched quickly, allowing researchers to spend valuable time performing research and writing reports instead of performing clerical tasks.
- *Selection or development and revision of a data collection tool.* Online literature searches help researchers locate developed data collection tools. If no suitable tool is found, researchers can develop their own tool using a word processing package and trial it by sending it out via e-mail or the Web.
- *Preparation of the grant/study proposal.* Word processing aids the writing process because revisions can be made quickly.
- *Budget preparation and maintenance.* Spreadsheets and financial planning software assist with this process.
- *Determination of appropriate sample size.* The ability to generalize study findings is related to the size of the sample. Power analysis is the process by which an appropriate sample size may be determined. Software is available for this purpose.
- *Data collection.* Computers aid in the collection of data in several ways. Data may be input into a computer through scanned questionnaires, direct entry of field observations, or the use of an online data collection tool. PDAs and notebook computers aid on-site entry of data eliminating note and paper tools (Hanberg & Brown, 2006).
- *Database utilization.* Databases allow organization and manipulation of collected data.
- *Statistical analysis/qualitative text analysis.* Statistical analysis software performs complex computations, while qualitative text analysis allows searches for particular words and phrases in text, noting frequency of appearance and context.
- *Preparation of the research findings for report.* Word processing and graphics programs enable researchers to present their findings without the need for clerical assistance or graphic artists.
- *Bibliographic database managers (BDMs).* This type of software aids the preparation of publications through the importation of references from literature databases without the need to rekey and format citations and reference lists according to the style selected.
- *Electronic dissemination of findings.* Online Journals, Web pages, and e-mail permit researchers to share their findings quickly. This contrasts with the traditional publication of study findings in print media that might take a year or more from the time of submission until distribution.

Literature Review

An exhaustive review of the literature can be time consuming. Without computer access to online or CD-ROM bibliographic databases, the researcher must wade through huge volumes of publications. The software programs that facilitate searches contain thesauruses so that the most appropriate terms can be selected. If the researcher determines that little has been published on the topic of interest, closely related terms and topics must also be searched. It is not unusual for a researcher to collect more than 100 pertinent research or theoretical references during the literature review. The increase in availability of full-text journal articles online has made the electronic literature search process even more productive.

Research Design

The design of a research study, including the choice of specific research method, is always driven by the research question. At the design stage the investigator determines whether the study will use a qualitative or quantitative approach, what instruments will be used to collect data, and the types of analyses that will be carried out on the data to answer the research questions. Computers may be used during this step to search the literature for instruments that have already been established or to design and test instruments that need to be developed for the particular study. In addition, the investigator would not likely select an instrument or design that requires extensive computer or mathematical analysis if such resources are not available.

Data Collection and Analysis

Once the types of data to be collected have been determined, the investigator will create forms on the computer for collecting the data. These may include the informed consent document, a tool to collect demographic data, and recording forms for research variables.

Research Dissemination

Research is of limited value if the findings are not widely dispersed to those health care providers who can use the findings to improve their practice. Computer word processing programs are used to author the final reports of research and to send the reports to various readerships. Many journals now require that manuscripts submitted for publication include both hardcopy and electronic versions; some require only an electronic version. As noted earlier in this concept, the number of electronic journals is increasing. Computers speed completion of a research project and the availability of the findings to the public. Computers are frequently used to present research at meetings. Using computer projectors to display screens of data and findings also allows the researcher to highlight, modify, and manipulate content in an instant. Computer conferencing, where researchers collaborate on a study from distant locations and can examine and analyze the data simultaneously on screen, is gaining in popularity.

RESEARCH ON THE WEB The expansion of guidelines for the ethical development of Internet sites has been ongoing since 1996, when Health on the Net Foundation (HON) became one of the very first websites to guide both clients and medical professionals to reliable sources of health care information on the Internet. HON's standards hold website developers to basic ethical standards in the presentation of information. The American Accreditation Healthcare Commission (2001) is also developing an accrediting process for health care websites. Tens of thousands of health-related websites exist, many new ones appearing and others becoming "dead links" daily. No standardized controls exist to ensure that the information provided is current or accurate. Nurses should evaluate health websites as they access them and assist clients in doing the same. Tools for doing this include (as of this publication) *Evaluating Internet Resources* from the State University of New York at Albany and *Criteria for Assessing the Quality of Health Information on the Internet—Policy Paper* from the Health Information Technology Institute of Mitretek Systems Health Summit Working Group (Box 46–9).

COMPUTERS IN NURSING ADMINISTRATION

The volume of data that nurses need to have available and the additional volume of data generated by nurses can and must be managed electronically. Nursing administrators require these data to develop strategic plans for the organization.

Human Resources

All employers must maintain a database, computerized or not, on each employee. In addition to the usual demographic and salary data, a database for licensed or certified health care personnel has unique fields for areas such as life support certification, health requirements (e.g., tuberculosis testing, hepatitis immunization, rubella titers), and performance appraisals. Administrators can use this human resources database to communicate with employees, examine staffing patterns, and create budget projections.

Medical Records Management

Costs are inherent in and reflected by medical records. It is expensive to keep records, but it is even more expensive not to be able to access them. Therefore, nurses require computer programs that allow client records to be searched for trends such as the most common presenting diagnoses, number of cases by diagnosis-related groups, most expensive cases, length of stay or total number of days the case was open, and client outcomes. Nurse informaticists can assist administrators with the design and implementation of systems that allow for such searches to be generated, analyzed, printed, and distributed.

Facilities Management

Many aspects of managing buildings and non-nursing services can be facilitated by computer. Heating, air conditioning, ventilation, and alarm systems are computer controlled. Security devices such as readers that scan identification cards, bar codes, or magnetic strips permit only authorized personnel to enter client or private areas. Computers also manage and report inventory, tracking everything from pillowcases to syringes.

Budget and Finance

Advantages of computerized billing are that claims are transmitted much more quickly and have a greater likelihood of being complete and accurate compared to handwritten documents. If this is the case, claims will be paid sooner and the agency will have better control over its financial status. Computers can also affect cost savings by reducing the clerical services time needed for accounts payable and receivable. In cases where nursing can directly bill and be reimbursed by payers, the same benefits of computerized accounting apply. The budget itself is generally a spreadsheet program. This software allows tracking as well as forecasting and planning. In uncertain times, the ability to perform "what if" calculations is especially valuable.

Quality Assurance and Utilization Reviews

Both internal and external stakeholders in health care organizations need to know that the services and activities of the organization have positive results. Once standards, pathways, key indicators, and other vital data have been identified and described, computers can facilitate the accumulation of data for individuals and groups of clients and analysis of the data. Quality is considered a process and not an end point. Applying this perspective, computerized systems are ideal for taking a snapshot view of the institution's quality indices at any time. Utilization review consists of examining trends and proposing advantageous disposition of resources (specifically, length of stay). For example, might clients who have had a fractured hip repaired have equivalent outcomes at lesser cost if transferred from the hospital to a skilled nursing facility sooner? Studies can be conducted with computer analyses to answer such questions.

Accreditation

The Joint Commission has mandated that hospitals have online mechanisms to monitor quality indicators, so as to reduce the difficulty and time involved in the accreditation process. Health care agencies must maintain databases of

policies and procedures, standards of care, and employee accomplishment of Joint Commission requirements such as continuing education and in-service trainings. The Joint Commission has also required a move to computer systems that assess outcomes rather than processes. Another aspect of accreditation review is demonstrating adequate staffing for the number and acuity of clients. Each agency, whether hospital, outpatient, or home care, must use a method of determining the number of hours of nursing care required for its current clients. This method can consider the severity of the clients' illnesses, length of time needed to perform certain procedures, training and expertise of the nursing staff, and any other parameters desired.

REVIEW Clinical Decision Support Systems

RELATE: LINK THE CONCEPTS

You are the staff nurse in a busy medical–surgical department at your community hospital. You and several of your colleagues believe that client anxiety has decreased in direct proportion to the amount of preoperative teaching that has been received.

Linking the exemplar of Clinical Decision Support Systems with the concept of Clinical Decision Making:
1. How would you go about researching this issue?
2. How would the findings support increased use of informatics in the work place?

REFER: GO TO MYNURSINGKIT

REFLECT: CASE STUDY

You are working the night shift at your local community hospital. Mrs. Prado, one of your clients, is newly diagnosed with a rare disorder that is unknown to you and your peers. Mrs. Prado is unable to sleep and is asking for more information about her diagnosis; she says she found a website that claims to have a cure for her disorder. Your unit has an Internet connection.
1. How would you respond?
2. How would you evaluate the quality of the information?

46.2 INDIVIDUAL INFORMATION AT POINT OF CARE

KEY TERMS

Electronic medical record, 2390
Nurse informaticist, 2391
Personal health information, 2391
Point of care, 2389

BASIS FOR SELECTION OF EXEMPLAR

Agency for Health Care Research and Quality
Institute for Healthcare Improvement
Institute of Medicine
NLN Competencies

LEARNING OUTCOMES

After reading about this exemplar, you will be able to:
1. Contrast the advantages and concerns of computer-based medical records.
2. Discuss HIPAA as it relates to electronic medical records at point of care.
3. Describe the uses of technology at point of care.

OVERVIEW

How might a computer assist individual nurses with their daily activities? Consider that the nurse providing client care may spend as much as one-third of the time recording data in the client's record. The nurse spends additional time trying to access data about the client that may be somewhere in the medical record or elsewhere in the health care agency.

There are several different types of computerized bedside data entry systems. These allow recording of client assessments, medication administration (Figure 46–4 ■),

progress notes, care plan updating, client acuity, and accrued charges. The terminal can be fixed and hardwired to the central system or cordless and handheld. In either case, the system may have the ability to transmit the data to distant sites. A slightly different type of bedside terminal is the **point-of-care** or point-of-service computer. In this case, the terminal is located near, but not necessarily at, the client. Point-of-care devices located at or near the site of client care can save time and promote efficiency (see the Evidence-Based Practice feature).

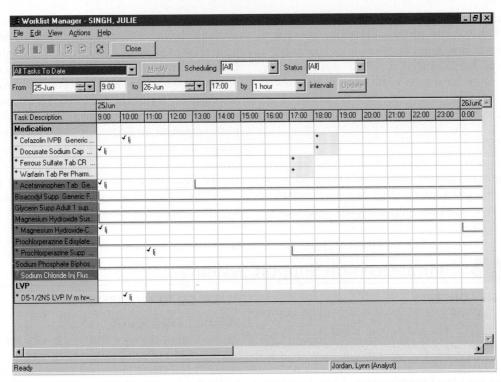

Figure 46-4 ■ This screen shows a MAR (medication administration record) for several regularly scheduled medications. The worksheet displays the next time the medications are scheduled to be administered.

Courtesy of Sutter Health.

> ### EVIDENCE-BASED PRACTICE   Does Point-of-Care Nursing Documentation Make a Difference?
>
> This article reports on five research studies aimed at determining whether or not bedside electronic charting made a difference in quality of documentation and nurses' satisfaction. The studies were diverse, ranging from a pilot examination of functionality, usefulness, and acceptability to a large chart review of compliance with accreditation charting standards. In each case, results indicated that electronic charting improved compliance with documentation standards. Time spent charting was decreased and nurse satisfaction increased. It should be recognized that these were early studies and resistance to change may influence reproducibility of the magnitude of the results in larger institutions.
>
> **Implications**
> Novel approaches to charting that reduce the time and effort of recording will likely be of broad interest to nurses. Anything that allows more time to be spent with clients and enhances the ease of documentation—especially the more routine and standard reports required—is a positive move. However, it is far too early to have complete confidence that satisfaction with electronic bedside charting will be maintained over time as the novelty wears off. Institutions are spending many dollars on new computer charting systems. At the minimum, the cost is well spent even if only for the consistency of charting and the ability to mine the data for outcomes assessment and quality improvement. However, much more research on the effects of online charting is needed.
>
> *Note:* From Langowski, C. (2005). The times they are a changing: Effects of online nursing documentation systems. *Quality Management in Health Care, 14,* 121–125.

COMPUTER-BASED CLIENT RECORDS

The **electronic medical record** permits electronic client data retrieval by caregivers, administrators, accrediting organizations, and other persons who require the data. The Computer-Based Patient Record Institute, established in 1992, identified four ways the EMR could improve health care: (a) constant availability of client health information across the life span, (b) ability to monitor quality, (c) access to warehoused (stored) data, and (d) ability for clients to share in knowledge and activities influencing their own health. Because of the way computers provide access to the EMR, providers easily retrieve specific

data such as trends in vital signs (Figure 46–5 ■), immunization records, and current problems. The system can be designed to warn providers about conflicting medications or client parameters that indicate dangerous conditions (Figure 46–6 ■). Sophisticated systems allow replay of audio, graphic, or video data for comparison with current status. All text is legible and can be searched for keywords.

There are several areas of concern with EMRs. Maintaining privacy and security of data is a significant issue. One way that computers can protect data is by user authentication via passwords or biometric identifiers (e.g., fingerprint

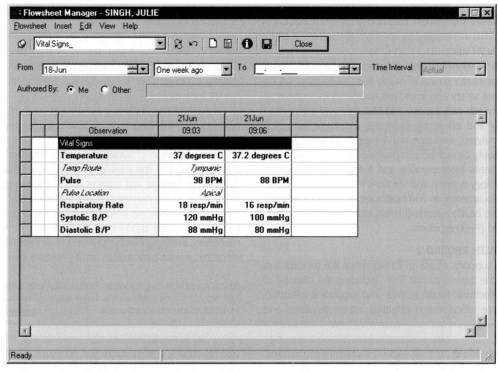

Figure 46–5 ■ This screen displays the client's vital signs. They can be entered by the nurse (or anyone with the security rights to do so) at the bedside, and they can then be displayed wherever needed.

Courtesy of Sutter Health.

or retinal scans)—only those persons who have a legitimate need to access the data receive the password. Additional policies and procedures for protecting the confidentiality of EMRs are evolving as the use of computer systems becomes more widespread. Following several previous reports, the ANA developed a position statement on privacy, confidentiality of medical records, and the nurse's role (Box 46–10). One role of the **nurse informaticist**, an expert who combines computer, information, and nursing science, is to develop policies and procedures that promote effective and secure use of computerized records by nurses and other health care professionals.

Prior to The Health Insurance Portability and Accountability Act of 1996 (HIPAA), there were no national standards for

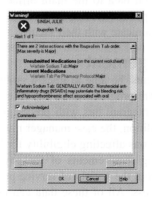

Figure 46–6 ■ One of the strengths of an electronic medical record is its ability to alert the clinician to potential drug interactions using warnings like the one displayed.

Courtesy of Sutter Health.

EMRs: not for the specific data that should be included nor for how the record should be organized. Nurses need to be involved in the design, implementation, and evaluation of EMRs to maximize their use and effectiveness.

HIPAA established legal requirements for the protection, security, and appropriate sharing of client **personal health information** (referred to as protected health information or PHI) through the following objectives (Haramboure, 1999; Hellerstein, 2000):

- To ensure the portability of health insurance
- To prevent health care fraud and abuse
- To ensure the security and privacy of health information
- To enforce health information standards that will improve the efficiency of health care delivery, simplify the exchange of data between health care entities, and reduce cost
- To reduce the paperwork associated with processing health care transactions.

Because PHI is now stored electronically, HIPAA regulations have mandated strict control over access and communication of HIS data. Each health care agency in which nurses work will orient them to the specific technological controls in place. The HIPAA privacy rule affects all organizations and individuals involved in the delivery of health care. Organizations, including hospitals, physician offices, home health agencies, and nursing homes and all individual clinicians, instructors, students, and volunteers, now have additional responsibilities and must examine current policies and practices to comply with the provisions of this legislation. Also affected are payers, employers, data services, clearinghouses, regulatory agencies, and information system vendors, Medicare, and Medicaid.

The nurse should consider the client's cultural and spiritual preferences when asking clients to make decisions about a procedure or treatment. For example, informed consent in the United States is based on the principle of autonomy—that is, each person has the right to make his or her own decisions regarding treatment, provided that he or she is conscious or competent to do so. In contrast to this individual perspective, people from other cultures (e.g., Southeast Asians and Native Americans) may have a group perspective regarding decision making. These clients may believe that another member of their family or group or tribe should make the decision. Although legally the client is the only person who has the authority to give consent, the nurse can provide culturally competent care by asking the client if he or she would like to have a family member or spiritual leader present during discussions regarding health care treatment.

indicates participation in the care or nonverbally takes actions that are consistent with the care. For example, clients who position their bodies for an injection or cooperate with the taking of vital signs infer implied consent.

COMPETENCY FOR CONSENT Competency is a legal presumption applied to individuals when they become adults. Competency gives adults the right to negotiate certain legal activities, such as making a will or entering into a contract. In most states, a person is considered to be competent at 18 years of age unless some evidence to the contrary persuades a court to declare that person incompetent.

Adults who have been declared legally incompetent through a court order are provided a legal guardian. The legal guardian will know to provide a copy of the court order giving him or her the authority to make health care decision on the other adult's behalf. Examples of adults who may be legally incompetent include those who have suffered a debilitating brain injury as a result of a motor vehicle accident and those who have profound intellectual disability.

An adult may be rendered temporarily incompetent by narcotic medication or accident, or an adult may gradually be rendered incompetent as a result of dementia. The nurse who has concerns about a client's level of competency should alert the primary care provider. If the primary care provider determines the client is not competent for the purposes of informed consent, he or she will determine if the emergency doctrine (see Consent in an Emergency) applies or if someone else can validly make health care decisions on the client's behalf. State laws regarding consent for adults who are rendered temporarily incompetent vary. Courts generally presume continuing competency of adults unless the health care facility can show the client is unable to understand the consequences of his or her actions (Guido, 2010). All health care staff, including nurses, should be familiar with their state's laws and with the policies and procedures of their employing agency. Nurses should recognize the effect of issues related to competency on providing nursing care, as the client has the right to decline nursing care as well as medical procedures.

CONSENT IN AN EMERGENCY In most states, the law assumes a person's consent to medical treatment when he or she is in imminent danger of loss of life or limb and unable to give informed consent. In other words, the emergency doctrine assumes that the person would reasonably consent to treatment if able to do so. This doctrine serves as a guiding principle that permits health care providers to perform potentially life-saving procedures under circumstances that make it is impossible or impractical to obtain consent. The emergency doctrine may not always apply. For example, it does not extend to allowing health care providers to implement a treatment or procedure to which the client would not reasonably consent if the client were able to do so. It also does not permit health care providers to provide a treatment or procedure which the client previously refused. For example, if a client has previously refused a procedure on religious grounds, health care providers may not implement the procedure if the client becomes unconscious. State laws provide for protection from liability for failure to obtain informed consent (Hartman, 1999).

CHILD PARTICIPATION IN HEALTH CARE DECISIONS For a minor child (under age 18), a parent or guardian must give informed consent for medical treatment. Specific legal exceptions do exist, however, including when the emergency doctrine applies; the child is an *emancipated minor* (one who is no longer under parental control and manages his or her own financial affairs); the child is a resident of a state that allows a *mature minor* to give valid consent (for example, 14- and 15-year-old adolescents who are able to understand treatment risks); a court order to proceed with treatment exists; or the law recognizes the minor as having the ability to consent to a specific treatment. In the majority of states, a minor who is the parent of a child may give informed consent for health care treatment of the child. Some states also permit teenagers of a certain age who are seeking certain types of care to do so without parental consent. Types of care that may not require parental permission include birth control, prenatal care, mental health counseling, diagnosis and treatment of sexually transmitted disease, and treatment of substance abuse (Anderson, Schaechter, & Brosco, 2005).

Mature minors are permitted in some states to give consent for treatment or to refuse treatment. In some cases, the minor must convince a judge that he or she is mature enough to make an independent judgment about consent for treatment. Nurses need to know the state and federal laws regarding consent as well as the agency's policies and procedures regarding informed consent. North Carolina law, for example, provides for all minors over the age of 12 to consent for contraceptive services, treatment of sexually transmitted diseases, and prenatal care. For an overview of minor consent laws in the United States, see Box 47–4.

CLINICAL EXAMPLE

Marvin, a 15-year-old boy with acute myelocytic leukemia, has come out of his second remission with an acute onset of fever, joint pain, and petechiae (Figure 47–2 ■). A bone marrow transplant is one of the few remaining therapeutic options. Although Marvin has agreed to a transplant if a suitable donor is found, he does not want to be resuscitated and placed on life-support equipment should he have a cardiac arrest. He has talked extensively with the hospital chaplain and social worker and feels comfortable with his decision. His parents want an all-out effort to sustain his life until a donor is located.

1. At what age can children make an informed decision about whether to accept or refuse treatment?
2. What happens when parents and children have conflicting opinions about treatment?

Controlled Substance Act

The **Controlled Substance Act (CSA)** is a federal law that requires drugs be classified based on the substance's medical use, potential for abuse, and safety risks. The classifications are referred to as Schedules and are numbered from I to V, with Schedules I and II having the highest potential for abuse (see Table 47–2). The CSA is enforced by the U.S. Drug Enforcement Agency, which regulates a closed system of distribution. This system provides for registration with unique identifiers for legitimate handlers of controlled substances and required record keeping that traces the flow of any drug from the time it is first imported or manufactured, through the distribution level, to the

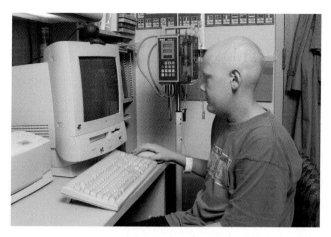

Figure 47–2 ■ Marvin, a 15-year-old with acute myelocytic leukemia.

pharmacy or hospital that dispenses it, and then to the actual client who receives it.

Good Samaritan Laws

Most states have **Good Samaritan laws** that encourage health care providers to help victims in an emergency. These laws are designed to protect the health care worker from potential liability when volunteering his or her skills outside of an employment contract. Nurses should review the Nurse Practice Act and the Good Samaritan Act in the state in which they work before volunteering their skills. To be protected by the Good Samaritan laws, the nurse must adhere to the standard of nursing care during all volunteer activities. The nurse should provide only care that is consistent with his or her level of training and licensure. Once the decision to render emergency care is made, the nurse is responsible for following through by providing the necessary care or safely placing the victim in the care of someone who can provide the appropriate care (Brooke, 2003).

Box 47–4 **Overview of Minor Consent Laws**

CONTRACEPTIVE SERVICES
Twenty-six states and the District of Columbia allow all minors (age 12 years and older) to consent to contraceptive services. Twenty-one states allow only certain categories of minors to consent to contraceptive services.

SEXUALLY TRANSMITTED INFECTIONS SERVICES
All states and the District of Columbia allow all minors to consent to services for sexually transmitted diseases.

PRENATAL CARE
Thirty-two states and the District of Columbia explicitly allow all minors to consent to prenatal care.

ADOPTION
Twenty-eight states and the District of Columbia allow all minor parents to choose to place their child for adoption.

MEDICAL CARE FOR A CHILD
Thirty states and the District of Columbia allow all minor parents to consent to medical care for their child. The remaining 20 states have no relevant explicit policy or case law.

ABORTION
Three states and the District of Columbia explicitly allow all minors to consent to abortion services. Twenty-two states require that at least one parent consent to a minor's request for an abortion, while 11 states require prior notification of at least one parent.

Source: Adapted from Guttmacher Institute. (2010). *An overview of minors' consent law.* Retrieved January 8, 2010, from http://www.guttmacher.org/statecenter/spibs/spib_OMCL.pdf

TABLE 47–2 U.S. Drug Schedules and Examples

DEPENDENCY POTENTIAL

DRUG SCHEDULE	ABUSE POTENTIAL	PHYSICAL DEPENDENCE	PSYCHOLOGICAL DEPENDENCE	EXAMPLES	THERAPEUTIC USE
I	Highest	High	High	Heroin, lysergic acid diethylamide (LSD), marijuana, and methaqualone	Limited or no therapeutic use
II	High	High	High	Morphine, phencyclidine (PCP), cocaine, methadone, and methamphetamine	Used therapeutically with prescription; some drugs no longer used
III	Moderate	Moderate	High	Anabolic steroids, codeine and hydrocodone with aspirin or Tylenol, and some barbiturates	Used therapeutically with prescription
IV	Lower	Lower	Lower	Dextropropoxyphene, pentazocine, meprobamate, diazepam, alprazolam	Used therapeutically with prescription
V	Lowest	Lowest	Lowest	OTC cough medicines with codeine	Used therapeutically without prescription

Box 47–5 Where to Go for Additional Information

REGULATION/ORGANIZATIONS (WITH RESEARCH LINKS)
NCSBN National Council State Boards of Nursing
http://www.ncsbn.org
State Boards of Nursing (contact information)
https//www.ncsbn.org/515.htm
National Nursing student's Association
http://www.nsna.org/
National Practitioner Data Bank
http://www.npdb-hipdb.hrsa.gov/

ADVANCE DIRECTIVES
Partnership for Caring
1620 Eye St. NW, Suite 202
Washington, DC 20007

1-800-658-8898
http://www.partnershipforcaring.org
Health in Aging Organization
http://www.nia.nih.gov/HealthInformation/ResourceDirectory.htm

CONTROLLED SUBSTANCE ACT
http://www.usdoj.gov/dea/pubs/csa.html

WHISTLEBLOWING
osha.gov/dep/oia/whistleblower

CREDENTIALING
http://www.nursingworld.org/MainMenuCategories/
CertificationandAccreditation/Certification.aspx

CONCLUSION

From medication administration to licensure requirements, the number of laws that impact nurses can be overwhelming. Nurses must rely on continuing education, workplace policies and procedures, state regulatory agencies, and professional organizations for information regarding changes in laws and requirements. Failure to keep up with changes in laws and regulations can endanger the client and place the nurse at risk for liability.

Box 47–5 provides links to organizations and websites with more information on various laws and regulations that impact nurses.

47.1 NURSE PRACTICE ACTS

OVERVIEW

The practice of nursing is regulated at the state level through a **nurse practice act (NPA)**. An NPA is a series of state statutes that define the scope of practice, standards for education programs, licensure requirements, and grounds for disciplinary actions. The law provides a framework for establishing nursing actions in the care of clients (Box 47–6). Laws set the boundaries for and maintain a standard of nursing practice (Figure 47–3 ■). For the registered nurse (RN), the provisions of the NPAs are quite similar from state to state. Greater variation exists in the scope of practice for the licensed practical nurse (LPN)/licensed vocation nurse (LVN). The nurse is held accountable to the specific standards for licensure and grounds for revocation in the state of employment.

Each state's NPA is enforced and administered by a state board of nursing (BON), though some states use other titles for this regulatory board. BONs were established some 100 years ago to standardize the education of nurses, establish standards for safe nursing practice, and issue licenses in order to protect the public from unprepared, unsafe practitioners. BONs have since

Box 47–6 **Anatomy of a Nurse Practice Act (NPA)**

Typically, the following components are addressed in an NPA. Each nursing student and practicing nurse should understand his or her state's NPA and how each component of the NPA affects practice. Components of an NPA include the following:

- Definition of nursing
- Requirements for licensure
- Penalty for practicing without a license
- Exemptions from licensure
- Licensure across jurisdictions.

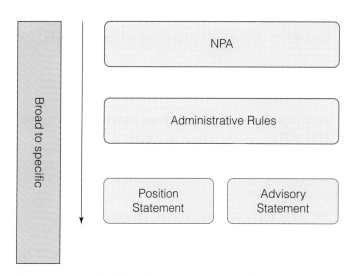

Figure 47–3 ■ Relationship among the Nursing Practice Act, Administrative Rules, and position/advisory statements.

expanded their functions to include activities such as programs for impaired nurses, remediation of practice issues, and participation in multistate licensure compacts. To achieve their mission of protecting the public health, BONs also serve as a forum for citizen complaints about nursing services and against individual nurses.

The members of the board of nursing are appointed according to the regulations in each state with the exception of North Carolina. North Carolina is the only state where licensed nurses serving on the board are elected by other licensed nurses, and members of the public who serve are appointed. The state's NPA dictates the membership of the state's BON, which usually includes a mix of RNs, LPNs/LVNs, advanced practice registered nurses (APRNs), and consumers.

LICENSURE

Licensure allows a nurse the legal privilege to practice nursing as defined in each state's NPA. Through the process of licensure, the BON ensures minimum standards of competency to provide safe nursing care to the public. Typically, BONs oversee licensure through the following activities:

- Establishing and monitoring educational standards for nursing education programs
- Defining professional standards
- Examining and renewing the licenses of duly qualified applicants
- Investigating violations of the NPA
- Sanctioning (to the point of initiating prosecution against) those who violate the NPA
- Holding disciplinary hearings for possible suspension or revocation of a license
- Establishing and overseeing diversity programs in some states.

Each BON oversees the administration of a licensure examination that measures the competencies needed to perform safely and effectively as a newly licensed, entry-level nurse. The National Council of State Boards of Nursing (NCSBN, 2010) has developed two licensure examinations, the National Council Licensure Examination for Registered Nurses (NCLEX-RN®) and the National Council Licensure Examination for Practical Nurses (NCLEX-PN®), for state and territory BONs to implement as part of their requirements for licensure.

Licenses are issued by the state or territory in which the applicant nurse wishes to practice. For licensed nurses at all levels of practice, the BON monitors compliance with state laws, including maintaining continuing competency and annual renewal of licensure. To maintain the privilege to practice afforded by the license, the individual nurse is required to demonstrate awareness and application of standards of nursing care and meet his or her responsibilities to both clients and the health care system. The board is also responsible for taking action against those nurses who have exhibited unsafe nursing practice or otherwise engaged in professional misconduct or who fail meet requirements for licensure renewal.

Each BON details what charges of professional misconduct may result in the revocation or suspension of a nurse's license. Typically, most BONs will take action against the nurse who is found guilty of charges that include the following:

- Giving false information or withholding material information from the board in procuring or attempting to procure a license to practice nursing.
- Being convicted of or pleading either guilty or nolo contendere to any crime that indicates the nurse is unfit or incompetent to practice or has deceived or defrauded the public. If a defendant pleads **nolo contendere**, the individual neither admits nor denies that he or she has committed the crime but agrees to a punishment (usually a fine or jail time) as if guilty. Usually, this type of plea is entered because it cannot be used as an admission of guilt if a civil lawsuit is initiated following the conclusion of a criminal trial.
- Engaging in conduct that endangers the public health.
- Being unfit or incompetent to practice by reason of deliberate or negligent acts or omissions, regardless of whether actual injury to the client is established.
- Engaging in conduct that deceives, defrauds, or harms the public in the course of professional activities or services.

A 2009 report by the NCSBN states that for the calendar years 1996–2006, the percentage of licensed nurses disciplined by BONs increased from 0.10% to 0.18%. Of the violations cited in the report, 25% were drug related (i.e., drug abuse, drug diversion [self], other drug related, alcohol abuse, drug use only,

---

Box 47–7 **Research Priorities of the NCSBN, 2009–2012**

CLIENT SAFETY

- NCSBN's Taxonomy of Error, Root Cause Analysis and Practice-responsibility (TERCAP®) project.

PRACTICE ROLE CLARITY, CHALLENGES (LPN/VN, RN, AND APRN)

- Investigating the practice of a wide range of personnel, from medication aides to the advanced practice nurse.
- Regulatory model for transition to practice for new graduate nurses.

INNOVATIONS IN NURSING EDUCATION AND CLINICAL

- Use of simulation in nursing education.

CONTINUED COMPETENCE OF REGISTERED NURSES PRACTICING BEYOND 5 YEARS

- Regulatory model for continued competence.

EFFECTIVE DISCIPLINE AND ALTERNATIVES TO DISCIPLINE

- Deterring misconduct, affirming professional standards and norms of reasonable conduct, and encouraging rehabilitation or remediation.
- Evaluating the effectiveness of alternative programs.

MODELS FOR STATE-BASED NURSING REGULATION TO SUPPORT NATIONAL AND INTERNATIONAL PORTABILITY AND DATA CONSISTENCY

- Workforce development and benchmarking. A portion of this research agenda is devoted to projects that are ongoing and provide information and data for member board use. These projects include member board profiles, workforce data collection, commitment to ongoing regulatory excellence, licensure statistics, NCLEX® candidate projections, and the Practice and Professional Issues surveys.

Source: National Council of State Boards of Nursing. (2010a). *Research agenda 2010.* Retrieved March 13, 2010, from https://www.ncsbn.org/169.htm

---

drug-related conviction, writing illegal prescriptions, presenting illegal prescriptions, wastage errors, and drug diversion), 9% were criminal, and 7% were related to medication administration. During that same period, 7,076 criminal violations by licensed nurses were reported; this included all levels of nurses, from LPN/LVN through APRN. Nurses who were disciplined during this period had an average of almost 12 years of experience.

NATIONAL COUNCIL OF STATE BOARDS OF NURSING

The NCSBN provides leadership to advance regulatory excellence for public protection. The membership of the NCSBN includes BONs in the 50 states, the District of Columbia, and four U.S. territories (Guam, Virgin Islands, American Samoa, and the Northern Mariana Islands). Four states have separate BONs for RNs and LPNs/LVNs (California, Georgia, Louisiana, and West Virginia).

The NCSBN provides support services to the member BONs and serves as a central repository of data. Perhaps the most

familiar activity of the NCSBN is the development of the initial competency licensure examinations for nurses (NCLEX-RN® and NCLEX-PN®). Other examinations developed by the NCSBN include the National Nurse Aide Assessment Program and the Medication Aide Certification Examination.

The NCSBN also conducts research on nursing practice issues and provides online continuing education opportunities through the e-learning community (Box 47–7). It maintains the Nursys® database, which coordinates national publicly available nurse licensure information, and it works with state boards to promote uniformity in the regulation of the practice of nursing. An outcome of these activities is the Nurse Licensure Compact.

NURSE LICENSURE COMPACT

The **mutual recognition model** of nurse licensure allows a nurse to have a single license that confers the privilege to practice in other states that are part of the Nurse Licensure Compact (Box 47–8). The nurse is held accountable for following the laws and rules of the state in which the nurse practices or where the

---

Box 47–8 **Mutual Recognition Model**

- Each state has to enter into an interstate compact, called the Nurse Licensure Compact (NLC), that allows nurses to practice in more than one state.
- Multistate licensure privilege means the authority to practice nursing in another state that has signed an interstate compact. It is not an additional license.
- A nurse must have a license in his or her primary state of legal residency if that state is an NLC state.
- The states continue to have authority in determining licensure requirements and disciplinary actions.
- The nurse is held accountable for knowing and practicing the nursing practice laws and regulations in the state where the client is located.

- Enactment does not change a state's nurse practice act.
- Complaints and/or violations are addressed by the home state (place of residence) and the remote state (place of practice).
- RNs and LPNs/LVNs are included in the interstate compact or NLC. Since 2002, there has been a separate APRN Compact. A state must be a member of the NLC for RNs and LPNs before entering into the APRN Compact. A state must adopt both compacts to cover LPNs/RNs and APRNs for mutual recognition.

Source: Nurse Licensure Compact Administrators. (2004). *Frequently asked questions regarding the National Council of State Boards of Nursing (NCSBN) Nurse Licensure Compact (NLC).* Retrieved April 29, 2006, from http://www.ncsbn.org/pdfs/FrequentlyAskedQuestions.pdf

client is located. Monitoring the nurse's license and any disciplinary action is the responsibility of the state issuing the license. It is similar to the driver's license model: A single license to drive is issued in the state of primary residency, but this license also allows the privilege to drive in other compact states.

In order to achieve mutual recognition, each state must enact legislation or regulations authorizing the Nurse Licensure Compact. States entering the compact also adopt administrative rules and regulations for implementation of the compact. (For information on states participating in the compact, go to https://www.ncsbn.org/158.htm.)

CREDENTIALING

While a nursing license grants the legal privilege to practice, **credentialing** is the formal identification of professionals who meet predetermined standards of professional skill or competence. The federal government has used the term **certification** to define the credentialing process by which a nongovernmental agency or association recognizes the professional competence of an individual who has met the predetermined qualifications specified by the agency or association. The American Nurses Credentialing Center (ANCC), a subsidiary of the American Nurses Association (ANA), provides credentialing programs to certify nurses in specialty practice areas, recognizes health care organizations for nursing excellence through the Magnet Recognition Program®, and accredits providers of continuing nursing education and nursing specialty organizations.

Federal organizations and federal guidelines, such as The Joint Commission and Centers for Medicare and Medicaid Services, impact on the standards of care the nurse is held accountable for practicing. Individual health care agencies must implement policies, procedures, and job descriptions to ensure that the nurses they employ follow all applicable regulations and guidelines. The nurse needs to know the employing institution's policies and procedures and the specific job descriptions of the licensed and unlicensed nursing personnel. The purpose of knowing the standards of care is to protect both the client and the nurse.

The impact of laws and standards on nurses is profound (Figure 47–4 ■). The professional nurse is held accountable for many standards and statutes. Knowledge of the laws that regulate and affect nursing practice enables the nurse to practice within current legal principles and be aware of his or her legal obligations and responsibilities.

NURSING STUDENTS

Each NPA addresses the duties and responsibilities of nursing students in that state. Typically, this includes language allowing nursing students the privilege to practice nursing without a license while engaged in the clinical practicum of an approved nursing education program under the supervision of qualified faculty. Nursing students have the ultimate **responsibility** (accountability for their actions that includes the obligation to answer for an act done and to repair any injury one may have caused) for their own actions. They are held accountable to the same standard of care as the licensed nurse (Box 47–9). Nursing faculty members are held accountable for appropriate assignment and supervision of the student.

PRACTICE ALERT

Students do not practice on a faculty member's license. The only person who can legally practice on a license is the individual whose name appears on the license.

Box 47–9 Clinical Performance Guidelines for Nursing Students

1. Client safety is always the first priority.
2. Know the facility's policies and procedures before undertaking any clinical assignment.
3. Ensure you are knowledgeable about the client's condition, interventions, medications, and treatments.
4. If you are unprepared for a clinical assignment, inform your instructor. Never perform care for which you are unprepared.
5. Seek help before beginning a procedure about which you are unsure. If the instructor is not readily available, allow the staff nurse to perform the intervention.

Source: Adapted from Guido, G. W. (2006). *Legal and ethical issues in nursing* (4th ed.). Upper Saddle River, NJ: Prentice Hall.

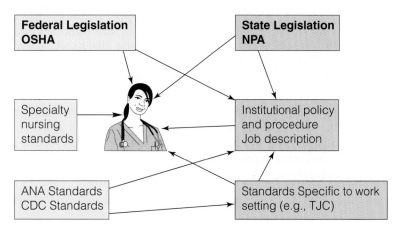

Figure 47–4 ■ Impact of laws and standards on the nurse.

STANDARDS OF PRACTICE

Nursing, as a profession, has a responsibility to self-regulate by defining the practice of nursing, researching and developing the practice, establishing standards of practice, and providing for the education and credentialing of nurses. The ANA, the largest professional nursing organization, has established Standards of Clinical Nursing Practice. These address both standards for nursing care and standards for professional performance (see Box 40–4, ANA Standards in Concept 40, Accountability).

47.2 ADVANCE DIRECTIVES

OVERVIEW

A **health care advance directive** is a legal document executed by an individual that expresses that individual's desires regarding medical treatment which may be used once the individual is no longer able to communicate his or her preferences directly. The client's right to use advance directives is guaranteed in the Patient Self-Determination Act. The **Patient Self-Determination Act** is a federal law requiring health care institutions that receive federal funding (but not individual health care providers) to do the following:

1. At the time of admission, give clients a written summary of:
   - Health care decision-making rights. (Each state has developed such a summary for hospitals, nursing homes, and home health agencies to use.)
   - The facility's policies with respect to recognizing advance directives.
2. Ask clients if they have an advance directive, and document the directive's existence in the medical record. (It is up to the client to provide a copy of the directive.)
3. Educate staff and community about advance directives.
4. Ensure that the individuals know that the facility never discriminates based on whether or not the individual has an advance directive.

Competent clients may execute advance directives at any time. Advance directives are formal, written documents that typically outline the client's desires regarding the following:
- Use or withholding of hydration and/or total parenteral nutrition
- Resuscitation or intubation in the event of a life-threatening emergency (do-not-resuscitate and do-not-intubate orders are discussed in Exemplar 5.2, End-of-Life Care)
- Who has the authority to make decisions on the client's behalf in the event the client is unable to do so (referred to as a health care surrogate).

Types of advance directives include the living will and the durable power of attorney for health care. A **living will** provides specific instructions about what medical treatment the client chooses to omit or refuse (e.g., ventilator support) in the event the client is unable to make such a decision. Through a **durable power of attorney for health care**, the client may designate another person (usually a family member, significant other, or close personal friend) as *health care surrogate* or *health care proxy*, and give that person power to make health care decisions on behalf of the client if the client is unable to do so. These may be combined into a single document or may be two separate documents.

ELEMENTS OF AN ADVANCE DIRECTIVE

A broadly drafted advance directive usually gives an agent/surrogate decision maker authority to
- Consent to or refuse any medical treatment or diagnostic procedure relating to physical or mental health of the individual, including artificial nutrition and hydration.
- Hire or discharge medical providers, and authorize admission to medical and long-term care facilities.
- Consent to measures for comfort care and pain relief.
- Have access to all medical records.
- Take whatever measures are necessary to carry out wishes, including granting releases or waivers to medical facilities and seeking judicial remedies if problems arise.

Each state, through legislation, determines the specific requirements for health care advanced directives. In most states, advance directives must be witnessed by two people and do not require review by an attorney. Many states require that a specific legislated form be used. The majority of states do not permit relatives, heirs, or primary care providers to serve as witnesses for advance directives. In some states, the client has the option to limit the authority of the health care agent as desired. Nurses working with a client who has advance directives should make sure they understand what the client's advance directives include, and should know the laws in their state related to self-determination as well as their employing agency's policies and procedures for following advance directives. Figure 47–5 ■ shows an example of an advance health care directive that combines a living will declaration and a durable power of attorney for health care. Samples of state-specific forms can be obtained from the National Hospice and Palliative Care Organization (http://www.nhpco.org).

POWER OF ATTORNEY FOR HEALTH CARE
(1) **DESIGNATION OF AGENT:** I designate the following individual as my agent to make health care decisions for me: _____

_____
(Name of individual you choose as agent)

_____
(address) (city) (state) (zip code)

_____
(home phone) (work phone)

OPTIONAL: If I revoke my agent's authority or if my agent is not willing, able, or reasonably available to make a health-care decision for me, I designate as my first alternate agent:

_____
(Name of individual you choose as first alternate agent)

_____
(address) (city) (state) (zip code)

_____
(home phone) (work phone)

OPTIONAL: If I revoke the authority of my agent and first alternate agent or if neither is willing, able, or reasonably available to make a health care decision for me, I designate as my second alternate agent:

_____
(Name of individual you choose as second alternate agent)

_____
(address) (city) (state) (zip code)

_____
(home phone) (work phone)

(2) **AGENT'S AUTHORITY:** My agent is authorized to make all health care decisions for me, including decisions to provide, withhold, or withdraw artificial nutrition and hydration, and all other forms of health care to keep me alive, **except** as I state here:

(3) **WHEN AGENT'S AUTHORITY BECOMES EFFECTIVE:** My agent's authority becomes effective when my primary physician determines that I am unable to make my own health care decisions unless I mark the following box. If I mark this box [ ], my agent's authority to make health care decisions for me takes effect immediately.

(4) **AGENT'S OBLIGATION:** My agent shall make health care decisions for me in accordance with this power of attorney for health care, any instructions I give below, and my other wishes to the extent known to my agent. To the extent my wishes are unknown, my agent shall make health care decisions for me in accordance with what my agent determines to be in my best interest. In determining my best interest, my agent shall consider my personal values to the extent known to my agent.

(5) **AGENT'S POSTDEATH AUTHORITY:** My agent is authorized to make anatomical gifts, authorize an autopsy, and direct disposition of my remains, except as I state here or elsewhere in this form:

INSTRUCTIONS FOR HEALTH CARE
Strike any wording you do not want.

(6) **END-OF-LIFE DECISIONS:** I direct that my health care providers and others involved in my care provide, withhold, or withdraw treatment in accordance with the choice I have marked below: **(Initial only one box)**
[ ] (a) **Choice NOT To Prolong Life**
I do not want my life to be prolonged if (1) I have an incurable and irreversible condition that will result in my death within a relatively short time, (2) I become unconscious and, to a reasonable degree of medical certainty, I will not regain consciousness, or (3) the likely risks and burdens of treatment would outweigh the expected benefits, **OR**
[ ] (b) **Choice To Prolong Life**
I want my life to be prolonged as long as possible within the limits of generally accepted health care standards.

(7) **RELIEF FROM PAIN:** Except as I state in the following space, I direct that treatment for alleviation of pain or discomfort should be provided at all times even if it hastens my death:

DONATION OF ORGANS AT DEATH
(8) Upon my death: (mark applicable box)
[ ] (a) I give any needed organs, tissues, or parts,
OR
[ ] (b) I give the following organs, tissues, or parts only: _____
[ ] (c) My gift is for the following purposes:
(strike any of the following you do not want)
(1) Transplant
(2) Therapy
(3) Research
(4) Education

(9) **EFFECT OF COPY:** A copy of this form has the same effect as the original.

(10) **SIGNATURE:** Sign and date the form here:

_____   _____
               (date)   (sign your name)

_____   _____
              (address)   (print your name)

_____   _____
                 (city)   (state)

(11) **WITNESSES:** This advance health care directive will not be valid for making health care decisions unless it is either: (1) signed by two (2) qualified adult witnesses who are personally known to you and who are present when you sign or acknowledge your signature; or (2) acknowledged before a notary public.

Figure 47–5 ■ Sample advance health care directive.

ROLE OF THE NURSE

Clients and families often have difficulty making advance treatment decisions for end-of-life matters. The nurse should reassure them that even if they make a decision and have an advance directive, they will have the option to change their decision when competent. For example, the client may have decided not to have ventilator support in the case of terminal illness, but when the situation occurs, the client has the right to change his or her mind or take more time to make the decision.

PRACTICE ALERT

Nurses can assist clients and their families by instructing clients to provide a copy of their advance directives to their next of kin, primary health care providers, and any health care facility to which they are admitted, including emergency departments, rehabilitations facilities, and senior living centers.

Nurses need to assess whether clients and families have an accurate understanding of life-sustaining measures. Clients and families may misunderstand what actions may sustain life and base their decisions on these misconceptions. Nurses need to incorporate teaching in this area and continue to be supportive of clients' decisions.

CLINICAL EXAMPLE

Mrs. King is a 53-year-old client who is hospitalized with a newly diagnosed inoperable malignant brain tumor. She has a signed advanced directive that indicates she does not want any extraordinary measures to keep her alive if she has an incurable or irreversible condition that will result in her death within a relatively short period of time. The neurosurgeon has presented her with palliative treatment options. Mrs. King refuses treatment for the tumor. Mr. King speaks to the neurosurgeon outside of his wife's room stating, "I want everything possible done! The children and I have discussed this and we don't agree with not treating the tumor."
1. What should happen with Mrs. King's treatment? Why?
2. How may the family's reaction affect implementing the advance directive?
3. When could the family member refuse or consent to treatment?
4. How should the nurse respond?
5. What law, rule, or policy describes the nurse's responsibility?

47.3 HEALTH INSURANCE PORTABILITY AND ACCOUNTABILITY ACT

OVERVIEW

The **Health Insurance Portability and Accountability Act (HIPAA)** of 1996 was enacted by Congress to minimize the exclusion of pre-existing conditions as a barrier to health care insurance, designate special rights for those who lose other health coverage, and eliminate medical underwriting in group plans. The Act includes the Privacy Rule, which creates a national standard for of the disclosure of private health information. This rule impacts all health care providers as well as health insurance plan providers.

PROTECTED HEALTH INFORMATION

The Privacy Rule protects all "individually identifiable health information" held or transmitted in any form or media, whether electronic, paper, or oral. The rule calls this information **protected health information** and delineates it further to include information that identifies the individual (e.g., name, address, birth date, and Social Security number) or for which reasonable basis exists to believe the information can be used to identify the individual as it relates to

- The individual's past, present, or future physical or mental health or condition.
- The provision of health care to the individual.
- The past, present, or future payment for the provision of health care to the individual.

The HIPAA also includes provisions for the protection of clients that address access to medical records, required notice of privacy practices and opportunity for confidential communications, limits on use of medical information beyond the sharing among health care providers directly involved in providing care, and prohibition of the use of personal information for marketing.

In the event a client feels that a health care plan or provider has violated his or her rights according to the HIPAA, the individual may file a formal complaint either directly to the entity or to the U. S. Department of Health and Human Services Office for Civil Rights. Information about how to file a complaint should be included in each entity's notice of privacy practices.

Nurses must maintain a current understanding of the law in order to protect the client's privacy and to avoid civil punitive damage and possible criminal charges. Nurses should be familiar with the particular policies of their employers. Box 47–10 provides examples of how HIPAA affects nursing practice.

Flores and Dodier (2005) report that despite the extensive time and money that have been expended by the health care industry, the general population remains confused about their actual rights, and some health care workers see HIPAA privacy compliance as frivolous. Ultimately, the burden of maintaining security of protected health information is for the protection of the most vulnerable populations, and personnel in covered entities will need to continue to learn and implement the HIPAA standards.

PRACTICE ALERT

Disclosure of client information is a breach of confidentiality that may subject a nurse to legal action. Disclosure of confidential information occurs when a client's condition—for example, a diagnosis of HIV infection—is discussed inappropriately with any third party. In addition, privacy must be provided when calling individuals in for office visits and in all provisions of care.

Box 47–10 Examples of HIPAA Compliance and Nursing Practice

- A client's name cannot be posted near or on the room door.
- Charts should be in a secure, nonpublic location to prevent the public from viewing or accessing confidential health information.
- Printed copies of protected health information should not be left unattended at a printer or fax machine.
- Access to protected health information is limited to those authorized to obtain the information.
- Health care providers will need a password to access a client's electronic chart.

- A notice informing clients of their rights regarding privacy and their health information should be posted and provided to clients upon their admission to the facility.
- Voice levels should be lowered to minimize disclosure of information (e.g., when discussing a client's condition over the telephone, giving a report, or reading information aloud from a computer screen or chart).
- Health care providers must stay current with HIPAA regulations.

PRIVACY VERSUS CONFIDENTIALITY

Privacy includes the right of individuals to keep their personal information from being disclosed. The individual decides with who, when, and where to share his or her health information. **Confidentiality** refers to the assurance the client has that private information will not be disclosed without the client's consent. Confidentiality refers to both the nature of the information the nurse obtains from the client as well as how the nurse treats client information once it has been disclosed to the nurse (Erickson & Millar, 2005).

- *Obtaining information.* Nurses should request and record only information pertinent to the health status of the individual as a client to whom the nurse is assigned. If, for example, the nurse runs into a neighbor in the emergency waiting room, it would be inappropriate for the nurse to ask the neighbor, "What are you doing here?" Doing so would inadvertently invite protected information that is not required for provision of health care.
- *Disclosing information.* Information obtained from the client should only be disclosed to those directly involved in providing that client's health care. Even the presence of the individual in the health care setting is protected information.

It would be a breach of confidentiality, for example, for the nurse to go home and tell her family that a state senator or representative, the family's pastor, neighbor, or anyone else was a client. Protection of client information, once disclosed, is one tenant of the nurse's responsibility as the client's advocate, and challenges to client privacy can include other members of the interdisciplinary team.

- *Advocating for confidentiality.* Nurses are professionally obligated not only to avoid participating in discussions of clients outside those communications directly related to providing care but also to curb others from participation. Gossiping at work seems to be a national past time, but it has no place in health care setting. Celebrity status, notoriety, and an unusual medical condition all add to the potential risks to confidentiality. If the nurse is in a coffee shop and hears another nurse or health care provider discussing a client, he or she is expected to redirect those professionals to maintain client privacy.

In addition to the actions and behaviors described here, nurses should be familiar with the specific policies and procedures for protecting client privacy and confidentiality for the health care agency in which they work.

47.4 MANDATORY REPORTING

OVERVIEW

The term **mandatory reporting** refers to a legal requirement to report an act, event, or situation that is designated by state or local law as a reportable event. Disclosure statutes mandate the reporting of certain types of health information, and all states mandate the reporting of certain vital statistics, including births and deaths. Many states also require health care providers to report abortions and neonatal deaths. Federal and state laws mandate the reporting of communicable diseases, including venereal diseases. This exemplar discusses types of acts, events, or situations that are reportable as well as the nurse's responsibilities related to mandatory reporting.

ABUSE OR NEGLECT OF MINORS AND OLDER ADULTS

Abuse or suspected abuse of vulnerable individuals is mandated to be reported in most states. As a general rule, the nurse reports the required information through the administrative chain of the institution, beginning with the nurse's immediate supervisor and the primary health care provider. All information reported is documented in the client record. In most states, mandatory reporters are required only to have a good faith suspicion, based on information disclosed by the client and/or on physical symptoms manifested by the client (e.g., glove-stocking burn injuries), that abuse has occurred. They are not required to conduct any type of investigation or otherwise confirm that abuse or neglect has, in fact, occurred. For definitions and manifestations of child and elder abuse, see Concept 31, Violence.

GOOD FAITH IMMUNITY

In every state health care workers are protected when they report suspected child abuse in good faith, even if the subsequent investigation does not make a determination of abuse. Guidelines regarding disclosure of health information as a mandatory reporter are presented in Box 47–11.

Box 47–11 Guidelines Regarding Disclosure of Health Information

Depending on the setting, the nurse may be the only professional with first-hand information necessary for making an accurate report. General guidelines that nurses should follow regarding reporting health-related information include the following:

- Know the federal and state laws concerning duty to report.
- Report the required information to the appropriate governmental agency promptly.

- Comply with reporting laws in good faith.
- Follow agency policy carefully when making a report.
- Avoid a breach of confidentiality, and report only the information mandated. Good faith immunity only applies to required information reported to the appropriate agency or office.

Source: Adapted from Guido, G. W. (2010). *Legal and ethical issues in nursing* (5th ed.). Upper Saddle River, NJ: Prentice Hall.

DEVELOPMENTAL CONSIDERATIONS   Reporting Abuse or Neglect of an Adult or Older Adult by a Caretaker

States have specific laws pertaining to the abuse and neglect of adults and older adults. These laws may be similar to those that govern the abuse and neglect of children. For example, many states generally offer good faith immunity to individuals reporting

suspected abuse or neglect of an older adult or an adult with a disability. Nurses should know the laws of their individual states and their agency's policies for reporting suspected abuse or neglect of an adult or older adult.

MANDATORY REPORTING OF NURSES IN VIOLATION OF THE NPA

Each state's Nurse Practice Act addresses the requirements for reporting nurses who are in violation of the act. For example, North Carolina's General Statutes (NCGS § 90-171.47) mandate that any person who has reasonable cause to suspect that a nurse is in violation of the NPA has the duty to report the relevant facts to the Board of Nursing (BON). The reporting individual is not expected to do any type of investigation.

Because BONs take these reports very seriously, their websites generally make reporting forms easily available. Typically, employers use a different reporting form than the general public. The NPA spells out any formal action the board may take, and it usually requires clear and convincing evidence that the nurse has violated state nursing laws or rules. The nature of alleged violations varies widely, and cases are decided on their own merits. Many complaints are resolved through informal processes. In other instances, a formal administrative hearing is held. BONs are required to respect each nurse's right to due process. This ensures that the nurse is informed of any allegations regarding his or her practice, that the nurse has an opportunity to respond to and defend against the allegations, and that the matter is heard by a fair and impartial body. An immunity clause protects individuals who make a report unless the reporting person knew the report was false or acted with reckless disregard, without concern for the validity of the allegations made in the report.

Nurses themselves have a legal obligation to report conduct that is incompetent, unethical, and illegal. This includes reporting violence, abuse, or neglect toward clients by other nurses and extends to reporting conduct involving third parties, including family members and other health care

providers. Nurses are in a position to identify and assess cases of violence, abuse, and neglect.

MANDATORY REPORTING OF CERTAIN INJURIES AND ILLNESSES

Each state has laws that require health care providers and hospitals to report certain types of injuries and illnesses. Those that usually fall under the reporting laws include the following:

- Bullet wounds, gunshot wounds, powder burns, or any other injuries arising or suspected of arising from the discharge of a gun or firearm
- Illnesses that appear to be caused by poisoning
- Injuries caused by, or appearing to be caused by, a knife or other sharp or pointed instrument if the physician or surgeon treating the individual suspects a criminal act may have been involved
- Any wound, injury, or illness resulting in bodily harm as a result of a suspected criminal act or act of violence
- Infectious diseases, such as tuberculosis, HIV/AIDS, and *Escherichia coli.*

The primary care provider or hospital staff member making the report shall provide the name, age, sex, race, residence, or present location of the client who is injured or ill as well as the nature and extent of the injuries or illness. Again, good faith immunity typically applies. Although the primary health care provider is mandated to report, most agencies have policy and procedure in place for routine reporting. Due to presenting circumstances, the emergency department typically reports injuries due to violence. A diagnosis of infectious disease may occur at any point in the health care interaction. The nurse needs to be familiar with the agency policy for reporting infectious diseases and ensure that the report is made.

Box 47–12 **Nationally Notifiable Infectious Conditions**

The Centers for Disease Control and Prevention have identified more than 50 infectious diseases in the United States that must be reported. These include the following:

- Anthrax
- Botulism
- Cholera
- Diphtheria
- Hepatitis
- HIV infection
- Influenza-associated pediatric mortality
- Meningoccal disease
- Shigellosis
- Syphilis.

A complete list of the 2010 Nationally Notifiable Infections Diseases and Conditions can be found at http://www.cdc.gov/ncphi/disss/nndss/PHS/infdis2010.htm.

Mandatory reporting of infectious conditions is a cornerstone of maintaining public health. Since 1878, the U.S. Public Health System has been collecting information on infectious conditions for the purpose of early identification and control of massive outbreaks, including, when necessary, instituting quarantines. High-profile diseases and threats of bioterrorism have brought renewed attention to this system of ongoing monitoring. Data are reported at the county level, with primary care providers reporting these diseases and conditions to local health departments (Box 47–12). Each county health department reports to the state's Department of Health, where data are managed and maintained. Data on many diseases and conditions are provided from the state level to the Centers for Disease Control and Prevention, which publish the *Morbidity and Mortality Weekly Report.* Although the law targets physician reporting, nurses need to be aware of the policies and procedures for reporting within their place of employment, especially those who are employed directly by their local health department. For diseases and conditions that are required to be reported within 24 hours, the initial report shall be made by telephone to the health department, with the written report being made within 7 days.

OTHER EXAMPLES OF MANDATORY REPORTING

In most states, child care workers, teachers, and other school personnel are mandated to report any suspicions of child abuse or neglect that involve children and families with whom they work. School principals and other administrators typically are required to report to law enforcement when they have knowledge that a crime has been committed on school property. Crimes that typically must be reported include the following:

- Assault (especially assault with a weapon or assault resulting in serious injury)
- Sexual assault
- Rape
- Kidnapping
- Indecent liberties with a minor
- Possession of a firearm on school property or in violation of the law.

Photo processors or computer technicians who, within the scope of their employment, come across images of a minor (or one who reasonably appears to be a minor) engaging in sexual activity typically are required to make a report to local law enforcement. These individuals often are afforded good faith immunity.

47.5 RISK MANAGEMENT

OVERVIEW

Risk management focuses on limiting a health care agency's financial and legal risk associated with the delivery of care, particularly in terms of lawsuits, hopefully before incidents occur. Risk management is a process that identifies, analyzes, and treats potential hazards within a setting for the purpose of identifying and rectifying the hazards, thus preventing harm.

Nurses participate in risk management every day when they ensure client safety and quality care. Typical areas for high risk of incidents include the following:

- Medication administration
- Falls
- Overall client safety
- Use of technology and equipment (e.g., ensuring that equipment is working correctly before using it)

- Assessment and communication of allergies
- Any action or intervention that might harm the client.

STRATEGIES FOR RISK MANAGEMENT

Facilities may have an individual or a team dedicated to risk management. In most cases, there will be a designated risk manager whose role is "to maintain a safe and effective health care environment and prevent or reduce loss to the health care organization" (Pike, Janssen, & Brooks, 2002, p. 3). Strategies that health care organizations use to minimize risk include the following:

- Purchasing insurance or self-insuring to protect against financial risk
- Identifying exposures, types, where they occur, frequency, and level of risk

- Implementing practices to protect against undue risk
- Implementing organizational programs to prevent occurrence of events that might increase financial risk (e.g., incident report system, staff education about risk and documentation, and data collection to assist in identifying potential problems)
- Investigating incidents that might result in a potential lawsuit as soon as possible after the incident occurs
- Monitoring strategies for prevention of risk.

Health care organizations must also consider the risks to anyone who enters the organization's facility, such as visitors, community members, and family members (e.g., a visitor falls in the hallway). For more information, see the Concept 48, Quality Improvement, and Concept 49, Safety.

Implementing a Physician's Orders

Nurses can minimize risk by analyzing procedures and medications ordered by the physician. It is the nurse's responsibility to seek clarification of ambiguous or seemingly erroneous orders from the prescribing physician. Clarification from any other source is unacceptable and is regarded as a departure from competent nursing practice.

If the order is neither ambiguous nor apparently erroneous, the nurse is responsible for implementing the order. For example, if the physician orders oxygen to be administered at 4 liters per minute, the nurse must administer oxygen at that rate, and not at 2 or 6 liters per minute. If the orders state that the client is not to have solid food after a bowel resection, the nurse must ensure that no solid food is given to the client.

There are several categories of orders that nurses must question to protect themselves legally:

- *Question any order a client questions.* For example, if a client who has been receiving an intramuscular injection tells the nurse that the doctor changed the order from an injectable to an oral medication, the nurse must recheck the order before giving the medication.
- *Question any order if the client's condition has changed.* The nurse is considered responsible for notifying the physician of any significant changes in the client's condition, whether the physician requests notification or not. For example, if a client who is receiving an intravenous infusion suddenly develops a rapid pulse, chest pain, and a cough, the nurse must notify the physician immediately and question continuance of the ordered rate of infusion. If a client who is receiving morphine for pain develops severely depressed respirations, the nurse must withhold the medication and notify the physician.
- *Question and record verbal orders to avoid miscommunications.* In addition to recording the time, the date, the physician's name, and the orders, the nurse documents the circumstances that occasioned the call to the physician, reads the orders back to the physician, and documents that the physician confirmed the orders as the nurse read them back.
- *Question any order that is illegible, unclear, or incomplete.* Misinterpretations in the name of a drug or in dose, for example, can easily occur with handwritten orders. The nurse is responsible for ensuring that the order is interpreted the way it was intended and that it is a safe and appropriate order.

Providing Competent Nursing Care

Nurses further minimize and manage risk by providing competent client care. Nurses need to provide care that is within the legal boundaries of their practice and within the boundaries of agency policies and procedures. Nurses therefore must be familiar with their various job descriptions, which may be different from agency to agency. Every nurse is responsible for ensuring that his or her education and experience are adequate to meet the responsibilities delineated in the job description.

Competency also involves care that protects clients from harm. Nurses need to anticipate sources of client injury, educate clients about hazards, and implement measures to prevent injury.

Application of the nursing process is another essential aspect of providing safe and effective client care. Clients need to be assessed and monitored appropriately and involved in care decisions. All assessments and care must be documented accurately. Effective communication can also protect the nurse from negligence claims. Nurses need to approach every client with sincere concern and include the client in conversations. In addition, nurses should always acknowledge when they do not know the answer to a client's questions, telling the client they will find out the answer and then follow through.

Methods of legal protection are summarized in Box 47–13.

Reducing Pediatric Medical Errors

Children are at a higher risk for medical error than other patients and also may be more vulnerable to harm from errors due to their immature physiology (Hughes & Edgerton, 2005). Reasons for increased medical error among children include the following (Hughes & Edgerton, 2005; Kozer, Berkovitch, & Koren, 2006):

- Medication dosage calculations are more complex. Many medications are produced in adult concentrations requiring dilution, or dosages must be calculated based upon weight or body surface area. This means the optimal dose is based on mg/kg and divided by number of doses to be given a day. An additional problem is that children often need suspensions or liquid preparations, adding to the dosage calculation complexity. Not only must the correct dose be calculated, but also the amount of liquid preparation with that dose. Errors in mathematical calculations are one of the most common causes of medication errors.
- The misplacement of a decimal in the medication dosage calculation can result in an overdose that can cause harm to the child or even death. This is particularly important for critically ill or injured children who do not have the reserves to deal with an overdose of medication.

Box 47–13 Guideline for Legal Protection for Nurses

- Function within the scope of your education, job description, and nurse practice act.
- Follow the procedures and policies of the employing agency.
- Build and maintain good rapport with clients.
- Always check the identity of a client to make sure it is the right client.
- Observe and monitor the client accurately. Communicate and record significant changes in the client's condition to the physician.
- Promptly and accurately document all assessments and care given.
- Be alert when implementing nursing interventions, and give each task your full attention and skill.
- Perform procedures correctly and appropriately.

- Make sure the correct medications are given in the correct dose, by the right route, at the scheduled time, and to the right client.
- When delegating nursing responsibilities, make sure that the person who is delegated a task understands what to do and that the person has the required knowledge and skill.
- Protect clients from injury.
- Report all incidents involving clients.
- Always check any order that a client questions.
- Know your own strengths and weaknesses. Ask for assistance and supervision in situations for which you feel inadequately prepared.
- Maintain your clinical competence. For students, this demands study and practice before caring for clients. For graduate nurses, it means continued study to maintain and update clinical knowledge and skills.

- Many drug preparations require dilution to achieve the small dosage required by infants.
- Medications are sometimes prescribed that are not yet approved by the Food and Drug Administration for use in children, and pediatric standard dosage guidelines have not been established.
- Young children cannot communicate well if they are having a reaction to the medication.

Another cause of potential medical error involves families with limited English proficiency. There is a risk for errors in interpretation between the health professional and the family member regarding care. For example, failure to obtain historical information about a drug allergy may lead to serious adverse effects. Even when using a hospital interpreter, errors such as omitting instructions on dose, route, frequency, and duration of medications have potential clinical consequences (Flores & Ngui, 2006).

INCIDENT REPORTS

As part of risk management, each health care organization has an incident reporting system (Pike et al., 2002). Nurses participate in this process by completing the required forms when involved in an incident and by following policies and procedures. Most incidents, however, do not result in a lawsuit.

An **incident report** is an agency record of an accident or incident occurring within the agency and is designed to collect adequate information to assist personnel in preventing future incidents or occurrences. Incident reports are also called variance reports or unusual occurrence reports. Examples of occurrences that would be reported include medication administration

variances (e.g., wrong medication, wrong dose, wrong route, wrong time, and omissions) and a client or visitor falling.

In some jurisdictions, incident reports may be used in discovery. **Discovery** is the legal process of obtaining information before a trial. A nurse completing an incident report should always fill out the report as though it is discoverable. No language admitting liability should be included. The report should completely and accurately document the facts without assumptions, conclusions, or blame. The report should include the client's account of the incident in direct quotes, and identify all witnesses to the incident. Incident reports generally include the following:

- Names and identifying information of any clients and health care personnel involved in the incident as well as information regarding witnesses (if any)
- The location, time, and date of the incident
- Equipment or medication involved (if medication, state the medication's name and dosage).

While the event which prompted the incident report is noted in the client's chart, there should be no entry in the client's chart to indicate that an incident report was completed. For example, if the client was given the wrong medication, the actual administration of the medication will be noted in the client's chart. If the client required any treatment as a result of the event, that also is noted in the client's chart (Guido, 2010).

Nurses engage in risk management by following ANA standards of care and practice, following their employing agency's policies and procedures, and by working collaboratively to ensure client safety is maintained at all times. Risk management is required of every nurse in the course of practicing nursing on a daily basis.

47.6 WHISTLEBLOWING

OVERVIEW

The Whistleblower Protection Act of 1989 establishes certain protections for individuals who report gross misconduct on the part of their employers to federal authorities. **Whistleblowing** is the action taken by a nurse who goes outside of the organization for the public's best interest when the organization fails to follow procedures regarding safety and client care (Lachman, 2008). The nurse who takes such action is called a

whistleblower. In order to qualify for protection under the Act, nurses must first make every effort to resolve the concern by following the internal reporting procedures of the agency that employs them. Additionally, an individual does not qualify for protection under the Act unless the employer has threatened or engaged in retaliation against the employee as a result of the employee addressing his or her complaint.

Not every act of misconduct will rise to the standard that it will qualify under the Whistleblower Protection Act. The activity or policy in question must violate a state or federal law or rule, and the employer must be aware that the activity or policy is a violation. A few examples of incidents to report, in addition to those that are legally mandated as discussed in Exemplar 47.4, are billing fraud, failure to maintain safety equipment, and chronic insufficient staffing. The nurse making the complaint must give the employer written notice and appropriate time to correct the issue. The nurse must also make or threaten to make a report to the appropriate state or federal agency.

Additional legislation supports individuals in reporting fraud. The False Claims Act encourages individuals to report medical and billing agency fraud. In March, 2010, new health care reform legislation strengthened the False Claims Act in order to ensure that health care providers and clients can report fraud under the Patient Protection and Affordable Care Act. The National Whistleblowers Center (http://whistleblowers.org/index.html) provides additional information and advocacy on this important and complex issue (National Whistleblowers Center, 2010).

PRACTICE ALERT

Reporting a coworker can be especially difficult, but it is critical that the nurse informs the supervisor about a possible problem with a coworker or another health care provider, especially if the individual's action reflects incompetence or is illegal or unethical.

CONSEQUENCES OF WHISTLEBLOWING

The nurse who makes a report outside of the employing agency should be prepared for potentially negative consequences. These may include losing the support of one's coworkers or even losing one's job. Failing to act, however, may jeopardize client care.

PRACTICE ALERT

The failure of a nurse to report illegal, unethical, or unsafe conduct may result in the nurse being sued by the client, action taken against the nurse's license, or termination by the employer (Monson, 2005).

Statutes exist to prevent recourse by the employer for reasonable, good faith reporting of illegal, unethical, or unsafe conduct in order to provide a safe, environment for clients. To help ensure that employees are free to participate in safety and health activities, Section 11(c) (The Whistleblower Protection Program) of the Occupational Safety and Health Act prohibits any person from discharging, or in any manner retaliating or discriminating against, any employee because that employee has exercised rights under the Act. Provided the whistleblower has done everything required prior to notifying the federal agency, the whistleblower's protected rights include making formal notification to the Occupational Safety and Health Administration (OSHA) and seeking an OSHA inspection, participating in an OSHA inspection, and participating or testifying in any proceeding related to an OSHA inspection. Discrimination by the employer includes the following actions:

- Firing or laying off
- Blacklisting
- Demoting
- Denying overtime or promotion
- Disciplining
- Denial of benefits
- Failure to hire or rehire
- Intimidation
- Reassignment affecting promotion prospects
- Reducing pay or hours.

To prevail in discrimination claim, the nurse must report the illegal activity before resigning from the place of employment. To file a complaint under Section 11(c), contact the nearest OSHA office within 30 days of the discrimination. Discrimination complaints cannot be filed online.

REVIEW Legal Issues

RELATE: LINK THE CONCEPTS

Linking the concept of Legal Issues with the concept of Assessment:

1. How does a thorough assessment of the client contribute to risk management?
2. What type of consent is necessary for the nurse to take the client's temperature and vital signs? For the client to undergo an x-ray if a broken leg is suspected?
3. What law or rule addresses the nurse's ability to assess a client and make nursing diagnoses based on that assessment?
4. What aspects of a client assessment are protected under the Privacy Rule?

Linking the concept of Legal Issues with the concept of Communication:

1. How does a change-of-shift report minimize the nurse's risk for professional negligence or malpractice?
2. How does accuracy in documentation contribute to risk management?
3. What type or types of communication result in the best quality client care and are therefore most likely to prevent the nurse from being accused of malpractice?
4. What aspects of communication impact whether or not a violation of federal or state laws may reported under the Whistleblower's Protection Act?

REFER: GO TO MYNURSINGKIT

REFLECT: CASE STUDY

Joanne, an RN coworker on your surgical unit, returned to work about 6 weeks ago following back surgery. Since her return, you have noticed that she is frequently and uncharacteristically late for work and has called in sick six times. Twice you have witnessed her "biting the head off" an unlicensed assistive person. Mrs. Glancy, a client who is 2 days postoperative, puts her light on and tells you that she is in severe pain and the pain medication she received didn't have any effect on the pain level. She states "It's the strangest thing; the pill never seems to work in the evenings like it does in the daytime and at night." You report Mrs. Glancy's pain to Joanne who is her primary nurse. At the end of the shift, you and an oncoming nurse are doing the narcotic count and notice that Joanne has given 6 doses of the same narcotic during the shift with 1 dose being documented as given to a client at 8 p.m. who had been discharged at 5 p.m.

1. What are your responsibilities? Should you take any action? If so, why?
2. What laws do you need to review? What policies?
3. What documentation will you need?

REFERENCES

American Nurses Association. Statement of purpose. Retrieved March 13, 2010, from http://www.nursingworld.org/FunctionalMenuCategories/AboutANA/WhoWeAre/ANAsStatementofPurpose.aspx

Anderson, S., Schaechter, J., & Brosco, J. (2006). Adolescent patients and their confidentiality: Staying within legal bounds. This article originally appeared in *Contemporary Pediatrics*. *Contemporary OB/GYN, 51*(5), 53–59. Retrieved from CINAHL with Full Text database.

Bolin, J. (2005). When nurses are reported to the National Practitioner Data Bank. *Journal of Nursing Law, 10*(3), 141–148.

Brooke, P. (2003). How good a Samaritan should you be? *Nursing, 33*(6), 46–47.

Brooke, P. (2008). Malpractice maladies: Awareness and initiative can help you avoid legal consequences. *Nursing Management, 39*(7), 20–26.

Croke, E., & Daguro, P. (2005). Liability for the health care provider: Non-implementation of patients' advanced directives. *Journal of Legal Nurse Consulting, 16*(2), 19–24.

Croke, E. (2006). Nursing malpractice: Determining liability elements for negligent acts. *Journal of Legal Nurse Consulting, 17*(3), 3–8.

Erickson, J., & Millar, S. (2005). Caring for patients while respecting their privacy: Renewing our commitment. *Online Journal of Issues in Nursing, 10*(2). Retrieved August 16, 2008, from CINAHL with Full Text database.

Flores, J., & Dodier, A. (2005). HIPAA: Past, present and future implications for nurses. *Online Journal of Issues in Nursing, 10*(2). Retrieved August 16, 2008, from CINAHL with Full Text database.

Flores, G., & Ngui, E. (2006). Racial/ethnic disparities and patient safety. *Pediatric Clinics of North America, 53*, 1197–1215.

Guido, G. W. (2006). *Legal and ethical issues in nursing* (4ᵗʰ ed.). Upper Saddle River, NJ: Prentice Hall.

Guido, G. W. (2010). *Legal and ethical issues in nursing* (5ᵗʰ ed.). Upper Saddle River, NJ: Prentice Hall.

Guttmacher Institute. (2010). *An overview of minors' consent law*. Retrieved January 8, 2010, from http://www.guttmacher.org/statecenter/spibs/spib_OMCL.pdf

Hartman.K & Liang, B. (1999). Exceptions to informed consent in emergency medicine. *Hospital Physician March*, 53–59.

Lachman, V. (2008). Ethics, law, and policy. Whistleblowers: Troublemakers or virtuous nurses? *MEDSURG Nursing, 17*(2), 128–134.

Monson, M. (2005). Legal checkpoints. What to know about duty to report. *Nursing Management, 36*(5), 14–16.

National Council of State Boards of Nursing. (2009). *Report of findings from an analysis of Nursys disciplinary data from 1996–2006.* (Research Brief Vol. 39). Chicago: Author.

National Council of State Boards of Nursing. (2010). NCLEX 2010. Retrieved March 13, 2010, from https://www.ncsbn.org/NCLEX.htm

National Council of State Boards of Nursing. (2010a). Research agenda 2010. Retrieved March 13, 2010, from https://www.ncsbn.org/169.htm

National Whistleblowers Center. (2010). Healthcare bill enhances whistleblower protections. Retrieved March 29, 2010, from http://www.whistleblowers.org/index.php?option=com_content&task=view&id=1062&Itemid=178

North Carolina Board of Nursing. (2009a). Nursing Practice Act ARTICLE 9A. Retrieved from http://www.ncbon.com/

North Carolina Board of Nursing. (2009b). 21 North Carolina Administrative Code, Chapter 36. Retrieved from http://www.ncbon.com/

NCBON. (2009c). Position Statement: Accepting an assignment §G.S. 90-171.20(7)&(8). Retrieved from http://www.ncbon.com/content.aspx?ID=682

Pike, Janssen, & Brooks. (2002). Role and function of a hospital risk manager. *Journal of Legal Nurse Consultants, 13*(2), 3–13. Retrieved from CINAHL with Full Text database.

Reasonable person. (2010). Law library. American law and legal information. Retrieved March 25, 2010, from http://law.jrank.org/pages/8780/Negligence-Reasonable-Person.html

Sager v. *Rochester General Hospital*, 647 NYS 2d 408 (1996).

Singh, T. (2007). Avoiding malpractice: Watch your medications!. *Nevada RNformation, 16*(1), 8. Retrieved from CINAHL with Full Text database.

Singh, T. (2006). Avoiding malpractice: Know the standard of care. *Nevada RNformation, 15*(1), 19. Retrieved from CINAHL with Full Text database.

Singh, T. (2006). Avoiding malpractice through proper documentation. *Nevada RNformation, 15*(4), 13. Retrieved from CINAHL with Full Text database.

Singh, T. (2005). Avoiding malpractice: Is insurance really necessary?. *Nevada RNformation, 14*(3), 21. Retrieved from CINAHL with Full Text database.

Weld, K., & Garmon Bibb, S. (2009). Concept Analysis: Malpractice and modern-day nursing practice. *Nursing Forum, 44*(1), 2–10. doi:10.1111/j.1744-6198.2009.00121.x. Retrieved March 13, 2010 from http://search.ebscohost.com.proxy054.nclive.org/login.aspx?direct=true&db=aph&AN=36335802&site=ehost-live

Quallich. S.A. (2004). The practice of informed consent. *Urologic Nursing, 24*(6), 513–515.

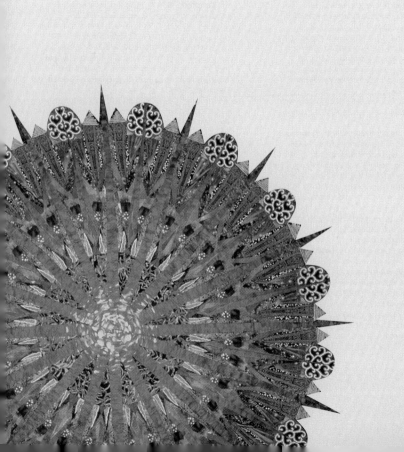

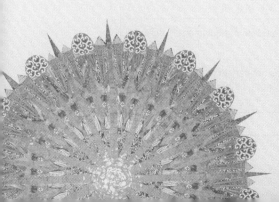

Quality Improvement

48

Concept at-a-Glance

About Quality Improvement, *2421*

BASIS FOR SELECTION OF CONCEPT

Institute of Medicine
The Joint Commission

Concept Learning Outcomes

After reading about this concept, you will be able to:

1. Differentiate quality improvement from quality management.
2. List and describe the components of a quality management program.
3. Contrast four quantifiable quality improvement systems.
4. Describe national incentives for quality improvement.
5. Summarize the impact of quality of care on cost of care.
6. Elaborate on how nurse staffing impacts quality of care.
7. Describe the nurse's role in reducing risk and improving quality.
8. Provide examples of sentinel events, and the resulting root cause analysis that would be required.

Concept Key Terms

Audit, *2426*
Benchmarking, *2425*
Breach of care, *2424*
Breach of duty, *2424*
Concurrent audit, *2426*
Continuous quality improvement (CQI), *2427*
Indicator, *2425*
Intradisciplinary assessment, *2425*
Lean Six Sigma, *2428*
Outcome standards, *2425*
Outcomes management, *2425*
Peer review, *2425*
Plan-Do-Study-Act (PDSA), *2427*

Process standards, *2425*
Quality, *2421*
Quality improvement, *2422*
Quality management, *2421*
Quality management plan, *2425*
Retrospective audit, *2426*
Root cause analysis, *2424*
Sentinel event, *2423*
Six Sigma, *2428*
Standards, *2425*
Structure standards, *2425*
Total quality management (TQM), *2426*
Utilization reviews, *2426*

About Quality Improvement

The Institute of Medicine (IOM) defines **quality** as "the degree to which health services for individuals and populations increase the likelihood of desired health outcomes and are consistent with current professional knowledge" (IOM, 2001). Nurses provide quality care to clients by following professional standards of care and practice and the ANA Code of Ethics for Nurses, by maintaining a current, evidence-based practice, and by participating in quality management programs and quality improvement efforts. **Quality management** can be defined as a preventive approach designed to address problems before they become crises. **Quality improvement** describes the systematic processes that health care organizations and professionals use to measure client outcomes, identify hazards and errors, and to improve client care. Quality improvement specifically attempts to avoid attributing blame and to create systems to prevent errors from happening (Wiseman & Kaprielian, 2005). ●

THE NEED TO IMPROVE THE QUALITY OF HEALTH CARE

In 2000, the landmark report by the Institute of Medicine, *To Err Is Human: Building a Safer Health System*, revealed that 98,000 deaths in hospitals each year resulted from preventable medical mistakes. The report stunned both health care providers and the public, and brought a critical focus to the need to improve client care and ensure client safety through quality improvement efforts.

The IOM report was, in part, stimulated by the efforts of the Presidential Advisory Commission on Consumer Protection and Quality in the Health Care Industry, a 32-member commission established by President Bill Clinton. The Presidential Advisory Commission, whose membership included three nurse leaders, published *Quality First: Better Health Care for all Americans* (The President's Advisory Commission on Consumer Protection and Quality in the Health Care Industry, 1999).

Another major report came from the Committee on the Quality of Health Care in America was *Crossing the Quality Chasm* (Institute of Medicine, 2001), which focused on developing a new health care system for the twenty-first century, one that improves care. This report concluded that the system is in need of repair, one of fundamental change. The report also emphasized the impact of the rapid change in the health care system: new medical science, new technology, rapid availability of information, and so on. The report described a system in which health care providers cannot keep up with the rapid

changes and in which "performance of the health care system varies considerably" (Institute of Medicine, 2001, p. 3). As was noted in *To Err Is Human*, the system is fragmented and poorly organized, and fails to make the best use of its resources.

Crossing the Quality Chasm also described the impact that the increase of chronic conditions has had on the system. With people living longer, mostly due to the advances in medical science and technology, more are living with chronic conditions. "Chronic conditions, defined as illnesses that last longer than 3 months and are not self-limiting, are now the leading cause of illness, disability, and health problems in this country, and affect almost half of the U.S. population" (Hoffman et al., 1996; as cited in Institute of Medicine, 2001, p. 27). Many clients with chronic conditions also have comorbid conditions. They have complicated problems and require collaborative treatment efforts, "involving the definition of clinical problems in terms that both patients and providers understand; joint development of a care plan with goals, targets, and implementations strategies; provision of self-management training and support services; and active, sustained follow-up using visits, telephone calls, e-mail, and Web-based monitoring and decision support programs" (Von Korff et al., 1997; as cited in Institute of Medicine, 2001, p. 27). *Crossing the Quality Chasm* concluded that the *complex*, fragmented, and disorganized health care system is ineffective in dealing with these problems.

To improve the health care system, *Crossing the Quality Chasm* outlined six aims for improvement—safe, effective, client-centered, timely, efficient, and equitable—which are identified in Figure 48–1 ■. It also recommended changes that were identified by Wagner, Austin, and Von Korff (1996):

1. Need for evidence-based, planned care
2. Reorganization of practices to meet the needs of clients who require more time, a broad array of resources, and closer follow-up

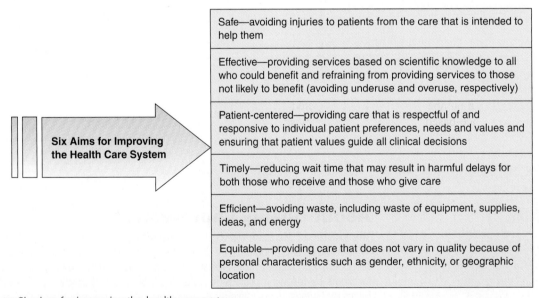

Figure 48–1 ■ Six aims for improving the health care system.

Source: Adapted from Finkelman, Anita W. Insitute of Medicine. (2001). Crossing the quality chasm. Washington DC: National Academy Press, pp. 5–6. Reprinted with permission.

3. Systematic attention to clients' need for information and behavioral change
4. Ready access to necessary clinical expertise
5. Use of supportive information systems.

NATIONAL INITIATIVES

Following these reports, the health care industry began to embrace quality improvement. The need to improve client safety and health outcomes and to implement changes to support these improvements was obvious to individuals working at every level of health care. Governmental agencies such as the Department of Health and Human Services, physicians groups such as the American Medical Association, and professional nursing organizations such as the American Nurses Association began to develop indicators of quality care and measures to document the quality of care. Three important efforts include the development of the National Database of Nursing Quality Indicators™, the publication of *Patient Safety and Quality: An Evidence-Based Handbook for Nurses*, and the development of National Patient Safety Goals by The Joint Commission.

In 1998, the American Nurses Association developed the National Database of Nursing Quality Indicators™ in an effort to build on existing studies and to gather the data necessary to document the benefits of nursing care on client outcomes. Currently more than 1,100 facilities participate, providing information on several quality indicators including falls, falls with injury, number of nursing care hours per patient day, and the prevalence of pressure ulcers. NDNQI provides important statistically valid and reliable data that may be used by organizations to improve client care and to identify relationships between nursing staffing levels and client outcomes. NDNQI has become an important tool in the development of nursing policy and efforts to improve nursing care (Montalvo, 2007).

Patient Safety and Quality: An Evidence-Based Handbook for Nurses is an effort by the Agency for Healthcare Research and Quality (AHRQ) to examine a broad range of issues related to providing high quality nursing care. This report recognizes that nurses are uniquely positioned to participate in quality surveillance measures and in efforts to prevent, minimize, and reduce errors and events that compromise client safety. The handbook examines a number of critical issues including the need for evidence-based practice among nurses, client-centered care issues such as injury prevention, and the need to reduce declining function among hospitalized older adults. Pediatric safety and quality and nursing work environments are also among the quality issues that this report addresses (AHRQ, 2008).

One development that has been critical in the improvement of client care has been the development of National Patient Safety Goals (NPSGs). The Joint Commission revises these goals on an annual basis and requires all accredited health care organizations to meet the goals that are designed for their specific type of facility. Types of facilities include critical care hospitals, long-term care facilities, and home

care agencies. Although the focus of the NPSGs is on system-wide solutions, the intent is that these solutions will improve client safety for each and every client that the health care organization serves. For more information on the NPSGs, see Concept 49, Safety.

In addition to efforts by the Institute of Medicine, the American Nurses Association, and The Joint Commission, the Institute of Healthcare Improvement (IHI) offers programs to assist organizations in improving the quality of care they provide (IHI, 2007). The Institute's goals are
■ No needless deaths
■ No needless pain or suffering
■ No helplessness in those served or serving
■ No unwanted waiting
■ No waste.

The work of these agencies provides information to organizations related to standards against which client care can be measured, tools for measurement, and means of improvement. These agencies provide the infrastructure that enables organizations to embrace and implement quality improvement.

IMPLEMENTING QUALITY IMPROVEMENT

Improving client care requires measurement of the status of care delivery. This requires understanding how quality can be measured and determining what aspects of care may not be measurable. This is not a simple task, and health care organizations struggle to arrive at the best methods. For example, measuring the quality of the nurse–client relationship quantitatively is challenging due to the many variables involved. Just the issue of personalities and communication methods make this a difficult task.

The concept of quality improvement moves health care from a mode of identifying failed standards and problems to a proactive attitude which anticipates and prevents problems and works to improve care and quality of care. This paradigm shift involves everyone in the organization and promotes problem solving and experimentation. In order to anticipate and identify changes that need to be made, health care organizations implement quality management programs.

Sentinel Events

The mission of The Joint Commission (Joint Commission, 2005a) is "To continuously improve the safety and quality of care provided to the public through the provision of health care accreditation and related services that support performance improvement in health care organizations." The Joint Commission has put great emphasis on the importance of what are called "sentinel events." Although each agency must define sentinel events for itself, the definition must be consistent with that given by The Joint Commission (2005b):
■ A **sentinel event** is an unexpected occurrence involving death or serious physical or psychological injury, or the risk thereof. Serious injury specifically includes loss of limb or function. The phrase "or the risk thereof" includes any

process variation for which a recurrence would carry a significant chance of a serious adverse outcome.

■ Such events are called "sentinel" because they signal the need for immediate investigation and response.

The Joint Commission has the authority to conduct a review of certain sentinel events that occur within accredited health care organizations. Types of events that are considered reviewable may be different for one type of facility than another. Examples of sentinel events that may be considered reviewable by The Joint Commission include the following:

■ Any event that results in an unanticipated death or loss of permanent function that did not occur as a result of the client's underlying condition

■ Unanticipated death of a full-term infant

■ Discharge of an infant to the wrong family

■ Rape that occurs on the facility's premises

■ Surgery on the wrong client or the wrong body part

■ Suicide of any client receiving care or services in a staffed 24-hour setting or within 72 hours of discharge (Joint Commission, 2007).

Health care facilities accredited by The Joint Commission are encouraged, but not required, to self-report all sentinel events. Regardless of whether or not a facility reports a sentinel event to The Joint Commission, the facility is expected to respond to the event using procedures consistent with The Joint Commission's requirements. This includes conducting a root cause analysis to determine the events or actions that led to the event (Joint Commission, 2007).

Root Cause Analysis

The Joint Commission requires health care organizations to respond to a sentinel event by assessing the cause, identifying a plan for intervention, and evaluating the results of the plan. Often, assessment involves a root cause analysis. **Root cause analysis** is a process for identifying the factors that bring about deviations in practices that lead to the event. A root cause analysis focuses primarily on systems and processes, not individual performance. It begins with examination of the single event but has the goal of determining which organizational improvements are needed to decrease the likelihood of such events occurring again. A root cause analysis may also be used to determine the circumstances leading to a breach of care.

Breach of Care

A **breach of care** or **breach of duty**, occurs when the nurse deviates from the standard of care. Guido (2010) writes that this occurs when the nurse does something that should not have been done (e.g., gives the incorrect medication) or does not do something that should have been done (e.g., fails to administer a scheduled medication) (Guido, p. 95).

The last 10 years have seen an increase in the number of malpractice suits against nurses or involving nurses as part of a lawsuit against a health care facility. Some of the most frequent breaches of duty that have resulted in lawsuits against nurses include medication errors, communication errors, failures to monitor and assess, working while impaired (due to

inadequate sleep or substance abuse), and negligent or inappropriate delegation or supervision (Domrose, 2007).

Quality improvement efforts seek to determine weaknesses in procedures and processes as well as organizational issues that can impact nurses' ability to provide nursing care consistent with established professional standards of care, as well as organizational protocols. In addition to the ways that nurses can minimize risk (discussed in Concept 37), nurses must also be aware of the need to report problems in care delivery (including questionable physician orders and suspicions of nurse impairment) to nursing supervisors. In short, nurses need to use the chain of command (Domrose, 2007).

Guido (2010) emphasizes the need for nurses to remain current in their skills and education and to base all care on the nursing process model, documenting "every step of the nursing care plan and the patient's responses to interventions" (Guido, p. 105). In doing so, nurses reduce the likelihood of committing a breach of care and, therefore, reduce the risk of an adverse event and resulting malpractice suit.

CLINICAL EXAMPLE

Two daughters of a U.S. veteran sued their state's Department of Veteran Affairs and the veterans' home where their father lived after he left the home in his wheelchair and subsequently died. According to the Associated Press, a security camera recorded the client leaving the home at 3:45 a.m., and the staff did not begin searching for him until 4:30 a.m. The weather outside was below freezing with a mixture of rain and snow. The client managed to get across a major highway and was eventually found 800 feet from his wheelchair. He died in the hospital 2 days later (Associated Press, 2010).

1. Based on the limited description of this sentinel event, what standards of nursing care may have been breached?

2. What procedures or practices do you think a root cause analysis might reveal as contributing to the client's death?

COMPONENTS OF QUALITY MANAGEMENT PROGRAMS

A quality management program is based on an integrated system of information and accountability. Clinical information systems (see Concept 46, Informatics) can provide the data needed to enable organizations to track activities and outcomes. For example, data from clinical information systems can be used to track client wait times from admitting to outpatient testing to admission in an inpatient care unit. If delays in the process are identified, appropriate staff and resources can be made available at the right time to decrease delays and increase efficiency and client satisfaction. Methods to discover problems in the system without blaming the "sharp end," the last individual in the chain to act (e.g., the nurse gives a wrong medication), must be accepted and used by the entire staff.

Quality management programs differ depending on the needs of the health care organization and the types of client care it provides. Despite these differences, a comprehensive quality management program generally includes the following four components.

A Comprehensive Quality Management Plan

A **quality management plan** is a systematic method to design, measure, assess, and improve organizational performance. Using a multidisciplinary approach, this plan identifies processes and systems that represent the goals and mission of the organization, identifies the customers, and specifies opportunities for improvement. Critical paths are an example of a quality management plan. Critical paths identify expected outcomes within a specific time frame. This allows care staff to track and account for variances from the expected outcomes. Most units follow a multidisciplinary plan that requires the cooperation of other departments as well as a unit-specific plan. A unit-specific plan usually focuses on activities identified as critical to that unit, such as determining if vital signs are measured and recorded within an hour of each client's admission.

Decision-making processes are guided by data collected, such as the number of postoperative infections or the number of return clinic visits. The team charged with evaluating the data and designing a plan for improvement maintains a focus on client outcomes, expectations, and satisfaction. Implementation of any plan or change is continually evaluated using a client satisfaction survey, which is just one method that can be used to monitor nursing care. For example, in some organizations nursing staff makes direct phone calls to clients following outpatient surgery to ensure clients understand discharge instructions and that their pain is controlled following discharge. Nurses conducting follow-up care with these clients refer any potential complications to the surgeon.

Benchmarking Standards

Standards are generally accepted levels or models of performance or a set of conditions determined to be acceptable by some authorities. **Benchmarking** is a method of comparing standards to actual performance. Standards relate to three major dimensions of quality care:

1. Structure
2. Process
3. Outcome.

Structure standards relate to the physical environment, organization, and management of an organization. An example of a structure standard would be the provision of equipment and the written policy that provides the expectation for care. **Process standards** are those connected with the actual delivery of care, such as the nursing in-services provided to teach nurses how to use new policies, procedures, or equipment. **Outcome standards** involve the end results of care that has been given, such as determining if all medications were given appropriately.

An **indicator** is a tool used to measure the performance of structure, process, and outcome standards. Indicators are measurable, objective, and based on current knowledge. Health care providers determine quality indicators and then use benchmarking to compare actual performance to indicators across institutions or disciplines. These comparisons yield information essential to quality improvement efforts. For example, the nursing unit decides to evaluate the quality of the care provided to newly admitted clients. They determine that the indicators for their study will be a completed initial assessment within 1 hour of admission, a documented and accurate nursing plan of care by the end of the shift, and accurate implementation of physician's orders. The indicators are then compared against each newly admitted client's medical records to benchmark the frequency with which the indicators were met. The nurses on the unit will be informed if the study indicates that the nursing care provided does not comply with the standards for the unit, for example, if less than 80% of newly admitted clients had a complete nursing care plan by the end of the shift.

In nursing, both generic and specific standards of care are available from the American Nurses Association or specialty organizations; however, each organization and each client care area must designate standards specific to the client population being served. These standards are the foundation on which all other measures of quality are based.

An example of a standard is that every client will have a written nursing care plan within 12 hours of admission.

Intradisciplinary Assessment and Improvement

There will always be a need for groups to assess, analyze, and improve their own performance.

Methods to assess performance should involve a single discipline, or intradisciplinary performance. Peer review, audits, and outcomes management are examples of **intradisciplinary assessment**.

PEER REVIEW **Peer review** occurs when practicing nurses assess and judge the performance of professional peers against predetermined standards. Peer review is an important method of assessment because nurses are the experts at determining the indicators of quality nursing care and when such care has been provided. Their expertise is especially useful in complicated cases; sometimes more than one expert's opinion is used for comparisons. For example, a hospital may bring together experienced nurses from the departments of obstetrics, gynecology, and reproductive services to evaluate the standards of care for high risk pregnancies.

OUTCOMES MANAGEMENT **Outcomes management** measures and evaluates costs and quality in order to improve clinical practice. Internal or external data from the literature or other health care providers are used as benchmarks against which process, quality, and financial goals can be set and achieved. Additionally, data from internal clinical information systems can be used to provide information about client care delivery and associated cost. Outcomes management assessments typically use research-based standardized practice models such as order sets or critical pathways as the standards against which client outcomes are measured. Outcomes data are gathered and analyzed. Care is redesigned based on the outcomes analysis and new processes implemented as necessary. Where client outcomes indicate quality care is being provided, outcomes data can provide information regarding how quality care is being achieved. For example, a large neonatal intensive care unit discovered that their client outcomes for infants requiring ventilatory support were far superior to national averages. As a result, they examined their processes as compared to others to determine what factor had the greatest significance in improving client outcomes.

AUDITS An **audit** is an examination of records or financial accounts to verify accuracy. An audit can be retrospective or concurrent. A **retrospective audit** is conducted after a client's discharge and involves examining records of a large number of cases. The client's entire course of care is evaluated and comparisons are made across cases. Recommendations for change can be based on the experiences of many clients with similar care problems as well as on the spectrum of care considered.

A **concurrent audit** is conducted during the client's course of care. Concurrent audits allow organizations to examine the care being given to achieve a desired outcome in the client's health and to evaluate the nursing care activities being provided. They allow for changes to be made if client outcomes indicate a need for changes. If the audit is focused only on nursing, it is used as an intradisciplinary assessment. If the audit is used across departments, it becomes an interdisciplinary tool. For example, an audit of the client's respiratory care as provided by nurses may focus on positioning, oxygen administration, and medication administration. An interdisciplinary audit may focus on timeliness of respiratory treatments, appropriate medical orders, as well as the proper delivery of nursing care.

Interdisciplinary Assessment and Improvement

Multidisciplinary, client-focused teamwork emphasizing collaboration, communication, coordination, and integration of care is the core of successful quality management programs. Utilization review is one method for assessing teamwork. Audits and peer reviews can be used as well. It is important to remember that interdisciplinary assessments do not take the place of intradisciplinary quality efforts such as infection control and surveying client satisfaction with care.

UTILIZATION REVIEW **Utilization reviews** are based on the appropriate allocation of resources and are mandated by The Joint Commission for organizations that it accredits. A utilization review is not specifically directed toward nursing care, but it may provide information on nursing practices that require further investigation. For example, a utilization review may reveal that safer client care on a particular unit requires a lower nurse to client ratio. The facility must then determine the availability of resources (nurses, operating budget) to meet the demand for greater staffing on this unit.

MEASURING QUALITY IMPROVEMENT

There are a number of quantifiable systems that measure performance against set standards. Four common programs are total quality management, continuous quality improvement, Six Sigma, and Lean Six Sigma. The system used will depend on the facility and the type of client care that it provides.

Total Quality Management

Total quality management (TQM) is a management philosophy that emphasizes a commitment to excellence throughout the organization. TQM was created by Dr. W. Edwards Deming. Dr. Deming based his system on principles of quality management that were originally applied to improve quality and performance in the manufacturing industry. These principles, or characteristics, are now widely used to improve quality and customer satisfaction in a number of service industries, including health care.

Four core characteristics of total quality management are:

1. It is customer/client focused.
2. It involves the total organization.
3. It uses quality tools and statistics for measurement.
4. It identifies key processes for improvement.

CUSTOMER/CLIENT FOCUS An important theme of quality management is to address the needs of both internal and external customers. Internal customers include employees and departments within the organization, such as nurses, laboratory technicians, and office staff. External customers of a health care organization include clients, visitors, physicians, managed-care organizations, insurance companies, regulatory agencies such as The Joint Commission, and public health departments.

Under the principles of TQM, nurses must know who the customers are and endeavor to meet their needs. Putting the customer first requires creative and innovative methods to meet the ever-changing needs of internal and external customers. Providing flexible schedules for employees, adjusting routines for a.m. care to meet the needs of clients, extending clinic hours beyond 5 p.m., and putting infant changing tables in restrooms are some examples of changes implemented in organizations using TQM.

TOTAL ORGANIZATIONAL INVOLVEMENT The goal of quality management is to involve and empower all employees to make a difference in the quality of service they provide. This means all nurses must understand the TQM philosophy as it relates to their job and the overall goals and mission of the organization. Knowledge of the TQM process breaks down barriers between departments. It eliminates the phrase "that's not my job" as departments work together as a team. In organizations that embrace TQM, one might find employees occasionally stepping beyond their ordinary job descriptions in an effort to increase productivity and meet customer needs. For example, one might see a nurse cleaning a bed for a new admission from the emergency room or an administrator transporting a client to the radiology department. Sharing processes across departments and client care functions increases teamwork, productivity, and positive client outcomes.

USING QUALITY TOOLS AND STATISTICS FOR MEASUREMENT A common management adage is "You can't manage what you can't (or don't) measure" (Chaiken & Holmquest, 2003). There are many tools, formats, and designs that can be used to build knowledge, make decisions, and improve quality. Tools for data analysis and display can be used to identify areas for process and quality improvement, and then to benchmark the progress of improvements. Deming applied the scientific method to develop a model he called the Plan-Do-Study-Act cycle (PDSA) depicted in Figure 48–2 ■.

Plan-Do-Study-Act (PDSA) When the nurse identifies a problem with the way things are normally done, it must consider a change to improve outcomes. Once the change is identified and put into action, the change must be evaluated to determine its effectiveness. The **Plan-Do-Study-Act (PDSA)** is one method of testing the effectiveness of the change. A plan to test the change is developed (Plan), then the plan is put into action (Do), and then the consequences of the changed process are collected (Study). Based on an analysis of the consequences of the changes made, the nurse determines what modifications are required (Act). See the Clinical Example that follows.

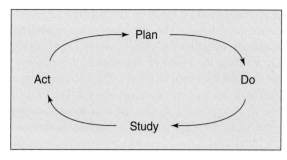

Figure 48–2 ■ PDSA cycle.
Source: Adapted from Schroeder, P. (1994). Improving quality performance. St. Louis, MO: Mosby.

CLINICAL EXAMPLE
At 6:30 a.m., 30 minutes before change of shift, Sue Ann Wong is finishing morning care for a client in the ICU. Sue Ann, a very experienced and reliable nurse, knows she still has charting to complete, new orders to transcribe, and that the client's room needs to be tidied before her replacement arrives. While thinking about all that needs to be done, Sue Ann mistakenly connects the client's tube feeding to the IV line and the IV line to the client's nasogastric tube. Fifteen minutes later Sue Ann notices what she has done and the client is already showing serious effects from the error. The infusing IV and tube feeding are discontinued, the doctor is notified and arrives at the client's bedside, and corrective action is put in place. Unfortunately, it is too late and the client dies several hours later.

The next day the nurse manager conducts a root cause analysis, a special process used to determine factors that contributed to the event, by sitting with Sue Ann and asking her to describe what happened, why she thinks it happened, and what the unit could do to prevent this error from ever occurring again. This analysis leads to the decision to purchase new tubing for feedings that will not fit into an IV line, thereby preventing a misconnection in the future. The nurse manager develops a plan to put a rush order in for the new tubing, orient staff to the new equipment, and ask the Standards and Practice Committee to research and revise the current procedure for tube feedings to incorporate the new tubing and caution against changing IV tubing and tube feed tubing at the same time (Plan). When the new procedure is written and the new tubing arrives, the nurse manager puts the plan into action, calling a mandatory staff meeting to share the new procedure and demonstrate how to use the new tubing (Act). The nurse manager surveys the nursing staff members over the course of the next month to determine their proficiency with both the new tubing and the new procedure. The nurse manager also reviews client charts to determine if any problems or complications arise (Study). The nurse manager and quality improvement team find that the new tubing that has been ordered often leaks. The nurse manager finds similar tubing with a better connector and replaces the old tubing to everyone's satisfaction (Act).

IDENTIFICATION OF KEY PROCESSES FOR IMPROVEMENT
All activities performed in an organization can be described in terms of processes. Processes within a health care setting can be

■ Systems-related (e.g., admitting, discharging, and transferring clients)
■ Clinical (e.g., administering medications, managing pain)
■ Managerial (e.g., risk management and performance evaluations).

Processes can be complex and may involve multidisciplinary or interdepartmental actions. Processes involving multiple departments must be studied in detail by members from each department involved in the activity. Careful study of processes allows team members to seek opportunities to reduce waste and inefficiencies, to minimize the potential for errors, and to develop ways to improve performance and promote positive outcomes.

CLINICAL EXAMPLE
Consider the many departments involved in the administration of medications. The physician must order the medication, the order must be accurately transcribed, and the order must be sent to the pharmacy where a pharmacist fills the order. A pharmacy clerk then delivers the medication to the unit, where he or she must place it in the correct client drawer. Finally, the nurse must prepare the medication and check the accuracy of the order before administering it to a client. All of these departments and people must work well together in order to deliver the right medication to the correct client while assuring that the dosage is correct, the medication is appropriate to treat the client's problem, and that the medication will not interact with other medications the client is taking.

Continuous Quality Improvement
TQM is an overall philosophy, whereas **continuous quality improvement (CQI)** is a process used to improve quality and performance. TQM and CQI often are used synonymously. In health care organizations, CQI is the process used to systematically investigate ways to improve client care. As the name implies, continuous quality improvement is a never-ending endeavor (Hedges, 2006).

CQI means more than just meeting standards and thresholds or solving problems. It involves evaluation, actions, and a mindset to strive constantly for excellence. This concept is sometimes difficult to grasp because client care involves the synchronization of activities in multiple departments. Therefore, the importance of developing and implementing a carefully designed process is key to a successful CQI implementation.

There are four major players in the CQI process:

1. Resource group
2. Coordinator
3. Team leader
4. Team.

The resource group is made up of senior management (e.g., CEO, vice presidents). The resource group establishes the organization's overall CQI policy, vision, and values, and actively involves the board of directors in this process. This ensures that the CQI program has sufficient emphasis and is provided with the training resources needed. The CQI coordinator is often appointed by the CEO to provide day-to-day management of the CQI process and related activities (e.g., training programs).

CQI teams are designated to evaluate and improve selected processes. These teams are formally established and supported by the resource group. CQI teams range in size from 5 to 10 people, and include representation from all major functions of the process being evaluated.

Each CQI team is headed by a team leader who is familiar with the process being evaluated. The leader organizes team meetings, sets meeting agendas, and guides the group through the discussion, evaluation, and implementation process. On the nursing unit, the team manager may be a middle manager or an experienced staff nurse. All nurses may be members of the team, or the team may be limited to those on the CQI committee. Regardless of the team's composition, all nurses on the unit contribute to the success or failure of the CQI effort.

One study integrated continuous quality improvement with client feedback (Hyrkas & Lehti, 2003). Results revealed that nurses and clients were more satisfied when their evaluations of the quality of care agreed. The researchers concluded that integrating CQI with team supervision improved the quality of client care as well.

Six Sigma

Six Sigma is another quality management program that uses quantitative data to monitor progress (Pande & Holpp, 2002). Six Sigma is a *measure*, a *goal*, and a *system of management*.

- *As a measure.* Sigma is the Greek letter—σ—for standard, meaning how much performance varies from a standard. This is similar to how CQI monitors results against an outcome measure.
- *As a goal.* One goal might be accuracy. How many times, for example, is the right medication given in the right amount to the right client at the right time by the right route?
- *As a management system.* Compared to other quality management systems, Six Sigma involves management to a greater extent in monitoring performance and ensuring favorable results.

The system has six themes:

1. Customer (client) focus
2. Data driven
3. Process emphasis
4. Proactive management
5. Boundary-free collaboration
6. Aim for perfection; tolerate failure.

The first three themes are similar to other quality management programs. The focus is on the object of the service, in nursing's case—the client. Data provide the evidence of results and the emphasis is on the processes used in the system.

The latter three themes, however, differ from other programs. Management is actively involved and boundaries breached (e.g., the disconnect between departments). More radically, Six Sigma tolerates failure (a necessary condition for creativity) while striving for perfection.

Lean Six Sigma

Lean Six Sigma focuses on improving process flow and eliminating waste (Martin, 2007). Waste occurs when the organization provides more resources than are required. For example, most managers respond to an increase in the number of clients served by adding staff but tend not to reduce staff when the number of clients declines (Caldwell, 2006). Because the goal of Lean Six Sigma is to identify and reduce waste, it provides tools that can be used with a Six Sigma management system.

IMPROVING THE QUALITY OF CARE

TQM, CQI, Six Sigma, and Lean Six Sigma are quantifiable systems that measure performance against set standards, but they are not a panacea for all of health care's problems. For example, in the 1970s, health maintenance organizations, following the example of Paul Ellwood, tried to "manage" health care with prepaid service. Elwood neglected, however, to account for unintended consequences. Although Elwood sought to encourage preventive care, the reverse happened: Physicians were motivated to limit or reduce care (Bruhn, 2004).

In contrast to Ellwood, Donald Berwick (2002) used an organizational approach to health care's problems by focusing on the client, not the physician. Similarly, Kaissi (2006) proposes that a culture of safety, rather than a culture of blame, characterizes an organization where everyone accepts responsibility for client safety. Errors are opportunities to improve by focusing on "what happened" as opposed to "who did it." Wojner (2002) agrees, stating that providers and administrators must partner to reduce errors and improve safety and that organizational transparency should be the goal of client safety initiatives.

How Quality Improvement Affects Costs

Quality measures can reduce costs by preventing misuse or waste of important resources (Nolan & Bisognano, 2006). Examples include the time nurses waste looking for missing supplies or lab results, the costs of overtime pay and agency nurses due to unfilled positions, and delay in client discharge due to lack of coordination or an adverse event (e. g., medication error).

Nurse Staffing

Evidence is growing that increased nurse staffing results in better client outcomes (American Nurses Association, 2007). A comprehensive review of studies from 1990 to 2006 in the United States and Canada found that a higher RN-to-client ratio resulted in reduced client mortality and shortened lengths of stay (Reeves, 2007). Likewise, another study reported that as the number of nurses rises, infection rates fall (Reeves, 2007).

Reducing Medication Errors

To reduce medication errors, the Institute of Medicine (2006) suggests that clients must become more involved in managing their own care and that providers must help educate clients as well as encourage clients to educate themselves. The IOM also advises using point-of-care technology to access drug reference information and that medication names be unique to avoid unnecessary confusion. Nurses can also provide education to clients and their families regarding proper medication administration and encourage them to ask their physician and pharmacist for clarification when they have questions regarding their medications.

RISK MANAGEMENT

Whereas quality management is a prevention-focused approach, risk management is problem focused. It is a component of quality management, but its purpose is to identify, analyze, and evaluate risks and then to develop a plan for reducing the frequency and severity of accidents and injuries. Risk management is a continuous daily program of detection, education, and intervention.

A risk management program involves all departments of the organization. It must be an organization-wide program, with the board of directors' approval and input from all departments. The program must have high-level commitment, including that of the chief executive officer and the chief nurse.

A risk management program:

1. Identifies potential risks for accident, injury, or financial loss. Formal and informal communication with all organizational departments and inspection of facilities are essential to identifying problem areas.
2. Reviews current organization-wide monitoring systems (incident reports, audits, committee minutes, oral complaints, client questionnaires), evaluates completeness, and determines additional systems needed to provide the factual data essential for risk management control.
3. Analyzes the frequency, severity, and causes of general categories and specific types of incidents causing injury or adverse outcomes to clients. To plan risk intervention strategies, it is necessary to estimate the outcomes associated with the various types of incidents.
4. Reviews and appraises safety and risk aspects of client care procedures and new programs.
5. Monitors laws and codes related to client safety, consent, and care.
6. Eliminates or reduces risks as much as possible.
7. Reviews the work of other committees to determine potential liability and recommend prevention or corrective action. Examples of such committees are infection, medical audit, safety/security, pharmacy, nursing audit, and productivity.
8. Identifies needs for client, family, and employee education.
9. Evaluates the results of a risk management program.
10. Provides periodic reports to administration, medical staff, and the board of directors.

The nurse plays a key role in the success of any risk management program. Nurses can reduce risk by viewing health and illness from the client's perspective. Usually, the nurse's understanding of quality differs from the client's expectations and perceptions. By understanding the meaning of the course of illness to the client and the family, the nurse will manage risk better because that understanding can enable the nurse to individualize client care. This individualized attention produces respect and, in turn, reduces risk.

A client incident or a client's or family's expression of dissatisfaction regarding care indicates an issue with quality of care and carries potential liability. A distraught, dissatisfied, complaining client is a high risk; a satisfied client or family is a low risk. A personal approach is required to reduce risk or liability. Many claims are filed because of a breakdown in communication between the health care provider and the client. In many instances, after an incident or bad outcome, a quick visit or call from an organization's representative to the client or family can soothe tempers and clarify misinformation.

Once an incident has occurred, the important factors in successful risk management are

- Recognition of the incident.
- Quick follow-up and action.
- Personal contact.
- Immediate restitution (where appropriate).

Most clients' and their family's concerns can and should be handled at the unit level. When the first line of communication breaks down, the nurse needs a resource—usually the nurse manager, risk manager, or nursing service administrator.

For more information on risk management, see Exemplar 47.5, Risk Management.

PRACTICE ALERT
The nurse sets the tone that contributes to a safe and low-risk environment. One of the most important ways to reduce risk is to instill a sense of confidence in both clients and families by emphasizing and recognizing that they will receive personalized attention and that their needs will be attended to with competence.

CREATING A BLAME-FREE ENVIRONMENT

Most errors in health care are due to system failures, according to the Institute of Medicine's 2000 report. Thus, reducing errors and preventing potential errors (near misses) requires a systemwide solution.

The goal of dealing with adverse events is to correct system failures, prevent future mistakes, and ensure client safety (Mace, 2005). Reprisal for mistakes, on the other hand, discourages reporting, which can lead to continuation of the problem area or exacerbation of the problem. Conversely, nurses should be encouraged to report adverse events and to help discover solutions to prevent mistakes in the future.

To create a blame-free environment the organization must put in place organization-wide, equitable policies for reporting. Mace (2005) recommends dealing with exceptions to the blame-free environment with a separate disciplinary policy.

EVIDENCE-BASED PRACTICE How Is Quality Improvement Being Conducted in Nursing Homes?

The purpose of this study, conducted in 35 nursing homes managed by the Veterans Administration, was to examine the association between quality improvement (QI) and client outcomes. Over 1,000 members of the nursing staff completed surveys on the culture of the setting, satisfaction, and specific information regarding implementation of pressure ulcer prevention guidelines. There were differences among the nursing homes in their implementation of QI practices, and QI appeared to be associated with employee satisfaction and the perception of providing better care. However, the results were inconclusive in terms of demonstrating an effect of QI on quality of care.

Implications

The results demonstrated the need for continued study before QI is widely promoted as a means for improving nursing home quality. The relationship between use of QI and satisfaction of the nursing staff is an optimistic sign. Quality improvement, as well as other interventions to improve care, is unlikely to be successfully implemented in nursing homes that are not suitably predisposed to making the necessary changes in how care is delivered.

Note: From Berlowitz, D. R., Young, G. J., Hickey, E. C., Saliba, D., Mittman, B. S., Czarnowski, E., et al. (2003). Quality improvement implementation in the nursing home. *Health Services Research, 38*(1 Part 1), 65–83.

Exceptions include failure to report an adverse event or error, criminal acts, false reporting, or refusing to participate in a system designed to prevent errors.

Managing and improving quality requires ongoing attention to systemwide processes and individual actions. The nurse is in a key position to identify problems and encourage a culture of safety and quality.

NURSING PRACTICE

All nurses, no matter where they are employed or what area they specialize in, must be involved in quality improvement. The nursing student demonstrates concern for quality by making a commitment never to perform an act which the student is uncertain how to perform, by showing accountability for his or her actions, and by admitting to errors if they occur. Each nurse, whether a nursing student or a practicing nurse, has the responsibility to know the policies and

procedures in the facility where clinicals are performed and to follow them exactly.

CONCLUSION

Measured standards are used extensively both to prevent and to reveal errors, but the same cannot be said when measuring human behavior, which can vary and still be effective (Borckardt et al., 2006). Embracing any system to the extent that variance is completely discouraged can reduce creativity (Harris & Zeisler, 2002). Absence of creativity may sacrifice improvement in quality at the expense of innovative ideas and processes, resulting in organizations that fail to allow input, become stagnant, and cease to be effective. This is the danger of all living systems that depend on outside input for survival. This is not to say that quality improvement systems are not essential. They are. Organizations must find ways to foster creativity and innovation without compromising quality management.

REVIEW Quality Improvement

RELATE: LINK THE CONCEPTS

Linking the concept of Quality Improvement with the concept of Collaboration:
1. How can the nurse use conflict management skills to resolve client or client's family member's dissatisfaction with care?
2. How does strong interdisciplinary team communication improve the outcomes of total quality management?

Linking the concept of Quality Improvement with the concept of Managing Care:
3. How does an effective quality improvement process reduce the cost of care?
4. How does proper care coordination improve the quality of care provided to clients?

REFER: GO TO MYNURSINGKIT

REFLECT: CASE STUDY

Jesus Hernandez is a newly graduated nurse who has successfully passed the NCLEX-RN® and has accepted a job working on a busy genitourinary unit in the local community hospital. During orientation,

he is working evening shift with a preceptor. On this particular evening, the unit has been very busy and the charge nurse asks Jesus's preceptor, Fred McFarlane, to take a few clients in addition to acting as a preceptor for Jesus with his assigned clients. Fred agrees and instructs Jesus to seek him out if he needs help or has any questions.

Quite by accident, Jesus notices that Fred makes a medication error when he fails to administer an ordered medication at an appropriate time to one of Fred's assigned clients. Jesus doesn't say anything because Fred acknowledges the error independently, but Jesus isn't sure what to do at the end of the shift when he realizes Fred is not going to fill out an incident report.
1. Should an incident report be filled out regarding Fred's late administration of a medication to the client if no harm resulted? Explain the rationale for your answer.
2. Who is responsible for completing an incident report, if one is required? Explain your answer.
3. What is Jesus's responsibility related to the sentinel event if he had no care responsibility related to the client who received the medication later than ordered?
4. How would you handle this situation if you were Jesus?

REFERENCES

American Nurses Association. (2007). Infections and deaths down, quality up: Evidence for having appropriate nurse staffing mounts. *American Journal of Nursing, 107*(4), 19.

Associated Press. (2010). Daughters sue veterans' home after dad wandered out into freezing cold and died. Retrieved April 30, 2010, from http://www.nola.com/crime/index.ssf/2010/02/daughters_sue_veterans_home_af.html

Berlowitz, D. R., Young, G. J., Hickey, E. C., Saliba, D., Mittman, B. S., Czarnowski, E., et al. (2003). Quality improvement implementation in the nursing home. *Health Services Research, 38*(1 Part 1), 65–83.

Berwick, D. M., Godfrey, A. B., & Roessner, J. (2002). *Curing health care: New strategies for quality improvement.* Hoboken, NJ: Jossey-Bass.

Borckardt, J. J., Nash, M. R., Hardesty, S., Herbert, J., Cooney, H., & Pelic, C. (2006). How unusual are the "unusual events" detected by control chart techniques in healthcare settings? *Journal for Healthcare Quality: Promoting Excellence in Healthcare, 28*(4), 4–9.

Bruhn, J. G. (2004). Leaders who create change and those who manage it: How leaders limit success. *The Health Care Manager, 23*(7), 132–140.

Caldwell, C. (2006). Lean Six Sigma: Tools for rapid cycle cost reduction. *Healthcare Financial Management, 60*(10), 96–98.

Domrose, C. (2007). Malpractice suits against nurses on the rise. Retrieved April 30, 2010, from http://news.nurse.com/apps/pbcs.dll/article?AID=2007708270302

Chaiken, B. P., & Holmquest, D. L. (2003). Patient safety: Modifying processes to eliminate medical errors. *Nursing Outlook, 51*(3), S21–S24.

Guido, G. W. (2010). *Legal and ethical issues in nursing.* Upper Saddle River, NJ: Pearson.

Harris, S. D., & Zeisler, S. (2002). Weak signals: Detecting the next big thing. *The Futurist, 36*(6), 21–28.

Hedges, C. (2006). Research, evidence-based practice, and quality improvement. *AACN Advanced Critical Care, 17*(4), 457–458.

Hyrkas, K., & Lehti, K. (2003). Continuous quality improvement through team supervision supported by continuous self-monitoring of work and systematic patient feedback. *Journal of Nursing Management, 11*(3), 177–188.

Institute for Healthcare Improvement. (2007). *About us.* Retrieved December 2007, from http://www.ihi.org/IHI

Institute of Medicine. (2000). *To err is human: Building a safer health system.* Washington, DC: National Academy Press.

Institute of Medicine. (2001). *Crossing the quality chasm: A new health system for the 21st century.* Washington, DC: National Academy Press.

Institute of Medicine. (2006). *Preventing medication errors.* Washington, DC: National Academy Press.

Joint Commission. (2007). Sentinel events policies and procedures. Retrieved April 5, 2010, from http://www.jointcommission.org/NR/rdonlyres/F84F9DC6-A5DA-490F-A91F-A9FCE26347C4/0/SE_chapter_july07.pdf

Joint Commission on Accreditation of Healthcare Organizations. (2005a). *Mission statement.* Retrieved April 16, 2006, from http://www.jointcommission.org/AboutUs/joint_commission_facts.htm

Joint Commission on Accreditation of Healthcare Organizations. (2005b). *Sentinel event policy and procedures.* Retrieved April 16, 2006, from http://www.jointcommission.org/SentinelEvents/

Kaissi, A. (2006). An organizational approach to understanding patient safety and medical errors. *The Health Care Manager, 25*(4), 292–305.

Mace, K. A. (2005). Is employee discipline the solution for patient safety? *Nursing Management, 36*(12), 57–59.

Martin, W. F. (2007). Quality models: Selecting the best model to deliver results. *The Physician Executive, 33*(3), 24–29.

Montalvo, I. (September 30, 2007). The national database of nursing quality indicators™ (NDNQI®). *OJIN: The Online Journal of Issues in Nursing, 12*(3), Manuscript 2. Retrieved from www.nursingworld.org/MainMenuCategories/ANAMarketplace/ANAPeriodicals/OJIN/TableofContents/Volume122007/No3Sept07/NursingQualityIndicators.aspx

Nolan, R., & Bisognano, M. (2006). Finding the balance between quality and cost. *Healthcare Financial Management, 60*(4), 67–72.

Pande, P., & Holpp, L. (2002). *What is Six Sigma?* New York: McGraw-Hill.

Reeves, K. (2007). New evidence report on nurse staffing and quality of patient care. *MEDSURG Nursing, 16*(2), 73–74.

The President's Advisory Commission on Consumer Protection and Quality in the Health Care Industry. (1999). *Quality first: Better health care for all Americans.* Washington, DC: U.S. Government Printing Office.

Von Korff, M., et al. (1997). Collaborative management of chronic illness. *Annals of Internal Medicine, 127*(12), 1097–1102.

Wagner, E., Austin, B., & Von Korff, M. (1996). Organizing care for patients with chronic illness. *Milbank Quarterly, 74*(4), 511–542.

Wiseman, B., & Kaprielian, V. S. (2005). Patient safety–quality improvement. Duke Center for Instructional Technology. Retrieved March 29, 2010, from http://patientsafetyed.duhs.duke.edu/module_a/module_overview.html

Wojner, A. W. (2002). Capturing error rates and reporting significant data. *Critical Care Nursing Clinics of North America, 14*(4), 375–384.

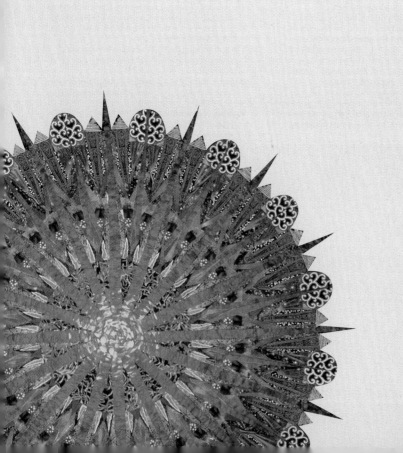

Safety

49

Concept at-a-Glance

About Safety, *2433*

49.1   Anticipatory Guidance, *2439*

49.2   Environmental Safety, *2442*

49.3   Injury and Illness Prevention, *2449*

49.4   National Patient Safety Goals, *2459*

49.5   Responsible Sexual Behavior, *2461*

Concept Learning Outcomes

After reading about this concept, you will be able to:

1. Describe the factors assessed for in determining the client's safety.

2. Apply appropriate nursing diagnoses to the client with potential risks to safety.

3. Describe nursing interventions to reduce the client's risk of injury.

4. Predict specific learning outcomes appropriate for evaluating the client's response to care related to safety.

5. Define standard precautions and describe how they reduce risk to nurses and clients.

Concept Key Terms

Awareness, *2434*

Hand-off communication, *2435*

Personal protective equipment, *2435*

Safety, *2433*

Standard precautions, *2435*

About Safety

Safety, defined as protection from harm or injury, has always been a fundamental concern of nurses in every setting. The landmark IOM report *To Err is Human: Building a Safer Health System* brought to light a number of issues related to client safety and stirred a nationwide effort by the entire health care industry to increase client safety and quality of care in health care facilities (IOM, 2000). Two more recent publications focus specifically on how nurses promote client safety: *Keeping Patients Safe: Transforming the Work of Nurses* and *Patient Safety and Quality: An Evidence-Based Handbook for Nurses*. These publications identify specific, evidence-based practices that nurses can use to provide safe, quality care for clients in the variety of health care settings.

More than any other group of health care professionals, nurses are "in a key position to improve the quality of health care through patient safety interventions and strategies" (Mitchell, 2008, p. 20). This concept discusses a number of preventive strategies and safety interventions that nurses can use to promote client safety and reduce client risk for illness or injury. Because nurses care for clients within the context of clients' own practices, beliefs, and environments, this concept also discusses factors that affect client safety and what constitutes a safe environment. •

FACTORS AFFECTING SAFETY

The ability of people to protect themselves from illness or injury is affected by many factors. Nurses need to assess each of these factors when planning care or teaching clients to protect themselves.

Age and Development

People learn to protect themselves from many illnesses and injuries through knowledge and accurate assessment of the environment. For the very young, learning about the environment is essential and requires a great deal of exploration. Appropriate parental supervision and teaching combined with personal experience help children learn what is potentially harmful.

Older adults can have difficulty with movement and diminished sensory acuity that contribute to the likelihood of injury. Specific age-related potential hazards and preventive measures are discussed in Exemplar 49.3, Injury and Illness Prevention. Selected hazards throughout the life span are discussed in the Developmental Considerations feature that follows.

Lifestyle

Lifestyle factors that place people at risk for injury include unsafe work environments; residence in neighborhoods with high crime rates; access to weapons, including firearms and ammunition; insufficient income to buy safety equipment or make necessary repairs; and access to illicit drugs, which may also be contaminated by harmful additives. Risk-taking behavior is a factor in some accidents.

Mobility and Health Status

People with impaired mobility due to paralysis, muscle weakness, poor balance, or coordination obviously are prone to injury. Clients with spinal cord injury and paralysis of both legs may be unable to move even when they perceive discomfort. Weakness resulting from illness or surgery can also place clients at risk for injury. Some disease processes affect mobility and balance. People with Parkinson's disease, for example, may develop a shuffling pattern of walking that increases their risk for tripping and falling or may fall due to a temporary inability to walk or move (National Parkinson Foundation, 2010).

Sensory-Perceptual Alterations

Accurate sensory perception of environmental stimuli is vital to safety. People with impaired touch perception, hearing, taste, smell, and vision are highly susceptible to injury.

Cognitive Awareness

Awareness is the ability to perceive environmental stimuli or body reactions and to respond appropriately through thought and action. Clients with impaired awareness include those who

- Suffer from sleep deficit
- Are unconscious or semiconscious
- Are disoriented and therefore may not understand where they are or what to do to help themselves
- Perceive stimuli that do not exist
- Experience alterations in judgment due to disease or medications such as narcotics, tranquilizers, hypnotics, and sedatives.

Clients with mild confusion may momentarily forget where they are, wander from their rooms, misplace personal belongings, and risk potential injury.

Emotional State

Extreme emotional states can alter a person's ability to perceive environmental hazards. Stressful situations can reduce level of concentration, cause errors of judgment, and decrease awareness of external stimuli. People with depression may think and react to environmental stimuli more slowly than usual.

Ability to Communicate

Individuals with diminished ability to receive and convey information are at risk for injury. This includes clients with aphasia, people with language barriers, and those who are

---

DEVELOPMENTAL CONSIDERATIONS | Selected Hazards Throughout the Life Span

- *Developing fetus:* Exposure to maternal smoking, alcohol consumption, addictive drugs, x-rays (first trimester), and certain pesticides
- *Newborns and infants:* Falling, suffocating in crib, choking from aspirated milk or ingested objects, burns from hot water or other spilled hot liquids, automobile accidents, crib or playpen injuries, electric shock, and poisoning
- *Toddlers:* Physical trauma from falling, banging into objects, or getting cut by sharp objects; automobile accidents; burns; poisoning; drowning; and electric shock

- *Preschoolers:* Injury from traffic, playground equipment, and other objects; choking, suffocation, and obstruction of airway or ear canal by foreign objects; poisoning; drowning; fire and burns; and harm from other people or animals
- *Adolescents:* Vehicular (automobile, bicycle) accidents, recreational accidents, firearms, and substance abuse
- *Older adults:* Falling, burns, and pedestrian or automobile accidents

unable to read. For example, the individual who is unable to interpret the sign "No Smoking—Oxygen in Use" could cause a fire if he or she lights a cigarette.

Culture

Culture can influence safety. Language barriers can prevent one from receiving and understanding information about all aspects of injury and illness prevention. Culture influences social and physical behaviors that impact health. Individuals from some cultures often have difficulty understanding where to go to seek health services or may face other barriers to access, such as lack of insurance.

Complementary and Alternative Medicine

Complementary and alternative medicine practices must be assessed for safety, including positive and negative effects, cost, efficacy, and clinical usefulness. The use of herbs and natural products raises many issues, such as safety and efficacy, interactions with medications or other herbs or supplements, and standardization of product ingredients among manufacturers. Nurses should assess clients' use of complementary and/or alternative medicine and help them determine potential side effects, risks, and other implications of the types of therapy they use.

The National Center for Complementary and Alternative Medicine lists the following safety considerations for herbal and dietary supplements (NCCAM, 2009):
- Read the label instructions.
- Understand that manufacturers do not have to prove consistency, quality, or efficacy of product.
- Understand that manufacturers are not required to follow truth in labeling—the amount of an active ingredient may be lower or higher than what is indicated on the label.
- Understand that terms like "natural" do not guarantee the safety of a product.

Safety Awareness

Information is crucial to safety. Clients in unfamiliar environments frequently need specific safety information. Lack of knowledge about unfamiliar equipment, such as medical equipment, is a potential hazard. Healthy clients need information about water safety, car safety, fire prevention, ways to prevent the ingestion of harmful substances, and many preventive measures related to specific age-related hazards.

HAND-OFF COMMUNICATION

Hand-off communication is conducted any time the nurse plans to be absent from the unit, whether for a break or the end of the shift. For more information on what to include in hand-off communication see Exemplar 36.4, Reporting.

STANDARD PRECAUTIONS

Standard precautions are one of the most important tools for lowering the risk for developing a contagious or nosocomial infection in any health care setting. **Standard precautions** are guidelines recommended by the Centers for Disease Control for reducing the risk of exposure to blood-borne pathogens and other pathogens common in hospital settings. Standard precautions include the major features of universal precautions and body substance isolation, both of which are discussed in detail in Concept 15, Infection. Recommended practices for standard precautions are shown in Box 49–1. Standard precautions should be used at all times when caring for clients in health care settings, regardless of the client's diagnosis infection status.

Personal Protective Equipment

Appropriate use of **personal protective equipment** (e.g., gloves, masks, gowns, goggles, and special resuscitative equipment) reduces the risk for injury to health care providers in health care settings. All health care providers must apply clean or sterile gloves, gowns, masks, and protective eyewear according to the risk of exposure to potentially infective materials. The U.S. Occupational Safety and Health Administration (OSHA) requires use of a HEPA-filtered respirator for protection against occupational exposure to tuberculosis. Surgical masks are ineffective to filter droplet nuclei, necessitating the use of protective devices capable of filtering bacteria and particles smaller than 1 micron.

Handwashing

Handwashing is a primary control measure for infections transmitted via respiratory secretions. *Effective handwashing is the single most important measure in infection control.* Although infections can also be transmitted by the airborne route, via contaminated equipment, and from the environment, these routes are less significant.

For routine client care, the World Health Organization (2005) recommends handwashing under a stream of water for at least 20 seconds using plain granule soap, soap-filled sheets, or liquid soap when hands are visibly soiled, after using the restroom, after removing gloves, before handling invasive devices (e.g., intravenous tubing), and after contact with medical equipment or furniture. A soap and water wash is recommended for visibly soiled hands.

Soap and water alone are inadequate to sufficiently remove pathogens. The Centers for Disease Control and Prevention (2002) recommends use of alcohol-based antiseptic hand rubs (rinses, gels, or foams) before and after direct client contact. Recently, placement of alcohol-based antiseptic hand rub dispensers has been approved for agency corridors (Centers for Medicare and Medicaid Services, 2005).

Antiseptic soaps and detergents are the next most effective agents, and nonantiseptic soaps are the least effective. Antimicrobial soaps are usually provided in high-risk areas, such as the newborn nursery, and are frequently supplied in dispensers at the sink. Studies have shown that the convenience of antimicrobial foams and gels, which do not require soap and water, may increase health care workers' adherence to hand cleansing. The Centers for Disease Control and Prevention recommend antimicrobial hand cleansing agents.

Box 49-1 **Standard Precautions**

- Designed for all clients in hospital.
- These precautions apply to (a) blood; (b) all body fluids, excretions, and secretions except sweat; (c) nonintact (broken) skin; and (d) mucous membranes.
- Designed to reduce risk of transmission of microorganisms from recognized and unrecognized sources.

1. Perform proper hand hygiene after contact with blood, body fluids, secretions, excretions, and contaminated objects whether or not gloves are worn.
   a. Perform proper hand hygiene immediately after removing gloves.
   b. Use a nonantimicrobial product for routine hand cleansing.
   c. Use an antimicrobial agent or an antiseptic agent for the control of specific outbreaks of infection.
2. Wear clean gloves when touching blood, body fluids, secretions, excretions, and contaminated items (e.g., soiled gowns).
   a. Clean gloves can be unsterile unless their use is intended to prevent the entrance of microorganisms into the body.
   b. Remove gloves before touching noncontaminated items and surfaces.
   c. Perform proper hand hygiene immediately after removing gloves.
3. Wear a mask, eye protection, or a face shield if splashes or sprays of blood, body fluids, secretions, or excretions can be expected.

4. Wear a clean, nonsterile gown if client care is likely to result in splashes or sprays of blood, body fluids, secretions, or excretions. The gown is intended to protect clothing.
   a. Remove a soiled gown carefully to avoid the transfer of microorganisms to other individuals (e.g., clients or other health care workers).
   b. Cleanse hands after removing gown.
5. Carefully handle client care equipment that is soiled with blood, body fluids, secretions, or excretions to prevent the transfer of microorganisms to other individuals and the environment.
   a. Ensure reusable equipment is cleaned and reprocessed correctly.
   b. Dispose of single-use equipment correctly.
6. Handle, transport, and process linen that is soiled with blood, body fluids, secretions, or excretions in such a manner to prevent contamination of clothing and the transfer of microorganisms to other individuals and to the environment.
7. Prevent injuries from used scalpels, needles, and other equipment, and place in puncture-resistant containers.

Source: Adapted from Garner J. S., & the Hospital Infection Control Practices Advisory Committee (HICPAC). (1996). Guidelines for isolation precautions in hospitals. *Infection Control Hospital Epidemiology, 17*, 53–80, and (1996). *American Journal of Infection Control, 24*, 24–52.

PRACTICE ALERT
Performing hand hygiene with either soap or alcohol-based cleansers can damage the skin through the drying effect of the detergents or chemicals. If the nurse develops dermatitis, the client may be at higher risk for infection, because handwashing does not decrease bacterial counts on skin with dermatitis. The nurse is also at higher risk because the normal skin barrier has been broken.

NURSING PROCESS

Nurses increase the client's safety and reduce risk for injury by adhering to the nursing process. Assessing for risk, diagnosing risks for injury, planning for safety, implementing precautions, and evaluating the effectiveness of these strategies are critical to providing safe nursing care.

Assessment

Assessing clients at risk for accidents and injury involves noting important indicators in the nursing history and physical examination, using specifically developed risk assessment tools, and evaluating the client's environment (e.g., residence, work, or community). Nurses should gather data about age and developmental level; general health status; mobility status; presence or absence of physiologic or perceptual deficits, such as olfactory, visual, tactile, taste, or other sensory impairments; altered thought processes or other impaired cognitive or emotional capabilities; lifestyle choices; any indications of

abuse or neglect; and any history of accident and injury. A safety history also needs to include the client's awareness of hazards, knowledge of safety precautions both at home and at work, and any perceived threats to safety (Figure 49–1 ■).

Assessing Risk
Assessing clients' safety risks can be challenging. For example, the questions the nurse asks during the nursing history will be different for the single mother with 2-year-old twins than for the older adult living at home alone. For the single mother, the nurse's assessment may include questions related to sleep patterns, stress levels, and child safety precautions such as the use of car safety seats and plug covers. For the older adult or the adult with impaired mobility, the nurse may ask questions about use of medications, home safety measures such as hand rails and smoke detectors, and risk for falling. The Minnesota Falls Prevention Initiative recommends that health care professionals regularly ask the following three questions of older adults (MFPI, n.d.):

1. Have you fallen in the past year?
2. How many times have you fallen in the past year?
3. Are you afraid of falling?

Home Hazard Appraisal
Hazards in the home are major causes of falls, fire, poisoning, suffocation, and other accidents. Improper use of household equipment, tools, and cooking utensils also creates a hazardous environment. These hazards are discussed in detail in Exemplar 49.3, Illness and Injury Prevention. See the following feature, Home Hazard Appraisal for Adults.

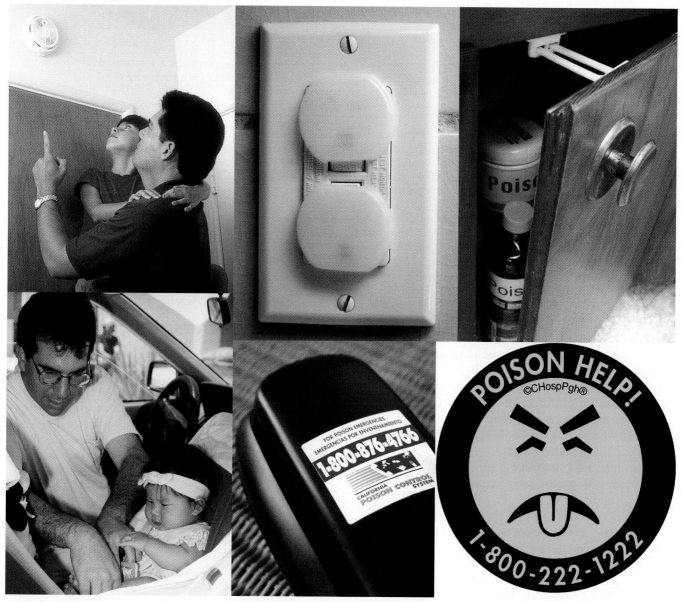

Figure 49–1 ■ Nurses need to teach clients about safety and how to prevent accidents such as using smoke detectors, safety covers for electrical outlets, childproof locks on drawers and cabinets, Mr. Yuk stickers on toxic substances, infant car seats, and by placing poison control information near or on the telephone.

Source: Top, courtesy of Tony Freeman/PhotoEdit; Jerry Marshall; Michael Newman/PhotoEdit. Bottom, Grantpix/Photo Researchers, Inc.; Geri Enberg; Children's Hospital Pittsburgh.

Diagnosis

NANDA offers a broad diagnostic label related to safety issues:
- Risk for Injury: A state in which the individual is at risk for injury as a result of environmental conditions interacting with the individual's adaptive and defense resources.

This broad label consists of seven subcategories that the nurse may use to describe a safety issue more specifically or to isolate safety interventions (Wilkinson, 2005):

1. Risk for Poisoning: Increased risk of accidental exposure to or ingestion of drugs or dangerous products in doses sufficient to cause poisoning.
2. Risk for Suffocation: Increased risk of accidental suffocation (inadequate air available for inhalation).
3. Risk for Trauma: Increased risk of accidental tissue injury (e.g., wound, burn, or fracture).
4. Risk for Latex Allergy Response: Risk of hypersensitivity to natural latex rubber products.
5. Risk for Contamination: Risk of exposure to environmental contaminants in doses sufficient to cause adverse health effects.
6. Risk for Aspiration: At risk for the entry of gastrointestinal secretions, oropharyngeal secretions, solids, or fluids into tracheobronchial passages.
7. Risk for Disuse Syndrome: At risk for deterioration of body systems as the result of prescribed or unavoidable musculoskeletal inactivity.

Home Care Assessment

Home Hazard Appraisal for Adults

- *Walkways and stairways (inside and outside):* Note uneven sidewalks or paths, broken or loose steps, absence of handrails or placement on only one side of stairways, insecure handrails, congested hallways or other traffic areas, and adequacy of lighting at night.
- *Floors:* Note uneven and highly polished or slippery floors and any unanchored rugs or mats.
- *Furniture:* Note hazardous placement of furniture with sharp corners. Note chairs or stools that are too low to get into and out of or that provide inadequate support.
- *Bathroom(s):* Note presence of grab bars around tubs and toilets, nonslip surfaces in tubs and shower stalls, handheld showerhead, adequacy of night lighting, need for raised toilet seat or bath chair in tub or shower, ease of access to shelves, and water temperature regulated at a maximum of 49°C (120°F).
- *Kitchen:* Note pilot lights (gas stove) in need of repair, inaccessible storage areas, and hazardous furniture.
- *Bedrooms:* Note adequacy of lighting, in particular the availability of night-lights and accessibility of light switches; ease of access to commode, urinal, or bedpan; and need for hospital bed or bed rails.
- *Electrical:* Note unanchored or frayed electrical cords and outlets that are overloaded or near water.
- *Fire protection:* Note presence or absence of smoke detectors, fire extinguisher, and fire escape plan, and improper storage of combustibles (e.g., gasoline) or corrosives (e.g., rust remover).
- *Toxic substances:* Note improperly labeled cleaning solutions.
- *Communication devices:* Note presence of method to call for help, such as a telephone or intercom in the bedroom and elsewhere (e.g., kitchen), and access to emergency telephone numbers.
- *Medications:* Note medications kept beyond date of expiration, adequacy of lighting for medication cabinet or storage, and method of disposal of sharp objects such as needles used for injections.

Other safety-related diagnoses the nurse may choose to use include the following:

- Deficient Knowledge (Accident Prevention): Inability to state or explain information or demonstrate a required skill related to safety of self and others.
- Latex Allergy Response: A hypersensitive reaction to natural latex rubber products.
- Contamination: Exposure to environmental contaminants in doses sufficient to cause adverse health effects.

Plan

When planning care to prevent accidents and injury, the nurse considers all factors affecting the client's safety, specifies desired outcomes, and selects nursing activities to meet these outcomes. The major goal for clients with safety risks is to prevent accidents and injury. To meet this goal, clients often need to change their health behavior and may need to modify their environment.

Desired outcomes reflect the client's acquisition of knowledge about hazards, behaviors that incorporate safety practices, and skills to perform in the event of certain emergencies. The nurse needs to individualize these for clients. Examples of desired outcomes include the following:

- The client will describe methods to prevent specific hazards (e.g., falls, suffocation, choking, fires, drowning, and electric shock).
- The client will describe home safety measures (e.g., proper handwashing techniques, fire safety measures, smoke detector maintenance, fall prevention strategies, burn prevention measures, poison prevention measures, safe storage of hazardous materials, firearm safety precautions, electrocution prevention, water safety precautions, bicycle safety, and motor vehicle safety).
- The client will alter his or her home physical environment to reduce the risk of injury.
- The client will describe emergency procedures for poisoning and fire.

Implementation

Implementation of the nursing plan of care directed toward safety may include preventative measures, such as padding side rails when the client is at risk for seizures, anticipatory guidance such as teaching the new mother the importance of always putting the baby in a car seat (Box 49–2) or educational activities such as teaching the older client how to reduce the risk of falls in the home. Implementations may take place in the facility (e.g., covering the top of the crib for a 2 year old to prevent a fall from trying to climb over the bars), in the home (e.g., removing throw rugs in the home of a client with reduced mobility), or in the community (e.g., teaching the importance of having working fire and carbon monoxide monitors in all homes).

PRACTICE ALERT

Nurses should use caution when teaching or assisting parents with infant car safety seats. Nurses who go beyond their level of expertise could face legal action if a subsequent car crash results in injury to the baby. Refer parents to a local trained child passenger safety technician for assistance, or use 1-866-SEAT-CHECK to find a car seat inspection location. You can also refer parents to the AAP car seat guide.

Box 49–2 Car Safety for the School-Age Child

- For children over 40 lb (generally 4–8 years old), use a belt-positioning, forward-facing booster seat located in the backseat. Always use both lap and shoulder belts. Make sure the lap belt fits low and tight across the lap/upper thigh area and the shoulder belt is snug across the chest and shoulder to avoid abdominal injuries.
- Children 4'9" and taller can sit in a regular car seat restrained with lap and shoulder belt that are snug and correctly located across the lap and chest. The backseat is preferred for all children and should be the only location used for children 12 years and younger.

Evaluation

Evaluating whether or not the client has been successful in decreasing risks for illness or injury includes determining whether or not the client implemented recommended safety measures. A client interview may be sufficient to make this evaluation, but in some cases a home appraisal or a review of the client's file may be indicated. Parents may report fewer cases of illness in the family following teaching their children proper handwashing and making soap and towels available at every sink in the house. Older adults may report that they move more easily and safely around the house after installing hand rails, clearing up clutter, and improving lighting.

NURSING PRACTICE

Everything the nurse does—whether giving medications, performing a procedure, assessing the client, or providing client teaching—is directed toward safety. Safety is the primary priority when planning and implementing care. In addition to reducing risk in the facility and helping clients reduce their risk at home, the nurse is also involved in community safety through political activism, community teaching, and recognition of potential hazards.

REVIEW About Safety

RELATE: LINK THE CONCEPTS

Linking the concept of Safety with the concept of Quality Improvement:

1. How does a thorough total quality management system contribute to the client's safety in the facility?
2. The facility has been noting a number of different sentinel events over the past month. How could the facility use its quality improvement program to address the safety concerns?

Linking the concept of Safety with the concept of Communication:

3. How can the nurse improve the client's safety through the use of strong communication skills?
4. What types of things will the nurse communicate to the newly admitted client to improve safety?

REFER: GO TO MYNURSINGKIT

REFLECT: CASE STUDY

Bill Smith, 14 years old, was admitted to the hospital following a bicycle accident that resulted in a compound fracture of the femur requiring 3 weeks in traction. Bill had a cast applied this morning and is very excited to finally be able to get out of bed. The nurse measures for properly sized crutches and enters the client's room to teach him how to use the crutches with a plan to allow him to move to the chair this morning and advance his mobility throughout the day.

1. What risks does Bill have for injury?
2. How can the nurse adapt the plan of care to reduce these risks?
3. What developmental factors contribute to Bill's risk for injury?
4. Why did the nurse choose to only allow the client to walk to the chair instead of allowing him free mobility this morning?

49.1 ANTICIPATORY GUIDANCE

KEY TERMS

Anticipatory guidance, 2439
Cosleeping, 2440

BASIS FOR SELECTION OF EXEMPLAR

Healthy People 2010
Standards of Nursing Practice

LEARNING OUTCOMES

After reading about this exemplar, you will be able to:

1. Describe the nurse's role in providing anticipatory guidance to the client.

OVERVIEW

Anticipatory guidance is most often used to describe client teaching for parents about developmental changes they can expect to see as their children reach specific ages. However, anticipatory guidance may be provided to clients across the life span. The definition of **anticipatory guidance** provided by the *Nursing Interventions Classification* is "preparation of a patient for an anticipated developmental and/or situational crisis" (Bulechek, Butcher, & Dochterman, 2008, p. 137). For example, the nurse may provide anticipatory guidance to older adults to help them recognize limitations secondary to illness so that they can overcome those limitations and maintain safety.

Anticipatory guidance may be provided at any interaction with the client. Some occasions when providing anticipatory guidance is especially appropriate include the following:

- Well-child exams
- Prenatal care visits
- When adolescents ask for information regarding sexual activity or birth control
- When helping older adults adapt to changes in lifestyle as a result of normal changes of aging.

The nurse provides anticipatory guidance in the form of client teaching (discussed in more depth in Concept 39, Teaching and Learning).

Because the time for each visit is limited, nurses should build upon clients' current knowledge and care practices and start with a topic in which the client expresses interest. Nurses using anticipatory guidance should not simply introduce new information, but should reinforce what the client and family are doing well and clear up any poorly understood concepts.

Nurses rely on resources in the community to enhance the guidance provided. For example, Bright Futures (http://www .brightfutures.org/) provides information for anticipatory guidance regarding children. State and local SAFE KIDS coalitions help inform families about injury prevention strategies. School health programs, such as the National Fire Prevention Association's "Risk Watch" (http://www.nfpa.org/categoryList .asp?categoryID=1050), may educate children about injury prevention; other school programs may educate students about smoking and drug avoidance. Nurses should stay informed about the types of health education provided in different settings within their communities in order to be able to reinforce concepts already being taught.

Each stage of development requires different anticipatory guidance. In addition, nurses providing anticipatory guidance should consider the client's health status and health literacy level. See Concept 7, Development; Concept 13, Health, Wellness and Illness; and in this concept, Exemplar 49.3, Injury and Illness Prevention.

DEVELOPMENTAL CONSIDERATIONS

Before giving anticipatory guidance, nurses must consider a number of factors, including age and developmental status.

Children and Adolescents

Anticipatory guidance for children focuses on providing their parents with information on topics such as growth and development; nutrition; oral health; mental health issues

Box 49–3 **Distracted Driving**

Distracted driving has become one of the most talked about safety awareness issues. In 2009, following extensive reviews of more than 50 peer-reviewed research reports, the National Safety Council called for a nationwide ban on all use of cell phones while driving. The NSC estimates that talking on cell phones increases the chances of a motor vehicle accident by four times, and that talking on a cell phone or texting while driving causes approximately 1.6 million accidents each year (Figure 49–2 ■). A number of states have enacted legislation to prevent drivers from using cell phones or texting while driving (National Safety Council, 2010).

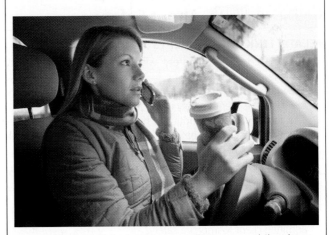

Figure 49–2 ■ Drivers who are talking on mobile phones are four times more likely to be involved in a motor vehicle crash.

DEVELOPMENTAL CONSIDERATIONS | **Sleep Safety for Newborns and Infants**

Newborns should not have pillows or stuffed animals in the crib while they sleep; these items may cause suffocation (American Academy of Pediatrics, 2005). Mattresses should fit snugly in a crib to prevent entrapment and suffocation, and the crib should be inspected regularly to determine whether it is in safe working order. Crib slats should be no more than 2 3/8 inches apart. Parents can be encouraged to attend infant cardiopulmonary resuscitation (CPR) classes, especially if there is a family history of SIDS or the infant requires special care. Parents should be discouraged from **cosleeping**, which increases the infant's risk for SIDS. For families who engage in cosleeping, nurses should provide the following guidelines:

■ Place the infant on a firm mattress, never on comforters, pillows, or a waterbed.
■ Never sleep with your infant if you have been using drugs or have become intoxicated.

■ Ensure that the infant is protected from rolling off the bed or becoming entrapped in the bed rails or a space between the frame and the mattress.
■ As with crib sleeping, remove all decorative pillows, stuffed animals, toys, or blankets that could impair the baby's breathing. Do not cover the baby with blankets, sheets, or down comforters.
■ Make sure the baby is sleeping on his or her back.
■ Ensure plenty of ventilation to the infant.
■ Avoid overdressing the infant because the parent's body heat will reduce the need for excess clothing.
■ Never smoke in bed with the infant. Family members should smoke outdoors and not in the household with the infant.
■ If additional children are sleeping in the bed, make sure they are not sleeping directly next to the infant.

EVIDENCE-BASED PRACTICE Bicycle Helmet Effectiveness and Use

Problem
About 900 children die of bicycle-related injuries annually in the United States. Although helmets can reduce injury, many times they are not worn or are worn incorrectly.

Evidence
A review of 22 studies on helmet use among children provides insight into which strategies are most likely to encourage use of this important safety equipment. Community-based information appears to be the most effective location for delivery of messages, while information provided in schools is slightly less successful. Provision of free helmets is also a positive factor in helmet use, and is more effective than partially subsidized helmets (Royal, Kendrick, & Coleman, 2005).

Implications
Interventions can significantly increase parental and child knowledge about benefits of helmets and their correct use. Interventions to increase helmet use can be integrated into schools, and perhaps more importantly, into community presentations. Providing free or low-cost helmets directly relates to helmet use, so strategies to fund such programs are important. Nurses should not assume that reports of safety precautions such as wearing helmets or seat belts mean that children use these measures correctly. Teach about the benefits of helmets at each health supervision visit. Ask for demonstrations and provide suggestions to improve technique as needed. Common injury causes such as car and bicycle crashes necessitate including at least these evaluations as part of health maintenance activities.

Critical Thinking Application
Where will you find information about helmet safety? What educational programs are available in your schools and communities? Are helmets made available for families that might not be able to afford their purchase? How do you determine if a child is wearing a helmet correctly? Plan educational materials and programs for children who bicycle.

---

such as child and parental mood; ways that families manage stress; risks of second hand smoke; sleep safety and patterns; administering medications and using sunscreen; automobile and bicycle safety; relationships among family members and between peers and classmates; supervising and limiting TV and video game time; the importance of disease prevention strategies, such as immunizations; and injury prevention strategies.

Adolescents may need anticipatory guidance on responsible sexual behavior, sleep patterns, alcohol and drug use, wearing safety equipment during sports activities, using problem solving skills, and automobile safety (Ball, Bindler, & Cowen, pp. 326–335). See Box 49–3, Distracted Driving.

Adults
Nurses provide anticipatory guidance for adults on a case-by-case basis. Appropriate topics may include injury prevention strategies for using electric tools and mechanical equipment; using sunscreen and sunglasses with UVA/UVB protection; and responsible sexual behaviors and drug and alcohol use.

Older Adults
Anticipatory guidance for older adults may include topics such as fall prevention; medication use and potential side effects; age-related changes in nutritional needs; safe driving evaluations; and the need for advance directives.

REVIEW Anticipatory Guidance

RELATE: LINK THE CONCEPTS
Linking the exemplar Anticipatory Guidance with the concept of Reproduction:
1. When caring for a mother preparing to take her first newborn home, what anticipatory guidance would you provide to reduce the risk of injury to the newborn?
2. When caring for a woman during her first prenatal visit, what anticipatory guidance will you provide the client to reduce the risk of injury to both the fetus and the client?

Linking the exemplar of Anticipatory Guidance with the concept of Advocacy:
3. How does the nurse's role as a client advocate blend with the need to provide anticipatory guidance?
4. A mother brings her 14-month-old son to the clinic with symptoms of an ear infection. While the nurse conducts the interview, the mother states, "He is just so stubborn (indicating the child). He refuses to use the potty and keeps wetting his diapers no matter what I do. I'm getting so frustrated!" How can the nurse advocate for the child by providing anticipatory guidance?

REFER: GO TO MYNURSINGKIT

REFLECT: CASE STUDY
The nurse is working in a Planned Parenthood clinic and admits a 14-year-old girl who is requesting birth control pills. The girl states she has been sexually active for about 2 weeks and doesn't want to get pregnant. She tells the nurse she is dating a "very popular" 16-year-old boy who goes to the same school and who claims to have had multiple sexual experiences.
1. What type of anticipatory guidance can the nurse provide this client?
2. Would it be appropriate for the nurse to encourage abstinence with this client? Explain your answer.
3. How can the nurse provide anticipatory guidance that is suitable for this client's developmental stage?

49.2 ENVIRONMENTAL SAFETY

KEY TERM

Adverse event, *2443*

Chemical restraints, *2446*

Error, *2443*

Physical restraints, *2445*

Restraints, *2445*

Safety, *2443*

Sentinel event, *2446*

BASIS FOR SELECTION OF EXEMPLAR

Healthy People 2010

OSHA

LEARNING OUTCOMES

After reading about this exemplar, you will be able to:

1. Provide strategies and client teaching appropriate to reducing risk for injury or illness in the home.

2. Provide strategies and client teaching appropriate to reducing risk for injury or illness in the workplace.

3. Provide strategies and client teaching appropriate to reducing risk for injury or illness in the community.

4. Provide strategies and client teaching appropriate to reducing risk for injury or illness in the health care setting.

5. Recommend strategies for promoting safety in the health care setting.

6. Identify nursing competencies important to promoting client safety and quality of care.

7. Recommend strategies for reducing procedure and equipment-related accidents.

8. Discuss the use and legal implications of restraints.

9. Describe alternatives to restraints.

OVERVIEW

Environmental safety is an issue in many settings. Depending on the client's situation, the nurse may need to assess the environment of the client's home, workplace, or community. Client safety is also affected in the health care setting, where nurses work to prevent incidental injuries and nosocomial infections.

CLIENT SETTINGS

Safety at home is important for all clients, but especially for those whose mobility is limited, those who have small children, or those who have a cognitive impairment. A safe home requires well-maintained flooring and carpets, a nonskid bathtub or shower surface, functioning smoke and carbon monoxide alarms that are strategically placed, and knowledge of fire escape routes. Outdoor areas, such as swimming pools, need to be safely secured and maintained. Adequate lighting, both inside and out, minimizes the potential for accidents. Hazards in the home are major causes of falls, fire, poisoning, suffocation, and other accidents, such as those caused by improper use of household equipment, tools, and cooking utensils.

PRACTICE ALERT

Nurses respond to safety hazards whether or not they are on duty. For example, when a nurse goes to the grocery store and sees water on the floor, the nurse reports it to the produce manager to prevent possible injury if someone slips and falls.

In the workplace, machinery, industrial belts and pulleys, and chemicals may create dangers (Figure 49–3 ■). Worker fatigue, noise and air pollution, or working at great heights or in subterranean areas may also create occupational hazards. Failure of a company to follow OSHA and other safety requirements may create life-threatening situations for employees. The work environment of the nurse may be unsafe as well, especially if employees fail to follow procedures. Health care workers need to maintain an awareness of the potential risks of their work environment.

In the community, adequate street lighting, safe water and sewage treatment, and regulation of sanitation in food buying and handling all contribute to a healthy, hazard-free community. A safe and secure community strives to be free of excess noise, crime, traffic congestion, dilapidated housing, or unprotected creeks and landfills.

CARE SETTINGS Preventing Medication Errors in the Home

The U.S. Pharmacopeia's Safe Medication Use Expert Committee (Santell and Cousins, 2004) reports that medication errors occurring in the home are the result of communication problems (21%), knowledge deficit (19%), and inadequate monitoring (4%). Ten percent of errors are caused by lack of access to information. Warfarin is the drug most frequently (9%) associated with medication errors in the home; next in frequency are insulin (7%), morphine (4%), and vancomycin (4%). Improper dosage (36%) and omission errors (28%) top the list of types of errors. In this study, the client, family, or caregiver is reported to be at fault in 39% of errors, the nurse in 36%, and the physician or pharmacist in 11%. The study points out the need for better client education, a role in which the nurse plays a large part.

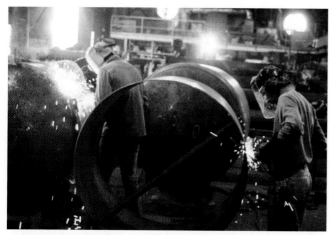

Figure 49–3 ■ Welders wear protective equipment to prevent burns and other injuries.

HEALTH CARE SETTINGS

The 2000 Institute of Medicine (IOM) report *To Err Is Human: Building a Safer Health System* estimated that 44,000–98,000 people die in the United States each year because of medical errors in hospitals. In 2004, HealthGrades released results of a study it conducted from 2000–2002 using Medicare data from all 50 states. In the study, HealthGrades examined 16 of the 20 AHRQ patient safety indicators. Based on this study, HealthGrades determined that approximately 195,000 deaths in hospitals each year result from medical errors (Medical News Today, 2004).

Client safety problems can include a variety of errors, such as medication errors, wrong-site surgery, restraint-related injuries or death, falls, burns, pressure ulcers, and mistaken identity (Figure 49–4 ■). The 2000 IOM report

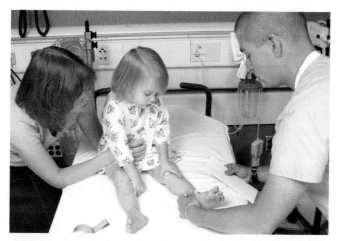

Figure 49–4 ■ An important client safety action is to verify the identity of the child prior to performing any procedure or administering medication. The nurse needs two forms of identification. In this case, the child's identification bracelet is compared to the name and birthdate on the laboratory test form, and the parent also confirms the child's identity.

defines **safety** as "freedom from accidental injury" (p. 58) and **error** as the "failure of a planned action to be completed as intended or the use of a wrong plan to achieve an aim" (p. 54).

As part of its research, the IOM reviewed many studies that investigated adverse events. An **adverse event** is an illness or injury caused by medical management rather than the underlying disease or condition of the client. The IOM noted that more than 50% of the adverse events studied were preventable. The report emphasized that while some of the errors were caused by incompetent or impaired providers, the majority could have been avoided had better systems of care been in place. Leonard, Frankel, Simmonds, and Vega (2004) echoed this belief by stating that an ever-increasing body of evidence indicates at least 80% of medical error is system derived—meaning that system flaws set good people up to fail. These same authors state that when people perform complex tasks, errors will occur.

The hospital environment is quite complex. Leonard et al. (2004) identified the following factors that increase the risk of human error:

■ *Limited short-term memory.* In busy hospital environments, nurses have rapidly changing information coming at them continuously. Systems that rely on human memory are prone to failure.

■ *Being late or in a hurry.* People start cutting corners when they are late or in a hurry. This may get the work done more quickly; however, it also contributes to the possibility of missing an important detail or piece of information that could cause client harm.

■ *Limited ability to multitask.* People perform better when performing only one task at a time.

■ *Interruptions.* Many interruptions occur in complex environments, such as a hospital. Frequent interruptions make it more difficult for the nurse to get back on task or to remember what he or she was thinking.

■ *Stress.* Stress causes anxiety, and anxiety affects performance. Also, stress affects a person's thinking by filtering information, which subsequently affects problem-solving ability. When people are stressed, they tend to hear only what they want to hear or to miss all of the information provided.

■ *Fatigue and other physiological factors.* Studies show that fatigue affects a person's ability to process complex information.

■ *Environmental factors.* Heat, noise, distractions, visual stimuli, and lighting can affect performance and lead to mistakes. Workplace design is a part of keeping clients and staff safe.

Another IOM report, *Keeping Patients Safe: Transforming the Work Environment of Nurses* (2004), established a link between nurses' work environment and client safety. The IOM found that the usual work environment of nurses is characterized by many serious threats to client safety. Examples in this report include inconsistent staffing levels, long work hours, work processes, and physical design of the workplace.

PROMOTING CLIENT SAFETY IN THE HEALTH CARE SETTING

As stated previously, the IOM report *To Err Is Human* provided proof that errors in the health care industry are at an unacceptably high level. Health care facilities and the health care system at large must make substantive changes and use quality improvement methods (see Concept 48) to improve client safety and care quality. Nurses who follow facility policies and procedures and maintain a current, evidence-based practice will be able to design appropriate plans of care and intervene appropriately to reduce their clients' risks for illness and injury.

System Changes to Promote Client Safety

Recent health care literature (Leonard et al., 2004; Page, 2004; Kohn et al., 2000) suggests that new systems to improve client safety are needed. Examples include the following:

- *Establishing a National Center for Patient Safety.* This center would provide leadership for safety improvements and expand the knowledge base for improving safety and preventing errors in health care (Kohn et al., 2000).
- *Establishing a reporting system.* This information would be used to design systems that are safer for clients. Literature discussions (Berntsen, 2004; Kohn et al., 2000) suggest both a mandatory reporting system for errors causing serious injury or death and a voluntary reporting system for errors that result in no harm (sometimes called "near misses" or "close calls").
- *Promoting effective teamwork and communication.* Health care practitioners are part of a team, and client safety may be at risk if critical, relevant information is not communicated appropriately. Successful communication between the nurse and other members of the health care team, especially the primary care provider, is critical.
- *Creating a culture of trust.* There is a need to change the culture in health care from placing blame to examining how to improve. Trust needs to be developed and sustained for people to feel open to discuss and share experiences about their safety near misses and/or errors.
- *Involving health care workers in the design of work processes and work spaces.* This would promote efficiency and safety.

Nursing Competencies Necessary for Promoting Safety and Quality Care

The Quality and Safety Education Project for Nurses was funded by the Robert Wood Johnson Foundation to "address the challenge of preparing future nurses with the knowledge, skills, and attitudes (KSA) necessary to continuously improve the quality and safety of the healthcare systems in which they work" (QSEN, 2010a).

The project identified six competencies necessary for nurses to improve the quality and safety of health care systems. The competencies are defined as follows (QSEN, 2010b):

- *Patient-centered care.* Recognize the patient or designee as the source of control and full partner in providing compassionate and coordinated care based on respect for patient's preferences, values, and needs.

- *Teamwork and collaboration.* Function effectively within nursing and inter-professional teams, fostering open communication, mutual respect, and shared decision-making to achieve quality patient care.
- *Evidence-based practice.* Integrate best current evidence with clinical expertise and patient/family preferences and values for delivery of optimal health care.
- *Quality improvement.* Use data to monitor the outcomes of care processes and use improvement methods to design and test changes to continuously improve the quality and safety of health care systems.
- *Informatics.* Use information and technology to communicate, manage knowledge, mitigate error, and support decision making.
- *Safety.* Minimizes risk of harm to patients and providers through both system effectiveness and individual performance.

Pilot schools throughout the country have been integrating these six competencies into their nursing programs. For each competency, the QSEN committee has defined the competency and developed guidelines regarding the knowledge, skills, and attitudes (KSAs) that should be expected of graduating nursing students. The competency KSAs can be found at http://www.qsen.org/ksas_prelicensure.php.

Selected Ways Nurses Can Promote Client Safety in the Health Care Setting

Nurses are at the front line of client care and safety. Evidence-based interventions in a number of areas can reduce errors and hazards and improve client health outcomes.

SIDE RAILS Although it may seem that raising the side rails on a bed is an effective method of preventing falls, rails should not be raised routinely for this purpose. Research has shown that persons with memory impairment, altered mobility, nocturia, and other sleep disorders are prone to becoming entrapped in side rails and may, in fact, be more likely to fall while trying to get out of bed by going around or over the raised rails (Marcy-Edwards, 2005).

PRACTICE ALERT
Nurses who work with clients in hospitals and other institutional settings should provide easy access to a bedpan, urinal, commode, or bathroom. Make sure that lighting is adequate and that pathways are free from obstacles for clients getting up to use the bathroom.

USE OF ELECTRONIC DEVICES Electronic devices are available to detect that clients are attempting to move or get out of bed. A bed or chair safety monitoring device has a position-sensitive switch that triggers an audio alarm when the client attempts to get out of the bed or chair.

PREVENTING PRESSURE ULCERS From 2003–2005, HealthGrades Patient Safety in American Hospitals reviewed client records from 5,000 hospitals. The study found that pressure ulcers had one of the highest occurrence rates. Although Florence Nightingale attributed the development of "bedsores" to a failure of nursing, many health care providers now believe that the development of pressure ulcers stems from a failure of cooperation among the entire health care team. A growing body of evidence suggests that Quality Improvement models combined with systematic care can prevent pressure ulcers in clients in all inpatient health care settings (Lyder and Ayello, 2008). Preventive measures for pressure ulcers, such as supportive surfaces and repositioning of clients, are discussed in Exemplar 30.3.

PREVENTING FUNCTIONAL DECLINE OF OLDER ADULTS

Functional decline is the leading complication of hospitalization of older adults. Functional decline includes changes in physical status as well as cognitive changes such as delirium. During hospitalization, the older adult experiences a decrease in exercise capacity due to the amount of time in bed rest. This negatively impacts a number of systems, including lower cardiac output and oxygen uptake. Hospitalized older adults can also experience accelerated bone loss which can increase their risk for injury (Kleinpell, Fletcher, and Jennings, 2008).

Nurses can help reduce the chances of functional decline in these clients by conducting a comprehensive geriatric assessment upon admission. Such an assessment should include assessing the client's sensory perception, cognitive status, mobility status, and ability to participate in Activities of Daily Living. The comprehensive assessment will provide important information for designing a plan of care intended to improve client health outcomes and reduce functional decline. Depending on client ability, appropriate interventions may include walking programs, progressive resistance strength training, and promotion of family participation in clients' activity plans (Kleinpell, Fletcher, and Jennings, 2008).

Procedure- and Equipment-Related Accidents

Risk assessment in the health care setting must include risks related to procedures and equipment. Whether giving a medication or assisting a client out of bed, nurses need to follow safeguards to prevent errors or accidents. Most health care agencies establish protocols that are designed to prevent accidents. When in doubt regarding a course of action, the nurse should consult the appropriate written guidelines before proceeding.

Nurses must also consider the client's developmental age when providing or planning care. Box 49–4 describes safety measures for the hospitalized child in relation to procedure- and equipment-related accidents, and Box 49–5 looks at long-term care considerations for safety measures related to the older adult.

When an accident or error does occur, most agencies require that the incident be reported. The nurse completes the report immediately after taking whatever action is required to safeguard the client and notifying the charge nurse. (Sentinel events, risk management, and quality improvement are discussed in greater detail in Concept 48, Quality Improvement.) Appropriate incident reporting helps to identify patterns that may indicate a need for changes in policies and procedures to promote client safety.

Using Restraints

Restraints are protective devices used to limit the physical activity of the client or a part of the body. They can be classified as physical or chemical. **Physical restraints** are any manual method or physical or mechanical device, material, or equipment attached to the client's body; they cannot be removed easily and they restrict the client's movement.

Box 49–4 Safety Measures for the Hospitalized Child

NEWBORN AND INFANT
- Use age-appropriate crib and bedding.
- Secure equipment cords under the infant's gown or shirt.
- Do not allow the infant to chew on cords.
- Properly dispose of syringe caps and other small items that may present a choking hazard.
- Establish with parents a list of persons who may visit the child.
- Keep crib rails up when a parent is not at the bedside.

TODDLER AND PRESCHOOLER
- Maintain bed in low position.
- Keep side rails up when a parent is not at the bedside.
- Do not allow the child to chew on cords.
- Keep room clutter-free.
- Remove all unnecessary equipment from the child's room.
- Properly dispose of syringe caps and other small items that may present a choking hazard.
- Latex balloons should not be permitted because of the risk of suffocation.
- If toddlers and preschoolers are curious about hospital equipment, provide them the opportunity to explore the equipment safely and with guidance (e.g., syringes without needles or blood pressure cuffs to satisfy curiosity).
- Keep in mind that these children are naturally curious and explorative.
- Instruct family members to inform staff when they are leaving the room to ensure that the toddler or preschooler is being observed.

SCHOOL-AGE CHILD
- Instruct the child to avoid manipulating hospital equipment such as intravenous fluid pumps, client-controlled analgesia (PCA) pumps, and oxygen gauges.
- Allow the child the opportunity to explore hospital surroundings and equipment with guidance.
- Instruct family members to inform staff when they are leaving the room to ensure that the child is being observed.

ADOLESCENT
- Address issues such as smoking in the room and consuming alcohol, because friends could possibly bring cigarettes or alcohol to the hospitalized adolescent.

Box 49–5 Long-Term Care Considerations: Preventing Falls in Health Care Agencies

- On admission, orient clients to their surroundings, and explain the call system.
- Carefully assess the client's ability to ambulate and transfer. Provide walking aids and assistance as required.
- Closely supervise the clients at risk for falls, especially at night.
- Encourage the client to use the call bell to request assistance. Ensure that the bell is within easy reach.
- Place beside tables and overbed tables near the bed or chair so that clients do not overreach and consequently lose their balance.
- Always keep hospital beds in the low position and with the wheels locked when not providing care so that clients can move in or out of bed easily.
- Encourage clients to use grab bars mounted in toilet and bathing areas and railings along corridors.
- Make sure nonskid bath mats are available in tubs and showers.
- Encourage the client to wear nonskid footwear.
- Keep the environment tidy. In particular, keep light cords from underfoot and furniture out of the way.
- Use individualized interventions (e.g., alarm sensitive to client position) rather than side rails for confused clients.

Chemical restraints are medications such as neuroleptics, anxiolytics, sedatives, and psychotropic agents used to control socially disruptive behavior. The purpose of restraints is to prevent the client from injuring self or others.

Restraints, however, can injure. In 1998, The Joint Commission sent out a sentinel event alert warning of the need to prevent restraint deaths (Joint Commission, 1998). This alert resulted after a tracking study of **sentinel events**, which are unexpected occurrences that resulted in death or serious injury. The results indicated that 20 clients who were being physically restrained had died, with the majority of deaths caused by asphyxiation and strangulation.

In addition to the physical safety concerns, many consider restraints to be demeaning and psychologically harmful. Some believe they limit a client's autonomy. The current focus in health care is to explore ways to prevent, reduce, and hopefully eliminate the use of restraints while protecting a client's safety, rights, and dignity. The American Nurses Association's position is that restraints should be used only when "no other viable option is available" (ANA, 2010).

LEGAL IMPLICATIONS OF RESTRAINTS Increasingly, determining the need for safety measures is viewed as an independent nursing function. However, because restraints restrict the individual's freedom, their use has legal implications. Nurses need to know their agency's policies and state laws about restraining clients. The U.S. Centers for Medicare and Medicaid Services (CMS) published revised standards for use of restraints in the United States in 2006 (CMS, 2006). These standards apply to all health care organizations and specify two standards for applying restraints: the behavior management standard when the client is a danger to self or others, and the acute medical and surgical care standard when temporary immobilization of a client is required to perform a procedure.

1. In the case of the behavior management standard, the nurse may apply restraints but the primary care provider or other licensed independent practitioner must see the client within 1 hour for evaluation. A written restraint order for an adult, following evaluation, is valid for only 4 hours. If the client must be restrained and secluded, there must be continual visual and audio monitoring of the client's status.
2. The medical surgical care standard permits up to 12 hours for obtaining the primary care provider written order for the restraints. All orders must be renewed daily. See Figure 49–5 ■ for an example of a restraint monitoring and intervention flow sheet.

Standards require that a primary care provider's order for restraints state the reason and time period. The use of a prn order for restraints is prohibited. In all cases, restraints should be used *only* after every other possible means of ensuring safety have been unsuccessful and documented. See alternatives to the use of restraints in Box 49–6. Restrained clients often become more restless and anxious as a result of the loss of self-control. Nurses must document that the need for the restraint was made clear both to the client and family.

Clients have the right to be free from restraints that are not medically necessary. As a result, there must be justification that the use of restraints will protect the client and that less restrictive measures were attempted and found not effective. Restraints *cannot* be used for staff convenience or client punishment. If the above conditions are met and restraints are needed, it is important for the nurse to be able to correctly apply restraints without endangering client safety.

SELECTING A RESTRAINT Before selecting a restraint, nurses need to understand its purpose clearly and measure it against the following five criteria:

1. It restricts the client's movement as little as possible. If a client needs to have one arm restrained, do not restrain the entire body.
2. It does not interfere with the client's treatment or health problem. If a client has poor blood circulation to the hands, apply a restraint that will not aggravate that circulatory problem.
3. It is readily changeable. Restraints need to be changed frequently, especially if they become soiled. Keeping other guidelines in mind, choose a restraint that can be changed with minimal disturbance to the client.
4. It is safe for the particular client. Choose a restraint with which the client cannot self-inflict injury. For example, a physically restrained person could be injured trying to climb out of bed if one wrist is tied to the bed frame. A jacket restraint would restrain the person more safely.
5. It is the least obvious to others. Both clients and visitors are often embarrassed by a restraint, even though they understand why it is being used. The less obvious the restraint, the more comfortable people feel.

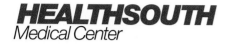

ACUTE MEDICAL/SURGICAL CARE
RESTRAINT FLOW SHEET

Restraint Initiated: Date: _____   Time: _____

Order Expires: Date: _____   Time: _____
                                    New verbal order required every 24 hours.

Assessment should be based on individual needs. Patients must be assessed at least every 2 hours.

		0700	0800	0900	1000	1100	1200	1300	1400	1500	1600	1700	1800	1900	2000	2100	2200	2300	2400	0100	0200	0300	0400	0500	0600
Restraints Removed																									
Skin & Circulation Assessed																									
Toileting Offered																									
Food/Fluids Offered																									
Range of Motion & Patient Repositioned																									
Patient Response	R=Restless C=Calm S=Sleeping U=Unaware																								
Effect of Restraint	A=Adequate I=Inadequate (explain)																								
Continued Need	Y=Yes N=No																								
Restraint Reapplied																									
Initials																									

Explain: _____

_____

INIT	SIGNATURE	TITLE

Figure 49–5 ■ Restraint monitoring and intervention flow sheet.

Box 49–6 **Alternatives to Restraints**

- Assign nurses in pairs to act as "buddies" so that one nurse can observe the client when the other leaves the unit.
- Place unstable clients in an area that is constantly or closely supervised.
- Prepare clients before a move to limit relocation shock and resultant confusion.
- Stay with a client using a bedside commode or bathroom if the client is confused or sedated or has a gait disturbance or a high risk score for falling.
- Monitor all the client's medications and, if possible, attempt to lower or eliminate dosages of sedatives or psychotropics.
- Position beds at their lowest level to facilitate getting in and out of bed.
- Replace full-length side rails with half- or three-quarter-length rails to prevent confused clients from climbing over rails or falling from the end of the bed.
- Use rocking chairs to help confused clients expend some of their energy so that they will be less inclined to wander.
- Wedge pillows or pads against the sides of wheelchairs to keep clients well positioned.
- Place a removable lap tray on a wheelchair to provide support and help keep the client in place.
- To quiet agitated clients, try a warm beverage, soft lights, a back rub, or a walk.
- Use "environmental restraints," such as pieces of furniture or large plants as barriers, to keep clients from wandering beyond appropriate areas.
- Place a picture or other personal item on the door to clients' rooms to help them identify their room.
- Try to determine the causes of the client's sundowner syndrome (nocturnal wandering and disorientation as darkness falls, associated with dementia). Possible causes include poor hearing, poor eyesight, or pain.
- Establish ongoing assessment to monitor changes in physical and cognitive functional abilities and risk factors.

KINDS OF RESTRAINTS There are several kinds of restraints. Among the most common for adults are jacket restraints, belt restraints, mitt or hand restraints, and limb restraints. Geri chairs, wheelchairs with lap trays, and bed rails can also be considered restraints. Restraints for infants and children include mummy restraints, elbow restraints, and crib nets.

When evaluating if a device is a restraint or not, determine the intended use (e.g., physical restriction), its involuntary application, and/or the client need for the restraint (Joint Commission, 2005). For example, if all of the bed's side rails are up and restrict the client's freedom to leave the bed, and the client did not voluntarily request all rails to be up, they are a restraint. If, however, one side rail is up to assist the client to get in and out of the bed, it is not a restraint. Also, if the client can release or remove a device, it would not be considered a restraint.

There are several types of vest restraints, but all are essentially sleeveless jackets or vests with straps (tails) that can be tied to the bed frame under the mattress. These body restraints are used to ensure the safety of confused or sedated clients in beds or wheelchairs. The U.S. Food and Drug Administration (FDA) advises that manufacturers place "front" and "back" labels on vest restraints.

Belt or safety strap body restraints (Figure 49–6 ■) are used to ensure the safety of all clients who are being moved on stretchers or in wheelchairs. Some wheelchairs have a soft, padded safety bar that attaches to side brackets that are installed under the arm rests. To prevent the person from slumping forward, the nurse then attaches a shoulder "Y" strap to the bar and over the client's shoulders to the rear handles. Other safety belt models have a three-loop design. One loop surrounds the person's waist and attaches to the rear handles. If such restraints are unavailable, the nurse can place a folded towel or small sheet around the client's waist and fasten it at the back of the wheelchair. Belt

restraints may also be used for certain clients confined to bed or to chairs.

A mitt or hand restraint (Figure 49–7 ■) is used to prevent confused clients from using their hands or fingers to scratch and injure themselves. For example, a confused client may need to be prevented from pulling at intravenous tubing or a head bandage following brain surgery. Hand or mitt restraints allow the client to be ambulatory and/or to move the arm freely rather than be confined to a bed or a chair. Mittens need to be removed on a regular basis to permit the client to wash and exercise the hands. The nurse also needs to take off the mitten to check the circulation to the hand.

Limb restraints (Figure 49–8 ■), which are generally made of cloth, may be used to immobilize a limb, primarily for therapeutic reasons (e.g., to maintain an intravenous infusion).

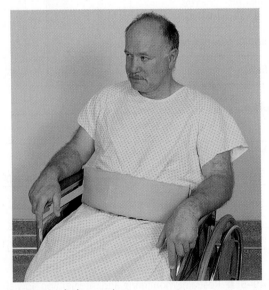

Figure 49–6 ■ A belt restraint.

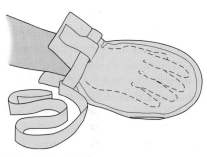

Figure 49–7 ■ A mitt restraint.

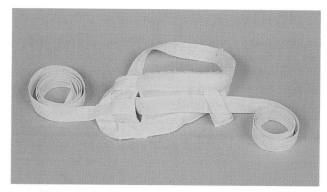

Figure 49–8 ■ A limb restraint.

REVIEW Environmental Safety

RELATE: LINK THE CONCEPTS

Linking the exemplar of Environmental Safety with the concept of Communication:

1. What departments in an acute care facility are most likely to notice a pattern of increased incidents of pressure ulcers? To whom would you report your concerns if you suspected that clients were developing pressure ulcers at an increased rate?
2. How does the facility communicate policies related to workplace safety to the nursing staff?

Linking the exemplar of Environmental Safety with the concept of Sensory Perception:

3. How would you recommend altering a client's home environment to optimize safety if they had an alteration in vision?
4. How would you recommend altering a client's home environment to optimize safety if they had an alteration in hearing?

READY: GO TO COMPANION SKILLS MANUAL

- Managing clients in restraints
- Applying a wrist or ankle restraint
- Applying a papoose board immobilizer
- Applying a mummy immobilizer

REFER: GO TO MYNURSINGKIT

REFLECT: CASE STUDY

Mr. Moore is a 72-year-old widower who is recovering from a fall in which he fractured his hip and underwent surgical repair 1 week ago. He will be staying with his son for 2 weeks after he is discharged from the hospital, but he is eager to return to his own home. Once Mr. Moore is home, his son will visit nightly after work, he will receive Meals on Wheels once a day, and a home health care attendant will visit weekly to assist him with hygienic care until he is more independent. Mr. Moore's wife died 3 years ago, but he has remained independent and continued his social functions. He lives in a small, single-level house with his dog and cat, and he enjoys gardening. Before fracturing his hip, he walked his dog daily. You will be his home health care nurse.

1. While hospitalized, Mr. Moore experienced some mild confusion during the night, but his nurses decided not to restrain him. What are the best reasons for avoiding the use of restraints for clients such as Mr. Moore?
2. What are some of the more obvious factors that may affect Mr. Moore's safety as he returns home?
3. What do you need to assess in regard to Mr. Moore's safety, and what suggestions can you make for enhancing his safety?
4. What strengths do you note about Mr. Moore that may protect him from injury when he returns home?

49.3 INJURY AND ILLNESS PREVENTION

KEY TERMS

Burn, *2450*
Carbon monoxide (CO), *2451*
Macroshock, *2453*
Plumbism, *2454*
Scald, *2450*
Suffocation, *2452*

BASIS FOR SELECTION OF EXEMPLAR

Healthy People 2010
National Institutes of Health
National Patient Safety Goals
The Joint Commission

LEARNING OUTCOMES

After reading about this exemplar, you will be able to:

1. Develop a nursing plan of care aimed at preventing injury and illness.
2. Conduct a risk assessment.
3. Describe specific nursing interventions aimed at reducing the risk of injury or illness.
4. Demonstrate client teaching aimed at reducing the risk of injury or illness.
5. Describe specific risks associated with different stages of the life span and developmentally appropriate teaching to reduce these risks.

OVERVIEW

The nurse plays a pivotal role in providing anticipatory guidance and teaching the client prevent injury and illness. In order for intervention to be effective, the nurse must assess the client for potential risks. Risk assessment takes into consideration factors such as development, age, gender, lifestyle choices, physical and psychosocial condition, and specific client concerns (Box 49–7).

Fires

Fires continue to be a constant risk in both health care settings and homes. Fires in health care agencies usually result from malfunctioning electric equipment or combustion of anesthetic gas. Fires in the home most frequently result from careless disposal of burning cigarettes or matches, from grease, or from faulty electric wiring.

AGENCY FIRES In health care settings, fire is particularly hazardous for clients who are incapacitated and unable to leave the building without assistance. This incapacity makes it extremely important for nurses to be aware of the fire safety regulations and fire prevention practices of the agency in which they work. The Joint Commission advocates that hospitals use the National Fire Prevention's Association Life Safety Code to ensure that their facilities meet certain fire safety requirements for brick-and-mortar issues such as electrical wiring and fire escapes (Joint Commission Resources, Inc., 2010).

Box 49–7 Extreme Sports

A growing number of children engage in "extreme" sports, those that carry a high degree of risk and have not traditionally been common. Some examples are mountain biking, three wheeling, ski racing, snowboarding through trees and on courses with pikes and other challenges, ice climbing, rock climbing, wakeboarding, and skateboarding. Nurses should know the typical risks for sports that are popular in their communities. For example, 60% of skateboard injuries involve children under age 15, and most of them are boys (AAOS, 2010). While the nurse is probably unable to dissuade youth from engaging in these activities, the nurse is able to emphasize appropriate safety measures (Figure 49–9 ■):

- Find out what protective gear the youth wears and what is recommended.
- Keep at hand examples of stories of youth who have been saved by use of such gear.
- Encourage the youth to engage in sports activities only when others are present and to have a plan for emergencies, including a working cell phone, leaving information with an adult about plans and expected return, and planning for harsh weather with items such as emergency blankets, gear, and food.
- Encourage the youth to talk with parents and other adults about the risks and responsibilities of these activities.

PREVENTING SPECIFIC HAZARDS

Critical aspects of nursing care include implementing measures to prevent specific hazards or injuries such as burns, fires, falls, poisoning, suffocation, electrocution, etc. Teaching clients about safety is another important aspect. Nurses usually have opportunities to teach clients while providing care.

Burns and Scalds

A **burn** results from excessive exposure to thermal, chemical, electric, or radioactive agents. Common causes of burns in the home include the following:

- Household cleaners and detergents
- Bleach
- Smoking materials, such as cigarettes and cigars
- Unattended cooking.

A **scald** is a burn from a hot liquid or vapor, such as steam. Common home hazards that can cause scalding include the following:

- Pot handles that protrude over the edge of a stove
- Electric appliances used to heat liquids or oils, especially those with dangling cords that are within reach of crawling infants and young children
- Excessively hot bath water.

In health care agencies, the risk of scalds and burns is greater for clients whose skin sensitivity to temperature is impaired. Scalds can occur from overly hot bath water; burns can occur from therapeutic applications of heat. It is important for the nurse to assess how well clients can protect themselves and what special precautions, if any, need to be taken.

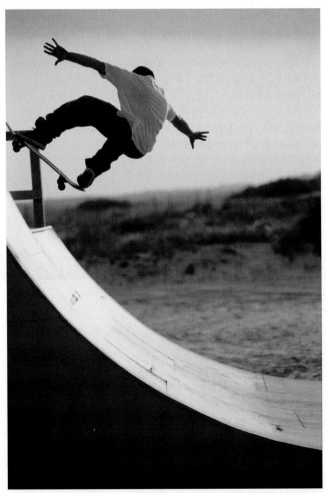

Figure 49–9 ■ This teenage skateboarder is at risk for fractures and head injury because he is not wearing protective equipment.

Knowing what to do in the event of a fire is the responsibility of every nurse. Many hospitals and health care facilities train nurses and other employees to use the RACE acronym when responding to a fire (Miller, 2010; UNC Healthcare, 2009):

1. **R**emove anyone from the immediate fire area.
2. **A**lert others and pull the manual fire alarm pull station.
3. **C**onfine the fire by closing doors.
4. **E**xtinguish or evacuate.

Extinguishing the fire requires knowledge of three categories of fire, classified according to the type of material that is burning:

- *Class A:* Paper, wood, upholstery, rags, ordinary rubbish
- *Class B:* Flammable liquids and gases
- *Class C:* Electrical.

The right type of extinguisher must be used to fight the fire. Extinguishers have picture symbols showing the type of fire for which they are to be used. Directions for use are also attached.

HOME FIRES Nursing interventions for home fires focus on teaching fire safety. Preventive measures include the following:

- Keep emergency numbers near the telephone or stored for speed dialing.
- Be sure the smoke alarms are operable and appropriately located.
- Change smoke alarm batteries annually on a special day, such as a birthday or January 1.
- Have a family "fire drill" plan. Every member needs to know the nearest exit from different locations of the home.
- Keep fire extinguishers available and in working order.
- Close windows and doors if possible. Cover the mouth and nose with a damp cloth when exiting through a smoke-filled area; and avoid heavy smoke by assuming a bent position with the head as close to the floor as possible.

As mentioned, fires in the home most frequently result from careless disposal of burning cigarettes or matches, from grease, or from faulty electric wiring.

Falls

People of any age can fall, but infants and toddlers and older adults are particularly prone to falling and serious injury as a result. Falls are the leading cause of injuries among older adults. They are also a major cause of hospital and nursing home admissions. Most falls occur in the home and are a major threat to the independence of older adults. Fear of falling is common in older adults, even in those who have not experienced a fall. This fear is of particular concern for those who live alone and who anticipate being helpless and unable to summon help after a fall. For these individuals, the nurse should encourage daily or more frequent contact with a friend or family member, installation of a personal emergency response system, and implement measures to maintain a physical environment that prevents falls. Risk factors and associated preventive measures are shown in Table 49–1.

> **PRACTICE ALERT**
> Along with breaking bones, falls can also break self-confidence, leading to fear of falling. This fear may result in decreased activity level and therefore decreased muscle strength. Each of these factors increases the risk of falling.

Weak leg muscles, weak knees, poor balance, and loss of flexibility contribute to falls in the older adults. The nurse can use an assessment tool called the Timed Up and Go (TUG) test, which is predictive of performance, in a hospital, subacute, or home setting (Bohannon, 2006). To perform the TUG test,

1. Use a standard armchair and place a line 10 feet from the chair.
2. Have the client wear customary shoes and use a customary walking aid.
3. Ask the client to rise from the chair, walk to the line on the floor, turn, return to the chair, and sit down.
4. Time the client from initial rising to return to sitting.
5. The normal time to complete the test is 7–10 seconds. Clients who cannot complete the task in that time are likely to have mobility and functional problems (Podsiallo & Richardson, 1991).

This quick assessment along with an assessment of the client's environment can help the nurse recommend safety measures to the client and family.

Prevention of falls in health care agencies is an ongoing concern (American Geriatrics Society, 2006). Health care environments are designed with many safety features to reduce the risk of falls, such as railings along corridors; call bells at each bedside; safety bars in toilet areas; locks on beds, wheelchairs, and stretchers; side rails on beds; night-lights; and so on. In addition, nurses can implement measures to decrease the incidence of falls.

> **PRACTICE ALERT**
> When a client falls, the nurse should assess the client for injuries and then notify the primary care provider.

Poisoning

Inadequate supervision and improper storage of household toxic substances are the major reasons for poisoning in children. Implementing poison prevention for children is focused on teaching parents to "childproof" the environment, including disposing of unused medications properly (see Box 49–8).

Carbon Monoxide Poisoning

Carbon monoxide (CO) is an odorless, colorless, tasteless gas that is very toxic. Exposure to CO can cause symptoms including headaches, dizziness, weakness, nausea, vomiting, or loss of muscle control. Prolonged exposure to CO can lead to unconsciousness, brain damage, or death. Preventing CO exposure is particularly important in the home because all gasoline-powered vehicles, lawn mowers, kerosene stoves, barbecues, and burning wood emit CO. Incomplete or faulty combustion of any fuel, including natural gas used in furnaces, also produces CO. By using these types of equipment and maintaining them according to manufacturer instructions, consumers can reduce the risk for CO exposure. Carbon monoxide detectors are available for the home.

TABLE 49-1 Risk Factors and Preventive Measures for Falls

RISK FACTOR	PREVENTIVE MEASURES
Poor vision	■ Ensure eyeglasses are functional. ■ Ensure appropriate lighting. ■ Mark doorways and edges of steps as needed. ■ Keep the environment tidy.
Cognitive dysfunction (confusion, disorientation, impaired memory, or judgment)	■ Set safe limits to activities. ■ Remove unsafe objects.
Impaired gait or balance and difficulty walking because of lower-extremity dysfunction (e.g., arthritis)	■ Wear shoes or well-fitted slippers with nonskid soles. ■ Use ambulatory devices as necessary (cane, crutches, walker, braces, wheelchair). ■ Provide assistance with ambulation as needed. ■ Monitor gait and balance. ■ Adapt living arrangements to one floor if necessary. ■ Encourage exercise and activity as tolerated to maintain muscle strength, joint flexibility, and balance. ■ Ensure uncluttered environment with securely fastened rugs.
Difficulty getting in and out of chair or in and out of bed	■ Encourage client to request assistance. ■ Keep the bed in the low position. ■ Install grab bars in bathroom. ■ Provide raised toilet seat.
Orthostatic hypotension	■ Instruct client to rise slowly from a lying to a sitting to a standing position, and then to stand in place for several seconds before walking.
Urinary frequency or receiving diuretics	■ Provide a bedside commode. ■ Assist with voiding on a frequent and scheduled basis.
Weakness from disease process or therapy	■ Encourage client to summon help. ■ Monitor activity tolerance.
Current medication regimen that includes sedatives, hypnotics, tranquilizers, narcotic analgesics, diuretics	■ Attach side rails to the bed if appropriate. ■ Keep the rails in place when the bed is in the lowest position. ■ Monitor orientation and alertness status. ■ Discuss how alcohol contributes to fall-related injuries. ■ Encourage client not to mix alcohol and medications and to avoid alcohol when necessary. ■ Encourage annual or more frequent review of all medications prescribed.

Suffocation or Choking

Suffocation, or asphyxiation, is lack of oxygen because of interrupted breathing. Suffocation occurs when the air source is cut off for any reason. One common reason is choking, which occurs when food or a foreign object becomes lodged in the throat. The universal sign of distress is the victim's grasping the anterior neck and being unable to speak or cough. The emergency response is the Heimlich maneuver, or abdominal thrust, which can dislodge the foreign object and reestablish an airway.

Other causes of suffocation are drowning, gas or smoke inhalation, accidental coverage of the nose and mouth by a piece of plastic, accidental strangulation by the shoulder harness of a seat belt, and being trapped in a confined space (e.g., a discarded refrigerator). If a person does not receive immediate relief from suffocation, the interrupted breathing leads to respiratory and cardiac arrest and death. Any obstruction to the air passages must be removed immediately and life support measures instituted when an arrest occurs.

Excessive Noise

Excessive noise is a health hazard. Depending on the overall level of noise, the frequency range of the noise, and the duration of exposure and individual susceptibility, excessive noise can cause hearing loss. Tolerance of noise is largely individual. When ill or injured, people are frequently sensitive to noises that normally would not disturb them. It is important for nurses to minimize noise in the hospital setting and to encourage clients to protect their hearing as much as possible.

Electrical Hazards

All electric equipment must be properly grounded. The electric plug of grounded equipment has three prongs. The two short prongs transmit the power to the equipment. The third, longer prong is the grounding device, which carries short circuits or stray electric current to the ground. Grounding prongs offer a path of least resistance to stray electric currents.

Box 49–8 Disposing of Unused Medications

Federal guidelines issued in 2007 recommend that consumers dispose of both over-the-counter and prescription medications by following directions given on the bottle or container. If no directions are given, drugs may be thrown out with household trash if they are first mixed with an undesirable substance such as coffee grounds or kitty litter. The drugs should then be placed in a sealed bag or container before being thrown away. Scratching personal information off prescription drug labels will help protect the consumer's identity and personal health information (FDA, 2009).

Adolescent and adult poisonings are usually caused by insect or snake bites and drugs used for recreation or in suicide attempts. Implementing poison prevention in these age groups focuses on providing information and counseling.

Poisoning in older adults usually results from accidental ingestion of a toxic substance (e.g., due to failing eyesight) or an overdose of a prescribed medication (e.g., due to impaired memory). Adverse reactions due to polypharmacy are also a concern for older adults. Implementing poison prevention with older adults focuses on safeguarding the environment and monitoring the underlying problems.

Older adults who have dementia are at particular risk for poisoning. Older adults who have dementia have the need to feel everything and will put anything in their mouths, including plants, flowers, candles, small objects, and medications. These and other potentially dangerous items need to be locked up or kept out of reach. A telephone number for the nearest poison control center should be readily available. These precautions are important whether the individual with dementia is being cared for at home or in an institution.

In response to the ever-increasing number of poison hazards, many countries have established poison control centers that provide accurate, up-to-date information about potential hazards and recommend treatment as needed. For certain poisons, specific antidotes or treatments are available; for many, there is no specific therapy.

Nurses intervene in community settings by educating the public about what to do in the event of poisoning:

1. Identify the specific poison by searching for an opened container, empty bottle, or other evidence.
2. Contact the poison control center, indicate the exact quantity of poison the person ingested, and state the person's age and apparent symptoms.
3. Keep the person as quiet as possible and lying on the side or sitting with the head placed between the legs to prevent aspiration of vomitus.

The Client Teaching feature that follows provides additional guidelines for teaching clients to prevent poisoning.

Faulty equipment, such as equipment with a frayed cord, presents a danger of electric shock or may start a fire. For example, an electric spark near certain anesthetic gases or a high concentration of oxygen can cause a serious fire. Actions to reduce electrical hazards are described in the Client Teaching feature that follows.

When major electrical injury (**macroshock**) does occur, the victim may sustain both superficial and deep burns, muscle contractions, and cardiac and respiratory arrest necessitating cardiopulmonary resuscitation and life support. Electric shock occurs when a current travels through the body to the ground rather than through electric wiring, or from static electricity that builds up on the body. Using machines in good repair, wearing shoes with rubber soles, standing on a nonconductive floor, and using nonconductive gloves can prevent macroshock. However, even with such precautions, the rescuer must know not to touch the victim until the electricity is shut off or the victim has been removed from contact with the electric current; otherwise, the rescuer may also receive electrical injury.

CLIENT TEACHING Preventing Poisoning

- Lock potentially toxic agents, including drugs and cleaning agents, in a cupboard, or attach special plastic hooks to the insides of cabinet doors to keep them securely closed. Unlatching these hooks requires firmer thumb pressure than small children can usually exert. Don't let children watch you open the latches. Kids learn fast!
- Avoid storing toxic liquids or solids in food containers, such as soft drink bottles, peanut butter jars, or milk cartons.
- Do not remove container labels or reuse empty containers to store different substances. Laws mandate that the labels of all poisons specify antidotes.
- Do not rely on cooking to destroy toxic chemicals in plants. Never use anything prepared from nature as a medicine or "tea."
- Teach children never to eat any part of an unknown plant or mushroom and not to put leaves, stems, bark, seeds, nuts, or berries from any plant into their mouths.
- Place poison warning stickers designed for children on containers of bleach, lye, kerosene, solvent, and other toxic substances.
- Do not refer to medicine as candy or pretend false enjoyment when taking medications in front of children; allow them to see the necessity of the medicine without glamorizing it.
- Read and follow label directions on all products before using them.
- Keep syrup of ipecac on hand at all times. Syrup of ipecac is a nonprescription emetic available in single-dose, 15-mL vials in all drugstores. Use it only after advice from the local poison control center or the family primary care provider.
- Do not keep poisonous plants in the home and avoid planting poisonous plants in the yard. The cooperative extension agency in your county can provide a list of poisonous plants.
- Display the phone number of the poison control center near or on all telephones in the home so that it is available to babysitters, family, and friends.

CLIENT TEACHING **Reducing Electrical Hazards**

- Check cords for fraying or other signs of damage before using an appliance. Do not use if damage is apparent.
- Avoid overloading outlets and fuse boxes with too many appliances.
- Use only grounded outlets and plugs.
- Always pull a plug from the wall outlet by firmly grasping the plug and pulling it straight out. Pulling a plug by its cord can damage the cord and plug unit.
- Never use electric appliances near sinks, bathtubs, showers, or other wet areas, because water readily conducts electricity.
- Keep electric cords and appliances out of the reach of young children.
- Place covers over wall outlets to protect young children.

- Have all noninsulated wiring in the home altered to meet safety standards.
- Carefully read instructions before operating electric equipment. Clients who do not understand how to operate the equipment should seek advice.
- Always disconnect appliances before cleaning or repairing them.
- Unplug any appliance that has given a tingling sensation or shock, and have an electrician evaluate it for stray current.
- Keep electric cords coiled or taped to the ground away from areas of traffic to prevent others from damaging the cords or tripping over them.

Firearms

Parents who bring a handgun into the home must accept full responsibility for teaching safety rules to any children who have knowledge of the presence of firearms. The following basic firearm safety rules must be implemented for any gun:
- Store all guns in sturdy, locked cabinets without glass, and make sure the keys are inaccessible to children.
- Store the bullets in a different location from the guns.
- Tell children never to touch a gun or stay in a friend's house where a gun is accessible.
- Teach children never to point the barrel of a gun at anyone.
- Ensure the firearm is unloaded and the action is open when handing it to someone else.
- Don't handle firearms while affected by alcohol or drugs of any kind, including pharmaceuticals.
- When cleaning or dry firing a firearm, remove all ammunition to another room, and double-check the firearm when you enter the room you will be using to clean the firearm.
- Have firearms that are regularly used inspected by a qualified gunsmith at least every 2 years.

Radiation

Radiation injury can occur from overexposure to radioactive materials used in diagnostic and therapeutic procedures. Clients being examined using radiography or fluoroscopy generally receive minimal exposure, and few precautions are necessary. However, nurses need to protect themselves when some clients are receiving radiation therapy. Exposure to radiation can be minimized by limiting the time near the source, providing as much distance as possible from the source, and using shielding devices (e.g., lead aprons) when near the source. Nurses need to become familiar with agency protocols related to radiation therapy.

PROMOTING SAFETY ACROSS THE LIFE SPAN

Measures to ensure the safety of people of all ages focus on observation or prediction of potentially harmful situations so that harm can be avoided and client education that empowers clients to protect themselves and their families from injury. Safety measures covering the life span from infancy to elders are listed in the accompanying Client Teaching feature.

Newborns and Infants

Accidents are a leading cause of death during infancy, especially during the first year of life. Infants are completely dependent on others for care; they are oblivious to such dangers as falling or ingesting harmful substances. Parents need to learn the amount of observation necessary to maintain infant safety. They need help to identify and remove common hazards in and around the home as well as first-aid information that includes cardiopulmonary resuscitation and interventions for airway obstruction. Common accidents during infancy include burns, suffocation or choking, automobile accidents, falls, and poisoning. Education and support of parents can make them more knowledgeable and better prepared to protect their children from accidents and injuries.

Toddlers

Toddlers are curious and like to feel and taste everything. They are fascinated by potential dangers, such as pools and busy streets, so they need constant supervision and protection. Parents prevent many accidents by "toddler-proofing" the home or other setting where the child will be (Figure 49–10 ■). This practice extends to the use of federally approved car restraints and removing or securing all items that can pose a safety hazard to the child in any setting.

It may be necessary to inspect for and remove sources of lead from the environment. Lead poisoning (**plumbism**) is a risk for children exposed to lead paint chips, fumes from leaded gasoline, certain hair dyes, soil, or any "leaded" substances. As of 2008, it was estimated that 310,000 children under the age of 6 had too much lead in their blood. The ingestion of lead-based paint chips is the most common cause of lead poisoning in children (National Safety Council, 2009).

CLIENT TEACHING **Safety Measures Throughout the Life Span**

NEWBORNS AND INFANTS

- Use a federally approved car seat at all times (including coming home from the hospital). It should be in the backseat, facing backward.
- Never leave the infant unattended on a raised surface.
- Check the temperature of the infant's bath water and formula before using.
- Hold the infant upright during feeding. Do not prop the bottle. Cut food in small pieces, and do not feed the infant peanuts or popcorn.
- Investigate the infant's crib for compliance with federal safety regulations: slats no more than 2 3/8 inches apart, lead-free paint, height of crib sides, tight fit of mattress to crib.
- Use a playpen with sides made of small-sized netting. Never leave playpen sides down.
- Provide large, soft toys with no small detachable or sharp-edged parts.
- Use guard gates on stairs and screens on windows.
- Supervise the infant in swings and high chairs.
- Cover electric outlets. Coil cords out of reach.
- Place plants, household cleaners, and wastebaskets out of reach. Lock away potential poisons, such as medicines, paint, and gasoline.

TODDLERS

- Continue to use federally approved car seats at all times. Place children in the backseat when traveling in a car.
- Teach children not to put objects in the mouth, including pills (unless given by parent).
- Keep objects with sharp edges out of children's reach.
- Place hot pots on back burners with handles turned inward.
- Keep cleaning solutions, insecticides, and medicines in locked cupboards.
- Keep windows and balconies screened.
- Supervise toddlers in the tub.
- Fence in pools, and supervise toddlers at all times when in or near pools. Do not overfill the bathtub. Do not let toddlers play near ditches or wells.
- Teach children not to run or ride a tricycle into the street.
- Obtain a low bed when the child begins to climb.
- Cover outlets with safety covers or plugs.

PRESCHOOLERS

- Do not allow children to run with candy or other objects in the mouth.
- Teach children not to put small objects in the mouth, nose, and ears.
- Remove doors from unused equipment, such as refrigerators or safes.
- Always supervise preschoolers crossing streets, and begin safety teaching about obeying traffic signals and looking both ways.
- Check Halloween treats before allowing children to eat them. Discard loose or open candy.
- Teach children to play in "safe" areas, not on streets and railroad tracks.
- Teach preschoolers the dangers of playing with matches and near charcoal, fire, and heating appliances.
- Teach children to avoid strangers and keep parents informed of their whereabouts.
- Teach preschoolers not to walk in front of swings and not to push others off playground equipment.

SCHOOL-AGE CHILDREN

- Teach children safety rules for recreational and sports activities: never swim alone, always wear a life jacket when in a boat, and wear a protective helmet and also knee and elbow pads when needed.
- Supervise contact sports and activities in which children aim at a target.
- Teach children to obey all traffic and safety rules for bicycling, skateboarding, and roller skating.
- Teach children to use light or reflective clothing when walking or cycling at night.
- Teach children safe ways to use the stove, garden tools, and other equipment.
- Supervise children when they use saws, electric appliances, tools, and other potentially dangerous equipment.
- Teach children not to play with fireworks, gunpowder, or firearms. Keep firearms unloaded, locked up, and out of reach.
- Teach children to avoid excavations, quarries, vacant buildings, and playing around heavy machinery.
- Teach children the health hazards of smoking. If you smoke, stop.
- Teach children the effects of drugs and alcohol on judgment and coordination.

ADOLESCENTS

- Have adolescents complete a drivers' education course, and take practice drives with them in various kinds of weather.
- Set firm limits on automobile use—namely, never to drive after drinking or using drugs, and never to ride with a driver who has done so. Encourage adolescents to call home for a ride if they have been drinking, assuring them they can do so without a reprimand.
- Restrict number of passengers in the car during the first year of driving.
- Teach adolescents to wear a safety helmet when riding motorcycles, scooters, and other sports vehicles. Teach safety rules for water sports.
- Encourage adolescents to use proper equipment when participating in sports. Schedule a physical examination before participation, and be certain there is medical supervision for all athletic activities.
- Encourage adolescents to swim, jog, and go boating in groups so they can obtain help in case of an accident.
- Teach safety measures for use of power tools.
- Teach rules for hunting and the proper care and use of firearms.
- Inform the adolescent of the dangers of drugs, alcohol, and unprotected sex. Include teaching about date rape prevention and defense.
- Teach dangers of sunbathing and tanning beds, as well as use of sun block and protective clothing when doing outdoor activities.
- Be alert to changes in the adolescent's mood and behavior. Listen to and maintain open communication with the adolescent. Open communication is a powerful preventive measure.
- Set a good example of behavior that the adolescent can follow.

YOUNG ADULTS

- Reinforce motor vehicle safety: Drive defensively, use "designated drivers" if alcohol is consumed, routinely check brakes and tires, and use seat and shoulder belts or car seats for all passengers.
- Remind the young adult to repair potential fire hazards, such as electric wiring.
- Reinforce water safety (e.g., know the depth of a pool or lake before diving); supervise backyard pools and other water activities.

(continued)

CLIENT TEACHING Safety Measures Throughout the Life Span (continued)

- Discuss evaluating the potential for workplace injuries or death when making decisions about a career or occupation. Encourage the young adult to participate actively in programs that reduce occupational hazards.
- Discuss avoiding excessive sun radiation by limiting exposure, using sun-blocking agents, and wearing protective clothing. Explain the skin changes that may indicate a cancerous condition.
- Encourage young adults who are unable to cope with the pressures, responsibilities, and expectations of adulthood to seek counseling.

MIDDLE-AGED ADULTS

- Reinforce motor vehicle safety: Use seat belts, and drive within the speed limit, especially at night. Test visual acuity periodically.
- Make certain that stairways are well lighted and uncluttered.
- Equip bathrooms with hand grasps and nonskid bath mats.
- Test smoke detectors and fire alarms regularly.
- Keep all machines and tools in good working condition at work and at home. Follow safety precautions when using machinery.
- Reinforce safety measures taught earlier in life, such as the hazards of excessive sun exposure.

OLDER ADULTS

- Encourage the client to have regular vision and hearing tests.
- Assist the client to have a home hazard appraisal.
- Encourage the client to keep as active as possible.

PREVENTIVE MEASURES

- Ensure eyeglasses are functional.
- Ensure appropriate lighting.
- Mark doorways and edges of steps as needed.

- Keep environment tidy and uncluttered.
- Set safe limits to activities.
- Remove unsafe objects.
- Wear shoes or well-fitted slippers with nonskid soles.
- Use ambulatory devices as necessary (cane, crutches, walker, braces, wheelchair).
- Provide assistance with ambulation as needed.
- Monitor gait and balance.
- Adapt living arrangements to one floor if necessary.
- Encourage exercise and activity as tolerated to maintain muscle strength, joint flexibility, and balance.
- Ensure uncluttered environment with securely fastened rugs.
- Encourage client to request assistance.
- Keep bed in the low position.
- Install grab bars in bathroom.
- Provide raised toilet seat.
- Instruct client to rise slowly from a lying to a sitting to a standing position, and then to stand in place for several seconds before walking.
- Provide a bedside commode as needed.
- Assist with voiding on a frequent and scheduled basis.
- Encourage client to summon help.
- Monitor activity tolerance.
- Attach side rails to the bed.
- Keep rails in place when the bed is in the lowest position.
- Monitor orientation and alertness status.
- Encourage annual or more frequent review of all medications prescribed.

PRACTICE ALERT

The remodeling and renovation of older homes (e.g., those built before 1978) accounts for most of the lead poisoning seen today. Nurses need to educate families living in older homes about their children's risk for lead poisoning and provide lead poisoning prevention advice.

Preschoolers

Children of preschool age are active and often very clumsy, making them susceptible to injury. Control of the environment must continue, with adults keeping hazards such as matches, medicines, and other potential poisons out of reach. Safety education for the child must begin at this time. Education of the preschooler involves learning how to cross streets, what traffic signals mean, and how to ride bicycles and other wheeled toys safely. Children must be cautioned to avoid hazards, such as busy streets, swimming pools, and other potentially dangerous areas. Parents must maintain careful surveillance; the developmental level of the preschooler does not allow for self-reliance in matters of safety (Figure 49–11 ■). Parents must also keep in mind that their child's cognitive and motor skills increase quickly; hence, safety measures must keep up with the acquisition of new skills.

CLINICAL EXAMPLE

Mrs. Howard is a 60-year-old woman. Her grown daughter was beaten by her boyfriend and will be in recovery for a number of weeks. Mrs. Howard is caring for her 3-year-old grandson. Because the assault occurred in her daughter's house while the boy was present, Social Services is involved and has asked the Health Department to send a child health nurse to conduct a home assessment. The nurse conducts the assessment and finds that many cleaning supplies are kept at floor level and that there is paint peeling around the windows and doors. The refrigerator is well-stocked with fresh foods and the home is clean and tidy.

1. What nursing diagnoses would be appropriate?
2. What client outcomes would you plan for Mrs. Howard and her grandson?
3. What resources are available in your community to assist you with intervening or advocating for these clients?

School-Age Children

By the time children attend school, they are learning to think before they act. They often prefer adult equipment to toys. They want to play with other children in such activities as bicycling, hiking, swimming, and boating. Although sensitive to peer pressure, the school-age child will respond to rules.

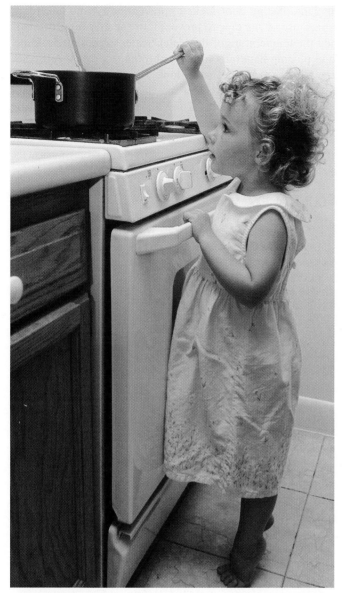

Figure 49–10 ■ Promoting safety (e.g., by placing hot pots on back burners with handles turned inward) is required to keep children from injury.

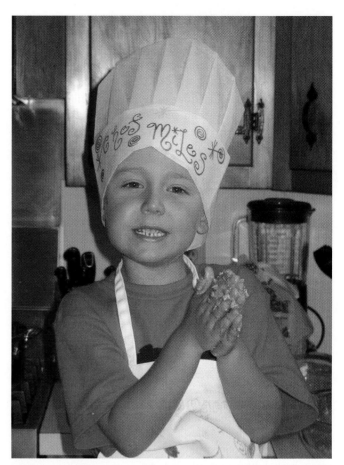

Figure 49–11 ■ Preschoolers enjoy imitating their parents, but they must be supervised carefully.

Children of this age engage in fantasy and magical thinking. They often imitate actions of parents and superheroes with whom they identify.

Injuries are the leading cause of death in school-age children. The most frequent causes of fatalities, in descending order, are motor vehicle crashes, drownings, fires, and firearms. School-age children are also involved in many minor injuries, frequently resulting from outdoor activities and recreational equipment, such as swings, bicycles, skateboards, and swimming pools.

Adolescents

Obtaining a driver's license is an important event in the life of an adolescent in United States, but the privilege is not always wisely handled. Teenagers may use driving as an outlet for stress, as a way to assert independence, or to impress peers. When setting limits on automobile use, parents need to assess the teenager's level of responsibility, common sense, and ability to resist peer pressure. The age of the teenager alone does not determine readiness to handle this responsibility.

Adolescents are at risk for sports injuries because their coordination skills are not fully developed. However, sports activities are important to the adolescent's self-esteem and overall development. In addition to providing beneficial exercise, sports activities enhance social and personal development. They help the adolescent experience competition, teamwork, and conflict resolution.

Suicide and homicide are two leading causes of death among teenagers. Adolescent males commit suicide at a higher rate than adolescent females, and African Americans commit homicide at a higher rate than European Americans. Suicides by firearms, drugs, and automobile exhaust gases are the most common. Factors influencing the high suicide and homicide rates include economic deprivation, family breakup, and the availability of firearms, which are the most frequently used weapons. Cutting or stabbing tools are the next most frequently used weapons.

Young Adults

Motor vehicle crashes are by far the leading cause of mortality for this group. Other causes of death for young adults include drowning, fires, burns, firearms, and suicide.

The nurse's role in the prevention of suicide includes identifying behaviors that may indicate potential problems: depression; a variety of physical complaints, including weight loss, sleep disturbances, and digestive disorders; and decreased interest in social and work roles along with an increase in isolation. A young adult identified as at risk for suicide should be referred to a mental health professional or a crisis center. Nurses can also reduce the incidence of suicide by participating in educational programs that provide information about the early signs of suicide.

One safety hazard for many young adults is exposure to natural radiation from sunbathing or outdoor activities. Exposure to the sun is directly related to skin cancer. Outdoor activities also may increase the young adult's risk of hyperthermia or hypothermia. Anticipatory guidance for athletes, for example, may include providing information about heat stroke and the importance of adequate hydration and rest between periods of heavy activity on hot days.

Middle-Aged Adults

Changing physiologic factors, as well as concern over personal and work-related responsibilities, may contribute to the injury rate of middle-aged persons. Motor vehicle crashes are the most common cause of accidental death in this age group. Decreased reaction times and visual acuity may make the middle-aged adult prone to accidents. Other unintentional causes of death for middle-aged adults include falls, fires, burns, poisonings, and drownings. Occupational injuries continue to be a significant safety hazard during the middle years.

Older Adults

Injury prevention is a major concern for older adults. Because their vision generally is limited, their reflexes are slower and their bones are thinning, older adults should use caution when climbing stairs, driving a car, and even walking. Driving, particularly night driving, requires caution, because accommodation of the eye to light is impaired and peripheral vision is diminished. Older adults need to learn to turn their head before changing lanes and should not rely on side vision, for example, when crossing a street or changing lanes. Driving in fog or other hazardous conditions should be avoided.

Fires are a hazard for the older adult with a failing memory. The older person may forget that the iron or stove has been left on or may not extinguish a cigarette completely. Because of reduced sensitivity to pain and heat, care must be taken to prevent burns when the person bathes or uses heating devices.

Older adults at risk for wandering as a result of dementia need to wear identification devices. They can also be registered with the local Alzheimer's Association's Wanderer's Alert Program. Strategies used to prevent injury to toddlers may be modified to provide a *safer* physical environment without infantilizing persons with Alzheimer's disease (Hurley et al., 2004). To make the home safer and decrease the chances of falls, fires, and burns the caregiver (with another person such as the visiting nurse or occupational therapist) should tour the home to identify safety issues and develop a plan to rectify them. Areas of importance include placing door locks to prevent entry into hazardous areas, use of rug tape to prevent loose scatter rugs, decreasing the temperature of the water heater to prevent scalding, and placing handrails in the bathroom to prevent falls. See the clinical example that follows.

Because older adults who take analgesics or sedatives may become lethargic or confused, they should be monitored regularly and closely. Other measures to induce sleep should be used whenever possible. The nurse teaches the importance of taking only prescribed medications and contacting a health professional at the first indication of medication intolerance.

CLINICAL EXAMPLE

Mr. Phillips is a 55-year-old man who suffered a stroke that has resulted in weakness on his left side. Following discharge from the hospital to a rehabilitation center, he has been working with a physical therapist because his gait is unsteady. Prior to discharge from the rehab center, his nurse conducts a home appraisal. There are several throw rugs in the house and the furniture is arranged so that there is not a clear path through any room. The bathroom does not have any grab bars.

1. What nursing diagnoses are appropriate based on the results of the home appraisal and Mr. Phillips' current condition?
2. What outcomes would you plan for Mr. Phillips?
3. What will be necessary for Mr. Phillips to meet these outcomes?

The incidence of suicide in older adults is increasing. A suicide attempt by the older adult may go unnoticed if the adult is attempting self-harm through hidden self-destructive behaviors, such as starvation, overdosing with medications, and noncompliance with medical care, treatments, and medications. In older individuals, the suicide attempt is usually more serious, because the adult truly intends to end his or her life and not just to get attention, as is often seen in other age groups.

Ebersole, Hess, Touhy, and Jett (2005) have listed important facts regarding suicide of the older adult. These include the following:

- White men are the most likely to commit suicide.
- Uncontrollable pain, loss of a loved one, and major life changes can be contributing factors.
- Major depression and social isolation increase the risk of suicide.
- Older adults rarely threaten to commit suicide; they just do it.

Nurses need to be aware of the symptoms and risk factors of suicide. They should direct the client to the appropriate professional or agency for treatment and counseling.

VIOLENCE HAZARDS ACROSS THE LIFE SPAN

Domestic violence is increasing at an alarming rate and involving individuals of all ages. It includes child abuse, intimate partner abuse, and elder abuse, and it affects the health and safety of families and the community. Statistics are inaccurate because of the underreporting of incidents. Nurses should be involved in working with all phases of domestic violence: prevention, screening, referrals for treatment, and follow-up care. This usually requires collaborative planning with primary care providers, law enforcement agencies, social services, and other community agencies.

Nurses also have the opportunity to become advocates on behalf of community support programs for domestic violence. They can also become involved with educating other professionals regarding prevention, screening, and treatment.

Domestic violence takes on extra importance, because people who were abused as children often display abusive behavior as adults. This points out the need for prevention and early intervention to prevent the cycle from continuing. Nurses can be of assistance in restoring dignity, health, and safety to vulnerable individuals. This subject is discussed in more detail in the Concept 31, Violence.

REVIEW Injury and Illness Prevention

RELATE: LINK THE CONCEPTS

Linking the exemplar of Injury and Illness Prevention with the concept of Addiction Behaviors:

1. What activities can the nurse implement to reduce the risk of injury and illness for the client with an addiction to cocaine? To alcohol?
2. The nurse is caring for a client who has just discovered she is pregnant and admits to smoking from 10 to 20 cigarettes a day. Describe a nursing plan of care to reduce risk to both the client and her fetus from her addiction behavior.

Linking the exemplar of Injury and Illness Prevention with the concept of Mobility:

3. How is the client with osteoarthritis at increased risk for injury or illness?
4. What are the priorities of nursing care for a client with altered mobility to reduce the risk of injury and illness?

REFER: GO TO MYNURSINGKIT

REFLECT: CASE STUDY

Norma James is a 65-year-old widow who lives alone. Although she has lived in the neighborhood for years, she is somewhat socially isolated. She has two adult sons with whom she has limited contact; they live out of the state and rarely call. She considers

only a few individuals friends; she does not particularly like many people and prefers the company of her six cats.

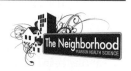

Mrs. James does not work; she has very limited savings and relies on Social Security benefits for income. She smokes about half a pack of cigarettes a day and has been a smoker since she was in her 20s. She drinks alcohol "a couple times a year, usually a glass of wine at a special dinner."

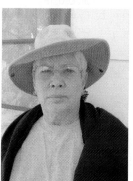

Mrs. James has a long history of type 2 diabetes mellitus and hypertension. In more recent years, she has been diagnosed with atrial fibrillation.

1. What risks does Mrs. James have for illness or injury?
2. What are your priorities for her nursing plan of care to reduce these risks for injury and illness?
3. Mrs. James has a history of evaluating information received from her health care provider rather skeptically. How can you increase the likelihood of her complying with your recommendations to reduce her risk of injury?

49.4 NATIONAL PATIENT SAFETY GOALS

KEY TERM
National Patient Safety Goals (NPSGs), *2459*

BASIS FOR SELECTION OF EXEMPLAR
Agency for Health Care Research and Quality
The Joint Commission

LEARNING OUTCOMES
After reading about this exemplar, you will be able to:

1. Explain the purpose of National Patient Safety Goals.
2. Apply National Patient Safety Goals to specific clinical activities.

OVERVIEW

As a result of IOM's 2000 report *To Err Is Human*, the health care industry and national organizations (e.g., National Patient Safety Foundation) increased their awareness of the need to improve client safety. For example, The Joint Commission requires its accredited agencies to meet specific **National Patient Safety Goals (NPSGs)** (Joint Commission, 2009a). National Patient Safety Goals have been designed based on type of facility, such as critical access hospitals, long-term care facilities, or home care agencies; the most recent versions can be

found online at http://www.jointcommission.org/patientsafety/ nationalpatientsafetygoals/.

It is important to remember that the focus of the NPSGs is on system-wide solutions (Joint Commission, 2009b). This is an important change from the traditional method of focusing on who made the error to analyzing systems to determine what events may have lead to the error and why the error was made. Joint Commission National Patient Safety Goals are revised and updated frequently based on identified needs. Box 49–9 details The Joint Commission's 2010 National Patient Safety Goals for Critical Access Hospitals.

Box 49–9 The Joint Commission 2010 National Patient Safety Goals for Critical Access Hospitals

IMPROVE THE ACCURACY OF PATIENT IDENTIFICATION
- Use at least two patient identifiers when administering medications, blood, or blood components; when collecting blood samples and other specimens for clinical testing; and when providing treatments or procedures. The patient's room number or physical location is not used as an identifier.
- Label containers used for blood and other specimens in the presence of the patient.

IMPROVE THE EFFECTIVENESS OF COMMUNICATION AMONG CAREGIVERS
- Develop written procedures for managing the critical results of tests and diagnostic procedures that address the following:
  a. The definition of critical results of tests and diagnostic procedures
  b. By whom and to whom critical results of tests and diagnostic procedures are reported
  c. The acceptable length of time between the availability and reporting of critical results of tests and diagnostic procedures.
- Implement the procedures for managing the critical results of tests and diagnostic procedures.
- Evaluate the timeliness of reporting the critical results of tests and diagnostic procedures.

IMPROVE THE SAFETY OF USING MEDICATIONS
- In perioperative and other procedural settings both on and off the sterile field, label medications and solutions that are not immediately administered. This applies even if there is only one medication being used. *Note:* An immediately administered medication is one that an authorized staff member prepares or obtains, takes directly to a patient, and administers to that patient without any break in the process.
- In perioperative and other procedural settings both on and off the sterile field, labeling occurs when any medication or solution is transferred from the original packaging to another container.
- In perioperative and other procedural settings both on and off the sterile field, medication or solution labels include the following:
  a. Medication name
  b. Strength
  c. Quantity
  d. Diluent and volume (if not apparent from the container)
  e. Preparation date
  f. Expiration date when not used within 24 hours
  g. Expiration time when expiration occurs in less than 24 hours. *Note:* The date and time are not necessary for short procedures, as defined by the critical access hospital.
- Verify all medication or solution labels both verbally and visually. Verification is done by two individuals qualified to participate in the procedure whenever the person preparing the education or solution is not the person who will be administering it.
- Label each medication or solution as soon as it is prepared, unless it is immediately administered. *Note:* An immediately administered medication is one that an authorized staff member prepares or obtains, takes directly to a patient, and administers to that patient without any break in the process.
- Immediately discard any medication or solution found unlabeled.
- Remove all labeled containers on the sterile field and discard their contents at the conclusion of the procedure. *Note:* This does not apply to multiuse vials that are handled according to infection control practices.
- All medications and solutions both on and off the sterile field and their labels are reviewed by entering and exiting staff responsible for the management of medications.

REDUCE THE RISK OF HEALTH CARE–ASSOCIATED INFECTIONS
- Comply with either the current Centers for Disease Control and Prevention (CDC) hand hygiene guidelines or the current World Health Organization (WHO) hand hygiene guidelines (CDC, 2002; WHO, 2005).
- Implement evidence-based practices to prevent health care–associated infections due to multidrug-resistant organisms in critical access hospitals. *Note:* This requirement applies to, but is not limited to, epidemiologically important organisms such as methicillin-resistant *Staphylococcus aureus* (MRSA), *Clostridium difficile* (CDI), vancomycin-resistant enterococci (VRE), and multidrug-resistant gram-negative bacteria.
- Implement evidence-based practices to prevent central line–associated bloodstream infections. *Note:* This requirement covers short- and long-term central venous catheters and peripherally inserted central catheter (PICC) lines.
- Implement evidence-based practices for preventing surgical site infections.

ACCURATELY AND COMPLETELY RECONCILE MEDICATIONS ACROSS THE CONTINUUM OF CARE
- A process exists for comparing the patient's current medications with those ordered for the patient while under the care of the critical access hospital. *Note:* This standard is not in effect at this time.
- When a patient is referred to or transferred from one critical access hospital to another, the complete and reconciled list of medications is communicated to the next provider of service, and the communication is documented. Alternatively, when a patient leaves the critical access hospital's care to go directly to his or her home, the complete and reconciled list of medications is provided to the patient's known primary care provider, the original referring provider, or a known next provider of service. *Note 1:* When the next provider of service is unknown or when no known formal relationship is planned with a next provider, giving the patient and, as needed, the family the list of reconciled medications is sufficient. *Note 2:* This standard is not in effect at this time.
- When a patient leaves the critical access hospital's care, a complete and reconciled list of the patient's medications is provided directly to the patient and, as needed, the family, and the list is explained to the patient and/or family. *Note:* This standard is not in effect at this time.
- In settings where medications are used minimally, or prescribed for a short duration, modified medication reconciliation processes are performed. *Note 1:* This requirement does not apply to critical access hospitals that do not administer medications. It may be important for health care organizations to know which types of medications their patients are taking because these medications could affect the care, treatment, and services provided. *Note 2:* This standard is not in effect at this time.

Source: © The Joint Commission (2009). *Accreditation Program: Critical Access Hospital National Patient Safety Goals.* Accessed April 2, 2010, from http://www.jointcommission.org/NR/rdonlyres/E6FF3F84-280A-48DB-AA67-B9CE7CA693FE/0/RevisedChapter_CAH_NPSG_20090924.pdf. Reprinted with permission.

REVIEW National Patient Safety Goals

RELATE: LINK THE CONCEPTS

Linking the exemplar of National Patient Safety Goals with the concept of Inflammation:

1. The nurse is working in the operating room and has just transferred the client to the operating table. What actions should the nurse perform in order to increase the client's safety according to National Patient Safety Goals?
2. The nurse working in the preoperative holding area will carry out what interventions to increase the client's safety according to National Patient Safety Goals?

Linking the exemplar of National Patient Safety Goals with the concept of Mobility:

3. The nurse is working in a long-term care facility and is preparing to help a client with altered mobility from the bed into a chair. The client's medical record indicates three people are required to assist this client, but the nurse can only find one other staff member to assist in the transfer. What should the nurse do, and why?

4. After admitting a new client to the unit, the nurse reviews the client's currently prescribed medications before determining the amount of assistance required in helping the client with altered mobility to make transfers. Why?

REFER: GO TO MYNURSINGKIT

REFLECT: CASE STUDY

Andy McKinney, aged 45, is admitted to the outpatient surgical center for repair of his torn right rotator cuff. Mr. McKinney takes medications for hypertension and high triglycerides and has a history of a mild allergy to latex. His wife, who is a nurse, asks the nurse who admits Mr. McKinney what interventions will be put in place to maintain his safety.

1. How will the nurse respond to Mrs. McKinney's question?
2. What actions will the surgical team take to assure that the proper shoulder is operated on?
3. What actions will the nurse take related to the client's latex allergy?

49.5 RESPONSIBLE SEXUAL BEHAVIOR

KEY TERMS

Date rape, *2462*
Dating violence, *2461*

BASIS FOR SELECTION OF EXEMPLAR

Healthy People 2010
National Institutes of Health

LEARNING OUTCOMES

1. Describe responsible sexual behavior.
2. Demonstrate client teaching to reduce the risk of sexually transmitted infections.

OVERVIEW

The increase in the incidence of sexually transmitted infections, especially human immunodeficiency syndrome/acquired immunodeficiency syndrome (HIV/AIDS) and genital herpes, has caused many people to modify their sexual practices and activities. Women frequently ask questions or voice concerns about these issues to the nurse in a clinic or ambulatory setting. The nurse working in these settings may need to assume the role of counselor on sexual and reproductive matters.

All sexually active individuals need to know how to reduce the spread of HIV and other sexually transmitted infections The only totally safe sex practices are abstinence, long-term mutually monogamous sexual relations between two uninfected people, or mutual masturbation without direct contact.

Responsible sexual behavior involves more than just the physical act of sex itself. It also involves knowing how to identify the warnings signs of, and how to protect oneself from, both dating violence and date rape.

SAFER SEX

Clients who do engage in sexual activity need to know and practice safer sex (Box 49–10). Reducing the number of sexual partners—for example, by entering into and remaining in a long-term mutually monogamous relationship with an uninfected partner—reduces the risk. Clients should not engage in unprotected sex, especially if the HIV status of the partner is unknown. Latex condoms have been shown to reduce the risk of transmitting HIV and other infections. Their effectiveness is improved when nonoxynol-9 (a spermicide) is used for lubrication; however, it may cause genital ulcers, which can facilitate transmission of bloodborne diseases, such as HIV and hepatitis. To be effective, condoms must be used with every sexual encounter involving vaginal, oral, or anal intercourse. They also need to be applied and removed properly. A female condom is also available for use.

DATING VIOLENCE

Dating violence is another type of intimate partner abuse; this type occurs in relationships among youth. Most dating violence is directed at females and studies have focused largely on girls. Over 9% of adolescent girls report being victims of dating violence. African American girls report dating violence more commonly than Hispanic or Caucasian girls (Howard, Wang, & Yan, 2007; MMWR, 2006). Girls who report dating violence were also more likely to report other risk behaviors, such as feeling sad, having attempted

Box 49–10 **Guidelines for Safer Sex**

- Practice mutual monogamy; if you are not in a mutually monogamous relationship, limit the number of sexual partners.
- Do not engage in unprotected sex, especially if the HIV status of your partner is unknown. (Remember that a person may be infected, and infective, for up to 6 months before converting to seropositive status.)
- When entering into a new monogamous relationship, both partners should undergo HIV testing initially. If both are negative, practice abstinence or safer sex for 6 months, followed by retesting. If results still indicate that both partners are negative, sexual activity can probably be considered safe.
- Use latex condoms for oral, vaginal, or anal intercourse; avoid natural or animal skin condoms, which allow passage of HIV.
- For vaginal or anal sex, lubricate the condom with the spermicidal agent nonoxynol-9 for additional protection.
- Do not use an oil-based lubricant such as petroleum jelly, which can result in condom damage; water-based lubricants are acceptable.

- Women should carry and use a female condom.
- Remember that use of other means of birth control, such as oral contraceptives, provide no protection against HIV; barrier protection with a condom is necessary.
- Engage in safer sexual practices that are less damaging to sensitive tissues (e.g., mutual masturbation, avoiding anal or oral sex).
- Do not use drugs or alcohol.
- Do not share needles, razors, toothbrushes, sexual toys, or other items that may be contaminated with blood or body fluids.
- If HIV positive:
  a. Do not engage in unprotected sexual activity.
  b. Inform all current and former sexual partners of HIV status.
  c. Inform all health care personnel—primary care providers, physicians, and dentists in particular—of HIV status.
  d. Do not donate blood, plasma, blood products, sperm, organs, or tissue.
  e. If female, do not become pregnant.

suicide, or having used substances such as tobacco and drugs. Early sexual activity, having a higher number of sex partners, and being less likely to use birth control are also associated with higher incidences of dating violence. A cluster risk profile may therefore put adolescents more at risk for dating violence. Box 49–11 lists early warning signs of teenage dating violence.

Date rape is a term used when dating violence takes the form of rape. This can be particularly harmful to females who often do not want to discuss the event or press charges against the attacker. See Exemplar 31.3, Rape-Trauma Syndrome.

Box 49–11 **Early Warning Signs of Teenage Dating Violence**

The teenage perpetrator:
- Believes that men should be in control and women should be submissive.
- Is jealous and possessive of his girlfriend, won't let her have friends, and checks up on her.
- Tries to control his girlfriend by giving orders and making all the decisions.
- Threatens his girlfriend with violence.
- Uses or owns weapons.
- Has a history of losing his temper quickly and fighting.
- Brags about mistreating others.
- Blames his girlfriend when he is violent; says she provoked him and made him do it.
- Has a history of abusive relationships.

REVIEW **Responsible Sexual Behavior**

RELATE: LINK THE CONCEPTS

Linking the exemplar of Responsible Sexual Behavior with the concept of Infection:
1. How can responsible sexual behaviors reduce the risk of infection?
2. How can the nurse teach responsible sexual behaviors with the geriatric client?

Linking the exemplar of Responsible Sexual Behavior with the concept of Ethics:
3. The nurse is caring for a client who is HIV/AIDS positive. The client says that it is not his responsibility to protect his sexual partners and that everyone needs to look out for themselves. How would you respond to this comment?
4. The nurse is caring for a male client who says he wants to be sexually responsible. What information would you provide this client based on his ethical concerns?

REFER: GO TO MYNURSINGKIT

REFLECT: CASE STUDY

Qualyndria Gunderson, 14 years old, comes to the doctor's office with her mother and requests to be seen alone while her mother sits in the waiting area. The nurse escorts Qualyndria back to the examination room. The client says she has become sexually active and would like a prescription for birth control pills but doesn't want her mother to know about it. She says her mother thinks she's here to discuss menstrual pain.

When the nurse goes out to the waiting room to escort another client into the examination area, Mrs. Gunderson asks to speak to the nurse. After escorting Mrs. Gunderson to an area where they can talk privately, the nurse learns that Mrs. Gunderson has been dodging questions from her daughter about sexuality. Mrs. Gunderson says she doesn't want her daughter to know about such matters until she is older, at least not until she is 18 years old. Mrs. Gunderson says she is warning the nurse because she thinks her daughter may ask these questions of the health care team, and she asks the nurse to avoid answering the questions or supplying her daughter with information about sex, explaining that she believes this information should come from her and that she'll provide it when she feels her daughter is old enough to understand.

1. How would you respond to this mother?
2. How would this mother's request impact what you teach Qualyndria about responsible sexual behavior?
3. What would you tell this mother about her daughter's sexual activity?

EXPLORE mynursingkit

MyNursingKit is your one stop for online chapter review materials and resources. Prepare for success with additional NCLEX®-style practice questions, interactive assignments and activities, web links, animations and videos, and more!

Register your access code from the front of your book at **www.mynursingkit.com**.

REFERENCES

American Academy of Pediatrics. (2005, November). Policy statement: The changing concept of sudden infant death syndrome: Diagnostic coding shifts, controversies regarding the sleeping environment, and new variables to consider in reducing risk. *Pediatrics, 116*(5), 1245–1255.

American Academy of Orthopaedic Surgeons. (2010). *Skateboarding safety.* Retrieved April 14, 2010, from http://orthoinfo.aaos.org/topic.cfm?topic=a00273

American Geriatrics Society. (2006). *Falls in older adults. Management in primary practice.* Retrieved June 18, 2006, from http://www.americangeriatrics.org/education/falls.shtml

American Nurses Association. (2010). Ethics and human rights. Retrieved April 30, 2010 from http://nursingworld.org/MainMenuCategories/HealthcareandPolicyIssues/ANAPositionStatements/EthicsandHumanRights.aspx

Ball, J.W., Bindler, R. C., & Cowen, K. J. (2010). *Child health nursing* (2nd ed.). Upper Saddle River, NJ: Pearson.

Berntsen, K. J. (2004). Valuable lessons in patient safety. Reporting near misses in health care. *Journal of Nursing Care Quality, 19*(3), 177–179.

Bohannon, R. W. (2006). Reference values for the timed up and go test: a descriptive meta-analysis. *Journal of Geriatric Physical Therapy, 29*(2), 64-68. Retrieved January 30, 2010, from http://www.geriatricspt.org/members/pubs/journal/2006/august/JGPTVol29No2-bohannon.pdf

Bulechek, G.M., Butcher, H.K., & Dochterman, J.M. (2008). *Nursing Interventions Classification (NIC)* (5th ed.). Philadelphia, PA: Mosby Elsevier.

Centers for Disease Control and Prevention. (2006). *Facts about botulism.* Retrieved February 12, 2010, http://emergency.cdc.gov/agent/botulism/factsheet.asp

Centers for Disease Control and Prevention. (2002). Guidelines for hand hygiene in health-care settings. *Morbidity and Mortality Weekly Report, 51*(RR-16), 1–56. Retrieved March 12, 2010, from http://www.cdc.gov/mmwr/preview/mmwrhtml/rr5116a1.htm

Centers for Medicare and Medicaid Services. (2005). Alcohol based hand rub solutions TIA 00-1 (101). *Federal Register, 70*(57), 15229–15239.

Centers for Medicare and Medicaid Services. (2006). Hospital conditions of participation: patients' rights; final rule 42 CFR part 482. *Federal Register, 71*(236), 71378-71428.

Ebersole, P., Hess, P., Touhy, T., & Jett, K. (2005). *Gerontological nursing & healthy aging* (2nd ed.). St. Louis, MO: Mosby.

Federal Drug Administration. (2009). How to dispose of unused medications. Retrieved April 11, 2010 from http://www.fda.gov/ForConsumers/ConsumerUpdates/ucm101653.htm

Hurley, A. C., Gauthier, M. A., Horvath, K. J., Harvey, R., Smith, S. J., Trudeau, S. A., et al. (2004). Promoting safer home environments for persons with Alzheimer's disease. *Journal of Gerontological Nursing, 30*(6), 43–51.

Howard, D. E., Wang, M. Q., & Yan, F. (2007). Psychosocial factors associated with reports of dating violence among U.S. adolescent females.. *Adolescence, 42*(166), 311–324. Retrieved April 11, 2010, from http://www.ncbi.nlm.nih.gov/pubmed/17849938

Institute of Medicine. (2000). *To err is human. Building a safer health system.* Washington, DC: National Academy of Sciences.

Institute of Medicine. (2004). *Keeping patients safe. Transforming the work environment of nurses.* Washington, DC: National Academies Press.

Joint Commission. (1998). Sentinel event alert: Accreditation committee approves examples of voluntary reportable sentinel events. Issue 4, May 11. Retrieved February 9, 2010, from http://www.jointcommission.org/SentinelEvents/SentinelEventAlert/sea_4.htm

Joint Commission. (2009a). *2010 critical access hospital: national patient safety goals.* Retrieved April 30, 2010, from http://www.jointcommission.org/NR/rdonlyres/E6FF3F84-280A-48DB-AA67-B9CE7CA693FE/0/RevisedChapter_CAH_NPSG_20090924.pdf

Joint Commission. (2009b). *Facts about 2010 National Patient Safety Goals.* Retrieved April 30, 2010, from http://www.jointcommission.org/PatientSafety/NationalPatientSafetyGoals/npsg_facts.htm

Joint Commission on Accreditation of Healthcare Organizations (JCAHO). (2005). *Restraint and seclusion.* Retrieved June 11, 2006, from http://www.jointcommission.org/AccreditationPrograms/BehavioralHealthCare/Standards/FAQs/Provision+of+Care+Treatment+and+Services/Restraint+and+Seclusion/Restraint_Seclusion.htm

Joint Commission Resources, Inc. (2010a). The life safety book: A guide to the Joint Commission life safety chapter and statement of conditions. Retrieved May 5, 2010, from http://www.jcrinc.com/Books-and-E-books/The-Life-Safety-Book/1620/

Kleinpell, R. M., Fletcher, K., and Jennings, B. M. (2008). Reducing functional decline in the hospitalized elderly. *Patient safety and quality: An evidence-based handbook for nurses.* Rockville: MD Agency for Healthcare Research and Quality.

Kohn, L. T., Corrigan, J. M., & Donaldson, M. S. (Eds.). (2000). *To err is human. Building a safer health system.* Washington, DC: National Academy Press.

Leonard, M., Frankel, A., Simmonds, T., & Vega, K. B. (2004). *Achieving safe and reliable health care.* Chicago: Health Administration Press.

Lyder, C. H., and Ayello, E. A. (2008). Pressure ulcers: A safety issue. *Patient safety and quality: An evidence-based handbook for nurses.* Rockville, MD: The Agency for Healthcare Research and Quality.

Marcy-Edwards, D. (2005). Bed rails: Is there an up side? *Canadian Nurse, 101*(1), 30–34.

Medical News Today. (2004). In hospital deaths from medical errors at 195,000 per year. Retrieved April 2, 2010, from http://www.medicalnewstoday.com/articles/11856.php

Miller, K. (2010). Memory prompts. Retrieved May 5, 2010, from http://www.jcrinc.com/Blog/2010/4/7/Memory-Prompts/

Minnesota Falls Prevention Initiative. (n.d.) Risk assessment tools. Retrieved April 9, 2010, from http://www.mnfallsprevention.org/professional/assessmenttools.html

Mitchell, P. H. (2008). Defining patient safety and quality care. *Patient safety and quality: An evidence-based handbook for nurses.* Rockville, MD: Agency for Healthcare Research and Quality.

MMWR. (2006). Youth risk behavior surveillance—United States. (2005). *Morbidity and Mortality Weekly Report, 55*(SS05), 1–108.

National Center for Complementary and Alternative Medicine. (2009). *Using dietary supplements wisely.* Retrieved April 9, 2010 from http://nccam.nih.gov/health/supplements/wiseuse.htm

National Parkinson Foundation. (2010). *Safety at home.* Retrieved April 9, 2010 from http://www.parkinson.org/Parkinson-s-Disease/Living-Well/Safety-at-Home

National Safety Council. (2010). Distracted driving. Retrieved April 9, 2010 from http://www.nsc.org/safety_road/Distracted_Driving/Pages/distracted_driving.aspx

National Safety Council. (2009). *Lead poisoning.* Retrieved April 12, 2010 from http://www.nsc.org/news_resources/Resources/Documents/Lead_Poisoning.pdf

Page, A. (Ed.). (2004). *Keeping patients safe. Transforming the work environment of nurses.* Washington, DC: National Academies Press.

Podsiallo, D. & Richardson, S. (1991). The timed up and go: a test of basic functional mobility for frail elderly persons. *Journal of the American Geriatrics Society, 39,* 142-148.

Quality and Safety Education for Nurses. (2010a). Project overview. Retrieved April 12, 2010, from http://www.qsen .org/overview.php

Quality and Safety Education for Nurses. (2010b). Competency KSAs (prelicensure). Retrieved April 12, 2010, from http:// www.qsen.org/ksas_prelicensure.php

Royal, S. T., Kendrick, D., & Coleman, T. (2005). Non-legislative interventions for the promotion of cycle helmet wearing by children. *Cochrane Database of Systematic Reviews, 2,* CD003985.

Santell, J.P., & Cousins, D. (2004). Preventing medication errors that occur in the home. *U.S. Pharmacist, 29*(9), 64–68.

UNC Healthcare. (2009). UNC hospitals fire emergency plan. Retrieved May 5, 2010, from http://labs.unchealthcare.org/ safety_manual/vi_a_fire_prevent.pdf

Wilkinson, J. M. (2005). *Nursing diagnosis handbook with NIC interventions and NOC outcomes* (8th ed.). Upper Saddle River, NJ: Prentice Hall Health.

World Health Organization. (2005). *WHO guidelines on hand hygiene in health care.* Geneva, Switzerland: World Health Organization.

Activity Intolerance
Activity Intolerance, Risk for
Activity Planning, Ineffective
Airway Clearance, Ineffective
Anxiety
Anxiety, Death
Aspiration, Risk for
Attachment, Risk for Impaired
Autonomic Dysreflexia
Autonomic Dysreflexia, Risk for
Bleeding, Risk for
Blood Glucose, Risk for Unstable
Body Image, Disturbed
Body Temperature: Imbalanced, Risk for
Bowel Incontinence
Breastfeeding, Effective
Breastfeeding, Ineffective
Breastfeeding, Interrupted
Breathing Pattern, Ineffective
Cardiac Output, Decreased
Caregiver Role Strain
Caregiver Role Strain, Risk for
Childbearing Process, Readiness for Enhanced
Comfort, Impaired
Comfort, Readiness for Enhanced
Communication: Impaired, Verbal
Communication, Readiness for Enhanced
Confusion, Acute
Confusion, Acute, Risk for
Confusion, Chronic
Constipation
Constipation, Perceived
Constipation, Risk for
Contamination
Contamination, Risk for
Coping: Community, Ineffective
Coping: Community, Readiness for Enhanced
Coping, Defensive
Coping: Family, Compromised
Coping: Family, Disabled
Coping: Family, Readiness for Enhanced
Coping (Individual), Readiness for Enhanced
Coping, Ineffective
Decisional Conflict
Decision Making, Readiness for Enhanced
Denial, Ineffective
Dentition, Impaired
Development: Delayed, Risk for
Diarrhea
Disuse Syndrome, Risk for
Diversional Activity, Deficient
Energy Field, Disturbed
Environmental Interpretation Syndrome, Impaired
Electrolyte Imbalance, Risk for
Failure to Thrive, Adult
Falls, Risk for
Family Processes, Dysfunctional
Family Processes, Interrupted
Family Processes, Readiness for Enhanced
Fatigue
Fear
Fluid Balance, Readiness for Enhanced
Fluid Volume, Deficient
Fluid Volume, Deficient, Risk for
Fluid Volume, Excess
Fluid Volume, Imbalanced, Risk for
Gas Exchange, Impaired
Gastrointestinal Motility, Dysfunctional
Gastrointestinal Motility, Risk for Dysfunctional
Grieving
Grieving, Complicated

Grieving, Risk for Complicated
Growth, Disproportionate, Risk for
Growth and Development, Delayed
Health Behavior, Risk-Prone
Health Maintenance, Ineffective
Health Management: Self, Ineffective
Home Maintenance, Impaired
Hope, Readiness for Enhanced
Hopelessness
Human Dignity, Risk for Compromised
Hyperthermia
Hypothermia
Immunization Status, Readiness for Enhanced
Infant Behavior, Disorganized
Infant Behavior: Disorganized, Risk for
Infant Behavior: Organized, Readiness for
   Enhanced
Infant Feeding Pattern, Ineffective
Infection, Risk for
Injury, Risk for
Insomnia
Intracranial Adaptive Capacity, Decreased
Knowledge, Deficient (Specify)
Knowledge (Specify), Readiness for Enhanced
Latex Allergy Response
Latex Allergy Response, Risk for
Liver Function, Impaired, Risk for
Loneliness, Risk for
Maternal/Fetal Dyad, Risk for Disturbed
Memory, Impaired
Mobility: Bed, Impaired
Mobility: Physical, Impaired
Mobility: Wheelchair, Impaired
Moral Distress
Nausea
Neonatal Jaundice
Neurovascular Dysfunction: Peripheral, Risk for
Noncompliance (Specify)
Nutrition, Imbalanced: Less than Body
   Requirements
Nutrition, Imbalanced: More than Body
   Requirements
Nutrition, Imbalanced: More than Body
   Requirements, Risk for
Nutrition, Imbalanced: Less than Body
   Requirements, Risk for
Nutrition, Readiness for Enhanced
Oral Mucous Membrane, Impaired
Pain, Acute
Pain, Chronic
Parenting, Impaired
Parenting, Readiness for Enhanced
Parenting, Risk for Impaired
Parental role Conflict
Perioperative Positioning Injury, Risk for
Personal Identity, Disturbed
Poisoning, Risk for
Post-Trauma Syndrome
Post-Trauma Syndrome, Risk for
Power, Readiness for Enhanced
Powerlessness
Powerlessness, Risk for
Protection, Ineffective
Rape-Trauma Syndrome
Relationship, Readiness for Enhanced
Religiosity, Impaired
Religiosity, Readiness for Enhanced
Religiosity, Risk for Impaired
Relocation Stress Syndrome
Relocation Stress Syndrome, Risk for
Resilience, Individual, Impaired

Resilience, Risk for Compromised
Resilience, Readiness for Enhanced
Role Conflict, Parental
Role Performance, Ineffective
Sedentary Lifestyle
Self-Care, Readiness for Enhanced
Self-Care Deficit: Bathing
Self-Care Deficit: Dressing
Self-Care Deficit: Feeding
Self-Care Deficit: Toileting
Self-Concept, Readiness for Enhanced
Self-Esteem, Chronic Low
Self-Esteem, Situational Low
Self-Esteem, Risk for Situational Low
Self Health Management, Readiness for Enhanced
Self-Mutilation
Self-Mutilation, Risk for
Self Neglect
Sensory Perception, Disturbed (Specify: Auditory,
   Gustatory, Kinesthetic, Olfactory Tactile, Visual)
Sexual Dysfunction
Sexuality Pattern, Ineffective
Shock, Risk for
Skin Integrity, Impaired
Skin Integrity, Risk for Impaired
Sleep Deprivation
Sleep pattern, Disturbed
Sleep, Readiness for Enhanced
Social Interaction, Impaired
Social Isolation
Sorrow, Chronic
Spiritual Distress
Spiritual Distress, Risk for
Spiritual Well-Being, Readiness for Enhanced
Spontaneous Ventilation, Impaired
Stress, Overload
Sudden Infant Death Syndrome, Risk for
Suffocation, Risk for
Suicide, Risk for
Surgical Recovery, Delayed
Swallowing, Impaired
Therapeutic Regimen Management: Family,
   Ineffective
Thermoregulation, Ineffective
Tissue Integrity, Impaired
Tissue Perfusion, Ineffective (Specify: Cerebral,
   Cardiac, Gastrointestinal, Renal)
Tissue Perfusion, Ineffective, Peripheral
Transfer Ability, Impaired
Trauma, Risk for
Vascular trauma, Risk for
Unilateral Neglect
Urinary Elimination, Impaired
Urinary Elimination, Readiness for Enhanced
Urinary Incontinence, Functional
Urinary Incontinence, Overflow
Urinary Incontinence, Reflex
Urinary Incontinence, Stress
Urinary Incontinence, Urge
Urinary Incontinence, Risk for Urge
Urinary Retention
Ventilatory Weaning Response, Dysfunctional
Violence: Other-Directed, Risk for
Violence: Self-Directed, Risk for
Walking, Impaired
Wandering

Source: NANDA International (2009).
Nursing Diagnoses: Definitions and classifications.
Chichester, West Sussex, United Kingdom:
Wiley-Blackwell. Used with permission.

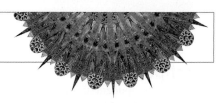

ACETAMINOPHEN (SERUM)

Reference Values

Adult: *Therapeutic:* 5–20 mcg/ml, 31–124 μmol/l (SI units). *Toxic:* greater than 50 mcg/ml, 305 μmol/l (SI units), greater than 200 mcg/ml possible hepatotoxicity.

Child: *Therapeutic:* Same as adult. *Toxic:* Similar to adult.

ACETONE, KETONE BODIES (SERUM OR PLASMA)

Reference Values

Adult: *Acetone:* Semiquantitative: Negative (less than 1 mg/dl); quantitative: 0.3–2.0 mg/dl, 51.63–44.0 μmol/l (SI units). *Ketones:* 0.5–4 mg/dl.

Child: *Newborn to 1 Week:* Slightly higher than adult. *Over 1 Week:* Same as adult.

ACETYLCHOLINE RECEPTOR ANTIBODY (ACHR) (SERUM)

Reference Values

Less than 0.02 to less than 0.03 nmol/l or negative.

ACID PHOSPHATASE (ACP) (SERUM)

Reference Values

Adult: Less than 2.6 ng/ml; 05 unit/l range, varies according to the method used; 0.2–13 international unit/l (SI units).

ADENOVIRUS ANTIBODY (SERUM)

Reference Values

Adult and Child: Negative. *Positive:* Fourfold titer increase.

ADRENOCORTICOTROPIC HORMONE (ACTH) (PLASMA)

Reference Values

7 a.m. to 10 a.m.: 8–80 pg/ml; highest levels occur in early morning.

4 p.m.: 5–30 pg/ml.

10 p.m. to Midnight: Less than 10 pg/ml; lowest levels occur at bedtime.

ALANINE AMINOTRANSFERASE (ALT) (SERUM)

Reference Values

Adult: 10–35 unit/l; 4–36 unit/l at 37°C (SI units). *Male:* Levels may be slightly higher.

Child: *Infant:* Could be twice as high as adult. *Child:* Similar to adult.

Elderly: Slightly higher than adult.

Description

Alanine aminotransferase (ALT)/serum glutamic pyruvic transaminase (SGPT) is an enzyme found primarily in the liver cells and is effective in diagnosing hepatocellular destruction. It is also found in small amounts in the heart, kidney, and skeletal muscle.

Serum ALT levels can be higher than levels of its sister transferase (transaminase), aspartate aminotransferase (AST)/serum glutamic oxaloacetic transaminase (SGOT), in cases of acute hepatitis and liver damage from drugs and chemicals, with its serum levels reaching to 200 to 4000 unit/l. ALT is used for differentiating between jaundice caused by liver disease and hemolytic jaundice. With jaundice, the serum ALT levels of liver origin can be higher than 300 units; from causes outside the liver, the levels can be less than 300 units. Serum ALT levels usually elevate before jaundice appears.

ALT/SGPT levels are frequently compared with AST/SGOT levels for diagnostic purposes. ALT is increased more markedly than AST in liver necrosis and acute hepatitis, while AST is more markedly increased in myocardial necrosis (acute myocardial infarction), cirrhosis, cancer of the liver, chronic hepatitis, and liver congestion. ALT levels are normal or slightly elevated in myocardial necrosis. The ALT levels return more slowly to normal range than AST levels in liver conditions.

Clinical Problems

Decreased Level: Exercise. *Drug Influence: Salicylates.*

Increased Level: *Highest Increase:* Acute (viral) hepatitis, necrosis of the liver (drug or chemical toxicity). *Slight or Moderate Increase:* Cirrhosis, cancer of the liver, congestive heart failure, acute alcohol intoxication. *Drug Influence:* Antibiotics (carbenicillin, clindamycin, erythromycin, gentamicin, lincomycin, mithramycin, spectinomycin, tetracycline), narcotics (meperidine [Demerol], morphine, codeine), antihypertensives (methyldopa, guanethidine), digitalis preparations, indomethacin (Indocin), salicylates, rifampin, flurazepam (Dalmane), propranolol (Inderal), oral contraceptives (progestin-estrogen), lead, heparin.

ALBUMIN (SERUM)

Reference Values

Adult: 3.5–5.0 g/dl; 52% to 68% of total protein.

Child: *Newborn:* 2.9–5.4 g/dl. *Infant:* 4.4–5.4 g/dl. *Child:* 4.0–5.8 g/dl.

Description

Albumin, a component of proteins, makes up more than half of plasma proteins. Albumin is synthesized by the liver. It increases osmotic pressure (oncotic pressure), which is necessary for maintaining the vascular fluid. A decrease in serum albumin will cause fluid to shift from within the vessels to the tissues, resulting in edema.

The *A/G ratio* is a calculation of the distribution of two major protein fractions, albumin and globulin. The reference value of A/G ratio is greater than 1.0, which is the albumin value divided by globulin value (albumin ÷ globulin). A high ratio value is considered insignificant; low ratio value occurs in liver and renal diseases. Protein electrophoresis is more accurate and has replaced the A/G ratio calculation.

ALCOHOL (ETHYL OR ETHANOL) (SERUM OR PLASMA)
Reference Values

No Alcohol: 00.0% *No Significant Alcohol Influence:* less than 0.05% or 50 mg/dl. *Alcohol Influence Present:* 0.05%–0.10% or 50–100 mg/dl. *Reaction Time Affected:* 0.10%–0.15% or 100–150 mg/dl. *Indicative of Alcohol Intoxication:* greater than 0.15% or greater than 150 mg/dl. *Severe Alcohol Intoxication:* greater than 0.25% or 250 mg/dl. *Comatose:* greater than 0.30% or 300 mg/dl. *Fatal:* greater than 0.40% or 400 mg/dl.

ALDOLASE (ALD) (SERUM)
Reference Values

Adult: Less than 6 unit/l, 38 unit/dl (Sibley-Lehninger), 22–59 milliunit/l at 37°C (SI units).
Child: *Infant:* 12–24 unit/dl (four times). *Child:* 6–16 unit/dl (two times).

Description

Aldolase is an enzyme present most abundantly in the skeletal and cardiac muscles. This enzyme is used to monitor skeletal muscle diseases such as muscular dystrophy, dermatomyositis, and trichinosis. It is not elevated in muscle disease of neural origin, such as multiple sclerosis, poliomyelitis, and myasthenia gravis.

Serum aldolase is helpful in diagnosing early cases of Duchennes muscular dystrophy before clinical symptoms appear. Progressive muscular dystrophy may cause elevated serum aldolase levels 10 to 15 times greater than normal. In late stages of muscular dystrophy, the enzyme level may return to normal or below normal. Serum aldolase is not the most effective diagnostic test for myocardial infarction (MI), because there is only a slight rise. Following an acute MI, it peaks (two times normal) in 24 hours and returns to normal in 4 to 7 days.

ALDOSTERONE (SERUM)
Reference Values

Adult: Less than 16 ng/dl (fasting); 4–30 ng/dl (sitting position).
Child (3–11 years): 5–70 ng/dl.
Pregnancy: 2 to 3 times higher than adult.

Description

Aldosterone is the most potent of all mineralocorticoids produced by the adrenal cortex. This hormone responds to various changes in the body. When there is a sodium loss and a water loss, aldosterone is secreted for reestablishing sodium and water balance. Renin promotes aldosterone secretion, which causes more sodium and water to be retained and body fluid to be increased. Stress will increase aldosterone secretion. Hypernatremia (serum sodium excess) inhibits aldosterone secretion.

Serum aldosterone is not the most reliable test, because there can be fluctuations caused by various influences. If the client is in a supine position, serum aldosterone will be lower than if he or she were in a sitting or standing position. A 24-hour urine test is considered more reliable than a random serum aldosterone collection. Several serum aldosterone levels may be requested.

ALDOSTERONE (URINE)
Reference Values

Adult: 6–25 mcg/24 hours

ALKALINE PHOSPHATASE (ALP) WITH ISOENZYME (SERUM)
Reference Values

Adult: 42–136 unit/l; ALP[1]: 20–130 unit/l; ALP[2]: 20–120 unit/l.
Child: *Infant and child (aged 0–12 years):* 40–115 unit/l. *Older child (13–18 years):* 50–230 unit/l.
Elderly: Slightly higher than adult.

Description

Alkaline phosphatase (ALP) is an enzyme produced mainly in the liver and bone; it is also derived from the intestine, kidney, and placenta. The ALP test is useful for determining liver and bone diseases. In cases of mild liver-cell damage, the ALP level may be only slightly elevated, but it could be markedly elevated in acute liver disease. Once the acute phase is over, the serum level will promptly decrease, whereas the serum bilirubin will remain increased. For determining liver dysfunction, several laboratory tests are performed (i.e., bilirubin, leucine aminopeptidase [LAP], 5′-nucleotidase [5′-NT], and gamma-glutamyl transpeptidase [GGTP]).

With bone disorders, the ALP level is increased because of abnormal osteoblastic activity (bone cell production). In children it is not abnormal to find high levels of ALP before and during puberty because of bone growth.

Isoenzymes of ALP are used to distinguish between liver and bone diseases, ALP[1] indicating disease of liver origin, and ALP[2], bone origin.

Purposes
- To determine the presence of a liver or bone disorder.
- To compare ALP results with other laboratory tests for confirmation of a liver or bone disorder.

ALPHA FETOPROTEIN (AFP) (SERUM AND AMNIOTIC FLUID)

Reference Values

Nonpregnancy: Less than 15 ng/ml.

Pregnancy:

SERUM		AMNIOTIC FLUID	
Weeks of Gestation	ng/ml	Weeks of Gestation	ng/ml
8–12	0–39	14	11.0–32.0
13	6–31	15	5.5–31.0
14	7–50	16	5.7–31.5
15	7–60	17	3.8–32.5
16	10–72	18	3.6–28.0
17	11–90	19	3.7–24.5
18	14–94	20	2.2–15.0
19	24–112	21	3.8–18.0
20	31–122		
21	19–124		

Description
Serum alpha fetoprotein (AFP), a screening test, is usually done between 16 and 20 weeks gestation to determine the probability of twins, or to detect low birth weight or serious birth defects, such as open neural-tube defect. If a high serum AFP level occurs, the test should be repeated one week later. Ultrasound and amniocentesis may be performed to confirm elevated serum levels and to diagnose neural-tube defects in the fetus.

Purpose
- To identify the probability of neural-tube defects, fetal death, or other anomalies in pregnancy (*see Clinical Problems*).

Clinical Problems
Decreased Level: Downs syndrome, absence of pregnancy.

Increased Level: *Nonpregnant:* Cirrhosis of the liver (not liver metastasis), hepatitis, germ-cell tumor of gonads, such as testicular cancer, metastases to liver. *Pregnant:* Neural-tube

NURSING IMPLICATIONS WITH RATIONALE
Alpa Fetoprotein

- Explain that the test is for screening purposes. If the test is positive, genetic counseling might be necessary.
- Be supportive of individuals and family.

CLIENT TEACHING
- Instruct the client that it is essential to give the correct gestation date of the pregnancy, if known, to avoid a laboratory test error. Inform the client that the test might be repeated in a week.
- If an ultrasound is performed, instruct the client that it is usually done to confirm gestational age or to confirm the positive serum AFP and amniocentesis result(s).

defects (spina bifida, anencephaly, myelomeningocele), fetal death, fetal distress, Turners syndrome, other anomalies (duodenal atresia, tetralogy of Fallot, hydrocephalus, trisomy 13), severe Rh immunization.

Procedure
- There is no food or fluid restriction.
- Collect 5 to 7 ml of venous blood in a red-top tube. Avoid hemolysis.

Factors Affecting Laboratory Results
- Fetal blood contamination could cause an elevated amniotic AFP level.
- Inaccurate recording of gestation week could affect results.
- Multiple pregnancy or fetal death could cause a false-positive test.
- Hemolysis of blood sample could affect results.
- Body weight may be a factor (although not definitely confirmed). A heavier female tends to have a lower serum AFP level.

AMINOGLYCOSIDES (SERUM)
Amikacin [Amikin], Gentamicin [Garamycin], Tobramycin [Nebcin]

Reference Values
Adult:

THERAPEUTIC RANGE			
Drug Name	Peak	Trough	Toxic Level
Amikacin	15–30 mcg/ml	<10 mcg/ml	>35 mcg/ml
Gentamicin	6–10 mcg/ml	<1.5 mcg/ml	>12 mcg/ml
Kanamycin	15–30 mcg/ml	14 mcg/ml	>35 mcg/ml
Netilmicin	0.5–10 mcg/ml	<4 mcg/ml	>16 mcg/ml
Tobramycin	5–10 mcg/ml	<2 mcg/ml	>12 mcg/ml

Child: Same as adult.

AMINO ACID (URINE)

Reference Values

Normal values are age dependent; 200 mg/24 h.

AMMONIA (PLASMA)

Reference Values

Adult: 15–45 mcg/dl, 11–35 µmol/l (SI units).
Child: *Newborn:* 64–107 mcg/dl. *Child:* 29–70 mcg/dl; 29–70 µmol/l (SI units).

Description

Ammonia, a by-product of protein metabolism, is formed from the bacterial action in the intestine and from metabolizing tissues. Most of the ammonia is absorbed into the portal circulation and is converted in the liver to urea. With severe liver decompensation or when blood flow to the liver is altered, the plasma ammonia level remains elevated.

Elevated plasma ammonia is best correlated with hepatic failure; however, other conditions that interfere with liver function (congestive heart failure [CHF], acidosis) may cause a temporary elevation of plasma ammonia.

AMNIOTIC FLUID ANALYSIS

Amniocentesis, Amnioscopy

Normal Finding

Clear amniotic fluid, no chromosomal or neural tube abnormalities.

Description

Amniotic fluid analysis is useful for detecting chromosomal abnormalities, such as Down syndrome or mongolism (trisomy 21); neural tube defects (spina bifida); and sex-linked disorders, such as hemophilia; and for determining fetal maturity. The amniotic fluid is obtained by amniocentesis. This procedure involves the insertion of a needle into the suprapubic area after the fetus has been located and manually elevated and the aspiration of 5 to 15 ml of amniotic fluid. Ultrasound may be used to locate the placenta and to determine fetal position so that needle contact can be avoided. Amniocentesis is performed during the 14th to 16th weeks of pregnancy. It usually is not done before the 14th week because of the insufficient amount of amniotic fluid or after the 16th week if a therapeutic abortion might be suggested.

Analyses of the amniotic fluid may also include color, bilirubin (present in the fluid until the 28th week but absent at full term), meconium (present during stress—e.g., in breech presentation), creatinine, lecithin/sphingomyelin (L/S) ratio (a decreased ratio can indicate respiratory distress syndrome), glucose, lipids, and alpha-fetoprotein (AFP).

Amnioscopy involves insertion of a fiberoptic lighted instrument (snioscope) into the cervical canal to visualize the amniotic fluid. The color of the amniotic fluid can indicate fetal hypoxia. This test is normally performed close to full term, because it requires cervical dilation. Because there is a risk of rupturing the amniotic membrane and of intrauterine infection, the test is rarely performed.

Foam Stability Test

This test determines if surfactant from mature fetal lungs is present in the amniotic fluid. When the test tube of amniotic fluid is shaken, bubbles appear around the surface if adequate amounts of surfactant are present.

Factors Affecting Diagnostic Results

■ A traumatic amniocentesis tap may produce blood in the amniotic fluid.

AMYLASE WITH ISOENZYMES (SERUM)

Reference Values

Adult: 60–160 Somogyi unit/dl, 30–170 unit/l (SI units).
Pregnancy: Slightly increased.
Child: Not usually done.
Elderly: Slightly higher than adult.
Serum Isoenzymes: *S (salivary) type:* 45–70%. *P (pancreatic) type:* 30–55%. Values may differ with method used.

Description

Amylase is an enzyme that is derived from the pancreas, the salivary glands, and the liver. Its function is to change starch to sugar. In acute pancreatitis, serum amylase is increased to twice its normal level. Its level begins to increase 2 to 12 hours after

---

NURSING IMPLICATIONS WITH RATIONALE
Amniotic Fluid Analysis

■ Recognize when amniocentesis for amniotic fluid analysis is indicated (i.e., with a familial history of sex-linked, genetic, or chromosomal disorders; with a history of previous miscarriages; and in advanced maternal age [greater than **35** years old]). It is not a screening test.

■ Be sure that the client urinates before the test and that the consent form is signed.

■ Be supportive of the woman and her partner. Be a good listener. Allow them time to ask questions and to express any concerns. Refer questions you cannot answer to the appropriate health professionals.

CLIENT TEACHING

■ Inform the client that normal results do not guarantee a normal infant, nor do they always predict sex correctly. The health care provider should tell the woman of potential risks, such as premature labor, spontaneous abortion, infection, and fetal or placental bleeding from the needle. These complications rarely occur, but the woman should be told of the risk factors.

■ Instruct the client to notify the health care provider immediately of any of the following: bleeding or leaking fluid from the vagina, abdominal pain or cramping, chills and fever, or lack of fetal movement.

■ Encourage the woman and her partner to seek genetic counseling, especially if a chromosomal abnormality has been determined. Usually the final decision about terminating a pregnancy rests with the pregnant woman and her partner.

onset, peaks in 20 to 30 hours, and returns to normal in 2 to 4 days. Acute pancreatitis is frequently associated with inflammation, severe pain, and necrosis caused by digestive enzymes (including amylase) escaping into the surrounding tissue.

Increased serum amylase can occur after abdominal surgery involving the gall-bladder (stones or biliary duct) and stomach (partial gastrectomy). Following abdominal surgery, some surgeons order a routine serum amylase for 2 days to determine whether the pancreas has been injured.

The urine amylase level is helpful in determining the significance of a normal or slightly elevated serum amylase, especially when the client has symptoms of pancreatitis. Amylase levels can also be obtained from abdominal fluid, ascitic fluid, pleural effusion, and saliva.

There are two types of amylase isoenzymes, P type (pancreatic origin) and S type (salivary origin). P-type elevation occurs more frequently in acute pancreatitis. Elevated S type can occur as a result of parotitis, and ovarian and bronchogenic tumors. Amylase isoenzymes are usually ordered to rule out a nonpancreatic source of the elevated serum amylase level. A pancreatic isoenzyme kit is commercially available.

AMYLASE (URINE)

Reference Values

Adult: 4–37 unit/ ½ h.

AMYLOID BETA PROTEIN PRECURSOR (CSF)

Alzheimers Disease Marker

Reference Values

Normal: 450 units/l cerebrospinal fluid (CSF).

Description

A CSF test that can aid in diagnosing Alzheimers disease is amyloid beta protein precursor test. It is found that the amyloid beta protein is present in the senile plaques within the brain. Amyloid can also be found in the meningeal blood vessels of clients with Alzheimers disease. It is believed that this type of protein may have neurotoxic effects on the brain cells. Small amounts of amyloid can be found in the CSF of most healthy persons; however, a higher value occurs in the CSF of clients with Alzheimers, and a somewhat higher value than normal may occur in an aged client with senile dementia.

ANGIOGRAPHY (ANGIOGRAM)

Arteriography: Cardiac [see Cardiac Catheterization], Cerebral Angiography, Pulmonary Angiography, and Renal Angiography

Description

The terms *angiography* (examination of the blood vessels) and *arteriography* (examination of the arteries) are used interchangeably. A catheter is inserted into the femoral, brachial, subclavian, or carotid artery, and a contrast dye is injected to allow visualization of the blood vessels. Normally the client feels a warm, flushed sensation as the dye is injected. Angiographies are useful for evaluating patency of blood vessels and for identifying abnormal vascularization resulting from neoplasms (tumors). This test may be indicated when computed tomography or radionuclide scanning suggests vascular abnormalities.

An embolus due to catheter clot formation is the most dangerous complication of angiography. Other complications include puncturing the site causing hematoma and/or hemorrhage, contrast media reactions, and infection.

CEREBRAL ANGIOGRAPHY Any of the three arteries (femoral, brachial, or carotid) can be used for access. The dye will outline the carotid artery, vertebral artery, large blood vessels of the circle of Willis, and small cerebral arterial branches.

PULMONARY ANGIOGRAPHY The catheter is inserted into the brachial artery (in the arm) or the femoral artery and is threaded to the pulmonary artery. The dye is injected for visualizing pulmonary vessels. During the test the client should be monitored for cardiac dysrhythmias.

RENAL ANGIOGRAPHY The catheter is inserted into the femoral artery and is passed upward through the iliac artery and the aorta to the renal artery. This test permits visualization of the renal vessels and the parenchyma. An aortogram is sometimes made with real angiography to detect any vessel abnormality and to show the relationship of the renal arteries to the aorta.

Purposes
- To detect aneurysms, thrombosis, emboli, space-occupying lesions, stenosis, plaques.
- To evaluate cerebral, pulmonary, and renal blood flow.

Clinical Problems

Type of Angiography	Indications/Purposes
Cerebral	■ To detect cerebrovascular aneurysm; cerebral thrombosis; hematomas; tumors from increased vascularization; cerebral plaques or spasm; cerebral fistula ■ To determine cerebral blood flow, cause of increased intracranial pressure (↑ ICP)
Pulmonary	■ To detect pulmonary embolism; tumors; aneurysms; congenital defects; vascular changes associated with emphysema, blebs, and bullae; heart abnormality ■ To evaluate pulmonary circulation
Renal	■ To detect renal artery stenosis; renal thrombus or embolus; space-occupying lesions (i.e., tumors, cysts); aneurysms ■ To determine the causative factor of hypertension, cause of renal failure ■ To evaluate renal circulation

Procedure

All Angiographies

- A consent form should be signed by the client or a designated family member.
- The client should be NPO for 8 to 12 hours before the angiogram. Anticoagulants (heparin) are usually discontinued.
- Record vital signs. Have client void before the test.
- Dentures and metallic objects should be removed before the test.
- The access site should be shaved.
- Premedications (i.e., a sedative or narcotic analgesic), if ordered, are administered an hour before the test. If the client has a history of severe allergic reactions to various substances or drugs, the health care provider may order steroids or antihistamines before and after the procedure as a prophylactic measure.
- Intravenous (IV) fluids may be started before the procedure so that emergency drugs, if needed, may be administered.

- The client lies in a supine position on an x-ray table. A local anesthetic is administered to the injection incisional site.
- The test takes approximately 1 to 2 hours.

RENAL   A laxative or cleansing enema is usually ordered the evening before the test.

PULMONARY   Electrocardiography electrodes are attached to the clients chest for cardiac monitoring (tracings of heart activity) during the angiography. Pulmonary pressures are recorded, and blood samples are obtained before the contrast dye is injected.

Factors Affecting Diagnostic Results

- Feces and gas can distort or decrease the visualization of the kidneys.
- Barium sulfate from a recent barium study can interfere with the test results.
- Movement during the filming can distort the x-ray picture.

NURSING IMPLICATIONS WITH RATIONALE   Angiography

PRETEST

- Obtain a client history of hypersensitivity to iodine, seafood, or contrast dye from other x-ray procedures (e.g., intravenous pyelography [IVP]). The health care provider should also know if the client is highly sensitive to other substances. Skin testing could be done before the test, or prophylactic medications (i.e., steroids, antihistamines) may be given prior to and/or following the test.
- Record baseline vital signs.
- Give a laxative or cleansing enema, if ordered. Explain to the client that it will cleanse the lower intestinal tract, allowing better visualization.
- Have the client void, wear a gown, and remove dentures.
- Administer premedications (sedative and narcotic analgesic) as ordered. Check that the consent form has been signed before giving premedications. The client should be in bed with the bed sides up after the premedications are given.
- Encourage the client to ask questions. This test can be frightening to clients, and they will need time to express any concerns.
- Assess for vasovagal reaction (common complication; i.e., decreased pulse rate and blood pressure [BP], cold and clammy skin). Give IV fluids and atropine IV. This reaction lasts about 15 to 20 minutes.

CLIENT TEACHING

- Explain the procedure to the client *(see Description and Procedure)*. Inform the client that the radiologist, surgeon, or health care provider will inject a contrast dye into an artery at the groin, elbow, or neck. The area will be numbed, and a catheter will be inserted and threaded with the guidance of fluoroscopy to the appropriate site.
- Inform the client that when the dye is injected he or she will most likely feel a warm, flushed sensation that should last for a minute or two. Explain to the client that the test should not cause pain but can cause some periodic discomfort during the procedure.

POSTTEST

- Apply pressure on the injection site for 5 to 10 minutes or longer (venous access) or 30 minutes or longer (arterial access) until bleeding has stopped. Check the injection site for bleeding when taking vital signs.

- Monitor vital signs as ordered, such as every 15 minutes for the first hour, every 30 minutes for the next 2 hours, and then every hour for the next 4 hours, or until stable. The temperature should be taken every 4 hours for 24 to 48 hours or as ordered.
- Enforce bed rest for 5 hours for venous access or 6 to 8 hours for arterial access or as ordered. Activities should be restricted for a day.
- Assess the injection site for swelling and for hematoma.
- Check peripheral pulses in the extremities (i.e., dorsalis pedis, femoral, and radial). Absence or weakness in pulse volume should be reported immediately.
- Note the temperature and color of the extremity. Report changes (e.g., colorpale, pain in the extremity, especially distal to access site) to the health care provider immediately. Arterial occlusion to the extremity could occur.
- Apply cold compresses or an ice pack to the injection site for edema or pain, if ordered.
- Monitor electrocardiogram tracings, urine output, and IV fluids. IV fluids and cardiac monitoring may be discontinued after the angiography.
- Inform the client that coughing usually is not abnormal following a pulmonary angiography.
- Assess for dysphagia and for respiratory distress if the carotid artery was used for cerebral angiography.
- Assess for weakness or numbness in an extremity, confusion, slurred speech, or visual changes following a cerebral angiography. These could be symptoms of a transient ischemic attack (TIA), known as a small stroke.
- Observe for a delayed allergic reaction to the contrast dye (i.e., tachycardia, dyspnea, skin rash, urticaria [hives], decreasing systolic BP, and decreased urine output).
- Be supportive of the client and his or her family. Answer questions, and explain your nursing implications.

ANGIOTENSIN-CONVERTING ENZYME (ACE) (SERUM)
Reference Values

Adult greater than 20 yrs: 8–67 unit/l.
Child and Adult less than 20 yrs: Test is NOT performed because they normally have elevated ACE levels.

Description

Angiotensin-converting enzyme (ACE) is found primarily in the lung epithelial cells and to a lesser extent in blood vessels and renal cells. The purpose of ACE is to regulate arterial blood pressure by converting angiotensin I to the vasoconstrictor angiotensin II, which increases blood pressure and stimulates the adrenal cortex to release aldosterone (sodium-retaining hormone). However, this test has little value for diagnosing hypertension.

High serum ACE levels are found primarily with active sarcoidosis. This test should not be performed for clients who are under 20 years of age because they normally have elevated ACE levels. Approximately 5% of the population has an elevated ACE level. The purpose for the ACE test is to diagnose and determine the severity of pulmonary sarcoidosis. Seventy to 90% of clients with active sarcoidosis have elevated serum ACE levels. Other conditions that have elevated ACE levels include Gauchers disease (disorder of fat metabolism), leprosy, alcoholic cirrhosis, active histoplasmosis, tuberculosis, pulmonary embolism, hyperthyroidism, and Hodgkins disease.

ANION GAP
Reference Values

Adult: 10–17 mEq/l (values differ from 7 to 20 mEq/l).

Description

The anion gap is the difference between electrolytes, the positive ions (cations), sodium and potassium, and the negative ions (anions), chloride and bicarbonate (serum CO_2) to determine if an acid–base imbalance is present. Unmeasured anions in the serum such as phosphates, sulfates, lactates, ketone bodies, and other organic acids contribute to metabolic acid–base imbalances (metabolic acidosis and alkalosis). Actually, the difference between the milliequivalents of cations and anions is referred to as the *anion gap*.

Serum levels of the cations, sodium and potassium, and the anions, chloride and bicarbonate, are applied to the formula:

$$\text{Anion gap} = (\text{sodium} + \text{potassium}) - (\text{chloride} + CO_2\ [\text{bicarbonate}])$$

An elevated anion gap (greater than 17 mEq/l) indicates metabolic acidosis; a decreased anion gap (less than 10 mEq/l) indicates metabolic alkalosis.

ANTIBIOTIC SUSCEPTIBILITY (SENSITIVITY)
Reference Values

Adult: Organism is sensitive or intermediate or resistant to antibiotics.
Child: Same as adult.

Description

It is important to identify not only the organism responsible for the infection but also the antibiotic(s) that will inhibit the growth of the bacteria. The health care provider orders a culture and sensitivity test (C and S) when a wound infection, urinary tract infection, or other types of infected secretions are suspected. The choice of antibiotic depends on the pathogenic organism and its susceptibility to the antibiotics.

Purpose

■ To check the effectiveness of selected antibiotics on a specific bacteria from a culture.

ANTICARDIOLIPIN ANTIBODIES (ACA) (SERUM)

Reference Value
Negative.

Description

Anticardiolipin antibodies (ACA) are autoantibodies found in some clients with systemic lupus erythematosus (SLE). They occur in 45% of clients with SLE and less than 7% of clients without SLE. These antibodies were originally found in clients with SLE and were called *lupus anticoagulants* (LA). Later it was determined that these antibodies did not act as anticoagulants and that they were found in health problems other than lupus. ACA and LA are members of the antiphospholipid (APA) family of immunoglobulins active against phospholipids. ACA may also be present in clients having thrombocytopenia, spontaneous or recurrent thrombosis, and fetal loss.

ANTICONVULSANTS (BLOOD, SERUM, PLASMA)

Reference Values

Adult:

THERAPEUTIC RANGE

Drug Name	mcg/ml	µmoL/l
Carbamazepine	4–12	16.9–50.8
(Child)	(Same as adult)	
Ethosuximide	40–100	283–708
(Child)	(2–4 per 1 mg/kg/day)	
Phenytoin	10–20	39.6–79.3
Primidone	5–12	23–55
(Child <5 years)	(7–10)	(30–45)
Valproic acid	50–100	347–693
(Child)	(Same as adult)	

TOXIC LEVEL

	mcg/ml	µmoL/l
Carbamazepine	>12–15	>50.8–69
(Child)	(Same as adult)	
Ethosuximide	>100	>708
(Child)	(Same as adult or higher)	
Phenytoin	>20	>79.3
Primidone	>1215	>55–69
(Child <5 years)	(>12)	(>55)
Valproic acid	>100	>693
(Child)	(Same as adult)	

ANTIDEPRESSANTS (TRICYCLICS) (SERUM)

Amitriptyline, Desipramine, Doxepin, Imipramine, Nortriptyline

Reference Values

Adult:

Drug Name	Therapeutic Range ng/ml	Toxic Level ng/ml
Amitriptyline HCl (Elavil)	75–225	>500
Desipramine HCl (Norpramin)	125–300	>500
Doxepin HCl (Sinequan)	150–300	>500
Imipramine HCl (Tofranil)	150–300	>500
Nortriptyline HCl (Aventyl)	75–150	>300

ANTIDIURETIC HORMONE (ADH) (PLASMA)

Reference Values

Adult: 1–5 pg/ml; 1–5 ng/l.

Description

Antidiuretic hormone (ADH) is produced by the hypothalamus and stored in the posterior pituitary gland (neurohypophysis). The primary function of ADH is in water reabsorption from the distal renal tubules in response to the serum osmolality. *Antidiuretic* means against diuresis. There is more ADH secreted from the posterior pituitary gland when the serum osmolality is increased to greater than 295 mOsm/kg (concentrated body fluids). More water reabsorption occurs, which dilutes the body fluid. When the serum osmolality is decreased to greater than 280 mOsm/kg, less ADH is secreted, and thus more water is excreted via the kidneys.

Syndrome (secretion) of inappropriate ADH (SIADH) is an excess secretion of ADH that is not influenced by the serum osmolality level. SIADH causes excess water retention. Stress, surgery, pain, and certain drugs (narcotics, anesthetics) contribute to SIADH.

ANTINUCLEAR ANTIBODIES (ANA) (SERUM)

Anti-DNA Antibody, Anti-DNP Antibody

Reference Values

Adult: Negative at 1:20 dilution.

Description

The antinuclear antibodies (ANA) test is a screening test for diagnosing systemic lupus erythematosus (SLE) and other collagen diseases. ANAs are immunoglobulins (IgM, IgG, IgA) that react with the nuclear part of leukocytes. They form antibodies against deoxyribonucleic acid (DNA), ribonucleic acid (RNA), and others. Two ANAs, anti-DNA and anti–D-nucleoprotein (Anti-DNP), are almost always present with SLE. Anti-DNA will fluctuate according to the disease process, with remission, and with exacerbation. It is normally present (95%) in lupus nephritis.

The total ANA level can also be elevated in scleroderma, rheumatoid arthritis, cirrhosis, leukemia, infectious mononucleosis, and malignancy. For diagnosing lupus, the ANA test should be compared with other tests for lupus.

ANTITHROMBIN III (PLASMA)

Reference Values

75% to 135% of normal/average

Description

Antithrombin III (AT-III) is suggested to evaluate clients who have a hypercoagulable state, and especially for clients with a history of thromboembolic disease. Some clients have a genetic deficiency of AT-III, thus this predisposes the client to thrombus formation. Also clients who are deficient in AT-III may be resistant to heparin and would require a larger dose of an anticoagulant. Usually heparin resistance does not occur unless the AT-III is less than 60%. Elevated AT-III levels may occur in clients with acute hepatitis and a deficiency in vitamin K.

ARTERIAL BLOOD GASES (ABGS) (ARTERIAL BLOOD)
Reference Values
Adult: pH: 7.35–7.45; $PaCO_2$: 35–45 mm Hg; PaO_2: 75–100 mm Hg; SaO_2: greater than 95%; SvO_2: greater than 70%; HCO_3: 24–28 mEq/l; base excesses (BE): +2 to −2 mEq/l.

Child: pH: 7.36–7.44. Other measurements are same as adult.

Description
Arterial blood gases (ABGs) are usually ordered to assess disturbances of acid–base (A–B) balance caused by a respiratory disorder and/or a metabolic disorder. The basic components of ABGs include the pH, $PaCO_2$, PaO_2, SO_2, HCO_3, and BE.

pH: The pH, the negative logarithm of the hydrogen ion concentration, determines the acidity or alkalinity of body fluids. A pH less than 7.35 indicates acidosis, either respiratory acidosis or metabolic acidosis. A pH greater than 7.45 indicates alkalosis, either respiratory or metabolic alkalosis.

$PaCO_2$: The partial pressure of carbon dioxide ($PaCO_2$) reflects the adequacy of alveolar ventilation. When there is alveolar damage, carbon dioxide (CO_2) cannot escape. Carbon dioxide combines with water to form carbonic acid ($H_2O + CO_2 = H_2CO_3$), causing an acidotic state. When the client has alveolar hypoventilation, the $PaCO_2$ is elevated, and respiratory acidosis results. Chronic obstructive lung disease is a major cause of respiratory acidosis. When the client has alveolar hyperventilation (blowing off CO_2 by rapid deep breathing), the $PaCO_2$ is decreased, and respiratory alkalosis results.

PaO_2: The partial pressure of oxygen (PaO_2) determines the amount of oxygen available to bind with hemoglobin. The pH affects the combining power of oxygen and hemoglobin, and with a low pH, there will be less oxygen in the hemoglobin. The PaO_2 is decreased in respiratory diseases, such as emphysema, pneumonia, and pulmonary edema; in the presence of abnormal hemoglobin (CO Hb, Meth Hb, Sulfa Hb); and in polycythemia.

SO_2: The oxygen saturation (SO_2) is the percentage of oxygen in the blood that combines with hemoglobin. It is measured indirectly by calculation of the PaO_2 and pH or measured directly by co-oximetry. The combination of oxygen saturation, partial pressure of oxygen, and hemoglobin indicates tissue oxygenation.

HCO_3 and BE: Bicarbonate ion (HCO_3) is an alkaline substance that comprises over half of the total buffer base in the blood. When there is a deficit of bicarbonate and other bases or an increase in nonvolatile acid such as lactic acid, metabolic acidosis occurs. If a bicarbonate excess is present, then metabolic alkalosis results. The bicarbonate plays a very important role in maintaining a pH of 7.35 to 7.45.

The base excess (BE) value is frequently checked with the HCO_3 value. A base excess of less than 2 is acidosis and greater than +2 is alkalosis.

Acid–Base Imbalances: To determine the type of A–B imbalance, the pH, $PaCO_2$, HCO_3, and BE are checked. The $PaCO_2$ is a respiratory determinant, and the HCO_3 and BE are metabolic determinants. The $PaCO_2$, HCO_3, and BE values are compared to the pH. A pH of less than 7.35 is acidosis and one of greater than 7.45 is alkalosis.

1. If the pH is less than 7.35, the $PaCO_2$ is greater than 45 mm Hg, and the HCO_3 and BE are normal, the A–B imbalance is respiratory acidosis.
2. If the pH is greater than 7.45, the $PaCO_2$ is less than 35 mm Hg, and the HCO_3 and BE are normal, the A–B imbalance is respiratory alkalosis.
3. If the pH is less than 7.35, the $PaCO_2$ is normal, the HCO_3 and BE are less than 24 mEq/l and less than −2, the A–B imbalance is metabolic acidosis.
4. If the pH is greater than 7.45, the $PaCO_2$ is normal, the HCO_3 and BE are greater than 28 mEq/l and greater than +2, the A–B imbalance is metabolic alkalosis.

Acid–Base (A–B) Imbalance	pH	$PaCO_2$	HCO_3	BE
Respiratory acidosis	↓	↑	N	N
Respiratory alkalosis	↑	↓	N	N
Metabolic acidosis	↓	N	↓	↓
Metabolic alkalosis	↑	N	↑	↑

Clinical Problems
Respiratory Acidosis (pH less than 7.35; $PaCO_2$ greater than 45 mm Hg): Chronic obstructive lung disease (emphysema, chronic bronchitis, severe asthma), acute respiratory distress syndrome (ARDS), Guillain-Barré syndrome, anesthesia, pneumonia. *Drug Influence:* Narcotics, sedatives.

Respiratory Alkalosis (pH greater than 7.45; $PaCO_2$ less than 35 mm Hg): Salicylate toxicity (early phase), anxiety, hysteria, tetany, strenuous exercise (swimming, running), fever, hyperthyroidism, delirium tremens, pulmonary embolism.

Metabolic Acidosis (pH less than 7.35; HCO_3 less than 24 mEq/l): Diabetic ketoacidosis, severe diarrhea, starvation/malnutrition, shock, burns, kidney failure, acute myocardial infarction.

Metabolic Alkalosis (pH greater than 7.45; HCO_3 greater than 28 mEq/l): Severe vomiting, gastric suction, peptic ulcer, potassium loss, excess administration of bicarbonate, hepatic failure, cystic fibrosis. *Drug Influence:* Sodium bicarbonate, sodium oxalate, potassium oxalate.

Factors Affecting Laboratory Results

- Improper handling of the blood sample, such as not using ice water, exposure of specimen to air, and not expelling all the heparin out of the collection syringe, causes inaccurate results.
- Hemolysis of the blood sample causes false results.
- Narcotics and sedatives can contribute to the respiratory acidotic state, and sodium bicarbonate could cause metabolic alkalosis.
- Inaccurate results can occur as a result of suctioning, changes in O_2 therapy, and ventilator use; exposure to carbon monoxide or nitrate; and blood transfusion.

ARTHROGRAPHY
Description

Arthrography is an x-ray examination of a joint using air, contrast media, or both in the joint space. The purposes are to detect abnormalities of the cartilage and/or ligaments (e.g., tears) and to visualize structures of the joint capsule.

Procedure

- Food and fluids are not restricted.
- Prepare the knee or shoulder area using aseptic technique.
- Local anesthetic is administered to puncture site.
- A needle is inserted into the joint space (e.g., knee), and synovial fluid is aspirated for synovial fluid analysis.
- Air and/or contrast medium is injected into the joint space, and x-rays are taken.
- The knee may be bandaged.

ARTHROSCOPY
Description

Arthroscopy is an endoscopic examination of the interior aspect of a joint (usually the knee) using a fiberoptic endoscope. Normally an *arthrography* is performed prior to arthroscopy. Arthroscopy may be used to diagnose meniscal, patellar, extrasynovial, and synovial diseases; to perform joint surgery; and to monitor disease process or the effects of medical or surgical therapeutic regimen. Frequently biopsy or surgery is performed during the test procedure. For a surgical procedure, spinal or general anesthesia is used and for visualization of the interior joint space, a local anesthetic. Arthroscopy is contraindicated if a wound or severe skin infection is present or if the client has severe fibrous ankylosis.

Procedure

- A consent form should be signed.
- There is no food or fluid restriction for local anesthetic. NPO after midnight for spinal and general anesthesia.
- Local, spinal, or general anesthesia is used, depending on the purpose and procedure for the test.
- Ace bandage and/or tourniquet may be applied to decrease blood volume in the leg.

- The arthroscope is inserted into the interior joint for visualization, for draining fluid from the joint, for biopsy, and/or for surgery.
- A dressing is applied to the incision site of the affected joint.

ASPARTATE AMINOTRANSFERASE (AST) (SERUM)
Serum Glutamic Oxaloacetic Transaminase (SGOT)

Reference Values

Adult: *Average range:* 8–38 unit/l 5–40 unit/ml (Frankel), 4–36 international unit/l, 16–60 unit/ml at 30°C (Karmen), 8–33 unit/l at 37°C (SI units). Female values may be slightly lower than those of males. Exercise tends to increase values (values can vary among institutions).
Child: *Newborns:* Four times the normal level. *Child:* Similar to adults. *Elderly:* Slightly higher than adults.

Description

Aspartate aminotransferase/serum glutamic oxaloacetic transaminase (AST/SGOT) is an enzyme found mainly in the heart muscle and liver, with moderate amounts in skeletal muscle, the kidneys, and the pancreas. Its concentration is low in the blood except when there is cellular injury, and then large amounts are released into circulation.

High levels of serum AST are found following an acute myocardial infarction (MI) and liver damage. Six to 10 hours after an acute MI, AST leaks out of the heart muscle and reaches its peak in 24 to 48 hours after the infarction. The serum AST level returns to normal 4 to 6 days later if there is no additional infarction. Serum AST is usually compared with other cardiac enzymes (creatine kinase [CK], lactate dehydrogenase [LDH]).

In liver disease, the serum level increases by 10 times or more and remains elevated for a longer period of time.

BARBITURATE (BLOOD)
Reference Values

Adult:

Barbiturate	Action	Therapeutic	Toxic
Secobarbital (Seconal)	Short acting	1–5 mcg/ml	>8 mcg/ml
Pentobarbital (Nembutal)	Short acting	1–5 mcg/ml	>8 mcg/ml
Amobarbital (Amytal)	Intermediate acting	5–14 mcg/ml	>20 mcg/ml
Phenobarbital	Long acting	10–30 mcg/ml	>60 mcg/ml
		20–40 mcg/ml (seizure control)	

Child: *Phenobarbital: Therapeutic:* 15–30 mcg/ml *Toxic:* greater than 35 mcg/ml.

BARIUM ENEMA
Lower Gastrointestinal Test, X-Ray Examination of the Colon

Description

The barium enema test is an x-ray examination of the large intestine (colon) to detect the presence of polyps, an intestinal mass, diverticuli, an intestinal stricture/obstruction, or ulcerations. Barium sulfate (single contrast) or barium sulfate and air (double contrast or air contrast) is administered slowly through a rectal tube into the large colon. The filling process is monitored by fluoroscopy, and then x-rays are taken. The colon must be free of fecal material so that the barium will outline the large intestine to detect any disorders. The double-contrast technique (barium and air) is useful for identifying polyps.

The barium enema test is indicated for clients complaining of lower abdominal pain and cramps; blood, mucus, or pus in the stool; changes in bowel habits; and changes in stool formation. The test can be performed in a hospital, in a clinic, or at a private laboratory.

Procedure

In most institutions the procedures for the barium enema are similar; however, they usually differ to some degree. Some institutions request that the client maintain a low-residue diet (tender meats, eggs, bread, clear soup, pureed bland vegetables and fruits, potatoes, and boiled milk) for 2 to 3 days before the test. Abdominal x-rays, ultrasound studies, radionuclide scans, and proctosigmoidoscopy should be done *before* the barium enema. It is important that the colon is free of fecal material.

Prepreparation

- Oral medications should not be given for 24 hours before the test, unless indicated by the health care provider. Narcotics and barbiturates could interfere with fecal elimination before and after the test.
- The client should be on a clear-liquid diet for 18 to 24 hours before the test. This would include broth, ginger ale, cola, black coffee or tea with sugar only, gelatin, and syrup from canned fruit. Some institutions permit a white chicken sandwich (*no* butter, lettuce, or mayonnaise) or hard boiled eggs and gelatin for lunch and dinner, then NPO after dinner.
- Encourage the client to increase water and clear liquid intake 24 hours before the test to maintain adequate hydration.
- Prescribe laxatives (castor oil or magnesium citrate) to be taken the day before the test in the late afternoon or early evening (4 p.m. to 8 p.m.).
- A cleansing enema or laxative suppository such as bisacodyl (Dulcolax) may be given the evening before the test.
- Saline enemas (maximum three enemas) should be given early in the morning (6 a.m.) until the returned solution is clear. Some private laboratories have clients use bisacodyl suppositories in the morning instead of the enemas.

- Black coffee or tea is permitted 1 hour before the test. Some institutions permit dry toast.

Postpreparation

- The client should expel the barium in the bathroom or bedpan immediately after the test.
- Fluid intake should be increased for hydration and to prevent constipation due to retained barium.
- A laxative, such as milk of magnesia or magnesium citrate, or an oil retention enema should be given to remove the barium from the colon. A laxative may need to be repeated the following day after the test.

Factors Affecting Diagnostic Results

- Inadequate bowel preparation with fecal material remaining in the colon could affect results.
- The use of barium sulfate in upper gastrointestinal and small bowel studies 2 to 3 days before the barium enema test could affect the results.

NURSING IMPLICATIONS WITH RATIONALE
Barium Enema

- Review the written procedure for that institution. Explain the procedure to the client. Procedures do differ from one institution to another. Usually the preparations for a barium enema have similarities (clear liquids, increased fluid intake, laxatives, and cleansing enemas). Fecal material in the large intestine (bowel or colon) should be completely eliminated.
- List the procedure step by step for the client. Most private laboratories and hospitals have written preparation slips. The procedure may be sent to the client at home.
- Emphasize the importance of following dietary restrictions and of bowel preparation. Adequate prepreparation is essential or the test may need to be repeated.
- Notify the health care provider if the client has severe abdominal cramps and pain prior to the test. The barium enema test should not be performed if the client has severe ulcerative colitis, suspected perforation, or tachycardia.

CLIENT TEACHING

- Explain to the client that he or she will be lying on a tilting x-ray table for positioning purposes to increase the barium flow into the colon. Explain that a technician will be with him or her and will explain each step of the procedure.
- Inform the client that the test takes approximately ½ to 1 hour to complete. Tell the client to take deep breaths through the mouth, which helps to decrease tension and to promote relaxation.
- Administer a laxative or cleansing enema after the test. Instruct the client to check the color of the stools for 2 to 3 days. Stools may be light in color because of the barium sulfate. Absence of stool should be reported. Retention of barium sulfate after the test could cause obstruction and/or fecal impaction.

BILIRUBIN (INDIRECT) (SERUM)

Reference Values

Adult: 0.1–1.0 mg/dl, 1.7–17.1 μmol/l (SI units).
Child: Same as adult.

Description

(See Bilirubin [total and direct].)

Indirect-reacting or unconjugated bilirubin is protein bound and is associated with increased destruction of red blood cells (hemolysis).

Elevated indirect bilirubin can occur in autoimmune- or transfusion-induced hemolysis, in hemolytic processes caused by sickle cell anemia, in pernicious anemia, and with malaria and septicemia. Internal hemorrhage into soft tissues and the body cavity can cause the bilirubin to rise in 5 to 6 hours. With certain clinical problems, congestive heart failure (CHF), and severe liver damage, both indirect and direct bilirubin levels will increase. Indirect bilirubin frequently increases because the damaged liver cells cannot conjugate normal amounts, which leads to increased, unconjugated bilirubin.

Levels of indirect serum bilirubin may increase in hemolytic disease, such as erythroblastosis fetalis, in newborns. The newborns liver is immature, and when extremely high levels of bilirubin occur, irreversible neurologic damage, referred to as kernicterus, could result.

BILIRUBIN (TOTAL AND DIRECT) (SERUM)

Reference Values

Adult: *Total:* 0.1–1.2 mg/dl, 1.7–20.5 μmol/l (SI units). *Direct (conjugated):* 0.1–0.3 mg/dl, 1.7–5.1 μmol/l (SI units).
Child: *Newborn: Total:* 1–12 mg/dl, 17.1–205 μmol/l (SI units). *Child:* 0.2–0.8 mg/dl.

Description

Bilirubin is formed from the breakdown of hemoglobin by the reticuloendothelial system and is carried in the plasma to the liver, where it is conjugated (directly) to form bilirubin diglucuronide and is excreted in the bile. There are two forms of bilirubin in the body: the conjugated, or direct-reacting (soluble), and the unconjugated, or indirect-reacting (protein bound). If the total bilirubin is within normal range, direct and indirect bilirubin levels do not need to be analyzed. If one value of bilirubin is reported, it represents the total bilirubin.

Direct or conjugated bilirubin is frequently the result of obstructive jaundice, either extrahepatic (from stones or tumor) or intrahepatic in origin. Conjugated bilirubin cannot escape in the bile into the intestine and thus backs up and is absorbed into the blood stream. Damaged liver cells cause a blockage of the bile sinusoid, increasing the serum level of direct bilirubin. With hepatitis and decompensated cirrhosis, both direct and indirect bilirubin may be elevated.

Serum bilirubin (total) in newborns can be as high as 12 mg/dl; the panic level is greater than 15 mg/dl. Jaundice is frequently present when serum bilirubin levels are greater than 3 mg/dl.

BILIRUBIN AND BILE (URINE)

Reference Values

Adult: *Negative:* 0.02 mg/dl.

Description

Bilirubin is not normally present in urine; however, a very small quantity could be present without being detected by routine test methods. Bilirubin is formed from the breakdown of hemoglobin and is transported to the liver, where it is conjugated and is excreted as bile. Conjugated or direct bilirubin is water soluble and is excreted in the urine when there is an increased serum level. Unconjugated or indirect bilirubin is fat-soluble and cannot be excreted in the urine.

Bilirubinuria (bilirubin in urine) indicates liver damage or biliary obstruction (e.g., stones), and a large amount has a characteristic dark-amber color. When the amber-colored urine is shaken, it produces a yellow foam. It can frequently be tested by the floor nurse with a dipstick or reagent tablet.

BIOPSY (BONE MARROW, BREAST, ENDOMETRIUM, KIDNEY, LIVER)

Description

Biopsy is the removal and examination of tissue from the body. Usually biopsies are performed to detect malignancy or to identify the presence of a disease process. Biopsies can be obtained by (1) aspiration by applying suction; (2) the brush method, using stiff bristles that scrape fragments of cells and tissue; (3) excision by surgical cutting at tissue site; (4) fine-needle or needle aspiration at tissue site with or without the guidance of ultrasound; (5) insertion of a needle through the skin; and (6) punch biopsy, using a punch-type instrument.

Biopsies are performed on various organs and body structures, such as bone marrow, the breast, endometrium of the uterus, kidney, and liver. The methods used for the biopsy tissues of various organs may differ.

BONE DENSITOMETRY

Bone Density (BD), Bone Mineral Density (BMD), Bone Absorptiometry

Normal Finding

Normal bone densitometry scan is determined according to the clients age, sex, and height.

NORMAL 1 standard deviation below peak bone mass level.

OSTEOPOROSIS greater than 2.5 standard deviations below peak bone mass level (WHO standard).

Description

The bones are made up of minerals and protein. Bone mass peaks when the person is in the mid-30s. After that, bone is lost at a rate somewhat greater than new bone is made. When a woman reaches menopause, bone loss accelerates to about 1 to 3 percent a year. After age 60, bone loss in women slows but it does not stop and as she gets older, bone mass loss could be between 35 and 50 percent. The risk of bone fracture is greater in women than men. Men lose bone also; however, it is at a lower rate than women; 3 to 5 percent a decade. Usually, men develop osteoporosis about a decade later than women.

Bone density test is to detect early osteoporosis by determining the density of bone mineral content. Clients who have a loss of bone mineral are readily prone to have fractures. The bones that are usually examined are the lumbar spine and the proximal hip (neck of the femur). Another bone site, the heel bone, can be evaluated according to the clients symptoms.

The dual energy x-ray absorptiometry, (DEXA) measures bone mineral density and only exposes the client to a minimal amount of radiation. Images from the detector/camera are computer analyzed to determine the bone mineral content. The computer can calculate the size and thickness of the bone.

BLEEDING TIME (BLOOD)
Reference Values

Adult: *Ivy Method:* 3–7 minutes. *Duke Method:* 1–3 minutes. SI units for the Ivy and Duke methods are the same. (Duke method is seldom performed.)

Description

Two methods, Ivy and Duke, are used to determine whether bleeding time is normal or prolonged. Bleeding time is lengthened in thrombocytopenia (decreased platelet count, less than 50,000). The test is frequently performed when there is a history of bleeding (easy bruising), familial bleeding, or preoperative screening. The Ivy technique, in which the forearm is used for the incision, is the most popular method. Aspirin and anti-inflammatory medications can prolong the bleeding time.

BLOOD UREA NITROGEN (BUN) (SERUM)
Reference Values

Adult: 5–25 mg/dl.
Child: *Infant:* 5–15 mg/dl. *Child:* 5–20 mg/dl.
Elderly: Could be slightly higher than adult.

Description

Urea is formed as an end product of protein metabolism and is excreted by the kidneys. An elevated blood urea nitrogen (BUN) level could be an indication of dehydration, prerenal failure, or renal failure. Dehydration from vomiting, diarrhea, and/or inadequate fluid intake can cause an increase in the BUN (up to 35 mg/dl). With dehydration, the serum creatinine level would most likely be normal or high normal. Once the client is hydrated, the BUN should return to normal; if it does not, prerenal or renal failure would be suspected. Nephrons (kidney cells) tend to decrease during the aging process, and so older persons may have a higher BUN. Digested blood from gastrointestinal (GI) bleeding is a source of protein and can cause the BUN to elevate. A low BUN value usually indicates overhydration (hypervolemia).

The **BUN/Creatinine Ratio** is a calculation with reference value of 10:1 to 15:1. A decreased BUN/creatinine ratio occurs with malnutrition, liver disease, low-protein diet, excessive IV fluids, dialysis, or overhydration. An elevated BUN/creatinine ratio, greater than 15:1, is found in renal disease, inadequate renal perfusion, shock, dehydration, GI bleeding, and drugs such as steroids and tetracyclines. See separate listing for BUN/creatinine.

BLOOD UREA NITROGEN/CREATININE RATIO (SERUM)
Urea Nitrogen/Creatinine Ratio

Reference Values

Adult: 10:1 to 20:1 (BUN:creatinine). *Average:* 15:1.

Description

The blood urea nitrogen (BUN)/creatinine ratio is an effective test primarily for determining renal function. BUN level can increase because of dehydration as well as renal dysfunction. The creatinine level does not increase with dehydration but definitely increases with renal dysfunction. This ratio test is more sensitive to the relationship of BUN to creatinine than separate tests of BUN and creatinine. However, liver function, dietary protein intake, and muscle mass may affect test result.

A decreased ratio can occur from acute renal tubular necrosis and low protein intake. The ratio may be increased because of reduced renal perfusion, glomerular disease, obstructive uropathy, or high protein intake.

BRONCHOGRAPHY (BRONCHOGRAM)
Description

Bronchography is an x-ray test to visualize the trachea, bronchi, and entire bronchial tree after a radiopaque iodine contrast liquid is injected through a catheter into the tracheobronchial space. The bronchi are coated with the contrast dye, and a series of x-rays is then taken. Bronchography may be done in conjunction with bronchoscopy.

Bronchography is contraindicated during pregnancy. This test should also not be done if the client is hypersensitive to anesthetics, iodine, or x-ray dyes.

Procedure
- A consent form should be signed.
- The client should be NPO for 6 to 8 hours before the test.
- Oral hygiene should be given the night before the test and in the morning. This will decrease the number of bacteria that could be introduced into the lungs.
- Postural drainage is performed for 3 days before the test. This procedure aids in the removal of bronchial mucus and secretions. An expectorant (i.e., potassium iodide) may be ordered for 1 to 3 days before the test to loosen secretions and could detect an allergy to iodine.
- A sedative and atropine are usually given 1 hour before the test. The sedative/tranquilizer is to promote relaxation; atropine is to reduce secretions during the test.
- A topical anesthetic is sprayed into the pharynx and trachea. A catheter is passed through the nose into the trachea, and a local anesthetic and iodized contrast liquid are injected through the catheter.
- The client is usually asked to change body positions so that the contrast dye can reach most areas of the bronchial tree.
- Following the bronchography procedure, the client may receive nebulization and should perform postural drainage to remove contrast dye. Food and fluids are restricted until the gag (cough) reflex is present.

Factors Affecting Diagnostic Results
- Secretions in the tracheobronchial tree can prevent the contrast dye from coating the bronchial walls.

NURSING IMPLICATIONS WITH RATIONALE **Bronchography**

PRETEST
- Explain the procedure to the client. Explanation is important to help allay the clients anxiety.
- Check that the consent form is signed and that the client has voided before administering premedications. One of the drugs usually administered is atropine, which causes dryness of the mouth.
- Check that dentures, contact lenses, and jewelry have been removed.
- Obtain vital signs (VS), and prepare a VS flow chart. Record admission and pretest vital signs, which will serve as baseline VS.
- Advise the client that the procedure takes about 1 hour.

CLIENT TEACHING
- Instruct the client to relax before and during the test. The premedications will aid in increasing relaxation and decreasing anxiety. Tell the client the health care provider will inform him or her of how the procedure is progressing. Bronchoscopy usually is performed under local anesthesia but could be performed under general anesthesia. The client should be told whether he or she will receive a local or a general anesthetic.
- Inform the client that the drugs will make him or her feel sleepy and the mouth feel dry. The client should remain in bed, and the bed sides should be up after premedications are given.
- Instruct the client to practice breathing in and out through the nose with the mouth opened. This is important if the bronchoscope is inserted through the mouth.
- Encourage the client to ask questions and give him or her time to express concerns. Inform the client that there may be some discomfort but that the spray will help to decrease it. Inform the client that he or she will receive adequate air exchange. Oxygen can be given through the side arm of the bronchoscope or rigid scope and by mask for fiberoptic scope.
- Inform the client that there may be hoarseness and/or a sore throat after the test.

POSTTEST
- Recognize the complications that can follow bronchoscopy (i.e., laryngeal edema, bronchospasm, pneumothorax, cardiac dysrhythmias, and bleeding from the biopsy site).
- Check VS until stable and as indicated.
- Elevate the head of the bed (semi-Fowler's position). If the client is unconscious, turn him or her on the side with the head of the bed slightly elevated.
- Assess for signs and symptoms of respiratory difficulty (i.e., dyspnea, wheezing, apprehension, and decreased breath sounds). Notify the health care provider at once.
- Check for hemoptysis (coughing up excessive bloody secretions) and, if found, notify the health care provider. Inform the client that some blood-tinged mucus may be coughed up and that this is not abnormal. It usually occurs following a biopsy or after a traumatic insertion of the bronchoscope.
- Assess the gag (cough) reflex before giving food and liquids. Ask the client to swallow or cough. It normally takes 2 to 8 hours before the gag reflex returns. Offer ice chips and sips of water before offering food.
- Offer the client lozenges or prescribed medication for mild throat irritation after the gag reflex is present.
- Be supportive of the client. Touch the clients hand or arm for reassurance, as necessary.

CLIENT TEACHING
- Instruct the client not to smoke for 6 to 8 hours. Smoking may cause the client to cough and start bleeding, especially after abiopsy.
- Inform the client that collection of postbronchoscopic secretions may be required for cytologic testing.

BRONCHOSCOPY

Description

Bronchoscopy is the direct inspection of the larynx, trachea, and bronchi through a standard metal bronchoscope or a flexible fiberoptic bronchoscope called a bronchofibroscope. The flexible fiberoptic bronchoscope has a lens and light at its distal end, and because of its smallness in width and its flexibility, it allows for visualization of the segmental and subsegmental bronchi.

Through the bronchoscope, a catheter brush, biopsy forceps, or biopsy needle can be passed to obtain secretions and tissues for cytologic examination. The two main purposes of bronchoscopy are visualization and specimen collection in the tracheobronchial tree. Other purposes include removal of the secretions and laser of the lesions.

Procedure

- A consent form for bronchoscopy should be signed by the client or an appropriate family member.
- The client should be NPO for 6 hours before the bronchoscopy and preferably for 8 to 12 hours.
- The client should remove dentures, contact lenses, jewelry.
- Obtain a history of hypersensitivity to analgesics, anesthetics, and antibiotics.
- Check vital signs and record.
- Administer premedications.
- Record vital signs, premedications, and when the client voided on the preoperative check list and the clients chart.
- The client will be lying on a table in the supine or semi-Fowler's position with the head hyperextended, or he or she will be seated in a chair. Local anesthetic will be sprayed in the clients throat and nose, and the bronchoscope will be inserted through the clients nose or mouth by the health care provider. It is frequently inserted through the mouth when using the rigid scope and is inserted through the nose when using the fiberoptic scope.
- Specimen containers should be labeled, and specimens should be taken immediately to the laboratory. The procedure takes about 1 hour.

Factors Affecting Diagnostic Results

- Improper labeling of the specimen.
- Failure to take specimens immediately to the laboratory.

CALCITONIN (HCT) (SERUM)

Reference Values

Adult: *Male:* Less than 40 pg/ml, less than 40 ng/I (SI units). *Female:* Less than 25 pg/ml, less than 25 ng/l (SI units). Child: *Newborn:* Usually higher than in adults. Child: Less than 70 pg/ml, less than 70 ng/l (SI units).

Description

Calcitonin, a potent hormone secreted by the C cells of the thyroid gland, aids in maintaining normal serum calcium and phosphorus levels. This hormone is secreted in response to an elevated serum calcium level. It inhibits calcium reabsorption by the osteoclasts and osteocytes of the bones and increases calcium excretion by the kidneys. Calcitonin acts as an antagonist to the parathyroid hormone (PTH) and vitamin D, lowering serum calcium levels to maintain calcium balance in the body.

Excess calcitonin secretion occurs in medullary carcinoma of the thyroid. A serum calcitonin level is frequently ordered to aid in the diagnosis of thyroid medullary carcinoma (greater than 500–2000 pg/ml [probable] and greater than 2000 pg/ml [definite]) and ectopic calcitonin-producing tumors of the lung and breast. Monitoring calcitonin levels after medullary carcinoma removal will help predict if the tumor recurs.

When the serum calcitonin level is slightly to moderately elevated (100–500 pg/ml), a *calcitonin stimulation test* might be performed in diagnosis of thyroid medullary carcinoma. This test consists of either a 4-hour calcium infusion or a 10-second pentagastrin infusion with measurement of serum calcitonin before and after the infusion.

CALCIUM (CA) AND IONIZED CALCIUM (SERUM)

Reference Values

Adult Total Ca: 4.5–5.5 mEq/l, 9–11 mg/dl, 2.3–2.8 mmol/l (SI units). *Ionized Ca:* 4.255.25 mg/dl, 2.2–2.5 mEq/l, 1.1–1.24 mmol/l.
Child: *Newborn:* 3.7–7.0 mEq/l, 7.4–14.0 mg/dl. *Infant:* 5.0–6.0 mEq/l, 1012 mg/dl. *Child:* 4.5–5.8 mEq/l, 9–11.5 mg/dl.

Description

Calcium is found most abundantly in the bones and teeth. Approximately 50% of the calcium is ionized, and only ionized calcium can be used by the body. Protein and albumin in the blood bind with calcium, thus decreasing the amount of free, ionized calcium. The ionized calcium level can be determined by using formulas that estimate the ionized calcium from total calcium. These formulas have been disputed. Only a few laboratories have the equipment to perform serum-ionized calcium levels. In acidosis, more calcium is ionized, regardless of the serum level, and in alkalosis, most of the calcium is protein bsound and cannot be ionized.

The *serum-ionized calcium* (iCa) level is not affected by changes in serum protein/albumin concentration, and it reflects calcium metabolism better than total calcium values. A decrease in ionized calcium, less than 2.2 mEq/l or less than

4.25 mg/dl, might lead to neuromuscular irritability or tetany symptoms (tingling, twitching, spasmodic contractions).

Calcium is necessary for the transmission of nerve impulses and contraction of the myocardium and skeletal muscles. It causes blood clotting by converting prothrombin into thrombin. It strengthens capillary membranes. With a calcium deficit, there is an increased capillary permeability, which causes fluid to pass through the capillary.

A low serum-calcium level is called *hypocalcemia,* and an increased level is called *hypercalcemia.* Calcium imbalances require immediate attention, for serum calcium deficit can cause tetany symptoms, unless acidosis is present, and serum calcium excess can cause cardiac dysrhythmias.

CALCIUM CHANNEL BLOCKERS (SERUM)

Verapamil (Calan, Isoptin), Nifedipine (Procardia), Diltiazem (Cardizem)

Reference Values

Adult:

Drug Name	Therapeutic Range	Toxic Level
Verapamil	100–300 ng/ml;	300 ng/ml;
	0.08–0.3 mcg/ml	0.3 mcg/ml
Nifedipine	50–100 ng/ml	100 ng/ml
Diltiazem	50–200 ng/ml	200 ng/ml

Note: Dosage is calculated according to mg/kg.

CARBON MONOXIDE, CARBOXYHEMOGLOBIN (BLOOD)

Reference Values

Adult: *Nonsmoker:* Less than 2.5% of hemoglobin. *Smoker:* 4–5% saturation of hemoglobin. *Heavy Smoker:* 5–12% saturation of hemoglobin. *Toxic:* Greater than 15% saturation of hemoglobin.
Child: Similar to adult nonsmoker.

Description

Carbon monoxide (CO) combines with hemoglobin to produce carboxyhemoglobin, which can occur 200 times more readily than the combination of oxygen with hemoglobin (oxyhemoglobin). When CO replaces oxygen in the hemoglobin in excess of 25%, CO toxicity occurs.

Carbon monoxide is formed from incomplete combustion of carbon-combining compounds, as in automobile exhaust, fumes from improperly functioning furnaces, and cigarette smoke. Continuous exposure to CO, increasing carboxyhemoglobin by greater than 60%, leads to coma and death. The treatment for CO toxicity is to administer a high concentration of oxygen.

CARDIAC CATHETERIZATION

Cardiac Angiography (Angiocardiography), Coronary Arteriography

Description

Cardiac catheterization is a procedure in which a long catheter is inserted into a vein and artery of the arm, groin or neck. This catheter is threaded to the heart chambers and/or coronary arteries with the guidance of fluoroscopy. Contrast dye is injected for visualizing the heart structures. During injection of the dye, cineangiography is used for filming heart activity. The terms *angiocardiography* and *coronary arteriography* are used interchangeably with the term *cardiac catheterization;* however, with coronary arteriography, dye is injected directly into the coronary arteries, and with angiocardiography, dye is injected into heart, coronary, and/or pulmonary vessels.

With *right-cardiac catheterization,* the catheter is inserted into the femoral vein or an antecubital vein and threaded through the inferior vena cava into the right atrium to the pulmonary artery. Right atrium, right ventricle, and pulmonary artery pressures are measured, and blood samples from the right side of the heart can be obtained. While the dye is being injected, the functions of the tricuspid and pulmonary valves can be observed.

For *left-cardiac catheterization,* the catheter is inserted into the brachial or femoral artery and is advanced retrograde through the aorta to the coronary arteries and/or left ventricle. Dye is injected. The patency of the coronary arteries and/or functions of the aortic and mitral valves and the left ventricle can be observed. This procedure is indicated before heart surgery.

The frequency of complications arising from cardiac catheterizations have decreased to less than 2%. The complications that can occur, although rare, are myocardial infarction, cardiac dysrhythmias, cardiac tamponade, pulmonary embolism, and cerebral embolism (CVA). Other rare complications include renal failure or anaphylactic reaction to contrast dye, blood clot at catheter site requiring anticoagulation, or significant internal bleeding near insertion site.

Purposes
- To identify coronary artery disease (CAD).
- To determine cardiac valvular disease.
- To determine pressure in pulmonary vessels or heart chambers.
- To obtain a biopsy of myocardium.

NURSING IMPLICATIONS WITH RATIONALE **Cardiac Catheterization**

PRETEST

- Explain to the client that the purpose of the test is to check the coronary arteries for blockage, to check for heart valve defects, and/or to measure pressures in the pulmonary vessels, heart chambers, or obtain a biopsy of heart tissue. This test is often done before heart surgery to determine if bypass or valvular surgery is necessary.
- Explain the procedure to the client. The cardiologist or cardiac surgeon should explain the risk factors to the client.
- Obtain a client history of allergic reactions to seafood, iodine, or iodine contrast dye used in other x-ray tests (e.g., intravenous pyelography). A skin test may be performed to determine the severity of the allergy. An antihistamine (e.g., diphenhydramine [Benadryl]) and steroids may be given the day before and/or the day of the test as a prophylactic measure.
- Record baseline VS, and monitor the VS during the procedure.
- Have the client void and remove dentures before the test. Check that the catheter insertion site has been prepped (shaved and cleansed with an antiseptic).
- Encourage the client to ask questions, and allow the client and family time to express any concerns. Refer questions you cannot answer to the cardiologist or other health professionals.
- Administer premedications ½ to 1 hour before the test. Make sure that the client has voided and that the consent form has been signed before giving the premedications.

CLIENT TEACHING

- Inform the client that he or she will be in a special cardiac catheterization room. Give information about the padded table, the ECG leads to monitor heart activity, the IV fluids, which will run slowly, the local skin anesthetic, and instructions that he or she may receive (such as to cough and to breathe deeply).
- Inform the client that there should be no pain, except some discomfort at the catheter insertion site and from lying on the back. Instruct the client to ask any questions he or she may have during the test. Tell the client to tell the health care provider of any chest pain or difficulty in breathing during the procedure. The clients ECG and VS are monitored.

- Tell the client that a hot, flushing sensation may be felt for a minute or two because of the dye. The reason for this is a brief vasodilation caused by the dye.
- Tell the client that the test takes approximately ½ to 3 hours.

POSTTEST

- Monitor VS (blood pressure, pulse, respirations) every 15 minutes the first hour, every 30 minutes until stable, or as ordered. Temperatures are monitored for several days.
- Watch for cardiac rhythm and rate disturbances.
- Assess client for complaints of chest heaviness, shortness of breath, and abdominal or groin pains.
- Observe the catheter insertion site for bleeding or hematoma. Change dressings as needed.
- Check peripheral pulses below the insertion site; if the femoral artery was used, then check the popliteal and dorsalis pedis pulses; if the brachial artery was used, then check the radial pulse. Note the strength of the pulse beat.
- Assess the clients skin color and temperature.
- Be supportive of the client and family. Answer questions, or refer them to the appropriate health professionals. Communicate with the client about the nursing care being given.
- Administer narcotic analgesics or analgesics as ordered for discomfort. Give antibiotics, if ordered.

CLIENT TEACHING

- Instruct the client that he or she is to remain on bed rest for 8 to 12 hours. The client can turn from side to side, and the bed may be elevated 30 degrees. The leg should be extended if the femoral artery was used. If the brachial artery was used, the head of the bed can be slightly elevated; however, the arm should be immobilized for 3 hours. Policy concerning positioning may differ among institutions.
- Encourage fluid intake after the test, unless contraindicated (e.g., in the case of congestive heart failure).

- To evaluate artificial valves.
- To angioplasty or stent an area resulting from coronary artery disease (CAD).

Procedure

- Obtain a signed consent form. Check that the health care provider has discussed possible risk factors before the consent form is signed.
- Food and fluids are restricted for 6 to 8 hours before the test, according to the hospitals policy. Some institutions permit clear liquids until 4 hours before the test.
- Antihistamines (e.g., diphenhydramine [Benadryl]) and steroids may be ordered the evening before and the morning

of the test if an allergic reaction is suspected, such as to iodine products.
- Medications are restricted for 6 to 8 hours before the test unless otherwise ordered by the health care provider. Oral anticoagulants are discontinued, or the dosage is reduced to prevent excessive bleeding. Heparin may be ordered to prevent thrombi.
- The injection site of the arm or groin is shaved and cleansed with antiseptics.
- The weight and height of the client should be recorded. These are used to calculate the amount of dye needed (i.e., 1 ml/kg of body weight).

- The client should void before receiving the premedications. Dentures should be removed unless this is not indicated.
- Record baseline VS. Note the volume intensity of pulses. VS should be monitored during the test.
- Premedications may be given ½ to 1 hour before the cardiac catheterization.
- The client is positioned on a padded table. Skin anesthetic is given at the site of catheter insertion. Client lies still during insertion of the catheter and filming.
- A 5% dextrose in water (D_5W) infusion is started at a keep-vein-open (KVO) rate for administering emergency drugs, if needed. Occasionally, a higher rate of IV infusion of Normal Saline solution (NSS) or ½ NSS is administered prior to and during catheterization to prevent renal failure from contrast dye.
- Electrocardiography (ECG) leads are applied to the chest skin surface to monitor heart activity.
- A local skin anesthetic is injected at the catheter insertion site. A cutdown to locate the vessel may be needed. The client will feel a hot, flushing sensation for several seconds to a minute as the dye is injected.
- Coughing and deep breathing are frequently requested by the health care provider. Coughing can decrease nausea and dizziness and possible dysrhythmia.
- The procedure takes ½ to 3 hours.

Factors Affecting Diagnostic Results
- Insufficient amount of contrast dye could affect results.
- Movement by the client could cause complications and interfere with the filming.

CATECHOLAMINES (PLASMA)
Reference Values

Epinephrine: *Supine:* Less than 50 pg/ml. *Sitting:* Less than 60 pg/ml. *Standing:* Less than 90 pg/ml.

Norepinephrine: *Supine:* 110–410 pg/ml. *Sitting:* 120–680 pg/ml. *Standing:* 125–700 pg/ml.

Dopamine: *Supine and Standing:* Less than 87 pg/ml.

Pheochromocytoma: *Total Catecholamines:* Greater than 1000 pg/ml.

CEREBROSPINAL FLUID (CSF)
[Color, Pressure, Cell Count, Protein, Chloride, Glucose, Culture] Spinal Fluid

Reference Values

	Color	Pressure (mm H$_2$O)	Cell Count (Leukocytes) (mm$_3$, µl)
Adult	Clear, colorless	75–175	0–8
Child	Clear, colorless	50–100	0–8
Premature infant			0–20
Newborn	Clear		0–15
1–6 months			

	Protein (mg/dl)	Chloride (mEq/l)	Glucose (mg/dl)
Adult	15–45	118–132	40–80
Child	14–45	120–128	35–75
Premature infant	<400		
Newborn	30–200	110–122	20–40
1–6 months	30–100		

Description

Cerebrospinal fluid (CSF), also known as spinal fluid, circulates in the ventricles of the brain and through the spinal cord. Of the 150 ml of CSF, approximately 100 ml are produced by the blood in the brain ventricles and are reabsorbed back into circulation daily.

Spinal fluid is obtained by a lumbar puncture (spinal tap) performed in the lumbar sac at L–34, or at L–45. First CSF pressure is measured, then fluid is aspirated and placed in sterile test tubes. Data from the analysis of the spinal fluid are important for diagnosing spinal cord and brain diseases.

The analysis of spinal fluid usually includes color, pressure, cell count (leukocytes, or white blood cells [WBCs]), protein, chloride, and glucose. In addition, the pH of the CSF is usually checked; it is usually slightly lower, about one tenth (0.1) of a point, than the pH of the serum. The CSF protein and glucose levels are lower than the blood levels; however, the CSF chloride level is higher than the serum chloride level. Normally a culture is done to detect any organism present in the fluid.

CSF Analysis

CSF	Decreased Level	Elevated Level	Comments
Color		Abnormal color: 1. Pink or red—subarachnoid or cerebral hemorrhage; traumatic spinal tap 2. Xanthochromia (yellow color)— previous subarachnoid hemorrhage	Yellow color indicates old blood (4 to 5 days after a cerebral hemorrhage), mixture of bilirubin and blood, or extremely elevated protein levels; fluid discoloration normally remains for 3 weeks.
Pressure	Dehydration, hypovolemia	Intracranial pressure due to meningitis, subarachnoid hemorrhage, brain tumor, brain abscess, encephalitis	Slight elevation can occur with holding breath or tensing of muscles.
Cell count (lymphocytes)		<500 mm^3 (μl): viral infections poliomyelitis, aseptic meningitis, syphilis of CNS; multiple sclerosis; brain tumor; abscess; subarachnoid hemorrhage (40% or more monocytes) >500 mm^3 (μl): ↑ granulocytes, purulent infection	WBC differential count may be ordered to identify the types of leukocytes.

Protein		Meningitis: tuberculosis, purulent, aseptic
		
		Guillain-Barré syndrome
		Subarachnoid hemorrhage
		Brain tumor
		Abscess
		Syphilis
		Drug influence:
		  anesthetics
		  acetophenetidin (phenacetin)
		  chlorpromazine (Thorazine)
		  salicylates (aspirin)
		  streptomycin
		  sulfonamides
			Protein and cell counts usually increase together.

Chloride	Tubercular meningitis Bacterial meningitis		IV saline or electrolyte infusion could cause an inaccurate result. Syphilis, brain tumors and abscess, and encephalitis do not affect the CSF chloride level.
Glucose	Purulent meningitis Presence of fungi, protozoa, or pyogenic bacteria Subarachnoid hemorrhage Lymphomas Leukemia	Cerebral trauma Hypothalamic lesions Diabetes (hyperglycemia)	Brain abscess or tumor and degenerative diseases have little effect on the CSF glucose. The CSF glucose is usually two thirds of the blood glucose. The blood glucose level is determined for comparative reasons.
Culture		Meningitis	Generally done when meningitis is suspected.

CHLAMYDIA (SERUM AND TISSUE SMEAR OR CULTURE)

Reference Values

Normal Titer: Less than 1:16.
Positive Titer: Equal or greater than 1:64.

Description

Chlamydia is a bacterialike organism and has some features of a virus. There are two species of chlamydia: *C. psittaci,* which can cause psitticosis in birds and humans, and *C. trachomatis,* which appears in three types (lymphogranuloma venereum [LGV, venereal disease], genital and other infections, and trachoma [eye disorder]).

The occurrence of *C. psittaci* is more common in persons working in pet stores who may have contact with infected birds such as parakeets, and in those working in the poultry industry who may come in contact with infected turkeys. A respiratory infection may result and could cause chlamydial pneumonia. Serologic testing or tissue culture may be performed for diagnosis.

The *C. trachomatis* strain, LGV, is transmitted through sexual intercourse. It can occur in both males and females, causing enlargement of the inguinal and pelvic lymph nodes. Pregnant women can pass chlamydia infection to the newborn during birthing. This can cause trachoma ophthalmia neonatorum in the infant, which may lead to blindness later if untreated. Untreated genital infections caused by *C. trachomatis* could lead to sterility.

With psitticosis and LGV, the serum titer level is greater than 1:64 (more than four times the reference value). The titer level for genital infection caused by *C. trachomatis* is usually between 1:16 and 1:64. Normally the general population has a titer level of less than 1:16. Tissue culture may be used to confirm test results with the titer level. Tetracycline and erythromycin not penicillin, are usually the antibiotics used to treat chlamydia.

CHLORIDE (CL) (SERUM)

Reference Values

Adult: 95–105 mEq/l, 95–105 mmol/l (SI units).
Child: *Newborn:* 94–112 mEq/l. *Infant:* 95–110 mEq/l. *Child:* 98–105 mEq/l.

Description

Chloride is an anion found mostly in the extracellular fluid. Chloride plays an important role in maintaining body water balance, osmolality of body fluids (with sodium), and acid-base balance. It combines with hydrogen ion to produce the acidity (hydrochloric acid [HCl]) in the stomach.

For maintaining acid-base balance, chloride competes with bicarbonate for sodium. When the body fluids are more acidic, the kidneys excrete chloride and sodium, and bicarbonate is reabsorbed. In addition, chloride shifts in and out of red blood cells in exchange with bicarbonate.

Most of the chloride ingested is combined with sodium (sodium chloride [NaCl] or salt). The daily required chloride intake is 2 g. *Hypochloremia* means serum chloride deficit; *hyperchloremia* means serum chloride excess.

CHLORIDE (SWEAT)

Screening (Silver Nitrate); Iontophoresis (Pilocarpine)

Reference Values

Adult: Less than 60 mEq/l.
Child: Less than 50 mEq/l; marginal: 50–60 mEq/l; abnormal: greater than 60 mEq/l (possible cystic fibrosis).

Description

Sodium and chloride concentrations in sweat are higher in persons with cystic fibrosis, even though there usually is not an increased amount of sweat. Sweat chloride is considered more reliable than sweat sodium for diagnostic Purposes. Some falsely negative sweat sodium levels have been reported in persons with cystic fibrosis.

Two types of sweat chloride tests are used: (1) screening tests, which use silver nitrate on agar or filter (special) paper and require contact with the hand (palm or fingers), and (2) iontophoresis, in which pilocarpine is placed on the forearm to increase sweat gland secretion. A positive screening test is usually validated with iontophoresis, because the chloride level in the palm of the hand is usually higher than anywhere else. Some health care providers believe that the screening should be routine in all children; however, others disagree.

Procedure

Screening Test (Silver Nitrate)
■ Wash the child's hand and dry it. For 15 minutes, keep the hand from contacting any other part of the body.
■ Moisten the test paper containing silver nitrate compound with distilled water *(not saline).*
■ Press the child's hand on the paper for 4 seconds.
■ A positive result occurs when the excess chloride combines with the silver nitrate to form white silver chloride on the paper.
■ A heavy hand imprint is left by the child with cystic fibrosis.
Iontophoresis (Pilocarpine): Usually performed by laboratory personnel.
■ There is no food or fluid restriction.
■ Electrodes are placed on the skin of the forearm to create a small electric current for transporting pilocarpine (a stimulating drug) into the skin to induce sweating.
■ Sweat is collected and weighed. Chloride is measured.

Factors Affecting Laboratory Results

■ Unwashed hands for the screening test affect test results.
■ Use of saline solution to moisten the test paper causes inaccurate test results.

NURSING IMPLICATIONS WITH RATIONALE
Chloride

- Explain the procedures (screening or iontophoresis or both) to the child and family. Answer questions if possible, or refer them to appropriate health professionals.
- Explain to the child and family that the tests are not painful.
- Remain with the child during the procedure. Give comfort and reassurance as needed.

INCREASED LEVEL

- Associate an elevated sweat chloride level with cystic fibrosis. With cystic fibrosis, sweat chloride levels could be two to five times greater than normal.
- Obtain a familial history of cystic fibrosis, when indicated.
- Determine whether the child has washed and dried his or her hands before the screening test is performed. Dried sweat can leave a chloride residue, thus causing a false-positive result.

CHOLANGIOGRAPHY (INTRAVENOUS, PERCUTANEOUS, T-TUBE CHOLANGIOGRAPHY)

Description

Intravenous (IV) cholangiography examines the biliary ducts (hepatic ducts within the liver, the common hepatic duct, the cystic duct, and the common bile duct) by radiographic and tomographic visualization. Often the gallbladder is not well visualized. The contrast substance, an iodine preparation such as iodipamide meglumine (Cholografin) is injected intravenously. Approximately 15 minutes later x-rays are taken. IV cholangiography is a tedious and time-consuming test, and reactions are commoner with the IV contrast substance than with the oral agents.

Percutaneous cholangiography is indicated when biliary obstruction is suspected. The contrast substance is directly instilled into the biliary tree. The process is visualized by fluoroscopy, and spot films are taken.

T-tube cholangiography, also known as postoperative cholangiography, may be done 7 to 8 hours after a cholecystectomy to explore the common bile duct for patency of the duct and to see if any gallstones are left. During the operation, a T-shaped tube is placed in the common bile duct to promote drainage. The contrast substance is injected into the T-tube. A stone or two could be missed during a cholecystectomy, causing occlusion of the duct.

CHOLESTEROL (SERUM)
Reference Values

Adult: *Desirable Level:* Less than 200 mg/dl. *Moderate Risk:* 200–240 mg/dl. *High Risk:* Greater than 240 mg/dl. *Pregnancy:* High risk levels but a return to prepregnancy values 1 month after delivery.

Child: *Infant:* 90–130 mg/dl. *Child (2–19 years); Desirable Level:* 130–170 mg/dl. *Moderate Risk:* 171–184 mg/dl. *High Risk:* Greater than 185 mg/dl.

Description

Cholesterol is a blood lipid synthesized by the liver and is found in red blood cells, cell membranes, and muscles. About 70% of cholesterol is esterified (combined with fatty acids), and 30% is in the free form. Cholesterol is used by the body to form bile salts for fat digestion and for the formation of hormones by the adrenal glands, ovaries, and testes. Thyroid hormones and estrogen decrease the concentration of cholesterol, and an oophorectomy increases it.

Serum cholesterol is used as an indicator of atherosclerosis and coronary artery disease. Hypercholesterolemia causes plaque deposits in the coronary arteries, thus contributing to myocardial infarction. High serum cholesterol levels can be due to a familial (hereditary) tendency, biliary obstruction, and/or dietary intake. Approximately one third of Americans have a serum cholesterol level below 200 mg dL, which is desirable.

Clinical Problems

Decreased Level: Hyperthyroidism, Cushings syndrome (adrenal hormone excess), starvation, malabsorption, anemias, acute infections. *Drug Influence:* Antilipids (Zocor, Mevacor, Lipitor), thyroxine, antibiotics (kanamycin, neomycin, parmomycin, tetracycline), nicotinic acid, estrogens, glucagon, heparin, salicylates (aspirin), colchicine, oral hypoglycemic agents.

Increased Level: Acute myocardial infarction; atherosclerosis, hypothyroidism, biliary obstruction; biliary cirrhosis; cholangitis; familial hypercholesterolemia; uncontrolled diabetes mellitus; nephrotic syndrome; pancreatectomy; pregnancy (third trimester); types II, III, and V hyperlipoproteinemia; heavy stress periods; high-cholesterol diet (animal fats). *Drug Influence:* Aspirin, corticosteroids, steroids (anabolic agents and androgens), oral contraceptives, epinephrine and norepinephrine, bromides, phenothiazines (chlorpromazine [Thorazine], trifluoperazine [Stelazine], vitamins A and D, sulfonamides, phenytoin (Dilantin).

Procedure

- Keep the client NPO (food, fluids, and medications) for 12 hours. The client may have water.
- Collect 3 to 5 ml of venous blood in a red-top tube. Avoid hemolysis.
- List drugs the client is taking that are not withheld on the laboratory slip.

Factors Affecting Laboratory Results

- Aspirin and cortisone could cause decreased or elevated serum cholesterol levels.
- A high-cholesterol diet before the test could cause elevated serum cholesterol levels.
- Severe hypoxia could increase the serum cholesterol level.
- Hemolysis of the blood specimen may cause an elevation of the serum cholesterol level.

NURSING IMPLICATIONS WITH RATIONALE
Cholesterol

INCREASED LEVEL

- Relate clinical problems and drugs to hypercholesterolemia. An elevated cholesterol level can indicate liver disease as well as coronary artery disease.
- Hold drugs that could increase the serum level for 12 hours before the blood is drawn, with the health care provider's permission.

CLIENT TEACHING

- Explain to the client and family what is considered a normal serum cholesterol level and the effects of an elevated cholesterol level.
- Encourage the client to lose weight if overweight and hypercholesterolemic. Losing weight if obese can decrease serum cholesterol level.
- Instruct the client with hypercholesterolemia to decrease the intake of foods rich in cholesterol (i.e., bacon, eggs, butter, fatty meat, certain seafood, coconut, and chocolate).
- Teach the client with severe hypercholesterolemia to keep medical appointments for follow-up care.

CHORIONIC VILLI BIOPSY (CVB)
Description

Chorionic villi sampling can detect early fetal abnormalities. Fetal cells are obtained by suction from fingerlike projections around the embryonic membrane, which eventually becomes the placenta. The test is performed between the eighth and tenth weeks of pregnancy. After the tenth week, maternal cells begin to grow over the villi.

The advantages of CVB over amniocentesis is that CVB may be performed earlier, and results can be obtained in a few days and not weeks. CVB can diagnose many chromosomal and biochemical fetal disorders. The disadvantage is that CVB cannot determine neural-tubal defects and pulmonary maturity.

NURSING IMPLICATIONS WITH RATIONALE
Chorionic Villi Biopsy

- Obtain a history of last menstrual period (LMP) from the client and a history of family genetic disorders.
- Assess for signs of spontaneous abortion resulting from procedure, such as cramping, bleeding.
- Assess for infection resulting from procedure, such as chills, fever.
- Be supportive of client and family. Be a good listener.

CLIENT TEACHING

- Explain to the client that she will be in a lithotomy position and that ultrasound is used during the procedure.
- Instruct the client to report if excessive bleeding or severe cramping occurs after the procedure.

Procedure

- A consent form should be signed.
- There is no food or fluid restriction.
- Place the client in the lithotomy position.
- Ultrasound is used to verify the placement of the catheter at the villi. Suction is applied, and tissue is removed from the villi.
- Test takes approximately 30 minutes.

Factors Affecting Diagnostic Results
- Performing test after 10 weeks of gestation.

COLONOSCOPY
Description

Colonoscopy, an endoscopic procedure, is an inspection of the large intestine (colon) using a long, flexible fiberscope (colonoscope). The instrument is inserted anally and is advanced through the rectum, the sigmoid colon, and the large intestine to the cecum.

This test is useful for evaluating suspicious lesions in the large colon, such as polyps which could later develop into cancerous tumors, tumor mass, and inflammatory tissue. Biopsy of the tissue or polyp can be obtained. The biopsy forcep passes through the scope to obtain the tissue specimen. Polyps can be removed with the use of an electrocautery snare.

Colonoscopy should not be done on pregnant women near term, after recent abdominal surgery, or in a confused/uncooperative client. Caution should be taken in performing a colonoscopy following an acute myocardial infarction, in acute diverticulitis, or in severe (active) ulcerative colitis. Rarely colon perforation is caused by the fiberscope. Bleeding may occur after a biopsy or polypectomy.

Screening for polyps for the client over the age of 50 is important. However, if the client has a familial history of colon cancer, a colonoscopy may be recommended before the age of 50. Colon cancer is usually caused by adenomatous polyps and if the polyps are removed early, cancer of the colon would be unlikely.

VIRTUAL COLONOSCOPY A virtual colonoscopy is an examination of the colon by computed tomography (CT) scanning of the entire large colon. It is currently not as accurate as the traditional colonoscopy for it is difficult with this procedure to detect small polyps. In a major study, virtual colonoscopy missed 45% of polyps that were 5 mm or smaller. Differentiation of stool from polyps can be difficult.

The client still has to undergo the same colon prep before a virtual colonoscopy as the person would with a traditional colonoscopy. Traditional colonoscopy is required to remove a polyp found on a CT scan of the colon. Virtual colonoscopy has advantages over traditional colonoscopy for no sedatives are required. The procedure is less invasive. Additional information outside the colon may also be found, for example, incidental renal cell cancer.

Procedure

- A consent form should be signed.
- Specific laboratory tests may be ordered, such as CBC, INR (if client has taken Coumadin).
- Withhold medications that interfere with coagulation, such as aspirin, NSAIDs (Advil, Motrin), iron medication, and alcohol, one week prior to the test.
- Barium sulfate from other diagnostic studies can decrease visualization; therefore, the colonoscopy should not be attempted within 10 days to 2 weeks of a barium study.
- Avoid using soapsuds enemas. These can irritate intestine.
- Emergency drugs and equipment should be available for hypersensitivity to medications (premedications and anesthetic).
- Specimen containers should be labeled with the clients name, date, and the type of tissue.
- Client should be accompanied by someone who can drive him/her home following the test.
- The procedure takes approximately 15 minutes to 1 hour.

Pretest Procedure:

- The day before the procedure, the client may have clear liquids only, which includes, water, tea, coffee (without milk), strained fruit juices without pulp (apple, white grape, lemonade), plain jello (without added fruits or toppings), clear broths or bouillon (chicken or beef without noodles or solids), Gatorade, carbonated and non-carbonated soft drinks. All red fluids should be avoided due to the color of the dye which can affect the visualization of the test.

PREPARATION A (USE OF GOLYTELY/COLYTE SOLUTION)

Day Before the Test:

- Client should prepare GoLytely or Colyte solution according to instructions, and refrigerate solution.
- Client should drink GoLytely/Colyte as instructed, usually 7 p.m. to 10 p.m.

PREPARATION B (USE OF 3 OUNCE BOTTLE OF FLEET PHOSPHO SODA (ORAL LAXATIVE)

- Purchase the bottle of Fleet Phospho Soda from the drug store.

Day Before the Test:

- Follow the pretest procedure concerning the clear liquid diet.
- Between 5 and 6 p.m. on the evening before the colonoscopy, add 1½ ounces (45 cc/ml) of Fleet Phospho Soda to one 8 ounce glass of cool water or any clear liquid and sip.
- Then drink one 8 ounce glass of water/clear liquid every 30 minutes for the next 3 hours.

Day of the Test:

- Four hours before arriving for the colonocscopy, add 1½ ounce (45 cc/ml) of Fleet Phospho Soda to an 8 ounce glass of clear liquid and drink.
- Then drink one 8 ounce glass of water/clear liquid every 30 minutes for the next 2 hours.
- Have nothing further to eat or drink until the colonoscopy is completed.

NURSING IMPLICATIONS WITH RATIONALE
Colonoscopy

PRETEST

- The client should follow the pretest preparation procedure.
- Explain the procedure of the test. The client lies in the Sims position or left lateral position. A lubricated colonoscope is inserted. Air will be insufflated for better visualization. Photos are usually taken of any abnormal tissue or polyps.
- Record baseline vital signs, and if available, pertinent laboratory values.
- Report anxiety and fears to the physician or health professional prior to the test.

CLIENT TEACHING

- Instruct the client to bring someone to drive him/her home.
- Instruct the client to breathe deeply and slowly through the mouth during the insertion of the colonoscope.
- Inform the client that the procedure takes approximately 15 minutes to 1 hour.

POSTTEST

- Monitor vital signs and report abnormal changes.
- Assess for anal bleeding, abdominal distention, severe pain, severe abdominal cramps, and fever, and report any of the signs or symptoms immediately.

MEDICATION PROCEDURE

- Intravenous fluids with diprivan (Propofol), midazolam (Versed), or meperidine (Demerol) for conscious sedation is given immediately prior to the test.

Factors Affecting Diagnostic Results

- A soapsuds enema can cause intestinal irritation.
- Barium sulfate from other diagnostic studies can decrease visualization; therefore, the study should not be attempted within 10 days to 2 weeks of a barium study.
- Inadequate bowel preparation with fecal material remaining in the colon will decrease visualization.

COLPOSCOPY

Description

Colposcopy is the examination of the vagina and cervix using a binocular instrument (colposcope) that has a magnifying lens and a light. This test is for identifying precancerous lesions of the cervix and can be performed in the gynecologists office or in the hospital. After a positive Papanicolaou (Pap) smear or a suspicious cervical lesion, colposcopy is indicated for examining the vagina and cervix more thoroughly. Atypical epithelium, leukoplakia vulvae, and irregular blood vessels can be identified with this procedure, and photographs and a biopsy specimen can be obtained.

Since this test has become more popular, there has been a decreased need for conization (surgical removal of a cone of tissue from the cervical os). Colposcopy is also useful for monitoring women whose mothers received diethylstilbestrol during pregnancy; these women are prone to develop precancerous and cancerous lesions of the vagina and cervix. Colposcopy is used to monitor female clients who have had cervical lesions removed.

Procedure

- A consent form should be signed.
- Food and fluids are not restricted.
- The clients clothes should be removed, and the client should wear a gown and be properly draped.
- The client assumes a lithotomy position (legs in stirrups). A speculum is inserted into the vagina, and a long, dry cotton swab applicator is used to clear away any cervical secretions. Another long cotton-swab applicator with saline may be used to swab the cervix for visualizing vascular patterns.
- Acetic acid (3%) is applied to the vagina and cervix. This produces color changes in the cervical epithelium and helps in detecting abnormal changes.
- A biopsy specimen of suspicious tissues and photographs may be taken. Pressure should be applied to control bleeding at the biopsy site, or cautery may be used.
- A vaginal tampon may be worn after the procedure.
- The test takes approximately 15 to 20 minutes.

Factors Affecting Diagnostic Results

- Mucus, cervical secretions, creams, and medications can decrease visualization.

COMPUTED TOMOGRAPHY (CT) SCAN, COMPUTED AXIAL TOMOGRAPHY (CAT)

CAT Scan, Computed Transaxial Tomography [CTT], EMI Scan

Description

The CT scanner produces a narrow x-ray beam that examines body sections from many different angles. The CT scanner can revolve around the client who is lying on a table. It produces a series of cross-sectional images in sequence that build up a two-dimensional (2D) picture of the organ or structure. The traditional x-ray takes a flat or frontal picture, which also gives a two-dimensional view. The CT scanner is about 100 times more sensitive than the x-ray machine in separating different soft tissue densities. Although it is a costly diagnostic test, CT scanning is popular because it can diagnose an early stage of disease.

The CT scan can be performed with or without iodine contrast media (dye). It is not an invasive test unless contrast dye is used. The contrast dye causes a greater tissue absorption and is referred to as *contrast enhancement.* This enhancement enables small tumors to be seen.

CT is capable of scanning the head (internal auditory canal, brain, eye orbits, sinuses, neck), abdomen (stomach, small and large intestines, liver, spleen, pancreas, bile duct, kidney, and adrenals), pelvis (bladder, reproductive organs, and small and large bowel within pelvis), chest (lung, heart, mediastinal structure) and bones and joints. Magnetic resonance imaging (MRI), a noninvasive test, has *not* replaced CT scans; see discussion of MRI on pages 559–562.

High-speed and ultrafast electron beam (EBCT) scans are CT terms that are often incorrectly used interchangeably. These terms describe two different CT scanners, high-speed and ultrafast (electron beam) scanners. Both of these scanners have the ability to perform helical scanning and three-dimensional reconstruction of images. Helical scanning, also known as spiral scanning, is made possible through the use of slip-ring technology. A slip ring has no direct wire connection to the x-ray tube, allowing it to rotate indefinitely in one direction (Bonk). These scanners differ in one very large aspect. The high-speed scanner uses radiographic exposures averaging 1 second, sufficient time to image most anatomy. The EBCT scanner uses radiographic exposures of 100 milliseconds (Wright). This short exposure time is important for it enables the EBCT to accurately image the heart and coronary vessels.

HEAD AND BRAIN CT   The CT of the brain/head provides two-dimensional views of the brain consisting of cross-sectional images of brain tissue layers. This procedure can differentiate between tumors, aneurysms, cerebral infarction, and intracranial hemorrhage and hematoma. Also this CT scan can detect ventricular displacement or enlargement. Visualization of the pathology can be enhanced with IV iodinated contrast dye.

CHEST (THORACIC) CT   CT of the chest gives a cross-sectional view of the chest to differentiate between various pathologic conditions: tumors, nodules, cysts, abscesses, hematomas, and aortic aneurysms. It can detect pleural effusion and enlarged lymph nodes in the chest area. The use of IV contrast media aids in highlighting blood vessels, thus identifying abnormalities of the vascular structures. CT of the chest can be useful in evaluating the effects of treatment therapy on the tumor and if metastasis has occurred.

ABDOMINAL CT   CT of the abdomen is useful for diagnosing tumors, obstructions, cysts, hematoma, abscesses, bleeding, perforation, calculi, fibroids, and other pathologic conditions that appear in the liver, biliary tract, pancreas, spleen, GI tract, gallbladder, kidneys, adrenals, uterus and ovaries, and prostate. IV contrast dye may be used to enhance visualization. The kidney and urinary flow is easily seen with the use of contrast dye. Oral contrast media may be used for scanning the GI tract. The CT scan is useful for staging tumors and monitoring the effects of treatment therapy on the tumor.

SPINE CT   CT scan of the spine gives cross-sectional images that are displayed as twodimensional views on a monitor. It can be reconstructed in the sagittal and coronal plane, or as a 3D surface rendering. It is mainly used to view the bony landmarks. Contrast dye may be injected into the spinal column via lumbar puncture for clearer visualization of nerve roots and disc herniation. MRI is the preferred study of the spine; however, if MRI is contraindicated or unavailable, then contrast CT would likely be ordered.

LONG BONES AND JOINTS CT Skeletal CT provides cross-sectional images of the bone. This procedure is useful to detect bone and soft tissue tumors and bone metastases. Joint abnormalities can be identified with this CT. Contrast dye may be ordered.

Procedure

General Preparation for All Scans
■ A consent form should be signed.
■ There is no food or fluid restriction if contrast dye is NOT used.
■ For IV contrast injection studies, usually there is NPO (nothing by mouth) 4 hours prior to the CT. Diabetics may be given orange juice instead of water; check with the health care provider or CT supervisor. Oral hypoglycemic agents (glucophage) are contraindicated to iodinated contrast. For PM scheduling: NPO after a liquid breakfast.
■ Prescribed medications may be given with a small amount of water prior to the CT scan; check with the health care provider or CT supervisor.
■ A mild sedative may be ordered for some clients to alleviate anxiety.
■ Client should remain still/motionless during the procedure.
■ If contrast media (dye) is ordered and the client is allergic to iodine products, steroids or antihistamines may be given before the scan or may be given IV during the CT scan.
■ IV infusion or heparin lock insertion may be required prior to test. Use a 19- or 20-gauge needle. Never insert the needle into the antecubital area (anterior bend of the elbow).
■ CT scanning usually takes 15 minutes.

Head CT
■ Remove hairpins, braids, clips, and jewelry (earrings) before the test.
■ Remove dentures prior to the use of contrast dye.
■ A mild sedative or analgesic may be ordered for restless clients or for those who have aches and pains of the neck or back.
■ Head is positioned in a cradle, and a wide, rubberized strap is applied snugly around the head to keep it immobilized during test.

Neck CT
■ IV contrast media is used. Check general preparation for scan for IV contrast injection studies.

Abdominal and Pelvic CT
■ Abdominal x-ray (including the kidneys, ureters, and bladder) may be requested before CT scan.
■ The gastrointestinal tract must be free from barium. An enema may be ordered.
■ Current laboratory reports of serum creatinine and blood urea nitrogen should be available to determine if there is kidney dysfunction and if so to what degree. These tests should be done 7 days prior to the CT scan with contrast injection.
■ For an a.m. abdominal/pelvic scan, give the oral contrast media (15 oz) between 8 p.m. and 10 p.m. the evening before the scan. NPO after 10 p.m. One hour prior to the CT, give ½ bottle of the oral contrast. One-half hour prior to the CT, give the remaining ½ bottle of oral contrast.

■ For a p.m. abdominal/pelvic scan, give 1 bottle (15 oz) of oral contrast media at 7 a.m. the morning of the scan. NPO after 7 a.m. One hour prior to the CT, give ½ bottle of the oral contrast. One-half hour prior to the CT, give ½ bottle of the oral contrast.

Chest CT
■ A chest x-ray may be requested before a chest scan.
■ IV contrast media is frequently given in the left arm.

Spine CT
■ NPO is not indicated, because contrast media is usually not ordered.
■ Spine x-rays taken prior to scan should be available. Spine CT should be done after myelography.

Bony Pelvis, Long Bone, and Joint CT
■ The nuclear medicine study to locate hot areas should be done before the CT scan of the bones and joints.

NURSING IMPLICATIONS WITH RATIONALE
Computed Tomography Scan

PRETEST
■ Explain the procedure to the client. The CT scanner is circular, with a doughnut-like opening. The client is strapped to a special table, with the scanner revolving around the body area that is to be examined. Clicking noises will be heard from the scanner. The radiologist or specialized technician is stationed in a control room and can observe and communicate with the client at all times through an intercom system. The test is not painful.
■ Inform the client that holding breath may be requested several times during an abdominal scan.
■ Inform the client that the CT of the head takes 5 minutes without contrast media and 10 minutes with use of contrast. For body CT, the test takes 5 to 15 minutes.
■ Obtain a history of allergies to seafood, iodine, and contrast dye from other x-ray tests. Contrast enhancement is not always done with CT, especially chest and spinal CT scanning.
■ Advise the client that if contrast dye is injected IV, a warm, flushed sensation may be felt in the face or body. A salty, "fishy," or metallic taste, and a sensation of urinating (does not occur) may be experienced. Nausea is not uncommon. These sensations usually last for 1 or 2 minutes.
■ Observe for signs and symptoms of a severe allergic reaction to the dye (i.e., dyspnea, palpitations, tachycardia, hypotension, itching, and urticaria). Emergency drugs should be available.

POSTTEST
■ Observe for delayed allergic reaction to the contrast dye (i.e., skin rash, urticaria, headache, vomiting and/or renal dysfunction). Increased creatinine level can follow IV contrast use. An oral antihistamine may be ordered for mild reactions.
■ If contrast dye has been used, instruct the client to increase fluid intake to enhance the excretion of the dye.
■ Be supportive of the client and family. The CT scan can be frightening. The major risk involved is an allergic reaction to the dye.

CLIENT TEACHING
■ Instruct the client to resume his or her usual level of activity and diet, unless otherwise indicated.

Factors Affecting Diagnostic Results

- Barium sulfate can obscure visualization of the abdominal organs. Barium studies should be performed 4 days before the CT or after the CT.
- Excessive flatus can cause client discomfort and may cause an inaccurate reading.
- Movement can cause artifacts.
- Metal plates in skull and metal bridges.
- Dental fillings.

COOMBS DIRECT (BLOOD [RBCS])

Direct Antiglobulin Test

Reference Values

Adult: Negative.
Child: Negative.

Description

The direct Coombs test detects antibodies attached to red blood cells (RBCs) that may cause cellular damage. This test can identify a weak antigen–antibody reaction even when there is no visible RBC agglutination. A positive Coombs test reveals antibodies present in RBCs, but the test does not identify the antibody responsible.

This test is useful for diagnosing early erythroblastosis fetalis (hemolytic disease of newborns), autoimmune hemolytic anemia, hemolytic transfusion reaction, and some drug sensitizations (i.e., to levodopa and methyldopa).

The direct Coombs test is also known as the direct antiglobulin test, a method of detecting in vivo sensitization of RBCs.

COOMBS INDIRECT (SERUM)

Reference Values

Adult: Negative.
Child: Negative.

Description

The Coombs indirect test can detect free circulating antibodies in the clients serum. This test is done in cross matching blood for transfusions to prevent transfusion reaction to incompatible blood caused by minor blood-type factors. As a result of previous transfusions, a recipients blood may contain specific antibody (antibodies) that could cause a transfusion reaction.

The indirect Coombs test is also known as the indirect antiglobulin test, a method of detecting in vitro sensitization of red blood cells (RBCs).

C-REACTIVE PROTEIN (CRP) (SERUM) AND N HIGH SENSITIVITY CRP (HS CRP)

Reference Values

Adult: Not usually present: *Qualitative:* Greater than 1.2 titer, *Positive:* Quantitative: 20 mg/dl.
Child: Not usually present.

N High Sensitivity CRP (hs CRP):

Adult: Less than 0.175 mg/l.

Description

C-Reactive protein (CRP) is produced in the liver in response to tissue injury and inflammation. It appears in the blood 6 to 10 hours after an acute inflammatory process and tissue destruction. Also it peaks within 48 to 72 hours. The serum CRP usually decreases after the third day of injury. Serum CRP is also found in many body fluids (i.e., pleural, peritoneal, and synovial fluids).

This type of protein is needed to fight injury and infection. Inflammation can cause the protein to become an inflammatory protein. Many references state that the inflammatory protein is an important factor in cardiovascular disease.

Chronic infection, fat cells, hypertension, smoking, cardiovascular and peripheral disease, stroke, and rheumatoid arthritis can produce these inflammatory proteins which weaken the fatty plaques and cause eruption. The pieces of plaques become clots which lead to decreased blood flow and even heart attacks. Higher levels of inflammatory proteins in the blood indicate a higher potential for atherosclerosis.

N HIGH SENSITIVITY CRP (HS CRP) This test is a highly sensitive test for detecting the risk of cardiovascular and peripheral vascular diseases. It is frequently combined with cholesterol screening. Approximately one-third of those who have had a heart attack have normal cholesterol levels and normal blood pressure. A positive hs CRP test may indicate that the client is at a high risk for coronary artery disease (CAD) and stroke. The CRP does not elevate in cases of angina pectoris. This test can detect an inflammatory process that is caused by the build-up of plaque (atherosclerosis) in the arterial system, particularly the coronary arteries. Positive serum hs CRP values are much lower than the standard serum CRP, which makes it a more valuable test for predicting coronary heart disease.

CREATINE PHOSPHOKINASE (CPK) (SERUM), CPK ISOENZYMES (SERUM)

Creatine Kinase (CK)

Reference Values

Adult: *Male:* 5–35 mcg/ml, 30–180 international unit/l, 55–170 unit/l at 37ºC (SI units). *Female:* 5–25 mcg/ml, 25–150 international unit/l, 30–135 unit/l at 37ºC (SI units). Child: *Newborn:* 65–580 international unit/l at 30ºC. *Child: Male:* 0–70 international unit/l at 30ºC. *Female:* 0–50 international unit/l at 30ºC.

CPK Isoenzymes:

CPK-MM:	94%–100%	(muscle)
CPK-MB:	0%–6%	(heart)
CPK-BB:	0%	(brain)

Most labs have replaced CPK isoenzymes with CPK-MB fraction only.

Description

Creatine phosphokinase (CPK), also known as creatine kinase (CK), is an enzyme found in high concentration in the heart and skeletal muscles and in low concentration in the brain tissue. Serum CPK/CK is frequently elevated by skeletal muscle disease, acute myocardial infarction (MI), cerebrovascular disease, vigorous exercise, intramuscular (IM) injections, and electrolyte imbalance-hypokalemia. CPK/CK has two types of isoenzymes: M, associated with muscle, and B, associated with the brain. Electrophoresis separates the isoenzymes into three subdivisions: MM (in skeletal muscle and some in the heart), MB (in the heart), and BB (in brain tissue). When CPK/CK is elevated, a CPK electrophoresis is done to determine which group of isoenzymes is elevated. Increased isoenzyme CPK-MB could indicate damage to the myocardial cells.

Serum CPK/CK and CPK-MB rise within 4 to 6 hours after an acute MI, reach a peak in 18 to 24 hours (greater than 6 times the normal value), and then return to normal within 3 to 4 days, unless new necrosis or tissue damage occurs. If medication for acute MI has to be given parenterally (for instance, morphine), it would be better to give it intravenously than intramuscularly so that mild muscle injury (from IM) would not elevate the CPK level; however, injections have little or no effect on CPK-MB. Draw blood for a serum CPK/CK level before giving an IM injection.

CREATININE (SERUM)
Reference Values

Adult: 0.5–1.5 mg/dl; 45–132.3 μmol/l (SI units). Females may have slightly lower values because of their lesser muscle mass.

Child: *Newborn:* 0.8–1.4 mg/dl. Infant: 0.7–1.7 mg/dl. *Child (26 years):* 0.3–0.6 mg/dl, 27–54 μmol/l (SI units). *Older Child:* 0.4–1.2 mg/dl, 36–106 μmol/l (SI units). Values increase slightly with age relative to muscle mass.
Elderly: May have decreased values relative to decreased muscle mass and decreased creatinine production.

Description

Creatinine, a by-product of muscle catabolism, is derived from the breakdown of muscle creatine phosphate. The amount of creatinine produced is proportional to the muscle mass. Creatinine is filtered by the glomeruli and it is excreted in the urine.

Serum creatinine is considered a more sensitive and specific indicator of renal disease than blood urea nitrogen (BUN). It rises later and is *not influenced by diet or fluid intake*. A slight BUN elevation could be indicative of hypovolemia (fluid volume deficit); however, a serum creatinine of 2.5 mg/dl could be indicative of renal impairment. BUN and creatinine are frequently compared. If BUN increases and serum creatinine remains normal, dehydration (hypovolemia) is present; and if both increase, then renal disorder is present. Serum creatinine is especially useful in evaluation of glomerular function.

CREATININE CLEARANCE (URINE)

Creatinine (urine)

Reference Values

Adult: 85–135 ml/min. Females may have somewhat lower values.
Child: Similar to adult.
Elderly: Slightly decreased values than adult due to decreased glomerular filtration rate (GFR) caused by reduced renal plasma flow.
Urine Creatinine: 12 g/24 hours.

Description

Creatinine is a metabolic product of creatine phosphate in skeletal muscle, and it is excreted by the kidneys. Creatinine clearance is considered a reliable test for estimating GFR. With renal insufficiency, the GFR is decreased, and the serum creatinine is increased. GFR decreases with age, and with the older adult, the creatinine clearance may be diminished to as low as 60 ml/minute.

The creatinine clearance test consists of a 12- or 24-hour urine collection and a blood sample.

The formula for calculating the creatinine clearance test is:

$$\text{Creatinine clearance} = \frac{\text{Urine creatinine (mcg/dl)} \times \text{Urine volume (dl)}}{\text{Serum creatinine (mcg/dl)}}$$

A creatinine clearance less than 40 ml/minute is suggestive of moderate to severe renal impairment.

CROSS MATCHING (BLOOD)

Blood Typing Tests, Compatibility Test for RBCs, Type and Cross Match

Reference Values

Adult: Compatibility; absence of agglutination (clumping) of cells.
Child: Same as adult.

Description

The four *major* blood types (A, B, AB, and O) belong to the ABO blood group system. Red blood cells (RBCs) have either antigen A, B, AB, or none on the surface of the cells. Type A has A antigen, B has B antigen, AB has A and B antigens, and O does not contain an antigen. These antigens are capable of producing antibodies. The AB blood person is the universal recipient (can accept all blood), because there are no antibodies; the O blood person is the universal donor (can give blood to all types).

ABO blood type and Rh factor are first determined, then the compatibility of donor and recipient blood is determined by major cross match. The major cross match is between the donors RBCs and the recipients serum, and the test is performed to determine if the recipient has any antibodies to destroy the donors RBCs.

Factors Affecting Laboratory Results

■ Previously received incompatible blood can make blood cross matching difficult.

CULTURES (BLOOD, SPUTUM, STOOL, THROAT, WOUND, URINE)

Reference Values

Adult: Negative or no pathogen.
Child: Same as adult.

Description

Cultures are taken to isolate the microorganism that is causing the clinical infection. Most culture specimens are obtained using sterile swabs with medium (solid or broth), a sterile container (cup) with a lid, and a sterile syringe with a sterile bottle of liquid medium. The culture specimen should be taken immediately to the laboratory after collection (no longer than 30 minutes), because some organisms will die if not placed in the proper medium and incubated.

Most specimens for culture are either blood, sputum, stool, throat secretions, wound exudate, or urine. It usually takes 24 to 36 hours to grow the organisms and 48 hours for the growth and culture report.

Purpose

■ To isolate the microorganism in body tissue or body fluid.

Clinical Problems

Specimen	Clinical Condition or Most Commonly Isolated Organism
Blood	Bacteremia, septicemia, postoperative shock, fever of unknown origin
Sputum	Pulmonary tuberculosis, bacterial pneumonia, chronic bronchitis, bronchiectasis
Stool	*Salmonella* species, *Shigella* species, enteropathogenic *Escherichia coli, Staphylococcus* species, *Yersinia*
Throat	Beta-hemolytic streptococci (rheumatic fever), thrush (*Candida* species), tonsillar infection, *Staphylococcus aureus*
Wound	*Staphylococcus* species: *S. aureus, Pseudomonas aeruginosa, Proteus* species, *Bacteroides* species, *Klebsiella* species, *Serratia* species
Urine	*Escherichia coli, Klebsiella* species, *Pseudomonas aeruginosa, Serratia* species, *Shigella* species, Yeasts: *Candida* species

Procedure

■ Hand washing is essential before and after collection of the specimen.

■ Send the specimen for culture to the laboratory *immediately* after collection.

■ Obtain the specimen before antibiotic therapy is started. If the client is receiving antibiotics, the drug(s) should be listed on the laboratory slip.

■ Collection containers or tubes should be sterile. Aseptic technique should be used during collection. Contamination of the specimen could cause false-positive results and/or transmission of the organisms.

■ Check with the laboratory for specific techniques used.

Blood: Cleanse the clients skin according to the institutions procedure. Usually the skin is scrubbed first with povidone-iodine (Betadine). Iodine can be irritating to the skin, so it is removed and an application of benzalkonium chloride or alcohol is applied. Cleanse the top(s) of the culture bottle(s) with iodine and leave it or them to dry. The bottle(s) should contain a culture medium. Collect 5 to 10 ml of venous blood and place in the sterile bottle. Special vacuum tubes containing a culture medium for blood may be used instead of a culture bottle.

Sputum: *Sterile Container or Cup:* Obtain sputum for culture early in the morning, before breakfast. Instruct the client to give several deep coughs to raise sputum. Tell the client to avoid spitting saliva secretion into the sterile container. Saliva and postnasal drip secretions can contaminate the sputum specimen. Keep a lid on the sterile container. The container *should not* be completely filled and should be taken immediately to the laboratory. The sputum sample should not remain for hours by the clients bedside unless one needs a 24-hour sputum specimen (in this case, an extra sterile container should be left). *Acid-Fast Bacilli (TB Culture):* Follow the instructions on the container. Collect 5 to 10 ml of sputum, and take the sample immediately to the laboratory or refrigerate the specimen. Three sputum specimens may be requested, one each day for 3 days. Check for proper labeling.

Stool: Collect an approximately 1-inch-diameter feces sample. Use a sterile tongue blade and place the stool specimen in a sterile container with a lid. The suspected disease or organism should be noted on the laboratory slip. The stool specimen should not contain urine. The client should not be given barium or mineral oil, which can inhibit bacteria growth.

Throat: Use a sterile cotton swab or a polyester-tipped swab. The sterile culture kit could be used. Swab the inflamed or ulcerated tonsillar and/or posphryngeal areas of the throat. Place the applicator in a culturette tube with its culture medium. Take the throat culture specimen immediately to the laboratory. Do *not* give antibiotics before taking the culture.

Wound: Use a culture kit containing a sterile cotton swab or a polyester-tipped swab and a tube with culture medium. Swab the exudate of the wound and place the swab in the tube containing a culture medium. Wear sterile gloves when there is an excess amount of purulent drainage.

NURSING IMPLICATIONS WITH RATIONALE
Collecting a Culture

PRETEST

- Obtain history concerning the presence of cystitis or prostatitis, which could result in sepsis.
- Explain the procedure to the client. Answer questions or refer questions you cannot answer to the urologist.
- Check with the urologist about the form of anesthesia the client will receive—local or general. Inform the client that a local anesthetic will be injected into the urethra several minutes before the cystoscope is inserted.
- Check that the consent form has been signed before administering the premedications. Normally the drugs are given 1 hour before the test.
- Check with the client concerning hypersensitivity to anesthetics.
- Assess urinary patterns, such as amount, color, odor, specific gravity of the urine.
- Take baseline vital signs.

CLIENT TEACHING

- Inform the client that there may be some pressure or burning discomfort during and/or following the test.

POSTTEST

- Recognize the complications that can occur as a result of the cystoscopy, such as hemorrhaging, perforation of the bladder, urinary retention, and infection.
- Monitor vital signs (VS). Compare with baseline VS. VS may be ordered every half hour until stable.
- Monitor the urinary output for 48 hours following a cystoscopy. If urine output is less than 200 ml in 8 hours, encourage fluid intake. Anuria could indicate urinary retention due to blood clots or urethral stricture. Report findings to the urologist. An indwelling catheter may be ordered.
- Report and record gross hematuria. Inform the client that blood-tinged urine is not uncommon after a cystoscopic examination.
- Observe for signs and symptoms of an infection (i.e., fever, chills, an increased pulse rate, and pain). Antibiotics may be given before and after the test as a prophylactic measure.
- Apply heat to the lower abdomen to relieve pain and muscle spasm as ordered.

CLIENT TEACHING

- Advise the client to avoid alcoholic beverages for 2 days after the test.
- Inform the client that a slight burning sensation when voiding for a day or two is considered normal. Usually the urologist leaves an order for an analgesic.

Urine: *Clean-Caught (Midstream) Urine Specimen:* Clean-caught urine collection is the commonest method for collecting a urine specimen for culture. There are noncatheterization kits giving step-by-step instructions. Catheterizing for urine culture is seldom ordered. Usually the client collects the urine specimen for culture, so a detailed explanation should be given, according to the instructions. The penis or vulva should be well cleansed. At times, two urine specimens (2 to 10 ml) are requested to verify the organism and in case of a possible contamination of the urine specimen. Collect a midstream

urine specimen early in the morning, or as ordered, in a sterile container. The lid should fit tightly on the container and the urine specimen should be taken immediately to the bacteriology laboratory or be refrigerated. Label the urine specimen with the clients name, the date, and the exact time of collection (e.g., 7/22/07 @ 8:00 a.m.). List any antibiotics or sulfonamides the client is taking on the laboratory slip.

Factors Affecting Laboratory Results
- Contamination of the specimen causes inaccurate results.
- Antibiotics and sulfonamides may cause false-negative results.
- Urine in the stool collection may cause false test results.

CYSTOSCOPY, CYSTOGRAPHY (CYSTOGRAM)

Description

Cystoscopy is the direct visualization of the bladder wall and urethra with the use of a cystoscope (a tubular lighted telescopic lens). Usually this diagnostic test is performed by a urologist. Small renal calculi can be removed from the ureter, bladder, or urethra with this procedure, and a tissue biopsy can be obtained. In addition, *retrograde pyelography* (injection of contrast dye through the catheter into the ureters and renal pelvis) may be performed during the cystoscopy.

Cystoscopy is performed in a cystoscopy room of a hospital or in a urologists office under general or local anesthesia. Premedications are administered an hour prior to the test.

Cystography is the instillation of a contrast dye into the bladder via a catheter. This procedure can detect a rupture in the bladder, a neurogenic bladder, fistulas, and tumors. The test is useful when x-rays are needed and a cystoscopy or retrograde pyelography is contraindicated.

Purposes
- To detect renal calculi and renal tumor.
- To remove renal stones.
- To determine the cause of hematuria or urinary tract infection (UTI).

Procedure
- A consent form should be signed.
- The client can have a full liquid breakfast the morning of the test if local anesthetic is used. Several glasses of water may be ordered. If general anesthesia is to be administered, the client should be NPO for 8 hours before cystoscopy.
- Record baseline vital signs.
- A narcotic analgesic (meperidine, morphine) may be ordered an hour before the cystoscopy. The procedure is done under local or general anesthesia.
- The client is placed in a lithotomy position (feet or legs in stirrups). A local anesthetic is injected into the urethra. Water may be instilled to enhance better visualization. A urine specimen may be obtained.
- The cystoscopy takes approximately 30 minutes to 1 hour.

D-DIMER TEST (BLOOD)
Fragment D-Dimer, Fibrin Degradation Fragment

Reference Values
Negative for D-Dimer fragments: Greater than 250 ng/ml: greater than 250 mcg/l (SI units).

Description
D-dimer, a fibrin degradation fragment, occurs through fibrinolysis. This test measures the amount of fibrin degradation that occurs. It confirms the presence of fibrin split products (FSPs) and is more specific for diagnosing disseminated intravascular coagulation (DIC) than FSPs. However, both D-dimer and FSP tests are frequently used to determine DIC in a client.

D-dimer levels are increased when a fibrin clot is broken down by the thrombolytic drug, tissue plasminogen activator (tPA), streptokinase.

DIGOXIN (SERUM)
Lanoxin

Reference Values
Therapeutic: *Adult:* 0.5–2 ng/ml; 0.5–2 nmol/l (SI units). *Infants:* 13 ng/ml. *Child:* Same as adult.
Toxic: *Adult:* Greater than 2 ng/ml; greater than 2.6 nmol/l (SI units). *Infants:* greater than 3.5 ng/ml. *Child:* Same as adult.

Description
Digoxin, a form of digitalis, is a cardiac glycoside agent given to increase the force and velocity of myocardial contraction. More than 75% to 95% of the drug is absorbed through the gastrointestinal (GI) tract, and a large amount of digoxin is excreted unchanged through the kidneys. The half-life of digoxin is 35 to 40 hours, with a shorter half-life in neonates and infants and a longer time in short-term infants/premature infants.

Serum plateau levels of digoxin occur 6 to 8 hours after an oral dose, 2 to 4 hours after IV administration, and 10 to 12 hours after IM administration. The most frequent routes used for administering digoxin are by mouth (oral) and IV.

Electrolyte imbalance (hypokalemia or hypomagnesemia), acid base disturbances, and certain drugs predispose the person to digitalis toxicity. Common signs and symptoms of digitalis toxicity include pulse rate less than 60 per minute, anorexia, nausea, vomiting, headaches, and visual disturbance.

Factors Affecting Laboratory Results
- Administering digoxin intramuscularly might cause the absorption rate to be erratic, especially in a debilitated or elderly person with poor tissue perfusion.
- A low serum potassium or magnesium level could cause digitalis toxicity, and a high serum calcium level could cause digitalis toxicity.
- Hypothyroidism, severe heart disease, and renal function abnormalities may predispose a client to digitalis toxicity.

ECHOCARDIOGRAPHY (ECHOCARDIOGRAM)
M-Mode, Two-Dimensional (2D), Spectral Doppler, Color Flow Doppler, Transesophageal, Contrast, and Stress Echocardiography*

Description
Echocardiography (echocardiogram) is a noninvasive ultrasound test used to identify abnormal heart size, structure, and function, and valvular disease. A hand-held transducer (probe) is moved over the chest in the area of the heart and other specified surrounding areas. The transducer sends and receives high-frequency sound waves. The sound waves that are reflected (echo) from the heart back to the transducer produce pictures. These pictures appear on a television-like screen and are recorded on videotape and moving graph paper.

There are several types of echocardiographic studies, which include M-mode, two-dimensional (2D), spectral doppler, color doppler, transesophageal, contrast, and stress echocardiography. Transesophageal echocardiography (TEE) is gaining popularity for diagnosing and managing a wide range of cardiovascular diseases, such as valvular heart dysfunction and aortic pathology. Stress echocardiography is a valuable tool for assessing myocardial ischemia at half the cost of other cardiac studies.

M-MODE ECHOCARDIOGRAPHY M-mode echocardiography, the earliest type of echocardiography, is used to record the motion of various heart structures (M is for *motion*). This test assesses the dimension of the left ventricle and its degree of dilatation and contractility related to myocardial disease or volume overload. It is useful for measuring the thickness of the right and left ventricles (hypertrophy). M-mode echocardiography is also used for assessing the cardiac valves and valvular movements for stenosis, regurgitation, or prolapse.

TWO-DIMENSIONAL (2D) ECHOCARDIOGRAPHY This test employs M-mode echocardiography, which records motion, and provides two-dimensional (cross-sectional) views of the heart structures. It is used to evaluate the size, shape, and movement of the chambers and valves of the heart and it is useful in detecting valvular disease and in assessing congenital heart disease.

SPECTRAL DOPPLER ECHOCARDIOGRAPHY Spectral doppler echocardiography measures the amount, speed, and direction of blood passing through the heart valves and heart chambers. A swishing sound is heard as the blood flows throughout the heart. This test can detect tubulent blood flow through the heart valves, which may indicate valvular disease. Septal wall defects may also be detected.

COLOR DOPPLER ECHOCARDIOGRAPHY Color doppler (red and blue) echocardiography shows the direction of blood flowing through the heart. It can identify leaking heart valves (regurgitation) or hardened valves (stenosis), malfunction of prosthetic valves, and the presence of shunts (holes) in the heart. The use of the color doppler compliments 2D echocardiography and the spectral doppler study.

TRANSESOPHAGEAL ECHOCARDIOGRAPHY With trans-esophageal echocardiography (TEE), a transducer (probe) is attached to an endoscope and is inserted into the esophagus to visualize adjacent cardiac and extracardiac structures with greater acuity than most echocardiography studies, including transthoracic (TTE). TEE can be used in the intensive care unit, emergency department, and operating room, as well as in cardiac testing facilities. This type of echocardiography is useful for diagnosing mitral and aortic valvular pathology; determining the presence of a possible intracardiac thrombus in the left atrium; detecting suspected acute dissection of the aorta and endocarditis; monitoring left ventricular function before, during, or after surgery; and evaluating intracardiac repairs during surgery.

This test is contraindicated if esophageal pathology (e.g., strictures, varices, trauma) exists. Also, TEE should not be performed if undiagnosed active gastrointestinal bleeding is occurring or if the client is uncooperative. A light sedative is frequently given prior to testing. TEE can be performed on an unconscious client. TEE is tolerated well, with approximately 1% of clients being intolerant of the esophageal probe. The rate of complications is less than 0.2%.

CONTRAST ECHOCARDIOGRAPHY This test assists in determining intracardiac communications, myocardial ischemia, and perfusion defects. Microbubbles are injected into the venous circulation for the purpose of recording showers of echoes by M-mode or 2D tests. The micro bubbles pass through the right atrium and ventricle, where they are absorbed in the lung; they do not pass to the left side of the heart. If the microbubbles are detected on the left side of the heart, an intracardiac communication or shunt is present. New contrast agents may allow visualization of the coronary arteries and perfusion to the myocardium with echocardiography.

STRESS ECHOCARDIOGRAPHY It may be necessary to evaluate the function of the left ventricle under stress. Physical exercise hampers good imaging, so the ventricle is stressed pharmacologically using the inotropic drugs dobutamine and dipyridamole (Persantine). Dobutamine is a most effective nonexercise stressor. The object of this test is to detect myocardial ischemia caused by coronary artery disease (CAD). To determine perfusion and wall motion abnormalities, dipyridamole and a contrast agent are used. Some facilities use a combination of dipyridamole and dobutamine for stress echocardiographic testing. This combination increases the effectiveness of detecting multivessel coronary artery disease (CAD) from 72% with one pharmacologic agent to 92% using both. Arbutamine is a new inotropic agent in use in Europe and being tested in the United States.

Procedure

- A consent form should be signed.
- There is no food or fluid restriction.
- No medications should be omitted before the test unless indicated by the institution or health care provider.

- The client undresses from waist up and wears a hospital gown. For the test, the client will be positioned on his or her left side or in the supine position.
- Vital signs are recorded. Three electrode patches are applied to the chest area to monitor heart rate and changes in cardiac rhythm.
- Water-soluble gel is applied to the skin areas that are to be scanned. The transducer (probe), with slight pressure, is moved over different areas of the chest. Some clients may require that pictures be taken under the neck.
- The 2D echo takes about 20 to 30 minutes and the 2D echo with Doppler studies takes approximately 30 to 45 minutes.
- The cardiologist interprets the test result and submits a report to the clients health care provider, who gives the test results to the client.

TRANSESOPHAGEAL ECHOCARDIOGRAPHY (TEE)
- The client should be NPO for at least 4 hours prior to test.
- A light sedative is given prior to the test.
- An IV sedative (e.g., Versed) is given.
- The endoscopic transducer is inserted into the esophagus.
- The test takes 15 to 30 minutes.
- The client is monitored (Dynamap) during recovery for 1 to 2 hours.

CONTRAST ECHOCARDIOGRAPHY
- An IV line is inserted for injection of contrast media.

STRESS ECHOCARDIOGRAPHY
- The client should be NPO for 4 hours before the test.
- The client may be placed on a treadmill or receive a pharmacologic agent.
- Images are acquired during rest (pretest) and then during stress or immediately following stress (posttest).

Factors Affecting Diagnostic Results
- Large body habitus may cause poor image quality.
- Severe respiratory disease may affect test results.

ELECTROCARDIOGRAPHY (ELECTROCARDIOGRAM—ECG OR EKG), VECTORCARDIOGRAPHY (VECTORCARDIOGRAM—VCG)

Description

An electrocardiogram (ECG or EKG) records the electrical impulses of the heart by the means of electrodes and a galvanometer (ECG machine). These electrodes are placed on the legs, arms, and chest. Combinations of two electrodes are called bipolar leads (i.e., lead I is the combination of both arm electrodes, lead II is the combination of the right-arm and left-leg electrodes, and lead III is the combination of the left-arm and left-leg electrodes). The unipolar leads are AVF, AVL, and AVR; the A means augmented, V is the voltage, and F is left foot, L is left arm, and R is right arm. There are at least six unipolar chest or precordial leads. A standard ECG consists of 12 leads: six limb leads (I, II, III, AVF, AVL, AVR) and six chest (precordial) leads (V_1, V_2, V_3, V_4, V_5, V_6).

NURSING IMPLICATIONS WITH RATIONALE
Electrocardiography

■ Record the list of medications the client is taking. The health care provider may want to compare ECG readings to check for improvement and changes; therefore, knowing the drugs the client is taking at the time of the ECG would be helpful.

CLIENT TEACHING

■ Instruct the client to relax and to breathe normally during the ECG procedure. Tell the client to avoid tightening the muscles, grasping bed rails or other objects, and talking during the ECG tracing.
■ Tell the client that the ECG should not cause pain or any great discomfort.
■ Inform the client to tell you if he or she is having chest pain during the ECG tracing. Mark the ECG paper at the time the client is having chest pain.
■ Allow the client time to ask questions. Refer questions you cannot answer to another health care provider, e.g., physician or cardiologist.
■ Inform the client that the ECG takes about 15 minutes.

POSTTEST

■ Remove the electropaste or jelly, if used, from the electrode sites when ECG is completed. Assist the client with dressing, if necessary.

With each cardiac cycle or heartbeat, the sinoatrial node (SA or sinus node) sends an electrical impulse through the atrium, causing atrial contraction or atrial depolarization. The SA node is called the pacemaker, because it controls the heart beat. The impulse is then transmitted to the atrioventricular (AV) node and the bundle of His and travels down the ventricles, causing ventricular contraction or ventricular depolarization. When the atria and the ventricles relax, repolarization and recovery occurs.

The electrical activity that the ECG records is in the form of waves and complexes: P wave (atrial depolarization); QRS complex (ventricular depolarization); and ST segment, T wave, and Unit wave (ventricular repolarization). An abnormal ECG indicates a disturbance in the electrical activity of the myocardium. A person could have heart disease and have a normal ECG as long as the cardiac problem did not affect the transmission of electrical impulses.

VECTORCARDIOGRAM (VCG) The VCG records electrical impulses from the cardiac cycle, making it similar to the ECG. However, it shows a three-dimensional view (frontal, horizontal, and sagittal planes) of the heart, whereas the ECG shows a two-dimensional view (frontal and horizontal planes). The VCG is considered more sensitive than the ECG for diagnosing a myocardial infarction. It is useful for assessing ventricular hypertrophy in adults and children.

Procedure
■ Food, fluids, and medications are not restricted, unless otherwise indicated.
■ Clothing should be removed to the waist, and the female client should wear a gown.

■ Nylon stockings should be removed, and trouser bottoms should be raised.
■ The client should lie in a supine position.
■ The skin surface should be prepared. Excess hair should be shaved from the chest if necessary.
■ Electrodes with electropaste or pads are strapped to the four extremities. The color-coded lead wires are inserted into the correct electrodes. Chest electrodes are applied. The lead selector is turned to record the 12 standard leads unless the ECG machine automatically records the lead strips.
■ The ECG takes approximately 15 minutes.

Factors Affecting Diagnostic Results
■ Body movement and electromagnetic interference during the ECG recording could distort the tracing.
■ Poor electrode-to-skin contact will distort tracing.

ELECTROENCEPHALOGRAPHY (ELECTROENCEPHALOGRAM—EEG)
Description
The electroencephalogram (EEG) measures the electrical impulses produced by brain cells. Electrodes, applied to the scalp surface at predetermined measured positions, record brain-wave activity on moving paper. EEG tracings can detect patterns characteristic of some diseases (i.e., seizure disorders, neoplasms, cerebral vascular accidents, head trauma, and infections of the nervous system). At times, recorded brain waves may be normal when there is pathology.

Another use for the EEG is to determine cerebral death. If the EEG recording gives a flat or straight line for many hours, this usually indicates severe hypoxia and brain death. The cardiovascular functions are usually being maintained through the use of life-support systems (e.g., a respirator, oxygen, and IVs). The neurologist interprets the EEG readings and gives suggestions.

Procedure
The procedure may be performed while the client is (1) awake, (2) drowsy, (3) asleep, or (4) undergoing stimuli (hyperventilation or rhythmic flashes of bright light), or (5) a combination of any of these.

Pretest
■ The hair should be shampooed the night before the test. Instruct the client not to use oil or hair spray on the hair.
■ The decision concerning withdrawal of medications before the EEG is made by the health care provider. Sleeping pills and other sedatives may not be given the night before the test because they can affect the EEG recording.
■ Food and fluids are not restricted except *no* coffee, tea, cola, and alcohol before the test.
■ The EEG tracing is usually obtained with the client lying down; however, the client could be seated in a reclining chair.

NURSING IMPLICATIONS WITH RATIONALE
Electroencephalography

- A consent form should be signed.
- Explain the procedure to the client, step by step. List the important steps on paper for the client if needed.
- Report if the client is taking medications that could change the EEG result.
- Check with the health care provider and/or EEG department in regard to the type or types of recordings ordered (i.e., awake, sleep, stimuli).
- Be supportive of the client. Answer questions and permit the client to express concerns.
- Report to the health care provider and inform the EEG laboratory if the client is extremely anxious, restless, or upset.
- Observe for seizures and describe the seizure activity—the movements and how long they last. Have a tongue blade by the bedside at all times. Chart all seizure activity and the time of its occurrence, because it is very important for the technologist and electroencephalographer to know this.

CLIENT TEACHING

- Inform the client that he or she will *not* get an electric shock from the machine (electroencephalograph) and that the machine does not determine the clients intelligence and cannot read the clients mind. Many clients are apprehensive and fearful of this test.
- Encourage the client to eat a meal before the test. Hypoglycemia should be prevented because it can affect normal brain activity. Coffee, tea, cola, and any other stimulants should be avoided. Alcohol is a depressant and can affect the test result.
- Inform the client that the test does not produce pain.
- Advise the client to be calm and to relax during the test. If rest and stimuli (flashing lights) recordings are ordered, inform the client that there will be a brief time when there are flashing lights. Prepare the client, but do not increase the clients apprehension, if possible.
- Inform the client that the test takes 1½ to 2 hours. The room is quiet where the EEG recording is made and is conducive to rest and sleep.
- Instruct the client, after the test, that normal activity can be resumed.

- For a sleep recording, keep the client awake 2 to 3 hours later the night before the test and wake the client up at 6 a.m. A sedative such as chloral hydrate may be ordered.
- The EEG test takes approximately 1½ to 2 hours. Flat electrodes will be applied to the scalp.

Posttest
- Remove the collodion or paste from the clients head. Acetone may be used to remove the paste.
- The client should resume normal activity unless he or she has been sedated.

Factors Affecting Diagnostic Results
- Drugs (i.e., sedatives, barbiturates, anticonvulsants, and tranquilizers) can affect test results.
- Alcohol could decrease cerebral impulses.
- Oily hair or the use of hair spray can affect test results.

ELECTROMYOGRAPHY (ELECTROMYOGRAMEMG)
Description
Electromyography (EMG) measures electrical activity of skeletal muscles at rest and during voluntary muscle contraction. A needle electrode is inserted into the skeletal muscle to pick up electrical activity, which can be heard over a loudspeaker, viewed on an oscilloscope, and recorded on graphic paper all at the same time. Normally there is no electrical activity when the muscle is at rest; however, in motor disorders abnormal patterns can occur. With voluntary muscle contraction there is a loud popping sound and increased electrical activity (wave) is recorded.

The test is useful in diagnosing neuromuscular disorders. The EMG can be used to differentiate between myopathy and neuropathy.

Procedure
- A consent form should be signed.
- Food and fluids are not restricted, with the exceptions of *no* coffee, tea, colas, or other caffeine drinks, and *no* smoking for at least 3 hours before the EMG.
- Medications such as muscle relaxants, anticholinergics, and cholinergics should be withheld before the test with the approval of the health care provider. If the client needs the specific medication, the time for the test should be rearranged.
- The client lies on a table or stretcher or sits in a chair in a room free of noise. The EMG takes 1 hour but could take longer if a group of muscles is to be tested.
- Needle electrodes are inserted in selected or affected muscles. If the client experiences pain, the needle should be removed and reinserted.
- If serum enzyme tests are ordered (i.e., AST [SGOT], CPK, LDH), the samples should be drawn before the EMG or 5 to 10 days after the test.

Posttest
- If residual pain occurs, analgesic may be given.

Factors Affecting Diagnostic Results
- Pain could cause false reports.
- Age of the client: electrical activity may be decreased in some elderly persons.
- Drugs: muscle relaxants, anticholinergics, and cholinergics could affect the results.
- Fluids that contain caffeine can affect results.

ERYTHROCYTE SEDIMENTATION RATE (ESR) (BLOOD)
Sedimentation (SED) Rate

Reference Values

Adult: *Westergren Method: Male:* less than 50 years: 0–15 mm/hour. *Female:* less than 50 years: 0–20 mm/hour. *Male:* greater than 50 years: 020 mm/hour. *Female:* greater than 50 years: 0–30 mm/hour. *Wintrobe Method: Male:* 0–9 mm/hour. *Female:* 0–15 mm/hour.

Child: *Newborn:* 0–2 mm/hour; *4–14 years:* 0–10 mm/hour.

Description
The erythrocyte sedimentation rate (ESR) (known also as the sedimentation rate or SED rate) is the rate at which red blood cells (RBCs) settle in unclotted blood in millimeters per hour (mm/hour). The ESR is nonspecific. The rate can be increased in acute inflammatory process, acute and chronic infections, tissue damage (necrosis), rheumatoid, collagen diseases, malignancies, and physiologic stress situations (e.g., pregnancy). To some hematologists, the ESR is unreliable, because it is non-specific and is affected by physiologic factors that cause inaccurate results.

The C-reactive protein (CRP) test is considered more useful than the ESR because CRP increases more rapidly during an acute inflammatory process and returns to normal faster than the ESR. The ESR is still an old standby used by many physicians as a rough estimate of the disease process and for following the course of illness. With an elevated ESR, other laboratory tests should be conducted to properly identify the clinical problem.

ESOPHAGOGASTRODUODENOSCOPY, ESOPHAGOGASTROSCOPY
Gastroscopy, Esophagoscopy, Duodenoscopy, Endoscopy

Description
Esophagogastroscopy includes gastroscopy and esophagoscopy. If duodenoscopy is included with the endoscopic examination, the term is *esophagogastroduodenoscopy.* A flexible fiberoptic endoscope is used for direct visualization of the internal structures of the esophagus, stomach, and duodenum. Biopsy forceps or a cytology brush can also be inserted through a channel of the endoscope. Suction can be applied for the removal of secretions and foreign bodies.

This test is performed under local anesthesia or IV sedation (benzodiazepine or narcotics), in a gastroscopy room of a hospital or clinic, usually by a gastroenterologist. This procedure can be done on an emergency basis for removal of foreign objects (a bone, a pin, etc.) and for diagnostic purposes. The major complications that can occur from esophagogastroduodenoscopy are perforation and hemorrhage.

Procedure
- A consent form should be signed.
- The client should be NPO for 8 to 12 hours before the test. When this procedure is used during an emergency and NPO cannot be enforced, the clients stomach is lavaged (suctioned) to prevent aspiration.
- The client may take prescribed medications at 6 AM on the day of the test. Check with laboratory or health care provider for any changes.
- A sedative/tranquilizer, a narcotic analgesic, and atropine may be given an hour before the test, or they can be titrated

intravenously immediately prior to the procedure and during the procedure as needed.
- A local anesthetic may be used.
- Dentures, jewelry, and clothing should be removed from the neck to the waist.
- Record baseline vital signs. The client should void before the procedure.
- Specimen containers should be labeled with the clients name, the date, and the type of tissue.
- Emergency drugs and equipment should be available for hypersensitivity to medications (premedications and anesthetic) and for severe laryngospasms.
- The test takes approximately 1 hour or less.
- The client should not drive self home following the test because of possible aftereffects of sedation.

Factors Affecting Diagnostic Results
- Barium from a recent gastrointestinal imaging series can decrease visualization of the mucosa. This test should not be performed within 2 days after such tests. An x-ray film of the abdomen can be taken to see if barium is in the stomach or duodenum.

ESTROGEN (SERUM)
Reference Values
Adult: *Female:* Early menstrual cycle: 60–200 pg/ml. Midmenstrual cycle: 120–440 pg/ml. Late menstrual cycle: 150–350 pg/ml. Postmenopausal: less than 30 pg/ml. *Male:* 40–115 pg/ml.
Child: 1–6 years: 3–10 pg/ml; 8–12 years: less than 30 pg/ml.

Description
Estrogens are produced by the ovaries, adrenal cortex, and testes. There are over 30 estrogens identified in the body, but only three measurable types of estrogens: estrone (E_1), estradiol (E_2), and estriol (E_3). Total serum estrogen reflects estrone, mostly estradiol, and some estriol. For fetal well-being during pregnancy, serum E_3 is used.

FERRITIN (SERUM)
Reference Values
Adult: *Female:* 10–235 ng/ml, 10–235 mcg/l (SI units). *Male:* 15–445 ng/ml, 15–445 mcg/l (SI units). *Postmenopausal:* 10–310 ng/ml.
Child: *1–16 years:* 8–140 ng/ml. *Infant:* 2–12 months: 30–200 ng/ml; 1 month: 200–550 ng/ml. Newborn: 20–200 ng/ml.

Description
Ferritin, an iron-storage protein, is produced in the liver, spleen, and bone marrow. The ferritin levels are related to the amount of iron stored in the body tissues. It will release iron from tissue reserve as needed and will store excess iron to prevent damage effects from iron overload. One

NURSING IMPLICATIONS WITH RATIONALE
Esophagogastroduodenoscopy

- Recognize that a gastroscopy test for visualizing the esophageal, gastric, and duodenal mucosa is actually an esophagogastroduodenoscopy. These names are frequently used interchangeably.
- Check that the clients dentures, eyeglasses, and jewelry are removed. Give the client a hospital gown.
- Have the client void. Take vital signs.
- Check that a consent form has been signed before giving the client premedications. Once the sedative and the narcotic analgesic are given, the client should remain in bed with the bed sides up. Tell him or her that these medications will cause drowsiness.
- Be a good listener. Allow the client time to ask questions and to express concerns or fears. Refer questions you cannot answer to the gastroenterologist or health care provider.

CLIENT TEACHING
POSTTEST

- Explain the procedure to the client. Inform the client that the instrument is flexible; the procedure will be done under local anesthesia (the throat will be sprayed); premedications will be given before the test and usually IV sedation is given with the test; dentures and jewelry should be removed; and food and fluids will be restricted for 8 to 12 hours before the test.
- Explain to the client that he or she may feel some pressure with the insertion of the endoscope and may feel some fullness in the stomach when air is injected for better visualization of the stomach and intestine areas.
- Check the gag reflex before offering food and fluids by asking the client to swallow or by touching the posterior pharynx with a cotton swab or tongue blade if the throat was sprayed with an anesthetic.
- Keep the client NPO for 2 to 4 hours after the test or as ordered.
- Monitor vital signs (blood pressure, pulse, respirations) as ordered.
- Give the client throat lozenges or analgesics for throat discomfort. Inform the client that he or she may have flatus or "burp-up gas," which is normal. This is caused by the instillation of air during the procedure for visualization Purposes.
- Observe the client for possible complications (e.g., perforation in the gastrointestinal tract from the endoscope). Symptoms could include pain (epigastric, abdominal, back pain), dyspnea, fever, tachycardia, and subcutaneous emphysema in the neck.
- Be supportive of the client and family.

nanogram per milliliter of serum ferritin corresponds to 8 mg of stored iron.

Serum ferritin level is useful in evaluating the total body storage of iron. It can detect early iron deficiency anemia and anemias due to chronic disease that resemble iron deficiency. Serum ferritin is not affected by hemolysis and drugs.

FETAL NONSTRESS TEST (NST) AND CONTRACTION STRESS TEST (CST)
Description
The fetal nonstress test (NST) and the contraction stress test (CST) are two diagnostic tests used to help evaluate fetal functioning and well-being in response to either fetal movement (NST) or to spontaneous or induced uterine contraction (CST). The **NST** is inexpensive, rapidly accomplished, lacks side effects, and is helpful in identifying at-risk fetuses of mothers who exhibit high-risk pregnancy conditions, including diabetes, intrauterine growth retardation, pregnancy induced hypertension, report by mother of decreased fetal movements, among others. Only minimal equipment is required (external transducer for fetal heart rate monitoring); testing occurs 1 to 2 times per week depending on the reason for doing the testing. The **CST** is also employed at 32 to 34 weeks in evaluating high-risk pregnancies, particularly pregnancy conditions which may place the fetus at risk if there is poor placental perfusion including diabetes, intrauterine growth retardation, and postterm gestation over 42 weeks. In addition, certain fetuses who exhibit a nonreactive NST in the presence of additional data may also have a CST performed. Contraindications to CST testing include presence of a classical uterine incision, presence of placenta previa, multiple gestation, and vaginal bleeding, among others. Equipment required for CSTs includes an external transducer (for FHR monitoring), together with a tocodynamometer (toco) for monitoring uterine contractions. The NST and CST are able to be performed in hospital, office, and clinic settings; the NST may also be conducted in the home care setting with supervision.

FETAL NONSTRESS TEST (NST) NST is a noninvasive test that monitors FHR with fetal movement. According to the ACOG, the FHR should increase by 15 bpm within a 20-minute interval. If there is no fetal movement or increased FHR in 20 minutes, the mothers abdomen may be rubbed or a loud noise made close to the abdomen to stimulate fetal movement. If after 40 minutes there is no acceleration of FHR, the NST is nonreactive and a CST may be ordered. With a nonreactive NST after 40 minutes, fetal distress may be considered; however, the fetus may be in a sleep cycle or the mother may have taken a CNS depressant drug. The NST is usually performed at 30 weeks of gestation to allow for sufficient CNS maturation after which heart rate accelerations in response to movement become more fully established.

CONTRACTION STRESS TEST (CST) There are two types of CST; the nipple stimulation test and the oxytocin challenge test (OCT). The nipple stimulation test is a noninvasive test that stimulates the hypothalamus which promotes the release of oxytocin. This can cause uterine contractions, and a normal result would be that the FHR does not show late deceleration. The OCT is somewhat noninvasive but could induce labor in some clients. Oxytocin, a uterine stimulant, is well diluted in IV fluids and thus does not cause continuous contractions. There should be 3 moderate contractions occurring within 10 minutes, and the FHR should not show any late deceleration. If there is a late deceleration of FHR with contractions, the test indicates that hypoxia may result during labor due to insufficient placental function. The CST with oxytocin is performed at 32 weeks, preferably 34 weeks of gestation. In case this test would induce labor, the fetus would have a better chance to survive.

HEMATOCRIT (HCT) (BLOOD)
Reference Values

Adult: *Male:* 40–54%, 0.40–0.54 (SI units). *Female:* 36–46%, 0.36–0.46 (SI units). *Panic Value:* less than 15% and greater than 60%.
Child: *Newborn:* 44–65%. *1 to 3 Years Old:* 29–40%. *4 to 10 Years Old:* 31–43%.

Description

The hematocrit (Hct) is the volume (in milliliters) of packed red blood cells (RBCs) found in 100 ml (1 dl) of blood, expressed as a percentage. For example, a 36% hematocrit would indicate that 36 ml of RBCs were found in 100 ml of blood, or 36 vol/dl. The purpose of the test is to measure the concentration of RBCs (erythrocytes) in the blood.

Low hematocrits are found frequently in anemias and leukemias, and elevated levels are found in dehydration (a relative increase) and polycythemia vera. The hematocrit can be an indicator of the hydration status of the client. As with hemoglobin, an elevated hematocrit could indicate hemoconcentration because of a decrease in fluid volume and an increase in RBCs.

Factors Affecting Laboratory Results

■ If blood is collected from an extremity that has an IV line, the hematocrit will most likely be low. Avoid using such an extremity.
■ If blood is taken to check the hematocrit immediately after moderate to severe blood loss and transfusions, the hematocrit could be normal.
■ Age of the clientnewborns normally have higher hematocrits because of hemoconcentration.

HEMOGLOBIN (HB OR HGB) (BLOOD)
Reference Values

Adult: *Male:* 13.5–17 g/dl. *Female:* 12–15 g/dl.
Child: *Newborn:* 14–24 g/dl. *Infant:* 10–17 g/dl.
Child: 11–16 g/dl.

Description

Hemoglobin (Hb or Hgb), a protein substance found in red blood cells (RBCs), gives blood its red color. Hemoglobin is composed of iron, which is an oxygen carrier. Abnormally high hemoglobin levels may be due to hemoconcentration resulting from dehydration (fluid loss). Low hemoglobin values are related to various clinical problems. The RBC count and hemoglobin level do not always increase or decrease equally. For instance, a decreased RBC count and a normal or slightly decreased hemoglobin level occur in pernicious anemia, and a normal or slightly decreased RBC and a decreased hemoglobin level occur in iron deficiency (microcytic) anemia.

Factors Affecting Laboratory Results

■ Drugs could increase or decrease hemoglobin (*see Drug Influence*).
■ Taking blood from an arm or hand receiving IV fluids could dilute blood sample.
■ Leaving the tourniquet on for more than a minute will cause hemostasis, which will result in a falsely elevated hemoglobin level.
■ Living in high altitudes will increase hemoglobin levels.
■ Decreased fluid intake or fluid loss will increase hemoglobin levels due to hemoconcentration, and excessive fluid intake will decrease hemoglobin levels due to hemodilution.

HEMOGLOBIN A_1c (HGB A_1c OR HB A_1c) (BLOOD)

Glycosylated Hemoglobin (Hgb A_1a, Hgb A_1b, Hgb A_1c, Glycohemoglobin)

Reference Values

Total Glycosylated Hemoglobin: 5.59% of total Hgb (Hb).
Adult: *Hgb (Hb) A_1c:* Nondiabetic: 25%; Diabetic Control: 2.56%; high average; 6.17.5%; Diabetic Uncontrolled: greater than 8%.
Child: *Hgb (Hb) A_1c:* Nondiabetic: 1.54%.

Description

Hemoglobin A (Hgb or Hb A) comprises 91 to 95% of total hemoglobin. Glucose molecule is attached to Hb A_1, which is a portion of hemoglobin A. This process of attachment is called *glycosylation* or *glycosylated hemoglobin* or *hemoglobin A_1*. There is a bond between glucose and hemoglobin. Formation of Hb A_1 occurs slowly over 120 days, the life span of red blood cells (RBCs). Hb A_1 is composed of three hemoglobin molecules, Hb A_1a, Hb A_1b, and Hb A_1c of which 70% Hb A_1c is 70% glycosylated (absorbs glucose). The amount of glycosylated hemoglobin depends on the amount of blood glucose available. When the blood glucose level is elevated over a prolonged period of time, the red blood cells (RBCs) become saturated with glucose; glycohemoglobin results.

A glycosylated hemoglobin represents an average blood glucose level during a 1- to 4-month period. This test is used mainly as a measurement of the effectiveness of diabetic therapy. Fasting blood sugar reflects the blood glucose level at a 1-time fasting state; whereas, the Hgb or Hb A_1c is a better indicator of diabetes mellitus control. However, a false decreased Hb A_1c level can be caused by a decrease in red blood cells.

An elevated Hb A_1c greater than 8% indicates uncontrolled diabetes mellitus, and the client is at a high risk of developing long-term complications, such as nephropathy, retinopathy, neuropathy, and/or cardiopathy. Total glycohemoglobin may be a better indicator of diabetes control for clients with anemias or blood loss.

Factors Affecting Laboratory Results
■ Anemias may cause a low value result.
■ Hemolysis of the blood specimen can cause an inaccurate test result.
■ Heparin therapy may cause false test result.

HOLTER MONITORING
Description
Holter monitoring (ambulatory electrocardiography) evaluates the clients heart rate and rhythm during normal daily activities, rest, and sleep over 24 hours (occasionally 48 hours). The Holter monitor consists of a continuous electrocardiogram (ECG) recording on a cassette tape that is boxed inside an approximately 1-lb monitor. After 24 hours, the monitor with the tape is returned to the cardiac center and is scanned or reviewed for abnormal findings such as cardiac dysrhythmias.

Holter monitoring began 30 years ago and it is widely used today. The Holter recorder contains a clock that is coordinated with the tape recorder and an event marker for the client to use when having symptom(s). The client is given a diary to record the symptoms such as palpitations, chest pain, shortness of breath, syncope, vertigo, and the time of the symptoms.

The primary purpose for Holter monitoring is to identify suspected and unsuspected cardiac dysrhythmias, which can be correlated between the recorder, event marking of symptoms, and transient symptoms marked in the diary. It is infrequently ordered for clients having Prinzmetals variant angina, a form of myocardial ischemia that results from spasms of the coronary arteries. Holter monitoring is more sensitive for identifying the cause of the symptoms than a routine ECG.

Procedure
■ A signed consent form may be required.
■ There is no food or fluid restriction.
■ The skin is cleansed and shaved as needed, and electrodes are placed over bony areas to eliminate artifacts that could be caused by skeletal muscle movements.
■ Five to seven electrode patches are placed on the chest. For a five-lead electrode placement, two negative electrodes are secured at the upper right and left manubrial border of the sternum, and two positive electrodes are placed below the sternum, one placed at 2 cm right of the xiphoid process on the rib margin and the second at the left anterior axillary line—6th rib. A ground electrode is secured at the lower right rib margin over the bone.
■ The client is given a diary to record what he or she was doing when symptom(s) such as palpitations, chest pain, and shortness of breath occured.
■ The client should not shower, take a bath, or swim until the electrodes are removed. Also avoid vigorous exercise and sweating.

Posttest
■ The client returns the Holter monitor the next day (24 hours later) with the diary.
■ The nurse/technician reviews the diary with the client for any needed clarification.
■ The tape is scanned (reviewed) and the cardiologist submits a written report to the personal health care provider. The clients health care provider explains the ECG monitoring results to the client.

HUMAN CHORIONIC GONADOTROPIN (HCG) (SERUM AND URINE)
Reference Values
Values may be expressed as international unit/ml or ng/ml. Check with your laboratory.

Adult: *Serum:* Nonpregnant female: less than 0.01 international unit/ml.

Pregnant (Weeks)	Values
1	0.01–0.04 IU/ml
2	0.03–0.10 IU/ml
4	0.10–1.0 IU/ml
5–12	10–100 IU/ml
13–25	10–30 IU/ml
26–40	5–15 IU/ml

Urine: Nonpregnant: negative; pregnant: 1–12 weeks: 6000–500,000 international unit/24 h. Many OTC pregnancy kits available. The woman is usually tested 5 to 14 days after missed menstrual period.

Description
Human chorionic gonadotropin (HCG) is a hormone produced by the placenta. In pregnancy HCG appears in the blood and urine 14 to 26 days after the conception, and the HCG concentration peaks in approximately 8 weeks. After the first trimester of pregnancy, HCG production declines. HCG is not found in nonpregnant women, in death of the fetus, or after 3 to 4 days postpartum.

The immunologic test for pregnancy using anti-HCG serum is more sensitive, more accurate, less costly, and easier to perform than the older pregnancy test, which used live animals. The Aschheim-Zondek test and the Friedman test are no longer used.

Certain tumors (such as the hydatidiform mole, chorionepithelioma of the uterus, and choriocarcinoma of the testicle) can cause a positive HCG test. HCG levels may be requested on males for the determination of testicular tumor.

Procedure

- There is no food restriction.
- Perform the pregnancy test 2 weeks (no earlier than 5 days) after the first missed menstrual period. There are several commercially prepared kits for the immunologic pregnancy test.

Serum

- Perform the pregnancy test no earlier than 5 days after the first missed menstrual period.
- Collect 3 to 5 ml of venous blood in a red-top tube. Avoid hemolysis.

Urine

- The client should be NPO of fluid for 8 to 12 hours; no food is restricted.
- Take a morning urine specimen (60 ml) with specific gravity greater than 1.010 to the laboratory immediately. A 24-hour urine collection may be requested.
- Instruct the client to follow directions when using a commercial kit.
- Avoid blood in the urine, as false-positive results could occur.

  Note: There are many commercial kits; follow the directions on kit.

Factors Affecting Laboratory Results

- Diluted urine (specific gravity less than 1.010) could cause a false-negative test result.
- Certain drug groups can cause false-positive test results *(see Drug Influence)*.
- Protein and blood in the urine could cause false-positive test results.
- During menopause, there may be an excess secretion of pituitary gonadotropin hormone, which could cause a false-positive result.

HUMAN IMMUNODEFICIENCY VIRUS TYPE-1 (HIV-1) OR HIV* (SERUM)

Reference Values

Antibody screening: *HIV-1/2 antibody screen (ELISA, EIA)*
Adult and Child: Seronegative for antibodies to HIV-1/2; nonreactive.*
Child: Seronegative for antibodies to HIV 1/2 nonreactive.

HIV-1 and HIV-2 Western blot (confirmatory test that directly detects HIV viral gene proteins).

Adult and Child: Negative.
Antigen screening: *HIV-1 p24 Antigen.*
Adult and Child: Negative for p24 antigen of HIV; nonreactive.

Note: There is no HIV-2 p24 antigen test; confirmatory test for the HIV-1 p24 antigen is a neutralization.

Viral load tests: Sensitive assay that measures levels of HIVs ribonucleic acid (RNA) in plasma (to predict disease course). Uses polymerase chain reaction (PCR) to amplify HIV RNA. Used as a marker for basing treatment decisions and evaluating effectiveness of anti-HIV drug therapy (rechecked 48 weeks after changes in drug therapy as monitor monitoring technique). Expressed as the number of copies of HIV RNA in a 1-ml sample of plasma.
Low numbers: Represents suppressed replication.
High numbers: Represents increased replication and disease progression.

Description

HIV viral antigen may become detectable within approximately two to three weeks after infection. The outcome is a decrease in CD4+ T lymphocyte count, increased viral load, and the stimulation of the body's immune response; as antibodies to HIV and new CD4+ T lymphocyte cells are produced, the amount of viral load decreases. During the period of initial infection, it is estimated that about half of infected individuals remain asymptomatic while others may experience an influenza-type illness (low-grade fever, muscle aches, sweating, rash, sore throat, headache, fatigue, swollen lymph nodes). The client recovers, but during this two to twelve week period, antibodies against HIV are formed as part of the immune response. The Centers for Disease Control and Prevention Counsel that the average length of time for production of antibodies to HIV is 25 days (some earlier and some later) but that most individuals will seroconvert by 3 months allowing for antibody detection using the ELISA, EIA antibody tests and Western Blot confirmatory test. Addition of the HIV-1 antigen test may identify HIV infection in an individual within twoweeks (approximately a week earlier than the Anti-HIV-1/2 test), thus narrowing the vulnerable period when the virus may be passed to others while antibody-based screening tests cannot detect it. Care is called for however, since a negative test may mean that there is a not yet detectable viral level.

IMMUNOGLOBULINS (IG) (SERUM)

Reference Values

	Total Ig (99% mg/dl)	IgG (80% mg/dl)	IgA (15% mg/dl)
Adult	900–2,200	650–1,700	70–400
6–16 yr	800–1,700	700–1,650	80–230
46 yr	700–1,700	550–1,500	50–175
13 yr	400–1,500	300–1,400	20–150
6 mo	225–1,200	200–1,100	10–90
3 mo	325–750	275–750	5–55
Newborn	650–1,450	700–1,480	0–12

	IgM (4% mg/dl)	IgD (0.2% mg/dl)	IgE (0.0002% U/ml)
Adult	40–350	0–8	<40
		(IgE 0120 mg/dl)	
6–16 yr	45–260		<62
46 yr	22–100		<25
13 yr	40–230		<10
6 mo	10–80		
3 mo	15–70		
Newborn	5–30		

INSULIN (SERUM), INSULIN ANTIBODY

Reference Values

Adult: *Serum Insulin:* 5–25 micro-unit/ml, 10–250 micro-international unit/ml. *Panic Value:* 7 unit/ml (7 μU/ml).
Insulin Antibody Test: less than 4% serum binding of pork and beef insulin.

Description

Insulin, a hormone from the beta cells of the pancreas, is essential in transporting glucose to the cells for metabolism. Increased glucose levels stimulate insulin secretion.

Serum insulin and blood glucose levels are compared to determine the glucose disorder. Serum insulin is valuable in diagnosing insulinoma (islet cell tumor) and islet cell hyperplasia and in evaluating insulin production in diabetes mellitus. In insulinoma the serum insulin is high, and blood glucose is less than 30 mg/dl. Hyperinsulinemia can occur in obesity as well as in insulinoma.

The **insulin antibody test** is ordered when a diabetic, taking pork or beef insulin, requires larger and larger insulin dosages. Insulin antibodies develop as the result of impurities in animal insulins. These antibodies are of immunoglobulin types (i.e., IgG [most], IgM, IgE). The IgG antibodies neutralize the insulin, thus preventing glucose metabolism. IgM antibodies can cause insulin resistance, and IgE could be responsible for allergic effects.

INTERNATIONAL NORMALIZED RATIO (INR) (PLASMA)

Reference Values

Oral Anticoagulant Therapy: 2.0–3.0 INR.
Higher Value for Mechanical Heart Value: 2.5–3.5 INR.

Description

The international normalized ratio (INR) was devised to monitor more correctly anticoagulant therapy for clients receiving warfarin (Coumadin) therapy. The World Health Organization (WHO) recommends the use of INR for a more consistent reporting of prothrombin time results. The INR is calculated by the use of a nomogram demonstrating the relationship between the INR and the prothrombin time (PT) ratio. Usually both PT and INR values are reported for monitoring Coumadin therapy.

INTRAVENOUS PYELOGRAPHY (IVP)

Description

Intravenous pyelography (IVP) is more properly called *excretory urography,* because it visualizes the entire urinary tract and not just the kidney pelvis. A radiopaque substance (sodium diatrizoate or meglumine diatrizoate [Renografin-60]) is injected intravenously and a series of x-rays are taken at specific times. The test usually takes 30 to 45 minutes.

Excretory urography is useful for locating stones and tumors and for diagnosing kidney diseases (i.e., polycystic kidney, renovascular hypertension). A few clients may be hypersensitive to the radiopaque iodine dye, especially if they have a history of allergy to many substances. Emergency drugs (epinephrine, vasopressors, etc.), a tracheostomy set, a suction machine, and oxygen should be available for treating anaphylactoid reaction if it should occur.

Procedure

- A consent form for IVP should be signed by the client or an appropriate member of the family.
- The client should be NPO for 8 to 12 hours before the test. In the morning the client may be slightly dehydrated; however, this will help the kidney to concentrate the dye.
- A laxative is ordered the night before, and a cleansing enema(s) is ordered the morning of the test. These preparations may vary, so check with the radiology department for exact preparations.
- An antihistamine or a steroid may be given prior to the test to clients who are hypersensitive to iodine, seafood, and contrast dye used in other diagnostic tests as well as to those who have histories of asthma and severe allergies.
- Baseline vital signs should be recorded.
- The client lies in the supine position on an x-ray table. X-rays are taken 3, 5, 10, 15, and 20 minutes after the dye is injected.
- Emergency drugs and equipment should be available at all times.
- The test takes approximately 30 to 45 minutes. A delay in visualizing the kidneys could indicate kidney dysfunction.
- The client voids at the end of the test and another x-ray is taken to visualize the residual dye in the bladder.

Factors Affecting Diagnostic Results

- Feces, gas, and barium in the intestinal tract can decrease visualization of the kidney, ureters, and bladder.

NURSING IMPLICATIONS WITH RATIONALE · Intravenous Pyelography

- Obtain a client history of known allergies. Notify the health care provider (HCP) if the client is allergic to seafood, iodine preparations, or contrast dye. As a precaution, an antihistamine or a steroid drug may be ordered if the client has an allergic reaction to drugs. A skin test may be performed to determine how hypersensitive the client is to the radiopaque contrast dye.
- Check the blood urea nitrogen (BUN). If BUN levels are greater than 40 mg/dl, notify the HCP. Normally the test would not be done.

CLIENT TEACHING

- Explain to the client that the purpose of the test is to detect any kidney disorder or to observe the size, shape, and structure of the kidney, ureters, and bladder.
- Explain the procedure to the client. As a reminder, the procedural steps could be listed for the client.
- Instruct the client that he or she is not to eat or drink after dinner. Mild dehydration usually occurs. This could be harmful to clients with poor renal output, especially the aged and the debilitated. Sips of water or a glass of water may be indicated to avoid complications.

- Inform the client that he or she may feel a transient flushing or burning sensation and a salty or metallic taste during or following the IV injection of the contrast dye.
- Encourage the client to ask questions and to express any concerns before and during the procedure to the nurse, radiologist, and technician.

POSTTEST

- Monitor vital signs and urinary output.
- Observe, report, and record possible delayed reactions to the contrast dye (i.e., dyspnea, rashes, flushing, urticaria [hives], tachycardia, and others).
- Check the site where the dye was injected (usually it is in the antecubital fossa vein). If pain, warmth, or redness at the injection site is present, apply warm compresses, with permission.
- Administer oral antihistamines or steroids as ordered to treat dye reactions.

IRON (Fe), TOTAL IRON BINDING CAPACITY (TIBC), TRANSFERRIN, TRANSFERRIN SATURATION (SERUM)

Reference Values

	Serum Iron	TIBC
Adult	50–150 mcg/dl	250–450 mcg/dl
	10–27 μmol/l (SI units)	
	Males slightly higher	
Elderly	60–80 mcg/dl	<250 mcg/dl
Child		
Newborn	100–270 mcg/dl	60–175 mcg/dl
Infant		100–400 mcg/dl
6 months–2 years	40–100 mcg/dl	100–135 mcg/dl
>2 years		40–100 mcg/dl

	Serum Transferrin	Transferrin Saturation
Adult	200–430 mg/dl	30–50% (male)
		20–35% (female)
Elderly		
Child		
Newborn	125–275 mg/dl	
Infant		
6 months–2 years		
>2 years		

Description

Iron is absorbed from the duodenum and upper jejunum; the amount absorbed usually covers the amount of iron that has been lost. The average daily iron intake is 10–20 mg.

Iron is coupled with the iron-transporting protein **transferrin**. Transferrin is responsible for transporting iron to the bone marrow for the purpose of hemoglobin synthesis (*see Transferrin*). The storage compound for iron is ferritin (*see Ferritin*). Serum iron levels are elevated when there is excessive red blood cell destruction (hemolysis), and levels are decreased in iron deficiency anemia.

Total iron-binding capacity (TIBC) measures the maximum amount of iron that can bind to the protein transferrin. The level of TIBC decreases with age. Usually, serum iron and TIBC are determined together.

Transferrin can be measured as serum and as a percent of saturation (transferrin saturation). The transferrin saturation is the ratio between serum iron and TIBC relating to the availability of transerrin in binding with iron. Transferrin saturation is given in percent.

Serum iron, TIBC, transerrin, and transferrin saturation values are needed to adequately diagnose iron deficiency anemia and other disorders. The table below gives the various tests used for diagnosing health problems related to iron and transferrin imbalances.

SERUM IRON, TIBC, TRANSFERRIN, AND TRANSFERRIN SATURATION

Serum Iron	TIBC	Transferrin
Low	High	High
Low	Low	Low
High	Normal or low	Low

SERUM IRON, TIBC, TRANSFERRIN, AND TRANSFERRIN SATURATION

Transferrin Saturation	Health Problems
Low	Iron deficiency anemia
Normal	Chronic illness: cancer, infection, cirrhosis
Very high	Iron therapy overload

LACTIC ACID (BLOOD)

Reference Values

Adult: *Arterial Blood:* 0.5–2.0 mmol/l (SI units), less than 11.3 mg/dl. *Venous Blood:* 0.5–1.5 mmol/l, 8.11–5.3 mg/dl. *Panic Range:* greater than 5 mEq/l, greater than 45 mg/dl.

Description

Blood lactic acid or lactate is an indicator of the presence of lactic acidosis. Lactic acidosis is suspected if the anion gap is greater than 17 mEq/l and pH is decreased.

Shock and severe dehydration cause cell catabolism (cell breakdown) and an accumulation of acid metabolites, such as lactic acid. Excess lactic acid can decrease pH and cause lactic acidosis.

LACTIC (LACTATE) DEHYDROGENASE (LD OR LDH), LDH ISOENZYMES (SERUM)

Reference Values

Adult: *Total LDH:* 100–190 international unit/l, 70–250 unit/l. Values can differ according to the method used.
Isoenzymes: LDH_1, 14–26%; LDH_2, 27–37%; LDH_3, 13–26%; LDH_4, 8–16%; LDH_5, 6–16%. Differences of 2% to 4% are considered normal.
Child: *Newborn:* 300–1500 international unit/l. *Child:* 50–150 international unit/l; 110–295 unit/l.

Description

Lactic dehydrogenase (LDH) is an intracellular enzyme present in nearly all metabolizing cells, with the highest concentrations in the heart, skeletal muscle, liver, kidney, brain, and red blood cells (RBCs). LDH has two distinct subunits—M (muscle) and H (heart). These subunits are combined in different formations to make five isoenzymes.

- LDH_1: cardiac fraction; H, H, H, H; in heart, RBCs, kidneys, brain (some).
- LDH_2: cardiac fraction; H, H, H, M; in heart, RBCs, kidneys, brain (some).
- LDH_3: pulmonary fraction; H, H, M, M; in lungs and other tissues; spleen, pancreas, adrenal, thyroid, lymphatics.
- LDH_4: hepatic fraction; H, M, M, M; liver, skeletal muscle, kidneys and brain (some).
- LDH_5: hepatic fraction; M, M, M, M; liver, skeletal muscle, kidneys (some).

Like other enzymatic tests, such as the creatine phosphokinase (CPK) and aspartate aminotransferase (AST) tests, serum LDH and LDH_1 are used for diagnosing acute myocardial infarction (MI). A high serum LDH (total) level occurs 12 to 24 hours after the infarction, reaches its peak in 2 to 5 days, and remains elevated for 6 to 12 days, making it a useful test for delayed diagnosis of MI. A flipped LDH_1/LDH_2 ratio, with LDH_1 the highest, indicates a myocardial infarction.

LDH_3 is linked to pulmonary diseases, and LDH_5 is linked to liver and skeletal muscle diseases. In acute hepatitis, total LDH rises, and the LDH_5 usually rises before jaundice develops and falls before the bilirubin level does.

LAPAROSCOPY

Description

Laparoscopy is the insertion of a laparoscope through the abdominal wall into the peritoneum to visualize the abdominal and pelvic organs. A light camera is usually attached to the scope for visualization, and the peritoneal cavity is filled with liters of carbon dioxide gas to increase the view and separate the abdominal wall from the organs.

The **laparoscopy and pelviscopy** are useful for diagnosing endometriosis, ovarian cyst, tubal pregnancy, uterine fibroids, benign and malignant tumors, pelvic inflammatory disease (PID), salpingitis, cause of infertility, and adhesions. Surgical procedure can be performed with laparoscopy, such as biopsy specimens, tubal ligation, release of adhesions, and laser treatment for endometriosis.

Peritoneoscopy is primarily prescribed to view the liver and to stage cancers including lymphomas. It can be used for surgical procedures such as cholecystectomy, appendectomy, hernia repairs including hiatal hernia, bowel resection, and biopsies. Laparoscopy and peritoneoscopy overlap somewhat with their surgical procedures. These tests are usually performed with general anesthesia.

Contraindications for a laparoscopy include advanced abdominal wall cancer, severe bleeding disorder, and severe respiratory and/or cardiac disorders.

Procedures

Pretest
- A signed consent form is required.
- Nothing by mouth after midnight or 8 to 12 hours prior to the test procedure.
- Anticoagulant therapy should be discontinued 5 to 7 days prior to the test.
- Laboratory tests ordered prior to the test.
- Cleansing enemas as ordered the night before the procedure and/or in the morning.
- Client should void before the procedure.

NURSING IMPLICATIONS WITH RATIONALE

Laparoscopy

- Obtain a history of the client's health problem. Relate findings to other health professionals.
- Check baseline vital signs. These vital signs are compared with those during the test procedure and during the posttest time.
- Report gas pains that remain beyond 24 to 36 hours and any frank bleeding from incision site.
- Follow the posttest procedure.

CLIENT TEACHING

- Explain to the client to take analgesics as ordered to relieve pain and discomfort due to the gas that was inserted in the abdomen. Inform the client that all the gas in the abdomen is not always released from the procedure; it may take 24 hours.
- Instruct the client to report pain that lasts for 48 hours or more and any bright bleeding that occurs at the incisional site.
- Answer the client's questions and if unable to, refer the questions to the primary health care provider or other professionals.

- IV infusion started. IV medications may be given through the IV line.

Test Procedure
- Small surgical incision is made below the umbilicus.
- The peritoneal cavity is filled with carbon dioxide gas so that the organs can easily be visualized.
- Laparoscope is inserted through a trocar.
- After the procedure, carbon dioxide escapes; however, not all of the gas is removed but will be slowly eliminated from the body over a period of 24 hours.

Posttest
- Vital signs are monitored and bleeding from the small incisional area is checked periodically.
- Analgesics for pain and for shoulder or subcostal discomfort caused by carbon dioxide gas may be given every 4 to 6 hours.
- Physical activity should be minimized for 4 to 7 days posttest or as instructed by the health care provider.

Factors Affecting Diagnostic Results
- Excessive adhesions.
- Severely obese.

LEAD (BLOOD)
Reference Values

Adult: *Normal:* 10–20 mcg/dl. *Acceptable:* 20–40 mcg/dl. *Excessive:* 40–80 mcg/dl. *Toxic:* 80 mcg/dl.
Child: *Normal:* 10–20 mcg/dl. *Acceptable:* 20–30 mcg/dl. *Excessive:* 30–50 mcg/dl. *Toxic:* 50 mcg/dl.

Description

Excessive lead exposure due to occupational contact is a hazard to adults; however, most industries will accept a 40-mcg/dl blood lead level as a normal value. Lead toxicity can occur in children from eating chipped, lead-based paint found in old houses. Sources of lead include leaded gasoline (fumes), lead-based paint, unglazed pottery, and "moonshine" whiskey prepared in lead containers.

Lead is usually excreted rapidly in the urine, but if excessive lead exposure persists, the lead will accumulate in the bone and soft tissues. Chronic lead poisoning is more common than acute poisoning. Lead colic (crampy abdominal pain) occurs in both acute and chronic lead poisoning.

LECITHIN/SPHINGOMYELIN (L/S) RATIO (AMNIOTIC FLUID)
Reference Values

Before 35 Weeks of Gestation: 1:1. *Lecithin (L):* 6–9 mg/dl. *Sphingomyelin (S):* 4–6 mg/dl.

After 35 Weeks of Gestation: 4:1. *Lecithin (L):* 15–21 mg/dl. *Sphingomyelin (S):* 4–6 mg/dl.

Description

The lecithin/sphingomyelin (L/S) ratio can be used to predict neonatal respiratory distress syndrome (also called hyaline membrane disease) before delivery. Lecithin (L), a phospholipid, is responsible mostly for the formation of alveolar surfactant. Surfactant lubricates the alveolar lining and inhibits alveolar collapse, thus preventing atelectasis. Sphingomyelin (S) is another phospholipid, the value of which remains the same throughout pregnancy. A marked rise in amniotic lecithin after 35 weeks (to a level three or four times higher than that of sphingomyelin) is considered normal, and so chances for having hyaline membrane disease are small. The L/S ratio is also used to determine fetal maturity in the event that the gestation period is uncertain. In this situation, the L/S ratio is determined at intervals of a period of several weeks.

Procedure
- Consent form should be signed.
- There is no food, fluid, or drug restriction.
- The physician obtains amniotic fluid by the method of amniocentesis. The specimen should be cooled immediately to prevent the destruction of lecithin by certain enzymes in the amniotic fluid. The specimen should be frozen if testing cannot be done at a specified time (check with the laboratory).
- Care should be taken to prevent puncture of the mothers bladder. If urine in the specimen is suspected, then the specimen should be tested for urea and potassium. If these two levels are higher than blood levels, the specimen could be urine and not amniotic fluid. Ultrasound is frequently used when obtaining amniotic fluid.

Factors Affecting Laboratory Results
- Maternal vaginal secretions or a bloody tap into the amniotic fluid may cause a falsely increased reading for lecithin.
- The amniotic fluid specimen should be tested immediately to prevent inaccurate results.

LIPASE (SERUM)

Reference Values

Adult: 20–180 international unit/l, 114–286 unit/l, 14–280 unit/l (SI units). Norms vary among laboratories.

Child: *Infant:* 9–105 international unit/l at 37°C. *Child:* 20–136 international unit/l at 37°C.

Description

Lipase, an enzyme secreted by the pancreas, aids in digesting fats. Lipase, like amylase, appears in the blood stream following damage to the pancreas. Acute pancreatitis is the commonest cause for an elevated serum lipase level. Lipase and amylase levels increase early in the disease, but serum lipase can be elevated for up to 14 days after an acute episode, whereas the serum amylase returns to normal after approximately 3 days. Serum lipase is useful for a late diagnosis of acute pancreatitis.

LIPOPROTEINS, LIPOPROTEIN ELECTROPHORESIS, LIPIDS (SERUM)

Reference Values

Adult: *Total:* 400–800 mg/dl, 4–8 g/l (SI units). *Cholesterol:* 150–240 mg/dl (see test on cholesterol). *Triglycerides:* 10–190 mg/dl (see test on triglycerides). *Phospholipids:* 150–380 mg/dl.
LDL: 60160 mg/dl. *Risk for CHD:* High: greater than 160 mg/dl. Moderate: 130159 mg/dl. Low: less than 130 mg/dl. Desirable: 100 mg/dl.
HDL: 29–77 mg/dl. *Risk for CHD:* High: less than 35 mg/dl. Moderate: 35–45 mg/dl. Low: 46–59 mg/dl. Very low: greater than 60 mg/dl.
Child: *See tests on cholesterol and triglycerides.*

Description

Lipoproteins are lipids bound to protein, and the three main lipoproteins are cholesterol, triglycerides, and phospholipids. The two fractions of lipoproteins—alpha (α), high-density lipoproteins (HDL), and beta (B), low-density lipoproteins (chylomicrons, VLDL, LDL)—can be separated by electrophoresis. The beta groups are the largest contributors of atherosclerosis and coronary artery disease. HDL, called "friendly lipids," are composed of 50% protein and do aid in decreasing plaque deposits in blood vessels.

Increased lipoproteins (hyperlipidemia or hyperlipoproteinemia) can be phenotyped into five major types (I, IIA and IIB, III, IV, V). Cholesterol and triglycerides are the two lipids in each type found in varying amounts. With type II, the cholesterol is highly elevated, and the triglycerides are slightly increased. With type IV, the triglycerides are highly elevated, and the cholesterol is slightly increased. Types II and IV are the commonest phenotypes and are the most prevalent in atherosclerosis and coronary artery disease (CAD).

LIPOPROTEIN CLASSIFICATION

Subgroup Classes of Lipoproteins	Protein Composition (%)	Cholesterol (%)
Chylomicrons	2	3
Very low-density (VLDL, pre-beta)	10	10
Low-density (LDL, beta)	25	45
High-density (HDL, alpha)	50	20

Subgroup Classes of Lipoproteins	Triglycerides (%)	Phospholipids (%)
Chylomicrons	90	5
Very low-density (VLDL, pre-beta)	70	10
Low-density (LDL, beta)	10	20
High-density (HDL, alpha)	Trace	30

Adapted from Henry, J. B. *Todd-Sanford-Davidsohn: Clinical diagnosis and management by laboratory methods* (17th ed., p. 183), Philadelphia: Saunders, 1984.

LIPOPROTEIN PHENOTYPE: HYPERLIPIDEMIA

Type	Lipid Composition*
I	Increased chylomicrons, increased triglycerides; rare pattern of hyperlipidemia
IIA	Increased beta (low-density) lipoproteins (LDL); increased cholesterol, slightly increased triglycerides or normal; common pattern of hyperlipidemia
IIB	Increased beta and pre-beta lipoproteins, both cholesterol and triglycerides are elevated; common pattern of hyperlipidemia
III	Moderately increased cholesterol and triglycerides; uncommon pattern of hyperlipidemia
IV	Increase of pre-beta (very low-density) lipoproteins (VLDL); slightly increased cholesterol and markedly increased triglycerides; common pattern of hyperlipidemia
V	Increased chylomicrons, VLDL, and triglycerides, and slightly increased cholesterol; uncommon pattern of hyperlipidemia

*Types II and IV are increased in atherosclerosis and coronary artery diseases.

LITHIUM (SERUM)

Eskalith, Lithobid, Esthalith CR, Lithotabs, Cibalith

Reference Values

Adult: *Normal:* Negative. *Therapeutic:* 0.8–1.2 mEq/l. *Toxic:* greater than 1.5 mEq/l. *Lethal:* greater than 4.0 mEq/l.
Child: Not usually given to children.

LUTEINIZING HORMONE (LH) (SERUM AND URINE)

Reference Values

Ranges vary among laboratories.

Serum: *Adult:* Female: Follicular phase: 5–30 milliinternational unit/ml. Midcycle: 50–150 milliinternational unit/ml. Luteal phase: 2–25 milliinternational unit/ml. *Postmenopausal:* 40–100 milliinternational unit/ml. Male: 5–25 milliinternational unit/ml. *Child:* 6–12 years: less than 10 milliinternational unit/ml; 13–18 years: less than 20 milliinternational unit/ml.

Urine: *Adult:* Female: Follicular Phase: 5–25 international unit/24 h. Midcycle: 30–90 international unit/24 h. Luteal phase: 2–24 international unit/24 h. Postmenopausal: greater than 40 international unit/24h. Male: 7–25 international unit/ml.

Description

Luteinizing hormone (LH), gonadotropic hormone secreted by the anterior pituitary gland, is needed (with follicle-stimulating hormone [FSH]) for ovulation to occur. After ovulation, LH aids in stimulating the corpus luteum in secreting progesterone. FSH values are frequently evaluated with LH values. In men, LH stimulates testosterone production, and with FSH, they influence the development and maturation of spermatozoa.

LH is usually ordered to evaluate infertility in women and men. High-serum values are related to gonadal dysfunction, and low serum values are related to hypothalamus or pituitary failure. Women taking oral contraceptives have an absence of midcycle LH peak until the contraceptives are discontinued. This test might be used to evaluate hormonal therapy for inducing ovulation.

LYMPHOCYTES (T AND B) (BLOOD)

T and B Lymphocytes; Lymphocyte Marker Studies; Lymphocyte Subset Typing

Reference Values

Adult: *T Cells:* 6080%, 6002400 cells/µl. *B Cells:* 4–16%, 50–250 cells/µl.

Description

The two categories of lymphocytes are T lymphocytes and B lymphocytes. The T lymphocytes are associated with cell-mediated immune responses (cellular immunity), such as rejection of transplant and graft, tumor immunity, and microorganism (bacterial and viral) death. If the surface of the hosts tissue cell is altered, the T cells might perceive that altered cell as foreign and attack it. This might be helpful if the altered surface is of tumor development; however, this T-cell attack might give rise to autoimmune disease.

The B lymphocytes, derived from bone marrow, are responsible for humoral immunity. The B cells synthesize immunoglobulins to react to specific antigens. An interaction between T and B lymphocytes is necessary for a satisfactory immune response.

Measurement of T and B lymphocytes is valuable for diagnosing autoimmune diseases (i.e., immunosuppressive diseases such as acquired immunodeficiency syndrome [AIDS], lymphoma, and lymphocytic leukemia). T and B cells can be used to monitor changes during the treatment of immunosuppressive diseases.

MAGNESIUM (Mg) (SERUM)

Reference Values

Adult: 1.5–2.5 mEq/l, 1.8–3.0 mg/dl.
Child: *Newborn:* 1.4–2.9 mEq/l. *Child:* 1.6–2.6 mEq/l.

Description

Magnesium is most plentiful in the cells (intracellular fluid). One third of the magnesium ingested is absorbed through the small intestine, and the remaining unabsorbed magnesium is excreted in the stools. The absorbed magnesium is eventually excreted through the kidneys.

As with potassium, sodium, and calcium, magnesium is needed for neuromuscular activity. Magnesium influences use of potassium, calcium, and protein, and when there is a magnesium deficit, there is frequently a potassium and calcium deficit. Magnesium is also responsible for the transport of sodium and potassium across the cell membranes. Another function of magnesium is its activation of enzymes for carbohydrate and protein metabolism.

Magnesium is found in most foods, so it would be difficult for a person who maintains a normal diet to have a magnesium deficiency. The daily required magnesium intake for an adult is 200 to 300 mg, or 0.2 to 0.3 g.

A serum magnesium deficit is known as hypomagnesemia, and a serum magnesium excess is called hypermagnesemia.

MAGNETIC RESONANCE IMAGING (MRI)

Description

Magnetic resonance imaging (MRI) produces images similar to those produced by computed tomography (CT), however, unlike CT, it does not use ionizing radiation and thus is free of the hazards presented by exposure to x-rays. The cost of MRI is approximately one-third more than the cost of CT.

The MRI scanner consists of a magnet encased in a large, doughnut-shaped cylinder. The client lies on a narrow table and is guided into the cylinder until the body part to be imaged is within the magnetic field. The hydrogen nuclei of the cells of the body respond like magnets to the magnetic field and align. When a radio frequency wave is applied, the protons in the nuclei resonate, and when the radio frequency wave is removed, the energy released by the protons as they relax is detected as a radio signal. This signal is interpreted by a computer and translated into cross-sectional images.

Since the introduction of MRI in 1983, the quality of images produced by this technique has greatly improved, and MRI is now the most sensitive technique for defining the structure of internal organs and for detecting edema, infarction, hemorrhage, blood flow, tumors, infections, and plaques on the myelin sheath that cause Multiple Sclerosis. Many of these conditions would be difficult to distinguish using CT or conventional x-rays. It can differentiate between edema and tumor. MRI excels in diagnosing pathologic problems associated with the central nervous system (CNS), such as tumors, hemorrhage, edema, cerebral infarction, and subdural hematoma. Early after an ischemic stroke, imaging can detect the stroke's location and extent, and can determine the severity of the damage to the brain tissue. MRI can visualize bone, joint, and soft tissue injuries. Bone artifacts do not occur and MRI can identify a tumor adjacent to or within bony structures (e.g., pituitary gland tumor).

Pacemakers, wires left in the chest from a previous pacemaker, aneurysm or surgical intracranial clips and certain hearing aids are contraindications to undergoing an MRI procedure. Jewelry, watches, keys, credit cards, and hair clips must be removed prior to the procedure. When an emergency situation occurs during imaging, the client must be moved from the MRI room so that resuscitation equipment can be used. MRI is difficult to use to study critically ill clients on life-support systems because of the effect of the magnet on the equipment.

MRI and CT can be used for similar tissue studies. MRI involves use of contrast media in certain circumstances, but the IV contrast for MRI is chemically unrelated to the iodinated contrast used in CT and conventional radiography. Presently the only commercially available contrast for MRI is gadolinium-DTPA. Gadolinium (Magnavist) and Ferodax are frequently used to evaluate problems of the brain, base of the skull, and spine. This contrast agent can cross the "leaky" blood-brain barrier. Imaging can occur 5 to 60 minutes after the start of the gadolinium infusion.

MAGNETIC RESONANCE OF THE BRAIN AND SPINE (INTRACRANIAL [IC] MRI) Intracranial MRI gives cross-sectional images of the brain and spine. It can detect neuropathology through the bone such as visualizing fluid (edema) within soft tissues. The IC-MRI can identify cerebral thrombosis caused by cerebral vascular accident (stroke), cerebral tumors, abscesses, or aneurysms, cerebral hemorrhage, and demyelinated nerve fibers (myelin sheaths) causing multiple sclerosis (MS). It can also detail the abnormalities of the spinal cord and degenerated discs.

MAGNETIC RESONANCE OF THE HEART AND CORONARY ARTERIES Cine MRI, or ultrafast MRI, is a fast-moving MRI procedure that can image the heart in a continuous motion. It is useful for perfusion imaging, and it can determine the patency of coronary arteries following coronary grafts. Also, it is used to detect the viability of the myocardium and to assess chambers' volumes. The echo-planar MRI (EPI), like cine MRI, is used for rapid imaging of the heart and coronary arteries.

MAGNETIC RESONANCE ANGIOGRAPHY Magnetic resonance angiography (MRA) is a noninvasive means of displaying vessels by imaging. It maximizes the signals in structures containing blood flow and reconstructs only the structures with flow. It is useful for evaluating vascular lesions. Other structures of lesser interest are subtracted from the image by the computer.

MAGNETIC RESONANCE SPECTROSCOPY This MRI uses a scanner that can evaluate and detect ischemic heart disease and the effects of cancer treatment on tumors. It allows biochemical sampling of the tissue that is being imaged so that one can distinguish between a demyelinating condition and a neoplasm versus an infection without need for a biopsy. It can also confirm the presence of Alzheimer's dementia, to determine the extent of head injury due to trauma and stroke, and to identify the cause of coma.

Procedure

- A consent form should be signed.
- Inform the client that there will be no exposure to radiation.
- Empty bladder prior to the test.
- Remove all jewelry, including watches, glasses, hearing aids, hairpins, cosmetics that may contain metallic fragments, and any metal objects. The magnetic field can damage watches. Those with pacemakers are not candidates for MRI; some with metal prosthetics, and those with nerve stimulating devices may not be candidates for MRI. Remove dentures as advised.
- Occupational history is important. Metal in the body, such as shrapnel or flecks of ferrous metal in eye, may cause critical injury, such as retinal hemorrhage.
- Contraindications include pregnancy and clients with epilepsy. MRI could cause excess heat in the amniotic fluid.
- With the closed MRI, the client must lie absolutely still on a narrow table with a cylinder-type scanner around the body area being scanned.
- Sedation may be needed if the client, receiving closed MRI, is extremely claustrophobic. A client receiving a sedative should not drive home, therefore, a family member or friend should be available to drive.
- Open MRI may be ordered for clients who are claustrophic, obese, confused, or a child; a family member or friend may be present. A mirror is available to see outside during the procedure. Clients need to remain still during the open MRI. Open MRI uses a lower-field magnet, whereas the closed MRI uses a higher-field magnet; hence lesser quality images are usually produced by open MRI.
- Certain MRI studies require a noniodinated contrast media (gadolinium Magnevist) which may be injected intravenously. Use of MR contrast media may be contraindicated for those with kidney dyfunction; the contrast media is excreted by the kidneys.
- There is no food or fluid restriction for adults. NPO for 4 hours for children.
- The procedure takes approximately 45 minutes to 1½ hours.

NURSING IMPLICATIONS WITH RATIONALE
Magnetic Resonance Imaging

- Elicit any problems with claustrophobia. Relaxation techniques or a sedative might be used.
- Ascertain from the client the presence of a pacemaker, wire left in the body from a previous pacemaker, any metal prosthetics, or shrapnel left in the body which could cause serious tissue injury as the result of the magnetic pull.
- Alert the physician or health care provider if client is on an IV pump. MRI can disrupt IV flow.
- Provide emotional support.

CLIENT TEACHING
- Explain the procedure. Inform the client that various loud noises (clicking, thumping) from the scanner will be heard. Ear plugs are available. Inform the client that the MRI personnel will be in another room but can communicate via an intercom system. With the open MRI, a family member or friend may be in the room with the client while the MRI scanning is taking place. This is also possible with closed MRI.
- Explain to the client that there is no exposure to radiation. The contrast media that might be used is not iodinated contrast.
- Instruct the client to remove watches, credit cards, hairpins, jewelry, and makeup. The magnetic field can damage a watch.
- Inform the client that the MRI procedure is painless. Encourage the client to relax during the testing.
- Caution clients with cardiac pacemakers not to approach the MRI unit.
- Inform the client who has metal fillings in teeth that a "tingling sensation" may be felt during imaging.

BLOOD FLOW: EXTREMITIES
- The limb to be examined is rested in a cradlelike support. Reference sites to be imaged are marked on the leg or arm, and the extremity is moved into a flow cylinder.
- The procedure takes approximately 15 minutes for arms and 15 minutes for legs.

Factors Affecting Diagnostic Results
- Movement during the procedure will distort the imaging.
- Ferrous metal in the body could cause critical injury to the client.
- Nonferrous metal may produce artifacts that degrade the images if in close proximity to the area being scanned.

MAMMOGRAPHY (MAMMOGRAM)
Description
Mammography is an x-ray examination of the breasts to detect cysts or tumors. Benign cysts are seen on the mammogram as well-outlined, clear lesions and tend to be bilateral, whereas malignant tumors are irregular and poorly defined and tend to be unilateral. A breast mass (neoplasm) cannot be clinically palpable until it is 1 cm in size, so it may take 5 years or longer to grow and be detectable. A mammogram can detect a breast lesion approximately 2 years before it is palpable.

The mammogram can detect approximately 90% of breast malignancies; however, the test carries a 10% false-positive rate. A positive test should be confirmed by biopsy.

There have been technical improvements in the equipment, mammographic units, and the recording system used for mammography. The use of radiographic grids has improved the imaging quality of mammograms by decreasing image density. With the use of grids, the visibilty of small cancers is increased. Also, the use of magnification mammography has improved the capability to identify cancers; however, the magnification increases the client's radiation dose by prolonging exposure time.

Procedure
- Food and fluids are not restricted.
- The client removes clothes and jewelry from the neck to the waist and wears a paper or cloth gown that opens in the front. Powder and ointment on the breast should be removed to avoid false-positive results. No deodorants should be used.
- The client is standing, and each breast (one at a time) rests on an x-ray cassette table. As the breast is compressed, the client will be asked to hold her breath while the x-ray is taken. Two x-rays are taken of each breast.
- The procedure usually takes 15 to 30 minutes.

Factors Affecting Diagnostic Results
- Previous breast surgery can affect the reading of the x-ray film.
- Jewelry, metals, ointment, and powder could cause false-positive results.

METHEMOGLOBIN (BLOOD)
Reference Values
Normal: less than 1.5% of the total hemoglobin; 0.06–0.24 g/dl; 9.2–37.0 µmol/l (SI units).
Positive: greater than 20–70%, complaints of headache, dizziness, fatigue, tachycardia; greater than 70%, death.

Description
Methemoglobin (Hb M) occurs when the deoxygenated heme (iron portion of hemoglobin) is oxidized to a ferric state. In the ferric state, the heme cannot combine with oxygen; thus, cyanosis without dyspnea or other cardiovascular problems may result. Methemoglobinemia may be acquired from chemicals, radiation, and such drugs as nitrites, nitrates, certain sulfonamides, antimalarials, local anesthetics, or inherited enzyme deficiency. Poisoning from occupational or environmental contact could cause methemoglobinemia. A deficiency in the glucose-6-phosphate dehydrogenase (G-6-PD) enhances the production of Hb M.

If newborns are cyanotic after oxygen has been given, the methemoglobin level should be checked. Infants are more prone to develop methemoglobinemia.

MYOGLOBIN (SERUM)
Reference Values

Adult: 12–90 ng/ml, 12–90 mcg/l
Female: 12–75 ng/ml, 12–75 mcg/l
Male: 20–90 ng/ml, 20–90 mcg/l

Description

Myoglobin is an oxygen-binding protein, similar to hemoglobin, that is found in skeletal and cardiac muscle cells. Myoglobin is released into circulation after an injury. Increased serum myoglobin occurs about 2 to 6 hours following muscle tissue damage. Serum myoglobin level reaches its peak following a myocardial infarction (MI) in approximately 8 to 12 hours. Elevated serum myoglobin (myoglobinemia) is short-lived; in 50% of persons having an MI, the serum level begins to return to normal range in 12 to 18 hours. Urine myoglobin may be detected for 3 to 7 days following muscle injury.

Because serum myoglobin is nonspecific concerning which muscle is damaged, myocardium or skeletal, cardiac enzymes should also be ordered. Creatine phosphokinase (CPK) and CPK isoenzyme, CPK-MB, should be checked because this enzyme rises early after an MI. Assessment of signs and symptoms of an acute MI need to be considered along with the blood tests. This test is not performed following cardioversion or after an angina attack.

OCCULT BLOOD (FECES)
Reference Values

Adult: Negative.
Child: Negative.

Note: A diet rich in meats, poultry, fish, and drugs (cortisone, aspirin, potassium) could cause a false-positive occult blood test.

Description

Occult (nonvisible or hidden) blood in the feces usually indicates gastrointestinal bleeding. Bright red blood from the rectum can be indicative of bleeding from the lower large intestine (e.g., hemorrhoids), and tarry black stools indicate blood loss of greater than 50 ml from the upper GI tract.

Occult blood in the feces may be present days or several weeks after a single bleeding episode. False-positive occult blood test results may be due to ingestion of meats, poultry, fish, and certain drugs.

Factors Affecting Laboratory Results

■ Drugs (*see Drug Influence*).
■ Foods: meats; poultry; fish; and green, leafy vegetables can cause a false-positive test result.
■ Urine and soap solution in the feces may affect the test result.

OSMOLALITY (SERUM)
Reference Values

Adult: 280–300 mOsm/kg.
Panic Values: less than 240 mOsm/kg and greater than 320 mOsm/kg.
Child: 270–290 mOsm/kg.

Description

Serum osmolality is an indicator of serum concentration. It measures the number of dissolved particles (electrolytes, urea, sugar) in the serum and is helpful in the diagnosis of fluid and electrolyte imbalances. Sodium contributes 85% to 90% of the serum osmolality; changes in osmolality usually result from changes in the serum sodium concentration. Double the serum sodium can give a rough estimate of the serum osmolality.

The hydration status of the client is usually determined by the serum osmolality. An increased value (greater than 300 mOsm/kg) indicates hemoconcentration due to dehydration; a decreased value (less than 280 mOsm/kg) indicates hemodilution due to overhydration, or water excess. An osmometer is used in laboratories to determine serum osmolality; however, if the serum sodium, urea, and sugar levels are known, the serum osmolality can be calculated by the nurse as follows.

$$\text{Serum osmolality} = 2 \times \text{Serum sodium} + \frac{\text{BUN}}{3} + \frac{\text{Sugar}}{18}$$

OSMOLALITY (URINE)
Reference Values

Adult: 50–1200 mOsm/kg/H_2O, average 200–800 mOsm/kg H_2O.
Child: *Newborn:* 100–600 mOsm/kg/H_2O. *Child:* Same as adult.

Description

The urine osmolality test is more accurate than the specific gravity in determining the urine concentration, because its value reflects the number of particles, ions, and molecules and is not unduly influenced by large molecules. Specific gravity measures the quantity and nature of the particles, such as sugar, protein, and IV dyes (these elevate specific gravity but have little effect on osmolality).

The urine osmolality fluctuates in the same way that the urine-specific gravity does, and it can be low or high according to the client's state of hydration. A dehydrated client with normal kidney function could have a urine osmolality of 1000 mOsm/kg H_2O or more. When hemoconcentration occurs as a result of acidosis, shock, or hyperglycemia, the serum osmolality is elevated, and so should the urine osmolality be elevated.

If serum hypoosmolality and hyponatremia occur with urine hyperosmolality, the problem is most likely the syndrome of inappropriate antidiuretic hormone secretion (SIADH). ADH causes water reabsorption from the kidney, thus diluting the serum.

OVA AND PARASITES (O AND P) (FECES)

Reference Values

Adult: Negative.

Child: Negative.

Description

Parasites may be present in various forms in the intestine, including the ova (eggs), larvae (immature form), cysts (inactive stage), and trophozoites (motile form) of protozoa. It is vitally important to detect parasites so that proper treatment can be ordered. Some of the organisms identified are amoeba, flagellates, tapeworms, hookworms, and roundworms. A history of recent travel outside the United States should be reported to the laboratory, because it may help in identifying the parasite.

PAPANICOLAOU SMEAR (PAP SMEAR)

Description

The Pap (Papanicolaou) smear is used for detecting cervical cancer and precancerous tissues. Because malignant tissue changes usually take many years, yearly examination of exfoliative cervical cells (cells that have sloughed off) allows detection of early, precancerous conditions. It is suggested that women from the age of 18 to 40 years have Pap smears every 2 years and that women from the age of 40 years on have yearly smears.

The Pap smear (cytology) results are reported by the Bethesda system. General categories of The Bethesda System (TBS) are as follows:

I. Within normal limits.
II. Abnormal changes
  A. Benign cellular changes
    1. Differentiates reactive or inflammatory changes from true dysplastic changes.
    2. Most important features of TBS. *Management:* Repeat smears yearly.
  B. Epithelial abnormalities
    1. Atypical cells of undetermined significance (ACUS): favoring a neoplastic process or a reactive process. *Management:* Repeat smears at closer intervals, recall for colposcopy and/or combine repeat cytology with cervicography or HPV-DNA type.
    2. Low-grade squamous intraepithelial lesion (LGSIL): shows the earliest abnormal nuclear changes; combines diagnosis of HPV and mild dysplagia. *Management:* Repeat cytology at close intervals, recall for colposcopy.

NURSING IMPLICATIONS WITH RATIONALE
Papanicolaou Smear

- Explain the procedure to the client. Emphasize to the client that she should not douche, insert vaginal suppositories, or have sexual intercourse for at least 24 hours (some say 48 hours) before the Pap smear. Douching could wash away the cervical cells.
- Obtain a client history regarding menstruation and any menstrual problems (i.e., the last menstrual period, bleeding flow, vaginal discharge, itching, and whether she is taking hormones or oral contraceptives).
- Answer the client's questions, and refer questions you cannot answer to other health professionals. Try to alleviate the client's anxiety, if at all possible. Be a good listener.
- Label the slide with the client's name and the date. The laboratory slip should include the client's age and the specimen site(s).

CLIENT TEACHING

- Inform the client that a manual examination of the vagina, lower abdomen, rectum, and breast may or will follow the Pap smear.
- Explain to the client that the test should be done yearly or more as determined by her health care provider. High-risk clients with a familial history of cervical cancer or dysphagia should have a Pap smear taken twice a year. Usually women over 40 years old should have a Pap smear once a year.
- Inform the client that test results should be back in 5 to 7 days. Physicians and health care providers differ in the way they report test results; some send cards to the client stating that the Pap smear is normal, while other send cards only if the test is abnormal.

3. High-grade squamous intraepithelial lesion (HGSIL): includes moderate and severe dysplastic changes. *Management:* Recall for colposcopy.
4. Squamous cell carcinoma: changes consistent with cancer. *Management:* Recall for colposcopy.
5. Glandular cell abnormalities
  a. Atypical cells of undetermined significance, atypical endocervical cells. *Management:* In young women, check for endocervicitis, repeat smear, refer for colposcopy; in older women, refer for colposcopy with endocervical sample.
  b. Cancer *Management:* Refer for colposcopy.

For suggestive or positive Pap smears, colposcopy and/or a cervical biopsy are frequently ordered to confirm the test results. Atypical cells can occur following cervicitis and after excessive or prolonged use of hormones.

Procedure

- Food and fluids are not restricted.
- The client should not douche, insert vaginal medications, or have sexual intercourse for at least 24 hours (preferably 48 hours) before the test. The test should be done between menstrual periods.
- The client is generally asked to remove all clothes, because the breasts are examined after the Pap smear is taken. A paper or cloth gown is worn.

- Instruct the client to lie on the examining table in the lithotomy position (heels in the stirrups).
- A speculum is inserted into the vagina. The speculum may be lubricated with warm running water.
- A curved spatula (Pap stick) is used to scrape the cervix. The obtained specimen is transferred onto a slide and is immersed immediately in a fixative solution or sprayed with a commercial fixation spray. Label the slide with the client's name and date.
- The Pap smear procedure takes approximately 10 minutes.

Factors Affecting Diagnostic Results

- Allowing cells to dry on the slide before using the fixative solution or spray.
- Douching, use of vaginal suppositories, or sexual intercourse within the 24 hours before the test.
- Menstruation can interfere with the test results.
- Drugs (i.e., digitalis preparations, tetracycline, female hormones) could change cellular structure.
- Lubricating jelly on the speculum can interfere with test results.
- Inadequate specimen.

PARATHYROID HORMONE (PTH) (SERUM)

Parathormone

Reference Values

Adult: *Intact PTH:* 11–54 pg/ml; *C-Terminal PTH:* 50–330 pg/ml; *N-Terminal PTH:* 8–24 pg/ml.

PARTIAL THROMBOPLASTIN TIME (PTT), ACTIVATED PARTIAL THROMBOPLASTIN TIME (APTT) (PLASMA)

Reference Values

Adult: Results vary in accordance with equipment and laboratory values. *PTT:* 60–70 seconds. *APTT:* 20–35 seconds. Child: Increased above adult level.
Anticoagulant Therapy: 1.5–2.5 times the control in seconds.

Note: Most laboratories do APTT only.

Description

The partial thromboplastin time (PTT) is a screening test used to detect deficiencies in all clotting factors except VII and XIII and to detect platelet variations. It is more sensitive than the prothrombin time (PT) in detecting minor deficiencies but is not as sensitive as the activated partial thromboplastin time (APTT).

The PTT is useful for monitoring heparin therapy. Heparin doses are adjusted according to the PTT test.

The APTT is more sensitive in detecting clotting factor defects than the PTT, because the activator added in vitro shortens the clotting time. By shortening the clotting time, minor clotting defects can be detected.

The APTT is similar to the PTT, except that the thromboplastin reagent used in the APTT test contains an activator (kaolin, celite, or ellagic acid) for identification of deficient factors. This test is commonly used to monitor heparin therapy.

PHENOTHIAZINES (SERUM)
Reference Values
Adult:

Drug	Therapeutic Range	Peak Time	Toxic Level
Chlorpromazine (Thorazine)	50–300 ng/ml	2 to 4 hours	>750 ng/ml
Prochlorperazine (Compazine)	50–300 ng/ml	2 to 4 hours	>1000 ng/ml
Thioridazine	100–600 ng/ml	2 to 4 hours	>2000 ng/ml
(Mellaril)	0.2–2.6 mg/l		>10 mg/l
Trifluoperazine (Stelazine)	50–300 ng/ml	2 to 4 hours	>1000 ng/ml

PHENYTOIN SODIUM (SERUM)
Reference Values

Therapeutic Range: *Adult:* As an anticonvulsant, 10–20 mcg/ml, 39.6–79.3 µmol/l (SI units). As an antiarrhythmic, 10–18 mcg/ml, 39.6–71.4 µmol/l (SI units). *In saliva:* 12 mcg/ml, 49 µmol/l.

Toxic Level: *Adult:* greater than 20 mcg/ml, greater than 79.3 µmol/l (SI units). *Child:* greater than 15–20 mcg/ml, 56–79 µmol/l (SI units).

PHOSPHORUS (P)—INORGANIC (SERUM)
Phosphate (PO_4)

Reference Values

Adult: 1.7–2.6 mEq/l or 2.5–4.5 mg/dl; 0.78–1.52 mmol/l (SI units).
Child: *Newborn:* 3.5–8.6 mg/dl. *Infant:* 4.5–6.7 mg/dl. *Child:* 4.5–5.5 mg/dl.
Elderly: Slightly lower than adult.

Description

Phosphorus is the principal intracellular anion; however, most of phosphorus exists in the blood as phosphate. From 80% to 85% of the total phosphates in the body are combined with calcium in the teeth and bones.

Phosphorus is the laboratory term used, because phosphates are converted into inorganic phosphorus for the test. Functions of phosphorus include metabolism of carbohydrates and fats, maintenance of the acid-base balance, use of B vitamins, promotion of nerve and muscle activity, and transmission of hereditary traits.

Phosphorus (P) metabolism is associated with calcium (Ca) metabolism. Both ions need vitamin D for their absorption from the gastrointestinal tract. Phosphorus and calcium concentrations are controlled by the parathyroid hormone. Usually there is a reciprocal relationship between calcium and phosphorus: when serum phosphorus levels increase, serum calcium levels decrease, and when serum phosphorus levels decrease, serum calcium levels increase. In certain neoplastic bone diseases, this relationship is no longer true, because both calcium and phosphorus are increased.

A high serum phosphorus level is called *hyperphosphatemia,* which is usually associated with kidney dysfunction (poor urinary output). *Hypophosphatemia* means a low serum phosphorus level.

PLATELET AGGREGATION AND ADHESIONS (BLOOD)

Reference Values

Adult: Aggregation in 3 to 5 minutes.

Description

Platelet aggregation test measures the ability of platelets to adhere to each other when mixed with an aggregating agent such as collagen, ADP, or ristocetin. This test is performed to detect abnormality in platelet function and to aid in diagnosing hereditary and acquired platelet deficiencies such as von Willebrands disease. Increased bleeding tendencies result from a decrease in platelet aggregation time.

The **platelet adhesion test**, like platelet aggregation, evaluates platelet function and helps to confirm hereditary diseases such as von Willebrands disease. This test is also performed on clients taking large doses of aspirin for several weeks and on persons having a prolonged bleeding time. It is not performed in many laboratories because of the difficulty in standardizing the technique.

PLATELET COUNT (BLOOD— THROMBOCYTES)

Reference Values

Adult: 150,000400,000 µl (mean, 250,000 µl) 0.150.4 × 10^{12}/l (SI units).
Child: *Premature:* 100,000–300,000 *Newborn:* 150,000–300,000 µl *Infant:* 200,000 475,000 µl (mm^3 or K/Ul may be used for ul).

Description

Platelets (thrombocytes) are basic elements in the blood that promote coagulation. Platelets are much smaller than erythrocytes. They clump and stick to rough surfaces and injured sites when blood coagulation is needed. A decrease in circulating platelets of less than 50% of the normal value will cause bleeding; if the decrease is severe (less than 50,000 µl), hemorrhaging might occur.

Thrombocytopenia means platelet deficiency or a low platelet count. It is commonly associated with leukemias, aplastic anemia, and idiopathic thrombocytopenic purpura. Increased platelet counts (thrombocytosis) occur in polycythemia, in fractures, and after splenectomy.

POSITRON EMISSION TOMOGRAPHY (PET)

Description

Positron emission tomography (PET), a relatively noninvasive test, measures areas of positron-emitting isotope concentration. Myocardial perfusion abnormalities can be determined at rest and after administration of dipyridamole (Persantine).

PET is used to study the lungs and abdominal organs, and for oncologic purposes. In oncology, PET has been approved for lung nodules and colorectal cancer imaging. PET's greatest advances have been in oncology. For brain studies, PET assesses normal brain function; regional cerebral blood flow and volume; glucose, protein, and oxygen metabolism; blood-brain barrier function, neuroreceptor-neurotransmitter systems; and the pathophysiology of neurologic and psychiatric disorders. For heart studies, PET assesses cardiac perfusion or blood flow; glucose and oxygen metabolism; and receptor functions. PET perfusion imaging provides information concerning the severity of coronary artery disease (CAD).

Most PET imagers have several radiation detector rings. Each detector group represents a profile or one-dimensional projection of the radioactivity distribution in a tomographic slice. These profiles are combined to produce a cross-sectional (tomographic) image. The two-dimensional (2D) PET images are reconstructed from projection data derived from the detector rings. Three-dimensional (3D) PET imaging is a new approach in which images are generated from the 2D images.

The client receives a substance tagged with a radionuclide (i.e., radioactive glucose, rubidium 82, oxygen 15, nitrogen 13). Flurodeoxyglucose (FDG) is the most common radioisotope used in PET. Tomographic slices from crosssections of tissue are detected and visually displayed by computer. PET is most effective in determining blood flow to the brain and heart. Radiation from PET is a quarter of that received from computed tomography.

Procedure

- A consent form should be signed.
- Nothing by mouth (NPO) 4 to 6 hours prior to the study.
- No coffee, alcohol, or tobacco is allowed for 24 hours before the test.
- CT or MRI scans less than 6 weeks old should be available for the purpose of comparison.

NURSING IMPLICATIONS WITH RATIONALE
Positron Emission Tomography

PRETEST
- Check that a consent form has been signed.
- Assess the IV site, monitor vital signs.
- Listen to the client's concerns.

CLIENT TEACHING
- Inform the client that instructions given during test should be followed.
- Inform the client that a head holder or velcro straps could be used for the restriction of body movement during imaging.

POSTTEST
- Continue to monitor vital signs.
- Avoid postural hypotension by slowly moving the client to upright position.
- Increase fluid intake to remove radioisotope from the bladder.

CLIENT TEACHING
- Explain to the client that the radiation from the test is short lived and that the test is considered to be a relatively noninvasive test.
- Encourage the client to remain relaxed and to avoid stress. The client should not sleep but should remain quiet and still.
- Instruct the client to take fluids posttest to help eliminate the radioactive substance.

- Any laboratory or biopsy reports should be available. Glucose levels are required if a study with fasting glucose is being performed.
- Start two IVs, one for radioactive substance and the second to draw blood gas samples.
- For certain brain studies, a blindfold may be used to keep the client from being distracted.
- For brain studies, the client's head is placed in a holder to restrict movement. For heart or abdominal studies, velcro straps are used to restrict body motion.
- No sedatives are given, since client needs to follow instructions.
- Empty the bladder 1 to 2 hours before the test if imaging the pelvis.
- Test takes 1 to 2 hours.

Factors Affecting Diagnostic Results
- Anxiety could interfere with test results.
- Sedatives given might prevent client from following directions.

POTASSIUM (K) (SERUM)
Reference Values

Adult: 3.5–5.3 mEq/l; 3.5–5.3 mmol/l (SI units).
Panic Values: less than 2.5 mEq/l and greater than 7.0 mEq/l.
Child: *Infant:* 3.6–5.8 mEq/l. *Child:* 3.5–5.5 mEq/l.

Description
Potassium is the electrolyte found most abundantly in intracellular fluids (cells). The serum potassium level has a narrow range, and cardiac arrest could occur if serum level is less than 2.5 mEq/l or greater than 7.0 mEq/l.

Eighty to 90% of the body potassium is excreted by the kidneys. When there is tissue breakdown, potassium leaves the cells and enters the extracellular fluid (interstitial and intravascular fluids). With adequate kidney functions, the potassium in the intravascular fluid (plasma/blood vessels) will be excreted, and with excessive potassium excretion, a serum potassium deficit (hypokalemia) occurs. However, if the kidneys are excreting less than 600 ml of urine daily, potassium will accumulate in the intravascular fluid and serum potassium excess (hyperkalemia) will occur.

The body does not conserve potassium, and the kidneys excrete an average of 40 mEq/l daily (the range is 25 to 120 mEq/l/24 h), even with a low dietary potassium intake. The daily potassium requirement is 3 to 4 g, or 40 to 60 mEq/l.

PROGESTERONE (SERUM)
Reference Values

Adult: *Female:* Follicular Phase: 0.1–1.5 ng/ml, 20–150 ng/dl. Luteal Phase: 2–28 ng/ml, 250–2800 ng/dl. Postmenopausal: less than 1.0 ng/ml, less than 100 ng/dl. *Pregnancy:* First Trimester: 9–50 ng/ml. Second Trimester: 18–150 ng/ml. Third Trimester: 60–260 ng/ml. *Male:* less than 1.0 ng/ml, less than 100 ng/dl.

Description
Progesterone, a hormone produced primarily by the corpus luteum of the ovaries and in a small amount by the adrenal cortex, peaks during the luteal phase of the menstrual cycle for 4 to 5 days and during pregnancy. It prepares the endometrium for implantation of the fertilized egg. Only a small amount of progesterone is detected in the blood, because most is metabolized in the liver to pregnanediol, a progesterone metabolite.

Serum progesterone is useful in evaluating infertility problems, in confirming ovulation, and in assessing placental functions in pregnancy. A urine pregnanediol might be ordered to verify serum progesterone results.

PROLACTIN (PRL) SERUM
Reference Value

Female: *Nonpregnant:* Follicular Phase: 0–23 ng/ml. Luteal Phase: 0–40 ng/ml. Postmenopausal: less than 12 ng/ml. *Pregnant:* First Trimester: less than 80 ng/ml. Second Trimester: less than 160 ng/ml. Third Trimester: less than 400 ng/ml.
Male: 0.1–20 ng/ml.
Pituitary Adenoma: greater than 100–300 ng/ml.

Description

Prolactin, a hormone secreted by the anterior pituitary gland, is necessary in the development of the mammary glands for lactation and for stimulating and maintaining lactation postpartum. If the mother does not breastfeed, serum prolactin falls to normal range.

Serum prolactin levels 100–300 ng/ml in nonpregnant females and in males may indicate a pituitary adenoma (tumor). Bromocriptine (Parlodel) decreases the serum prolactin level and slows tumor growth until the pituitary tumor can be removed.

Prolactin levels may be monitored to determine the effects of surgery, chemotherapy, and/or radiation for treating prolactin-secreting tumors.

PROSTATE-SPECIFIC ANTIGEN (PSA) (SERUM)
Reference Values

Male: *No Prostatic Disorder:* 0–4 ng/ml. *Benign Prostatic Hypertrophy (BPH):* 4–19 ng/ml. *Prostate Cancer:* 10–120 ng/ml (depends on the stage of prostatic cancer).

Description

Prostate-specific antigen (PSA), a glycoprotein from the prostatic tissues, is increased in both benign prostatic hypertrophy (BPH) and prostatic cancer; however, it is markedly increased in prostatic cancer. The PSA value may also be increased after a rectal examination and prostate surgery. PSA is more sensitive than prostatic acid phosphatase (PAP), also known as acid phosphatase (ACP), in early detection of prostatic cancer. The use of PSA and PAP, along with rectal examination, assists with making an accurate diagnosis.

An annual PSA test should be started at the age of 50, but it should be started at the age of 40 if the male has a familial history of prostate cancer or is African-American. A digital rectal exam (DRE) should be done along with a PSA test. With an abnormal DRE, a biopsy of the prostate gland usually is performed regardless of whether the PSA test is normal or elevated. If the PSA is over 10, there is a 70% chance that the prostate gland is malignant. If the PSA is less than 4, the chance of a cancerous prostate is very small, but not zero. Also, an elevated PSA could be due to an enlarged prostate gland (benign prostatic hyperplasia [BPH]) or prostatitis which is inflammation of the prostate gland from a bacterial infection or other causes.

PSA may be used to diagnose or monitor the effect of prostatic cancer treatment with chemotherapy or radiation, determine disease process and prognosis, and detect a recurrence of the tumor. Repeating the PSA test may be necessary.

PROTEIN (TOTAL) (SERUM)
Reference Values

Adult: 6.0–8.0 g/dl.
Child: *Premature:* 4.2–7.6 g/dl. *Newborn:* 4.6–7.4 g/dl. *Infant:* 6.0–6.7 g/dl. *Child:* 6.2–8.0 g/dl.

Description

The total protein is composed mostly of albumin and globulins *(see Protein electrophoresis)*. The use of the total serum protein test is limited unless the serum albumin, A/G ratio, or protein electrophoresis test is also performed.

The protein level needs to be known to determine the significance of its components. With certain disease entities (i.e., collagen diseases, cancer, and infections), the total serum protein levels may be normal when the protein fractions are either decreased or elevated.

PROTEIN (URINE)
Reference Values

Random Specimen: *Negative:* 0–5 mg/dl. *Positive:* 6–2000 mg/dl (trace to +2).
24-Hour Specimen: 25–150 mg/24 h.

Description

Proteinuria is usually caused by renal disease due to glomerular damage and/or impaired renal tubular reabsorption. With a random urine specimen, protein can be detected using a reagent strip or dipstick, such as Combistix. Normally albumin is measured with the dipstick, because it is sensitive to reagent strip. A positive urine specimen (proteinuria) suggests that a 24-hour urine specimen be obtained for quantitative analysis of protein.

The amount of proteinuria in 24 hours is an indicator of the severity of renal involvement. Minimal proteinuria (less than 500 mg or 0.5 g/24 h) may be associated with chronic pyelonephritis; moderate proteinuria (500 to 4000 mg or 0.5 to 4 g/24 h) may be associated with acute or chronic glomerulonephritis or toxic nephropathies (i.e., use of aminoglycosides [gentamicin) and marked proteinuria (greater than 4000 mg or greater than 4 g/24 h) may be associated with nephrotic syndrome.

Emotions and physiologic stress may cause transient proteinura. Newborns may have an increased proteinuria during the first 3 days of life.

PROTHROMBIN TIME (PT) (PLASMA)
Reference Values

Adult: 10–13 seconds (depending on the method and reagents used) or 70–100%. *For Anticoagulant Therapy:* 1.5–2.0 times the control in seconds or 20–30%. INR: 2.0–3.0.
Child: Same as adult.

Description

Prothrombin (factor II of the coagulation factors) is synthesized by the liver and is an inactive precursor in the clotting process *(see Factor Assay)*. Prothrombin is converted to thrombin by the action of thromboplastin, which is needed to form a blood clot.

The prothrombin time (PT) measures the clotting ability of factors I (fibrinogen), II (prothrombin), V, VII, and X. Alterations of factors V and VII will prolong the PT for about 2 seconds, or 10% of normal. In liver disease the PT is usually prolonged, because the liver cells cannot synthesize prothrombin.

The major use of the PT is to monitor oral anticoagulant therapy (i.e., with bishydroxycoumarin [dicumarol] and warfarin sodium [Coumadin]).

INTERNATIONAL NORMALIZED RATIO (INR)   It has been recommended that the PT be reported as an International Normalized Ratio (INR). The INR was devised to improve the monitoring process for warfarin anticoagulant therapy. A clients response to the same dose of warfarin varies, thus the INR is used because it is an internationally standardized test for PT. The INR is designed for long-term warfarin therapy, and should only be used after the client has been stabilized on warfarin. Stabilization takes at least one week. The INR should not be used when the client is beginning warfarin therapy in order to avoid misleading test results. The target INR range for a client having heart valve replacement is 2.5 to 3.5.

PULMONARY FUNCTION TESTS

Normal Findings

Normal values according to clients age, sex, and height; greater than 80% of the predicted value. 95% confidence levels are also being used, these confidence ranges give a normal and a low or minimal normal value. This is done to account for physiologic differences in body types.

Description

Pulmonary function tests (PFTs) are useful in differentiating between obstructive and restrictive lung diseases and in quantifying the degree (mild, moderate, or severe) of obstructive or restrictive lung disorders. Other

Purposes for PFTs include establishing baseline test results for comparison with future tests; evaluating pulmonary status before surgery; determining pulmonary disability for insurance; tracking the progress of lung disease; assessing the response to therapy; pulmonary evaluation; determining pulmonary status before rehabilitation; and post rehabilitation to document outcomes.

In pulmonary physiology testing, the lungs are monitored by many complex devices and tests. The most basic device is the spirometer; it is used to measure flows, volumes, and capacities.

A number of pulmonary tests are conducted, because no single measurement can evaluate pulmonary performance. The most frequently performed PFTs are the slow vital capacity tests; lung-volume tests; forced vital capacity, flow-volume loop, and diffusion-study tests; bronchodilator response studies; exercise studies; and nutritional studies.

PULMONARY FUNCTION TESTS

1. Slow Vital Capacity (SVC) Tests
   - *Tidal volume (TV, V_t):* The amount of air inhaled and exhaled during rest or quiet respiration or normal breathing.
   - *Inspiratory capacity (IC):* The maximal inspired amount of air from endexpiratory tidal volume in normal breathing.
   - *Expiratory reserve volume (ERV):* The maximal amount of air that can be exhaled from end-expiratory tidal volume in normal breathing.
   - *Inspiratory reserve volume (IRV):* The maximal amount of air that can be inspired from end-inspiratory tidal volume in normal breathing.
   - *Vital capacity (VC):* The maximal amount of air exhaled after a maximal inhalation:

$$VC = ERV + IC$$

Note: These pulmonary measurements are done slowly, without force. Individuals with obstructive lung disease will be able to expire more volume with this test than during the forced vital capacity maneuver that may lead to early airway closure.

2. Lung Volume Studies
   - *Lung volume tests using indicator gas:* Helium dilution and nitrogen washout are special studies that use the data generated in the slow vital capacity test to obtain the lung volumes. Tracer gases such as 10% helium or 100% oxygen is required. Using one of the gases, the person breathes in and out as the tracer gas is equilibrated in the lung; the functional residual capacity (FRC) is calculated from the changes. This method will tend to underestimate persons with advanced obstructive lung disease. This under estimation is a result of the trapped air in the lung which does communicate with the airways.
   - *Lung volumes by plethysmography method:* Lung volumes can be obtained by total body plethysmography. Body plethysmography uses a device that resembles an air-tight telephone booth in which the subject sits. This method is a more accurate means to measure total volume of the lungs than the tracer gas method. Volumes measured in the box will be larger than by the indicator gas method. The body plethysmography is able to measure trapped air that does not communicate with the airways.
   - *Residual volume (RV):* The amount of air that remains in the lungs after maximal expiration.

$$RV = FRC - ERV$$

   - *Functional residual capacity (FRC):* The amount of air left in the lungs after tidal or normal expiration.

$$FRC = ERV + RV$$

In obstructive disorders, FRC is increased because of hyperinflation and/or air trapping in the lungs. This value may normalize in clients with asthma post exacerbation but will not for clients with COPD. In classical restrictive disorders, FRC, TLC, and RV are all reduced.

   - *Total lung capacity (TLC):* The total amount of air that is in the lungs at maximal inspiration.

$$TLC = VC + RV \text{ or } TLC = FRC + IC$$

3. Lung Volumes and Capacity
   - *Forced vital capacity (FVC):* The maximal amount of air which can be forced out of the lungs as hard, as fast, and as long as possible before a forceful inspiration. In obstructive lung disease, the FVC is decreased; in restrictive lung disease, the FVC is normal or decreased.

$$FVC = IC + ERV$$

   - *Forced inspiratory volume (FIV):* The greatest amount of air inhaled after a maximal expiration.
   - Forced expiratory volume timed (FEV_T): This value reflects the air flow through the bronchial tubes from the greatest to the smallest. It is reported as a time-based value as in 0.5 second $FEV_{.5}$, 1 second FEV_1, 2 seconds FEV_2, and 3 seconds FEV_3. A new American Thoracic Society (ATS) has suggested reporting the FEV_6 which is the amount of air expired in 6 seconds. This reflects the minimum exhalation time suggested for a force vital capacity maneuver. The parameter of choice for evaluation of asthmatics and other obstructive lung disease and to evaluate the response to bronchodilator therapy is still FEV_1. An improvement of greater than 15% after bronchodilator therapy is considered significant and indicates the presence of reversible airway obstruction, such as bronchospasm.

4. Flow-Volume Loop (FVL)
   Another method to visualize FVC measurement is by graphing flow versus volume. This test yields the same basic information as the FVC test but in addition provides the following useful visual information, such as small-airway disease and upper-airway obstruction. Its usefulness in screening people with some types of sleep disorder problems has been recently documented. It is used as a non-invasive tool to evaluate clients who may have some type of upper-airway obstruction from thermal injury, polyps on the vocal cords, vocal cord paralysis, edema of the epiglottis, scar tissue from old tracheotomy site, and floppy trachea.
   - *Peak expiratory flow (PEF):* The highest flow rate achieved at the beginning of the FVC; reported in liters per second. *Note:* Peak flow meters measure in liters per minute.
   - *Peak inspiratory flow (PIF):* The highest flow rate achieved at the beginning of the forced inspiratory capacity.
   - *Forced expiratory flow (FEF):* The FEF looks at flow at the 25%, 50%, and 75% of the FVC and evaluates flow in various size airways. It can evaluate the effectiveness of bronchodilator therapy. FEF 25% reflects flow through large airways; FEF 50% reflects flow through medium airways; and FEF 75% reflects flow through small airways. Decreased FEF 75% indicates small-airway disease.

5. Diffusion Capacity Test
   Diffusion tests can be done using number of techniques. The most commonly used is the single breath test. This requires the client to inspire from RV to TLC. The gas inhaled is a mixture of helium 10%, carbon monoxide 0.3%, oxygen 21%, and balance of gas is nitrogen. The client holds their breath for 10 seconds prior to expiration. After the first 750 ml is discarded to wash out dead-space gas, an alveolar sample is collected in a bag and analyzed for helium and carbon monoxide concentration. Results of this reflect the state of the alveolar capillary barrier.

   Decreased diffusing capacity occurs in such disease states as interstitial fibrosis, pulmonary edema, and emphysema. It will also decrease in persons with abnormal hemoglobin, such as occurs in anemias including methemoglobin and increased carboxyhemoglobin in smokers. Cardiac output can affect this result. Increased DLCO values can be caused by pulmonary hemorrhage.

6. Bronchial Provocation Studies
   Inhalation of pharmacological and antigenic substances is used to test the sensitivity or hyperreactivity of the airways. Types of challenge would include; methacholine, histamine, ASA, cold air, hypertonic saline, antigens, and others. Serial spirometry tests are performed to document the amount or degree of reactivity (a drop in FEV_1 greater than 20% of baseline spirometry). A baseline test followed by a challenge substance is given first, followed by a bronchodilator to assure reversal. Indications for these tests are; (1) normal spirometry test, (2) a history of symptoms such as wheezing, or coughing without a cause, and (3) symptoms related to exposure to industrial substances.

   Methacholine chloride is usually the testing drug of choice because it causes bronchoconstriction rapidly. The client inhales progressively larger doses of the drug until all levels are administered without change in FEV_1 or a drop of 20% of baseline FEV_1 is reached. The drug is then reversed by administration of a bronchodilator.

7. Exercise Studies
   Pulmonary function studies are done at a resting or static state. Exercise studies evaluate the client during an active or dynamic state. These tests are performed by having the subject walk on a treadmill or pedal an ergometer to a set protocol to stimulate activity at progressive workloads. During this test, the heart rate and rhythm is monitored by a 12-lead electrocardiogram (ECG). The client will also be breathing through a mouthpiece during the test to measure ventilation, expired carbon dioxide (VCO_2) and oxygen consumption (VO_2). Blood gases may be drawn at rest and at peak exercise. Pulse oximetry may also be monitored, as well as blood pressure. These tests are used to determine the amount of disability and to evaluate persons with exertion dyspnea. This information can have an exercise prescription for activities for fitness programs, pulmonary, and cardiac rehabilitation.

Types of exercise testing can be designed to simulate activity related problems, of which *exercise induced bronchospasm (EIB)* is an example. A common complaint of clients active in sport activities is bronchospasm. Several theories suggestive of the cause include allergy-triggered airway, production of nitric oxide by the airway hyper-reactivity in association with physical activity and mouth breathing required when the participant increases activity. When the individual breathes rapidly in and out through the mouth, the nose, which warms and filters air, is bypassed. This dry air causes chilling of the airway, leading to instability of the airways and can lead to bronchoconstriction in some persons.

8. Pulse Oximetry (POX)

This is a noninvasive procedure to measure the oxygen saturation (SaO$_2$) of the blood. The device measures the SaO$_2$ by passing two wavelengths of infrared light through an extremity such as a finger. The device (sensor probe) measures the saturation of oxyhemoglobin in the pulsatile fraction of blood. This method is an excellent noninvasive trending device; when values vary, a blood gas analysis of the partial pressure of oxygen (PO$_2$) and/or CO-oximetry to measure oxyhemoglobin (%HbO$_2$) and SaO$_2$ should be done to validate the results. A note of caution: Blood gas analyses normally do not measure SaO$_2$; they are calculated. Check with your blood gas laboratory for this information.

Pulse oximetry is a very useful test but it has some drawbacks. It should be trusted after direct comparison to CO-oximetry is done. Abnormal hemoglobin levels (i.e., carboxyhemoglobinemia, methemoglobinemia, and sulfhemoglobinemia) could fool the device. These abnormal levels are detected at the same infrared wavelengths as O$_2$ and may falsely be interpreted by the oximeter to be oxygen. Impeded blood flow to an area will also affect the pulse oximetry. Correlation with the clients true pulse will assist in correcting this problem. Light sources may also affect the results; thus the area should be guarded against external light sources.

9. Nutritional studies

Indirect calorimetry is the measurement of oxygen consumption (VO$_2$) to derive energy expenditure (EE) and carbon dioxide production (VCO$_2$) allowing us to derive respiratory quotient (RQ). Respiratory quotient obtained from the calorimetry yields the type and amount of substrate used in metabolism (carbohydrate, protein, fats). It is calculated as:

$$RQ = VO_2/VCO_2$$

This noninvasive test gives useful information as to the resting energy expenditure (REE), the amount of calories needed for minimal existence expressed in kilocalories per 24 hours. What it measures is the output side of the nutrition question since we know and measure the input side. The RQ will indicate the type of fuel substrates being metabolized. For example, a RQ of 1.0 indicates carbohydrates; RQ of 0.80 indicates mixed carbohydrates, fats, and protein; where an RQ 0.75 indicates lipids metabolism; and an RQ of 0.65 could be seen in an individual in ketosis. If 24 hour urine urea nitrogen is known, non protein R can be calculated along with the actual amount of carbohydrates, fats, and protein metabolized in grams and percent of EE.

10. Body Plethysmography (body box)

Body plethysmography is a method to measure the exact amount of air in the thorax. This is accomplished by having the subject sit inside an airtight box and breathe through a flow-measuring device. A panting maneuver is employed, and a shutter is closed to measure pressure at the mouth, and a second pressure measures the changes of the box. By measuring the mouth and box pressure, the measurements can be applied to Boyle's Law. The thoracic gas volume (TGV), which correlates to functional residual capacity, (FRC) can be measured. The compliance of the lungs can be measured but it requires the subject to swallow an esophageal balloon. This device can also measure airway resistances of the lung. Advantages are that the body box measures all air in the thorax that causes volumes to be larger in box studies than by other methods. Disadvantages to the body box test are that some clients have claustrophobia, and persons with perforated eardrums will tend to have readings much higher than normal which could be misleading. Obese clients may not be able to be tested due to weight limitations of the equipment. This test requires total client cooperation and ability to follow commands.

RED BLOOD CELL INDICES (MCV, MCH, MCHC, RDW) (BLOOD)
Reference Values

	Adult	Newborn
RBC count (million/μl × 10^{12}/l [SI units])	Male: 4.6–6.0	4.8–7.2
	Female: 4.0–5.0 4.6–6.0 × 10^{12} l	4.8–7.2 × 10^{12} l
MCV (μm^3 [conventional]) or fl [SI units])	80–98	96–108
MCH (pg [conventional and SI units])	27–31	32–34
MCHC (% or g/dl [conventional] or SI units)	32–36%	32–33%
	0.32–0.36	0.32–0.33
RDW (coulter S)	11.5–14.5	

	Child
RBC count (million/µl × 10¹²/l [SI units])	3.8–5.5
	$3.8–5.5 \times 10^{12}$ 1
MCV (µm³ [conventional]) or fl [SI units])	82–92
MCH (pg [conventional and SI units])	27–31
MCHC (% or g/dl [conventional] or SI units)	32–36%
	0.32–0.36
RDW (coulter S)	

Anemias: RDW AND MCV Values

RBC Disorder	RDW	MCV
Early factor deficiency (iron, folate, vitamin B_{12})	High	Normal
Iron-deficiency anemia	High	Low
Folic-acid-deficiency anemia	High	High
Vitamin B_{12} deficiency (pernicious anemia)	High	High
Hemolysis (RBC fragmentation)	High	Low
Hemolysis (autoimmune) anemia	High	High
Sickle cell anemia	High	Normal
Sickle cell trait	High	Normal

Description

Red blood cell (RBC) indices include the RBC count, RBC size (MCV: mean corpuscular volume), weight (MCH: mean corpuscular hemoglobin), hemoglobin concentration (MCHC: mean corpuscular hemoglobin concentration), and size differences (RDW: RBC distribution width). Other names for RBC indices are *erythrocyte indices* and *corpuscular indices*. To identify the types of anemias, the health care provider depends on the following RBC indices:

- *MCV:* MCV indicates the size of RBC: microcytic (small size), normocytic (normal size), and macrocytic (large size). A decreased MCV, or microcyte, might be indicative of iron-deficiency anemia and thalassemia. An example of an increased MCV, or macrocytosis, is pernicious anemia and folic acid anemia. MCV value can be calculated if the RBC count and hematocrit (Hct) are known.

$$MCV = \frac{Hct \times 10}{RBC\ count}$$

- *MCH:* MCH indicates the weight of hemoglobin in the RBC regardless of the size. In macrocytic anemias, the MCH is elevated, and it is decreased in hypochromic anemia. The MCH is derived by dividing the RBC count into 10 times the hemoglobin (Hb) value.

$$MCH = \frac{Hb \times 10}{RBC\ count}$$

- *MCHC:* MCHC indicates the hemoglobin concentration per unit volume of RBCs. A decreased MCHC can indicate a hypochromic anemia. The MCHC can be calculated from MCH and MCV or from hemoglobin and hematocrit.

$$MCH = \frac{MCH \times 100}{MCV} \quad OR \quad MCHC = \frac{Hb \times 100}{Hct}$$

- *RDW:* The RBC distribution width (RDW) is the size (width) differences of RBCs. RDW is the measurement of the width of the size distribution curve on a histogram. It is useful in predicting anemias early, before MCV changes and before signs and symptoms occur. An elevated RDW indicates iron deficiency, folic acid deficiency, and vitamin B_{12} deficiency anemias. RDW and MCV are used to differentiate among various RBC disorders (*see Anemias: RDW and MCV Values*).

RETICULOCYTE COUNT (BLOOD)
Reference Values

Adult: 0.5–1.5% of all RBCs, 25,000–75,000 µl (microliter).

Reticulocyte count = reticulocytes (%) × RBC count

Child: *Newborn:* 2.5–6.5% of all RBCs. *Infant:* 0.5–3.5% of all RBCs. *Child:* 0.5–2.0% of all RBCs.

Description

The reticulocyte count is an indicator of bone marrow activity and is used for diagnosing anemias. Reticulocytes are immature, nonnucleated red blood cells (RBCs) that are formed in the bone marrow and passed into circulation. Normally there are a small number of reticulocytes in circulation; however, an increased number (count) indicates RBC production acceleration. An increased count could be due to hemorrhage or hemolysis or to treatment of iron deficiency, vitamin B_{12} deficiency, or folic-acid-deficiency anemia. This test is also done to check on persons working with radioactive material or receiving radiotherapy. A persistently low count could be suggestive of bone marrow hypofunction or aplastic anemia.

Giving a percentage is not always the most accurate way of reporting the reticulocyte count, especially when the total RBC (erythrocyte) count is *not* within normal range. Both the RBC count and the reticulocyte count should be reported.

NURSING IMPLICATIONS WITH RATIONALE Retrograde Pyelography

PRETEST

- Record baseline vital signs.
- Obtain a client history of allergies to seafood, iodine, and/or radiopaque dye used in other diagnostic tests.
- Administer laxatives, cleansing enemas, and premedications as prescribed. If the client is not hospitalized, check that the prescribed orders were completed at home or in another institution. Check that the consent form has been signed before giving premedications.

CLIENT TEACHING

- Explain to the client that the purpose of the test is to identify kidney stones or to determine the cause of his or her kidney problems, or give a similar response related to the symptoms.
- Explain the procedure to the client. Explain to the client that he or she will be placed in stirrups. If the client is having the test done under local anesthesia, tell the client that he or she will most likely feel pressure and the urge to urinate with insertion of the cystoscope.
- Inform him or her that there should be little to no pain or discomfort. Tell the client that the test takes about 1 hour.

- Inform the client that food and fluids are restricted for 8 hours before the test. Some health care providers may not restrict water unless the client is to have general anesthesia. Check for symptoms of dehydration (i.e., dry mouth and mucous membranes, poor skin turgor, decreased urine output, and fast pulse and respirations). Report symptoms to the health care provider and record them on the clients chart.

POSTTEST

- Monitor vital signs until stable or as ordered.
- Observe for allergic reactions to the contrast dye (i.e., skin rash, urticaria [hives], flushing, dyspnea, and tachycardia).
- Monitor urinary output. Report and record gross hematuria. Blood-tinged urine usually is normal. Report to the health care provider if the client has not voided in 8 hours or the urinary output is less than 200 ml in 8 hours.
- Give an analgesic for discomfort or pain. Report severe pain.
- Observe for signs and symptoms of infection (sepsis; i.e., fever, chills, abdominal pain, tachycardia, and, later, hypotension).
- Be supportive of the client and family. Answer the client's questions, or refer them to urologist or appropriate health professional.

RETROGRADE PYELOGRAPHY (RETROGRADE PYELOGRAM)

Description

A retrograde pyelography test may be performed after or in place of intravenous pyelography (IVP). The contrast dye is injected through a catheter into the ureters and the renal pelvis. The visualization of the urinary tract is exceptionally good because the dye is injected directly. Usually this test is done in conjunction with cystoscopy.

Although retrograde pyelograms are not done too frequently today, this test is still performed when there is a suspected nonfunctioning kidney, an unlocated calculus, or an allergy to IV contrast dye. Only a small amount of the dye that is injected directly into the ureters will be absorbed through the membranes.

Procedure

- A consent form should be signed.
- The client should be NPO for 8 hours before the retrograde pyelography. The client should not be dehydrated before the test.
- Laxatives and cleansing enemas may be ordered prior to the test.
- Baseline vital signs should be recorded.
- Sedatives/tranquilizers and narcotic analgesics are given approximately 1 hour before the test.
- The client is usually placed in the lithotomy position (feet and legs in stirrups).
- Radiopaque contrast dye is injected through a ureteral catheter into the renal pelvis and x-rays are taken. As the catheter is removed, additional x-rays may be taken.

- This procedure is usually done under local or general anesthesia, and the test takes approximately 1 hour.

Factors Affecting Diagnostic Results

- Barium in the gastrointestinal tract could interfere with good visualization. Barium studies should be done after a retrograde pyelogram.

RHEUMATOID FACTOR (RF), RHEUMATOID ARTHRITIS (RA) FACTOR, RA LATEX FIXATION (SERUM)

Reference Values

Adult: less than 1:20 titer; less than 1:40 chronic inflammatory disease; 1:20–1:80 positive for rheumatoid arthritis and other conditions; greater than 1:80 positive for rheumatoid arthritis.
Child: Not usually done.
Elderly: Slightly increased.

Description

The rheumatoid factor (RF) or rheumatoid arthritis (RA) factor test is a screening test used to detect antibodies (IgM, IgG, or IgA) found in the serum of clients with rheumatoid arthritis. RF occurs in 53–94% (average 76%) of clients with rheumatoid arthritis, and if the test is negative, it should be repeated.

The RF tests can be positive in many of the collagen diseases. The RF tests should not be used for monitoring follow-up or treatment stages of RA, because RF tests often remain positive when clinical remissions have been achieved. It also takes approximately 6 months for a significant elevation of titer. For diagnosing and evaluating RA, the ANA and the C-reactive protein agglutination tests are frequently used.

SIGMOIDOSCOPY
Description
Sigmoidoscopy is an examination of the anus, rectum, and sigmoid colon using a flexible sigmoidoscope to visualize the descending colon. This test is usually performed for screening for colon polyps and can be performed in a physician's office, clinic, or hospital. It may be part of an annual physical examination. Sigmoidoscopy may be requested when the client does not want a colonoscopy. With this procedure the rectum and distal sigmoid colon can be visualized, and specimens can be obtained with biopsy forceps or a snare.

Procedure
- A consent form should be signed.
- The client should follow the pretest preparation given by the physician or health care provider. The client is usually allowed a light dinner the night before the test and then NPO afterwards. Usually heavy meals, vegetables, and fruits are prohibited within 24 hours of the test.
- No barium studies should be performed within 3 days of the test.
- Fleet enema(s) (hypertonic salt enema(s)) are given the morning of the test. If enemas are contraindicated, then a rectal suppository such as bisacodyl (Dulcolax), may be prescribed. Fecal material must be evacuated before the examination. Preparation with GoLytely could be used. Oral cathartics are seldom used, because they may increase fecal flow from the small intestine during the test.

- The client should assume a Sims (side-lying) position.
- A lubricated flexible endoscope is inserted into the rectum. The client should be instructed to breathe deeply and slowly. Air may be injected into the bowel to improve visualization.
- Specimens can be obtained during the procedure.
- The procedure takes approximately 15 to 30 minutes.

Factors Affecting Diagnostic Results
- Barium can decrease the visualization, and so barium studies should be performed a week before the test or afterwards.
- Fecal material in the lower colon can decrease visualization.

SLEEP STUDIES
Description
Normal sleep is composed of 2 phases; 4 stages of nonrapid eye movement (NREM) sleep and rapid eye movement (REM) sleep. Both NREM and REM occur cyclically during sleep at approximately 90 minute intervals.

A sleep disorder such as insomnia occurs more frequently in women and increases with age. Older adults have a decrease in stages 3 and 4 of NREM sleep and have frequent waking periods. Children have few REM sleep periods and longer periods of stage 3 and 4 NREM sleep. REM sleep periods become longer during the sleep process and if the person is aroused from REM sleep, he or she may recall a vivid, bizarre dream. Sleepwalking or nightmares occur in children most frequently during NREM sleep. Sleep disorders occur in 75% of psychiatric clients which also include those clients with anxiety, and mood and panic problems.

Sleep studies, primarily called polysomnography (PSG), determine the cause of sleep disorders, including daytime sleepiness, obstructive sleep apnea (OSA) which is also

---

NURSING IMPLICATIONS WITH RATIONALE **Sigmoidoscopy**

- Explain the purpose of the sigmoidoscopy to the client. The test could be a part of the routine physical examination for preventive health care, or the cause of symptoms such as, bright blood or mucus in stools, constipation, bowel changes.
- Explain the procedure to the client.
- Check the chart to determine if the client has had a barium study. If so, notify the physician.
- Obtain a client's history in regard to health problems and pregnancy. Caution should be taken with some health problems such as ulcerative colitis.
- Record baseline vital signs before the test and following the test.
- Allow the client time to ask questions and express concerns. Refer questions you cannot answer to a physician or to the appropriate health professional.

CLIENT TEACHING
- Inform the client that the procedure may cause some discomfort but should not cause severe pain. Encourage the client to breathe deeply and slowly and to relax during the test. Explain that there

may be some gas pains if a small amount of air is injected during the procedure for better visualization.

POSTTEST
- Monitor vital signs as indicated.
- Observe for signs and symptoms of bowel perforation, i.e., pain, abdominal distention, and rectal bleeding. These problems rarely occur. Report all symptoms immediately to the physician or health care professional.
- Be supportive of the client and his or her family.

CLIENT TEACHING
- Encourage the client to rest for several hours or as indicated after the test. This procedure may be done in a physicians office, clinic, or hospital. If the test is done on an outpatient basis, the client should rest for 1 hour before leaving.

NURSING IMPLICATIONS WITH RATIONALE
Sleep Study

- Obtain a history from the client in regards to medications, past stroke, head injury, headaches, seizures.
- Review the sleep log that the client has given.
- Check vital signs. Note if there is respiratory distress.

CLIENT TEACHING

- Explain to the client that electrodes will be attached to the head, chest, and legs.
  ECG: selected leads attached.
  EEG: 2 sets of electrodes to the scalp.
  EOG: 1 electrode to canthus eye.
  EMG: electrodes attached to the leg muscles.
  Pulse oximeter: attached to the finger to determine heart rate and oxygen saturation.
- Answer client's questions or refer the questions to other health professionals.

called sleep disordered breathing, insomnia, nocturnal awakening, and snoring problems. OSA occurs when there is no ventilation for 10 seconds. It may be attributed to oxygen desaturation, cardiac dysrhythmia, or sleep interruption. Also PSG is indicated for persons having difficulty staying awake during the day who fall asleep at inappropriate times, pregnancy-associated sleep disorders, short sleepers (hyposomniac-sleep duration less than 5 hours), and long sleepers (hypersomniac-sleep duration greater than 10 hours).

Testing for sleep disorders is performed in a sleep laboratory at night over an 8-hour period of time. The client is monitored during the night by electrocardiogram (ECG or EKG), pulse oximetry to determine heart rate and oxygen saturation, electroencephalogram (EEG), electrooculogram (EOG), electromyogram (EMG), airflow monitoring, and snoring sensor. All these testing devices may not be indicated.

Procedure

- A consent form should be signed.
- Keep a sleep log for 1–2 weeks prior to the PSG test.
- Avoid caffeine products, alcohol, sedatives, and naps 1–2 days before testing.
- Omit prescribed medications until the sleep studies are completed, if indicated.
- Sleep studies are scheduled in the sleep laboratory at night usually 10 or 11 p.m. until 6 or 7 a.m. (8-hour period of time).
- Attach electrodes for ECG, EEG, EMG.
- Attach the pulse oximetry.
- Place a commode by the bedside. Electrode leads may inhibit bathroom use.
- Lights are turned off.
- In the a.m., have the client evaluate his/her sleep experience.

Factors Affecting Diagnostic Results

- Defective electrodes or those that become loose or fall off.
- Inability to sleep.
- Drugs such as sedatives, caffeine taken prior to the test.

SODIUM (Na) (SERUM)
Reference Values

Adult: 135–145 mEq/l, 135–145 mmol/l (SI units).
Child: *Infant:* 134–150 mEq/l. *Child:* 135–145 mEq/l.

Description

Sodium (Na) is the major cation in the extracellular fluid (ECF), and it has a water-retaining effect. When there is excess sodium in the ECF, more water will be reabsorbed from the kidneys.

Sodium has many functions. It helps to maintain body fluids, is responsible for conduction of neuromuscular impulses via the sodium pump (sodium shifts into cells as potassium shifts out for cellular activity), it is involved in enzyme activity, and it regulates acid-base balance by combining with chloride or bicarbonate ions.

The body needs approximately 2–4 g of sodium daily. The American people daily consume approximately 6–12 g (90 to 240 mEq/l) of sodium in the form of salt (NaCl). A teaspoon of salt contains 2.3 g of sodium.

The names for sodium imbalances are *hyponatremia* (serum sodium deficit) and *hypernatremia* (serum sodium excess). When the serum sodium level is 125 mEq/l, sodium replacement with normal saline (0.9% NaCl) should be considered, and if the serum sodium level is 115 mEq/l or lower, concentrated saline solutions (3 or 5% NaCl) might be ordered. When rapidly replacing sodium loss, assessment for overhydration is important.

SODIUM (Na) (URINE)
Reference Values

Adult: 40–220 mEq/l/24 h.
Child: Similar to adult.

Description

Sodium excretion varies according to the sodium intake, aldosterone secretion, urine volume, and disease entities, such as chronic renal failure, adrenal gland dysfunction (Addisions disease and Cushings syndrome), cirrhosis of the liver, and congestive heart failure.

When the urine sodium level is less than 40 mEq/24 h, the decreased sodium excretion could be due to sodium retention or decreased sodium intake. The body could be retaining sodium even with a low serum sodium level.

The urine sodium level should be monitored when edema is present and the serum sodium level is low or normal.

STRESS/EXERCISE TESTS: TREADMILL EXERCISE ELECTROCARDIOLOGY, EXERCISE MYOCARDIAL PERFUSION IMAGING TEST (THALLIUM/ TECHNETIUM STRESS TEST), NUCLEAR PERSANTINE (DIPYRIDAMOLE) STRESS TEST, NUCLEAR DOBUTAMINE STRESS TEST

Normal Finding

Normal electrocardiogram (ECG) with little or no ST-segment depression with exercise. Normal myocardial perfusion.

Description

Treadmill stress testing is based on the theory that clients with coronary artery disease (CAD) will have marked ST-segment depression on the ECG when exercising. Depression of the ST segment and depression or inversion of the T wave indicate myocardial ischemia. In 1928 Fiel and Siegel reported on the relationship of exercising and ST-segment depression in clients complaining of angina. Master used an exercise test (two-step) in 1929 to demonstrate ischemia but used only pulse and blood pressure (BP) to note changes. In 1931 Wood and Wolferth felt exercise was a useful tool for diagnosing coronary disease but that it could be dangerous. Later it was discovered that ST-segment depression usually occurred before the onset of pain and was still present for some time after the pain had subsided. Mild ST-segment depression after exercise can occur without CAD.

TREADMILL AND BICYCLE ELECTROCARDIOLOGY In 1956 Bruce established guidelines for performing stress testing on a treadmill. Masters Step Test (1955) was also accepted as a method for stress testing. Another method used today is the bicycle ergometer test; however, the treadmill seems to be the choice for testing cardiac status. The body muscles do not seem to tire with the treadmill method as much as leg muscles do with the bicycle ergometer. For clients who cannot walk (i.e., paraplegics, amputees), an arm ergometer or pharmacologic stress testing (to be discussed later) can be used. With the treadmill stress test, the work rate (load) is changed every 3 minutes by increasing the speed slightly and the degree of incline (grade) by 3% each time (3%, 6%, 9%). The clients will exercise until they are fatigued, develop symptoms, or reach their maximum predicted heart rate (MPHR).

EXERCISE THALLIUM PERFUSION TEST The radioisotope thallium 201, which accumulates in the myocardial cells, is used during the stress test to determine myocardial perfusion during exercise. With severe narrowing of the coronary arteries, there is less thallium accumulation in the heart muscle. If a coronary vessel is completely occluded, no uptake of thallium will occur at the myocardial area that the vessel supplies. The presence of thallium is most effective for assessing myocardium viability.

Clients with coronary artery disease (CAD) may have normal thallium perfusion scans at rest; however, during exercise, when the heart demands more oxygen, myocardial perfusion decreases. The client returns in 2 or more hours to take a second scan of the heart at rest. Frequently second scans are done to differentiate between an ischemic area and an infarcted or scarred area of the myocardium. This test could be normal even with moderately narrowed coronary arteries when adequate collateral circulation to the heart is present.

Uses for the stress/exercise test or the exercise myocardial perfusion test include screening for CAD, evaluating myocardial perfusion, evaluating the work capacity of cardiac clients, and developing a cardiac rehabilitation program.

EXERCISE TECHNETIUM PERFUSION TEST For detection of myocardial ischemia, technetium Tc-99m-laced compounds, such as Tc-99m-sestamibi (cardiolite), are commonly used for perfusion scanning because they are trapped in the myocardium and do not redistribute. Technetium compounds provide more clinical information by allowing the assessment of perfusion, wall motion, and ejection fraction in one test procedure. Other technetium agents approved by the U.S. Food and Drug Administration (FDA) are Tc-99m-teboroxime and Tc-99m-tetrofosmin. Tc-99m-furifusion is a new technetium agent whose approval by the FDA is still pending.

Cardiolite imaging is perhaps the most useful noninvasive test for diagnosing and following CAD at the present time. Positive stress cardiolite scanning should be considered strong presumptive evidence of CAD. The more markedly abnormal the scan, the more likely the client has serious CAD. It is important to correlate the scan findings with the ECG, the exercise stress test, and the clients symptoms. The use of gated single positron emission (SPECT) (gated refers to the synchronizing of images with the computer and the clients heart rhythm) greatly improves the sensitivity and specificity of the cardiolite scan.

NUCLEAR PERSANTINE (DIPYRIDAMOLE) STRESS TEST This is an alternative stress test usually ordered when the client is not physically able to exercise or to walk on a treadmill. Persantine is administered intravenously to dilate the coronary arteries and increase blood flow to the myocardium. Arteries that have become narrowed because of CAD cannot expand like normal arteries. Thallium, cardiolite, or other Tc-based compounds, administered intravenously, detect decreased blood flow to the heart muscle (myocardium). The isotope is administered 3 minutes after the 4-minute IV Persantine infusion.

The client must avoid foods, beverages, and medications containing xanthines (caffeine and theophyllines), such as colas, chocolate, and tea, 24 hours prior to the test, and theophylline preparations 36 hours prior to the test.

Nuclear Persantine stress testing is contraindicated for clients who have severe bronchospastic lung disease, such as asthma, or advanced atrioventricular heart block. Additional unfavorable conditions in which this test is not indicated includes acute myocardial infarction within 48 hours of the test, severe aortic or mitral stenosis, resting systolic blood pressure less than 90 mm Hg, and allergy to dipyridamole.

NUCLEAR DOBUTAMINE STRESS TEST Dobutamine is an adrenergic (sympathomimetic) drug that increases myocardial contractility, heart rate, and systolic blood pressure, which increases the myocardial oxygen consumption and thus increases coronary blood flow. If the client has heart block or asthma and takes a theophylline preparation daily, this test may be ordered instead of the nuclear Persantine (dipyridamole) stress test. Dobutamine is an alternative stressor test.

Nuclear dobutamine stress testing can identify clients with CAD and identify those who are at high risk for severe ischemic changes prior to vascular surgery. Currently this test is not FDA approved; it is considered an investigational drug test.

Contraindications for nuclear dobutamine stress testing include clients having acute myocardial infarction within 10 days, acute myocarditis or pericarditis, unstable angina pectoris (prolonged episodes, episodes at rest), ventricular or atrial dysrhythmias, severe hypertension or hypotension, severe aortic or mitral stenosis, hyperthyroidism, and acutely severe infections. Propranolol (Inderal) should be available for any possible adverse reaction to the dobutamine infusion.

Procedure

- A consent form should be signed by the client.
- The client should be NPO 2 or 3 hours before the test. The client should not consume alcoholic and caffeine-containing drinks and should avoid smoking for 2 to 3 hours before the test. Milk could cause nausea.
- Medications should be taken, unless otherwise indicated by the health care provider.
- Comfortable clothes should be worn (i.e., shorts or slacks with a belt and sneakers or tennis shoes with socks). Most bedroom slippers are not suitable.
- The chest is shaved as needed, and the skin is cleansed with alcohol.
- Electrodes are applied to the chest according to the lead selections.
- Baseline ECG, pulse rate, and BP are taken and then are monitored throughout the test.
- The test is stopped if the client becomes dyspneic, suffers severe fatigue, complains of chest pain, has a rapid increase in pulse rates and/or BP, or develops life-threatening arrhythmias (i.e., ventricular tachycardia, premature ventricular contractions [PVCs] greater than 10 PVC in 1 minute).
- Usually the test is not stopped abruptly unless this is necessary. Vital signs and ECG tracings are recorded at the end of the testing or the recovery stage.
- The test takes approximately 30 minutes, which includes up to 10 to 15 minutes of exercising.

TREADMILL STRESS TEST Usually there are five stages. In the first stage the speed is 2 mph at a 3% grade or incline for 3 minutes. In the second stage the speed is 3.3 mph at a 6% grade for another 3 minutes. Normally the speed does not go beyond 3.3 mph. With each stage the grade is increased 3% and the time is increased by 3 minutes, unless fatigue or adverse reactions occur. The power-driven treadmill has support rails to help the client maintain balance.

BICYCLE ERGOMETER TEST The client is instructed to pedal the bike against an increased amount of resistance. The bike handlebars are for maintaining balance and should not be gripped tightly for support. The client should not shower or take a hot bath for 2 hours after testing.

EXERCISE THALLIUM PERFUSION TEST An IV line is inserted. Exercise time for the stress test is determined. The client obtains the maximal exercise level, and thallium is injected intravenously 1 minute before the test ends. The client continues to exercise for 1 to 2 more minutes. A scan is then taken by gamma camera, which visualizes thallium perfusion of the myocardium.

Client returns in 2 or more hours for a second scan.

EXERCISE TECHNETIUM PERFUSION TEST With the cardiolite stress test, the client receives two injections intravenously, one at rest and one at stress. The client should be NPO for 2 to 3 hours prior to the test. Any medications that may affect the blood pressure or heart rate should be discontinued 24 to 48 hours prior to the test (unless the test is being performed to evaluate the efficacy of cardiac medications). The client should be physically able to exercise on a treadmill. The total time for the test is 3 hours, which is shorter than thallium imaging.

PERSANTINE (DIPYRIDAMOLE) STRESS TEST The client remains NPO after midnight except for water. A diabetic client may have a light breakfast of juice and toast and one-half of the insulin dose, but should first check with the health care provider. Caffeine-containing drugs, food, and beverages such as colas must be avoided 24 hours prior to the test. Decaffeinated beverages should also be avoided. Theophylline preparations (TheoDur, Theolair-SR, Bronkodyl, Elixophyllin SR, and others) should be stopped 36 hours before the test.

The client is in a supine position during the test. The client receives a total of 0.56 mg/kg/dose of IV Persantine (dipyridamole) over a period of 4 minutes. Three minutes after the Persantine infusion, the isotope (thallium, cardiolite, or other Tc-based compound) is injected intravenously. Aminophylline should be available to reverse any adverse reaction to Persantine. Imaging procedure begins 15 to 30 minutes after the isotope infusion. Heart rate, blood pressure, and ECG will be monitored before and during the test.

The test is terminated if any of the following occur: ventricular tachycardia, second degree (heart block, severe ST-segment depression, severe hypotension [less than 90 mm Hg], and severe wheezing). The asthmatic client may use the beta-agonist inhaler if necessary during the procedure.

NUCLEAR DOBUTAMINE STRESS TEST The client remains NPO after midnight except for water. Beta blockers, calcium channel blockers, and angiotensin-converting enzyme (ACE) inhibitors should be discontinued 36 hours prior to the test. Nitrates should not be taken 6 hours before the test. Dobutamine is administered intravenously using an infusion pump. The dobutamine is mixed in a liter of normal saline solution and the dose and infusion rate is increased until the client's heart rate reaches approximately 85% of his or her maximum predicted heart rate. If the heart rate is less than 110 beats/min, IV atropine sulfate may be given. The isotope is injected when the maximum heart rate is achieved.

The test is terminated if any of the following occur: atrial or ventricular tachycardia, atrial flutter or fibrillation, severe ST-segment depression, progressive anginal pain, severe hypotension (less than 90 mm Hg systolic), and severe hypertension (greater than 220 mm Hg systolic or greater

NURSING IMPLICATIONS WITH RATIONALE Stress/Exercise Tests

- Recognize when the stress/exercise test is contraindicated (i.e., with recent myocardial infarction; severe, unstable angina; uncontrolled cardiac dysrhythmias; congestive heart failure; or recent pulmonary embolism).
- Check that the consent form has been signed.
- Recognize whether a treadmill stress test or pharmacological stress test is appropriate.
- Review medications that may interfere with test, for example, beta blockers to decrease heart rate.

TREADMILL STRESS TEST—CLIENT TEACHING

- Explain the procedure to the client in regard to NPO 2 to 3 hours prior to test; not smoking, continuing with medications; the clothing and shoes that should be worn; shaving and cleansing the chest area; electrode application; continuous monitoring of the ECG, pulse rate, and BP; and not leaning on the rails of the treadmill or the handlebars of the bike.
- Instruct the client to inform the cardiologist or technician if he or she experiences chest pain, difficulty in breathing, or severe fatigue. The risk of having a myocardial infarction during the stress test is less than 0.2%.
- Inform the client that after 10 to 15 minutes of testing or when the heart rate is at a desired or an elevated rate, the test is stopped. It will be terminated immediately if there are any severe ECG changes (i.e., multiple PVCs, ventricular tachycardia).
- Allow the client to ask questions. Refer questions you cannot answer to other appropriate health professionals (i.e., a cardiologist, a specialized technician, or a nurse in the stress test laboratory).
- Instruct the client to continue the walking exercise at the completion of the test for 2 to 3 minutes to prevent dizziness. The treadmill speed will be decreased. Tell the client that he or she may be perspiring and may be "out of breath." Profuse diaphoresis, cold and clammy skin, severe dyspnea, and severe tachycardia are not normal and the test will be terminated.
- Inform the client that an ECG and vital signs are taken 5 to 10 mintes after the stress test (recovery stage).
- Encourage the client to participate in a cardiac/exercise rehabilitation program as advised by the health care provider/cardiologist. Tell the client of the health advantages—constant heart monitoring, improved collateral circulation, increased oxygen supply to the heart, and dilating coronary resistance vessels.
- Discourage the client over 35 years of age from doing strenuous exercises without having a stress/exercise test or a cardiac evaluation.
- Inform the client that he or she can resume activity as indicated.
- Explain to the client that a written report is submitted to the clients personal physician from the cardiologist. The client should check with the health care provider for the test results.

EXERCISE THALLIUM PERFUSION TEST—CLIENT TEACHING

- Explain the procedure for the test (see Procedure). Explain that the difference between the routine stress test and the exercise thallium perfusion test is an injection of thallium 201 during the routine stress test followed by scans and/or x-rays. Nursing implications are the same for both tests.
- Instruct the client to return for additional pictures in 2 to 4 hours as indicated by the technician or cardiologist.

EXERCISE TECHNETIUM PERFUSION TEST—CLIENT TEACHING

- Explain the procedure (see Procedure)
- The client should lie quietly for approximately 30 minutes during the imaging.
- Inform the client that the test should last no more than 3 hours.
- Instruct the client taking medications that affect the blood pressure or heart rate to check with the health care provider about discontinuing the medications for 24 to 48 hours prior to testing.

NUCLEAR PERSANTINE (DIPYRIDAMOLE) STRESS TEST— CLIENT TEACHING

- Explain the procedure for the test to the client (see Procedure). The client should be NPO after midnight except for water.
- Instruct the client to avoid food, beverages, and drugs that contain caffeine. Beverages and foods rich in caffeine include colas (Coke and Pepsi), Dr. Pepper, Mountain Dew, Tab, chocolate (syrup and candy), tea, and coffee. Decaffeinated coffee and tea should also be avoided. Drugs containing caffeine include Anacin, Excedrin, NoDoz, Wigraine, Darvon compound, cafergot, fiorinal. Theophylline preparations should be avoided 36 hours before the test; the client should check with the health care provider in case it is not possible to discontinue the theophylline drug for that period of time.
- Explain to the client that first Persantine will be given intravenously and then an isotope. The client is positioned under a camera with his or her left arm over the head. The camera will be moving very close to the chest for taking pictures (imaging). The imaging takes approximately 20 to 30 minutes.
- Instruct the client to return for additional pictures in 2 to 4 hours as indicated by the technician or cardiologist.
- Explain to the client that a written report is submitted to the clients personal health care provider from the cardiologist.

NUCLEAR DOBUTAMINE STRESS TEST—CLIENT TEACHING

- Explain the procedure for the test to the client (see Procedure). The client should be NPO after midnight except for water.
- Instruct the client to discontinue drugs that are beta blockers, calcium channel blockers, or ACE inhibitors for 36 hours prior to the test with the health care providers approval. Give the client the date and time for stopping the drug. Nitrates should not be taken 6 hours before the test unless necessary (check with the health care provider).

than 120 mm Hg diastolic). Nitroglycerin may be given for angina pain. Propranolol (Inderal) should be available for adverse reaction to dobutamine. Imaging procedure occurs 15 minutes after the completion of the dobutamine infusion.

Factors Affecting Diagnostic Results

- Certain drugs (e.g., digitalis preparations) can cause a false-positive test result.
- Leaning on support rails of the treadmill or the handlebars of the bicycle.

NUCLEAR PERSANTINE (DIPYRIDAMOLE) STRESS TEST

- Taking theophylline preparations within 24 hours of the test.
- Ingesting caffeine products (beverages, chocolates) 6 hours before the test.
- Ingesting decaffeinated beverages 4 hours before the test.

NUCLEAR DOBUTAMINE STRESS TEST

- Taking beta blockers, calcium channel blockers, ACE inhibitors, 24 hours before the test.
- Taking nitrates 4 hours before the test.
- Ingesting a full meal 4 hours before the test.

THEOPHYLLINE (SERUM)

Reference Values

Therapeutic Range: *Adult:* 5–20 mcg/ml, 28–112 μmol/l (SI units). *Elderly:* 5–18 mcg/ml. *Premature Infant:* 7–14 mcg/ml. *Neonate:* 3–12 mcg/ml. *Child:* Same as adult. Toxic Level: *Adult:* greater than 20 mcg/ml, greater than 112 µmol/l (SI units). *Elderly:* Same as adult. *Premature Infant:* greater than 14 mcg/ml. *Neonate:* greater than 13 mcg/ml. *Child:* Same as adult.

Description

Theophylline, a xanthine derivative, relaxes smooth muscle of the bronchi and pulmonary blood vessels; reduces pulmonary hypertension; stimulates the central nervous system; stimulates myocardium, resulting in an increase in the force of contraction and cardiac output; increases renal blood flow, causing diuresis; and relaxes smooth muscles of the gastrointestinal tract. Usually theophylline products are given to control asthmatic attacks and to treat acute attack. Oral theophylline preparations are well absorbed from the gastrointestinal tract.

Ninety percent of theophylline is metabolized in the liver, with about 60% bound to plasma protein and 40% free. Ten percent of the drug is excreted unchanged in the urine. The half-life of theophylline is 5 to 10 hours in a non-smoker, 3 ½ to 5 hours in a smoker, and 3 ½ in children. Peak blood levels after an orally administered dose of theophylline occurs in 1 to 2 hours.

Persons with heart failure or liver disease or who are either very young or elderly could develop theophylline toxicity quickly. Serum theophylline levels in these persons should be monitored frequently.

Early signs and symptoms of theophylline toxicity are anorexia, nausea, vomiting, abdominal discomfort, nervousness, jitters, tachycardia, and cardiac arrhythmias. If severe theophylline toxicity occurs (greater than 30 mcg/ml) cardiac

dysrhythmias, seizures, respiratory arrest, and/or cardiac arrest might result.

THYROID-STIMULATING HORMONE (TSH) (SERUM)

Reference Values

Adult: 0.35–5.5 microinternational unit/ml, (μIU/ml), less than 3 ng/ml.
Newborn: less than 25 microinternational unit/ml (μIU/ml) by the third day.

Description

The anterior pituitary gland (anterior hypophysis) secretes thyroid-stimulating hormone (TSH) in response to thyroid-releasing hormone (TRH) from the hypothalamus. TSH stimulates the secretion of thyroxine (T_4) produced in the thyroid gland. The secretion of TSH is dependent on the negative-feedback system—a decreased T_4 level promotes the release of TRH, which stimulates TSH secretion. An elevated T_4 level suppresses TRH release, which suppresses TSH secretion.

TSH and T_4 levels are frequently measured to differentiate pituitary from thyroid dysfunctions. A decreased T_4 level and a normal or elevated TSH level can indicate a thyroid disorder. A decreased T_4 level with a decreased TSH level can indicate a pituitary disorder.

THYROXINE (T_4) (SERUM)

Reference Values

Adult: *Reported as Serum Thyroxine:* T_4 by column: 4.5–11.5 mcg/dl. T_4 (RIA): 5–12 mcg/dl. Free T_4: 1.0–2.3 ng/dl. *Reported as Thyroxine Iodine:* T_4 by column: 3.2–7.2 mcg/dl.
Child: *Newborn:* 11–23 mcg/dl. *1 to 4 Months Old:* 7.5–16.5 mcg/dl. *4 to 12 Months Old:* 5.5–14.5 mcg/dl *1 to 6 Years Old:* 5.5–13.5 mcg/dl. *6 to 10 Years Old:* 5–12.5 mcg/dl.

Description

Thyroxine (T_4) is the major hormone secreted by the thyroid gland and is at least 25 times more concentrated than triiodothyronine (T_3). The serum T_4 levels are commonly used to measure thyroid hormone concentration and the function of the thyroid gland. The use of protein-bound iodine (PBI) is considered obsolete, and this test is seldom performed.

In some institutions the T_4 test is required for all newborns (as is the phenylketonuria [PKU] test) to detect a decreased thyroxine secretion, which could lead to irreversible mental retardation.

TORCH SCREEN TEST

Reference Values

Maternal: *IgG Titer Antibodies:* Negative. *IgM Titer Antibodies:* Negative.
Infant: Same as maternal; infant should be under 2 months of age.

Arthroscopy A surgical procedure in which an arthroscope (a thin tube that is lighted and has a camera in one end) is inserted into a joint.

Ascites Excess fluid in the peritoneal cavity.

Asepsis The absence of disease-causing organisms.

Assault An attempt or threat to touch another person unjustifiably.

Assertive behavior Behavior that consists of expressing one's wishes and opinions, or taking care of oneself, but not at the expense of others.

Assertive communication A style of communication in which the sender declares and affirms his or her own rights while respecting the rights of others.

Assessment A systematic method of collecting data about a client for the purpose of determining the client's current and ongoing health status, predicting risks to health, and identifying health-promoting activities.

Assignment A downward or lateral transfer of the responsibility for completing an activity from one individual to another.

Assimilation The process of adapting to and integrating characteristics of the dominant culture as one's own; The process by which humans encounter and react to new situations by using the mechanisms they already possess.

Associative play A stage of play in which children play together or share tasks during play.

Astereognosis The inability to identify objects by touch.

Asthma A chronic inflammatory disease of the lungs characterized by recurrent episodes of wheezing, breathlessness, chest tightness, and coughing.

Asystole Cardiac standstill.

Atelectasis Collapse of lung tissue following obstruction of the bronchus or bronchioles.

Atheist An individual who does not believe in God.

Atherosclerosis A form of **arteriosclerosis** in which deposits of fat and fibrin obstruct and harden the arteries.

Atrial gallop A heart sound produced by atrial contraction and ejection of blood into the ventricle during late diastole. Also called the fourth heart sound.

Atrial kick An extra bolus of blood delivered to the ventricles before they contract.

Atrial natriuretic factor (ANF) A peptide-hormone released from cells in the atrium of the heart in response to excess blood volume and stretching of the atrial walls.

Atrial septal defect An opening in the atrial septum that permits left-to-right shunting of blood.

Atrioventricular (AV) canal defect A combination of defects in the atrial and ventricular septa and portions of tricuspid and mitral valves. A complete AV canal defect allows blood to travel freely among all four chambers of the heart.

Atrophy The wasting away or decrease in size of an organ, muscle, or tissue.

Attention deficit disorder (ADD) A variation in central nervous system processing characterized by developmentally inappropriate behaviors involving inattention. When hyperactivity

and impulsivity accompany inattention, the disorder is called **attention deficit hyperactivity disorder (ADHD)**.

Attention impairment A condition marked by an inability to process information and respond to such information appropriately; a client with attention impairment will have poor concentration and be easily distracted.

Attentive listening Listening actively, using all senses, as opposed to listening passively with just the ear.

Audiologist A health care professional specializing in identifying, diagnosing, treating, and monitoring disorders of the auditory and vestibular portions of the ear.

Audit An examination of records or financial accounts to verify accuracy.

Aura An olfactory or visual sensory sensation that may provide an early warning sign of a seizure.

Auscultation The process of listening to sounds produced within the body.

Authoritarian decision making A process in which one person makes a decision requiring others to conform, usually without input from those whom the decision affects. An example is when the employer decides on a policy that the nurse is expected to follow.

Authority The right to act or to complete a task.

Autistim spectrum disorders (ASDs) This term described three of the pervasive developmental disorders that share a number of similarities: autism, Asperger syndrome, and pervasive developmental disorder not otherwise specified (PDD-NOS).

Autoantibodies Antibodies that react to the individual's own tissues.

Autocratic (authoritarian) leader A **leader** who makes decisions for the group, based on a belief that individuals are externally motivated (their driving force is extrinsic, they desire rewards from others) and are incapable of independent decision making.

Autografting A procedure performed in the surgical suite in which part of the client's healthy skin is removed and used to effect permanent skin coverage over the wound area.

Autoimmune disorder/disease Failure of immune system to recognize itself, resulting in normal host tissue being targeted by immune defenses.

Autologous bone marrow transplant Bone marrow transplant using a client's own bone marrow.

Automatism A reaction that occurs automatically, without conscious thought.

Autonomic dysreflexia An exaggerated sympathetic response that occurs in clients with spinal cord injuries at or above the T6 level. Also called *autonomic hyperreflexia*.

Autonomy The state of being independent and self-directed without outside control. **Autonomy** refers to the right to make one's own decisions.

Autosomal chromosomes Genetic material found in the cell nucleus that determines physical characteristics (excluding gender) of the individual.

Autosome A single chromosome from any one of the 22 pairs of chromosomes not involved in sex determination (X or Y); humans have 22 pairs of autosomes.

Avian Influenza Also known as "bird flu," it is a form of influenza that commonly infects birds. This virus has not yet demonstrated the ability to spread between humans; however, concerns are that it will mutate to allow person-to-person spread. This viral strain has a mortality rate of greater than 50% in people who have been infected due to close association with infected birds.

Avoidant personality disorder (APD) One of 11 types of **personality disorders** recognized by the *DSM-IV*, APD is characterized by a pattern of social withdrawal along with a sense of inadequacy, fear, and hypersensitivity to potential rejection or shame.

Avolition The inability to persist in goal-directed activities.

Awareness The ability to perceive environmental stimuli and body reactions and to respond appropriately through thought and action.

Axial loading The application of vertical force to the spinal column.

Azotemia Increased levels of nitrogenous wastes in the blood.

B Lymphocytes Integral to specific immune response, they are activated and mature into either plasma cells, which secrete antibodies, or memory cells.

Bacilli Rod-shaped bacteria.

Bacteremia The presence of bacteria in the blood.

Bacteria The most common category of infection-causing microorganisms.

Bactericidal agent Destroys bacteria.

Bacteriostatic agent Prevents the growth and reproduction of some bacteria.

Balloon tamponade The inflation of the balloon tip of a multiple-lumen nasogastric tube to control bleeding.

Barotrauma Lung injury caused by alveolar overdistention.

Barrel chest An increase in the anteroposterior chest diameter resulting from air trapping and hyperinflation.

Basal cell carcinoma An epithelial tumor believed to originate either from the basal layer of the epidermis or from cells in the surrounding dermal structures.

Basal metabolic rate The amount of energy expended by the body at rest.

Base excess (BE) A calculated value also known as *buffer base capacity*. The BE measures substances that can accept or combine with hydrogen ions. It reflects the degree of acid–base imbalance by indicating the status of the body's total buffering capacity.

Bases (or **alkalis**) Substances that accept hydrogen ions in solution.

Basic research A form of **scientific research** that is concerned with generating new knowledge.

Battery The willful or negligent touching of a person (or the person's clothes or even something the person is carrying), which may or may not cause harm.

Behavioral therapy A form of therapy in which clients learn techniques to modify or change maladaptive behaviors.

Behaviorist theory A theory of learning that promotes the immediate identification of and reward for correct responses.

Belief system The way in which a culture explains the mysteries of the universe and life.

Benchmarking A method of comparing standards to actual performance.

Beneficence The act of doing good.

Benign prostatic hypertrophy (BPH) Age-related, nonmalignant enlargement of the prostate gland that decreases the outflow of urine by obstructing the urethra, causing difficult urination.

Bereavement The subjective response experienced by the surviving loved ones after the death of a person with whom they have shared a significant relationship.

Bias A negative belief or preference that is generalized about a group that leads to prejudgment.

Bilevel ventilator (BiPAP) Mechanical ventilation that provides inspiratory positive airway pressure as well as airway support during expiration.

Biliary colic A severe, steady pain in the epigastric region or right upper quadrant of the abdomen.

Binge drinking A form of alcoholism in which the addict frequently drinks copious amounts of alcohol in a single session.

Binge eating The ingestion of huge amounts of food (about 3,500 kcal) within a short time (about 1 hour).

Binge eating disorder An eating disorder characterized by recurring episodes of **binge eating**, a sense of lack of control and negative feelings about oneself, but without intervening periods of behavior such as self-induced vomiting, purging by laxatives, fasting, or prolonged exercise.

Binuclear family A postdivorce family in which the biologic children are members of two nuclear households, both that of the father and that of the mother, and the children alternate between the two homes.

Bioethics The application of ethics to issues of human life or health (e.g., to decisions about abortion or euthanasia).

Biological rhythm A cyclical event or function that consists of repeated occurrences and repeated, regular intervals between occurrences.

Bioterrorism The deliberate release of a virus, bacteria, or other microbes used to cause illness or death in people, animals, or plants.

Bipolar disorder A mood disorder characterized by alternating depression and elation, with periods of normal mood in between; also called manic–depressive disorder.

Bisexual An individual who is attracted to members of both sexes.

Bisphosphonates Drugs used to treat osteoporosis that inhibit bone resorption by suppressing osteoclast activity.

Blackouts A form of amnesia about events that occurred during the drinking period, which is seen in the early stages of alcoholism.

Bladder training Gradually increases the bladder capacity by increasing the intervals between voidings and resisting the urge to void.

Blended family A family formed after the death or divorce of a parent, may include stepparents on both sides, stepchildren, half-siblings.

Blepharism Spasms that cause the eye to blink continuously.

Blood flow The volume of blood transported in a vessel, in an organ, or throughout the entire circulation over a given period of time.

Blood pressure The force that blood exerts against the walls of the arteries as it is pumped from the heart.

Blood urea nitrogen (BUN) A measure of blood level of urea, the end product of protein metabolism.

Bloodborne pathogens Microorganisms carried in blood and body fluids that are capable of infecting others with serious and difficult to treat viral infections.

Body fluid Any fluid that is essential to homeostasis; water is the primary body fluid.

Body image The image of physical self.

Body mass index (BMI) A method of comparing weight to height as an indirect measure of body fat.

Body substance isolation (BSI) System that employs generic infection control precautions for all clients, except those with the few airborne diseases.

Body surface area (BSA) The relationship between height and weight measured in square meters.

Bone marrow transplant The treatment of disease by infusing a client with his or her own bone marrow or that of a healthy donor.

Borborygumus Hyperactive, high-pitched, tinkling, rushing, or growling bowel sounds heard in diarrhea or at the onset of bowel obstruction.

Borderline personality disorder (BPD) One of 11 **personality disorders** defined in the *DSM-IV*, it is marked by unstable interpersonal relationships, self-image, affect, and impulsivness.

Boundaries The invisible lines that define the amount and kind of contact allowable among members of the family and between the family and outside systems.

Boutonnière deformity A flexion deformity of the PIP joints with extension of the DIP joint.

Brachytherapy Radiation treatment given by placing radioactive material directly in or near the target, which is often a tumor.

Bradykinesia Slowed movements due to muscle rigidity.

Bradyphrenia Slowed thinking and a decreased ability to form thoughts, to plan, or to make decisions.

Brain death The cessation and irreversibility of all brain functions, including the brainstem.

Brainstem Contains the midbrain, pons, and medulla oblongata. Located between the cerebrum and spinal cord, the brainstem connects pathways between the higher and lower structures. Ten of the 12 pairs of cranial nerves originate in the brainstem.

Brainstorming A method of group decision making in which several people in a group generate ideas about a subject for the group as a whole to comment on, discuss, improve upon, select, or reject.

Braxton Hicks contractions Intermittent painless uterine contractions that may occur every 10–20 minutes and occur more frequently near the end of pregnancy.

Breach of duty A deviation from the standard of care owed the client.

Breakthrough pain A sudden flare or increase in pain despite comfort with or without baseline analgesia.

Breast Mammary gland.

Breast cancer The unregulated growth of abnormal cells in breast tissue.

Brief psychotic disorder Rapid onset of at least one of the following psychotic symptoms: delusions, hallucinations, disorganized speech, or disorganized behavior. The episode lasts at least 1 day but less than 1 month, after which the person returns to the premorbid level of functioning.

Bronchiectasis Chronic dilation of the bronchi and bronchioles.

Bronchiolitis A lower respiratory tract illness that occurs when an infecting agent (virus or bacterium) causes inflammation and obstruction of the small airways.

Bronchogenic carcinomas Tumors of the airway epithelium.

Bruits Blowing sound sometimes heard due to restriction of blood flow through the vessels.

Buffers Substances that prevent major changes in pH by releasing hydrogen ions.

Bulimia nervosa A type of **eating disorder** characterized by cycles of binge eating followed by purging.

Bureaucratic leader A **leader** who relies on the organization's rules, policies, and procedures to direct the group's work efforts.

Burn An injury resulting from exposure to heat, chemicals, radiation, or electric current.

Burn shock Hypovolemic shock resulting from the shift of a massive amount of fluid from the intracellular and intravascular compartments into the interstitium following burn injury.

Burnout A complex syndrome of behaviors that manifests as physical and emotional depletion, a negative attitude and self-concept, and feelings of helplessness and hopelessness.

Cachexia Physical wasting from weight loss and loss of muscle mass due to the rapid growth and reproduction of cancer cells and their need for increased nutrients.

Caffeine A stimulant that increases the heart rate and acts as a diuretic.

Calcium oxalate A chemical compound from which kidney stones may form.

Calcium phosphate A chemical compound from which kidney stones may form.

Calculi Renal stones.

Cancellous bone The spongy tissue of bone.

Cancer A family of complex diseases with manifestations that vary according to body system and type of tumor cells.

Cancer pain Pain that may result from the direct effects of the disease and its treatment, or it may be unrelated to the disease and its treatment in individuals with cancer.

Candidiasis A common, opportunistic fungal infection in clients with AIDS.

Cannabis sativa The plant source of marijuana.

Capitation A system of health care reimbursement in which health care providers are paid a fixed dollar amount per person for providing an agreed-upon set of health services to a defined population for a specific period of time.

Carbon monoxide (CO) Odorless, colorless, tasteless gas that is very toxic.

Carcinogen A substance that causes cancer.

Carcinogenesis The production or origin of cancer.

Cardiac arrest The cessation of heart function.

Cardiac cycle One contraction and relaxation of the heart; a single heartbeat.

Cardiac index The cardiac output adjusted for the client's body size.

Cardiac output The amount of blood pumped by the ventricles into the pulmonary and systemic circulations in 1 minute.

Cardiac reserve The heart's ability to respond to the body's changing need for cardiac output.

Cardinal ligament Major ligament of the uterus containing the uterine artery and vein.

Cardiogenic shock Shock that occurs when the heart's pumping ability is compromised to the point that it cannot maintain cardiac output and adequate tissue perfusion.

Cardiomyopathy Primary abnormality of the heart muscle that affects its structural or functional characteristics.

Cardiopulmonary resuscitation (CPR) A mechanical attempt to maintain tissue perfusion and oxygenation using oral resuscitation and external cardiac compressions.

Care management model A model of care delivery that focuses on the needs of the integrated delivery system.

Care map A standardized plan that outlines the expected outcomes and care required for clients with common, predictable—usually medical—conditions. Such plans, also referred to as **critical pathways, multidisciplinary care plans** and **collaborative care plans**, sequence the care that must be given on each day during the projected length of stay for the specific type of condition.

Caring Intentional action that conveys physical and emotional security and genuine connectedness with another person or group of people.

Caring practice Nursing care that includes connection, mutual recognition, and involvement.

Carpal spasm Involuntary contraction of the hand and fingers due to decreased calcium levels.

Carrier Human or animal reservoir of a specific infectious agent that usually does not manifest any clinical signs of the disease.

Case management A range of models for integrating health care services for individuals or groups; a method for delivering nursing care in which the nurse is responsible for a caseload of clients across the health care continuum.

Caseation necrosis A process in which tissue infected with **mycobacterium tuberculosis** dies and forms a cheeselike center in the infectious **bacilli**.

Cast A rigid device applied to immobilize injured bones and promote healing.

Catabolism The breakdown of body proteins.

Cataract An opacification (clouding) of lens of the eye.

Catatonic excitement A positive symptom of **schizophrenia** characterized by hyperactivity and bizarre behavior.

Catatonic inhibition A negative symptom of **schizophrenia** that involves decreased activity level; limited speech; minimal self-care; and, at times, a trancelike state.

Cation An **ion** that carries a positive charge.

Causation The act of causing something to happen; in legal terms, a breach of duty by a nurse or professional that caused injury or harm to the client.

Cavitation Formation of a cavity or bubble.

Cell-mediated (cellular) immune response Direct or indirect inactivation of antigen by lymphocytes.

Cellulitis An acute bacterial **infection** of the dermis and underlying connective tissue. Cellulitis is characterized by red or lilac, tender, warm, edematous skin that may have an ill-defined, nonelevated border.

Central nervous system (CNS) One of two principal parts of the neurologic system, the central nervous system consists of the brain and the spinal cord.

Central nervous system depressants Drugs that act to slow brain function, decreasing levels of alertness and awareness. CNS depressants include including barbiturates, benzodiazepines, paraldehyde, meprobamate, and chloral hydrate.

Central pain A type of pain related to a lesion in the brain that may spontaneously produce high-frequency bursts of impulses that are perceived as pain.

Cephalocaudal Growth that proceeds in the direction from head to toe.

Cerebellum Located below the cerebrum and behind the brainstem, it coordinates stimuli from the cerebral cortex to provide precise timing for skeletal muscle coordination and smooth movements.

Cerebral palsy (CP) A group of chronic conditions affecting body movement, coordination, and posture that results from a nonprogressive abnormality of the immature brain.

Cerebrum The largest portion of the brain.

Certification The **credentialing** process by which a nongovernmental agency or association recognizes the professional competence of an individual who has met the predetermined qualifications specified by the agency or association.

Cerumen Earwax.

Cervical cap A latex cup-shaped device, used with spermicidal cream or jelly, that fits snugly over the cervix and is held in place by suction.

Cervix The narrow neck of the uterus.

Chain of command The hierarchy of authority and responsibility within an organization.

Chancre A painless ulceration formed during the first stage of syphilis.

Change-of-shift report A report given to nurses on the next shift.

Channel The medium a sender uses to convey a message; for example, talking face to face.

Charismatic leader One whose leadership is characterized by an emotional relationship between the leader and the group members.

Chart A formal, legal document that provides evidence of a client's care. Also called the **client record**.

Charting The process of making an entry on a **client record**.

Charting by exception (CBE) A documentation system in which only significant findings or exceptions to norms are recorded.

Cheilosis Cracking of lips.

Chemical restraints Medications such as neuroleptics, anxiolytics, sedatives, and psychotropic agents used to control socially disruptive behavior.

Chemotherapy Cancer treatment involving the use of cytotoxic medications to decrease tumor size, adjunctive to surgery or radiation therapy; or to prevent or treat suspected metastases.

Chief complaint The symptoms reported that are the reason for admission or treatment of the client.

Childless family (also *child-free family*) A family without children.

Chlamydias A group of sexually transmitted infections caused by *Chlamydia trachomatis.*

Chloasma (melasma gravidarum) Brownish pigmentation over the bridge of the nose and the cheeks during pregnancy and in some women who are taking oral contraceptives. Also called *mask of pregnancy.*

Cholangitis Duct inflammation.

Cholecystitis Inflammation of the gallbladder.

Cholelithiasis The formation of stones (*calculi* or *gallstones*) in the gallbladder or biliary duct system.

Chromosomes Tightly coiled strands of DNA within the nucleus that contain genetic information.

Chronic bronchitis A disorder of excessive bronchial mucous secretion.

Chronic fatigue Profound fatigue of long duration that is not improved by rest.

Chronic fatigue syndrome A complex disorder in which the client experiences unrelenting fatigue and associated symptoms that are not alleviated by substantial rest and cannot be otherwise explained for a period of six months or longer.

Chronic illness An alteration in health or function that lasts for an extended period of time, usually six months or longer, and often for the duration of the individual's life.

Chronic infection An **infection** that develops slowly and persists for months or sometimes years.

Chronic intermittent colitis A recurrent form of **ulcerative colitis** characterized by insidious onset, few systemic manifestations, and attacks lasting 1–3 months, which occur at intervals of months to years.

Chronic lymphocytic leukemia (CLL) A disorder characterized by the proliferation and accumulation of small, abnormal, mature lymphocytes in the bone marrow, peripheral blood, and body tissues.

Chronic myeloid leukemia (CML) A disorder characterized by abnormal proliferation of all bone marrow elements.

Chronic obstructive pulmonary disease (COPD) A specific progressive disorder that slowly alters the structures of the respiratory system over time, irreversibly affecting lung function.

Chronic pain Prolonged pain, usually lasting longer than 6 months. It is not always associated with an identifiable cause and is often unresponsive to conventional medical treatment.

Chronic renal failure A type of **renal failure** that progresses slowly with few symptoms until the kidneys are severely damaged and unable to meet the excretory needs of the body.

Chronic venous insufficiency A disorder of inadequate venous return over a prolonged period of time.

Chvostek's sign Facial grimacing caused by repeated contractions of the facial muscle.

Cirrhosis A progressive, irreversible disorder, eventually leading to liver failure; the end stage of chronic liver disease.

Civil law Laws that define and address the rights and duties of private persons or citizens.

Clara Barton A schoolteacher who volunteered as a nurse during the Civil War. Most notably, she organized the American Red Cross, which linked with the International Red Cross when the U.S. Congress ratified the Geneva Convention in 1882.

Clean A state of **medical asepsis** in which almost all microorganisms are absent.

Client A person who engages the advice or services of another person who is qualified to provide this service.

Client advocate One who acts to protect the client and defend the client from harm. Client advocacy is a primary role for every nurse.

Client record See **chart**.

Client-focused care A delivery model that brings all services and care providers to the clients. The idea is that if activities normally provided by various members of the health care team are moved closer to the client, the number of personnel involved and the number of steps involved to get the work done are decreased.

Clinical decision support (CDS) Describes a system that provides health care providers with knowledge or specific information that is intelligently filtered, presented at appropriate times, and that enhances health and health care. Decision support systems aid in and strengthen the selection of viable options for care using the information of an organization.

Clinical information systems (CISs) Large, computerized database management systems that support several types of activities that may include provider order entry, result retrieval, documentation, and decision support across distributed locations.

Clinical nursing research Nursing research involving clients or studies that have the potential for affecting the care of clients, such as studies with animals or with so-called normal subjects.

Clonic phase Typically the second phase in a generalized or tonic-clonic seizure, characterized by alternating muscular contraction and relaxation.

Closed fracture A bone fracture in which the skin remains intact; also known as a simple fracture.

Closed questions Restrictive questions that generally require only "yes" or "no" or short factual answers giving specific information.

Club drugs Substances popular among adolescents and young adults who frequent dance clubs and "raves," the most common of which is MDMA (methylenedioxymethamphetamine), better known as Ecstasy.

Coaching A personal, performance-focused conversation designed to help an employee renew his or her commitment to self-sufficiency, organizational goals and values, and improve performance.

Coarctation of the aorta Narrowing or constriction in the descending aorta, often near the ductus arteriosus or left subclavian artery, which obstructs the systemic blood outflow.

Cocaine A powerful stimulant of natural origin that acts at the nerve terminals to prevent the reuptake of dopamine and norepinephrine, which in turn results in vasoconstriction, tachycardia, and hypertension.

Code of ethics A general guide for a profession's membership and a social contract with the public that it serves.

Codependence A cluster of maladaptive behaviors exhibited by significant others of a substance-abusing individual that serves to enable and protect the abuse at the expense of living a full and satisfying life.

Cognition The process by which an individual learns, stores, retrieves, and uses information.

Cognitive development The manner in which people learn to think, reason, and use language.

Cognitive domain The "thinking" domain; it includes six intellectual abilities and thinking processes beginning with knowing, comprehending, and applying and progressing to analysis, synthesis, and evaluation.

Cognitive skills Intellectual skills or thought processes that include problem solving, decision making, critical thinking, and creativity.

Cognitive theory Theory of cognitive development that recognizes developmental levels of learners and acknowledges the influence of the learner's motivation and environment.

Cohesiveness The attachment group members feel toward each other, the group, and the task. When there is a high level of cohesiveness, group members feel greater satisfaction.

Coinsurance The percentage share (usually 20%) of the cost of health insurance that is paid by the client or individual; the remaining percent is paid by the plan.

Coitus interruptus A method of contraception in which the male withdraw from the female's vagina when he feels that ejaculation is impending.

Colectomy Surgical resection and removal of the colon.

Collaboration Two or more people working toward a common goal by combining their skills, knowledge, and resources while avoiding duplication of effort.

Collaborative care plan A standardized plan that outlines the care required for clients with common, predictable—usually medical—conditions. Such plans, also referred to as

multidisciplinary care plans and **critical pathways**, sequence the care that must be given on each day during the projected length of stay for the specific type of condition.

Collaborative interventions Actions the nurse carries out in collaboration with other health care team members, such as physical therapists, social workers, dietitians, and physicians.

Colloid osmotic pressure A pulling force exerted by colloids that helps maintain the water content of blood by pulling water from the interstitial space into the vascular compartment.

Colloids Substances such as large protein molecules that do not readily dissolve into true solutions.

Colon cancer Cancer of the third segment of the large bowel.

Colonization The process by which strains of microorganisms become resident flora, capable of growing and multiplying.

Colorectal cancer Cancer of the colon or rectum.

Colostomy A surgical opening into the colon.

Combined oral contraceptives A combination of estrogen and progestin. Also called birth control pills.

Comfort To ease the grief or trouble of others; to give hope.

Commitment The state or an instance of being obligated or emotionally impelled (motivated).

Communicable disease An illness that is transmitted directly from one person or animal to another by contact with body fluids, or that is indirectly transmitted by contact with contaminated objects or **vectors**.

Communication Any means of exchanging information or feelings between two or more people. It is a basic component of human relationships, including nursing.

Communicator style The manner in which one communicates, including the way in which one interacts with others.

Community Emergency Response Team (CERT) Program Provided training to individuals on expectations, decision-making skills, rescuer safety, and organization in order for individuals charged with responding during emergencies to be better prepared to do so.

Comorbidity The presence of one or more additional disease processes.

Compartment syndrome Condition in which the tissue pressure in a muscle compartment exceeds microvascular pressure, interrupting cellular perfusion.

Compassion An awareness of and concern for others' suffering.

Competence Possession of the necessary knowledge and skills to perform one's job appropriately and safely on a daily basis.

Compliance The relationship between the volume of the intracranial components and intracranial pressure; the amount of distention or expansion the ventricles can achieve to increase stroke volume; An individual's desire to learn and to act on learning.

Complicated grief A form of **grief** in which the individual's strategies to cope with the loss are maladaptive.

Compromised host An individual who is at increased risk of infection.

Computer vision syndrome Eye and vision problems that result from work done in close proximity such as occurs when using a computer for long periods of time.

Concept map A visual tool in which ideas or data are enclosed in circles or boxes of some shape, and relationships between these are indicated by connecting lines or arrows.

Concrete thinking A type of thinking characterized by a focus on facts and details and an inability to generalize or think abstractly.

Concurrent audit A type of **audit** that is conducted during the client's course of care; it examines the care being given to achieve a desired outcome in the client's health.

Condom A sheath of synthetic material that covers the penis to prevent conception or disease.

Confabulation Making up information to fill memory gaps; used as defensive mechanism to protect the person's attempt to protect self-esteem when confronted with memory loss.

Confidentiality The assurance the client has that private information will not be disclosed without the client's consent. Confidentiality refers to both the nature of the information the nurse obtains from the client as well as how the nurse treats client information once it has been disclosed to the nurse.

Conflict Tension that arises when the action of one person frustrates the ability of the other to achieve a goal.

Confusion An alteration in cognition that makes it difficult to think clearly, focus attention, or make decisions.

Congenital cataracts A type of **cataract** that may appear in a child at birth or in childhood, usually in both eyes.

Congenital heart defect A defect of the heart or great vessels that is present at birth.

Congruent communication Occurs when the verbal and nonverbal aspects of the message match.

Conjugate vera The true conjugate, which extends from the middle of the sacral promontory to the middle of the pubic crest.

Conjunctiva The thin, transparent membrane that covers the anterior surface of the eye and lines the inner surfaces of the eyelids.

Conjunctivitis Inflammation of the **conjunctiva**. The most common eye disease, conjunctivitis is usually caused by a bacterial or viral infection.

Connective tissue Tissue made of fiber that forms the framework for support of the body's tissue and organs.

Consciousness A condition in which the person is aware of self and environment and is able to respond appropriately to stimuli. Full consciousness requires both normal arousal and full cognition.

Consensus decision making A process in which the emphasis is on including others in the decision making, even if an individual must make the final decision. Also referred to as **participative decision making**.

Consequence-based (teleological) theories Theories that look to the outcomes (consequences) of an action in judging whether that action is right or wrong.

Constipation Fewer than three bowel movements per week or the difficult passage of stools.

Constructivism A collection of theories with a common thread of individuals actively constructing knowledge to solve realistic problems, often in collaboration with others.

Consumer An individual, a group of people, or a community that uses a service or commodity.

Contact precautions Used for clients who are known to have or suspected of having serious illnesses that are easily transmitted by direct contact with the client or by contact with items in the environment, such as *shigella*.

Contingency contracts A reinforcement process. Congingency contracts operate by "if-then" rules. If the client performs a targeted response, such as abstinence from the addictive behavior (gambling, drug use, cutting, etc.), then the client receives desired reinforcers.

Contingency planning A type of planning in which a manager identifies and manages the many problems that interfere with getting work done. Contingency planning may be *reactive*, in response to a crisis, or *proactive*, in anticipation of problems or in response to opportunities.

Continuance commitment The awareness of costs associated with leaving a profession that develops when negative consequences of leaving, such as loss of income, are seen as reasons to remain.

Continuous positive airway pressure (CPAP) Mechanical ventilation that applies positive pressure to the airways of a client who is breathing spontaneously. Breathing is client-triggered and pressure controlled. CPAP is used to help maintain open airways and alveoli, decreasing the work of breathing.

Continuous quality improvement (CQI) A process used to improve quality and performance.

Continuous renal replacement therapy (CRRT) A form of **dialysis** in which blood is continuously circulated through a highly porous hemofilter from artery to vein or vein to vein.

Contractility The inherent capability of the cardiac muscle fibers to shorten.

Contracture Permanent shortening of connective tissue.

Contralateral deficit Loss or impairment of sensorimotor functions on the side of the body opposite the side of the brain that is damaged by stroke.

Controlled Substance Act A federal law that requires drugs be classified based on the substance's medical use, potential for abuse, and safety risks.

Controlling A management function that involves comparing actual results with projected results, similar to the evaluation step in the nursing process.

Convergence The medial rotation of the eyeballs so that each is directed toward the viewed object.

Cooperative play The stage of play in which children work together to contribute to a unified whole, such as forming a sports team or dancing in an ensemble.

Cor pulmonale Right-sided heart failure.

Corneal abrasion Disruption of the superficial epithelium of the cornea.

Corneal reflex Closure of eyelids (blinking) due to corneal irritation.

Corpus The upper triangular portion of the uterus, also called the uterine body.

Corpus luteum A small yellow body that develops within a ruptured ovarian follicle.

Corrective action Steps taken to overcome a job performance problem.

Coruna The elongated portion of the uterus where the fallopian tubes enter.

Coryza Inflammation of the mucous membranes lining the nose usually associated with nasal discharge.

Couplet Two premature ventricular contractions in a row.

Couvade In some cultures, the male's observance of certain rituals and taboos to signify the transition to fatherhood.

Covert conflict Conflict that is not is not discussed openly by those who are in conflict.

Covert data Information that is apparent only to the person affected; can be described or verified only by that person. Examples include itching, pain, feelings, and values. May be referred to as **subjective data** or **symptoms**.

Creatinine clearance A test that uses 24-hour urine and serum creatinine levels to determine the glomerular filtration rate; a sensitive indicator of renal function.

Creativity Thinking that results in the development of new ideas and products.

Credentialing Formal identification of professionals who meet predetermined standards of professional skill or competence.

Credibility The quality of being truthful, trustworthy, and reliable.

Crepitation A grating sound.

Crime An act prohibited by statute or by common law principles.

Criminal law Law that defines conduct that is harmful to another individual or to society as a whole and that may be punishable by fines or imprisonment.

Critical analysis The application of a set of questions to a particular situation or idea to determine essential information and ideas and discard superfluous information and ideas.

Critical pathway A standardized plan that outlines the expected outcomes and care required for clients with common, predictable—usually medical—conditions. Such plans, also referred to as **care maps**, **multidisciplinary care plans**, and **collaborative care plans**, sequence the care that must be given on each day during the projected length of stay for the specific type of condition.

Critical thinking A cognitive process during which an individual reviews data and considers potential explanations and outcomes before forming an opinion or making a decision.

Crohn's disease (also known as regional enteritis) A chronic, relapsing **inflammatory bowel disorder** affecting the GI tract.

Cross-dressing Occurs when an individual of one gender (typically male) dresses in clothing specific to the opposite gender.

Crystalloids Salts that dissolve readily into true solutions.

Cues Subjective or objective data that can be directly observed by the nurse; that is, what the client says or what the nurse can see, hear, feel, smell, or measure.

Cultural deprivation A lack of culturally assistive, supportive, or facilitative acts.

Cultural groups Racial, ethnic, religious, or social groups with specific group behaviors and characteristics that are learned and shared, including language, customs, beliefs, and values.

Cultural values Preferred ways of behaving or thinking that are sustained over time and used to govern a cultural group's actions and decisions.

Culture The patterns of behavior and thinking that people living in social groups learn, develop, and share.

Cultures Laboratory cultivations used to identify probable microorganisms by their characteristics, such as shape, growth patterns, and Gram-staining qualities.

Curling's ulcers Acute ulcerations of the stomach or duodenum that form following a burn injury.

Cyanosis Gray to blue or purple skin color caused by deoxygenated hemoglobin.

Cyclothymic disorder A type of **bipolar disorder** characterized by chronic, fluctuating mood disturbances involving numerous periods of hypomanic symptoms and numerous periods of depressive symptoms.

Cystitis Inflammation of the urinary bladder.

Cytokines Proteins that carry messages for immune system function.

Damages Money paid as compensation for loss or injury.

Database All information about a client, including nursing health history and physical assessment, physician history, physical examination, and laboratory and diagnostic test results.

Dating violence A type of intimate partner abuse occurring between individuals who are dating, but not married or otherwise related.

Dawn phenomenon A rise in blood glucose between 4 a.m. and 8 a.m. that is not a response to hypoglycemia.

Dead space Areas of the lung that are ventilated but not perfused.

Death anxiety Worry or fear related to death or dying.

Debridement The process of removing necrotic material, including all loose tissue, wound debris, and eschar (dead tissue), from a wound.

Decibels Units of loudness.

Decision making A critical-thinking process for choosing the best actions to meet a desired goal.

Declarative memory Memory related to people and facts, is consciously accessible, and can be verbally expressed.

Decode To relate the message perceived to the receiver's storehouse of knowledge and experience and to sort out the meaning of the message.

Decompensation Loss of effective compensation.

Deductible The amount of money a client is required to pay for health care services before insurance coverage begins to pay for care.

Deductive reasoning Making specific observations from a generalization.

Deep venous thrombosis (DVT) A blood clot that forms along the intimal lining of a large vein.

Defecation The expulsion of feces from the anus and rectum.

Defibrillation An emergency procedure that delivers an electrical shock to stop ventricular fibrillation and return to a rhythm that promotes cardiac output sufficient to sustain life.

Defining characteristics Client signs and symptoms that must be present to validate a nursing diagnosis.

Deformation The alteration of the spinal cord and soft tissues caused by abnormal movement.

Dehiscence An unintended separation of wound margins due to incomplete healing.

Dehydration A condition that occurs when a body does not take in as much water as it loses or lacks sufficient reserves to maintain proper function.

Delayed union The prolonged healing of bones beyond the usual time period.

Delegate One who assumes responsibility for the actual performance of a task or procedure.

Delegation The transference of responsibility and authority for an activity to a competent individual.

Delegator One who assigns a task to another but retains accountability for the outcome.

Delirium An acute disorder of cognition that affects functional independence.

Delirium tremens A medical emergency usually occurring 3–5 days following alcohol withdrawal and lasting 2–3 days. Characterized by paranoia, disorientation, delusions, visual hallucinations, elevated vital signs, vomiting, diarrhea, and diaphoresis. Also known as **alcohol withdrawal delirium**.

Delphi technique A method of group decision making that requires participants to maintain their anonymity, which eliminates peer pressure. Data are gathered through interviews or questionnaires in a series of rounds in which an initial question is posed. Once the responses are returned, they are compiled and redistributed. The participants do not know who said what: The comments or ratings are gathered for a compiled listing and are rated through averaging or statistical analysis. With the Delphi technique, agreement is reached as the process continues, either by consensus, voting, or mathematical average.

Delusion Firm idea or belief not founded in reality.

Democratic leader A **leader** who encourages group discussion and decision making.

Demography The study of population, including statistics about distribution by age and place of residence, mortality (death), and morbidity (incidence of disease).

Denominations Groups of members that adhere to the same practices and beliefs.

Dental caries Cavities.

Deoxyribonucleic acid (DNA) One of two types of nucleic acid made by cells, DNA contains the genetic instructions for the development and functioning of human beings.

Dependent functions Therapies, interventions, and treatments provided by the nurse that are dependent on orders from a physician or instructions from another health care provider, such as a physical therapist.

Dependent interventions Activities carried out under the physician's orders or supervision, or according to specified routines.

Dependent personality disorder (DPD) A **personality disorder** marked by a pervasive, excessive, and unrealistic need to be cared for; fear of separation; lack of self-confidence; an inability to make decisions; and an inability to function independently.

Depersonalization A feeling of strangeness or unreality about the self.

Depolarization The rapid inflow of sodium ions, causing an electrical change in which the inside of a cell becomes positive in relation to the outside; the phase in which the heart contracts as a result of ion channel functions.

Depo-Provera A long-acting progesterone that provides highly effective birth control for 3 months when given as a single injection.

Derealization A feeling of disconnection from the environment.

Dermatome An area of skin innervated by the cutaneous branch of one spinal nerve.

Desaturated blood Blood that is low in oxygen.

Desire phase The first phase of the sexual response cycle; the arousal of sexual interest.

Detrusor muscle The smooth muscle layers of the bladder wall, the detrusor muscle allows the bladder to expand as it fills with urine and contract as it releases urine during voiding.

Development An increase in the complexity and function of skill progression, the individual's capacity and skill to adapt to the environment. Related to **growth**.

Developmental disability Any of a variety of chronic conditions characterized by mental and/or physical impairment.

Developmental stage A level of achievement for a particular segment of a person's life.

Developmental task A skill or behavior pattern learned during stages of development.

Diabetes mellitus Group of chronic disorders of the endocrine pancreas, all categorized under a broad diagnostic label. The condition is characterized by inappropriate hyperglycemia caused by a relative or absolute deficiency of insulin or by a cellular resistance to the action of insulin.

Diabetic ketoacidosis A form of metabolic acidosis induced by stress in a person with type 1 diabetes.

Diabetic nephropathy Disease of the kidneys in clients with diabetes that is characterized by the presence of albumin in the urine, hypertension, edema, and progressive renal insufficiency.

Diabetic neuropathy A disorder of the peripheral nerves and the autonomic nervous system in clients with diabetes, which manifests in one or more of the following: sensory and motor impairment, muscle weakness and pain, cranial nerve disorders, impaired vasomotor function, impaired gastrointestinal function, and impaired genitourinary function.

Diabetic retinopathy The collective name for the changes in the retina that occur in the person with diabetes. The retinal capillary structure undergoes alterations in blood flow, leading to retinal ischemia and a breakdown in the blood retinal barrier.

Diagnosis A statement or conclusion regarding the nature of a phenomenon.

Diagnosis-related groups (DRGs) A Medicare system for paying hospitals and physicians that establishes fees according to diagnosis.

Diagnostic label Title used in writing a nursing diagnosis; taken from the North American Nursing Diagnosis Association (NANDA) standardized taxonomy of terms.

Diagonal conjugate Distance from the lower posterior border of the symphis pubis to the scaral promontory.

Dialysate Dialysis solution.

Dialysis A process by which fluids and molecules pass through a semipermeable membrane from an area of higher solute concentration to one of lower solute concentration according to the rules of osmosis.

Diaphragm A flexible disk that covers the cervix to prevent conception.

Diaphysis The shaft of the bone.

Diarrhea The passage of liquid feces and an increased frequency of defecation.

Diastole The phase of ventricular relaxation between heartbeats.

Diastolic blood pressure The minimum pressure within the arteries during **diastole**.

Diathermy Treatment with heat generated by high-frequency electrical currents.

Diet recall Client history of intake over a specified period of time.

Differentiated practice A system in which the best possible use of nursing personnel is based on their educational preparation and resultant skill sets.

Differentiation A process occurring over many cell cycles that allows cells to specialize in certain tasks.

Diffusion The continual intermingling of molecules in liquids, gases, or solids brought about by the random movement of the molecules.

Digital rectal examination An examination to detect for abnormalities in the rectum that can be detected through palpation.

Dihydrotestosterone (DHT) Formed in the prostate from testosterone, DHT is the androgen that mediates prostatic growth at all ages.

Dilated cardiomyopathy The most common form of **cardiomyopathy**, in which the heart chambers dilate and ventricular contraction is impaired.

Directing The process of getting the work of an organization done.

Directive interview A highly structured interview that uses closed questions to elicit specific information.

Dirty In **medical asepsis**, a term used to indicate that microorganisms are likely to be present.

Disaster A public emergency necessitating assistance from outside the affected community.

Discharge planning The process of anticipating and planning for client needs after discharge.

Discipline A method of teaching children the rules for how to behave in society and what is expected in different circumstances.

Discovery The legal process of obtaining information before a trial.

Discrimination The differential treatment of individuals or groups based on categories such as race, age, weight, gender, or social class, that occurs when an individual acts on prejudice and denies other people one or more of their fundamental rights.

Discussion An informal oral consideration of a subject by two or more health care personnel to identify a problem or establish strategies to resolve a problem.

Disease A detectable alteration in body function resulting from infection by microorganisms that causes a reduction of capacities or a shortening of the normal life span.

Disease surveillance Monitoring patterns of disease occurrence from cases of infections and communicable diseases reported by health care workers to state officials.

Disenfranchised grief Occurs when a person is unable to acknowledge the loss to other persons.

Disinfectants Agents that destroy pathogens other than spores.

Diskectomy The removal of the nucleus pulposus of an intervertebral disk.

Dismissal Termination from employment.

Dissatisfaction problems Issues that arise from unmet sexual needs and expectations.

Disseminated intravascular coagulation (DIC) A complication resulting from prolonged retention of the dead fetus in the mother's womb.

Distributive shock Shock which results from widespread vasodilatation and decreased peripheral resistance. Also called **vasogenic shock.**

Diuresis (polyurea) The production of abnormally large amounts of urine.

Diuretics Pharmacologic agents that increase urine formation and secretion.

Diversity The unique variations among and between individuals, variations that are informed by genetics and cultural background, but that are refined by experience and personal choice.

Diverticula Saclike projections of mucosa through the muscular layer of the colon.

Documenting The process of making an entry in a **client record.**

Do-not-intubate (DNI) order Usually written by the physician for the client who has a terminal illness or is near death, this order is usually based on the wishes of the client and family that no life-saving measures are provided once the client stops breathing.

Do-not-resuscitate (DNR or "no-code") order Usually written by the physician for the client who has a terminal illness or is near death, this order is usually based on the wishes of the client and family that no cardiopulmonary resuscitation be performed for respiratory or cardiac arrest.

Dormant Temporarily inactive but not dead.

Double depression A condition in which individuals experience **dysthymic disorder** in combination with **major depressive disorder**.

Down Syndrome A condition associated with mental retardation; Down Syndrome results when an individual is born with an extra chromosome.

Dramatic play The stage of play in which children use props to act out the drama of human life.

Droplet nuclei Residue of evaporated droplets emitted by an infected host; can remain in the air for long periods of time.

Droplet precautions Used for clients who are known to have or suspected of having serious illnesses transmitted by particle droplets larger than 5 microns, such as pertussis or pneumonia.

Dullness In percussion, a thudlike sound produced by dense tissue such as the liver, spleen, or heart.

Duodenal ulcer A **peptic ulcer** occurring in the duodenum.

Durable health care power of attorney A written directive made by an individual that designates who may make decisions about the individual's health care in the event the individual is unable to do so.

Durable power of attorney A document that can delegate the authority to make health, financial, and/or legal decisions on a person's behalf.

Duration In auscultation, the length of time that a sound is heard.

Duty A legally enforceable obligation to conform to a particular standard of conduct.

Dwarfism Excessively short stature, typically resulting from a genetic abnormality.

Dysfunctional uterine bleeding (DUB) Vaginal bleeding that is usually painless but abnormal in amount, duration, or time of occurrence.

Dysmenorrhea Painful menstruation.

Dysparenuria Painful intercourse.

Dysphagia Difficulty swallowing.

Dysplasia A loss of DNA control over differentiation occurring in response to adverse conditions.

Dyspnea Shortness of breath or difficulty breathing.

Dysrhythmias Abnormal heart rate or rhythm.

Dysthymic disorder A chronic disorder in which periods of depressed mood are interspersed with normal mood.

Dystonias Severe muscle spasms, particularly of the back, neck, tongue, and face.

Dysuria Difficult or painful urination.

Eating disorder A set of maladaptive responses to stress or anxiety characterized by obsessions with food and weight, often to the extent that daily functioning is impaired and physical and psychological health are threatened.

Echolalia The compulsive parroting of a word or phrase just spoken by another.

Echopraxia The compulsive imitation of the movements of another.

Eclampsia A major complication of pregnancy characterized by hypertension, albuminuria, oliguria, tonic and clonic convulsions, and coma.

Ecologic theory A theory of development that emphasizes the presence of mutual interactions between the individual and all of life's settings.

Ecomap Visual representation of how the family unit interacts with the external community environment, including schools, religious institutions, occupational duties, and recreational pursuits.

Ectopic beats Impulses originating outside normal conduction pathways of the heart.

Edema Swelling caused by excess fluid trapped in bodily tissue.

Effectiveness A measure of the quality or quantity of services provided.

Efficiency A measure of the resources used in the provision of nursing services.

Ego The realistic part of the individual that balances the gratification demands of the **id** with the limitations of social and physical circumstances.

Ego-syntonic The perception that one's difficulties in dealing with other people are external.

E-health The provision of health information, services, and products via the Internet.

Ejection fraction The fraction or percent of the diastolic volume that is ejected from the heart during systole.

Elderspeak A speech style similar to baby talk that gives the message of dependence and incompetence to older adults. The characteristics of elderspeak include diminutives (inappropriate terms of endearment), inappropriate plural pronoun use, tag questions, and slow, loud speech.

Elective surgery Performed when surgical intervention is the preferred treatment for a condition that is not imminently life threatening (but may ultimately threaten life or well-being) or to improve the client's life.

Electrocardiogram (ECG) A graphic record of the heart's activity.

Electrocardiography A diagnostic test of cardiac function.

Electroconvulsive therapy (ECT) A treatment procedure during which an electric current is passed through the brain; it is useful to clients with severe depression, acute mania, some psychotic conditions, and those who are acutely suicidal.

Electroencephalogram (EEG) Measures and records the brain's electrical activity.

Electrolyte Charged ion capable of conducting electricity.

Electronic communication Communication involving computers and technology (i.e., e-mail).

Electronic health record Electronic file containing integrated client health data. This term is sometimes used specifically to refer to the client's lifetime electronic health record.

Electronic medical record Legal record of a client created in a health care agency that is used to inform the client's **electronic health record**.

Elimination The secretion and excretion of body wastes from the kidneys and intestines.

Embolus Debris that obstructs a blood vessel.

Embryo The early stage of development of the young of any organism. In humans the embryonic period is from about 2 to 8 weeks' gestation and is characterized by cellular differentiation and predominantly hyperplastic growth.

Embryonic membranes The amnion and chorion.

Emergency A sudden, often unforeseen, event that threatens health or safety.

Emergency preparedness The act of making plans to prevent, respond to, and recover from emergencies.

Emergency response The coordinated response to meet the needs of the individuals in the community affected by an emergency or disaster.

Emergency surgery Surgery that is performed immediately to preserve function or the life of the client.

Emigration The movement of leukocytes through the blood vessel wall into affected tissue spaces in response to illness or injury.

Emotional availability The quality of parent–child interactions, including parental sensitivity, structuring, and degree of intrusiveness and hostility.

Emotions Feeling responses to a wide variety of emotional stimuli.

Emphysema A progressive pulmonary disease characterized by destruction of the walls of the alveoli, with resulting enlargement of abnormal air spaces.

Empirical data Data that can be gathered (observed or experienced) through the sense organs.

Empirical knowing Knowledge that comes from science; ranges from factual, observable phenomena to theoretical analysis.

Empyema Accumulation of purulent (infected) exudate in a space, e.g., the pleural cavity or the gallbladder.

Enabling behavior Any action by a person that consciously or unconsciously facilitates substance dependence.

Encapsulated Enclosed.

Encoding The selection of specific signs or symbols (codes) to transmit the message, such as which language and words to use, how to arrange the words, and what tone of voice and gestures to use.

Encopresis Abnormal elimination pattern characterized by recurrent soiling or passage of stool at inappropriate times.

Enculturation The process by which children learn culture from adults.

Endocardial cushions Fetal growth centers for mitral and tricuspid valves and AV septum.

End-of-life The final weeks of life when death is imminent.

End-of-life care The nursing care provided to a client who is dying or who is near death.

Endogenous insulin Insulin that is produced by the body.

Endogenous Developing from within.

Endometrium The innermost mucosal layer of the uterus.

Endotoxins Found in the cell wall of gram-negative bacteria, endotoxins are released only when the cell is disrupted. They act as activators of many human regulatory systems, producing fever, inflammation, and potentially clotting, bleeding, or hypotension when released in large quantities.

End-stage renal disease (ESRD) The final stage of **chronic renal failure**, when the kidneys are unable to excrete metabolic wastes and regulate fluid and electrolyte balance adequately.

Engrossment The characteristic sense of absorption, preoccupation, and interest in the infant demonstrated by fathers during early contact.

Enophthalmos Sunken appearance of the eyes.

Entropion Inversion of the eyelid.

Enuresis Involuntary passing of urine in children after bladder control is achieved.

Eosiniphil A type of leukocyte found in large numbers in the respiratory and gastrointestinal tracts. Eosinophils are thought to be responsible for protecting the body from parasitic

worms. They also play a role in hypersensitivity response by inactivating some of the inflammatory chemicals released during the inflammatory response.

Epidemic Widespread outbreak of infectious disease with many infected people.

Epilepsy A chronic disorder characterized by recurrent, unprovoked seizures secondary to a central nervous system (CNS) disorder.

Erectile dysfunction (ED) The inability of the male to attain and maintain an erection sufficient to permit satisfactory sexual intercourse.

Ergonomics The study and design of a work environment that maximizes productivity by reducing operator fatigue and discomfort.

Error Failure of a planned action to be completed as intended; the use of a wrong plan to achieve an aim.

Erythema A reddening of the skin.

Eschar Hard, leathery crust that covers a burn wound and harbors necrotic tissue.

Escharotomy Surgical removal of eschar from the torso or extremity to prevent circumferential constriction.

Esotropia Momentary turning inward of the eyes.

Estrogen The primary hormone responsible for female sex characteristics.

Ethical knowing Knowledge that focuses on matters of obligation or what ought to be done.

Ethics A system of moral principles or standards governing human conduct.

Ethnic groups Group of individuals that have common racial characteristics and share a cultural heritage.

Etiology The causal relationship between a problem and its related or risk factors.

Eustachian tube Connects the middle ear with the nasopharynx to help equalize the pressure in the middle ear with the atmospheric pressure.

Euthanasia From the Greek for painless, easy, gentle, or good death, now commonly used to signify a killing prompted by a humanitarian motive.

Euthyroid A normal thyroid state.

Evaluating/Evaluation The fifth and final phase of the **nursing process**; a planned, ongoing, purposeful activity in which clients and health care professionals determine (a) the client's progress toward achievement of goals/outcomes and (b) the effectiveness of the nursing care plan.

Evaluation statement A statement written by the nurse after evaluating if a client's goal has been met. Evaluation statements consist of two parts: a conclusion and supporting data. The *conclusion* is a statement that the goal/desired outcome was met, partially met, or not met. The *supporting data* are the list of client responses that support the conclusion.

Evidence-based practice (EBP) This means that nurses make clinical decisions based on the best research evidence, their clinical expertise, and the health care preferences of their clients.

Evisceration Protrusion of body contents through a surgical wound.

Exacerbation A reappearance of symptoms of a chronic illness; sometimes referred to as a *flare.*

Excitement phase The second phase of the sexual response cycle, marked by an increase in the blood flow to various body parts resulting in erection of the penis and clitoris and swelling of the labia, testes, and breasts.

Exercise A type of physical activity defined as a planned, structured, and repetitive bodily movement performed to improve or maintain one or more components of physical fitness.

Exercise intolerance Decreased ability to participate in activities using large skeletal muscles because of fatigue or dyspnea.

Exogenous Developing from outside sources.

Exogenous insulin Insulin from a source outside the body.

Exophthalmos Protruding eyes.

Exotoxins Soluble proteins that microorganisms secrete into surrounding tissue. Exotoxins are highly poisonous, causing cell death and dysfunction.

Expectorate To expel or spit out.

Expert systems Computer systems that use artificial intelligence to model a decision that experts in the field would make. Unlike decision support systems that provide several options from which the user may choose, expert systems provide the best decision based on criteria that experts would use.

Expressed consent An oral or written agreement.

Expressive jargon Using unintelligible words with normal speech intonations as if truly communicating in words.

Expressive speech The ability to speak and be understood by others.

Extended family The relatives of **nuclear** families, such as grandparents, aunts, and uncles.

Extended-kin network family A form of **extended family** in which two nuclear families of primary or unmarried kin live in close proximity to each other and share a social support network, goods, and services.

Extracapsular extraction A surgical treatment for **cataracts** in which the anterior capsule, nucleus, and cortex of the lens are removed, leaving the posterior capsule intact.

Extracapsular fracture A hip fracture involving the trochanteric region.

Extracellular fluid (ECF) Fluid found outside the cells and accounts for about one-third of total body fluid. It is subdivided into compartments. The two main compartments of ECF are intravascular and interstitial.

Extracorporeal shock wave lithotripsy (ESWL) A noninvasive technique for fragmenting kidney stones using shock waves generated outside the body.

Extrapulmonary tuberculosis Results when the disease spreads through the blood and lymph system to other organs.

Extrapyramidal side effects (EPS) A particularly serious set of adverse reactions to antipsychotic drugs. **EPS** include acute dystonia, akathisia, Parkinsonism, and tardive dyskinesia.

Exudate Material, such as fluid and cells, that has escaped from blood vessels during the inflammatory process and is deposited in tissue or on tissue surfaces.

Failure to thrive (FTT) A syndrome in which an infant falls below the fifth percentile for weight and height on a standard growth chart or is falling in percentiles on a growth chart.

Faith To believe in or be committed to something or someone.

Fallopian tubes Tubes that extend from the lateral angle of the uterus and terminate near the ovary. Also called oviducts and uterine tubes.

False imprisonment The unjustifiable detention of a person without legal warrant to confine the person.

False pelvis The portion of the pelvis above the linea terminalis, which supports the enlarged pregnant uterus.

Family Individuals who are joined together by marriage, blood, adoption, or residence in the same household.

Family burden The overall level of distress experienced by the family as a result of a family member's mental illness.

Family-centered care Health care that is provided in partnership with the client and family.

Family-centered nursing Nursing that considers the health of the family as a unit in addition to the health of individual family members.

Family cohesion The emotional bonding between family members.

Family communication Includes listening, speaking, self-disclosure, and the abilities of the family as a group.

Family coping mechanisms The behaviors families use to deal with stress or changes imposed from either within or without the family.

Family development The dynamics or changes a family experiences over time, including changes in relationships, communication patterns, roles, and interactions.

Family flexibility The amount of change in a family's leadership, role relationships, relationship rules, and the family's ability to respond to stress.

Family recovery Family response to a member's mental illness.

Family support Support from family members as they care for other family members, e.g., one sister relieves another to care for their aging mother over the weekend.

Family therapy A form of therapy in which the family system is treated as a unit and the focus is on family dynamics.

Fasciectomy (fascial excision) Process of excising the wound to the level of fascia.

Fat Embolism Syndrome (FES) Occurs when fat globules lodge in the pulmonary vascular bed or peripheral circulation.

Fatigue A condition characterized by a lack of energy and motivation that may or may not be accompanied by drowsiness.

Febrile seizures Generalized seizures that usually occur in children as the result of rapid temperature rise above 39°C (102°F), usually in association with an acute illness. No evidence of intracranial infection or other defined cause is found.

Fecal impaction A mass or collection of hardened feces in the folds of the rectum.

Fecal incontinence The loss of voluntary ability to control fecal and gaseous discharges through the anal sphincter.

Feces (stool) Body wastes and undigested food eliminated from the bowel.

Feedback The response or message that the receiver returns to the sender during communication; the mechanisms by which some of the output of a system is returned to the system as input.

Female orgasmic disorder A sexual arousal cycle that stops before orgasm.

Female reproductive cycle (FRC) The monthly rhythmic changes in sexually mature women; composed of the ovarian cycle, during which ovulation occurs, and the uterine cycle, during which menstruation occurs.

Female sexual arousal disorder Discomfort or pain during sexual intercourse caused by a lack of vaginal lubrication.

Fertility awareness-based methods Contraception based on an understanding of the changes that occur throughout a woman's ovulatory cycle. Also called *natural family planning*.

Fertilization The process by which a sperm fuses with an ovum to form a new diploid cell, or zygote.

Fetal alcohol syndrome A form of mental retardation that results when the developing fetus is exposed to ethyl alcohol.

Fetal demise Intrauterine fetal death (IUFD) occurs after 20 weeks' gestation.

Fetal heart rate (FHR) The number of times the fetal heart beats per minute; normal range is 120 to 160.

Fetal lie Relationship of the cephalocaudal axis (spinal column) of the fetus to the cephalocaudal axis (spinal column) of the woman. The fetus may be in a longitudinal or transverse lie.

Fetal position Relationship of the landmark on the presenting fetal part to the front, sides, or back of the maternal pelvis.

Fetal tachycardia A fetal heart rate of 160 beats per minute or more during a 10-minute period of continuous monitoring.

Fetoscope An adaptation of a stethoscope that facilitates auscultation of the fetal heart rate.

Fetoscopy A technique for directly observing the fetus and obtaining a sample of fetal blood or skin.

Fetus The child in utero from about the seventh to ninth week of gestation until birth.

Fibrin degradation products Potent anticoagulants.

Fibromyalgia A chronic disorder characterized by widespread musculoskeletal pain, fatigue, and multiple **tender points**.

Fidelity A moral principle that obligates the individual to be faithful to agreements and responsibilities one has undertaken.

Filtration A process whereby fluid and solutes move together across a membrane from one compartment to another.

Filtration pressure The pressure in the compartment that results in the movement of the fluid and substances dissolved in fluid out of the compartment.

Fimbria A funnel-like enlargement of the Fallopian tube with many fingerlike projections (fimbriae) reaching out to the ovary.

First heart sound The heart sound produced by the closure of the AV valve, characterized by the syllable "lub."

5 P's of neurovascular assessment Pain, pulse, pallor, paralysis/paresis, paresthesia.

Fixation The immobilization or inability of the individual to proceed to the next developmental stage because of anxiety.

Flaccidity Absence of muscle tone; hypotonia.

Flatness In percussion, an extremely dull sound produced by very dense tissue, such as muscle or bone.

Flatulence The presence of excessive amounts of gas in the stomach or intestines.

Flatus Gas or air normally present in the stomach or intestines.

Flight of ideas Rapidly changing, fragmentary thoughts.

Florence Nightingale Considered the founder of modern nursing, she was influential in developing nursing education, practice, and administration.

Flow sheet A record of the progress of specific or specialized data such as vital signs, fluid balance, or routine medications, often charted in graph form.

Fluid resuscitation The administration of intravenous (IV) fluids to restore the circulating blood volume during the acute period of increasing capillary permeability.

Fluid volume deficit (FVD) (hypovolemia) Loss of both water and electrolytes in similar proportions from the extracellular fluid.

Fluid volume excess (FVE) (hypervolemia) The retention of both water and sodium in similar proportions to normal extracellular fluid (ECF).

Focal seizures (also known as *partial seizures*) Seizures that are caused by abnormal electrical activity in one hemisphere or in a specific area of the cerebral cortex, most often the temporal, frontal, or parietal lobes. The seizure may spread regionally, and the symptoms are related to the region of the cortex that is affected.

Focus charting A method of charting that uses key words or foci to describe what is happening to the client.

Follicle-stimulating hormone (FSH) Hormone produced by the anterior pituitary during the first half of the menstrual cycle, stimulating development of the graafian follicle.

Foramen ovale An opening between the atria of the fetal heart.

Foraminotomy An enlargement of the opening between the disk and the facet joint to remove bony overgrowth.

Forced expiratory volume in 1 second (FEV1) The amount of air that can be exhaled in 1 second as measured by a spirometer.

Formal group A type of **group** that exists to carry out a task or goal rather than to meet the needs of group members.

Formal leader A **leader** selected by an organization and given official authority to make decisions and act.

Formal nursing care plan A written or computerized guide that organizes information about the client's care.

Forseeability A reasonable expectation that certain events will cause specific results.

Foster family A family consisting of one or more adults caring for one or more children from other families when the children can no longer live with their birth parents.

Fourth heart sound A heart sound produced by atrial contraction and ejection of blood into the ventricle during late diastole. Also called **atrial gallop**.

Fracture A break in the continuity of a bone.

Fragile X syndrome A form of mental retardation caused by a single recessive gene abnormality on the X chromosome.

Frank–Starling mechanism An increase in venous return increases ventricular filling and myocardial stretch, which increases the force of contraction.

Friend support Support or assistance from non-family members, such as friends or coworkers, for a family during a time of illness or stress.

Fulguration A procedure that destroys tissue with electrical current.

Full-thickness burn A burn that involves all layers of the skin, including the epidermis, the dermis, and the epidermal appendages.

Fulminant colitis An acute form of **ulcerative colitis** that involves the entire colon; manifestations include severe bloody diarrhea, acute abdominal pain, and fever.

Functional assessments Typically a combination of assessments that includes observations of child behavior, responses, and abilities that is used to assess how a child functions on a daily basis in his or her environment and to determine if the child has any developmental delays or special needs.

Functional nursing A task-oriented system of nursing care delivery in which tasks requiring the least skill are assigned to workers with the minimum skills required to perform them.

Functional strength The body's ability to perform work.

Fundus The rounded uppermost portion of the uterus.

Fungi A type of microorganism capable of producing infection. Yeasts and molds are common types of fungi.

Gallstone ileus A large gallstone.

Gamete Female or male germ cell; contains a haploid number of chromosomes.

Gametogenesis The process by which germ cells are produced.

Gastric lavage Irrigation of the stomach with large quantities of normal saline.

Gastric outlet obstruction Obstruction of the pyloric region of the stomach and duodenum that impairs gastric outflow; a potential complication of peptic ulcer disease.

Gastric ulcer A **peptic ulcer** occurring in the stomach.

Gender identity One's self-image as a female or male.

Gender-role behavior The outward expression of a person's sense of maleness or femaleness.

Generalized seizures The result of diffuse electrical activity that often begins in both hemispheres of the brain simultaneously, then spreads throughout the cortex into the brainstem. As a result, movements and spasms displayed by the client are bilateral and symmetric.

Generational cohort People born in the same general time span who share key life experiences, including historical events, public heroes, pastimes, and early work experiences.

Genital herpes A sexually transmitted disease caused by the herpes simplex virus.

Genital intercourse (coitus) Penetration of the vagina by the penis.

Genital warts A sexually transmitted disease caused by the human papillomavirus.

Genogram Visual representation of gender showing lines of birth descent through the generations.

Genotype The pattern of genes on chromosomes.

Geragogy The process of stimulating and helping older adults to learn.

Gestation Period of intrauterine development from conception through birth; pregnancy.

Gingiva The gum.

Gingivitis Red, swollen gingiva.

Glaucoma A condition characterized by optic neuropathy with gradual loss of peripheral vision and, usually, increased intraocular pressure of the eye.

Global self The collective beliefs and images one holds about oneself.

Global self-esteem How much one likes oneself as a whole.

Glomerular filtration rate (GFR) The rate at which fluid is filtered through the kidneys.

Glomerulonephritis Inflammation of the glomerular capillary membrane.

Glomerulus Found in the nephrons of the kidneys, a tuft of capillaries surrounded by Bowman's capsule.

Glucagon A hormone that stimulates the breakdown of glycogen in the liver, the formation of carbohydrates in the liver, and the breakdown of lipids in both the liver and adipose tissue.

Gluconeogenesis The formation of glucose from fats and proteins.

Glucosuria The excretion of glucose in the urine.

Glycogenolysis The breakdown of liver glycogen.

Glycosuria The excretion of carbohydrates into the urine.

Goals/desired outcomes A part of a care plan that describes, in terms of observable client responses, what the nurse hopes to achieve by implementing the nursing interventions.

Goiter An enlarged thyroid gland.

Gonadotropon-releasing hormone (GnRH) A hormone secreted by the hypothalamus that stimulates the anterior pituitary to secrete follicle-stimulating hormone (FSH) and leutenizing hormone (LH).

Good Samaritan laws Laws that are designed to protect the health care worker from potential liability when volunteering his or her skills outside of an employment contract.

Goodpasture's syndrome A rare autoimmune disorder of unknown etiology. It is characterized by formation of antibodies to the glomerular basement membrane.

Governance The establishment and maintenance of social, political, and economic arrangements by which practitioners control their practice, self-discipline, working conditions, and professional affairs.

Graafian follicle The ovarian cyst containing the ripe ovum, which secretes estrogens.

Graft-versus-host disease A series of immunologic reactions in response to transplanted cells.

Gram stain A diagnostic test conducted to identify the infecting organisms in urine by shape and characteristic.

Granulation tissue Young connective tissue with new capillaries formed in the healing process.

Grave's disease An autoimmune disorder marked by an enlarged thyroid and the signs of hyperthyroidism.

Grief The total response to the emotional experience related to loss.

Group Three or more individuals who have a common purpose, interact with each other, influence each other, and are interdependent.

Group decision making A process that allows people with multiple ideas and experiences to come together to form a decision.

Groupthink A type of decision making characterized by a group's failure to critically examine their own processes and practices. Groupthink may also occur when members of a group fail to recognize and respond to change.

Growth Physical change and increase in size.

Guillain-Barré syndrome (GBS) An acute inflammatory demyelinating disorder of the peripheral nervous system characterized by an acute onset of motor paralysis (usually ascending).

Gynecomastia Abnormal enlargement of the breast(s) in men.

H1 receptors Cellular histamine receptors that are present in the smooth muscle of the vascular system, the bronchial tree, and the digestive tract. Stimulation of these receptors results in itching, pain, edema, bronchoconstriction, and other characteristics symptoms of inflammation and allergy.

H1N1 influenza A form of the influenza virus that consists of avian genes, human genes, and genes from flu viruses typically found in pigs from Asia and Europe. Once mistakenly called "swine flu," it can be spread through human to human transmission.

H2 receptors Cellular histamine receptors present primarily in the stomach; their stimulation results in the secretion of large amounts of hydrochloric acid.

Habit training Attempts to keep clients dry by having them void at regular intervals.

Hallucination The perceptions of seeing, hearing, or feeling something that is not there.

Hardware The physical parts of a computer or computer system.

Harriet Tubman Known as the "Moses of Her People" for her work with the Underground Railroad; during the Civil War she nursed the sick and suffering of her own race.

Hashimoto's thyroiditis An autoimmune disorder in which antibodies destroy thyroid tissue.

Health A state of complete physical, mental, and social well-being.

Health beliefs Concepts about health that an individual believes are true, regardless of whether or not they are founded in fact.

Health care information system A group of computer systems used by a hospital or organization to support and enhance health care.

Health care surrogate An individual selected to make medical decisions when a person is no longer able to make them for himself or herself.

Health Insurance Portability and Accountability Act (HIPAA) A law enacted by Congress to minimize the exclusion of preexisting conditions as a barrier to health care insurance, designate special rights for those who lose other health coverage, and eliminate medical underwriting in group plans. The act includes the Privacy Rule, which creates a national standard for of the disclosure of private health information. This rule impacts all health care providers as well as health insurance plan providers.

Health literacy The ability to read, understand, and act on health information; includes such tasks as comprehending prescription labels, interpreting appointment slips, completing health insurance forms, and following instructions for diagnostic tests.

Health maintenance organization (HMO) A group health care agency that provides health maintenance and treatment services to voluntary enrollees. A fee is set without regard to the amount or kind of services provided.

Health policy Actions and decisions by government bodies or professional organizations that influence the actions and decisions of organizations and individuals within the health care system.

Health promotion Any activity undertaken for the purpose of achieving a higher level of health and well-being.

Health promotion diagnosis A clinical judgment of the motivation and desire of an individual, family, or community to increase well-being and actualize human health potential as expressed by a readiness to enhance specific health behaviors.

Heart block A block in the normal electrical conduction of the heart.

Heart failure The inability of the heart to pump adequate blood to meet the metabolic demands of the body.

Heart murmur Harsh, blowing sounds caused by disruption of blood flow into the heart, between the chambers of the heart, or from the heart into the pulmonary or aortic systems.

Heaving Lifting of the chest wall during contraction.

Helper T cells Play a vital role in normal immune system function, recognizing foreign antigens and infected cells and activating antibody-producing B cells. They are the primary cells infected by the **human immodeficiency virus**.

HELPP syndrome A cluster of changes including hemolysis, elevated liver enzymes, and low platelet count, sometimes associated with preeclampsia.

Hemanopia The loss of half of the visual field of one or both eyes.

Hematochezia Bright blood in the stool.

Hematocrit A laboratory test that measures the proportion of cells and plasma in blood.

Hematogenous spread Describes the spread of infection or disease through the blood.

Hematopoiesis Blood cell formation.

Hematuria The presence of blood in the urine.

Hemiarthroscopy The surgical replacement of the femoral head with a smooth metal sphere.

Hemiparesis Weakness of the left or right half of the body.

Hemiplegia Paralysis of the left or right half of the body.

Hemodialysis A process by which the client's blood flows through vascular catheters, passes by the **dialysate** in an external machine, and then returns to the client.

Hemodynamics The study of forces involved in blood circulation.

Hemoglobin The oxygen-carrying molecule within red blood cells; a laboratory test to measure the amount of hemoglobin.

Hemoglobinopathy A disorder of hemoglobin.

Hemolysis The destruction of red blood cells; releases hemoglobin into the circulation.

Hemolytic anemia A disorder that results from the premature destruction of red blood cells.

Hemoptysis Bloody sputum.

Hemorrhage Rapid or excessive bleeding.

Hemosiderosis The storage of excessive iron in tissues and organs.

Hemotympanum Bleeding into or behind the tympanic membrane.

Hernia A protrusion (such as of the intestine through the inguinal wall or canal).

Herniated intervertebral disk A rupture of the cartilage surrounding the intervertebral disk with protrusion of the nucleus pulposus.

Heroin An illicit CNS depressant narcotic that alters perception and produces euphoria.

Heterograft (xenograft) Skin used for transplantation that was obtained from an animal, usually a pig.

Heterosexism The view that heterosexuality is the only correct sexual orientation.

Heterosexual An individual who is attracted to members of the opposite sex.

Hip fracture A fracture of the femur at the head, neck, or trochanteric regions.

Histamine A key chemical mediator of inflammation.

Histrionic personality disorder (HPD) One of the 11 types of **personality disorder**, it is characterized by a lifelong tendency for dramatic, egocentric, attention-seeking response patterns.

Holism Best defined as considering more than the physiological health status of a client. Holism includes all factors that impact the client's physical and emotional well-being. In a holistic approach, the nurse recognizes that developmental, psychological, emotional, family, cultural, and environmental factors will affect immediate and long-term actual and potential health goals, problems, and plans.

Holosystolic Term used to describe the sounds heard during the entire phase of systole.

Holy day A day set aside for special religious observance.

Homan's sign Pain in the calf when the foot is dorsiflexed.

Homeostasis The body's tendency to maintain a state of physiologic balance in the presence of constantly changing conditions.

Homograft (allograft) Human skin that has been harvested from cadavers.

Homologous chromosomes The pair of chromosomes that are inherited, one from each parent.

Homophobia The fear, hatred, or mistrust of gays and lesbians often expressed in overt displays of discrimination.

Homosexual An individual who is attracted to members of the same sex.

Hope To expect or desire with confidence.

Hormone replacement therapy Administration of hormones, usually estrogen and a progestin, to alleviate the symptoms of menopause.

Hormones Chemical messengers secreted by various glands that exert controlling effects on the cells of the body.

Hospice care The support and care for persons in the last phase of an incurable disease so that they may live as fully and comfortably as possible.

Human chorionic gonadotropin (hCG) A hormone produced by the chorionic villi that is found in the urine of pregnant women. Also called prolan.

Human dignity The quality or state of being worthy of esteem or respect.

Human Immunodeficiency Virus (HIV) A primary immunodeficiency disorder, which is spread primarily through sexual contact with an infected person. HIV is the virus that causes **acquired immunodeficiency syndrome (AIDS)**.

Humanistic learning theory Focuses on self-development and achieving full potential; it is most likely to occur when is the information or skill being learned is relevant to the learner.

Humoral immune response Hyperreactive response of B cells characteristic of **systemic lupus erythematosus (SLE)**.

Hyaluronic acid (HA) A lubricating substance in cartilage and joint synovial fluid.

Hydronephrosis Accumulation of urine in the renal pelvis as a result of obstructed outflow.

Hydrostatic pressure The pressure a fluid exerts within a closed system on the walls of its container. The hydrostatic pressure of blood is the force blood exerts against the vascular walls (e.g., the artery walls). The principle involved in hydrostatic pressure is that fluids move from the area of greater pressure to the area of lesser pressure.

Hydroureter Distention of the ureter with urine.

Hyperalgesia Increased response to a pain stimulus because of peripheral sensitization.

Hypercalcemia Elevated blood levels of calcium.

Hypercapnia A condition that results when $PaCO_2$ rises above 45mmHg.

Hyperchloremia Elevated chloride levels in the blood.

Hypercyanotic episode A potentially life-threatening episode of hypoxia.

Hyperemia Increased blood flow to an area.

Hyperextension Forcible backward bending.

Hyperflexion Forcible forward bending.

Hyperglycemia Elevated glucose levels.

Hyperkalemia Elevated potassium levels in the blood.

Hypermagnesemia Elevated magnesium levels in the blood.

Hypernatremia Elevated sodium levels in the blood.

Hyperopia Farsightedness.

Hyperosmolar hyperglycemic state (HHS) A disorder characterized by a plasma osmolarity of 340 mOsm/L or greater, greatly elevated blood glucose levels, and altered levels of consciousness.

Hyperphosphatemia Increased blood levels of phosphate.

Hyperplasia An increase in the number or density of normal cells.

Hyperresonance A sound not produced in the normal body. It is described as booming and can be heard over an emphysematous lung.

Hyperresponsiveness An exaggerated response, as with bronchoconstriction in asthma.

Hypersensitivity An overreaction of the immune system to an antigen or antigens.

Hypersomnia The inability to stay awake during the day, despite obtaining sufficient sleep at night.

Hypertension Excess pressure in the arterial portion of the circulatory system.

Hypertensive emergency A systolic pressure is greater than 180 mmHg and the diastolic pressure higher than 120 mmHg. Also called malignant hypertension.

Hypertensive encephalopathy A syndrome characterized by extremely high blood pressure, altered level of consciousness, increased intracranial pressure, papilledema, and seizures.

Hyperthyroidism A disorder caused by excessive delivery of thyroid hormone to the peripheral tissues. Also called thyrotoxosis.

Hypertonic Refers to solutions that have a higher osmolality than body fluids; 3% sodium chloride is a hypertonic solution.

Hypertonic dehydration (or hypernatremic dehydration) Occurs when sodium loss is proportionately less than water loss.

Hypertrophic cardiomyopathy A disorder characterized by decreased compliance of the left ventricle and hypertrophy of the ventricular muscle mass.

Hypertrophic scar An overgrowth of dermal tissue that remains within the boundaries of the wound.

Hypertrophy Enlargement of glandular cells or muscles.

Hyperventilation Unusually fast respirations, or overbreathing.

Hypervolemia (Fluid volume excess) The retention of both water and sodium in similar proportions to normal extracellular fluid (ECF).

Hyphema Bleeding into the anterior chamber of the eye.

Hypoactive sexual desire disorder A deficiency in or absence of sexual fantasies and persistently low interest or a total lack of interest in sexual activity.

Hypocalcemia Decreased blood levels of calcium.

Hypocapnia A condition that results when $PaCO_2$ falls below 35 mmHg.

Hypochloremia Decreased blood levels of chloride.

Hypogeusia Diminished sense of taste.

Hypoglycemia Diminished glucose levels.

Hypokalemia Decreased blood levels of potassium.

Hypomagnesemia Decreased blood levels of magnesium.

Hypomania A less extreme form of mania that is not severe enough to markedly impair functioning or require hospitalization.

Hyponatremia Decreased blood levels of sodium.

Hypoperfusion Decreased blood flow.

Hypophosphatemia Decreased blood levels of phosphate.

Hypoplastic left heart syndrome One of the most severe congenital heart defects, characterized by absence or stenosis of mitral and aortic valves, an abnormally small left ventricle, a small aorta, and aortic or mitral stenosis or atresia.

Hyposmia Diminished sense of smell.

Hypothyroidism A disorder resulting when the thyroid gland produces an insufficient amount of thyroid hormone.

Hypotonic Refers to solutions that have a lower osmolality than body fluids, such as one-half normal saline (0.45% sodium chloride).

Hypotonic dehydration (or hyponatremic dehydration) This occurs when fluid loss is characterized by a proportionately greater loss of sodium than water.

Hypovolemia (Fluid volume deficit) Loss of both water and electrolytes in similar proportions from the extracellular fluid.

Hypovolemic shock Shock caused by a decrease in intravascular volume.

Hypoxemia A condition that results when PaO_2 falls below 80 mmHg.

Iatrogenic infection A type of **infection** that results directly from diagnostic or therapeutic procedures.

Id In Freudian terms, the source of instinctive and unconscious psychologic urges.

Ideal self How the individual thinks he/she should be or would prefer to be.

Ileostomy A surgical opening made in the ileum of the small intestine.

Ileus A condition that causes a temporary cessation of the passage of material through the intestines.

Illness A state in which the individual's physical, emotional, intellectual, social, developmental, or spiritual functioning is diminished.

Illness behavior A coping mechanism that includes the ways that an individual describes, monitors, and interprets symptoms, and the individual's ability to take remedial action and use the health care system.

Illusion A distorted perception of actual sensory stimuli.

Imitation The process by which individuals copy or reproduce what they have observed.

Immunity The body's natural or induced response to infection and the conditions associated with its response.

Immunization Introduces an **antigen** into the body, allowing **immunity** against a disease to develop naturally.

Immunocompetent Term used to describe clients who have an immune system that identifies antigens and effectively destroys or removes them.

Immunodeficiency A condition that develops when the immune system is incompetent or unable to respond effectively.

Immunoglobulin (Ig) A protein that functions as an antibody.

Immunosuppression Inability of the immune system to respond to an antigen. Occurs in response to disease or medications; may be intentional to prevent rejection of transplants or a side effect of some medications.

Implementing/Implementation The phase of the nursing process in which the nursing care plan is put into action.

Implied consent An agreement that is inferred by another's actions. For example, when a nurse asks a client for permission to administer an injection and the client rolls up his or her sleeve and turns his or her arm toward the nurse.

Impotence Inability to achieve or maintain an erection.

Impulse conduction The transmission of an impulse along the nerve pathways to the spinal cord and directly to the brain.

Impulsiveness or **Impulsivity** Acting without considering the consequences of one's behavior.

In vitro fertilization A process in which a woman's eggs are collected from her ovaries, fertilized in the laboratory, and then placed into her uterus after normal embryo development has begun.

Incident pain A type of breakthrough pain that is predictable because it is precipitated by an event or activity such as coughing or changing position.

Incident report An agency record of an accident or incident occurring within the agency and is designed to collect adequate information to assist personnel in preventing future incidents or occurrences.

Independent functions Areas of health care unique to nursing, and separate and distinct from medical management.

Independent interventions Those activities that nurses are licensed to initiate on the basis of their knowledge and skills. They include physical care, ongoing assessment, emotional support and comfort, teaching, counseling, environmental management, and making referrals to other health care professionals.

Indicator An observable client state, behavior, or self-reported perception or evaluation; a tool used to measure the performance of structure, process, and outcome standards.

Individual conflict **Conflict** that takes place within a single individual.

Individual decision When a person decides what to do on his or her own behalf.

Individualized care plan A plan tailored to meet the unique needs of a specific client—needs that are not addressed by the standardized plan.

Inductive reasoning Making generalizations from specific data.

Infection An invasion of the body tissue by microorganisms with the potential to cause illness or disease.

Infectious disease Any communicable disease that is caused by microorganisms that are commonly transmitted from one person to another or from an animal to a person.

Inferences Interpretations or conclusions made based on **cues** or observed data.

Infertility A lack of conception despite unprotected sexual intercourse for at least 12 months.

Inflammation or **Inflammatory response** An adaptive response to what the body sees as harmful, such as an allergen, illness, or injury. Inflammation typically is characterized by pain, heat, redness, and swelling.

Inflammatory bowel disease (IBD) Chronic inflammation of the bowel common to a group of conditions that includes Crohn's disease and ulcerative colitis.

Influenza A highly contagious viral respiratory disease characterized by **coryza** (inflammation of the mucous membranes lining the nose usually associated with nasal discharge), fever, cough, and systemic symptoms such as headache and **malaise** (vague feeling of physical discomfort).

Informal group A type of **group** that contributes to individual members' education or cultural values, but in which group members are not dependent on each other. Friendship groups and hobby groups are examples of informal groups.

Informal leader A **leader** who is not officially appointed to direct the activities of others but, because of seniority, age, or special abilities, is recognized by the group as a leader and plays an important role in influencing colleagues, coworkers, or other group members to achieve the group's goals.

Informal nursing care plan A strategy for action that exists in the nurse's mind.

Informatics The science of computer information systems.

Informed consent The client's legal and ethical rights to be informed of and give permission for any health care procedure or treatment.

Infundibulopelvic ligament A ligament that suspends and supports the ovaries.

Inhalants Substances inhaled to produce euphoria. Categorized into three types: anesthetics, volatile nitrites, and organic solvents.

Input Information, material, or energy that enters a system.

Insensible fluid loss Fluid loss that is not perceptible to the individual.

Insomnia The inability to fall asleep or remain asleep.

Inspection Visual examination; assessment by using the sense of sight. The nurse inspects with the naked eye and with a lighted instrument such as an otoscope (used to view the ear). In addition to visual observations, olfactory (smell) and auditory (hearing) cues are noted.

Insubordination Willful refusal to complete an assigned task or to follow instructions.

Insulin A hormone that facilitates the uptake and use of glucose by cells and prevents an excessive breakdown of glycogen in the liver and muscle.

Insulin reaction Low blood glucose levels, or hypoglycemia. Also called insulin shock.

Integrated health care system One that makes all levels of care available in an integrated form—primary care, secondary care, and tertiary care.

Integrity Acting in accordance with an appropriate code of ethics and accepted standards of practice.

Intensity The loudness or softness of a sound; amplitude.

Intergroup or **organizational conflict** **Conflict** that occurs between groups, e.g., units or services.

Intermittent claudication A cramping or aching pain in the calves of the legs, the thighs, and the buttocks that occurs with a predictable level of activity.

Interpersonal conflict **Conflict** that occurs between people.

Interpersonal skills All of the activities, verbal and nonverbal, people use when interacting directly with one another.

Intersex Ambiguous gender.

Interstitial fluid Accounts for approximately 75% of extracellular fluid; intersticial fluid surrounds the cells.

Interview A planned communication or a conversation with a purpose.

Intimacy A relationship that entails commitment, affective intimacy, cognitive intimacy, physical intimacy, and mutuality.

Intimate distance Describes a distance between individuals that is 1½ feet or less.

Intracapsular fracture A hip fracture involving the head or neck of the femur.

Intracellular fluid (ICF) Fluid found within the body cells, also called *cellular fluid.*

Intracranial hypertension A sustained state of **increased intracranial pressure** that is potentially life threatening.

Intracranial regulation The processes that affect intracranial compensation and adaptive neurologic function.

Intractable seizures Seizures that continue to occur even with optimal medical management.

Intradiscal electrothermal therapy (IDET) The use of thermal energy to treat pain from a bulging spinal disk.

Intradisciplinary assessment A type of performance evaluation that measures the performance of individuals from a single discipline.

Intragenerational family A family in which more than two generations live together.

Intranet A private computer network that uses Internet protocols and technologies, including Web browsers, servers, and languages, to facilitate collaborative data sharing.

Intrapartum The time from the onset of true labor until the birth of the infant and expulsion of the placenta.

Intrauterine device (IUD) A small plastic or metal form that is placed in the uterus to prevent implantation of a fertilized ovum.

Intrauterine fetal death (IUFD) Death of a fetus that occurs after 20 weeks' gestation; often referred to as **stillbirth** or **fetal demise.**

Intravascular fluid or **plasma** Accounts for approximately 20% of the **extracellular fluid** and is found within the vascular system.

Intravenous pyelography A diagnostic test used to evaluate the structure and excretory function of the kidneys, ureters, and bladder.

Intuition The understanding or learning of things without the conscious use of reasoning.

Involuntary admission The detention of a client in a psychiatric or medical facility against the client's will, normally reserved for cases in which the client is a danger to himself or others.

Ion Electrically charged particle.

Iron deficiency anemia A disorder that results when the supply of iron in the body is insufficient for the formation of red blood cells.

Ischemia Insufficient blood supply.

Ischemic Deprived of oxygen.

Ischial spines Prominences that arise near the junction of the ilium and ischium and jut into the pelvic cavity.

Isoelectric line A straight line on an electrocardiograph that indicates the absence of electrical activity.

Isokinetic exercises Resistive exercises that involve muscle contraction or tension against resistance; can be either isotonic or isometric.

Isometric exercises Exercises in which muscles contract without moving the joint.

Isotonic A solution that has the same osmolality as body fluids.

Isotonic dehydration (or isonatremic dehydration) A type of fluid imbalance that occurs when fluid loss is not balanced by intake and the losses of water and sodium are in proportion.

Isotonic exercises Exercises in which the muscle shortens to produce muscle contractions and active movement.

Isotonic fluid volume deficit A type of fluid imbalance that occurs when electrolytes are lost along with fluid.

Isotonic imbalance A fluid imbalance that occurs when water and electrolytes are lost or gained in equal proportions, so that the osmolality of body fluids remains constant.

Isthmus That portion of the uterus between the internal cervical os and the endometrial cavity.

Joint arthroplasty The reconstruction or replacement of a joint.

Joint custody Occurs when two parents who are not married have equal responsibility and legal rights for their shared children.

Justice Fairness; reward in accordance with honor, standards, or law.

Juvenile Rheumatoid Arthritis (JRA) A chronic inflammatory autoimmune disease diagnosed in children that is characterized by joint inflammation, resulting in decreased mobility, swelling, and pain.

Kaposi's sarcoma (KS) Often the presenting symptom of AIDS, it remains the most common cancer associated with the disease. Kaposi's sarcoma is caused by a virus called the Kaposi sarcoma-associated herpesvirus, also known as human herpesvirus 8.

Kardex The trade name for a method that makes use of a series of cards to concisely organize and record client data and instructions for daily nursing care—especially care that changes frequently and must be kept up-to-date.

Karyotype A pictorial analysis of chromosomes.

Keloid A scar that extends beyond the boundaries of the original wound.

Keratotic basal cell carcinoma A type of skin cancer.

Ketonuria The presence of ketones in the urine.

Ketosis An accumulation of ketone bodies produced during oxidation of fatty acids.

Kindling Long-term changes in brain neurotransmission that occur after repeated detoxifications.

Kinesthesia The ability to perceive movement and sense of position.

Kinesthetic A term referring to awareness of the position and movement of body parts.

Korsakoff's psychosis A condition typically seen in alcoholics that is characterized by intact intellectual functioning but an inability to retrieve long-term memory events or retain new information.

Kosher Acceptable or prepared according to Jewish law.

Kussmaul's respirations Deep, rapid respirations associated with compensatory mechanisms.

Labyrinthitis Inflammation of the inner ear. Also called **otitis externa**.

Laënnec's cirrhosis A progressive, irreversible liver disorder resulting from excessive alcohol consumption. Also called alcoholic cirrhosis.

Laissez-faire leader A **leader** who is less directive and more permissive than other types of leaders. The laissez-faire leader presupposes that the group is internally motivated.

Laminectomy The removal of a part of the vertebral lamina.

Laparoscopic cholecystectomy Removal of the gallbladder using an endoscope.

Law The sum total of the rules and regulations by which a society is governed.

Laxatives Medications that stimulate bowel activity and assist in fecal elimination.

Lead An insulated wire that connects an electrocardiograph to the electrodes attached to the patient.

Leader Anyone who uses interpersonal skills to influence others to accomplish a specific goal.

Leading question A question that influences the client to give a particular answer.

Lean Six Sigma A quality improvement program that focuses on improving process flow and eliminating waste.

Learning A change in human disposition or capability that persists and that cannot be solely accounted for by growth. Learning is represented by a change in behavior; in other words, the learner is able to apply or demonstrate what has been learned.

Learning disabilities Neurological conditions in which the brain cannot receive or process information normally.

Learning need A desire or a requirement to know something that is presently unknown to the learner.

Lesbian A woman who prefers relationships with other women.

Leukemia A group of chronic malignant disorders of white blood cells (WBCs) and WBC precursors.

Leukocytes The primary cells involved in both nonspecific and specific immune system responses. Also known as white blood cells (WBCs).

Leukocytosis An increase in the number of leukocytes in the blood (above 10,000/mm^3) in response to infection or inflammation.

Leukopenia A decrease in the number of circulating leukocytes.

Liability The state of being legally obliged and responsible.

Libido The psychic energy that, according to Freud, provides the underlying motivation to human development.

Lifestyle A person's general way of living, including living conditions and individual patterns of behavior that are influenced by sociocultural factors and personal characteristics.

Limit setting Establishing clear and consistent rules or guidelines for child or client behavior.

Line authority A type of **authority** in which the supervisor directs the activities of the employees that he or she supervises.

Lipoatrophy Atrophy of subcutaneous tissues.

Lipodystrophy Excessive growth of subcutaneous tissue.

Lithiasis Stone formation.

Lithotripsy The preferred treatment for urinary calculi, uses sound or shock waves to crush a stone.

Living will A document that provides written directions about life-prolonging procedures to provide instructions when a person can no longer communicate in a life-threatening situation.

Local Emergency Management Agency (LEMA) State agency with expertise in public safety, emergency medical services, and management, that helps local communities coordinate disaster preparedness, mitigation, and response activities.

Local infection Invasion by a microorganism that is limited to the specific part of the body where the microorganism remains.

Localized responses More common manifestations of type I hypersensitivity, they are typically atopic responses; that is, they have a strong genetic predisposition. Atopic reactions are the result of localized, rather than systemic, IgE-mediated responses to an **allergen**. They are prompted by contact of the allergen with IgE in the bronchial tree, nasal mucosa, and conjunctival tissues.

Locked-in syndrome A state of consciousness in which the client is alert and fully aware of the environment and has intact cognitive abilities but is unable to communicate through speech or movement because of blocked efferent pathways from the brain. Motor paralysis affects all voluntary muscles, although the upper cranial nerves (I through IV) may remain intact, allowing the client to communicate through eye movements and blinking.

Locus of control (LOC) A concept about whether clients believe their health status is under their own or others' control.

Long-term memory The repository for information stored for periods longer than 72 hours and usually weeks and years.

Loose association An indication of disordered thinking characterized by the shifting of verbal ideas from one topic to another, with no apparent relationship between thoughts, and the person speaking being unaware that the topics are unconnected. Commonly seen in **schizophrenia**.

Loss An actual or potential situation in which something that is valued becomes altered or no longer available.

Lower-body obesity Identified by a waist-to-hip ratio of less than 0.8; more commonly seen in women. Also called peripheral obesity.

Lung abscess A local area of necrosis and pus formation within the lung.

Lupus nephritis Inflammation of the kidneys resulting from **systemic lupus erythematosus** (SLE).

Lutenizing hormone (LH) Anterior pituitary hormone responsible for stimulating ovulation and for development of the **corpus luteum**.

Lymphadenopathy The enlargement of lymph nodes (over 1 cm) with or without tenderness. It may be caused by inflammation, infection, or malignancy of the nodes or the regions drained by the nodes.

Lymphangitis **Inflammation** of a lymph vessel.

Lymphocytes Account for 20–40% of circulating leukocytes. Lymphocytes are the principal effector and regulator cells of specific immune responses to protect the body from microorganisms, foreign tissue, and cell mutations or alterations.

Lyse Disintegrate.

Macrophages Large phagocytes that are important in the body's defense against chronic infections.

Macroshock Major electrical injury.

Major depressive disorder A mood disorder characterized by loss of interest in life and unresponsiveness, moving from mild to severe, severe lasting at least 2 weeks; also called unipolar disorder.

Major depressive episode Characterized by a change in several aspects of a person's life and emotional state consistently over a period of 14 days or longer.

Malaise Vague feeling of physical discomfort.

Male erectile disorder When a man has erection problems during 25% or more of his sexual interactions.

Male orgasmic disorder Difficulty of a male client to ejaculate.

Malignant Term used to refer to a cell or growth which, if not treated, will recur, continue to grow, and spread to other sites in the body, ending in death.

Malnutrition (also known as **undernutrition**) Health effects due to insufficient nutrient intake or stores.

Malpractice Conduct deviating from the standard of practice dictated by a profession.

Managed care A method of organizing care delivery that emphasizes communication and coordination of care among all health care team members.

Manager An individual employed by an organization who is responsible and accountable for efficiently accomplishing the goals of the organization.

Mandatory health insurance A system of health care in which the government of a country requires its citizens to carry health insurance.

Mandatory reporting A legal requirement to report an act, event, or situation that is designated by state or local law as a reportable event.

Mania An abnormal and persistently elevated, expansive, or irritable mood lasting at least one week, significantly impairing social or occupational functioning, and generally requiring hospitalization.

Manipulation Controlling behavior used to exploit others for personal gain.

Margination The accumulation of **leukocytes** along the inner surface of blood vessels. Occurs as part of the inflammatory process.

Mary Mahoney The first African American professional nurse.

Massage therapy The scientific manipulation of the soft tissues of the body for the purposes of promoting healing and wellness.

Mast cells Cells that detect foreign agents or injury and respond by releasing histamine, thereby activating the inflammatory process.

Masturbation The self-stimulation of one's genitals for sexual pleasure.

Maternal role attainment The process by which a woman learns mothering behaviors and becomes comfortable with her identity as a mother.

McDonald's sign A probable sign of pregnancy characterized by an ease in flexing the body of the uterus against the cervix.

Mean arterial pressure (MAP) The average pressure in the arterial circulation throughout the cardiac cycle.

Meatus A body passage or opening.

Meconium The first fecal material passed by the newborn, normally up to 24 hours after birth.

Medicaid A U.S. federal public assistance program paid out of general taxes and administered through the individual states to provide health care for those who require financial assistance.

Medical asepsis All practices intended to confine a specific microorganism to a specific area, thus limiting the number, growth, and transmission of the microorganism.

Medicare A national and state health insurance program for U.S. residents older than 65 years of age.

Medigap policy A type of private health insurance that is designed to supplement Medicare; also called Medicare Supplement Insurance.

Meditation The act of focusing one's thoughts or engaging in self-reflection or contemplation.

Meiosis A reductive division of sex cells, producing ova or sperm with a half set (haploid) of chromosomes.

Melanoma A type of malignant skin cancer.

Melasma gravidarum See chloasma.

Mendelian inheritance Traits that are passed on by a single gene.

Meninges Three connective tissue membranes that cover, protect, and nourish the **central nervous system**.

Menorrhagia Excessive or prolonged menstruation.

Menstrual cycle The cyclic phases of **menstruation** that occurs about every 28 days.

Menstruation The periodic shedding of the uterine lining in a woman of childbearing age who is not pregnant.

Mental retardation Significant limitation in intellectually functioning and adaptive behavior.

Mentor A competent, experienced professional who develops a relationship with a novice for the purpose of providing advice, support, information, and feedback in order to encourage development of the individual.

Message What a sender conveys through speaking or writing, the body language that accompanies the sender's words, and how the words are transmitted.

Metabolic acidosis (bicarbonate deficit) A disorder characterized by a low pH (< 7.35) and a low bicarbonate (< 22 mEq/L). It may be caused by excess acid in the body or loss of bicarbonate from the body.

Metabolic alkalosis (bicarbonate excess) A disorder characterized by a high pH (> 7.45) and a high bicarbonate (> 26 mEq/L). It may be caused by loss of acid or excess bicarbonate in the body.

Metabolic syndrome A disorder characterized by the presence of three or more of the following: increased waist circumference, hypertension, elevated blood triglycerides and fasting blood glucose, and low HDL cholesterol.

Metabolism The process of biochemical reactions occurring in the body's cells that are necessary to sustain life.

Metaphysic The portion of the bone between the diaphysis and the epiphysis.

Metaplasia A change in the normal pattern of differentiation such that dividing cells differentiate into cell types not normally found at that location in the body.

Metastasis The process by which spreading of malignant neoplasms occurs; the transfer of disease from one organ or part to another.

Metrorrhagia Bleeding between menstrual periods.

Microalbuminuria A low but abnormal level of albumin in the urine.

Microstaging The assessment of the level of invasion of a malignant melanoma and the maximum tumor thickness.

Micturition Releasing urine from the urinary bladder (voiding).

Middle ear effusion Results when negative pressure in the middle ear causes sterile serous fluid to move from the capillaries into the space.

Miliary tuberculosis Results from **hematogenous spread** (through the blood) of the bacilli throughout the body.

Milieu therapy A therapeutic recovery environment that supports behavior changes, teaches new coping skills, and helps the client move from addiction to sobriety.

Milliequivalent The chemical combining power of the ion, or the capacity of cations to combine with anions to form molecules.

Miscarriage The loss of a fetus prior to 20 weeks' gestation.

Mitigation Actions taken to prevent or reduce the harmful effects of a disaster on human health or property. Mitigation involves future-oriented activities to prevent subsequent disasters or to minimize their effects.

Mitosis The process of cell division.

Modeling The process by which a person learns by observing the behavior of others.

Monoamine oxidase inhibitor (MAOIs) Drug inhibiting monoamine oxidase, an enzyme that terminates the actions of neurotransmitters such as dopamine, norepinephrine, epinephrine, and serotonin.

Mononeuropathies Isolated peripheral neuropathies that affect a single nerve.

Monophasic A term used to describe **rheumatoid arthritis** when it occurs for a limited time and then improves.

Monopolizing The domination of a discussion by one member of a group.

Monosomy Absence of a chromosome.

Monotheism The belief in the existence of one God.

Monro-Kellie hypothesis States that if the volume of any of the three intracranial components (the brain, cerebral spinal fluid, and blood) increases, the volume of the others must decrease to maintain normal pressures in the cranial cavity.

Mood A sustained emotional state and how one feels subjectively.

Mood stabilizers Drugs used for bipolar disorder because they moderate extreme shifts in emotions between mania and depression.

Moral behavior The way in which a person perceives and responds to society's requirements.

Moral development The process of learning to tell the difference between right and wrong and of learning what ought and ought not to be done; the pattern of change in moral behavior that occurs with age.

Moral rules Specific prescriptions for actions.

Morality The requirements necessary for people to live together in society.

Morbid obesity Greater than 200% of ideal body weight.

Morning sickness A term that refers to the nausea and vomiting that a woman may experience in early pregnancy. This lay term is sometimes used because these symptoms frequently occur in the early part of the day and disappear within a few hours.

Morpheaform basal cell carcinoma A type of skin cancer.

Morula Developmental stage of the fertilized ovum in which there is a solid mass of cells.

Mosaicism The expression of two cell lines, each with a different chromosomal number, in an individual.

Motivation The desire to learn.

Mourning The behavioral process through which grief is eventually resolved or altered; it is often influenced by culture, spiritual beliefs, and custom.

Multiculturalism Characterized by many subcultures coexisting within a given society in which no one culture dominates.

Multidisciplinary care plan A standardized plan that outlines the care required for clients with common, predictable—usually medical—conditions. Such plans, also referred to as **collaborative care plans** and **critical pathways**, sequence the care that must be given on each day during the projected length of stay for the specific type of condition.

Multifocal A term used to describe premature ventricular contractions that arise from different **ectopic** sites.

Multigravida Woman who has been pregnant more than once.

Multipara Woman who has had more than one pregnancy in which the fetus was viable.

Multiple pregnancy More than one fetus in the uterus at the same time.

Multiple sclerosis (MS) A chronic demyelinating neurologic disease of the central nervous system associated with an abnormal immune response to an environmental factor.

Mural thrombi Blood clots in the heart wall.

Mutual recognition A model of nurse licensure that allows a nurse to have a single license that confers the privilege to practice in other states that are part of the Nurse Licensure Compact.

Mutual respect When two or more people show or feel honor or esteem toward one another.

Mycobacterium tuberculosis The bacteria that causes **tuberculosis**.

Mydriasis Abnormal or excessive dilation of the pupil of the eye, usually caused by a disease or drug.

Myelin sheath The fatty, segmented wrappings that normally protect and insulate nerves.

Myocardial hypertrophy An increase in the size of muscle cells of the myocardium.

Myometrium The middle muscular layer of the uterus.

Myopia Nearsightedness.

Myringotomy An incision of the tympanic membrane.

Myxedema The hypothyroid state, with characteristic accumulation of nonpitting edema in the connective tissues throughout the body.

Myxedema coma A life-threatening complication of long-standing, untreated hypothyroidism, usually triggered by an acute illness or trauma.

Narcissism Self-centered behavior in which the individual feels entitled to special favors due to a mistaken perception being the "center of the universe."

Narcissistic personality disorder (NPD) One of the 11 types of **personality disorders**, it is marked by in a pattern of grandiosity, difficulty regulating self-esteem, and the need for admiration and attention from others.

Narcolepsy A disorder characterized by daytime sleep attacks or excessive daytime sleepiness.

Narrative charting A descriptive record of client data and nursing interventions, written in sentences and paragraphs.

Natural killer cells (NK cells) Large, granular cells found in the spleen, lymph nodes, bone marrow, and blood. They constitute 15% of circulating lymphocytes. NK cells provide immune surveillance and resistance to infection, and they play an important role in the destruction of early malignant cells.

Nature The genetic or hereditary capability of the individual.

Negative feedback Output of a system that returns to the system as input and which inhibits system change.

Negative symptom A loss of normal function normally seen in mentally healthy adults, such as the ability to care for one's self, commonly seen in **schizophrenia**.

Neglect syndrome A disorder of attention that can result from stroke.

Negligence Conduct that deviates from what a reasonable person would perform in a particular circumstance.

Neonatal anemia A disorder caused by blood loss, hemolysis, and impaired red blood cell production related to birth.

Neoplasm A mass of new tissue.

Nephrectomy Removal of a kidney.

Nephritis Inflammation of the kidneys.

Nephrolithiasis The formation of stones in the kidney.

Nephrolithotomy A procedure for removal of a staghorn calculus that invades the calyces and renal parenchyma.

Nephrotoxins Substances which damage nerves or nerve tissue.

Nerve block A chemical interruption of a nerve pathway, affected by injecting a local anesthetic into the nerve.

Networking A process by which people develop linkages throughout the profession to communicate, share ideas and information, and offer support and direction to each other.

Neurofibrillary tangles Seen in Alzheimer's clients, they are thick, insoluble clots of protein inside the damaged brain cells or neurons.

Neurogenic bladder Interference with the normal mechanisms of urine elimination in which the client does not perceive bladder fullness and is unable to control the urinary sphincters; the result of impaired neurologic function.

Neurogenic shock The result of an imbalance between parasympathetic and sympathetic stimulation of vascular smooth muscle.

Neuron The basic cell of the nervous system.

Neuropathic pain Experienced by people who have damaged or malfunctioning nerves.

Neutral question An open-ended question that does not direct the client to answer in a certain way, such as "How do you feel?"

Newborn Infant from birth through the first 28 days of life.

Nicotine A highly addictive chemical that is found in tobacco and enters the body via the lungs (cigarettes, pipes, and cigars) and oral mucous membranes (chewing tobacco as well as smoking).

Nicotine replacement therapy (NRT) A pharmacologic therapy designed to relieve some of the physiologic effects of withdrawal, including cravings, for clients trying to quit smoking or using tobacco. NRT transdermal patches and gums are available over the counter; nicotine inhalers and nasal sprays are available by prescription only.

Nicotinic receptors Found in the hippocampus and involved with new sensory information and memory formation, they are thought to be impaired in clients with **schizophrenia**.

Nidation The cyclical preparation of the uterine lining by steroid hormones for implantation of the embryo.

Nociceptors The nerve receptors for pain.

Nocturia Voiding two or more times at night.

Nocturnal emissions Orgasm and emission of semen during sleep.

Nocturnal enuresis Bed-wetting; involuntary urination at night after bladder control is achieved.

Nocturnal frequency The need for older adults to arise during the night to urinate.

Nodular basal cell carcinoma A type of skin cancer.

Nolo contendere A type of plea in a court of law in which an individual neither admits nor denies that he or she has committed the crime but agrees to a punishment as if guilty.

Nominal group technique A method of group decision making in which the individuals meet as a group, but they write their responses without discussion. The ideas are then collected and an open discussion proceeds.

Nondirective interview An interview using open-ended questions and empathetic responses to build rapport and learn client concerns.

Noninvasive ventilation (NIV) Ventilator support using a tight-fitting face mask, thus avoiding intubation.

Nonmaleficence The duty to do no harm.

Non-Mendelian inheritance Traits that are passed on by the influence of multiple genes.

Non-programmed decision A type of decision that must be made in a situation that represents a new experience for the nurse. Non-programmed decisions typically require more time, data collection, and critical thinking than **programmed decisions**.

Non-small-cell carcinoma Lungs cancers other than small-cell carcinoma.

Nonunion Failure of the ends of the fracture to heal together.

Nonverbal communication Communication other than words, including gestures, posture, and facial expressions.

Norm A generally accepted measure, rule, model, or pattern; also referred to as a **standard**.

Normal sinus rhythm The normal heart rhythm, in which impulses originate in the SA (sinus) node and travel through all normal conduction pathways without delay.

Normative commitment A feeling of obligation to continue in a profession.

Nosocomial infections Also known as health care-associated infections (HAIs), infections that are associated with the delivery of health care services in a facility such as a hospital or nursing home.

NREM Sleep Non-rapid-eye-movement sleep; occurs when activity in the **reticular activating system** is inhibited.

Nuclear family A family structure consisting of a husband and wife and their biological children.

Nucleation The formation of a crystal from a liquid.

Nuclectomy The surgical removal of the nucleus pulposus.

Nulligravida A woman who has never been pregnant.

Nullipara A woman who has not given birth to a viable fetus.

Nurse informaticist An expert who combines computer, information, and nursing science, and develops policies and procedures that promote effective and secure use of computerized records by nurses and other health care professionals.

Nurse Practice Act A series of state statutes that define the scope of practice, standards for education programs, licensure requirements, and grounds for disciplinary actions. Nurse Practice Acts provide a framework for establishing nursing actions in the care of clients and set the boundaries for and maintain a standard of nursing practice.

Nursing diagnosis A statement or conclusion made by the nurse about the client's health problem. The statement consists of the **diagnostic label** and, frequently, the **etiology** of the health problem.

Nursing ethics Ethical issues that occur in nursing practice.

Nursing informatics The science of using computer information systems in the practice of nursing.

Nursing intervention Any treatment, based on clinical judgment and knowledge, that a nurse performs to enhance client outcomes.

Nursing Interventions Classification (NIC) A **taxonomy** of nursing actions each of which includes a label, a definition, and a list of activities.

Nursing Outcomes Classification (NOC) A **taxonomy** for describing client outcomes that respond to nursing interventions.

Nursing research The systematic, objective process of analyzing phenomena of importance to nursing.

Nurture The effects of the environment on an individual's performance.

Nutrients Substances found in food that are used by the body to promote growth, maintenance, and repair.

Nutrition The process by which the body ingests, absorbs, transports, uses, and eliminates nutrients in food.

Nutritional health The physical result of the balance between **nutrient** intake and nutritional requirements.

Nystagmus Involuntary rapid eye movement.

Obesity An excess of adipose tissue.

Objective data Also referred to as **signs** or overt data, are detectable by an observer or can be measured or tested against an accepted standard. They can be seen, heard, felt, or smelled, and are obtained by observation or physical examination. Examples of objective data include a discoloration of the skin and a blood pressure reading.

Objective family burden Actual, identifiable family problems associated with the mental illness of a family member.

Obligatory losses Essential fluid losses required to maintain body functioning.

Observational learning The acquisition of new skills or the alteration of old behaviors simply by watching other children and adults.

Obsessive–compulsive personality disorder (OCPD) One of 11 types of **personality disorders**, it is marked by fear and anxiety concerning loss of control over situations, objects, or people.

Obstetric conjugate The distance from the middle of the sacral promontory to an area approximately 1 cm below the pubic crest.

Obstructive shock Shock caused by an obstruction in the heart or great vessels that either impedes venous return or prevents effective cardiac pumping action.

Occult blood Hidden blood.

Occupational exposure Skin, eye, mucous membrane, or parental contact with blood or other potentially infectious materials that may result from the performance of an employee's duties.

Oliguria The production of abnormally small amounts of urine by the kidney.

Oncogenes Genes that promote cell proliferation and are capable of triggering cancerous characteristics.

Oncology The study of cancer.

Oncotic pressure A pulling force exerted by colloids that helps maintain the water content of blood by pulling water from the interstitial space into the vascular compartment.

On-the-job instruction The most widely used method of educating new staff, it often involves assigning new employees to experienced nurse peers, preceptors, or the nurse manager.

Oogenesis The process that produces the female gamete, called an ovum (egg).

Open-angle glaucoma The most common form of **glaucoma**, it is a chronic, gradually progressive disease that typically affects both eyes.

Open-ended questions Questions that invite clients to discover and explore, elaborate, clarify, or illustrate their thoughts or feelings. An open-ended question specifies only the broad topic to be discussed, and invites answers longer than one or two words.

Open fracture A fracture in which the skin integrity is disrupted. Also known as a compound fracture.

Open reduction and internal fixation (ORIF) The insertion of nails, screws, plates, or pins to hold fractured bones in place.

Opportunistic infection An invasion of the body tissue by microorganisms appearing in an individual with **immunodeficiency** that would normally not affect an individual with an intact immune system.

Opportunistic pathogen A microorganism that causes disease only in susceptible individuals.

Optimism A continuing belief or sense that things will work out for the best.

Oral-genital sex Kissing, licking, or sucking of the genitals for sexual pleasure.

Orchiectomy Surgical removal of the testes.

Organizational chart A graphical representation of an organization's hierarchical structure and the flow of responsibility within the organization.

Organizational commitment The relative strength of an individual's relationship and sense of belonging to an organization.

Organizational conflict Conflict that occurs between groups, e.g., units or services.

Organizing The process of coordinating work to be done.

Orgasmic phase The third phase of the sexual response cycle, marked by the involuntary release of sexual tension accompanied by physiological and psychological release.

Orientation A series of planned activities designed to acclimate new employees to the work place.

Orthopnea Difficulty breathing when supine.

Orthopneic position A body position with the head and arms supported on the overbed table to facilitate breathing.

Orthotic devices Orthopedic devices that may include splints or braces applied to reduce strain on a joint.

Osmolality A measure of the concentration of solutes in body fluids. Osmolality is determined by the total solute concentration within a fluid compartment and is measured as parts of solute per kilogram of water.

Osmolar imbalance A fluid imbalance that involves the loss or gain of only water, so that the osmolality of the serum is altered.

Osmosis The movement of water across cell membranes, from the less concentrated solution to the more concentrated solution.

Osmotic pressure The power of a solution to draw water across a semipermeable membrane.

Ossification The development of bone.

Osteoarthritis The most common form of arthritis in older adults. It is caused by chronic degenerative changes in the cartilage and synovial membranes of the joints.

Osteoblasts Cells that form bone.

Osteoclasts Cells that resorb bone.

Osteocytes Cells that maintain bone matrix.

Osteodystrophy A complex bone disease process of chronic kidney disease in which there is increased resorption of bone caused by chronic hyperparathyroidism.

Osteophytes Boney spurs that form when cartilage deteriorates.

Osteoporosis A metabolic bone disorder characterized by loss of bone mass, increased bone fragility, and increased risk of fractures.

Osteotomy An incision into or transection of the bone.

Otitis externa Inflammation of the ear canal. It is often called "swimmer's ear" because it is most frequently found in people who spend significant time in the water.

Otitis interna (also called **labyrinthitis**) An inflammation of the inner ear.

Otitis media Inflammation of the middle ear.

Otoscope A hand-held instrument with a light and a cone-shaped attachment known as the "ear speculum."

Outcome standards Standards related to the end results of care that has been given.

Outcomes management A type of performance assessment that measures and evaluates costs and quality in order to improve clinical practice.

Output Energy, material, or information that a system gives out as a result of its processes.

Ovarian cycle The three cyclical phases of oogenesis that occurs about every 28 days.

Ovarian ligaments Ligaments that anchor the lower pole of the ovary to the uterus.

Ovaries Female sex glands in which the ova are formed and in which estrogen and progesterone are produced. Normally, there are two ovaries.

Overdelegation Occurs when the delegator loses control over a situation by providing the delegate with too much authority or too much responsibility.

Overnutrition Health effects of excesses in nutrient intake or stores; can be manifested in conditions such as obesity, hypertension, hypercholesterolemia, or toxic levels of stored vitamins or minerals.

Profession An occupation that requires extensive education or a calling that requires special knowledge, skill, and preparation.

Professional behaviors Those actions by the nurse that invite trust and inspire confidence.

Professional support Assistance provided by professionals in the community who exhibit a nonblaming and respectful attitude towards families and clients, and who provide information and help locating community resources.

Professionalism A set of attributes; a way of life that implies responsibility and commitment.

Professionalization The process of becoming professional; acquiring characteristics considered to be professional.

Progesterone Hormone produced by the corpus luteum, adrenal cortex, and placenta whose function is to stimulate proliferation of the endometrium to facilitate growth of the embryo.

Programmed decisions Repetitive, routine decisions. Programmed decisions are often those that relate to or follow a policy or procedure.

Progress notes Chart entries made by a variety of methods and by all health professionals involved in a client's care for the purpose of describing a client's problems, treatments, and progress toward desired outcomes.

Prone Face-down.

Propioception The body's sense of its position.

Proptosis Forward displacement of the eye.

Prostaglandins (PGs) Complex lipids compounds synthesized by many cells of the body.

Prostate specific antigen (PSA) A protein produced in the cells of the prostate gland.

Prostatectomy Surgical removal of part or all of the prostate gland.

Prostatitis Inflammation of the prostate gland.

Prostatodynia A condition in which the client experiences the symptoms of prostatitis, but shows no evidence of inflammation or infection.

Protected health information Individually identifiable health information held or transmitted in any form or media, whether electronic, paper, or oral.

Protein-calorie malnutrition Problem of clients with long-term deficiencies in caloric intake; characteristics include depressed visceral proteins (e.g., albumin), weight loss, and visible muscle and fat wasting.

Proteinuria Excess protein in urine.

Protocols Predetermined and preprinted plans specifying the procedure to be followed in a particular situation.

Proxemics The study of distance between people in their interactions.

Proximodistal Growth that proceeds from the center of the body outward.

Pseudoaddiction A term applied to clients who display drug-seeking behaviors but differ from addicts in that they have true underlying pain for which they are seeking relief. These behaviors will generally stop when adequate pain control is achieved.

Psychiatric (psychosocial) rehabilitation The development of skills and support necessary for successful living, learning, and working in the community.

Psychogenic pain Pain that is experienced in the absence of any diagnosed physiologic cause or event.

Psychomotor domain The "skill" domain, it includes motor skills such as the fine motor skills required to give an injection.

Psychomotor retardation A state in which thinking and body movements are noticeably slowed and speech is slowed or absent.

Psychosis (or psychotic disorder) A mental health condition characterized by **delusions** (firm ideas and beliefs not founded in reality), **hallucinations** (perceptions of seeing, hearing, or feeling something that is not there), **illusions** (distorted perceptions of actual sensory stimuli), disorganized behavior, and a difficulty relating to others.

Psychosocial skills Skills which enable a person in crisis to maintain relationships with family and friends throughout and after a crisis period.

Psychostimulants A class of stimulants including cocaine and amphetamines that have a high potential for abuse.

Ptosis Drooping of the eyelid.

Puberty The stage during which an individual reaches sexual maturity.

Pubis Pertaining to the pubes or pubic area.

Public distance Describes a distance between individuals that is 12–15 feet.

Public insurance Insurance financed by the government.

Puerperium That time immediately following childbirth during which physiologic changes that occurred during pregnancy begin to return to normal.

Pulmonary atresia The absence of communication between the right ventricle and the pulmonary artery.

Pulmonary circulation Consists of the right side of the heart, the pulmonary artery, the pulmonary capillaries, and the pulmonary vein.

Pulmonary edema An abnormal accumulation of fluid in the interstitial tissue and alveoli of the lung.

Pulmonary embolism The obstruction of blood flow in part of the pulmonary vascular system by an **embolus**.

Pulmonary vascular resistance The force or resistance of the blood in the pulmonary circulation.

Pulse pressure The difference between the systolic and diastolic pressure.

Punctual On time.

Punishment Action taken to enforce rules when a child misbehaves.

Pupillary light reflex Reflex in which the pupil contracts in response to a bright light.

Purging Self-induced vomiting or misuse of laxatives, diuretics, or enemas.

Pursed-lipped breathing Exhaling through a narrow opening between the lips to prolong the expiratory phase in an effort to promote more alveolar emptying while maintaining open alveoli.

Pyelolithotomy An incision into and removal of a stone from the kidney pelvis.

Pyelonephritis Inflammation of the renal pelvis and parenchyma, the functional kidney tissue.

Pyorrhea Advanced **periodontal disease**.

Pyuria Cloudy or pus-filled urine.

Quadriplegia Loss of function of the arms, trunk, legs, and pelvic organs.

Qualifiers Words that have been added to some NANDA labels to give additional meaning to the diagnostic statement.

Quality A subjective description of a sound (e.g., whistling, gurgling); the degree to which health services for individuals and populations increase the likelihood of desired health outcomes and are consistent with current professional knowledge.

Quality improvement The systematic processes that health care organizations and professionals used to measure client outcomes, identify hazards and errors, and to improve client care.

Quality management A preventive approach designed to address problems before they become crises.

Quickening The mother's perception of fetal movement.

Race A term used to described socially defined populations that share genetically transmitted physical characteristics, such as skin color and bone structure.

Radiation cataracts A type of **cataract** that may result from long-term exposure to radiation.

Range of Motion The degree to which a joint can be moved; a measurement of flexon and extension.

Rapport A relationship of mutual trust and understanding between two people.

Rationale The scientific principle given as the reason for selecting a particular nursing intervention.

Readiness to learn The demonstration of behaviors or cues that reflect the learner's motivation to learn at a specific time.

Receiver A person or group who receives a message from another.

Receptive speech The ability to understand the spoken word.

Receptor A nerve cell acts as a receptor by converting the **stimulus** to a nerve impulse. Most receptors are specific, that is, sensitive to only one type of stimulus.

Record Written or computer-based communication.

Recording The process of making an entry in a client record. Also called **charting** or **documenting**.

Recovery A period of time following an emergency or disaster in which restoration, reconstitution, and mitigation take place; return to (or exceed) pre-illness levels of functioning.

Recurrence A later recurrence of a disorder after recovery.

Red blood cell (RBCs, *erythrocytes*) Blood cells shaped like a biconcave disk that contain hemoglobin required for oxygen transport to body tissues; the most common type of blood cell.

Referred pain Pain that is perceived in an area distant from the site of the stimuli.

Reflection Thinking from a critical point of view, analyzing why one acted in a certain way, and assessing the results of one's actions.

Reflexes Stimulus–response activities of the body, reflexes are fast, predictable, unlearned, innate, and involuntary reactions to stimuli.

Reflux A backward flow of acidic secretions into the lower esophagus.

Refraction The bending of light rays as they pass from one medium to another medium of different optical density.

Refractory hypoxemia The decrease of particle arterial oxygen despite administration of oxygen at high flow rates.

Refractory period A phase during which myocardial cells resist stimulation.

Refractory septic shock A persistently low mean arterial blood pressure despite vasopressor therapy and adequate fluid resuscitation.

Regeneration The replacement of destroyed tissue cells by cells that are identical or similar in structure and function.

Reinfection The development of a new infection with a different pathogen following successful treatment.

Relapse Return of a disorder soon after recovery.

Relationships-based (caring) theories Theories that stress courage, generosity, commitment, and the need to nurture and maintain relationships.

Relaxation response A healthful physiologic state that can be elicited through deep relaxation breathing with emphasis on a prolonged exhalation phase.

Religion A set of doctrines accepted by a group of people who gather together regularly to worship and that offer a means to relate to God or a higher power; an organized system of beliefs and practices.

REM Sleep Rapid-eye-movement sleep; occurs during sleep about every 90 minutes and lasts 5–30 minutes.

Remission A period during a chronic illness in which the symptoms of the illness disappear; sustained recovery lasting 8 weeks or more.

Renal colic Acute, severe flank pain on the affected side; develops when a stone obstructs the ureter, causing ureteral spasm.

Renal failure A condition in which the kidneys are unable produce urine, resulting in altered fluid, electrolyte, and acid–base balance.

Renal insufficiency Decrease in the kidneys' ability to conserve sodium and concentrate the urine.

Renin-angiotensin-aldosterone system System initiated by specialized receptors in the juxtaglomerular cells of the kidney nephrons that respond to changes in renal perfusion.

Repetitive motion disorders Injuries or disorders that result from using the same muscle groups over and over again without rest. Carpal tunnel syndrome is an example of a repetitive motion disorder.

Replication studies Research studies that involve repeating a study with all the essential elements of the original study held intact. Different samples and settings may be used.

Repolarization The process that returns the cell to its resting, polarized state.

Report An oral, written, or computer-based communication intended to convey information to others.

Reporting The act of communicating specific information to a person or group of people.

Research process A formalized, logical, systematic approach to solving problems.

Research utilization Knowledge that is only based upon evidence generated from research. It is different from **evidence-based practice** in that it does not include a critical review of the research findings as they are related to nursing care and it does not take client values and preferences into consideration.

Reservoir A source of microorganisms.

Residual urine Urine that remains in the bladder after voiding.

Resilience/resiliency The ability to function with healthy responses, even when experiencing significant stress or adversity.

Resolution phase The fourth and final phase of the sexual response cycle, marked by the return to the unaroused state.

Resonance A hollow sound, such as that produced by lungs filled with air.

Resource allocation Term used to describe how a resource is allocated, or provided, to clients or communities when there are not enough of the resource for every one who needs it.

Respiratory acidosis A condition caused by an excess of dissolved carbon dioxide, or carbonic acid. It is characterized by a pH less than 7.35 and a $PaCO_2$ greater than 45 mmHg.

Respiratory alkalosis A condition that results when pH rises above 7.45 and $PaCO_2$ falls below 35 mmHg. It is always caused by **hyperventilation** (unusually fast respiration, or overbreathing), leading to a carbon dioxide deficit.

Respiratory syncytial virus (RSV) A highly contagious respiratory infection that affects almost all children before 2 years of age.

Responsibility The specific accountability or liability associated with the performance of duties of a particular role.

Rest pain Cramping or aching pain in the calves of the legs, the thighs, and the buttocks that occurs while at rest.

Restraints Protective devices used to limit the physical activity of the client or a part of the body.

Restrictive cardiomyopathy A disorder characterized by rigid ventricular walls that impair diastolic filling.

Retinal detachment Separation of the retina or sensory portion of the eye from the choroid.

Retrograde conduction Cardiac conduction against the normal flow or pattern.

Retrospective audit A type of **audit** that is conducted after a client's discharge and involves examining records of a large number of cases.

Reverse delegation Occurs when someone with a lower rank delegates to someone with more authority.

Reverse triage A method of triage implemented during mass casualty incidents in which the most severely injured or ill victims who require the greatest resources are treated last to allow the greatest number of victims to receive medical attention.

Reward deficiency syndrome The decreased ability to experience pleasure. Reward deficiency syndrome drives the person to seek external forms of gratification through the use of substances, pathological gambling, or other high-risk behaviors.

Rheumatoid arthritis (RA) A chronic systemic autoimmune disease that causes inflammation of connective tissue, primarily in the joints.

Rhinorrhea A runny nose.

Ribonucleic acid (RNA) One of two types of nucleic acid made by cells. Ribonucleic acid is made up of ribose rather than deoxyribose and contains information that has been copied from DNA (the other type of nucleic acid).

Risk Factor A practice, behavior, or environmental factor that has potentially negative affects on individual health or causes a client to be vulnerable to developing a health problem.

Risk nursing diagnosis A clinical judgment that a problem does not exist, but the presence of risk factors indicates that a problem is likely to develop unless the nurse intervenes.

Role A set of expectations about how the person occupying one position behaves.

Role ambiguity Occurs when expectations are unclear, and when people do not know perform their roles and are unable to predict the reactions of others to their behavior.

Role conflict Conflict that occurs when there is incompatibility between one or more role expectations.

Role development Socialization into a particular role.

Role mastery Occurs when an individual's behaviors meet social expectations.

Role performance How a person in a particular role behaves related to the behaviors expected of that role.

Role strain The stress or strain experienced by an individual when incompatible behavior, expectations, or obligations are associated with a single social role.

Root cause analysis A process for identifying the factors that bring about deviations in practices that lead to a **sentinel event**.

Round ligaments The ligaments that hold the ovaries in place.

Sacral promotory A projection into the pelvic cavity on the anterior upper portion of the sacrum, which serves as a landmark for pelvic measurements.

Safety Protection from harm or injury.

Saline 0.9% sodium chloride, an isotonic solution.

Satiety The sensation of fullness.

Scald A **burn** from a hot liquid or vapor, such as steam.

Scapegoat An individual who has been selected to take the blame for another individual or for a group.

Scheduled toileting Toileting at regular intervals.

Schistocytes Fragmented red blood cells.

Schizoaffective disorder A psychotic disorder with features of both schizophrenia and mood disorders.

Schizoid personality disorder One of 11 types of **personality disorders**, it is characterized by a lifelong pattern of indifference to others and social isolation.

Schizophrenia The most common psychotic disorder, schizophrenia is a combination of disordered thinking, perceptual disturbances, behavioral abnormalities, affective disruptions, and impaired social competency.

Schizophreniform disorder A disorder with rapid onset of psychotic symptoms, very similar to schizophrenia, lasting less than 6 months.

Schizotypal personality disorder One of 11 types of **personality disorders**, it is characterized by a pattern of disturbed interpersonal relationships, thought patterns, appearance, and behavior.

Sciatica Lumbar back pain that radiates down the posterior leg to the ankle.

Scientific research A type of research that uses systematic, orderly, and objective methods of seeking information. The scientific method uses **empirical data** and requires that the researcher obtain data or facts in an unbiased manner.

Scleral buckling A surgical procedure to correct **retinal detachment**.

Seasonal affective disorder (SAD) A mood disorder characterized by depression during fall and winter and normal mood or hypomania during spring and summer.

Second heart sound Produced by closure of the semilunar valves, characterized by the syllable "dub."

Secondary cataracts Can form after surgery to treat another eye disorder, such as glaucoma, or as an effect of medication or another primary disorder.

Secondary group A type of group that is generally larger, more impersonal, and less sentimental than a **primary group**. Examples are professional associations, task groups, ad hoc committees, political parties, and business groups.

Secondary hypertension Elevated blood pressure resulting from an identifiable underlying process.

Secondary infertility The inability to conceive after one or more successful pregnancies, or the inability to sustain a pregnancy.

Secondary prevention Activities designed for early diagnosis and treatment of disease or illness.

Seizures Periods of abnormal electrical discharges in the brain that cause involuntary movement as well as behavior and sensory alterations.

Selective perception The process of filtering out unnecessary and distracting information in order to focus on what is important at any given moment.

Selective serotonin reuptake inhibitor (SSRI) A drug that selectively inhibits the reuptake of serotonin into nerve terminals; used mostly for depression.

Selectively permeable Refers to membranes separating body fluid compartments across which solutes can move with relative ease.

Self-awareness The relationship between an individual's perception of himself or herself and others' perceptions of him or her.

Self-concept One's mental image of oneself.

Self-esteem One's judgment of one's own worth.

Self-help group A **group** comprised of individuals who come together to face a common problem or difficulty.

Semen Sperm mixed with seminal fluid, ejaculated during sexual activity.

Semiformal group A type of **group** with a formal structure and voluntary membership. Aspects of a semiformal group may meet members' social or ego needs. Examples include churches, synagogues, social clubs, and parent–teacher organizations.

Sender A person or group who wishes to convey a message to another.

Sensitization An increased reaction to pain over time, or a reduced threshold for reaction to painful stimuli.

Sensory memory The momentary perception of stimuli from the environment.

Sensory overload An overabundance of sensory stimulation.

Sensory perception The conscious organization and translation of external data or stimuli into meaningful information.

Sensory reception The process of receiving external stimuli or data. External stimuli are **visual** (sight), **auditory** (hearing), **olfactory** (smell), **tactile** (touch), and **gustatory** (taste).

Sentinel event An unexpected occurrence involving death or serious physical or psychological injury, or the risk thereof.

Sepsis 1) The whole body inflammatory process resulting in acute illness; 2) The state of infection.

Septal defect A **congenital heart defect** that connects the right and left side of the heart.

Septic shock Altered perfusion resulting from a systemic infection that manifests with hypotension, delayed capillary refill, and inadequate perfusion and oxygenation of vital body tissues.

Septicemia A systemic infection caused by **bacteremia**.

Seroconversion Antibody response to a disease or vaccine.

Serum bicarbonate (HCO$_3^-$) reflects the renal regulation of acid–base balance. The normal HCO$_3^-$ value is 22–26 mEq/L.

Serum sickness A systemic type III hypersensitivity response, usually in response to a drug such as penicillin or a sulfonamide.

Sex chromosomes Genetic material found in the cell nucleus that determines the individual's gender.

Sexual aversion disorder A disorder characterized by severe distaste for sexual activity or the thought of sexual activity.

Sexual health The integration of the somatic, emotional, intellectual, and social aspects of sexual being, in ways that are positively enriching and that enhance personality, communication, and love.

Sexual orientation The preference of a person for one sex or the other.

Sexual self-concept How one values oneself as a sexual being.

Shared leadership A form of leadership that recognizes that a professional workforce is made up of many leaders. No one person is considered to have knowledge or ability beyond that of other members of the work group.

Shared psychotic disorder A condition that results when a person who is in a close relationship with another person who is delusional comes to share the delusional beliefs.

Shock A clinical syndrome characterized by a systemic imbalance between oxygen supply and demand.

Short-term memory Information held in the brain for immediate use; what one has in mind at a given moment.

Shunt A natural or artificially created tunnel or passage that allows blood to flow through an area.

Sickle cell anemia An inherited chronic anemia marked by defective hemoglobin and the irregular crescent shape of red blood cells.

Sickle cell crisis Severe episodes of fever and intense pain that are the hallmark of sickle cell disease.

Sickle cell disorder A hereditary **hemoglobinopathy**, a type of disorder characterized by replacement of normal hemoglobin with abnormal hemoglobin S (Hgb S) in RBCs.

Sickle cell trait Carrying one copy of the defective sickle cell gene, which can be passed on to children but not usually causing illness.

Signs Also referred to as **objective data** or overt data, are detectable by an observer or can be measured or tested against an accepted standard. They can be seen, heard, felt, or smelled, and they are obtained by observation or physical examination. Examples of objective data include a discoloration of the skin and a blood pressure reading.

Single-parent family Family in which only one parent resides in the home and is the primary caretaker and provider for the family.

Situational depression A maladaptive reaction to an identifiable psychosocial stressor or stressors that occurs within 3 months after the onset of the stressor and has persisted for no longer than 6 months.

Six Sigma A quality management program that uses quantitative data to monitor progress.

Sleep An altered state of consciousness in which the individual's perception and reaction to the environment are decreased.

Sleep apnea A disorder characterized by frequent short breathing pauses during sleep.

Sleep architecture The basic organization of normal sleep.

Sleep hygiene Interventions used to promote sleep.

Small cell carcinoma A highly malignant cancer usually associated with the lung.

SOAP An acronym for a charting method that follows a recording sequence of *subjective* data, *objective* data, *assessment*, and *planning.*

Sobriety The state of habitual refrain from using alcohol or drugs.

Social distance Describes a distance between individuals that is between 4–12 feet.

Social Justice The upholding of moral, legal, and humanistic principles.

Socialization A process by which a person learns the ways of a group or society in order to become a functioning participant.

Socialized insurance A system of health care in which all medically necessary services are covered, including physician care, hospital services, and to some extent prescription drugs.

Socialized medicine A system of health care in which the state or country owns and controls health care services.

Socratic questioning A technique one can use to look beneath the surface, recognize and examine assumptions, search for inconsistencies, examine multiple points of view, and differentiate what one knows from what one merely believes.

Software The instructions, or programs, that make a computer work for the user.

Sojourner Truth An abolitionist, Underground Railroad agent, preacher, and women's rights advocate; she was a nurse for more than 4 years during the Civil War and worked as a nurse and counselor for the Freedman's Relief Association after the war.

Solitary play A stage of play in which the infant still plays primarily alone, but enjoys the presence of others.

Solutes Substances that dissolve in liquid.

Solvent The component of a solution that can dissolve a **solute**.

Somatic cells Cells that make up the tissue of the body, with a full complement (diploid) of chromsomes, as opposed to sex cells.

Somatic pain Pain arising from nerve receptors originating in the skin or close to the surface of the body.

Somatization The process by which psychological distress is experienced and communicated in the form of somatic symptoms.

Somatostatin A substance (believed to be a neurotransmitter) that inhibits the production of both glucagon and insulin.

Somnology The study of sleep.

Somogyi phenomenon A combination of hypoglycemia during the night with a rebound, morning rise in blood glucose to hyperglycemic levels.

Source-oriented clinical record A record in which each person or department makes notations in a separate section or sections of the client's chart.

Spasticity Increased muscle tone (hypertonia), usually with some degree of weakness.

Specific defenses Immune system responses directed against identifiable bacteria, viruses, fungi, or other infectious agents.

Specific gravity An indicator of urine concentration that can be performed quickly and easily by nursing personnel.

Specific self-esteem How much one approves of a certain part of oneself.

Spermatogenesis The process by which mature spermatozoa are formed.

Spermicide A cream, jelly, foam, vaginal film, and suppository that is inserted into the vagina before intercourse to destroy sperm and prevent conception.

Spinal cord A continuation of the medulla oblongata, it has the ability to transmit impulses to and from the brain via the ascending and descending pathways.

Spinal cord injury Trauma to the spinal cord that results from excessive force to the spinal column.

Spinal cord stimulation (SCS) A form of therapy used with persistent pain that has not been controlled with less invasive therapies. SCS involves the insertion of an electrode (may be a single channel or multichannel device) adjacent to the spinal cord in the epidural space. The electrode(s) is attached to an impulse-generator (external or implanted) that sends electric impulses to the spinal cord to control pain.

Spinal fusion The insertion of a wedge-shaped piece of bone or bone chips between the vertebrae to stabilize them.

Spinal shock The temporary loss of reflex function due to injury.

Spiritual distress A challenge to the spiritual well-being or to the belief system that provides strength, hope, and meaning to life; a feeling of being separated from interconnectedness with others or with a higher power.

Spiritual skills Skills which help the individual find meaning in and understand the personal significance of an unexpected event.

Spiritual support Assistance to clients and families in providing meaning and sustaining courage during difficult times.

Spiritual well-being A feeling of inner peace and of being generally alive, purposeful, and fulfilled; the feeling is rooted in spiritual values and/or specific religious beliefs.

Spirituality The part of being human that seeks meaningfulness through personal connection, which may includebelief in or relationship with some higher power, creative force, driving being, or infinite source of energy.

Splitting The inability to integrate contradictory experiences.

Spontaneous abortion The loss of a fetus prior to 20 weeks' gestation; also called **miscarriage**.

Sprain A tearing of ligaments.

Sputum Mucus or mucopurulent matter expectorated from the lungs.

Squamous cell carcinoma A malignant tumor of the squamous epithelium of the skin or mucous membranes.

Staff authority A type of **authority** consisting of an advisory relationship in which the person in authority recommends or offers advise to the employee but is not responsible for assigning work activities.

Staghorn stones See **struvite stones**.

Staging A system of classifying cancer according to the size of the tumor, involvement of lymph nodes, and metastasis to distant sites.

Standard A generally accepted measure, rule, model, or pattern; also called a **norm**.

Standardized care plan A formal plan that specifies the nursing care for groups of clients with common needs (e.g., all clients with myocardial infarction).

Standards of care The skills and learning commonly possessed by members of a profession. The term also may be used to refer to policies or standards that describe nursing actions for clients with similar medical conditions rather than individuals, and they describe achievable rather than ideal nursing care.

Standards of practice Descriptions of the responsibilities for which nurses are accountable.

Standards of professional performance Set by the American Nurses Association (ANA), they describe behaviors expected in the professional nursing role.

Standing order A written document about policies, rules, regulations, or orders regarding client care.

State Children's Health Insurance Program (SCHIP) This program provides insurance coverage for poor and working-class children by expanding coverage for children under Medicaid and subsidizing low-cost state insurance alternatives.

Status asthmaticus A severe, prolonged form of asthma that is difficult to treat.

Status epilepticus A continuous seizure that lasts for more than 30 minutes or a series of seizures during which time consciousness is not regained.

Steatorrhea Excess fat in the feces.

Stem cell transplant The infusion of immature stem cells to replenish a client's blood cell lines, as an alternative to bone marrow transplantation.

Stenosis Narrowing of the valve, valve area, or great artery above the valve.

Step-down therapy A gradual reduction in the dosage and number of drugs used in a therapeutic regimen.

Stepfamily Consists of a biologic parent with children and a new spouse who may or may not have children.

Stereogenesis The ability to perceive and understand an object through touch.

Stereotaxic thalamotomy An x-ray taken during neurosurgery to guide the insertion of a needle into a specific area of the brain.

Stereotyping The act of generalizing that all people in a group are the same.

Stereotypy Rigid and obsessive behavior.

Sterile field An area free of microorganisms.

Sterile technique Practices that keep an area or object free of all microorganisms. Also known as **surgical asepsis**.

Sterilization A process that destroys all microorganisms, including spores and viruses; surgical procedures to permanently prevent pregnancy.

Stigma A collection of negative attitudes and beliefs that lead people to fear, reject, avoid, and discriminate against people with mental illness.

Stillbirth Intrauterine fetal death (IUFD) occurs after 20 weeks' gestation.

Stimulus The agent or act that stimulates a nerve receptor.

Stoma An artificial opening in the abdominal wall; it may be permanent or temporary.

Strategic planning The process of continual assessment, planning, and evaluation to guide the future of an organization.

Stress fracture A fracture that results from disease that has weakened the bone.

Striae Whitish-silver stretch marks seen in obesity and during or after pregnancy.

Stroke A condition in which neurologic deficits result from a sudden decrease in blood flow to a localized area of the brain. Also known as cerebrovascular accident.

Stroke volume Difference between the end-diastolic volume and the end-systolic volume.

Structural-functional theory Focuses on family structure and function, examining family relationships and how they effect the functions of the family and relationships with other systems.

Structure standards **Standards** related to the physical environment, organization, and management of an organization.

Struvite stones A type of calculi associated with UTI caused by urease-producing bacteria such as *Proteus*. These stones can grow to become very large, filling the renal pelvis and calyces. They are often called **staghorn stones** because of their shape.

Subculture groups Minority groups characterized by specific norms, beliefs, and values that coexist with a dominant culture.

Subdermal implant Capsules implanted within the skin that slowly release medication, such as for contraception.

Subfertility Occurs when both partners of a couple have reduced fertility.

Subjective data Information that is apparent only to the person affected; can be described or verified only by that person. Examples include itching, pain, feelings, and values. May be referred to as **symptoms** or **covert data**.

Subjective family burden The psychological distress of family members in relation to the **objective family burden** of having a family member with a mental illness.

Substance abuse Refers to the use of any chemical in a fashion inconsistent with medical or culturally defined social norms despite physical, psychological, or social adverse effects.

Substance dependence A condition in which the client can no longer control use of the substance, continues to use despite adverse effects, and experiences withdrawal symptoms without continued use of the substance.

Subsystem A component of a larger system.

Suctioning Aspirating secretions through a catheter connected to a suction machine or wall suction outlet.

Sudden cardiac death (SCD) Unexpected death occurring within 1 hour of the onset of cardiovascular symptoms.

Sudden infant death syndrome (SIDS) The sudden death of an apparently healthy infant that remains unexplained after other possible causes have been ruled out through autopsy, death scene investigation, and review of the medical history.

Suffocation A lack of oxygen because of interrupted breathing; also referred to as asphyxiation.

Sundowning A behavioral change commonly seen in dementia clients, characterized by increased agitation, time disorientation, and wandering behaviors during afternoon and evening hours; it is accelerated on overcast days.

Superego The conscience of personality, the ego ideal; the source of feelings of guilt, shame, and inhibition.

Superficial basal cell carcinoma A type of skin cancer.

Superficial burn A burn that involves only the epidermal layer of the skin.

Supersaturated urine A condition that results when the concentration of an insoluble salt in the urine is very high.

Supine On the back.

Supplemental Security Income (SSI) Special payments for people with disabilities, those who are blind, and people who are not eligible for Social Security; these payments are not restricted to health care costs.

Suprasystem An overarching system to which smaller systems or subsystems belong. For example, the family is the suprasystem of the individual.

Surge capacity A community's ability to rapidly meet the increased demand for qualified personnel and resources, including health care resources, in the event of a disaster.

Surgical asepsis or **sterile technique** Practices that keep an area or object free of all microorganisms.

Surgical debridement The process of excising a wound to the level of fascia (fascial excision) or sequentially removing thin slices of a burn wound to the level of viable tissue (sequential excision).

Swan-neck deformity Caused by **rheumatoid arthritis**, it is characterized by hyperextension of the proximal interphalangeal (PIP) joints joint with compensatory flexion of the distal interphalangeal (DIP) joints.

Switching A term used in disorders of mood and affect to describe a new illness phase (manic or depressed) without recovery.

Sympathetic tone A state of partial smooth muscle contraction around arteries and veins.

Symphysis pubic Fibrocartilaginous joint between the pelvic bones in the midline.

Symptoms Information that is apparent only to the person affected; can be described or verified only by that person. Examples include itching, pain, feelings, and values. May be referred to as **subjective data** or **covert data**.

Synchronized cardioversion Delivery of direct electrical current synchronized with the client's heart rhythm.

Syncope Transient loss of consciousness and muscle tone after exercise or activity.

Syndrome diagnosis A diagnosis that is associated with a cluster of other diagnoses.

Synovectomy Excision of synovial membrane, this procedure is used as a treatment for **rheumatoid arthritis**.

Synovitis Inflammation of the synovial membrane lining the articular capsule of a joint.

Syphilis A complex systemic sexually transmitted infection caused by the spirochete *Treponema pallidum*.

System A set of interacting identifiable parts or components.

Systematized delusions A manifestation of **schizophrenia** characterized by an extensively developed central delusional theme from which conclusions are deduced.

Systemic arthritis A form of **juvenile rheumatoid arthritis** that characteristically is manifested by high fever, polyarthritis, and rheumatoid rash. Systemic arthritis also affects internal organs and joints.

Systemic circulation Consists of the left side of the heart, the aorta and its branches, the capillaries that supply the brain and peripheral tissues, the systemic venous system, and the vena cava.

Systemic infection Occurs when an invading microorganism spreads and damages different parts of the body.

Systemic inflammatory response syndrome (SIRS) Describes the body's response to a critical illness that can result from an infectious or noninfectious cause precipitating a whole-body inflammatory process.

Systemic lupus erythematosus (SLE) A chronic inflammatory connective tissue disease.

Systemic vascular resistance The force or resistance of the blood in the body's blood vessels that helps return blood to the heart.

Systems theory The study of how a system operates, including how it interacts with other systems and how its components interact with each other within the system itself.

Systole The phase of ventricular contraction.

Systolic blood pressure The maximum pressure exerted within the arteries when the heart compresses.

T lymphocyte A type of **leukocyte** that matures in the thymus gland and is integral to the specific immune response.

Tachypnea Rapid respirations.

Tangential excision The sequential removal of thin slices of the burn wound to the level of viable tissue.

Tardive dyskinesia A condition characterized by unusual tongue and face movements such as lip smacking and wormlike motions of the tongue.

Tartar A visible, hard deposit of **plaque** and dead bacteria that forms at the gumlines.

Tau A protein found in the neurons.

Taxonomy A classification system or set of categories, such as nursing diagnoses, arranged on the basis of a single principle or consistent set of principles.

Teaching A system of activities intended to produce learning.

Team nursing The delivery of individualized nursing care to clients by a team led by a professional nurse.

Technical skills Purposeful, "hands-on" skills such as manipulating equipment, giving injections, bandaging, moving, lifting, and repositioning clients.

Telecommunications The transmission of information from one site to another, using equipment to transmit information in the forms of signs, signals, words, or pictures by cable, radio, or other system.

Telehealth The use of telecommunication technologies and computers to exchange health care information and to provide services to clients at remote locations.

Temperament The combination of biological and physical characteristics that is specific to each individual and influences personality and behavior.

Tender points Refers to tenderness that occurs in precise, localized areas, particularly in the neck, spine, shoulders, and hips.

Tendonitis Inflammation of a tendon.

Teratogen Any chemical that has the potential to harm the fetus, including pesticides, viruses, and medications.

Terminal weaning The gradual withdrawal of mechanical ventilation when survival without assisted ventilation is not expected.

Territoriality A concept of the space and things that an individual considers as belonging to the self.

Tertiary prevention Activities designed to restore individuals with disabilities to their optimal level of functioning.

Testosterone The primary male sex hormone produced by the testes.

Tetany Tonic muscle spasms.

Tetralogy of Fallot Consists of four defects—pulmonic stenosis, right ventricular hypertrophy, ventricular-septal defect, and an overriding aorta.

Tetraplegia Loss of function of the arms, trunk, legs, and pelvic organs.

Thalassemia Inherited disorder of hemoglobin synthesis in which either the alpha or beta chains of the hemoglobin molecule are missing or defective.

Therapeutic communication An interactive process between nurse and client that helps the client overcome temporary stress, to get along with other people, to adjust to the unalterable, and to overcome psychologic blocks that stand in the way of self-realization.

Therapeutic insemination The deposition of semen at the cervical os or in the uterus by mechanical means.

Therapeutic relationship The relationship that develops between the nurse and the client that is characterized by (a) the development of trust and acceptance between the nurse and the client and (b) an underlying belief that the nurse cares about and wants to help the client.

Third heart sound Sometimes heard after the second heart sound in children, young adults, and pregnant females during the third trimester. Also called a **ventricular gallop**.

Third spacing A shift of fluid from the vascular space into an area where it is not available to support normal physiologic processes.

Thoracentesis Needle insertion into the pleural space to remove fluid accumulation.

Threshold potential The point at which an action potential is capable of being generated.

Thrill A palpable vibration over the precordium or an artery.

Thromboemboli Blood clots.

Throughput The process by which information, energy, or material that enters a system (input) is used by the system.

Thyroid storm An extreme state of hyperthyroidism, also called thyroid crisis.

Thyroidectomy Surgical removal of the thyroid gland.

Thyroiditis Inflammation of the thyroid gland.

Thyrotoxosis A disorder caused by excessive delivery of thyroid hormone to the peripheral tissues.

Tine test A multiple-puncture device is used to introduce tuberculin into the skin.

Tinea pedis Fungal infection of the feet; aka "athlete's foot."

Tinnitus The perception of sound or noise in the ears without stimulus from the environment.

Token economies Formalized programs of contingency contracts.

Tolerance State in which a particular dose elicits a smaller response than it formerly did. With increased tolerance, the individual needs higher and higher doses to obtain the desired response.

Tone The amount of tension or resistance to movement in a muscle.

Tonic phase Initial phase of a generalized seizure, manifested by unconsciousness and continuous muscular contraction.

Tonic-clonic seizures Alternating contraction (tonic phase) and relaxation (clonic phase) of muscles during seizure activity.

Tonicity The osmolality of a solution. Solutions may be termed **isotonic**, **hypertonic**, or **hypotonic**.

Torsades de pointes A type of ventricular tachycardia associated with a prolongation of the QT interval.

Tort A civil wrong committed against a person or a person's property.

Total anomalous pulmonary venous return The pulmonary veins empty into the right atrium, or into veins leading to the right atrium, rather than into the left atrium.

Total lymphoid irradiation A procedure sometimes used in the treatment of **rheumatoid arthritis**; it decreases total lymphocyte levels.

Total quality management (TQI) A management philosophy that emphasizes a commitment to excellence throughout the organization.

Toxic multinodular goiter A tumor characterized by small, discrete, independently functioning nodules in the thyroid gland tissue that secrete excessive amounts of thyroid hormone.

Toxoplasmosis Space-occupying lesions common in clients with AIDS that may cause headache, altered mental status, and neurologic deficits.

Trachoma A chronic conjunctivitis caused by *Chlamydia trachomatis,* is a significant preventable cause of blindness worldwide.

Traction The application of a straightening or pulling force to return or maintain the fractured bones in normal anatomic position.

Traditional family An autonomous unit in which both parents reside in the home with their children, the mother assuming the nurturing role and the father providing the necessary economic resources.

Transactional leader A **leader** whose relationship with followers is based on an exchange for some resource valued by the follower.

Transcellular fluid One of the components of **extracellular fluid**. Examples of transcellular fluid are cerebrospinal, pericardial, pancreatic, pleural, intraocular, biliary, peritoneal, and synovial fluids.

Transcendence Person's recognition that there is something other or greater than the self and a seeking and valuing of that greater other, whether it is an ultimate being, force, or value.

Transformational leader A type of **leader** who inspires others with a clear, attractive, and attainable goal and enlists them to participate in attaining the goal.

Transfusion reaction A type II or cytotoxic hypersensitivity reaction to blood of an incompatible type.

Transgenderism Gradations of human characteristics running from female to male.

Transient ischemic attack (TIA) A brief period of localized cerebral ischemia that causes neurologic deficits lasting for less than 24 hours. Also called a mini-stroke.

Transjugular intrahepatic portosystemic shunt (TIPS) An expandable metal stent inserted through a transcutaneous needle to channel blood from the portal vein into the hepatic vein, bypassing the cirrhotic liver.

Transplacental immunity **Passive immunity** transferred from mother to infant.

Transposition of the great arteries A congenital heart defect in which the pulmonary artery, which is the outflow tract for the left ventricle, and the aorta, which is the outflow tract for the right ventricle, are switched (transposed).

Transsexual An individual who feels his or her sexual anatomy is not consistent with his or her gender identity.

Transverse diameter The largest diameter of the pelvic inlet; helps determine the shape of the inlet.

Traumatic cataracts A type of **cataract** that may result from an injury to the eye.

Triage Means "sorting." Triage is a continuous process in which client priorities are reassigned as needed treatments, time, and the condition of the clients change.

Tricuspid atresia The absence of the tricuspid valve.

Tricyclic antidepressant (TCA) A class of drugs used in the pharmacotherapy of depression.

Triglycerides Substances formed from dietary fats and carbohydrates in fat cells to store energy.

Triplet Three premature ventricular contractions in a row.

Tripod position A position of sitting and leaning forward.

Trisomy An extra chromosome.

Trousseau's sign Contraction of the hand and fingers in response to occlusion of the blood supply by a blood pressure cuff; caused by decreased blood calcium levels.

True pelvis The portion that lies below the **linea terminalis**, made up of the inlet, cavity and outlet.

Truncus arteriosus A heart defect in which a single large vessel empties both ventricles and provides circulation for the pulmonary, systemic, and coronary circulations.

Tubal ligation A surgical procedure to clip, tie off, band, or plug the fallopian tubes to effect sterilization of a female client.

Tubercle A granulomatous lesion (a sealed-off colony of bacilli) formed from **mycobacterium tuberculosis**.

Tuberculosis (TB) A chronic, recurrent infectious disease caused by **Mycobacterium tuberculosis**. TB usually affects the lungs, but any organ can be affected.

Two-career family A family in which both partners are employed by choice or necessity. A two-career family may or may not have children.

Tympanic membrane A thin, tense membrane which separates the middle ear from the external auditory canal, protecting the middle ear from the external environment.

Tympany A musical or drumlike sound produced from an air-filled stomach.

Ulcer A break in the GI mucosa which develops when the mucosal barrier is unable to protect the mucosa from damage by hydrochloric acid and pepsin, the gastric digestive juices.

Ulcerative colitis A chronic inflammatory bowel disorder that affects the mucosa and submucosa of the colon and rectum.

Ultrafiltration Removal of excess body water using a hydrostatic pressure gradient.

Unconscious mind The part of the individual's mental life of which he or she is unaware.

Underinsured Individuals who have health care insurance coverage that is insufficient to meet their needs.

Undernutrition (also known as **malnutrition**) Health effects due to insufficient nutrient intake or stores.

Unifocal When ventricular impulse arises from one ectopic site.

Unilateral decision A decision made by one person without input from others, especially those who might be affected by the decision. An example is when the nurse decides how to intervene for a client without input from the client.

Unilateral lobar pneumonia A pattern of **pneumonia** in which bacteria tend to be distributed evenly throughout one or more lobes of a single lung.

Uninsured Individuals who have no health care insurance.

Universal precautions (UP) Techniques used to decrease the risk of transmitting unidentified pathogens.

Unlicensed assistive personnel (UAP) Health care staff who assume delegated aspects of basic client care, such as bathing, assisting with feeding, and collecting specimens. UAPs include certified nurse assistants, hospital attendants, nurse technicians, and orderlies.

Unresolved bacteriuria The presence of bacteria in urine that fails to resolve with treatment.

Upper body obesity Identified by a waist-to-hip ratio of greater than 1 in men or 0.8 in women. Also called central obesity.

Uremia Excessive amounts of urea in the blood.

Ureteral stent A thin catheter inserted into the ureter to provide for urine flow and ureteral support.

Ureterolithotomy An incision in the affected ureter to remove a calculus.

Ureteroplasty The surgical repair of a ureter.

Urgency The sudden, strong desire to **void**.

Uric acid stones Develop when the urine concentration of uric acid is high.

Urinary calculi Stones in the urinary tract.

Urinary drainage system Those organs required to drain urine from the kidneys, including the ureters, urinary bladder, and urethra.

Urinary frequency The need to urinate often.

Urinary hesitancy A delay and difficulty in initiating voiding; often associated with dysuria.

Urinary incontinence Involuntary urination due to the temporary or permanent inability of the external sphincter muscles to control the flow of urine from the bladder.

Urinary reflux Backward flow of urine.

Urinary retention The accumulation of urine in the bladder and inability of the bladder to empty itself, resulting in overdistention of the bladder.

Urinary stasis Stagnation of urinary flow.

Urination Releasing urine from the urinary bladder (voiding).

Uroflowmetry Measures urine flow rate.

Urolithiasis The formation of stones in the urinary tract.

Uterosacral ligaments Ligaments that provide support for the uterus and cervix at the level of the ischial spines.

Uterus The hollow muscular organ in which the fertilized ovum is implanted and in which the developing fetus is nourished until birth.

Utilitarianism A form of consequentialist theory that views a good act as one that brings the most good and the least harm for the greatest number of people. This is called the principle of **utility**.

Utility See **utilitarianism**.

Utilization reviews Interdisciplinary assessments based on the appropriate allocation of resources. Utilization reviews are mandated by The Joint Commission for organizations that it accredits.

Uveitis Inflammation of the middle layer of the eye called the uvea.

Vaccine Suspensions of whole or fractionated bacteria or viruses that have been treated to make them nonpathogenic; introduced by **immunization** to provoke **active immunity**.

Vagina The muscular and membranous tube that connects the external genitals with the uterus.

Vaginismus The involuntary spasm of the outer one-third of the vaginal muscles, making penetration of the vagina painful and sometimes impossible.

Validation The act of "double-checking" or verifying data to confirm that it is accurate and factual.

Valsalva maneuver Forced exhalation against a closed glottis.

Values The standards that influence behavior; personal beliefs about the truth and the worth of thoughts, objects, or behaviors.

Variance A variation or deviation from a critical pathway or expected standard; goals not met or interventions not performed appropriately or according to the time frame.

Vasectomy A procedure to surgically sever the vas deferens on both sides of the scrotum to permanently prevent pregnancy.

Vasogenic shock Shock that results from widespread vasodilatation and decreased peripheral resistance. Also called distributive shock.

Venous stasis The collection and stagnation of blood in the lower extremities.

Venous thrombectomy Surgical removal of a blood clot.

Venous thrombosis A condition in which a blood clot (thrombus) forms on the wall of a vein, accompanied by inflammation of the vein wall and some degree of obstructed venous blood flow.

Ventilation The exchange of oxygen and carbon dioxide.

Ventricular bigeminy A premature ventricular contraction following each normal beat.

Ventricular gallop Sometimes heard after the second heart sound in children, young adults, and pregnant females during the third trimester. Also called the **third heart sound**.

Ventricular septal defect An opening in the ventricular septum causes increased pulmonary blood flow.

Ventricular trigeminy A premature ventricular contraction every third beat.

Veracity A moral principle that holds that one should tell the truth and not lie.

Verbal abuse Malicious, repeated, harmful mistreatment of an individual with whom one works, regardless of whether that person is an equal, a superior, or a subordinate; also referred to as workplace bullying.

Verbal communication The use of verbal language to send and receive messages.

Vertical transmission Perinatal transmission of an infection, such as the **human immunodeficiency virus**, from mother to infant.

Very-low-calorie diets A program providing a protein-sparing modified fast (400–800 kcal/day or less) under close medical supervision.

Vesicoureteral reflux A condition in which urine moves from the bladder back toward the kidney; a common risk factor in children who develop **pyelonephritis** that may also be seen in adults whose bladder outflow is obstructed.

Vestibulitis Pain of the outer portion of the vagina upon touch or attempted penetration.

Vibration A series of vigorous quiverings produced by hands that are placed flat against the client's chest wall.

Virchow's triad Three factors associated with thrombophlebitis; stasis of blood, vessel damage, and increased blood coagulability.

Virions Virus able to grow and reproduce outside a host.

Virulence The ability of a microorganism to produce disease.

Virus A type of microorganism that must enter living cells in order to reproduce.

Visceral Of or relating to any large organ in the body.

Visceral pain Pain arising from body organs. It is dull and poorly localized because of the low number of nociceptors.

Viscosupplementation A treatment for osteoarthritis of the knee, involving injecting lubricating substances directly into the knee.

Voiding Releasing urine from the urinary bladder (urinating).

Volatile acid Acids eliminated from the body as a gas.

Volkmann's contracture The impaired mobility of the arm and inability to extend the arm completely, which is a common complication of elbow fractures.

Voluntary admission The detention of a client in a psychiatric or medical facility at the client's request.

Voluntary health insurance Exists in countries that do not require citizens to carry health insurance and that do not provide health care to all people.

Vulnerable populations Social groups with inadequate access to health care because they lack resources and are exposed to more risk factors.

Vulva The female external genitals.

Vulvodynia Constant, unremitting burning that is localized to the vulva with an acute onset.

Weaning The process of removing ventilator support and reestablishing spontaneous, independent respirations; the process of discontinuing breastfeeding and accustoming an infant to another feeding method.

Well-being A subjective perception of feeling well that can be described objectively and measured.

Wellness A state of well-being that encompasses self responsibility, dynamic growth, nutrition, physical fitness, emotional health, preventive health care, and the whole being of the individual.

Wellness diagnosis A term that describes human responses to levels of wellness in an individual, family, or community that have a readiness for enhancement. For example, Readiness for Enhanced Coping.

Wernicke's encephalopathy A condition typically seen in alcoholics which is characterized by ataxia (lack of coordination), abnormal eye movements, and confusion.

Whistleblower A nurse who goes outside the organization for the public's best interest when the organization fails to follow procedures regarding safety and client care.

Whistleblowing Action taken by a nurse who goes outside of the organization for the public's best interest when the organization fails to follow procedures regarding safety and client care.

Work ethic A moral value that places high value on hard work and diligence.

World view The way in which people in a culture perceive ideas and attitudes about the world, other people, and life in general.

Xenophobia The fear or dislike of people different from one's self.

Xerostomia Dry mouth.

Zollinger-Ellison syndrome A form of **peptic ulcer disease** caused by a gastrinoma, or gastrin-secreting tumor of the pancreas, stomach, or intestines.

Zygote A fertilized egg.

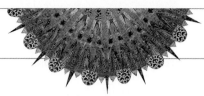

A

AA (Alcoholics Anonymous), 37, 37*t*
AACN. *See* American Association of Colleges of Nursing (AACN), 2367
Abacavir, 712*t*
Abbreviated grief, 601
Abbreviations, 2196–2198*t*
ABCD rule, 189*t*
ABC codes (Alternative Billing Concept codes), 2386
Abdominal assessment, 428*t*, 469*f*
Abdominal hysterectomy, 1751
Abducens, 1628*t*
Abducens nerve, 942*t*
ABGs. *See* Arterial blood gases
Abilify, 243, 244*t*, 1173*t*
Abortion:
  bioethics and, 2313, 2313*t*, 2314*t*
  controversy over, 1734
  definition, 1559*t*
  medical, 1734
  nursing care, 1735*t*
  reasons for, 2314*t*
  second trimester, 1734
  surgical, 1734
Abrasions, 1880*t*
Abruptio placentae, 1533
Abstinence, 30*t*, 1726
Abuse:
  client, 2301–2302
  intimate partner, 2461–2462, 2462*t*
  mandatory reporting of, 2413, 2414*t*
  verbal, 2131–2132
  assessment, 1940
  Assessment Interview, 1958*t*
  caring interventions, 1942–1943
  Case Study, 1962
  child. *See* Child abuse
  of children with mental retardation, 206*t*
  collaborative care
    domestic violence shelters, 1957
    working with children, 1957
  definition, 1937, 1944
  diagnostic tests, 1941–1942
  elder. *See* Elder abuse
  etiology
    gender-bias factors, 1951
    interpersonal history, 1950
    neurobiology, 1950
    social learning theory, 1950–1951
  laws dealing with, 1943
  manifestations, 1953, 1954–1955*t*, 1955–1957
  nursing diagnoses and interventions
    risk for caregiver role strain, 1960
    risk for decisional conflict, 1960
    risk for hopelessness, 1960
    risk for other directed violence, 1959–1960
    treating the abuser, 1960
    working with victims of abuse, 1960
  nursing process
    assessment, 1957–1959
    diagnosis, 1959
    evaluation, 1962
    planning and implementation, 1959–1960, 1962

overview, 1944–1945
  physical, 1945
  in pregnancy, 1950
  prevention, 1938–1939, 1939*t*
  risk factors
    age and physiologic status, 1951
    cultural, 1952
    gender, 1951
    other, 1953
    psychological, 1952
    socioeconomic, 1952–1953
    substance abuse, 1953
  screening and intervention triage for, 1941*t*
  sexual, 1947–1949
  types
    child. *See* Child abuse
    elder. *See* Elder abuse
    intimate partner violence, 1949–1950
Abuses of power:
  defined, 2228
  improper use of authority, 2229
  intimidation, 2229, 2229*t*
  sexual harassment, 2228–2229
Academic Center for Evidence-Based Nursing, 2335
Academic dishonesty, 2316, 2316*t*
Academy of Medical-Surgical Nurses, 2367
Acceptance, 2158
Acceptance stage of grief, 602*t*
Accessory nerve, 942*t*, 1628*t*
Accident, 1937
Accidental death, 2457–2458
Accidents:
  procedure- or equipment-related, 2445
Accommodation, 347, 1631, 2129
Accountability, 1778, 2144, 2237
  about, 2279–2280
  Case Study, 2284
  criteria of profession and, 2280–2281
  factors influencing
    consumer demands, 2282–2283
    demography, 2283–2284
    economics, 2282
    information and telecommunications, 2283
    legislation, 2283
    science and technology, 2283
  nursing practice and, 2284, 2326
Accreditation, 2366, 2389
Accrediting bodies, 2366
Acculturation, 322
ACE inhibitors. *See* Angiotensin-converting enzyme (ACE) inhibitors
Acetaldehyde dehydrogenase inhibitor, 39*t*
Acetaminophen, 1861*t*
  consumption parameters, 275*t*
  for increased intracranial pressure, 960*t*, 964
  mechanism of action, 275
  for pain management, 275
  in specific conditions
    osteoarthritis, 1127
Acetazolamide (Diamox), 1671*t*
Acetazolamide, 1670
Acetylcholine, 217, 666–667, 1670
Acetylcholinesterase inhibitors, 210
Acetylcysteine, 842
Acid phosphatase (ACP), 129*t*

Acid–base balance:
  about, 3–10
  alterations, 5–8
  assessment, 5
  disorders
    acidosis, 4
    alkalosis, 4
    classification, 5
    compensation, 8, 8*t*
  caring interventions, 8
  diagnostic tests, 8, 9*t*
  pharmacologic therapies, 8–10, 10*t*
  normal presentation, 5
  regulation of, 4–5
    buffer systems, 4
    renal system, 5
    respiratory system, 4–5
Acidosis:
  definition, 4
  metabolic, 4
  osteoporosis and, 1035
  pharmacotherapy, 8–9, 9*t*
  respiratory, 4
Acids, 3
  nonvolatile, 4
  volatile, 4
Acoustic nerves:
  functions, 1628*t*
Acoustic reflex testing, 1646
ACP. *See* Acid phosphatase (ACP)
Acquaintance phase, 1198
Acquaintance rape, 1970
Acquired hemolytic anemia, 100–101
Acquired immunity, 679
Acquired immunodeficiency syndrome (AIDS):
  antiretroviral therapy and, 703
  bioethics and, 2313
  Case Study, 725, 725*t*
  collaborative care
    diagnostic tests, 709–710
    overview, 708–709
  description of, 676, 693
  evidence-based practice, 716
  history of, 696–697
  home care of newborn with, 720*t*
  incidence and prevalence of, 697–699
  manifestations of
    AIDS dementia complex, 703–704, 707
    Kaposi's sarcoma, 705–706, 705*f*
    neurologic effects, 703–704
    opportunistic infections, 704–706
    overview, 702*t*, 706–707
    pediatric, 705, 707, 708*t*
    secondary cancers, 705
  Nursing Care Plan
    critical thinking, 724*t*
    diagnosis, 723*t*
    evaluation, 723*t*
    planning and implementation, 723*t*
  nursing diagnoses and interventions
    address ineffective sexual patterns, 722
    ineffective coping, 721
    knowledge deficit, 724
    maintain skin integrity, 721–722

manage imbalanced nutrition, less than body
    requirements, 722
  prevent infection, 717–720
  promote adherence to medication regimen, 720
  nursing process
    assessment, 715–716
    diagnosis, 716–717
    evaluation, 724
    planning and implementation, 717–724t
  pathophysiology and etiology, 697–701
  pneumonia and, 836
  risk factors, 701–703
Acquired immunodeficiency syndrome (AIDS). See
    also Human immunodeficiency virus (HIV)
  sensory neuropathies and, 1680
Acral lentiginous melanoma, 185
Acrosomal reaction, 1525
ACT (assertive community treatment), 245
ACTH. See Adrenal corticosteroid hormone;
    Adrenocorticotropic hormone
ACTH. See Adrenocorticotropic hormone
Actigall, 904
Actinic keratosis, 186–188
Actinomyces, 770
Action potential, 1305–1306, 1306f
Action verbs, 2087t
Actiq, 287t
Active chronic hepatitis, 693t
Active euthanasia, 2314
Active immunity, 682
Active learning, 2249, 2249f
Active listening, 2177t
Active transport, 521, 522f, 1533
Active transport pumps, 86t
Activities of daily living (ADLs), 651, 1067
Activity tolerance, 652
Activity-exercise patterns, 651
Actual diagnosis, 2065
Actual loss, 600
Acupressure wristbands, 1575f
Acupuncture, 245, 280
  anxiety disorders and, 1816t
  for herniated disk, 1084
  for mood disorders, 1177
  post-traumatic stress disorder and, 1845
Acute angle-closure, 1669
Acute angle-closure glaucoma, 815t
Acute chest syndrome, 178t
Acute cholecystitis, 902
Acute confusion, 226
Acute conjunctivitis, 815t
Acute coronary syndrome (ACS):
  definition, 1361
  description, 1362–1363
  manifestations, 1367, 1367t
Acute fatigue, 301
Acute hydronephrosis, 468t
Acute illness, 638
Acute lactic acidosis:
  causes, 11
Acute lymphoblastic leukemia, 148, 149f
Acute lymphocytic leukemia (ALL), 150–151,
    150t, 151f
Acute lymphocytic leukemia (ALL). See
    also Leukemia
Acute myeloid leukemia (AML), 148–149,
    150f, 150t

Acute myeloid leukemia (AML). See also
    Leukemia
Acute myocardial infarction (AMI):
  clinical therapies, 1376
  complications
    cardiogenic shock, 1369
    dysrhythmias, 1368–1369
    infarct extension, 1369
    pericarditis, 1369
    pump failure, 1369
    structural defects, 1369
  deep venous thrombosis and, 1391
  definition, 1361
  manifestations, 1367–1369, 1367t, 1368t
  medications for, 1375–1376
  Nursing Care Plan
    assessment, 1387t
    critical thinking, 1388t
    diagnoses, 1387t
    evaluation, 1387t
    planning and implementation, 1387t
  in older adults, 1368t
  pathophysiology, 1363–1364
  symptoms
    in older adults, 1311–1312
    in women, 1368t
Acute otitis media. See Otitis media
Acute pain:
  characteristics, 262–263
  vs. chronic pain, 257t
  clinical therapies, 267t
  definition, 257
  description, 259t
  in older adults, 273
  recurrent, 263
  referred, 263, 263f
  somatic, 263
  treatment, 259t
  visceral, 263
  Acute pain. See also Pain
Acute postinfection glomerulonephritis:
  manifestations, 925
Acute postinfectious glomerulonephritis (APIGN),
    923, 924f, 928f
Acute postinfectious, 924f
Acute postinfectious glomerulonephritis:
  prognosis, 928t
Acute postinfectious glomerulonephritis (APIGN).
    See also Nephritis
Acute psychoses, 232
Acute renal failure (ARF):
  Case Study, 551
  collaborative care
    diagnostic tests, 540
    fluid management, 542–543
    goals, 539–540
    nutrition, 543, 550
    pharmacologic therapies, 540, 541t, 542, 542t
    renal replacement therapy, 543–546
  course and manifestations
    in children, 538–539, 539t
    initiation phase, 537
    maintenance phase, 537–538
    in older adults, 539t
    recovery phase, 538–539
  definition, 534
  description, 528t

  incidence, 537
  intrinsic (intrarenal), 534, 534t
  Nursing Care Plan
    assessment, 549t
    critical thinking, 549t
    diagnoses, 549t
    evaluation, 549t
    planning and implementation, 549t
  nursing diagnoses and interventions, 550
  nursing process
    assessment, 547
    diagnosis, 548
    evaluation, 550
    overview, 546
    planning and implementation, 548, 550
  in older adults, 537t, 539t
  overview, 533–534
  pathophysiology and etiology, 534–537, 535t
  postrenal, 534, 534t
  prerenal, 534, 534t
  risk factors, 537
  treatment, 528t
Acute respiratory acidosis, 18–19, 19t, 21t
Acute respiratory distress syndrome (ARDS), 1895
  associated conditions, 1235t
  Case Study, 1252
  collaborative care
    artificial airways, 1243–1245
    mechanical ventilation, 1238–1243
    pharmacologic therapies, 1238
    positioning and management strategies, 1246
    suctioning, 1245
    treatment of infection, 1246
  community-based care, 1251
  end-stage, 1237f
  etiology, 1235
  manifestations, 1235, 1238t
  Nursing Care Plan
    assessment, 1250t
    critical thinking, 1250t
    diagnoses, 1250t
    evaluation, 1250t
    planning and implementation, 1250t
  nursing diagnoses and interventions
    anxiety, 1251
    decreased cardiac output, 1248
    dysfunctional ventilatory weaning response,
      1248–1249
    impaired spontaneous ventilation, 1248
    ineffective airway clearance, 1247–1248
  nursing process
    assessment, 1247
    diagnosis, 1247
    evaluation, 1251
    planning and implementation, 1247
  overview, 1234
  pathogenesis, 1235f
  pathophysiology, 1234, 1236f
  risk factors, 1235
  treatment, 1220t
Acute retroviral syndrome, 702t
Acute stress disorder:
  manifestations, 1814
Acute tubular necrosis (ATN), 534–535, 536f, 537
Acute uveitis, 815, 815t

Acyclovir:
herpes simplex virus infections of the eye and, 815–816
Ad hoc committees, 2140
ADA. *See* Americans with Disabilities Act
Adalimumab, 749
Adaptability:
in verbal communication, 2150
Adaptation, 347
and transactional model of stress and coping, 1799
definition, 1794
Adaptation model, 2059, 2060t
Adaptation phase, 350
Adaptive functioning, 201
Adaptive mechanisms, 343
ADD. *See* Attention deficit disorder
ADD (Administration on Developmental Disabilities), 205
Addenbrooke's Cognitive Examination, 207t
Adderall, 373t
Addiction behavior. *See also* Substance abuse
about, 27–39
alterations, 29–31
assessment, 31–32, 32t
caring interventions, 32–38
definition, 27
vs. dependence, 28
diagnostic tests, 32
explanations for, 28–29
normal presentation, 28–29
pharmacologic therapies, 38, 39t
to prescription drugs, 73
process, 28, 29t, 68
recovery from, 32
support groups, 36–37
terminology, 29, 30t
Addicts, 28
Addison's disease, 693t
Adenohypophysis (anterior pituitary), 978
definition, 978
hormones, 979f
Adenoidectomy, 315
Adenoids, 682
Adenosine, 1449, 1450t
Adenosine triphosphate (ATP), 1593
Adenotonsillectomy, 314t
ADH (aldehyde dehydrogenase), 41
ADH. *See* Antidiuretic hormone (ADH)
ADHD. *See* Attention deficit hyperactivity disorder
ADHD Rating Scale, 371t
Adherence, 650, 2245
Adjustment disorder:
definition, 1159
Adjustment phase, 350
Adjustment reaction to depressed mood, 1200
Administration for Children and Families, 2364
Administration on Developmental Disabilities (ADD), 205
Administration on Aging, 2364
Administrative agencies, 2398
Administrative information systems, 2375
Administrative laws, 2398
Administrative systems, 2378, 2378t
Admission assessment, 2193, 2376
ADNAase B, 926

Adolescence, 341t
developmental tasks in, 1581t
enhancing self-esteem in, 1591t
growth and development in, 364–366
sexual development in, 1692t, 1693
Adolescent family, 486
Adolescent mothers, 498t
Adolescent pregnancy:
factors contributing to
high-risk behaviors, 1554
psychosocial factors, 1554
socioeconomic and cultural factors, 1553–1554
family and social network reactions to, 1557
partners of adolescent mothers, 1556–1557
reaction to, 1555t, 1557t
risks to child, 1556
risks to mother
physiologic risks, 1554
psychologic risks, 1555
sociologic risks, 1555–1556
Adolescents:
anticipatory guidance for, 2440, 2441t
assessment of, 2009, 2017
advance care planning and, 294t
caffeine use in, 71
communication with, 2155t
dating violence and, 2461–2462, 2462t
depression in, 1190t
grief and loss in, 610t
group therapy for, 36
health promotion in, 641t
interventions for general population, 2018t
interventions for high-risk population, 2018t
leading causes of death, 2018t
mood disorders in, 1180
pain perception and behavior, 269t
promotion of oral health in, 659
recommended screenings and immunizations, 643t
safety measures, 2455t, 2457
sleep patterns and requirements, 668
smoking by, 56t
STIs in, 1693, 1755
substance abuse risk factors in, 70t
with seizure disorders, 974t, 975
with terminal illness, 613
Adoption:
coparent, 488
Adrenal cortex, 978t, 980, 1423
Adrenal corticosteroid hormone (ACTH):
in specific conditions
multiple sclerosis, 1120, 1121t
Adrenal glands:
definition, 980
pregnancy and, 1545
Adrenal medulla, 978t, 980
Adrenal tumor:
clinical therapies, 581t
manifestations, 581t
Adrenalcorticosteroids:
in specific conditions
multiple sclerosis, 1121t
Adrenaline, 980
Adrenergic antagonists, 1670, 1671t
administration, 1493t
mechanism of action, 1331t
nursing considerations, 1331t

Adrenergic stimulants, 1259, 1259t
Adrenocorticotropic hormone (ACTH), 129t, 137t, 978, 980
Adrenomedullin, 1423
Adult children of alcoholics, 31, 37
Adult learning theory, 2245, 2246t
Adult protective services (APS), 1962
Adult survivors:
of sexual abuse, 1948–1949
Adulthood:
developmental tasks in, 1581t
enhancing self-esteem in, 1591t
stages of, 346–347, 366–368
Adults:
anticipatory guidance for, 2441
interventions for general population, 2019t
interventions for high-risk populations, 2019t
leading causes of death, 2019t
middle, 366, 368t
older, 367–368, 369t
promotion of oral health in, 659
sleep patterns and requirements, 668
young, 366, 366t
See also Middle-aged adults; Older adults; Young adults
Advance directives, 289–290
elements of, 2410
ethical issues of, 2314
overview, 2410
role of nurse and, 2412
sample, 2411f
Advanced age-related macular degeneration. *See also* Macular degeneration
Advanced emergency medical technicians (AEMTs), 2358t
Adverse events, 2443
Advil. *See* Ibuprofen
Advisory Committee on Immunization Practices (ACIP), 683
Advocacy, 225
about, 2297–2298
advocate's role, 2298–2302
Case Study, 2303
for children and families, 2300
clinical example, 2300t
defined, 2297
dimensions of, 2299
educating providers and others, 2299
empowering the client, 2299
illegal, immoral, and unethical activities and, 2302
interventions, 2302
for the mentally ill, 250
nursing practice, 2302
professional and public, 2300
for vulnerable populations, 2300–2302
Advocates, 2298–2302, 2306
AEDs (Antiepileptic drugs), 959, 960t
Aenocarcinomas, 161t
Aerobic exercise, 652
Aesthetic knowing, 2031
Afebrile, 1854, 1859
Affect, 211
comparison of, in mood disorders, 1181f
definition, 1157
descriptors of, 239t, 1158, 1158t
suicide and, 1982
See also Mood

Affective commitment, 2231, 2231*f*
Affective domain, 2247
AFP. *See* Alpha-fetoprotein (AFP)
African Americans:
  adolescent pregnancy and, 1553
  blindness in, 1658*t*
  breast cancer in, 111*t*
  cancer risk and incidence, 116
  culture-specific assessment, 2010*t*
  glaucoma in, 1669
  gonorrhea prevalence, 1760
  homicide and, 1964
  hypertension in, 1425, 1426*t*
  kidney disease and, 562
  pain responses, 268*t*
  sickle cell disorder in, 177
  stroke and, 1501*t*
  views on older adults, 402*t*
  vision impairment in, 1649*t*
Afterload, 1304, 1405
Age:
  body temperature and, 1853
  diversity and, 401, 401–402*t*
  influence of, on health, 644
  osteoporosis and, 1034
Age-related macular degeneration (ARMD),
    1649*t*, 1676
  See also Macular degeneration
Ageism, 401, 622
Agency fires, 2450–2451
Agency for Healthcare Research and Quality
    (AHRQ), 2335, 2347, 2364, 2423
Ages & Stages Questionnaire (ASQ), 2013*t*
Aggravated assault, 1964
Aggressive behavior, 1169, 1963, 1965–1966
Aggressive communicators, 2179, 2179*t*
Aging:
  cardiovascular changes and, 1310–1312, 1311*f*
  cognitive abilities and, 199
  effect on skin, 1875, 1876*t*, 1877*t*
  hypertension and, 1426
  myths and realities of, 401*t*
  normal cognitive changes vs. Alzheimer's
    disease, 214*t*
  physical changes, 369*t*
  of population, 2342
  pressure ulcers and, 1916
  theories of, 345–347
  urinary system changes and, 415–416
Agnosia, 1502
Agnostics, 1771
Agonist analgesics, 276
Agonist-antagonist analgesics, 276
Agoraphobia:
  manifestations, 1836–1837
Agraphia, 215
AIDS dementia complex, 703–704, 707
AIDS. *See* Acquired immunodeficiency
    syndrome (AIDS)
Airway hyperresponsiveness, 1253
Airway remodeling, 1252
Airway resistance, 1253
Akathisia, 207*t*, 243
Al-Anon, 31, 37
Alanine aminotransferase (ALT), 129*t*
alarm reaction, 1794
  countershock phase, 1794, 1795*f*
  shock phase, 1794, 1795*f*

Alaska Natives:
  homicide and, 1964
  otitis media in, 1634*t*
  respiratory syncytial virus (RSV) and, 1281*t*
Albumin, 129*t*, 1884
  in acute renal failure, 542
  in plasma, 518
Albuterol sulfate, 841
Alcohol:
  abuse
    assessment, 45–46
    binge drinking, 40
    Case Study, 51
    chronic or situational low self-esteem, 48
    co-occurring disorders, 40
    co-occurring substances, 41*t*
    collaborative care, 44
    comorbid disorders, 1159
    costs of, 40
    deficient knowledge, 48
    depression and, 1192
    diagnosis, 46
    diagnostic tests, 44
    disturbed sensory perceptions, 50
    disturbed thought processes, 50
    health problems associated with, 662
    imbalanced nutrition, less than body
      requirements, 48
    ineffective coping, 48
    ineffective denial, 48
    legal issues, 50
    manifestations, 41, 42*t*, 43
    multisystemic effects, 43, 43*t*
    Nursing Care Plan, 49*t*
    nursing diagnosis and interventions, 46, 48, 50
    nursing process, 45–46, 48, 50
    other drugs used with, 41*t*
    pathophysiology and etiology, 40
    pattern of dependence, 40
    in pregnancy, 59, 61, 62*t*
    prevalence, 40
    relapse, 50*t*
    risk factors, 41, 41*t*
    risk for injury and violence, 46, 48
    safety issues, 50
    schizophrenia and, 236
    treatment, 44–45, 62*t*
  addiction
    description, 29*t*
    treatment, 29*t*
  consumption
    behavioral changes, 44*t*
    coronary artery disease and, 1373
    effect on fetus, 58*t*
    fetal alcohol syndrome and, 202
    cancer risk and, 121–122
    hypertension and, 1426, 1429
    sexual functioning and, 1701*t*
    social acceptability of, 40
    underage, 40
  during pregnancy, 341
  overdose, 44
  sleep and, 669
  street names, 74*t*
  withdrawal, 42*t*, 43–45
Alcohol dependence, 40
Alcohol poisoning, 44
Alcohol withdrawal delirium, 30*t*, 43

Alcohol withdrawal syndrome, 43
Alcoholic cirrhosis:
  definition, 1016
  Nursing Care Plan, 1023*t*
  pathophysiology, 1016
Alcoholic dementia, 43
Alcoholic ketoacidosis:
  pharmacologic therapies, 12
Alcoholic neuropathy, 1680
Alcoholics Anonymous (AA), 37, 37*t*
Alcoholism:
  definition, 40
  disease model of, 69
  types of, 40
Alcott, Louisa May, 2288
Aldehyde dehydrogenase (ADH), 41
Aldosterone, 411, 980, 1405
Aleve. *See* Naproxen
Alfuzosin (Uroxatral), 434
Alkaline phosphatase (ALP), 129*t*
  in musculoskeletal system assessment, 1077*t*
Alkalis, 3
Alkalosis:
  definition, 4
  metabolic, 4
  pharmacotherapy, 10, 10*t*
  respiratory, 4
  symptoms, 8
Alkylating agents, 95*t*
Allergens:
  hypersensitivity and, 725–726
  patch testing for, 1913
Allergic asthma, 734
Allergic contact dermatitis, 1912
Allergic rhinitis, 734
Allergies:
  characteristic findings in children with, 735*t*
  conjunctivitis and, 814
  hypersensitivity and, 725–726
  substances triggering, 728*t*
  See also Hypersensitivity
Allocation of resources:
  Case Study, 2351
  examples of, 2349–2350
  nurses and, 2350
  overview, 2349
AlloDerm, 1903
Allogeneic bone marrow transplant, 155
Allografts, 1903
Alloimmunization, 179
Alogia, 237
Alopecia, 1883*t*
ALP. *See* Alkaline phosphatase (ALP)
Alpha cells, 980, 989
5-alpha reductase inhibitors, 434*t*
  for benign prostatic hypertrophy, 434
Alpha-adrenergic agents:
  BPH and, 434, 434*t*
Alpha-adrenergic blockers, 1430*t*
Alpha-blockers, 1432, 1701*t*
Alpha-fetoprotein (AFP), 129*t*
Alpha-interferon:
  human immunodeficiency virus (HIV) and, 713
Alpha2-adrenergic agonists:
  for glaucoma, 1650*t*
Alphagan, 1671*t*
Alprazolam, 1814–1815
ALS. *See* Amyotrophic lateral sclerosis (ALS)

ALT. *See* Alanine aminotransferase (ALT)
Alternative (complimentary) care
  providers, 2116*t*
Alternative therapies. *See* Complementary and
  alternative medicine (CAM)
Altruism, 2306
ALU (arithmetic logic unit), 2374
Aluminum hydroxide, 542, 558–559
Alupent. *See* Metaproterenol
Alveolar macrophages, 678, 773
Alveoli:
  anatomy, physiology, and functions,
    1216–1217
  pediatric differences in, 837
Alzheimer's disease:
  alternative therapies, 217–219
  caregivers and, 211
  Case Study, 225
  causes, 206*t*
  characteristics of, 211
  collaborative care, 217
  communicating with client with, 221*t*
  community-based care, 224
  cultural variations, 213*t*
  familial, 214
  genetic factors, 214
  incidence, 211, 213
  interventions
    anxiety, 222, 222*t*
    caregiver role strain, 222, 224
    chronic confusion, 221
    decreasing risk for falls, 221
    hopelessness, 222
    impaired memory, 220
    risk for injuries, 221, 222*t*
  legal issues, 225
  manifestations, 214–216, 216*t*
  vs. normal aging, 214*t*
  Nursing Care Plan
    assessment, 223*t*
    critical thinking in the nursing process, 224*t*
    diagnosis, 223*t*
    evaluation, 224*t*
    implementation, 223*t*
    planning, 223*t*
    nursing process
    assessment, 219
    diagnosis, 220
    evaluation, 225
    implementation, 220
    plan, 220
  pathophysiology and etiology, 211–214
  patient advocacy, 225
  pharmacologic therapies, 210, 217, 218*t*
  protective factors, 214
  risk factors, 214
  safety considerations, 225
  sporadic, 214
  stage 1, 215
  stage 2, 215
  stage 3, 215
  warning signs, 214
Amantadine, 821
Ambien, 313
Ambiguity, 2108
Ambulation:
  assistive devices
    canes, 1078–1079

crutches, 1078
  walkers, 1078
  nursing interventions, 1078
AMD. *See* Macular degeneration
Amenorrhea, 1748
  pregnancy and, 1546, 1546*t*
American Accreditation Healthcare
  Commission, 2388
American Assembly for Men in Nursing
  (AAMN), 2367*t*
American Assisted Living Nurses Association, 2367
American Association of Colleges of Nursing
  (AACN), 2330, 2367
American Association of Colleges of Nursing
  (AACN) Magnet designation, 2386
American Burn Association, 1890, 1892, 1892*t*
American Civil War, 2288
American College of Nurse Midwives, 2294
American Hospital Association (AHA):
  list of patient rights, 2318
American Medical Informatics Association, 2385
American Nurses Association (ANA):
  Bill of Rights for Registered Nurses, 2310
  Code of Ethics for Nurses, 2183,
    2308–2312, 2310*t*
  definition of health, 636
  health policy and, 2362
  National Database of Nursing Quality
    Indicators, 2423
  nursing definition of, 2291
  on roles of health care professionals, 2114
  position statement on education for participation
    in nursing research, 2330*t*
  position statement on electronic health
    records, 2392*t*
  purpose of, 2366
  standard of professional nursing, 2115*t*
  Standards of Clinical Nursing Practice, 2402,
    2403*t*, 2410
  Standards of Practice, 2293, 2293*t*
  Standards of Professional Performance, 2244,
    2244*t*, 2327, 2328*t*
American Nurses Association Research and
  Studies Commission, 2333
American Nurses Credentialing Center (ANCC),
  2293, 2409
American Nurses Credentialing Center Magnet
  Recognition Program, 2310
American Red Cross, 2290
American Sign Language (ASL), 1655*t*
American Society of Addiction Medicine, 40
Americans with Disabilities Act (ADA), 205, 2301
Amino-glycosides:
  medication administration, 807
Aminophylline, 841
Amiodarone, 1336
Amish, 1784*t*
Ammonium chloride, 10, 10*t*
Amnion, 1528
Amniotic fluid:
  functions, 1528–1530
Amniotic sac, 1528
Amoxicillin:
  in specific conditions
    otitis media, 828
Amphetamine salts, 373*t*
Amphetamines, 72–73
  effect on fetus, 58*t*

sexual functioning and, 1701*t*
  street names, 74*t*
  use of, 68
Ampicillin:
  urinary tract infections and, 876
Amprenavir, 713
Amputation:
  phantom pain and, 264
Amsler grid, 1676*f*, 1677
Amygdala:
  mood disorders and, 1161
Amyl nitrate:
  sexual functioning and, 1701*t*
Amyl nitrite, 74
Amyloid plaques, 212
Amyloid precursor protein (APP), 212
Amyotrophic lateral sclerosis (ALS), 1076*t*
Amytal, 58*t*
ANA. *See* American Nurses Association
ANA Cabinet on Nursing Research, 2332
ANA Council of Nurse Researchers, 2330
ANA Standards of Practice, 2402, 2403*t*, 2410
Anabolic steroids:
  sexual functioning and, 1701*t*
Anabolism, 1597
Anaerobic exercise, 652
Anaerobic metabolism, 1362
Anal intercourse, 1697
Anal stimulation, 1697
Analgesics. *See also* specific drugs
  categories and examples, 274*t*
  home provision of, 287*t*
  for inflammation, 892*t*
  medication administration, 807
  for musculoskeletal disorders, 1079*t*
  overview, 807*t*
  for pain management, 274
  for myocardial infarction, 1375
Anaphylactic shock, 1489–1490, 1492*t*
Anaphylaxis:
  definition, 887
  hypersensitivity and, 725–726, 728*t*, 737, 739
  symptoms and treatment, 888*t*, 889*t*
Anaplasia, 88
Anaphylaxis:
  definition, 889*t*
Anaprox. *See* Naproxen
Anasarca, 582
ANCC. *See* American Nurses Credentialing Center
  Androgen deprivation therapy, 172–173
Andragogy, 2245
Androgens, 432, 1687
  prostate cancer and, 169
Androgyny, 1696
Anemia:
  in acute renal failure, 538*t*, 543
  Case Study, 106
  causes, 97*t*, 100*t*
  characteristics, 97*f*
  in chronic renal failure, 556
  Client Teaching, 104*t*
  clinical therapies, 557*t*
  collaborative care
    blood transfusion, 102
    complementary therapies, 102
    diagnostic tests, 101
    nutrition, 102
    pharmacologic therapies, 102

definition, 96
incidence, 97
manifestations, 97–101, 303t, 557t
multisystem effects, 98f
Nursing Care Plan
  assessment, 105t
  critical thinking, 105t
  diagnoses, 105t
  evaluation, 105t
  planning and implementation, 105t
nursing diagnoses and interventions
  activity intolerance, 103–104
  impaired oral mucous membrane, 104
  risk for decreased cardiac output, 104–105
  self-care deficit, 105
nursing process
  assessment, 103
  diagnosis, 103
  evaluation, 106
  planning and implementation, 103–105
  pathophysiologic mechanisms of, 96t
pathophysiology and etiology, 96–97
risk factors, 97
systemic lupus erythematosus (SLE) and, 759–760
types
  aplastic, 101, 102t
  blood loss, 97
  folic acid deficiency, 99–100, 102t
  hemolytic, 100–101, 102t
  iron deficiency, 97, 99, 102t
  megaloblastic, 99
  neonatal, 101
  nutritional, 99–100
  pernicious, 99
  physiologic anemia of infancy, 101
  sickle cell. See Sickle cell anemia
  vitamin B$_{12}$ deficiency, 99, 102t
Anergy, 1188
Anesthetics, 1913t
Anger management, 1967t, 1968
Anger stage:
  of grief, 602t
Angina pectoris:
  cardiomyopathy and, 1335t
  definition, 1361
  ischemia and, 1362
  manifestations, 1366–1367, 1367t
  medications for, 1375
  Prinzmetal's, 1362
  stable, 1362, 1367t
  unstable, 1362
Angiography, 1465
  in cancer, 128
Angioplasty, 1354t
Angiotensin, 980
Angiotensin II receptor blockers, 1330t, 1413,
    1414t, 1430t, 1432
Angiotensin-converting enzyme (ACE) inhibitors:
  administration, 217, 1414t, 1430t
  mechanism of action, 1330t
  nursing considerations, 1330t
  in specific conditions
    coronary artery disease, 1374–1375
    glomerular disorders, 927
    heart failure, 1413
    hypertension, 1430t, 1432
    myocardial infarction, 1376

Angiotensinogen, 980
Angle-closure glaucoma, 1669–1670, 1669t. See
    also Glaucoma
Anglicans, 1784t
Anhedonia, 29, 238, 1188
Animal-assisted therapy, 219
  for mood disorders, 1177
Animism, 360t
Anions, 518, 519f
Anisoylated plasminogen streptokinase activator
    complex (APSAC), 1376
Ankle-brachial blood pressure index (ABI), 1370
Ankylosing spondylitis, 889t
Anointing of the Sick, 1774
Anomia, 207t
Anorexia:
  in dying client, 618
  fluid volume deficit and, 577
Anorexia nervosa. See also Eating disorders
  binge-eating/purging type, 1599t
  vs. bulimia, 1585
  clinical therapies, 1601t
  definition, 1584, 1599
  diagnostic criteria, 1599t
  incidence, 1599
  manifestations, 1599–1600, 1601t
  pharmacologic therapies, 1592
  restricting type, 1599t
  theories on
    family factors, 1598
    genetics, 1598
    neurobiology, 1598
Anorexia-cachexia syndrome, 123, 124t
Anorgasmia, 1709
Anosmia, 1645t
Anovulation, 1748
ANP. See Atrial natriuretic peptide (ANP)
Ansaid. See Flurbiprofen
Antabuse, 45
Antacids, 934–935, 1020
Antagon, 1735t
Antegrade pyelography, 540
Antepartum:
  definition, 1559t
Antepartum care, 1558, 1558t
Anterior cavity, 1631
Anterior pituitary (adenohypophysis), 978t
  definition, 978
  female reproductive cycle and, 1521–1522
  hormones of, 979f
Anterior syndrome, 1145t
Anthracyclines, 90
Anthrax, 2357, 2357t
Anthropometric measurements:
  in children, 2009
Anthropometry, 1028
Anti-DNA antibody testing:
  systemic lupus erythematosus (SLE) and, 760
Anti-inflammatories:
  for asthma, 1262
  medication administration, 807
Anti-streptolysin O antigen titer, 1353t
Antianemics, 95t
Antianxiety agents:
  sexual functioning and, 1701t
  effect on fetus, 58t
  medications, 1807–1808, 1807t, 1814–1815

for sleep disorders, 313–314
in specific conditions
  burns, 1900
Antibiotics, 1861
  antitumor, 95t
  medication administration, 807
  overview, 807t
  peak and trough levels, 805
  for skin disorders, 1913t
  in specific conditions
    appendicitis, 894
    COPD, 1272–1273
    glomerular disorders, 926
    peptic ulcer disease, 933
    urinary tract infections, 876
Antibodies:
  in immune response, 680
  immunizations and, 682
  monoclonal. See Monoclonal antibodies
  primary immune response and, 680f
  production of, 677t
Antibody-mediated (humoral) immune response:
  immune system function and, 676
  immunoglobulins and, 680
  systemic lupus erythematosus (SLE) and, 756
Anticholinergic agents:
Anticholinergics, 1259, 1259–1260t
  in specific conditions
    multiple sclerosis, 1120
    for urinary elimination, 423t
    Parkinson's disease, 1139t
Anticipatory guidance, 2439–2440
  for adults, 2441
  Case Study, 2441
  for children and adolescents, 2440, 2441t
  developmental considerations, 2440, 2440t
  for older adults, 2441
Anticipatory grief, 601
Anticipatory loss, 600
Anticoagulants:
  Medication Administration, 1393t
  in specific conditions
    cardiomyopathy, 1335
    deep venous thrombosis, 1392
    myocardial infarction, 1376
    pulmonary embolism, 1479
    stroke, 1506
Anticonvulsants, 959, 960t, 971
  for bipolar disorders, 1182
  sexual functioning and, 1701t
Antideoxyribonuclease B (ADNAase B), 926
Antidepressants:
  atypical, 1173
  classes of, 1170
  for depression, 1190
  developmental considerations, 1174
  for eating disorders, 1602
  effects of, 1170
  for fatigue, 303t
  sexual functioning and, 1701t
  in specific conditions
    anxiety disorders, 1807t
    Parkinson's disease, 1137
    suicide and, 1983
    suicide risk and, 1190
  for substance abuse, 39t
  tricyclic. See Tricyclic antidepressants

use by young adults, 1831t
uses of, 1170
warnings about, 1170, 1190
Antidiarrheal agents, 431t
　for specific conditions
　　IBD, 916
Antidiuretic hormone (ADH), 137t, 410–411, 416, 524f
　antidiuretic hormone, 523, 978
　blood pressure and, 1423
　heart failure and, 1405
Antidysrhythmics, 1376, 1416, 1449, 1450t
Antiepileptic drugs (AEDs), 959, 960t, 971
Antiflatulent agents, 431t
Antifungals:
　medication administration, 807
　overview, 807t
Antigen presenting cells (APCs), 680f
Antigen-antibody complex:
　systemic lupus erythematosus (SLE) and, 760
Antigen-presenting cells (APCs), 678
Antigenic determinant sites, 679
Antigenic drift, 819t
Antigenic shift, 819t
Antigens:
　characteristics of, 680
　detection methods, 805
　hypersensitivity and, 725
　immune response to, 679–681
　immune system function and, 676, 677t
　as tumor markers, 127
　Antihelminthic:
　medication administration, 808
　overview, 808t
Antihistamines:
　hypersensitivity and, 737
　sexual functioning and, 1701t
　in specific conditions
　　anxiety disorders, 1807t
　　conjunctivitis, 815
Antihypertensives:
　administration, 1430–1431t
　in chronic renal failure, 558
　mechanism of action, 1330t
　nursing considerations, 1330t
　sexual functioning and, 1701t
　sites of drug action, 1432t
　in specific conditions
　　glomerular disorders, 927
Anti-inflammatory agents, 210
Antilipemic agents, 1376
Antimalarials:
　medication administration, 807
　overview, 807t
Antimetabolites, 95t
Antimicrobials:
　antibiotics. See Antibiotics, 770
　antifungals. See Antifungals, 770
　antivirals. See Antivirals, 770
　for burns, 1900
　classification, 807–808t
　sepsis and, 852
Antioxidants, 210, 217, 1677
Antiplatelet medications, 1376, 1377t, 1506
Antipsychotics, 217, 242–244, 244t
　for bipolar disorders, 1173t, 1181
　developmental considerations, 1174

sexual functioning and, 1701t
side effects, 1181
in specific conditions
　anxiety disorders, 1815
Antipyretics, 960t, 964, 1861
　medication administration, 807
　overview, 807t
Antiretrovirals, 703
　medication administration, 808
　overview, 808t
Antiseizure medications, 39t, 1174t
Antiseptics:
　chain of infection and, 777
　common, 778t
Antisocial behavior, 1964–1965
Antisocial personality disorder:
　characteristics, 1617
　diagnostic criteria, 1614t
　family factors and, 1609
　genetic factors in, 1608
　manifestations, 1611t
　neurobiology and, 1608
Antispasmodics, 1149, 1079t, 1149t
Antistreptokinase (ASK), 926
Antistreptolysin O (ASO) titer, 926
Antithrombotics, 1506–1507
Antithyroid agents, 987t
Antituberculosis medications, 863, 863–864t
Antitumor antibiotics, 95t
Antivirals:
　in specific conditions
　　influenza, 821
　　respiratory syncytial virus (RSV)/ bronchiolitis, 1283
Anuria, 416, 417t, 541t
Anxiety:
　in Alzheimer's disease, 222, 222t
　in children, 24t
　definition, 1808
　frequently prescribed antianxiety medications
　　antidepressants, 1807t
　　antihistamine, 1807t
　　azapirone, 1807t
　　benzodiazepines, 1807t
　hyperventilation and, 23
　manifestations, 303t
　medical conditions associated with, 1806t
　in respiratory acidosis, 20–21
　successful nursing interactions with anxious clients, 1805t
Anxiety disorders:
　Case Study, 1818–1819
　collaborative care
　　cognitive behavior therapy, 1815–1816
　　complementary and alternative therapies, 1816
　　diagnostic tests, 1814
　　pharmacologic therapies, 1814–1815
　comorbidity with, 1158
　coping toolkit, 1815t
　developmental considerations, 1814t
　manifestations, 1812t
　　acute stress disorder, 1814
　　generalized anxiety disorder, 1811–1812
　　panic disorder, 1813–1814
　　separation anxiety disorder, 1812–1813
　Nursing Care Plan, 1817t

nursing diagnoses and interventions
　encouraging health promotion strategies, 1818
nursing process
　assessment, 1816–1817
　diagnosis, 1817
　evaluation, 1818
　planning and implementation, 1817–1818
overview, 1808
pathophysiology and etiology, 1808, 1810
risk factors, 1810–1811
schizophrenia and, 236
theories of
　cognitive-behavioral theories, 1809–1810
　developmental theories, 1810
　neurobiological theories, 1809
　neurochemical theories, 1809
　psychodynamic theories, 1809
　transactional model, 1810
　anxiolytics, 210
Aorta:
　coarctation of, 1347–1348, 1424
　Aortic stenosis (AS), 1347t
Aortocaval compression, 1542–1543
AP format, 2187
Apathy, 2139
Aphakia, 1662
Aphasia, 207t, 1504
Apical pulse, 1307, 1316t, 1319–1320, 1319f, 1320f
Apical-radial pulse, 1320
APIE format, 2187, 2188f
APIER format, 2187
APIGN (acute postinfectious glomerulonephritis), 923
Aplastic anemia, 101, 102t
Aplastic crises, 178t
Apligraf, 1903
Apnea:
　definition, 1221
　pneumonia and, 840
　respiratory syncytial virus (RSV)/Bronchiolitis and, 1281
Apoproteins, 1361
APP (amyloid precursor protein), 212
Appearance:
　as component of professionalism, 2226–2227, 2227f
Appendectomy, 893f, 894
Appendicitis, 889t, 890
　Case Study, 901
　chronic, 894, 894t
　classification of, 893
　collaborative care
　　diagnosis, 894
　　pharmacologic therapies, 894
　　surgery, 894
　community care, 899t
　complications, 894
　definition, 893
　incidence, 893
　manifestations, 893, 894t
　Nursing Care Plan
　　assessment, 900t
　　critical thinking in the nursing process, 900t
　　diagnosis, 900t
　　evaluation, 900t
　　overview, 900t

nursing diagnoses and interventions
  acute pain, 899, 899t
  anxiety, 900
  discharge planning and home care teaching, 901
  risk for deficient fluid volume, 899
  risk for infection, 900
nursing process
  assessment, 899, 899t
  diagnosis, 899
  evaluation, 901
  planning and implementation, 899–901
pathophysiology and etiology, 893
perioperative nursing care, 894–895, 895t
risk factors, 893
treatment, 894t
Appendicular skeleton, 1056
Appendix, 681f
Applied research, 2329
Approximated, 1927
Apraclonidine, 1670, 1671t
Apraxia, 215, 1502
Apresoline. See Hydralazine, 676
Aqueous humor, 1668
Arab Americans:
  infertility treatments and, 1738t
  pain responses, 268t
Arava. See Leflunomide
ARDS. See Acute respiratory distress syndrome
Areflexia, 1146
ARF. See Acute renal failure
Aricept, 217
Aripiprazole, 243, 244t, 1173t
Arithmetic logic unit (ALU), 2374
Arizona State University Center for the Advancement
    of Evidence-Based Practice, 2335
Arlington National Cemetery, 2288, 2289f
Aromatherapy, 245
Arousal, 946
Arrhythmias, 1319. See also Dysrhythmias
Arrhythmogenic, 1368
Arrogance, 2238
Art therapy, 363t
Arterial blood gases (ABGs):
  normal values, 1226t
  purpose and description, 1226–1227
  in specific conditions
    acid–base balance assessment, 5, 8, 9t
    acute renal failure, 540
    chronic obstructive pulmonary disease
        (COPD), 1272
    congenital heart defects, 1353t
    coronary artery disease, 1371
    heart failure, 1411
    lung cancer, 164
    metabolic acidosis, 6t, 7t, 9t
    metabolic alkalosis, 6t, 7t, 9t
    pneumonia and, 841
    pulmonary embolism, 1479
    respiratory acidosis, 6t, 9t, 19
    respiratory alkalosis, 6t, 9t
    sepsis and, 852
Arterial blood pressure, 1308
  definition, 1422
  factors affecting, 1423–1424, 1423f
  in specific conditions
    shock, 1490
Arterial ulcers, 1464t

Arteriosclerosis, 1308
  definition, 1462
Arteriovenous (AV) fistula, 545, 545f
Arteriovenous graft, 546
Arthritis:
  exercise guidelines for older people with, 1128t
  osteoarthritis. See Osteoarthritis (OS)
  rheumatoid. See Rheumatoid arthritis
  symptoms, 890
Arthrodesis, 750
Arthroplasty, 750
Arthroscopy, 1076, 1129
Artificial airways:
  endotracheal tubes, 1243, 1244f
  nasopharyngeal airways, 1243, 1244f
  oropharyngeal airways, 1243, 1243f
  tracheostomies, 1243–1244, 1244f, 1245f
Artificial insemination. See Therapeutic
    insemination
Artificial nutrition and hydration (ANH), 297
Artificial teeth, 660
Ascending contract venography, 1391
Ascites, 582, 1017, 1022
Ascorbic acid, 1262
  recommended daily intake, 1596t
ASD. See Autism spectrum disorders, 378
Asepsis:
  definition of, 771
Aseptic technique, 422
Asian Americans:
  culture-specific assessment, 2010t
  glaucoma in, 1669t
  mood disorders and, 1180t
  pain responses, 268t
ASK (antistreptokinase), 926
ASL (American Sign Language), 1655t
Aspartate aminotransferase (AST), 129t
  DSM-IV-TR diagnostic criteria, 381t
Asperger syndrome, 378
  cognitive functioning and, 380
  language abilities and, 379
  manifestations, 379t
  therapies, 379t
Aspergillosis, 706. See Austin spectrum disorders
Asphyxiation, 2452
Aspiration:
  cirrhosis and, 1022
Aspiration biopsy:
  in breast cancer, 109f
Aspirin, 11
  for pain management, 275
  in specific conditions
    rheumatoid arthritis, 748, 749t
Aspirin therapy:
  acute myocardial infarction and, 1374
  for angina, 1375
  diabetes mellitus and, 1005
ASQ (Ages & Stages Questionnaire), 2013t
Assault, 2401
  aggravated, 1964
  Case Study, 1969
  collaborative care
    violence prevention programs for children, 1966
  definition, 1963
  description, 1939t
  nursing diagnoses and interventions
    anger management for children, 1968

  care of gunshot wounds, 1969
  facilitating self-responsibility, 1968
  improving socialization, 1968
  setting limits, 1968
nursing process
  assessment, 1967
  diagnosis, 1967
  evaluation, 1969
  planning and implementation, 1967–1969
pathophysiology and etiology, 1963–1964
risk factors
  age, 1964
  culture, 1964
  occupation, 1964
  socioeconomic factors, 1964–1965
  treatment/prevention, 1939t
  weapons and, 1964
Assertive behavior, 1169
Assertive communication, 2180
  benefits of, 2180
  Case Study, 2182
  communication styles, 2179–2180, 2180t
  overview, 2179
  techniques for, 2181
Assertive communicators, 2179–2180, 2179t
Assertive community treatment (ACT), 245
Assertiveness training, 1583t
Assessment:
  about, 1999–2000
  adolescents, 2009, 2017
  Case Study, 2008
  children, 2013–2017, 2064t
    cultural considerations, 2010t
    special considerations, 2009–2012, 2012t
  data collection, 2052, 2054–2059, 2054t, 2056t
  data organization, 2059–2061, 2061t
  data validation, 2064–2065, 2064t
  decision making and, 2045
  defined, 2052
  growth and development, 2012, 2013t
  holistic, 2008–2024, 2010t, 2011f, 2016t,
      2018–2020t, 2023t
  infants, 2013–2014
  interpretation of findings, 2006–2007
  life span stages and, 2012
  middle-aged adults, 2018–2019
  nursing practice, 2007–2008
  in nursing process, 2050t, 2052, 2052f,
      2053–2054t, 2054–2061, 2057–2058t,
      2060–2061t, 2064, 2064t
  older adults, 2020–2023, 2020t
    environment evaluation, 2021
    health and lifestyle considerations, 2022–2023
    health history accuracy, 2021–2022
    home environment, 2020t
    instruments for, 2024t
    Minimum Data Set, 2022
    social history, 2022
  parent–child attachment, 2012, 2014
  physical, 2059
  physical examination, 2000–2005
  preschoolers, 2015
  reassessment, 2101
  toddlers, 2014
  types, 2000, 2000t, 2052
  young adults, 2017–2018
Assessment data:
  validation of, 646

Assessment Interview:
  learning needs, 2257t
Assignment, 2092, 2218
Assimilation, 322, 347
Assist-control mode ventilation, 1239, 1240t
Assisted embryo hatching, 1738
Assisted reproduction:
  other techniques, 1737
  preimplantation genetic diagnosis, 1737–1738
  therapeutic insemination, 1735–1736
  in vitro fertilization, 1736–1737
Assisted suicide, 2314
Association, 2247t
Association of Pediatric Oncology Nurses, 2367
Associative play, 360
Assumptions, 2106
AST. See Aspartate aminotransferase (AST), 85
Astereognosis, 215
Asthenospermia, 1735
Asthma, 1258–1262
  airway diameter, 1254f
  Case Study, 1267
  changes in bronchioles, 1254f
  collaborative care
    diagnostic tests, 1258
    pharmacologic therapy, 1258
      stepwise approach, 1258t, 1259t, 1260t,
        1261t, 1262t
  common causes, 1254t
  complementary therapies, 1262–1263
  developmental considerations, 1258t, 1262t, 1264t
  management, stepwise approach to
    bronchodilators, 1258
  manifestations, 1255, 1255–1256t
  Medication Administration, 1260–1262t
  medications, 1258–1262
    anti-inflammatory agents, 1262
    bronchodilators, 1259–1262
    leukotriene modifiers, 1262
  Nursing Care Plan
    assessment, 1265t
    critical thinking, 1265t
    diagnoses, 1265t
    evaluation, 1265t
    planning and implementation, 1265t
  nursing diagnoses and interventions
    activity intolerance, 1266
    anxiety, 1264
    disease monitoring, 1256
    ineffective airway clearance, 1263–1264
    ineffective breathing pattern, 1264
    pediatric asthma, 1257
    pregnancy, 1258
    preventative measures, 1256–1257
  nursing process
    assessment, 1263
    diagnosis, 1263
    evaluation, 1266
    planning and implementation, 1263
  overview, 1252
  pathogenesis, 1253f
  pathophysiology and etiology, 1252–1254
  pediatric differences, 1253–1254
  pregnancy and, 1258
  risk factors, 1254
  treatment, 1220t
Asymptomatic bacteriuria (ASB), 873

Ataxia, 207t, 386t, 956t
Atelectasis, 822, 841
  acute respiratory distress syndrome (ARDS), 1246
  definition, 1222t
  respiratory syncytial virus (RSV)/bronchiolitis
    and, 1281
Atheists, 1771
Atheromas, 1362
Atherosclerosis:
  definition, 1361, 1462
  etiology, 1364
  peripheral, 1463t, 1464t
  progression of, 1361–1362
Athetosis, 386t
Athletic heart syndrome, 1438
Ativan, 971, 1815
Atomoxetine, 373t
Atorvastatin, 1374
ATP. See Adenosine triphosphate (ATP)
Atria, 1294–1295
Atrial fibrillation, 1391, 1442t, 1445
Atrial flutter, 1442t, 1445
Atrial gallop, 1296
Atrial kick, 1438
Atrial natriuretic factor (ANF), 523
Atrial natriuretic peptide (ANP), 1405, 1411, 1423
Atrial rhythms, 1440
Atrial septal defect (ASD), 1340–1341t
Atrioventricular (AV) canal, 1341–1342t
Atrioventricular (AV) conduction blocks,
    1443–1444t, 1446–1448
Atrioventricular (AV) dissociation, 1447–1448
Atrioventricular (AV) valves, 1295
Atrophy, 1060
  skin, 1879t
Attachment, 2012
  assessment, 2014
Attendance, 2236–2237
Attention deficit hyperactivity disorder (ADHD):
  in adults, 370, 372
  alternative therapies, 373t
  behavior management plans for, 376
  behavior therapy, 373
  case study, 377
  collaborative care, 371
  community-based care, 376
  definition, 370
  DSM-IV diagnostic criteria, 372t
  emotional support for, 376
  environmental distractions, 374
  environmental supports, 372
  incidence, 370
  manifestations, 370–371
  Nursing Care Plan
    assessment, 375t
    critical thinking, 375t
    evaluation, 375t
    implementation, 375t
    planning, 375t
  nursing process
    assessment, 374
    diagnosis, 374
    evaluation, 377
    implementation, 374, 376–377
    plan, 374
  pathophysiology and etiology, 370
  pharmacologic therapy, 372, 373t

  risk factors, 370
  school suggestions for children with, 377t
  screening tests, 371t, 372
  self-esteem promotion, 376
  stigma of, 376t
Attention impairment, 240
Attentive listening, 2165–2166, 2166t
Attitude, 2228, 2238
Atypical antidepressants, 1173
Atypical antipsychotics, 243, 244t
Audiologic testing, 828
Audiologist, 828
Audiometric testing:
  tuberculosis and, 862
Audiometry, 1646
Auditory canal, 1632, 1644t
Auditory hallucinations, 238
Auditory Processing Disorder, 1634
Auditory stimuli, 1628
Audits, 2426
  of health agencies, 2183
Aura, 970
Auranofin, 750t
Auricles, 1632, 1644t
Aurothioglucose, 750t
Auscultation, 1216, 2004–2005
Auscultatory gap, 1322
Authoritarian decision making, 2039
Authoritarian parents, 490, 491t
Authoritative parents, 490–491
Authority, 2126, 2144, 2218
Autism:
  DSM-IV-TR diagnostic criteria, 381t
  Hispanics and, 380t
  incidence, 378
Autism Behavior Checklist, 382t
Autism Diagnostic Interview—Revised, 382t
Autism Diagnostic Observation Schedule—
    Generic (ADOS-G), 382t
Autism spectrum disorders (ASDs):
  adults with, 380t
  alternative therapies, 382, 383t
  case study, 385
  collaborative care, 380
  diagnostic tests, 380
  DSM-IV-TR diagnostic criteria, 381t
  interventions
    care in the community, 384–385
    enhance communication, 384
    maintain safe environment, 384
    provide anticipatory guidance, 384
    provide supportive care, 384
    stabilize environmental stimuli, 384
  manifestations, 378–380, 379t
  nonverbal communication and, 2151t
  nursing process
    assessment, 383
    diagnosis, 383
    evaluation, 385
    implementation, 383–385
    plan, 383
  overview, 378
  pathophysiology and etiology, 378
  risk factors, 378
  screening tests, 382t
  therapies, 379t, 380, 382

Autistic disorder:
  manifestations, 379t
  therapies, 379t
Autoantibodies:
  immune system function and, 693
Autocratic (authoritarian) leaders, 2233–2234, 2234t
  systemic lupus erythematosus (SLE) and, 756
Autografting, 1901–1902
Autografts, 1902f
Autoimmune disorders:
  dendritic cells and, 678
  immune system function and, 676
  overview, 693t
Autoimmune hemolytic anemia, 729
Autologous bone marrow transplant, 155
Autolytic debridement, 1926
Automated documentation, 2376–2377
Automaticity, 1438
Automobile safety, 2440f, 2440t, 2455t, 2457
Autonomic dysreflexia, 1147
Autonomic hyperreflexia, 1147
Autonomic nervous system:
  diabetes mellitus and, 998
Autonomy, 639, 1777, 2248, 2281, 2306,
    2308–2309, 2315t, 2317, 2317t, 2404t
Autosomal chromosomes, 340
Autosomal dominant inheritance, 1723
Autosomal recessive inheritance, 1723–1724
Autosomes, 87, 1720
Avian influenza, 818–819, 819t
  See also Influenza
Avodart, 434, 434t
Avoidance, 2129
Avoidant personality disorder:
  characteristics, 1618
  diagnostic criteria, 1618t
  manifestations, 1611t
Avolition, 241
Avulsion fractures, 1094
Awareness, 1629, 2434
    Axial loading, 1144, 1144f
Axial skeleton, 1056
Axilla temperature, 1855
Axillary node dissection, 110
Axillary temperature, 1856
Ayurveda, 336
Azapirone, 1807t
Azathioprine, 561–562, 761, 761t
    Azopt, 1671t
Azotemia, 534
AZT. See Zidovudine
Azulfidine, 914, 915t
    Azulfidine. See Sulfasalazine

B

B cells. See B lymphocytes (B cells)
B lymphocytes (B cells):
  immune response and, 677t, 678–681, 679f, 680f
  systemic lupus erythematosus (SLE) and, 756
B-cell (humoral) function, 692f
B-DAST (Brief Drug Abuse Screening Test), 46, 78
B-estradiol, 1519
B-subunit radioimmunoassay (RIA), 1570
Babinskis reflex, 958t
Baby boomers, 2238, 2239t
Bacille Calmette-Guérin (BCG) vaccine, 862

Back problems:
  backpack use and pain, 1081t
  Case Study, 1092
  causes, 1065, 1080
  during pregnancy, 1575t, 1576–1577
  evidence-based practice, 1081t
  herniated disk. See Herniated disk
  low back pain. See Low back pain
  overview, 1080
  in pregnancy, 1082–1083t
  scoliosis. See Scoliosis
Back to Sleep campaign, 1289t
Bacteremia:
  definition of, 771
  infectious diseases and, 787
  pneumonia and, 840
  septic shock and, 850
Bacteria, 786t
  antibiotic-resistant, 789–790
  definition of, 771
  nosocomial infections and, 787
Bactericidal agent:
  definition of, 777
Bacteriostatic agent:
  definition of, 777
Bacteriuria:
  persistent, 882
  unresolved, 882
  urinary tract infections and, 872–875
Bacteroides, 770
Balanced suspension traction, 1100
Balanced translocation carrier, 1722
Balanitis, 1704t
Balloon tamponade, 1024
Balloon urethroplasty, 435
Balloon valvuloplasty, 1354t
Ballottement, 1548
Ballottement test, 1074, 1074t
BALs (blood alcohol levels), 43. See Blood
    alcohol levels
Bandura, Albert, 347–348
Barbiturates, 71
  effect on fetus, 58t
  sexual functioning and, 1701t
  street names, 74t
  bargaining stage:
  of grief, 602t
Bariatric surgery, 1029–1030
Baroreceptors, 1424
Barr body, 1722
Barrel chest:
  emphysema and, 1270
Barrier protection, 682
Bartholin's glands, 1687, 1688t, 1708t
Barton, Clara, 2288, 2290, 2290f
Basal body temperature (BBT) method, 1725
Basal cell cancer, 185–186, 186f, 186t, 189t
    See also Skin cancer
Basal metabolic rate (BMR), 1025, 1852
Base excess (BE):
  definition, 5
  normal value, 5
BASE jumpers, 28
Bases, 3
Basic research, 2329
Basopenia, 891t
Basophilia, 891t

Basophils, 677, 677t, 678f
BAT (brown adipose tissue), 1866
Battelle Developmental Inventory, 2013t
Battering, 1949
Battery, 2401
Baumrind, Diana, 490
BE. See Base excess
Beck Depression Inventory, 1165–1166, 1192
Becoming a mother (BAM), 1197
Bed-wetting, 414
Bedsores. See Pressure ulcers
Behavior change:
  promotion of, 648, 649f, 649t
Behavior modification, 1029, 2265–2266
Behavior skills, 34
Behavioral activation, 1175
Behavioral theory:
  eating disorders and, 1598
Behavioral therapy, 34–35
Behaviorism, 347
Behaviorist theory, 2246
Bejerot, Nils, 28
Belief systems, 329–330
Beliefs, defined, 2306
Belmont Report, The (1979), 2333
Belonging, 1591t
Belt restraints, 2448, 2448f
Benadryl. See Diphenhydramine
Benchmarking, 2425
Beneficence, 1777, 2308, 2315t, 2334
Benign, 117
Benign neoplasms, 117, 117t
Benign prostatic hyperplasia, 433f
Benign prostatic hypertrophy (BPH), 445
  alternative therapies, 435
  Case Study, 440–441
  collaborative care, 434
  definition, 432
  diagnostic tests, 434
  manifestations, 433, 433t
  Nursing Care Plan
    assessment, 438t
    critical thinking in the nursing process, 438t
    diagnosis, 438t
    evaluation, 438t
    overview, 438t
    planning and implementation, 438t
  nursing process
    assessment, 436
    diagnosis, 436
    evaluation, 440
    planning and implementation, 436–440, 439t
  pathophysiology and etiology, 432–433
  pharmacologic therapies, 434, 434t
  risk factors, 433
  surgery for, 435
  treatment, 433t
Benzodiazepines, 44, 71, 1807t, 1808,
    1814–1815, 1838
  street names, 74t
Benztropine (Cogentin), 243
Bereavement, 601
  literature, 630f
  in older adults, 623–624
  phases of, 603t
Berwick, Donald, 2428
Beta cells, 980, 989
Beta-adrenergic blockers, 1430–1431t, 1670, 1671t

Beta-androgenic blockers, for glaucoma, 1650*t*
Beta-blockers:
  sexual functioning and, 1701*t*
  in specific conditions
    angina pectoris, 1375
    cardiomyopathy, 1335–1336
    dysrhythmias, 1450
    heart failure, 1413
    hypertension, 1429, 1432
    myocardial infarction, 1376
Betaxolol (Betoptic), 1671*t*
Bethanechol Chloride, 423*t*
Bextra, 275
Bias, 398
Bible, 1782
Bibliographic database managers (BDMs), 2387*t*
Bibliographic databases, 2335
Bicarbonate (HCO$_3^-$):
  function, 525*t*
  in metabolic acidosis, 6*t*
  in metabolic alkalosis, 6*t*
  regulation, 525*t*, 526
  serum levels
    in metabolic acidosis, 5, 7*t*
    in metabolic alkalosis, 5, 7*t*
Bicarbonate–carbonic acid buffer system, 4
Bicycle helmets, 2441*t*
Bicuspid valve, 1295
BiDil, 1415
Biekerdyke, Mother, 2288
Bile acid sequestrants, 1374*t*
Bilevel ventilators (BiPAP), 1241
Biliary cirrhosis:
  definition, 1016
Biliary colic, 902
Biliary stasis, 903
Bilirubin, 129*t*
Bilirubin levels, 904*t*
Bilking agents, 455
Bill of Rights (U.S. Advisory Commission on
    Consumer Protection and Quality in the
    Health Care Industry), 2319*t*
Bill of Rights for Registered Nurses, 2310
Billing, 2388
Billings method, 1725
Bimatoprost (Lumigan), 1671*t*
Binge drinking, 40
Binge eating, 1600
Binge-eating disorder, 1585
  clinical therapies, 1601*t*
  diagnostic criteria, 1601*t*
  manifestations, 1601, 1601*t*
Binuclear family, 487
Biobrane, 1903
Bioethics, 2313
  abortion, 2313, 2313*t*, 2314*t*
  AIDS, 2313
  definition, 1776
  end-of-life issues, 2313–2315, 2313*t*
  organ transplantation, 2313
Biofeedback therapy:
  for fecal incontinence, 459
Biolectrical impedance, 1028
Biological dressing, 1903–1904
Biological rhythms, 666
  definition, 1162
  mood disorders and, 1162, 1164*t*
Biological variations, 327–328

Biopsy:
  kidney, 926
  in lung cancer, 164
Biopsy urease test, 933
Biopsychosocial model:
  of addiction, 28
Biosynthetic dressing, 1903–1904
Biot's respirations, 1221
Bioterrorism, 2357, 2357*t*, 2358*t*
Biotin, 1597*t*
BiPAP ventilator, 314
Bipolar disorders:
  alternative therapies, 1182
  bipolar I disorder, 1160
  bipolar II disorder, 1160
  Case Study, 1186
  classification, 1160
  collaborative care, 1181
  comorbidity with, 1158
  cyclothymic disorder, 1177, 1178*t*
  definition, 1160, 1160*t*, 1177
  diagnostic criteria, 1177, 1178*t*
  genetic links, 1161
  hypomanic episodes, 1178*t*
  manifestations
    in children and adolescents, 1180
    cyclothymic disorder, 1180
    depressed episodes, 1179, 1180*t*, 1197*t*, 1199*t*
    mania and hypomania, 1178*t*, 1179, 1179*f*, 1180*t*
    mixed episodes, 1180
    mixed episodes, 1178*t*
  Nursing Care Plan
    assessment, 1184*t*
    critical thinking, 1184*t*
    diagnosis, 1184*t*
    evaluation, 1184*t*
    planning and implementation, 1184*t*
  nursing diagnoses and interventions
    enhancing rest and sleep, 1185
    enhancing socialization, 1184
    promoting client safety, 1183
    promoting improved self-care, 1185
    promoting reality-based thinking, 1183–1184
    setting limits, 1185
  nursing process
    assessment, 1182
    diagnosis, 1182
    evaluation, 1185
    planning and implementation, 1183–1185, 1183*t*
  pharmacologic therapies, 1173, 1173*t*, 1174*t*, 1181–1182
  potential nurse reactions to clients with, 1183*t*
  rapid cycling, 1160
  relapse rates, 1158
  suicide risk and, 1158
  treatments, 1160*t*
Birth centers, 1198
Birth control pills. *See* Oral contraceptives
Bisexuals, 400, 1696
Bismuth compounds, 934
Bisphosphonates:
  mechanism of action, 988*t*
  nursing considerations, 988*t*
  osteoporosis and, 1037
Bivalving, 1107*f*
Black cohosh, 1744*t*
Blackouts, 43

Bladder:
  age-related changes in, 416
  assessment, 419*t*
  distention, 433
  female, 412*f*
  function of, 411
  male, 412*f*
  neurogenic, 417
  overdistention of, 445
Bladder distention:
  after prostatectomy, 439
Bladder neck suspension, 443*t*
Bladder stones, 468*t*
Bladder training, 445, 450
Blame-free environments, 2429–2430
Blast injuries, 2352*t*
Blastocyst, 1527
Blastomere analysis, 1737
Blastomere biopdy, 1737
Blastomeres, 1527
Bleeding time, 129*t*
Blended family, 487
Blepharism, 1665
Blinding, 2328*t*
Blindness, 1658*t*. *See also* Glaucoma
  macular degeneration, 1676
  prevalence of, 1635
Block to polyspermy, 1525
Blood:
  desaturated, 1309
  infusion, 1495
  Blood alcohol levels (BALs), 43–44, 44*t*, 1942
  Blood coagulation studies, 1884
  Blood colloid pressure, 580
Blood cultures, 709, 852
Blood flow, 1422
Blood glucose homeostasis, 989–990, 990*f*
Blood glucose monitoring, diabetes mellitus
    and, 1001
Blood hemoglobin, 1490
Blood hydrostatic pressure, 580
Blood loss anemia, 97
Blood pressure. *See also* Hypertension
  arterial, 1308
  assessment, 1320–1324
  classification, 1422*t*
  definition, 1422
  determinants of, 1308
  developmental considerations, 1323*t*
  diastolic, 1422
  diastolic pressure, 1308
  factors affecting, 1309, 1423–1424, 1423*f*
  hypotension, 1323–1324
  measurement, 1308
  pulse pressure, 1308
  sites, 1322
  systolic, 1308, 1422
Blood pressure cuff, 1320–1321, 1320*f*
Blood products, 1495
Blood transfusions:
  in specific conditions
    anemia, 102
    sickle cell disorder, 179–180
Blood type, 926, 1941–1942
Blood urea nitrogen (BUN), 416
  abnormal, possible causes, 129*t*
  renal function and, 553*f*

in specific conditions
  acute renal failure, 540
  sepsis and, 852
in specific conditions
  burns, 1900
  chronic renal failure, 558
  fluid volume deficit, 575
  heart failure, 1411
  shock, 1490
  systemic lupus erythematosus (SLE) and, 760
Blood viscosity, 1308
Blood volume, 1308
  in children, 1489t
Bloodborne pathogens, definition of, 778
Blu-ray, 2375
Blue Cross and Blue Shield Association, 2335
Blunt trauma, 1938, 2352t
Blunted affect, 238
BMI (body mass index), 1026–1028
BMR (basal metabolic rate), 1025, 1852
BMT. See Bone marrow transplant (BMT)
BNP. See Brain natriuretic peptide (BNP)
Boards of nursing (BONs), 2406–2407
Body, of interview, 2058–2059
Body fluids. See also Fluids and electrolytes
  acidity, 3
  composition, 519f
  composition of, 518–519
  distribution, 518–519
  extracellular, 518
  factors affecting balance of, 526–528
  intracellular, 518
  movement
    active transport, 521, 522f
    diffusion, 520–521, 521f
    filtration, 521, 521f
    osmosis, 519–520, 520f
  regulation
    antidiuretic hormone, 523, 524f
    atrial natriuretic factor, 523
    fluid intake, 521–522
    fluid output, 522–523
    kidneys, 523
    maintaining homeostasis, 523
    renin-angiotensin-aldosterone system, 523
    thirst mechanism, 522
Body heat:
  pressure ulcers and, 1916
Body image, 1582, 1582f, 1589, 1695
  hyperthyroidism and, 1047
Body image stressors, 1589t
Body language, 2151–2152, 2151f
Body of knowledge, 2280
Body mass index (BMI), 1026–1028
Body parts, mechanical devices for reducing
    pressure on, 1924t
Body preoccupation, 346
Body substance isolation (BSI):
  definition of, 778–779
Body surface area (BSA), 526, 1304–1305
Body systems model, 2060
Body temperature:
  alterations, 1854
  definition, 1851
  developmental considerations, 1858t
  factors affecting, 1853–1854
  hyperthermia. See Hyperthermia
  hypothermia. See Hypothermia

measurement of, 1854–1855, 1857
  normal range of, 1852
  range of, 1853
  regulation of, 1853
  types of, 1852
Body transcendence, 346
Bone density, weight-bearing exercise and, 652
Bone density examinations, 1076
Bone marrow, human immunodeficiency virus
    (HIV) and, 708t
Bone marrow examination, 153
Bone marrow transplant (BMT), 154–155
Bone mass, osteoporosis and, 1034–1035
Bone(s):
  age-related changes, 1063, 1063t
  compact, 1056, 1057f
  fractures. See Fractures
  functions, 1056
  ossification, 1058
  pediatric differences in, 1062
  remodeling in adults, 1058
  shapes, 1057
    classification according to, 1057f
    flat, 1058
    long, 1057, 1058f
    short, 1058
  of skeleton, 1056, 1056f
  spongy, 1056
  structure, 1056
Bony pelvis, 1516–1518, 1516f, 1519f, 1520f
Book of Common Prayer, 1783
Borborygmus, 428t
Borderline personality disorder:
  characteristics, 1614
    affective instability, 1615
    distortions of reality, 1616
    feelings of emptiness and aloneness, 1615
    identity diffusion, 1615
    impulsivity, 1614
    intense anger, 1615
    self-damaging acts, 1616
    unstable interpersonal relationships, 1615
  diagnostic criteria, 1614t
  family factors and, 1609
  manifestations, 1611t
  neurobiology and, 1608
  Nursing Care Plan
    assessment, 1623t
    critical thinking in the nursing process, 1623t
    diagnosis, 1623t
    evaluation, 1623t
    planning and implementation, 1623t
Bottom-up sampling, 1162f
Botulism, 2357t
Boundaries, family, 494–495
Boutonniére deformities, 744, 744t
Bowel cancer, treatment, 427t
Bowel elimination:
  in adolescents, 424
  alterations
    bowel cancer, 427t
    constipation, 427t
    diarrhea, 426, 427t
    flatulence, 427
    impaction, 427t
    obstruction, 427t
    assessment, 427, 428–429t, 430

Assessment Interview, 430t
Client Teaching, 462t
collaborative care, 460
diagnostic tests, 430
disorders
  constipation, 454–457, 457t
  encopresis, 457
  fecal impaction, 458
  fecal incontinence, 458, 460–462, 464
  overview, 454
factors affecting
  activity, 425
  anesthesia and surgical procedures, 426
  defecation habits, 426
  developmental factors, 424–425
  diagnostic procedures, 426
  diet, 425
  fluid intake, 425
  medications, 426
  pain, 426
  pathologic conditions, 426
  psychologic factors, 426
incontinence. See Fecal incontinence
in infants and newborns, 424, 425f
NANDA, NIC, and NOC linkages, 461t
normal presentation, 423–424
Nursing Care Plan
  assessment, 463t
  critical thinking in the nursing process, 463t
  diagnosis, 463t
  evaluation, 463t
  planning and implementation, 463t
nursing diagnoses and interventions, 461t
  bowel training programs, 464
  digital removal of fecal impaction, 462
  fecal incontinence pouch, 464
  promoting regular defecation, 461–462
nursing history, 430
nursing interventions, 430
nursing process
  assessment, 460
  diagnosis, 460
  evaluation, 464
  planning and implementation, 461–462, 464
in older adults, 424–425
overview, 423
pharmacologic therapies, 430, 431t
physical examination, 430
in pregnancy, 424
in school-age children, 424
in toddlers, 424
Bowel obstruction, in Crohn's disease, 916
Bowel strictures, 916
Bowel training programs, 464
Bowman's capsule, 410
BPH. See Benign prostatic hypertrophy
Brachial pulse, 1319, 1319f
Brachytherapy, 165
Braden Scale for Predicting Pressure Sore
    Risk, 1920f
Bradycardia:
  in children, 1309
  definition, 1319
Bradydysrhythmia, 1369
Bradykinesia, 1066, 1134–1135, 1136t
Bradykinin, 265, 887t
Bradyphrenia, 1136

Bradypnea, 1221
Brain:
  anatomy, physiology, and functions
    brainstem, 941
    cerebellum, 941
    cerebrum, 940
    diencephalon, 940
    meninges, 940
Brain death, 948–949
Brain function, deterioration of, 945t
Brain injury, 201
Brain natriuretic peptide (BNP), 1405, 1411, 1423
Brain oxygenation, monitoring of, 964
Brain tumors, increased intracranial pressure
    from, 962
Brainstem, 941
Brainstorming, 2040, 2136, 2138t
Bravelle, 1735t
Braxton Hicks contractions, 1533, 1542, 1547
Breach of care, 2424, 2424t
Breach of duty, 2400, 2424, 2424t
Breakthrough pain, 264
Breast cancer:
  Case Study, 115
  causes, 107
  Client Teaching, 115t
  collaborative care
    diagnostic tests, 109
    pharmacologic therapies, 110
    radiation therapy, 111–112
    surgery, 110–111
  definition, 106
  evidence-based practice, 111t
  mammography to detect, 109
  manifestations, 108–109, 108t, 109t
  Nursing Care Plan
    assessment, 114t
    critical thinking, 114t
    diagnoses, 114t
    evaluation, 114t
    planning and implementation, 114t
  nursing diagnoses and interventions
    anxiety, 112
    decisional conflict, 112
    disturbed body image, 115
    grief, 113
    risk for infection, 113
    risk for injury, 113, 115
  nursing process
    assessment, 112
    diagnosis, 112
    evaluation, 115
    planning and implementation, 112–115
  in older women, 107t
  pathophysiology and etiology, 106–107
  risk factors, 108
  screening guidelines, 132t
  staging, 107, 107t
  treatments
    chemotherapy, 110
    surgery, 110–111
  types
    adenocarcinomas, 107
    inflammatory, 107
    Paget's disease, 107
Breast reconstruction, 110–111, 111f
Breast self-examination, 109t
Breast tenderness, 1546t, 1574t

Breastfeeding, psychotropic medication use
    during, 1174, 1201
Breasts:
  assessment, 1705–1706t
  female, 1691
  male, 1687
  pregnancy and, 1542, 1546
Breath sounds:
  adventitious
    crackles, 1222t
    rhonchi, 1222t
    stridor, 1222t
    wheezing, 1222t
  normal presentation
    bronchovesicular, 1216
    tubular, 1216
    vesicular, 1217
Breckinridge, Mary, 2291
Brevity, of speech, 2150, 2150t
Brewster, Mary, 2290
Brief Drug Abuse Screening Test (B-DAST), 46
Brief psychotic disorder, 235
Brigance Screens, 2013t
Bright Futures, 2440
Brimonidine, 1670, 1671t
Brinzolamide (Azopt), 1671t
British Sign Language (BSL), 1655t
Bromocriptine, 1735t
Bronchi, 1216
Bronchiectasis, 837
Bronchiolitis, 1281. See also Respiratory syncytial
    virus/bronchiolitis
Bronchodilator drugs, 20
Bronchodilators, 20, 841, 1259–1262, 1273
Bronchogenic carcinomas, 161, 163
Bronchoplastic reconstruction, 165t
Bronchopleural fistula, tuberculosis and, 860
Bronchopneumonia, 834–836, 835t, 837t
Bronchoscopy:
  in lung cancer, 164
  purpose and description, 1229
brown adipose tissue (BAT), 1866
Brown-Séquard's syndrome, 1145t
Brudzinski's sign, 957t
Bruises, 1882t
Bruits, 428t
Brushing teeth, 660
Bruxism, 311t
Bryant traction, 1106t
BSL (British Sign Language), 1655t
Buccal cavity, 655
Buck traction, 1099–1100, 1106t
Buddhism, 1776t, 1784, 1784t
Budgets, 2388
Buffer base capacity, 5
Buffers, 4
Bulge sign, 1074
Bulge test, 1074t
Bulimia nervosa. See also Eating disorders
  vs. anorexia, 1585
  clinical therapies, 1601t
  definition, 1584
  diagnostic criteria, 1600t
  diagnostic tests, 1602
  incidence, 1599
  manifestations, 1600, 1601t
  neurobiology and, 1598

  nonpurging type, 1600t
  Nursing Care Plan
    assessment, 1605t
    critical thinking in the nursing process, 1605t
    diagnosis, 1605t
    evaluation, 1605t
    planning and implementation, 1605t
  purging type, 1600t
Bullae, 1878t
Bumetanide, 541t
Bumex. See Bumetanide, 517
BUN. See Blood urea nitrogen (BUN)
Bunions, 1070
Bupropion, 1173, 1190
Bureaucratic caring, theory of, 2028–2029, 2030f
Bureaucratic leaders, 2234
Burn centers, 1897t
Burn prevention, 2450t
Burnout, 2232
Burn shock, 1894–1895
Burns:
  Case Study, 1911
  causative agents, 1887t
  in children, 1887, 1888t, 1905f, 1905t, 1908t
  chemical, 2353t
  classification
    American Burn Association, 1892t
    depth, 1888–1889, 1888f
    extent, 1890
    full-thickness, 1889, 1889f, 1894t
    partial-thickness, 1889, 1889f, 1894t
    rule of nines, 1890
    superficial, 1888, 1894t
  Client Teaching, 1909t
  collaborative care
    burn team, 1896
  definition, 1886
  diagnostic tests, 1900
  eye, 1662, 1663t, 1664
  fluid loss from, 570
  incidence, 1887
  major, 1892, 1897–1898
  manifestations, 1892, 1894t
  minor, 1892, 1896–1897
  Nursing Care Plan
    assessment, 1910t
    critical thinking in nursing process, 1910t
    diagnoses, 1910t
    evaluation, 1910t
    planning and implementation, 1910t
  nursing diagnoses and interventions
    acute pain, 1907
    deficient fluid volume, 1906, 1907t
    imbalanced nutrition, less than body
      requirements, 1908
    impaired physical mobility, 1907–1908
    impaired skin integrity, 1905–1906
    powerlessness, 1908
    risk for infection, 1907
  nursing process
    assessment, 1904–1905
    diagnosis, 1905
    evaluation, 1908
    implementation, 1905–1908, 1907t, 1909t
    interventions by stage, 1909t
    plan, 1905
  in older adults, 1906t
  pathophysiology and etiology, 1886–1887

recovery from, 1908*t*
risk factors, 1887–1888
rule of nines, 1890*f*
systemic effects
cardiac rhythm alterations, 1895
cardiovascular system, 1894–1895
gastrointestinal system, 1895
hypovolemic shock, 1894–1895
immune system, 1896
integumentary system, 1892–1893
metabolism, 1896
overview, 1892
peripheral vascular compromise, 1895
respiratory system, 1895
urinary system, 1896
treatment, 1894*t*, 1896
acute stage, 1898
biologic and biosynthetic dressings,
1903–1904
debridement, 1897
dressing the wound, 1902–1903
emergency and acute, 1899–1900
emergent/resuscitative stage, 1897
fluid resuscitation, 1899
infection control, 1900–1901
infection prevention, 1898
litargirio, 1896*t*
major burns, 1897–1898
medications, 1900–1901
minor burns, 1896–1897
nutrition therapy, 1898
nutritional support, 1904
pain control, 1900
pain management, 1898
prehospital client management, 1898–1899
pressure garments, 1903*f*
rehabilitative stage, 1898
respiratory management, 1899–1900
stop burning process, 1898
support vital function, 1898–1899
surgery, 1901–1902
wound care, 1898
wound dressing, 1902*f*
wound management, 1902
types of injury
chemical, 1886, 1887*t*, 1898
electrical, 1886–1887, 1887*f*, 1898
radiation, 1887, 1898
thermal, 1886, 1886*f*, 1898
wound healing, 1890
inflammation, 1890
proliferation, 1890
remodeling, 1892
Bursae, 1061
Bursitis, 1068*f*
BuSpar, 210, 217, 1815
Buspirone, 210, 217, 1815
Butyl nitrite, 74
Bypass grafts, 1378–1379

C

C-reactive protein, 129*t*, 890, 1353*t*, 1370
Ca²⁺. *See* Calcium
Cabergoline, 1735*t*
Cachexia, 108*t*, 123
Cadet Nurse Corps, 2288

Caffeine, 71
sleep and, 669
use in pregnancy, 59
CAGE questionnaire, 46
Calcitonin, 129*t*, 137*t*, 979
Calcium (Ca²⁺):
abnormal, possible causes, 129*t*
excess, and dementia, 210
function, 525*t*
imbalances. *See* Hypercalcemia; Hypocalcemia
in body fluid compartments, 520*t*
in musculoskeletal system assessment, 1077*t*
osteoporosis and, 1035
recommended daily intake, 1597*t*
regulation, 525, 525*t*
Calcium carbonate, 558
Calcium chloride, 542*t*
Calcium gluconate, 542*t*
Calcium oxalate, 466
Calcium phosphate, 466
Calcium stones, 466, 467*t*
Calcium-channel blockers:
administration, 1431*t*, 1450*t*
for angina, 1375
mechanism of action, 1331*t*
nursing considerations, 1331*t*
in specific conditions
dysrhythmias, 1450
hypertension, 1431*t*, 1432
Calculi, 420
development and location of, 466*f*
urinary tract infections and, 876
Caldwell-Moloy pelvic types, 1518, 1520*f*
CAM (Confusion Assessment Method), 207*t*,
227, 228*t*
Campylobacter jejuni, 1679
Canadian Center for Evidence-Based Practice, 2335
Canasa, 916
Cancellous bone:
osteoporosis and, 1034
Cancer:
acquired immunodeficiency syndrome (AIDS)
and, 705
assessment
developmental, of children, 91–92
physical, 91
Assessment Interview, 131
Case Study, 141
childhood
Client Teaching, 134*t*
hair loss and, 135*t*
oncologic emergencies, 88–90
psychosocial needs, 90
special considerations, 93–94
survival, 90–91
Client Teaching, 134*t*
definition, 116
diagnostic tests, 92, 125–130
cytologic examination, 125–126
direct visualization, 128
laboratory tests, 128–129, 129–130*t*
oncologic imaging, 127–128
tumor markers, 126–127
etiology, 119–120
grading and staging, 125–126
incidence, 116*t*

manifestations
anorexia-cachexia syndrome, 123, 124*t*
disruption of function, 122
hematologic alterations, 122
hemorrhage, 122
infection, 122, 124*t*
pain, 123–124, 124*t*
paraneoplastic syndrome, 123, 124*t*
physical stress, 124
psychologic stress, 125
Nursing Care Plan
assessment, 139*t*
critical thinking, 140*t*
diagnoses, 139*t*
evaluation, 140*t*
overview, 139*t*
planning and implementation, 139–140*t*
nursing diagnoses and interventions
activity intolerance, 92
anticipatory grieving, 135–136
anxiety, 133–134
disturbed body image, 134–135
imbalanced nutrition, less than body
requirements, 136–138
impaired tissue integrity, 138
manage treatment side effects, 93
nutrition and hydration, 92
pain management, 92
provide psychosocial support, 93–94
risk for infection, 136
risk for injury, 136
nursing process
assessment, 131–132
diagnosis, 132
evaluation, 138
planning and implementation, 132–138
oncologic emergencies
hematologic emergencies, 89–90
metabolic emergencies, 89
space-occupying lesions, 90
ontologic imaging, 127–128
overview, 116
pathophysiology, 117–119
risk factors
age, 120
alcohol use, 121–122
diet, 121
gender, 120
heredity, 120
infection, 121
obesity, 122
occupation, 121
poverty, 121
recreational drug use, 122
stress, 121
sun exposure, 122
tobacco use, 121
screening guidelines, 132*t*
secondary, 90
staging, 107
stress and, 94*t*
theories of carcinogenesis
cellular mutation, 119
oncogenes, 119
tumor suppressor genes, 119
treatment
pharmacologic therapies, 94, 95*t*, 130–131

radiation therapy, 131
side effects, 93
surgery, 130
types
breast. *See* Breast cancer
cervical. *See* Cervical cancer
colorectal. *See* Colorectal cancer
leukemia. *See* Leukemia
lung. *See* Lung cancer
prostate. *See* Prostate cancer
skin. *See* Skin cancer
of urinary system, 418*t*
when to call for help, 137*t*
Cancer pain, 257, 264
causes, 124
types, 123–124
Candida albicans, 770
Candidiasis, acquired immunodeficiency
syndrome (AIDS) and, 704, 706*t*, 714*t*
Canes, 1078–1079
Cannabis sativa, 71
Capacitation, 1525
Capsaicin, 1262
Car safety, for school-age children, 2438*t*
Carbamazepine, 217, 1174, 1174*t*
Carbohydrates, 1593, 1593*t*
Carbon dioxide, 4
Carbon dioxide narcosis, 18
Carbon monoxide (CO), 2451
Carbon monoxide detectors, 2451
Carbon monoxide poisoning, 1895, 2451
Carbonic acid, 4–5
Carbonic anhydrase inhibitors, 1650*t*, 1670, 1671*t*
Carcinoembryonic antigen (CEA), 129*t*
Carcinogenesis, 119
Carcinogens, 119–120
Cardiac arrest:
in children, 1309
definition, 1454
Cardiac auscultation, 1317*t*
Cardiac catheterization:
in congenital heart defects, 1352*t*
procedure, 1354*t*
Cardiac complications:
hyperthyroidism and, 1045
Cardiac conduction system, 1438
Cardiac cycle, 1302–1305, 1303*f*
Cardiac dysrhythmias. *See* Dysrhythmias
Cardiac functioning, pediatric differences, 1309
Cardiac glycosides, 1331*t*
Cardiac index, 1304–1305
Cardiac mapping, 1454
Cardiac markers, 1371, 1371*t*
Cardiac monitoring:
continuous, 1448
for dysrhythmias, 1448
home, 1448
indications for, 1448*t*
Cardiac muscle, 1060
Cardiac output (CO):
aging and, 1312
clinical indicators of, 1304–1305
definition, 1303, 1405, 1484
determinants of, 1303
heart rate and, 1405
ranges of, 1304

Cardiac rate, 1316*t*
Cardiac rehabilitation, 1382–1383, 1388*t*
Cardiac reserve, 1304, 1406
Cardiac rhythm alterations, in burns, 1895
Cardiac tamponade, 1380
Cardiac transplantation, 1336, 1416–1417
Cardiogenic shock, 1369, 1488–1489, 1491*t*
Cardiomyopathy:
Case Study, 1338
classification
dilated, 1333, 1333*t*
hypertrophic, 1333, 1333*t*
peripartum, 1334
restrictive, 1333–1334, 1333*t*
Client Teaching, 1337*t*
collaborative care
diagnostic tests, 1335
overview, 1334
pharmacologic therapies, 1335–1336
surgery, 1336
definition, 1332
description, 1314*t*
etiology, 1334
heart failure and, 1407
manifestations, 1334, 1335*t*
nursing diagnoses and interventions
activity intolerance, 1337–1338
decreased cardiac output, 1336–1337
deficient knowledge, low-sodium diet, 1338
excess fluid volume, 1337
nursing process
assessment, 1336
diagnosis, 1336
evaluation, 1338
planning and implementation, 1336–1338
physiology, 1332–1334
risk actors, 1334
treatment, 1314*t*
Cardiomyoplasty, 1417
Cardiopulmonary bypass (CPB) pump, 1378
Cardiopulmonary resuscitation (CPR), 297,
1455, 1456*t*
Cardiotonics, sexual functioning and, 1701*t*
Cardiovascular assessment, anatomic landmarks
for, 1307, 1307*f*
Cardiovascular disease:
acute myocardial infarction. *See* Acute
myocardial infarction (AMI)
age-related, 1313, 1313*t*
cardiomyopathy. *See* Cardiomyopathy
caring interventions, 1326
chronic renal failure and, 556
congenital. *See* Congenital heart defects
coronary artery disease. *See* Coronary
artery disease
diagnostic tests, 1326
dialysis and, 560
dysrhythmia. *See* Dysrhythmia
heart failure. *See* Heart failure
pediatric, 1313
smoking and, 52
stroke and, 1501
sudden cardiac death. *See* Sudden cardiac
death (SCD)
valve disease. *See* Valve disease
Cardiovascular system. *See also* Heart
assessment, 1315, 1316–1318*t*

Assessment Interview, 1324
benefits of exercise for, 653, 653*t*
developmental aspects
changes during pregnancy, 1309–1310
normal changes of aging, 1310–1312, 1311*f*
pediatric differences, 1309
diabetes mellitus and, 997–998
effects of shock on, 1485
fetal development, 1536*t*
genetic considerations, 1326
health assessment interview, 1324–1325
pregnancy and, 1542–1543
Cardura, 434, 434*t*
Care coordination:
application of, 2209
barriers to effective, 2208
Case Study, 2209
overview, 2208
skills needed for, 2208, 2209*t*
Care management model, 2121
Care maps, 2123. *See also* Critical pathways
Care plan conferences, 2201
Care plan meetings, 2040*t*
Care plans, 2078, 2187
Caregiver, nurse as, 2294*t*
Caregiver role strain, in Alzheimer's disease, 211,
222, 224
Caring, 2158
aspects of, 2028
compassion and, 2033
defined, 2028
nursing theories on, 2028–2031
bureaucratic caring, 2028–2029, 2030*f*
caring as human mode of being, 2029
culture care diversity and universality, 2028
nursing as caring, 2030
primacy of caring, 2031
theory of human care, 2030
professionalization of, 2028
six Cs of, 2029*t*
Caring encounters, 2032–2033, 2034*t*
Caring for self, 2034–2035
Caring interventions, about, 2027–2028
Caring practice, 2028, 2031, 2034–2035
Caring presence, 2032–2033
Caring theories, 1777
Carotid angioplasty, 1507
Carotid endarterectomy, 1507, 1507*f*
Carotid pulse, 1319*f*
Carpal spasm, 986*t*
Carpal tunnel syndrome, 1069*f*, 1575*t*, 2383
Carphologia, 207*t*
Carrier, 1723
definition, 772
Carteolol (Cartrol, Ocupress), 1671*t*
Cartilage, 1065
Cartilaginous joints, 1061
Case management, 2191–2192, 2192*f*, 2343–2344
Case Study, 2125
computerized, 2392
critical pathways, 2123, 2123–2124*t*, 2125*t*
defined, 2206
implementation of, 2122
overview, 2121–2122
Case managers, 2116*t*, 2121–2122, 2121*t*, 2122*f*,
2294*t*, 2343
Case method, 2206

Case Studies:
abuse, 1962
accountability, 2284
acute renal failure, 551
acute respiratory distress syndrome (ARDS), 1252
ADHD, 377
advocacy, 2303
alcohol abuse, 51
Alzheimer's disease, 225
anemia, 106
anticipatory guidance, 2441
anxiety disorders, 1818–1819
appendicitis, 901
assault, 1969
assertive communication, 2182
assessment, 2008
asthma, 1267
autism spectrum disorders, 385
back problems, 1092
benign prostatic hypertrophy, 440–441
bipolar disorders, 1186
breast cancer, 115
burns, 1911
cancer, 141
cardiomyopathy, 1338
care coordination, 2209
caring interventions, 2036
case management, 2125
cataracts, 1661
cellulitis, 812
cerebral palsy, 391
chain of command, 2127
chronic obstructive pulmonary disease
    (COPD), 1280
chronic renal failure, 568
client education, 2268
clinical decision making, 2046
clinical decision support systems, 2389
collaboration, 2121
colorectal cancer, 148
communication, 2164
competence, 2286
conflict resolution, 2133
confusion, 231
congenital heart defects, 1360
conjunctivitis, 816
coronary artery disease, 1389
cost-effective care, 2216
crisis, 1827
critical thinking, 2111
culture, 337
death and dying, 621
deep venous thrombosis, 1397
delegation, 2224
depression, 1195
diabetes mellitus, 1015
disseminated intravascular coagulation, 1403
diversity, 406
documentation, 2200
dysrhythmias, 1461
eating disorders, 1606
emergency preparedness, 2359
end-of-life care, 301
environmental safety, 2449
erectile dysfunction, 1716
ethics, 2320
evidence-based practice, 2336
eye injuries, 1667

failure to thrive, 394
family planning, 1741
family response to health alterations, 514
fatigue, 305
fibromyalgia, 308
fluid and electrolyte imbalances, 596
fractures, 1110
gallstones, 908–909
glaucoma, 1675
grief and loss, 625
health care access, 2348
health care systems, 2344–2345
hearing impairment, 1656t
heart failure, 1421t
heath policy, 2370
hip fractures, 1117
HIV/AIDS, 725t
hypersensitivity, 741
hypertension, 1437
increased intracranial pressure, 967
inflammatory bowel disease, 923
influenza, 824
informatics, 2385
injury prevention, 2459
leadership, 2236
legal issues, 2419
leukemia, 160
liver disease, 1024
lung cancer, 168–169
macular degeneration, 1678
managing care, 2208
menopause, 1746
menstrual dysfunction, 1754
mentoring, 2271
metabolic acidosis, 14
metabolic alkalosis, 17
morality, 1781
motor vehicle crashes, 1993
multiple sclerosis, 1124
nephritis, 930
nursing process, 2103–2104
obsessive-compulsive disorder, 1835
osteoarthritis, 1133
osteoporosis, 1040
otitis media, 832
pain, 287
Parkinson's disease, 1142
peptic ulcer disease, 937
perinatal loss, 633
peripheral neuropathy, 1683
peripheral vascular disease, 1468
personality disorders, 1624
phobias, 1842
pneumonia, 849
postpartum depression, 1207
post-traumatic stress disorder, 1848
pregnancy-induced hypertension, 1475
prenatal substance exposure, 65–66
pressure ulcers, 1926t
professional behaviors, 2229–2230
professional commitment, 2232
prostate cancer, 175
pulmonary embolism, 1483
quality improvement, 2430
rape, 1977
religion, 1788
reporting, 2202
resource allocation, 2351

respiratory acidosis, 22
respiratory alkalosis, 25
respiratory syncytial virus (RSV)/
    Bronchiolitis, 1286
rheumatoid arthritis, 756
safety, 2439
schizophrenia, 252
seizure disorders, 975
sepsis, 855
sexually transmitted infections, 1766
shock, 1498–1499
sickle cell disorder, 183
situational depression, 1211
skin cancer, 194
sleep disorders, 318
smoking, 57
spinal cord injury, 1155
spiritual distress, 1791
staff education, 2275
stroke, 1513
substance abuse, 82
sudden infant death syndrome (SIDS), 1290
suicide, 1986
systemic lupus erythematosus (SLE), 765
teaching and learning, 2253
therapeutic communication, 2178
tuberculosis, 870
urinary calculi, 480
urinary tract infection, 882
work ethic, 2241
wound healing, 1933
Case Western Reserve University Sarah Cole
    Hirsch Institute, 2335
Caseation necrosis, 856
Casein-free diets, 382
Cassells and Redman model of ethical decision
    making, 2311t
Casts, 1100, 1101t, 1102f, 1107
CAT scans, 2392
Cat-cry syndrome, 1721t, 1722
Catabolism, 550, 1597
Cataracts, 1637t, 1638, 1642t, 1658f
    Case Study, 1661
    in children, 1657t
    collaborative care
        alternative therapies, 1659
        surgery, 1658–1659, 1660t
    definition, 1657
    manifestations, 1658
    Nursing Care Plan
        assessment, 1674t
        diagnosis, 1674t
        evaluation, 1674t
        overview, 1674t
        planning and implementation, 1674t
    nursing diagnoses and interventions
        community-based care, 1660
        decisional conflict, cataract removal, 1660
        risk for ineffective therapeutic regimen, 1660
    nursing process
        assessment, 1659
        diagnosis, 1659
        evaluation, 1660
        planning and implementation, 1659–1660
    pathophysiology and etiology, 1657
    risk factors, 1657
    types
        congenital, 1657

radiation, 1657
 secondary, 1657
 traumatic, 1657
Catatonia, 237–238
Catatonic excitement, 237
Catatonic inhibition, 237
Catecholamines, 978t, 980
Categorization, 2248
Category A medications, 1573
Category B medications, 1573
Category C medications, 1573
Category D medications, 1573
Category X medications, 1573
Catheter ablation, 1454
Catheterization:
 home care, 449t
 nosocomial infections and, 788
 urinary tract infections and, 874–875, 880
Catholicism, end-of-life care and, 293
Cations, 518, 519f
Causation, 2400
Cavitation, 857
CBE. See Charting by exception
CBI (continuous bladder irrigation), 439
CBT. See Cognitive-behavioral therapy (CBT)
CCU. See Critical care units (CCU)
CD4 cell count, 709–710
CD4 cells, 697, 698f, 699f, 704, 708t
CDC. See Centers for Disease Control and
 Prevention (CDC)
CEA. See Carcinoembryonic antigen (CEA)
Ceftriaxone:
 conjunctivitis and, 815
 urinary tract infections and, 876
Celexa, 210, 217, 1585
Cell cycle, 88
Cell membrane, 86
Cell mutations, 1524
Cell-mediated (cellular) immune response:
 hypersensitivity and, 730
 in burns, 1896
 immune system function and, 676, 681
 pediatric, 692
 systemic lupus erythematosus (SLE) and, 756
Cell phones, driving and, 2440f, 2440t
Cells:
 alterations
  anaplasia, 88
  dysplasia, 88
  hyperplasia, 88
  metaplasia, 88
 cell cycle
  differentiation, 88
  meiosis, 88
  mitosis, 88
 malignant, 117–119, 118t
 meiosis, 1523–1524
 metastatic, 118–119
 mitosis, 1523
 shapes, 86
 somatic, 88, 1720
 specialization, 85
 structure
  cell membrane, 86
  chromosomes, 87
  cytoplasm, 86
  DNA, 87–88
  endoplasmic reticulum, 86–87

Golgi apparatus, 87
 lysosomes, 87
 mitochondria, 87
 nucleus and nucleolus, 86, 87t
 ribosomes, 86
Cellular casts, systemic lupus erythematosus
 (SLE) and, 760
Cellular immune response. See Cell-mediated
 (cellular) immune response
Cellular immunity, 680f
Cellular multiplication, 1527
Cellular mutation, 119
Cellular regulation. See also Cancer
 about, 85–95
 alterations, 88–91
 assessment, 91–92
 caring interventions, 92–94
 diagnostic tests, 92
 normal presentation, 86–88
 pharmacologic therapies, 94, 95t
Cellular transportation, methods, 86t
Cellulitis:
 appearance of, 809f
 Case Study, 812
 collaborative care
  clinical therapy, 810
  diagnostic tests, 810
 definition, 808
 etiology, 809
 manifestations, 809–810, 810t
 Nursing Care Plan
  assessment, 811t
  critical thinking, 811t
  diagnoses, 811t
  evaluation, 811t
  planning and implementation, 811t
 nursing process
  assessment, 810
  diagnosis, 810
  evaluation, 812
  planning and implementation, 812
 pathophysiology, 808–809
 risk factors, 809
 treatments, 801
Celsius, conversion to Fahrenheit, 1854
Cementum, 656
Center for Outcomes and Effectiveness Research
 (COER), 2210
Centers for Disease Control and Prevention
 (CDC), 2364, 2415
 H1N1 vaccine distribution by, 2350
 on emergency preparedness, 2351
Centers for Medicare and Medicaid Services
 (CMS), 2364, 2368, 2381
Central apnea, 310
Central nervous system (CNS):
 abnormalities in schizophrenia, 233t
 brain, 940–941
 components, 940
 function of, 940
 pathways of destruction, 213t
 pregnancy and, 1544
 reflexes, 941
 spinal cord, 941
Central nervous system (CNS) depressants, 71
Central obesity, 1026
Central pain, 264
Central processing unit (CPU), 2374

Central syndrome, 1145t
Central venous catheterization, 1490
Central venous pressure (CVP), 1412
Centrally acting sympatholytics, 1431t
Centration, 360t, 2015
Cephalocaudal growth, 340, 340f
Cephalosporins:
 medication administration, 807
 pneumonia and, 841
Cerebellar function, assessment, 956–957t
Cerebellum, 941
Cerebral blood flow, 961
Cerebral cortex, 940–941
Cerebral dysfunction, manifestations, 944, 945t
Cerebral edema, 961
Cerebral hemispherectomy, 972
Cerebral microdialysis catheters, 964
Cerebral palsy (CP):
 case study, 391
 characteristics, 386t
 collaborative care, 387
 community-based care, 391t
 definition, 385
 diagnostic tests, 387
 early intervention programs, 388
 interventions
  foster parental knowledge, 389
  maintain skin integrity, 389
  promote growth and development, 389
  promote physical mobility, 389
  promote safety, 389
  provide adequate nutrition, 389
  provide emotional support, 389
 manifestations, 386–387, 387t
 Nursing Care Plan
  assessment, 390t
  critical thinking in the nursing process, 391t
  diagnosis, 390t
  evaluation, 390t
  implementation, 390t
  planning, 390t
 nursing process
  assessment, 388, 388t
  diagnosis, 388–389
  evaluation, 389
  planning and implementation, 389, 391t
 pathophysiology and etiology, 385–386
 risk factors, 386
 surgical interventions, 388
 therapies, 387t, 388
Cerebral perfusion pressure (CPP), 964
Cerebrospinal fluid, 940
Cerebrospinal fluid (CSF) analysis, 1120
Cerebrum, 940
Certification, 2409
Cerumen (earwax), 1632, 1636t
Cervical cancer:
 acquired immunodeficiency syndrome (AIDS)
  and, 705
 HPV infection and, 1758
 race/ethnicity and, 1700t
 screening guidelines, 132t
Cervical cap, 1729, 1729f
Cervical disks:
 manifestations of ruptured, 1082
Cervical injury, 1149t
Cervical mucus method, 1725

Ciprofloxacin, 770, 876, 916
Circadian rhythms, 666, 1162, 1853
Circulatory system, fetal, 1534–1535, 1535f
Circumcision:
  female, 1699
  male, 1700
Circumplex model, 496f
Cirrhosis, 42t
  alcoholic, 1016
  biliary, 1016
  Case Study, 1024
  clinical therapies, 581t, 1017t
  collaborative care
    diagnostic tests, 1019–1020
    nutritional therapies, 1020
    pharmacologic therapies, 1020
    surgery, 1020
  definition, 1016
  manifestations, 581t, 1016–1019, 1017t
    ascites, 1017, 1022
    esophageal varices, 1019, 1022, 1024
    hepatorenal syndrome, 1019
    portal hypertension, 1017
    portal systemic encephalopathy, 1019
    splenomegaly, 1017
    spontaneous bacterial peritonitis, 1019
  Multisystem Effects, 1018t
  Nursing Care Plan
    assessment, 1023t
    critical thinking, 1023t
    diagnosis, 1023t
    evaluation, 1023t
    planning and implementation, 1023t
  nursing diagnoses and interventions
    disturbed thought processes, 1021
    excess fluid volume, 1021
    imbalanced nutrition, less than body
      requirements, 1022
    impaired skin integrity, 1022
    ineffective protection, 1021
    management of complications, 1022, 1024
  nursing process
    assessment, 1020
    diagnosis, 1020–1021
    implementation, 1021
    planning, 1021
  nutrition and, 1022
  overview, 1015–1016
  pathophysiology and etiology, 1016
  posthepatic, 1016
  risk factors, 1016
  treatment, 983t
  types of, 1016
Citalopram, 210, 217, 1585
Civil law, 2398
Civil War, 2288, 2288f
CIWA-Ar (Clinical Institute Withdrawal
  Assessment for Alcohol—Revised), 46
CK-MB, 1371
CK. See Creatine kinase
Cl–. See Chloride
Clarifying, 2169, 2169t, 2175, 2177t
Clarity, of speech, 2150, 2150t
Clavicles, 1307
Clean wounds, 1879
Clean-contaminated wounds, 1879
Cleavage, 1527
Client abuse, 2301–2302

Client advocacy, 2306
Client advocacy. See Advocacy, 2297
Client advocate, 2297
  nurse as, 2294t, 2331–2332
  role of, 2298–2302
Client autonomy, 2317, 2317t
Client care decisions, 2040
Client care information systems, 2375
Client confidentiality, 2317
Client contracting, 2265
Client education, 670–673
  areas for, 2254t
  Case Study, 2268
  clinical example, 2268t
  computer applications for, 2393
  documentation of teaching process, 2268
  family inclusion in, 2267t
  learning styles and, 2255
  low literacy skills and, 2259t
  nursing process, 2254
    assessment, 2254–2259, 2256–2257t, 2258t,
      2259t, 2259t
    diagnosis, 2258–2260
    evaluation, 2267–2268
    implementation, 2262, 2264–2267
    plan, 2260–2262, 2261t, 2262t
  overview, 2254, 2254t
  teaching clients and families, 2254
Client goals, establishing, 2054, 2085–2087,
    2085f, 2089
Client monitoring, computerized, 2392
Client outcomes:
  desired outcomes, 2054
  nursing delivery models and, 2207t
  revision of, 2101
Client privacy, 2317
Client records:
  computerized, 2183, 2189–2190, 2192t,
    2390–2393, 2391f
    ANA position statement on, 2392t
  definition, 2183
  ethical and legal considerations, 2183
  problem-oriented medical records, 2185–2187
  purposes of, 2183–2184
  recording guidelines, 2195–2199,
    2196–2198t, 2199t
  as source of data, 2055
  source-oriented records, 2184–2185, 2185t
Client rights, 250
Client safety:
  maintaining, 2401
  promotion of, 2444–2446, 2445t, 2446t,
    2448, 2448t
Client support systems, 2255
Client Teaching:
  anemia, 104t
  asthma, 1259t
  breast cancer, 115t
  burn care, 1909t
  cancer, 134t
  cardiac rehabilitation, 1388t
  cardiomyopathy, 1337t
  chronic obstructive pulmonary disease
    (COPD), 1270t
  cirrhosis, 1022t
  deep breathing and progressing relaxation, 1841t
  deep venous thrombosis, 1395t
  diabetes mellitus, 1003t, 1011t

  disseminated intravascular coagulation, 1403t
  dysfunctional uterine bleeding, 1751t
  dysrhythmias, 1457t
  eating disorders, 1604t
  effective communication styles, 248
  erectile dysfunction, 1716t
  eye injuries
    health education, 1667t
    prevention and first aid, 1665t
  fall prevention in older adults, 1104t
  foot care for peripheral atherosclerosis, 1464t
  foot care for peripheral vascular disease, 1466t
  glaucoma, 1673t
  heart failure, 1420t
  home care after spinal surgery, 1091t
  home care for fractures, 1110t
  hypertension, 1435t
  low-sodium diet, 586
  malignant melanoma, 192t
  MAOIs, 1173
  mood stabilizers, 1173
  obsessive-compulsive disorder, 1834t
  Parkinson's disease, 1140t
  proper body mechanics, 1084t
  prostate cancer home care, 175t
  pulmonary embolism, 1480t
  reducing dry skin and relieving pruritus, 1914t
  self-care of systemic lupus erythematosus, 764
  sickle cell disorder, 181t
  SSRIs, 1172
  substance abuse, 81t
  sudden cardiac death, 1458t
  sudden infant death syndrome (SIDS), 1289t
  tricyclic antidepressants, 1171
  typical human responses to traumatic
    events, 1847t
Client values, 2307–2308
Client-focused care, 2206, 2344
Clients, 2292
  death of, 2034
  determining strengths of, 2071
  disabled, advocacy for, 2301, 2301t
  education levels of, 402
  effects of staff and organizational conflict on, 2132
  empowering, 2033, 2033f, 2299
  homeless, 403
  with intellectual disabilities, 403
  low-literacy, 402–403
  managing conflicts with, 2130
  misidentification of, 2401
  reassessment of, 2096
  rights of, 2298
  as source of data, 2054
  understanding, 2032, 2032t
  from vulnerable populations, 403–404
Climacteric period, 1742
Clinical Care Classification (CCC), 2386
Clinical data warehouse (CDW), 2375
Clinical decision making:
  about, 2037–2045, 2039t, 2041t, 2044t
  Case Study, 2046
  Decision making, 2037
  Evidence-Based Practice, 2044t
  nursing process and, 2045–2047
Clinical decision support (CDS) systems:
  Case Study, 2389
  nursing administration and, 2388–2389
  overview, 2385–2386

research and, 2386–2388, 2387t, 2388t
uniform languages and, 2386
Clinical errors, 2334
Clinical information systems (CISs), 2375, 2424
Clinical Institute Withdrawal Assessment for Alcohol (CIWA-Ar), 45
Clinical Institute Withdrawal Assessment for Alcohol—Revised (CIWA-Ar), 46, 47f
Clinical manifestations. *See* Manifestations
Clinical nurse specialist, 2294
Clinical nursing research, 2326
Clinical Opiate Withdrawal Scale (COWS), 78
Clinical pelvimetry, 1570
Clinical Practice Guidelines—Early Intervention Program of the New York State Department of Health, 382t
Clinical questions, 2334
Clinical research, 2328t
Clinoril. *See* Sulindac
Clitoris, 1687–1688, 1688t, 1707t
Clofibrate, 1374
Clomid, 1735t
Clomiphene citrate, 1735t
Clonic phase, 970
Closed awareness, 298
Closed fractures, 1093, 1095t
Closed questions, 2056, 2057t, 2170
Closing, of interview, 2059
Clostridium, 770
Clostridium difficile, 790
Clozapine, 243, 244t, 1815
Clozaril, 243, 244t, 1815
Club drugs, 60, 68, 73
Clubbed nail beds, 1218–1219
CNS. *See* Central nervous system
Co-management, 2118
Co-occurring disorders, 30t
    definition, 67
    with substance abuse, 67
Co-occurring substances, 41t
Coaches, 2271t
Coaching, 2270, 2275
Coagulation studies, 1479
Coanalgesics, for pain management, 274, 277–278
Coarctation of the aorta (COA), 1347–1348t, 1424
COAs (children of alcoholics), 31
Cocaine:
    acute myocardial infarction and, 1364
    effect on fetus, 58t
    sexual functioning and, 1701t
    street names, 74t
    therapies, 62t
    use in pregnancy, 59, 71
    use of, 68, 71–72
Cocaine Anonymous, 37
Coccugeus, 1517t
Coccyx, 1517–1518
Cochlea, 1633
Cochlear implants, 1654
Cochrane Database of Systematic Reviews, 2335
Cochrane, Archie, 2324
Code of Academic and Clinical Conduct, 2282t
Code of Ethics for Nurses (ANA), 1778, 2227
Codes of ethics, 2281, 2308–2312, 2309–2310t
Codeine, 276, 277t
Codependency, 30–31, 30t
Coding systems, 2375
Coenzyme Q10, 1417

COER. *See* Center for Outcomes and Effectiveness Research
Cogentin, 243
Cognition:
    about, 197–210
    aging and, 199
    alterations, 200–207
    assessment, 207, 208–210t
    definition, 197, 946
    factors influencing, 198
    normal presentation, 198–200
    pharmacologic therapies, 210
    senses and, 207
Cognitive appraisal:
    primary appraisal, 1796
    reappraisal, 1796
    secondary appraisal, 1796
Cognitive assessment, 207, 208–209t, 210t
Cognitive awareness, 2434
Cognitive development, 198, 347, 348t, 2247
    in adolescence, 364
    infancy, 354–355
    preschool years, 360
    school-age children, 362
    toddlerhood, 358
Cognitive disorders:
    in children, 201–205
    confusion, 226–227, 228–229t, 230–231
    dementia, 206–207
    learning disabilities, 200–201
    mental retardation, 201–205, 206t
    nursing management, 201–205
    pediatric, 200
    pharmacologic therapies, 210
    schizophrenia, 239–241
Cognitive domain, 2247
Cognitive factors, influencing health, 645
Cognitive function:
    benefits for exercise for, 654
    in older adults, 199–200
Cognitive impairments, assessment of, 2160, 2160t
Cognitive learning processes, 2247t
Cognitive modification, 1175
Cognitive skills, 34, 2096
Cognitive theories, 198
Cognitive theory, 1162, 1164t, 2246–2247, 2247t
    eating disorders and, 1598
    nursing practices and, 198
Cognitive-behavioral therapy (CBT), 1175, 1189t, 1190
    anxiety disorders and, 1815–1816
    phobias and, 1839
    stress and, 1806–1807
    for methamphetamine addiction, 73
    for personality disorders, 1619
    for sleep disorders, 315
Cogwheel rigidity, 1135
Cohabiting family, 487
Cohesiveness, group, 2138, 2139t
Coinsurance, 2211, 2368
Coitus interruptus, 1726
Cold zones, 2356t
Colectomy:
    definition, 916
    total, 916
Colesevelam, 1374
Colestipol, 1374

Collaboration, 2177t, 2444
    about, 2113–2114, 2114t
    benefits of, 2118
    case management, 2121–2123, 2123–2124t, 2125, 2125t
    Case Study, 2121
    chain of command, 2126–2127
    characteristics and beliefs of collaborative health care, 2114t
    characteristics of effective, 2118
    collaborative practice, 2117–2118
    competencies
        communication skills, 2118–2119
        decision making, 2119–2120, 2120t
        feedback, giving and receiving, 2119
        mutual respect and trust, 2119
    for conflict resolution, 2129
    continuum of, 2118f
    coordination and, 2208
    definition of, 2113–2114
    factors leading to need for increased, 2120
    groups, 2133–2141, 2135t, 2136t, 2137t, 2138t, 2141t
    health care for chronically ill older adults, 2117t
    management theories, 2142–2145
    members of health care team, 2116–2117t
    nurses and, 2114–2115, 2115t
    nursing practice and, 2120
    physician-nurse, 2118t
Collaborative care plans, 2081
Collaborative decision making, 2115
Collaborative health care teams, 2117
Collaborative interventions, 2090
Collaborative problems, 2067, 2068t, 2072f, 2073, 2073t
Collagen, 1875, 1928
Collegial relationships, 2131
Collateral channels, 1361
Colloid osmotic pressure, 520
Colloid solutions, 1494, 1494t
Colloids, 519, 533t
Colon cancer, 141. *See also* Colorectal cancer
Colonization, definition of, 771
Colony-stimulating factors (CSFs), 154
Colorectal cancer:
    Case Study, 148
    collaborative care
        chemotherapy, 144–145
        diagnostic tests, 143
        radiation therapy, 144
        screening, 143
        surgery, 143–144
    Crohn's disease and, 914
    distribution and frequency, 141f
    incidence, 142
    manifestations, 142–143, 143t
    Nursing Care Plan
        assessment, 147t
        critical thinking, 147t
        diagnoses, 147t
        evaluation, 147t
        planning and implementation, 147t
    nursing diagnoses and interventions
        acute pain, 145
        anticipatory grieving, 146

imbalanced nutrition, less than body
    requirements, 145–146
  risk for sexual dysfunction, 146
nursing process
  assessment, 145
  diagnosis, 145
  evaluation, 146
  planning and implementation, 145–146
overview, 141
pathophysiology and etiology, 141–142
risk factors, 142, 142t
screening guidelines, 132t
TNM staging system, 142–143t
ulcerative colitis and, 914
Colostomy, 144, 144f
Coma, 946t
  assessment, 949t
  irreversible, 948
  prognosis, 949
Combined oral contraceptives (COCs), 1731–1732
Comfort:
  about, 255–261
  alterations, 256–258, 259t
  assessment, 259–260
  Assessment Interview, 298t
  caring interventions, 260
  diagnostic tests, 260
  in end-of-life care, 297t
  healing and, 256
  normal presentation, 256
  pharmacologic therapies, 260, 261t
  spiritual and emotional, 298
Comminuted fractures, 1095t
Commission on Collegiate Nursing Education
    (CCNE), 2366
Commitment, 250, 2029t
  affective, 2231, 2231f
  continuance, 2231
  defined, 2230
  normative, 2231
  organizational, 2230
  professional, 2230–2232
  stages of development, 2231–2232
  types of, 2231
Committee on the Quality of Health Care in
    America, 2422
Committees, 2140
Communal family, 487
Communicable disease. See also Infectious disease
  definition of, 770
  pediatric, 791
Communication, 2006
  about, 2147–2149
  in adolescence, 365
  assertive, 2179–2182, 2180t
  barriers to, 2158–2159, 2159t, 2162–2163
  Case Study, 2164
  with children, 2155t
  clients with dementia and, 2161t
  congruent, 2157
  defined, 2148
  documentation, 2182–2187, 2185t, 2189,
    2191–2197, 2195t, 2199–2200, 2199t, 2199t
  family, 493–494
  hand-off, 2435
  by infants, 357

intrapersonal, 2148, 2148f
language issues and, 334
modes of, 2149–2154, 2150t, 2151t
  electronic communication, 2150, 2152–2153
  nonverbal, 2157t
  nonverbal communication, 2149, 2151–2152,
    2151f, 2157t
  verbal communication, 2149–2151, 2161, 2161t
  written communication, 2153–2154
nursing interventions
  avoid potential cultural barriers to
    communication, 2162–2163
  educate client and support persons, 2163
  employ measures to enhance
    communication, 2162
  manipulation of environment, 2162
  provide support, 2162
nursing practice, 2163
nursing process
  assessment, 2158–2160, 2161t
  diagnosis, 2161
  evaluation, 2163
  implementation, 2161–2163
  plan, 2161
and nursing transaction model of stress,
    1796–1797
with parents, 335t
in preschool years, 361t
with older adults, 2160t
process, 2149, 2149f
  factors influencing, 2155–2158
  message, 2149
  receiver, 2149
  response, 2149
  sender, 2149
reporting, 2200–2203, 2201t
by school-age children, 363
style, 2160
therapeutic, 2164–2179, 2166–2168t, 2169t,
    2171t, 2174t, 2175t, 2177t, 2178t
by toddlers, 358–359
use of effective, 2402
Communication skills, 2118–2119
Communication styles, 2119
Communicator, nurse as, 2294t
Communited fractures, 1094
Community Emergency Response Team (CERT)
    Program, 2355
Community health care, computers and, 2392
Community health centers, 2348
Community health education, 671
Comorbid disorders, 1158–1159, 2422
Compact bone, 1057
Compact discs (CDs), 2375
Compartment syndrome, 1895
  acute, 1094
  definition, 1094, 1105
  interventions, 1095
  manifestations, 1096t
Compassion, 2029t, 2033
  as component of professionalism, 2228, 2228f
Competence, 2029t, 2033, 2034t
  areas of competency, 2285
    caring for the dying, 2285
    health and wellness promotion, 2285

health restoration, 2285
illness prevention, 2285
Case Study, 2286
defined, 2285
nursing process and, 2286
promoting lifelong, 2286
Competency, 2226, 2404
Competition, 2129, 2214
Complement, 887t
Complement assays, 736
Complementary and alternative medicine
    (CAM), 1383
  acupuncture, 280, 1084, 1177
  ADHD, 373t
  alcoholism, 45
  Alternative therapies:
  Alzheimer's disease, 217–219
  anemia, 102
  animal-assisted therapy, 1177
  anxiety disorders, 1816
  art therapy, 363t
  asthma, 1262–1263
  autism spectrum disorders, 382, 383t
  back problems, 1084
  benign prostatic hypertrophy, 435
  bipolar disorders, 1182
  cataracts, 1659
  chiropractic therapy, 1084
  chronic renal failure, 562
  conjunctivitis, 816
  COPD, 1274
  culture and, 336
  in end-of-life care, 297
  fatigue, 304
  fibromyalgia, 307
  gallstones, 905
  guided imagery, 315
  heart failure, 1417
  herbal laxatives, 457t
  herbal supplements. See Herbal
    supplements/therapy
  hypertension, 1433, 1433t
  immune system, 696
  inflammatory bowel disease, 919
  leukemia, 156
  lung cancer, 165t
  massage, 280, 297, 1084, 1816
  meditation, 1816
  menopause, 1743, 1744t
  mood disorders, 1175–1176
  morning sickness, 1576t
  music therapy, 363t, 1177
  osteoarthritis, 1130
  otitis media, 829
  pain control, 1900t
  pain, 266t, 280
  peripheral neuropathy, 1681
  peripheral vascular disease, 1465
  personality disorders, 1619, 1620t
  PMS, 1752
  pneumonia, 844
  relaxation techniques, 1620t
  rheumatoid arthritis, 751
  safety issues, 2435
  schizophrenia, 245

seizure disorders, 972
sickle cell anemia, 180
skin lesions, 1885*t*
sleep disorders, 315
smoking cessation, 53
systemic lupus erythematosus (SLE), 761
touch therapy, 1816
transcendental meditation, 1433*t*
transcranial magnetic stimulation, 1175
urinary incontinence, 444
urinary tract infections, 877–878
vagus nerve stimulation, 1176
yoga, 1176, 1816
Complete blood count (CBC):
　human immunodeficiency virus (HIV) and,
　　709–710
　in specific conditions
　　acute renal failure, 540
　　burns, 1900
　　chronic obstructive pulmonary disease
　　　(COPD), 1272
　　chronic renal failure, 558
　　congenital heart defects, 1353*t*
　　coronary artery disease, 1371
　　disseminated intravascular coagulation, 1399
　　fluid imbalances, 531
　　leukemia, 153
　　lung cancer, 164
　　otitis media, 828
　　pneumonia, 841
　systemic lupus erythematosus (SLE) and, 760
Complex regional pain syndrome, 264
Compliance, 961, 1307, 2245
Complicated grief, 601, 606, 608*t*, 623
Complicated grief treatment (CGT), 608*t*
Comportment, 2029*t*
Compound fractures, 1093
Compressed fractures, 1094
Compression fractures, 1095*t*
Compromised host:
　definition of, 773
　nosocomial infections and, 787
Compulsion, 1828
Computed tomography (CT), 841
　acute renal failure, 540
　cancer, 127
　eye assessment, 1646
　increased intracranial pressure, 963
　kidneys, 469
　lung cancer, 164
　traumatic injury, 1942
Computer information systems, 2375
Computer literacy, 2374
Computer terminology, 2374–2375
Computer use, locations of, 2253*t*
Computer vision syndrome (CVS), 2383
Computer-assisted instruction, 2265
Computer-based patient record (CPR), 2378
Computer-Based Patient Record Institute, 2390
Computerized axial tomography (CAT) scans, 2392
Computerized care plans, 2081
Computerized diagnostics, 2392
Computerized medical records, 2378–2379, 2380*t*,
　　2389–2393, 2391*f*, 2392*t*
Computerized provider order entry (CPOE),
　　2375, 2385
Computerized records, 2183, 2189–2190, 2192*t*

Computers:
　community and home health and, 2392
　components of, 2374*f*
　in nursing administration, 2388–2389
in nursing research, 2386–2387, 2387*t*
COMT (catechol-O-methyltransferase)
　　inhibitors, 1138*t*
Concept formation, 2247*t*
Concept maps, 2081, 2082*f*
Conception:
　cellular differentiation, 1528
　fertilization, 1524–1526
　implantation, 1527–1528
　meiosis, 1523–1524, 1525*f*
　mitosis, 1523
　oogenesis, 1524
　preembryonic development, 1527–1530
　spermatogenesis, 1524
Concerta, 372, 373*t*
Concrete operations stage, 348
Concrete thinking, 240
Concurrent audit, 2426
Conditioning behavioral responses, 2246
Condoms, 1697, 2461
　application, 1727
　effectiveness, 1727
　female, 1728, 1728*f*
　STIs and, 1728
Conduction, 1852–1853
Conduction system, of heart, 1305–1307, 1305*f*
Conductivity, 1438
Condyloma acuminata, 1758
Confabulation, 43
Confidence, 2029*t*, 2107
Confidentiality, 2183, 2309, 2317, 2413
Conflict:
　causes of, 2128–2129
　covert, 2128
　definition of, 2127
　effects of staff and organizational, on clients, 2132
　gender issues in, 2130–2131
　individual, 2127
　intergroup, 2129*t*
　interpersonal, 2127
　management, 2144
　managing, 2130
　organizational, 2128
　overt, 2128
　in physician–nurse relationship, 2131
　preventing, 2129
　responding to, 2129
　role, 2127
　types of, 2127–2128
　verbal abuse and, 2131–2132
Conflict resolution:
　Case Study, 2133
　overview, 2127–2128
　strategies, 2130*t*
Confrontations, 2171–2172, 2175
Confucianism, 1776*t*
Confusion, 946*t*
　in Alzheimer's disease, 221
　clinical manifestations, 227
　definition, 226
　nursing care
　　assessment, 227
　　diagnosis, 227

　　evaluation, 230
　　implementation, 227, 230
　　plan, 227
　nursing process
　pathophysiology and etiology, 226–227
　therapeutic environment for, 230*t*
Confusion Assessment Method (CAM), 207*t*,
　　227, 228*t*
Congenital cataracts, 1657
Congenital heart defects:
　aortic stenosis, 1347*t*
　atrial septal defect, 1340–1341*t*
　atrioventricular (AV) canal, 1341–1342*t*
　Case study, 1360
　in children, 1309, 1313
　clinical therapies, 1340–1349*t*
　coarctation of the aorta (COA), 1347–1348*t*
　collaborative care
　　clinical interventions, 1351, 1354–1355*t*
　　diagnostic tests, 1351, 1352–1353*t*
　　pharmacologic therapies, 1351
　　surgery, 1354–1355*t*
　definition, 1339
　etiology, 1349
　hypoplastic left heart syndrome (HLHS),
　　1348–1349*t*
　manifestations, 1340–1349*t*, 1350*t*
　　defects decreasing pulmonary blood flow,
　　　1350–1351
　　defects increasing pulmonary blood flow, 1350
　　defects obstructing systemic blood flow, 1351
　　heart murmurs, 1349–1350
　　mixed defects, 1351
　Nursing Care Plan
　　assessment, 1358*t*
　　critical thinking, 1358*t*
　　diagnoses, 1358*t*
　　evaluation, 1358*t*
　　planning and implementation, 1358*t*
　nursing diagnoses and interventions
　　activity, 1357
　　discharge planning and postsurgical home care,
　　　1357, 1359
　　manage fluids and nutrition, 1357
　　pain management, 1357
　　postoperative care, 1357
　　preparation for surgery, 1357
　　presurgical home care, 1357
　　promote respiratory function, 1357
　　psychosocial support, 1356–1357
　nursing process
　　assessment, 1355, 1356*t*
　　diagnosis, 1355–1356
　　evaluation, 1359
　　planning and implementation, 1356–1359
　patent ductus arteriosus, 1340*t*
　pathophysiology, 1340–1349*t*
　physiology
　　defects decreasing pulmonary blood flow,
　　　1339, 1342
　　defects increasing pulmonary blood flow, 1339
　　defects obstructing systemic blood flow, 1342
　　mixed defects, 1342
　pulmonary atresia, 1344*t*
　pulmonic stenosis, 1343*t*
　risk factors, unique to women, 1366
　tetralogy of Fallout, 1343–1344*t*
　total anomalous pulmonary venous return, 1346*t*

transposition of the great arteries, 1345*t*
tricuspid atresia, 1344*t*
truncus arteriosus, 1345–1346*t*
ventricular septal defect, 1341*t*
Congenital nevi, 184
Congestive heart failure, 1404. *See also* Heart failure
  clinical therapies, 581*t*
  manifestations, 581*t*
Congruent communication, 2157
Conjugate vera, 1517
Conjunctiva, 1630
Conjunctivitis:
  acute, 815*t*
  Case Study, 818
  collaborative care
    complementary therapies, 816
    diagnostic tests, 815
    medical treatment, 815
    pharmacologic therapies, 815, 816*t*
  complementary and alternative therapies and, 816
  definition, 813
  etiology of, 814
  manifestations, 813*f*, 814, 814*f*
  nursing diagnoses and interventions
    home care, 817
    risk for disturbed sensory perception, 817
    risk of infection, 817
  nursing process
    assessment, 816
    diagnosis, 817
    evaluation, 817
    planning and implementation, 817
  pathophysiology, 813–814
  risk factors, 814
  treatments, 801, 815–816
Connective tissue, systemic lupus erythematosus
    (SLE) and, 757
Connors' Parent and Teacher Rating Scales—
    Revised—Long Form, 371*t*
Consciousness:
  definition, 946
  level of, 946–949, 946*t*
Consensus decision making, 2039
Consent. *See also* Informed consent
  competency for, 2404
  defined, 2403
  in emergency, 2404
  expressed, 2403
  implied, 2403
Consequence-based theories, 1777
Conservation, 360*t*, 362
Constant data, 2054
Constant fever, 1859
Constipation:
  alternative therapies, 457*t*
  causes, 455*t*
  characteristics, 454*t*
  childhood, 456–457, 456*t*
  definition, 454
  developmental considerations, 456–457
  during pregnancy, 1574*t*
  manifestations, 455
  in older adults, 424–425, 454, 456*t*
  opioid use and, 277*t*, 278*t*
  pathophysiology, 454
  in pregnancy, 454
  risk factors, 454

treatment, 427*t*, 455
  enemas, 456
  medications, 455
  nutrition, 456
Constituent member associations (CMAs), 2366
Constructivism, 2248
Consultation, 2118
Consumer demands, 2282–2283
Consumer-driven health care plan (CDHP), 2369
Consumerism, 2212
Consumers, 2282, 2292
Consumption coagulopathy, 626
Contact dermatitis, 730
  allergic, 1912
  causes of, 1912*t*
  collaborative care, 1913
  distribution of lesions, 1913*t*
  irritant, 1912
  manifestations, 1912–1913
  nursing process
    assessment, 1913
    diagnosis, 1914
    evaluation, 1914
    planning and implementation, 1914
  overview, 1912
  pathophysiology and etiology, 1912
  risk factors, 1912
Contaminated wounds, 1879
Contamination, 2438
Context, 2109
Continent ileostomy, 917*f*
Contingency contracts, 35
Contingency planning, 2143
Contingency plans, 2237
Contingency theory, 2234
Continuance commitment, 2231
Continuing education, 2324
Continuity theory, 347
Continuous ambulatory peritoneal dialysis
    (CAPD), 560
Continuous arteriovenous hemodialysis
    (CAVHD), 545*t*
Continuous arteriovenous hemofiltration
    (CAVH), 545*f*, 545*t*
Continuous bladder irrigation (CBI), 439
Continuous cardiac monitoring, 1448
Continuous cyclic peritoneal dialysis (CCPD), 560
Continuous positive airway pressure (CPAP), 310,
    314, 315*f*, 1239, 1240*t*
Continuous quality improvement (CQI), 2427–2428
Continuous renal replacement therapy (CRRT),
    543–545, 545*t*
Continuous venovenous hemodialysis
    (CVVHD), 545*t*
Contraception:
  barrier methods
    condoms, 1727–1728
    diaphragm and cervical cap, 1728–1729, 1729*f*
    vaginal sponge, 1730
  coitus interruptus, 1726
  decisions about, 1717
  discontinuing, 1734
  douching, 1727
  emergency postcoital, 1733, 1733*t*
  fertility awareness methods, 1725–1726, 1726*t*
  hormonal
    benefits, 1732

  combined estrogen-progestin, 1731
  contraindications, 1731
  long-acting progestin, 1732–1733
  minipill, 1732
  side effects, 1731*t*
  skin patch, 1732
  vaginal ring, 1732
  intrauterine devices, 1730–1731, 1730*f*
  male, 1734
  operative sterilization
    definition, 1733
    tubal ligation, 1733
    vasectomy, 1733
  oral contraceptives, 1711*t*
  situational, 1726
  spermicides, 1727
  vaginal sponge, 1730, 1730*f*
Contract management systems, 2378*t*
Contractility, 1304, 1405, 1438
Contractures, 1889, 1889*f*, 1902
Contralateral deficit, 1500
Control groups, 2328*t*
Control unit, 2374
Controlled Substance Act (CSA), 68, 2405
Controlling, 2144
Contusions, 1880*t*
Convenience groups, 2135
Convention, definition, 1853
Conventional stage, 352*t*
Convergence, 1632
Cooperative play, 363
Coordination, 2118, 2208. *See also* Care
    coordination
Coparent adoption, 488
Copayments, 2369
COPD. *See* Chronic obstructive pulmonary disease
Coping:
  alterations from normal coping
    generalized anxiety disorder, 1804*t*
    obsessive-compulsive disorder (OCD), 1804*t*
    phobias, 1804*t*
    post-traumatic stress disorder (PTSD), 1804*t*
    treatments for, 1804*t*
  and transactional model of stress, 1796,
    1798–1799
  Assessment Interview, 1805*t*
  coping toolkit, 1815*t*
  crisis and, 1821
  definition, 1794
  with diabetes mellitus, 1012–1014
  factors affecting stress response, 1798*t*
  with rape, 1976–1977
  types of coping
    appraisal-focused coping, 1799, 1799*t*
    approach-coping, 1799, 1799*t*
    avoidance-coping, 1799, 1799*t*
    emotion-focused coping, 1799, 1799*t*
    problem-focused coping, 1799, 1799*t*
Coping mechanisms, 497
Copper, recommended daily intake, 1597*t*
Cor pulmonale, 1270
Cordotomy, 279
Core temperature, 1852
Cornea, 1630, 1635, 1636*t*, 1642*t*
Corneal abrasion, 1661
Corneal reflex, 1630
Cornell Depression Scale (CDS), 1193

Cornell Scale for Depression in Dementia, 207t
Coronary arteries, 1361
Coronary artery bypass grafting, 1378–1379, 1379f, 1380–1382t
Coronary artery disease (CAD):
    acute myocardial infarction. See Acute myocardial infarction (AMI)
    Case Study, 1389
    Client Teaching, 1388t
    clinical therapies, 1369t
    collaborative care
        cardiac rehabilitation, 1382–1383
        clinical therapies, 1376
        complementary therapies, 1383
        diagnostic tests, 1370–1372
        invasive procedures, 1382
        pharmacologic therapies, 1373–1375
        revascularization procedures, 1376–1382
        risk factor management, 1372–1373
        treatment goals, 1370
    description, 1314t
    diabetes mellitus and, 997
    etiology, 1364
    heart failure and, 1407
    manifestations, 1369t
        acute coronary syndrome, 1367
        acute myocardial infarction, 1367–1369
        angina pectoris, 1366–1367
    nursing diagnoses and interventions
        acute pain, 1385
        fear, 1386
        imbalanced nutrition, more than body requirements, 1384–1385
        ineffective coping, 1386
        ineffective health maintenance, 1385
        ineffective tissue perfusion, 1385–1386
        ineffective tissue perfusion, cardiac, 1386, 1388
        risk for ineffective therapeutic regimen management, 1388
    nursing process
        assessment, 1383–1384
        diagnosis, 1384
        evaluation, 1388–1389
        overview, 1383
        planning and implementation, 1384–1388
    overview, 1360–1361
    pathophysiology, 1361–1364
        acute coronary syndrome, 1362–1363
        acute myocardial infarction, 1363–1364
        atherosclerosis, 1361–1362
        ischemia, 1362
    rheumatoid arthritis and, 745, 747
    risk factors
        cigarette smoking, 1365–1366
        diabetes mellitus, 1365, 1373
        diet, 1366
        emerging, 1366
        homocysteine, 1366
        hyperlipidemia, 1365
        hypertension, 1364–1365, 1373
        metabolic syndrome, 1366
        modifiable, 1364–1366
        nonmodifiable, 1364
        obesity, 1366
        physical inactivity, 1366
    surgery
        coronary artery bypass grafting, 1378–1379

    minimally invasive coronary artery surgery, 1379
    transmyocardial laser revascularization, 1382
    treatment, 1314t
Coronary circulation, 1298, 1300, 1301f
Corpus luteum, 1519, 1522, 1534, 1690–1691
Corrective action, 2237
Corticosteroids, 960t, 1913t
    administration of, 915t
        asthma, 1260t, 1262
        COPD, 1273
        glomerular disorders, 927
        hypersensitivity, 737
        IBS, 914
        osteoarthritis, 1127
        rheumatoid arthritis, 748
        stroke, 1507
        systemic lupus erythematosus (SLE), 761
Corticotropic cells, 978
Cortisol, 915t, 980
Cortisone, 342, 980
Corynebacterium xerosis, 770
Coryza, influenza and, 818
Cosleeping, 2440t
Cost effectiveness, of nursing care, 2326
Cost-effective care:
    Case Study, 2216
    cost-containment strategies, 2214–2215
    international perspective on, 2212–2213, 2213t
    nursing economics, 2215–2216
    overview, 2210
    payment sources in U.S., 2210–2212
Cotton applicators, 2005t
Cotyledons, 1531
Coumadin:
    administration, 1393t
    for pulmonary embolism, 1479
Counseling sessions, 648
Counselor, nurse as, 2294t
Counterirritants, 1127
Countershock, 1449
Countertransference, 2140
Couplet, 1446
Couvade, 1552t
Covert conflict, 2128
COWS (Clinical Opiate Withdrawal Scale), 78
COX (cyclooxygenase), 275
COX-2, 275
COX-2 inhibitors, 210, 1127. See also Nonsteroidal anti-inflammatory drugs (NSAIDs)
CP. See Cerebral palsy
CPK (creatine phosphokinase), 1900
CPR. See Cardiopulmonary resuscitation (CPR)
CPU (central processing unit), 2374
CQI. See Continuous quality improvement
Crack, use in pregnancy, 59
Crackles, 1222t
Cranial nerves, 941, 942f, 942t, 952–954t, 1630f
    assessment, 957t, 1645t
    functions, 1628t
Creams, 1913t
Creatine, 129t
Creatine clearance, 926
Creatine clearance test, 422
Creatine kinase (CK), 1077t, 1371
Creatine phosphokinase (CPK), 1900
Creatinine, 540, 926

Creatinine clearance, 558
Creativity, 2105
Credentialing, 2409
Credès method, 966
Credibility, 2150
Crepitation, 1071t
Cri du chat syndrome, 1721t, 1722
Crime, 2398
Crimean War, 2288
Criminal law, 2398
Crinone, 1735t
Crisis:
    Assessment Interview
        sociocultural assessment, 1824
    balancing factors
        coping mechanisms, 1821
        perception of the event, 1820
        situational supports, 1821
    caring interventions, 1820
    Case Study, 1827
    characteristics of crisis, 1820t
    collaborative care
        art therapy, 1823
        pharmacologic therapies, 1823
        prayer and faith, 1823
    communicating painful information, 1822t
    communication do's and don'ts, 1825t
    crisis connection, 1823t
    crisis intervention, 1821–1822
    manifestations, 1821t
    Nursing Care Plan
        assessment, 1826t
        critical thinking, 1826t
        diagnosis, 1826t
        evaluation, 1826t
        planning and implementation, 1826t
    nursing diagnoses and interventions
        anticipatory guidance, 1826
        assisting with environmental change, 1826
        communication strategies, 1825
        helping to develop social supports, 1826–1827
    nursing process
        assessment, 1824
            individual assessment, 1823–1825
        diagnosis, 1825
        evaluation, 1827
        planning and implementation, 1825
    overview, 1819
    pathophysiology and etiology, 1819–1820
    resilience, 1820
    risk factors, 1820t
        disaster assessment, 1820–1821
    types of
        maturational crisis, 1820
        situational crisis, 1820
Crisis counseling:
    ABCs of crisis counseling, 1827t
    description, 1822
Crisis intervention, 33–34
Critical analysis, 2105
Critical care units (CCU), deaths in, 289t
Critical paths, 2425
Critical pathways, 2081, 2121, 2123, 2123–2124t, 2125t, 2191–2192, 2192f, 2376–2378

Critical thinking:
application of, 2091*t*
to nursing practice, 2110–2111, 2110*t*
to nursing process, 2103
attitudes that foster, 2106–2108
Case Study, 2111
compared with decision making and problem
solving, 2041*t*
creativity and, 2105
decision making and, 2044*t*
defined, 2038, 2068, 2104
developing attitudes and skills for, 2108
in diagnostic process, 2068
importance of, 2105*t*
in nursing process, 2052*t*
overview, 2104–2105
problem solving and, 2044
skills in, 2105–2106
standards of, 2109, 2109*t*, 2110*t*
use of, 2104–2105
Crohn's and Colitis Foundation of America, 921*t*
Crohn's disease, 889*t*. *See also* Inflammatory
bowel disease
characteristics, 910*t*
complications, 914, 916
definition, 909
incidence, 909
manifestations, 909, 912*t*, 914
pathophysiology and etiology, 910
progression of, 911*f*
Cromolyn sodium, 737, 1262
Cross-dressers, 400, 1697
Cross-tolerance, 30*t*
Crossing the Quality Chasm (Institute of
Medicine), 2422
Crossing the Quality Chasm (IOM), 2324, 2386
Crown, 656
CRP. *See* C-reactive protein
Crusades, 2287
Crusts, skin, 1879*t*
Crutches, 1078
Crypts of Lieberkuhn, 911*f*
Crystalloid fluids, 1899
Crystalloid solutions, 1494
Crystalloids, 519, 533*t*
CSA. *See* Controlled Substance Act (CSA)
CSFs. *See* Colony-stimulating factors (CSFs)
Cuboid bones, 1058
Cued speech, 1655
Cues, 2064
clustering, 2068–2069
comparing against standards, 2069*t*
Cultural barriers, to learning, 2251
Cultural bias, 322
Cultural characteristics, 322
Cultural competence, 331–336
Cultural deprivation, 1634
Cultural differences, in views of older adults, 402*t*
Cultural factors, impacting assessment, 2007
Cultural groups, 322
Cultural influences, on development, 342
Cultural model, of addiction, 28
Cultural sensitivity, 332
Cultural stereotypes, eating disorders and, 1599
Cultural values/beliefs, 327–328

Culturally and linguistically appropriate services
(CLAS), national standards on, 2154*t*
Culturally congruent care, 2028
Culturally sensitive nursing, 2029*t*
Culture. *See also* Focus on Diversity and Culture
about, 321–328
affect on sensory perception, 1634
alternative health care and, 336
aspects of, 322–324
assault and, 1964
case study, 337
child behaviors and, 2010*t*
client education and, 2255
communication and, 2156
definition, 322
differences among, 326–327
families and, 485
gender roles and, 399
health beliefs and, 650
influence on grief, 604, 604*t*
influence on grief and loss, 611
nursing process
assessment, 331
evaluation, 335
implementation, 333–335
planning, 331–333
nutritional health and, 663*t*
personal space and, 2156–2157, 2156*f*
personality and, 1587*t*
physical assessment and, 327–328
pregnancy and, 1553
safety issues and, 2435
sexuality and, 1699
social supports and, 646*t*
in United States, 324–325, 324*f*
Cultured epithelial autografting, 1901
Cultures:
conjunctivitis and, 815
in infection, 804
otitis media and, 828
pneumonia and, 841
tuberculosis and, 862
urinary tract infections and, 875
Cumulative Index of Nursing and Allied Health
Literature (CINAHL), 2375
Cunnilingus, 1697
Cuprimine. *See* D-penicillamine
Curanderism, 336
Curative factors, of group therapy, 35, 36*t*
Curling's ulcer, 1896, 1901
Curiosity, 2108
Cutting, 32
CVP (central venous pressure), 1412
Cyanide gas, 1895
Cyanocobalamin, recommended daily intake, 1596*t*
Cyanosis, 1218, 1309, 1339, 1350
pneumonia and, 839
Cycle of violence, 1937, 1937*t*
Cyclins, 88
Cyclooxygenase (COX), 275
Cyclooxygenase 2 (COX-2) inhibitors, 210
Cyclophosphamide, 761, 761*t*
Cyclosporine, 561–562, 761*t*
Cyclothymic disorder:
diagnostic criteria, 1177, 1178*t*
manifestations, 1180

Cymbalta, 1173
Cystine stones, 467*t*
Cystitis:
manifestations of, 874*t*, 875
Nursing Care Plan
assessment, 879*t*
critical thinking, 879*t*
diagnoses, 879*t*
evaluation, 879*t*
planning and implementation, 879*t*
urinary tract infections and, 872
Cystoscopy, 469, 876
Cysts, 1878*t*
Cytokines, 155, 681, 708*t*
Cytologic examination, 125–126, 164
Cytomegalovirus (CMV), 706*t*, 714*t*
Cytoplasm, 86
Cytotoxic cells, 677*t*, 679, 679*f*, 681. *See also*
T lymphocytes (T cells)
Cytoxan. *See* Cyclophosphamide

D

Damages, 2400
Darkness, sleep and, 666
DASH diet, 1429, 1429*t*
Data:
clustering, 2068–2069
comparing against standards, 2068, 2069*t*
comparing with outcomes, 2099
constant, 2054
identifying gaps or inconsistencies in, 2069
objective, 2054, 2054*t*
organization, 2059–2061, 2061*t*
sources, 2054–2055
subjective, 2054, 2054*t*
types of, 2054
validation, 2064–2065, 2064*t*
Data analysis, 2068–2069, 2387
Data collection, 2052, 2054–2055, 2054*t*, 2387
for evaluation, 2099
methods, 2055–2059, 2056*t*
Database, 2052
of POMR, 2186
Date rape, 1950, 1970–1971, 2462
Dating violence, 2461–2462, 2462*t*
Dawn phenomenon, 992
Daypro. *See* Oxaprozin
Daytrana, 373*t*
DBT. *See* Dialectical behavior therapy
DC1s, 678
DC2s, 678
Deaconess groups, 2287
Dead space, 1477
Death and dying. *See also* End-of-life care; Grief
and loss
accidental, 2457–2458
approaching, 298
Assessment Interview, 298*t*
beliefs related to, 1774
caring for the, 2034, 2285
Case Study, 621
children, 293–296
children's experience of, 613
books for, 612*t*
by developmental age, 613

factors influencing family response, 611–612
of friend, 611
other significant losses, 611
children's response to
assessment, 613–614
Assessment Interview, 614t
diagnosis, 614
evaluation, 614
planning and implementation, 614
comfort for dying patient, 618t
due to medical errors, 2443
Dying Person's Bill of Rights, 290t
faith-based beliefs and, 612
family response, 615
of grandparent, 611
leading causes of, 289
adolescents, 2018t
children, 2016t
older adults, 2023t
loss from, 600
of loved one, 600
manifestations, 617t, 619, 619t
as natural process, 257
nurse's response to, 615–617, 619
nursing diagnoses and interventions
fear, 620–621
risk for compromised dignity, 620
nursing process
assessment, 620
diagnosis, 620
evaluation, 621
planning and implementation, 620–621
overview, 615
of parent, 609, 611
physiological changes in dying client
altered level of consciousness, 619
anorexia, nausea, and dehydration, 618
dyspnea, 618
hypotension, 619
pain, 618
postmortem care, 619
related to substance abuse, 68
spiritual beliefs and, 612
state of awareness about, 298
support for client and family, 619
traumatic injury leading to, 1941
Death anxiety, 299, 613
Debridement, 1897, 1924
definition, 886
Decade of Behavior, 2332
Decerebrate posturing, 957t
Decibels, 1651
Decidua, 1528
Deciduous teeth, 657
Decision making, 2119–2120, 2120t
about, 2037–2038
assessment process and, 2045
barriers to, 2042
compared with critical thinking and problem
solving, 2041t
conditions, 2041–2042
decision-making process, 2040–2043, 2041t, 2043t
compared with nursing process, 2043t
steps in, 2043
defined, 2037
developmental considerations and, 2042t

diagnosis and, 2045
ethical, 2308, 2311, 2311f, 2311t
evaluation and, 2046
group, 2039–2040
identifying need for, 2040, 2041t
implementation phase and, 2045–2046, 2046t
individual, 2039
nursing practice and, 2046
planning and, 2039, 2045
processes, 2425
as response to change, 2038–2039
styles, 2039, 2039t
Decision support systems. See Clinical decision
support (CDS) systems
Decision-making methods, 2136, 2138, 2138t
Decisions, types of, 2040
Declaration of Patient Rights, 2318–2319t
Declarative memory, 240
Decode, 2149
Decompensation, 1404
Decorticate posturing, 957t
Decubitus ulcers. See Pressure ulcers
Deductibles, 2211
Deductive reasoning, 2106
Deep brain stimulation, 1137
Deep coma, 946t
Deep palpation, 2002–2003, 2003f
Deep sleep, 666
Deep venous thrombosis:
Case Study, 1397
Client Teaching, 1395t
collaborative care
clinical therapies, 1394
diagnostic tests, 1391
pharmacologic therapies, 1392
prophylaxis, 1392
surgery, 1392
definition, 1096, 1390
etiology, 1390–1391
locations, 1390f
manifestations, 1097, 1391, 1391t
Nursing Care Plan
assessment, 1396t
critical thinking, 1396t
diagnosis, 1396t
evaluation, 1396t
planning and implementation, 1396t
nursing diagnoses and interventions
impaired physical mobility, 1395
ineffective protection, 1395
ineffective tissue perfusion, peripheral,
1394–1395
pain, 1394
risk for ineffective tissue perfusion,
cardiopulmonary, 1395, 1397
nursing process
assessment, 1394
diagnosis, 1394
evaluation, 1397
planning and implementation, 1394–1397
physiology, 1390
precursors, 1097t
risk factors, 1391, 1391t
treatment, 1097
Defecation:
definition, 423

Defense mechanisms, 34, 343
Defensive responses, 2159t
Defibrillation, 1449, 1449f
Deficient knowledge, 2258, 2438, 2258–2260
Defining characteristics, 2066
Deformation, 1144
Degenerative joint disease. See Osteoarthritis (OS)
Dehiscence, 898, 1929
Dehydration. See also Fluid volume deficit
in children, 570–571, 574–575, 574t
definition, 521, 569
in dying client, 618
hypertonic, 570
hypotonic, 569
isotonic, 569
risk factors, 571, 572t
symptoms, 572t
Dehydroepiandrosterone (DHEA), 219
Delavirdine, 713
Delayed grief, 606
Delayed union, 1097
Delegate:
acceptance of delegation by, 2220–2221
defined, 2217
unwilling, 2222
Delegated care, supervision of, 2098
Delegation, 2092
acceptance of, 2220–2221
vs. assignment, 2218
benefits of, 2218–2219
Case Study, 2224
clinical example, 2220
decision tree for, 2223f
defined, 2217
vs. dumping, 2218
factors affecting, 2220–2222
ineffective, 2222
key behaviors for, 2220t
liability and, 2222–2224
obstacles to, 2221, 2221t
delegator insecurity, 2221–2222
nonsupportive environment, 2221
unwilling delegate, 2222
overview, 2217
principles of, 2217–2218
principles used to decide whether to use, 2218t
process, 2219
decide on the delegate, 2219
describe the task, 2219
determine the task, 2219
monitor performance and provide feedback, 2220
reach agreement, 2219
reverse, 2222
skills, 2208
tasks that may and may not be delegated, 2218t
tools for successful, 2217t
Delegator, 2217
Delirium, 206, 226
alcohol withdrawal, 30t, 43
clinical manifestations, 227
compared with dementia, 211, 212t
Nursing Care Plan, 229t
assessment, 229t
critical thinking and nursing process, 230t
diagnosis, 229t
ethical dilemma, 229t

evaluation, 229t
    expected outcomes, 229t
    planning and implementation, 229t
  nursing process
    assessment, 227
  risk factors, 226
  therapeutic environment for, 230t
Delirium tremens (DTs), 29t, 30t, 42t, 43
Delphi technique, 2137, 2138t
Delta cells, 980, 989
Delta sleep, 666
Delta-9-tetrahydrocannabinol (THC), 71
Delusions, 232, 239, 240
  types of, 240t
Delusions of control, 240
Delusions of grandeur, 240
Delusions of persecution, 240
Demadex. See Torsemide
Dementia:
  alcoholic, 43
  Alzheimer's type. See Alzheimer's disease
  causes, 206, 206t
  characteristics of, 211
  communication and, 2161t
  compared with delirium, 211, 212t
  compared with depression, 216t
  deficits associated with, 207t
  definition, 206
  frontotemporal, 206t
  incidence, 206
  Lewy body, 206t
  in Parkinson's disease, 1136, 1136t
  pathophysiology and etiology, 226–227
  sleep disorders and, 312
  vascular, 206t
Dementia Symptoms Scale, 207t
Demerol, 1866
Deming, W. Edwards, 2426
Democratic leaders, 2234, 2234t
Demographics, changes in, and health care
    delivery, 2342
Demography, 2283–2284
Dendritic cells, 678
Denial, 34
Denial stage, of grief, 602t
Denominations, 1783
Dental caries, 656, 658t, 659
Dentin, 656
Dentists, 2116t
Dentures, 660
Denver II, 2013t
Denver Developmental Screening Test II
    (DDSTII), 958t
Deontological theories, 1777
Deoxyribonucleic acid (DNA), 86–88
Depade, 45
Depakene, 1174t
Depakote, 217, 1174
Department of Health and Human Services
    (DHHS), 2333, 2340, 2362, 2364, 2364t
Depen Titratable. See D-penicillamine
Dependence, 28
Dependent functions, 2067
Dependent interventions, 2089
Dependent personality disorder:
  characteristics, 1619
  diagnostic criteria, 1618t
  manifestations, 1611t

Depersonalization, 1613, 1843
Depo-Provera, 1733
Depolarization, 1305–1306
Depressed episodes, 1179, 1180t, 1197t, 1199t
Depressed fractures, 1094f, 1095t
Depression:
  alcoholism and, 40
  in Alzheimer's disease, 215
  caring interventions
    assertive behavior, 1169
    minimizing maladaptive dependence, 1169
    preventing suicide and promoting safety,
      1169, 1169t
  Case Study, 1195
  in children and adolescents, 1190t, 1193
  collaborative care, 1190
  comorbidity with, 1158
  compared with dementia, 216t
  definition, 1160t
  developmental considerations, 1190t
  diabetes mellitus and, 999
  diagnostic criteria, 1187–1188t
  double, 1159
  dysthymic disorder. See Dysthymic disorder
  gender differences in, 1163
  vs. grief, 1167t
  life events and, 1163f
  major. See Major depressive disorder (MDD)
  manifestations, 1186
  measures
    Beck Depression Inventory, 1165–1166
  nonpharmacologic therapies
    alternative therapies, 1175–1177
    cognitive-behavioral therapy, 1175, 1189t, 1190
    electroconvulsive therapy, 1189t,
      1191–1192, 1191t
    interpersonal psychotherapy, 1191
    psychotherapy, 1174, 1190
  Nursing Care Plan
    assessment, 1194t
    critical thinking, 1194t
    diagnosis, 1194t
    evaluation, 1194t
    planning and implementation, 1194t
  nursing diagnoses and interventions
    hopelessness, 1195
    self-esteem, 1194–1195
  nursing process
    assessment, 1192–1193, 1193t
    diagnosis, 1193
    evaluation, 1195
    planning and implementation, 1193, 1195
  in older adults, 207, 1190t
  overview, 1186
  in Parkinson's disease, 1136
  pharmacologic therapies
    antidepressants, 1170–1171, 1190
    MAOIs, 1172–1173
    SSRIs, 1171–1172, 1189t
  physical complaints and, 1192t
  postpartum. See Postpartum depression
  risk factors, 1186
    childhood sexual abuse, 1163
    gender, 1163
  seasonal affective disorder, 1189
  seasonal pattern, 1188t
  situational. See Situational depression
  sleep disorders and, 311–312

theories of
    genetic links, 1160
    overview, 1160
    treatments, 1160t
Depression stage, of grief, 602t
Derealization, 1613
Dermatitis, 1885t
  contact. See Contact dermatitis
Dermatomes, 263, 943, 944f, 1362
Dermis, 1875
Deroxat, 1201
DES (diethylstilbstrol), 1709t
Desaturated blood, 1309
Desire phase, 1697
Desired outcome statements, 2087
Desired outcomes:
  for client, 2088t
  components of, 2087, 2088t
  defined, 2085
  deriving from nursing diagnoses, 2085t
  goals, 2085
  guidelines for writing, 2089
  identification of, 2090–2091t, 2102–2103t
  indicators and, 2086
  NOCs and, 2086
  purposes of, 2086, 2098
  relationship to nursing diagnoses, 2087
  revision of, 2101
Desyrel, 217
Detached retina, 1662, 1663t
Detection of Autism by Infant Sociability
    Interview (DAISI), 382t
Detoxification, 30t
Detrol, 443
Detrusor muscles, 411, 433
Development, 339
  about, 339–369
  across age span, 2012
  adolescence, 364–366
  in adulthood, 366–368
  cognitive, 2247
  communication skills and, 2155
  definition, 340
  differentiated, 340
  infants, 354–357, 355t
  influences on
    cultural, 342
    environment, 342
    family and parenting, 342
    genetics, 340, 341
    health, 342
    nutrition, 342
    prenatal, 341
    psychosocial, 343
  instruments to assess, 2013t
  middle age, 2012
  moral, 350–353, 352t
  preschool age, 359–361
  puberty, 2012
  school-age children, 362–364
  spiritual, 353, 353t, 354t
  stages of, 340, 341t
  theories of
    adult, 345–346
    application to nursing practice, 368
    behaviorism, 347
    continuity theory, 347
    disengagement theory, 347

ecologic theory, 350, 351f
Erikson, 344–345, 344t
Freudian, 343t, 343–344
Gould, 346
Havigurst, 345, 346t
Jung, 347
Peck, 345–346
Piaget's theory of cognitive development, 347, 348t, 360t
psychosocial, 345–347
resiliency theory, 350
social learning theory, 347–348
temperament theory, 349–350
Vygotsky, 345
toddlers, 357–359
young adulthood, 2012
Developmental Checklist-Early Screen (DBC-ES), 382t
Developmental considerations:
anticipatory guidance, 2440t
assessment of children, 2064t
communicating with children, 2155t
communicating with older adults, 2160t
diagnosis, 2076t
establishing rapport with children, 2176t
evaluation, 2101t
hazards throughout life span, 2434t
health care decisions, 2042t
long-term care, 2194t
nursing care plans, 2095t
Developmental Disabilities Act, 205
Developmental disability, 201
Developmental factors, impacting assessment, 2006
Developmental losses, 600
Developmental milestones, 354, 2009
adolescence, 364t
infancy, 355t, 2014
preschool age, 359t
school-age years, 362t
toddlerhood, 357t
Developmental stages, 340
Developmental tasks, 345, 346t
Developmental theories, 2061
Dexamethasone suppression test, 129t
Dexedrine, 373t
DextroStat, 373t
DHA (docosahexaenoic acid), 892t
DHEA (Dehydroepiandrosterone), 219
DHSS. See Department of Health and Human Services (DHHS)
DHT (dihydrotestosterone), 432
Diabetes mellitus:
blood glucose homeostasis, 989–990, 990f
cardiovascular system and, 997–998
Case Study, 1015
in children, 1008, 1009t
collaborative care
blood glucose monitoring, 1001–1002
diagnostic tests, 1000–1002
exercise, 1007
management monitoring, 1000–1001
nutrition, 1005–1006
pharmacologic therapies, 1002–1005, 1002t, 1003t
sick-day management, 1006–1007
surgery, 1007–1008
complications, 993t, 994t
acute, 992–997

chronic, 997–1000
neuropathy, 1679
coping and, 1012–1014
coronary artery disease and, 1365, 1373
definition, 989
description, 983t
developmental considerations, 1009t
gestational, 989, 992, 1002
hyperglycemia
dawn phenomenon, 992
diabetic ketoacidosis, 993t, 995–996, 995f
hyperosmolar hyperglycemic state (HHS), 996
Somogyi phenomenon, 995
hypoglycemia, 993t, 996–997
Multisystem Effects, 994t
Nursing Care Plan
assessment, 1013t
critical thinking, 1014t
diagnosis, 1013t
evaluation, 1013t
planning and implementation, 1013t
nursing diagnoses and interventions
ineffective coping, 1012, 1014
risk for impaired skin integrity, 1010–1011
risk for infection, 1011
risk for injury, 1012
sexual dysfunction, 1012
nursing process
assessment, 1008
diagnosis, 1009
evaluation, 1014
implementation, 1009–1014
planning, 1009
older adults and, 1008, 1009t
overview, 989–990
risk of infection and, 775–776
role of hormones in, 989
sexual dysfunction and, 1694
stroke and, 1501
type 1. See Type 1 diabetes mellitus
type 2. See Type 2 diabetes mellitus
types of, 989
Diabetic ketoacidosis (DKA), 993t, 995–996, 995f
causes, 11
pharmacologic therapies, 12
Diabetic nephropathy:
chronic renal failure and, 553t
nephritis and, 924
Diabetic neuropathies, 998–999
Diabetic retinopathy, 998
ethnicity and, 1649t
Diagnosis. See also Nursing diagnosis
decision making and, 2045
defined, 2065
developmental considerations, 2076t
nursing diagnoses, 2065
in nursing process, 2050t, 2065–2069, 2065f, 2071–2074, 2076, 2076t
Diagnosis-related group (DRG) codes, 2184
Diagnosis-related groups (DRGs), 2081, 2122, 2184, 2211, 2282, 2343
Diagnostic and Statistical Manual of Mental Disorders (DSM-IV-TR), 66
Diagnostic labels, 2065–2066
Diagnostic peritoneal lavage, 1942
Diagnostic process:
analyzing data, 2068–2069
critical thinking in, 2068

formulating diagnostic statements, 2071–2073
identifying health problems, risks, and strengths, 2071
use of, 2068
Diagnostic reasoning, avoiding errors in, 2074
Diagnostic Review Committee, 2076
Diagnostic statements:
evaluating quality of, 2073
formulating, 2071–2073
guidelines for writing, 2074t
one-part, 2072–2073
revision of, 2101
three-part, 2072, 2073t
two-part, 2071–2072, 2072t
variations on, 2073
Diagnostic tests:
acid–base imbalances, 8, 9t
acute renal failure, 540
alcohol abuse, 44
anemia, 101
anxiety disorders, 1814
appendicitis, 894
asthma, 1258
for benign prostatic hypertrophy, 434
bowel elimination, 430
breast cancer, 109
burns, 1900
cancer, 92, 125–130
cardiac disorders, 1326
cardiomyopathy, 1335
cellulitis, 810
chlamydias, 1760
chronic obstructive pulmonary disease (COPD), 1272
chronic renal failure, 558
cirrhosis, 1019–1020
colorectal cancer, 143
congenital heart defects, 1351, 1352–1353t
conjunctivitis, 815
coronary artery disease, 1370–1372
deep venous thrombosis, 1391
discomfort, 260
disseminated intravascular coagulation, 1399
dysrhythmias, 1448–1449
eating disorders, 1602
endocrine system, 987
erectile dysfunction, 1714
fatigue, 302
fibromyalgia, 306–307
fluid and electrolyte balance, 531
fluid volume deficit, 575
fluid volume excess, 582
fractures, 1098
gallstones, 903–904, 904t
genital herpes, 1758
glaucoma, 1670
gonorrhea, 1760
heart failure, 1411
herniated disk, 1082
hip fractures, 1112
HIV/AIDS, 709–710
hypersensitivity, 735–736
hypertension, 1427–1428
hyperthyroidism, 1044
hypothyroidism, 1050
immune system, 695
for increased intracranial pressure, 963
infectious diseases, 804–805

infertility, 1734
inflammation, 890, 891t
inflammatory bowel disease, 914
leukemia, 153, 154t
lung cancer, 164
macular degeneration, 1677
melanoma, 188
menopause, 1743
menstrual dysfunction, 1749
mental retardation, 202
metabolic alkalosis, 16
mood disorders, 1170
multiple sclerosis, 1120
musculoskeletal system, 1076–1077, 1077t
for nephritis, 926
neurologic system, 958–959
for nutritional assessment, 662
obsessive-compulsive disorder, 1831
osteoarthritis, 1127
osteoporosis, 1036
otitis media, 828
pain, 273
Parkinson's disease, 1137
for peptic ulcer disease, 933
peripheral neuropathy, 1681
peripheral vascular disease, 1464–1465
pneumonia, 841
pregnancy, 1570, 1571t
prostate cancer, 170
pulmonary embolism, 1479
rape, 1973
respiratory acidosis, 19
respiratory syncytial virus (RSV)/bronchiolitis,
    1282–1283
rheumatoid arthritis, 748
scoliosis, 1087
seizure disorders, 970
sensory perception, 1645
sepsis, 852
sexuality, 1710
shock, 1490
sickle cell disorder, 179
for skin, 1884
spinal cord injury, 1148
stroke, 1505
substance abuse, 32, 75
syphilis, 1762
systemic lupus erythematosus (SLE), 760
trauma, 1941–1942
for urinary calculi, 468–469
urinary system, 420, 421–422t
urinary tract infections, 875–876
Diagnostics, computerized, 2392
Diagonal conjugate, 1517
Dialectical behavior therapy (DBT), 1619
Dialogue, 2109
Dialysate, 543
Dialysis:
  in chronic renal failure, 559–560
  complications, 560
  continuous renal replacement therapy,
      543–545, 545t
  definition, 416, 543
  evidence-based research, 567
  hemodialysis, 416, 543–544, 543f, 559–560, 567
  nursing care, 544t, 547t

peritoneal, 416, 543, 546, 547t, 559–560
  vascular access, 545–546
Diamox, 1670, 1671t
Diaphysis, 1728–1729, 1729f
Diaphysis:
  osteoporosis and, 1034
Diarrhea:
  causes, 427t
  definition, 426
  dehydration from, 571
  in inflammatory bowel disease, 920
  treatment, 427t
Diastasis recti, 1544
Diastole, 1296, 1302–1303
Diastolic blood pressure, 1308, 1422
Diathermy, 1131
Diazepam, 959, 971, 1814–1815
DIC (disseminated intravascular coagulation), 626
DIC. See Disseminated intravascular coagulation
    (DIC)
Dickens, Charles, 2289
Diclofenac, 749t
Didanosine, 712t
Diencephalon, 940
Diet:
  blood pressure and, 1424
  cancer risk and, 121
  coronary artery disease and, 1366, 1372–1373,
      1373t, 1383
  cultural influences on, 663t
  hypertension and, 1429
  low-residue, 918t
  obesity and, 1029
  religious beliefs concerning, 1773
  sleep and, 669
Diet recall, 663
Dietary guidelines, 1593t
Dietary Guidelines for Americans, 663
Dietary reference intakes (DRIs), 1595
Diethylstilbestrol (DES), 1709t
Dieticians, 2116t
Differentiated practice, 2206
Differentiation, 88
Diffusion, 520–521, 521f
  cellular transportation method of, 86t
  simple, 1533
Digital rectal examination (DRE), 436
Digitalis:
  administration, 1414–1415t
  in specific conditions
    heart failure, 1415
Digoxin, 1331t, 1414–1415t, 1449, 1450t
Dihydrotestosterone (DHT), 432
Dilantin, 959, 971
Dilated cardiomyopathy, 1333–1334, 1333t
Dilation and curettage (D&C), 1734, 1750
Diphenhydramine, 737, 739
Diphtheria vaccine, 687
Diplegia, 386t
Diploid number, 1720
Diphtheria, in children, 791t
Direct auscultation, 2004
Direct Coombs' test, 736
Direct percussion, 2003, 2004f
Direct-purchase health insurance, 2369

Directing, 2143
Directive interviews, 2056
Dirty wounds, 1879
Disaccharides, 1593
Disalcid. See Salsalate, 676
Disaster plans, 2354
Disaster-related eye injuries, 2352t
Disasters:
  defined, 2351
  site-specific disaster zones, 2356
  types of, 2352t, 2353t
Discharge instructions, 2376
Discharge planning, 2077
Discipline, 492
Discoid lesions:
  systemic lupus erythematosus (SLE) and, 757, 760
Discomfort. See also Comfort; Pain
  definition, 256
  therapies for, 260, 261t
Discovery, 2417
Discovery-oriented learning, 2248
Discovery/problem-solving technique, 2265
Discrimination, 398
  based on age, 401
  based on sexual orientation, 400
Discussion, 2182
Disease:
  cultural views on, 791
  definition, 638
  vs. illness, 638
Disease model of addiction, 28
Disease prevention:
  vs. health promotion, 641
  vs. health protection, 640
Disease surveillance, 791
Disease susceptibility, 327
Disease-modifying drugs, 748–749, 750t
Disease-modifying osteoarthritis drugs
    (DMOADs), 1127
Disenfranchised grief, 606, 622t
Disengaged families, 495
Disengagement theory, 347
Disinfectants:
  chain of infection and, 777
  common, 778t
Diskectomy, 1083
Dismissal, 2237
Disorientation, 946t
Disruptive Behavior Disorder Scale, 371t
Dissatisfaction problems, 1703
Disseminated intravascular coagulation (DIC), 626
  Case Study, 1403
  Client Teaching, 1403t
  collaborative care
    clinical therapies, 1399, 1400t
    diagnostic tests, 1399
  definition, 1398
  etiology, 1398
  manifestations, 1399, 1400t
  Nursing Care Plan
    assessment, 1402t
    critical thinking, 1402t
    diagnoses, 1402t
    evaluation, 1402t
    planning and implementation, 1402t

nursing diagnoses and interventions
  fear, 1402–1403
  impaired gas exchange, 1401
  ineffective tissue perfusion, 1401
  pain, 1401–1402
nursing process
  assessment, 1401
  diagnosis, 1401
  evaluation, 1403
  overview, 1399
  planning and implementation, 1401–1403
physiology, 1398, 1398f
risk factors, 1398–1399, 1399t
Dissociation, 1948
Dissociative identity disorder (DDI), child sexual abuse and, 1948
Dissonance, 2108
Distorted thought, corrective statements for, 1623t
Distracted driving, 2440f, 2440t
Distributive shock, 1489, 1492t
Disulfiram (Antabuse), 45
Ditropan, 443
Diuresis, 416, 538
Diuretics, 533t
  administration, 1414t
  for increased intracranial pressure, 959t, 963, 963t
  mechanism of action, 1330t
  nursing considerations, 1330t
  sexual functioning and, 1701t
  in specific conditions
    acute renal failure, 541t
    cirrhosis, 1020
    glaucoma, 1670
    heart failure, 1413
    hypertension, 1429
  for urinary elimination, 423, 423t
Diurnal enuresis, 417
Divalproex, 1174
Diversity, 397–398
  about, 397–406
  case study, 406
  as concept in provision of health services, 405–406t, 406
  definition, 398
  factors contributing to, 398
    age, 401, 401–402t
    education, abilities, and life experiences, 402–403
    gender, 399–400
    sexual orientation, 400–401
  Nursing Care Plan, 405t
    assessment, 405t
    critical thinking in the nursing process, 406t
    diagnosis, 405t
    evaluation, 405t
    implementation, 405t
    planning, 405t
  race and, 404
  sources of, 398–399
Diverticula, 433
Dix, Dorothea, 2288
Dizygotic twins, 1530, 1531f
DKA (diabetic ketoacidosis), 993t, 995–996, 995f
DMOADs. See Disease-modifying osteoarthritis drugs (DMOADs)

DMSA scanning:
  urinary tract infections and, 876
DNA (deoxyribonucleic acid), 86–87. See also Genetics
DNRs. See Do-not-resuscitate orders (DNRs)
Do Not Use list, 2196, 2198t
Do-not-intubate (DNI) orders, 296
Do-not-resuscitate orders (DNRs), 290, 290t, 296, 2314
Dobutamine, 1943
Dock, Lavinia L., 2291
Docosahexaenoic acid (DHA), 892t
Document holder, 2384t
Documentation:
  automated, 2376–2377
  Case Study, 2200
  do's and don'ts of, 2199t
  ethical and legal considerations, 2183
  Evidence-Based Practice, 2199t
  facility specific, 2194–2195, 2195t
  home care, 2195, 2195t
  long-term care, 2194–2195, 2194t, 2195t
  nursing, 2402
  of nursing activities, 2098, 2192–2194, 2193t
  overview, 2182–2183
  purposes of client records, 2183–2184
  recording guidelines, 2195–2199, 2196–2198t, 2199t
  systems, 2184
    case management, 2191–2192, 2192f
    charting by exception, 2189, 2189f
    computerized, 2189–2190, 2192t
    focus charting, 2187, 2188f, 2189
    PIE model, 2187
    problem-oriented medical records, 2185–2187
    source-oriented records, 2184–2185, 2185t
  of teaching process, 2268
  variance, 2192f
Documenting, 2182
Domestic partners, 2369
Domestic violence shelters, 1957
Domestic violence, 2458–2459. See also Intimate partner violence
Donepezil (Aricept), 217
Dong quai, 1744t
Dopamine, 666–667, 1608
  addiction and, 28
  nicotine and, 51
  in specific conditions
    acute renal failure, 542
    heart failure, 1415t
    myocardial infarction, 1376
    traumatic injury, 1943
  substance abuse and, 67
Dopamine agonists:
  in specific conditions
    Parkinson's disease, 1138t
Dopamine system stabilizers, 243
Dopaminergics, 1138t
Dopar, 243
Doppler ultrasound, 1465
Doppler ultrasound stethoscope (DUS), 1318, 1318f, 1321
Dorsal recumbent position, 2002t
Dorzolamide (Trusopt), 1670, 1671t

Dostinex, 1735t
Double-blind research, 2328t
Double depression, 1159
Doulas, 1200
Down syndrome, 201–202, 202t, 203t
  characteristics, 1720, 1721t, 1722f
  incidence, 1721t
  structural abnormalities and, 1722
Downregulation, 28
Doxazosin (Cardura), 434
Dramatic play, 361
DRD2 A1 allele gene, 41
DRE (digital rectal examination), 436
DRGs. See Diagnosis-related groups (DRGs)
Dreams, 667
Dressler syndrome, 1369
DRIs. See Dietary reference intakes (DRIs)
Droplet nuclei:
  transmission of infection and, 773
  tuberculosis and, 857
Drug Abuse Warning Network (DAWN), 73
Drug Enforcement Administration, 68
Drug schedules, 2406t
Dry powder inhaler (DPI), 1259, 1259t, 1273
Dry skin, 1914t
DSM-IV-TR diagnostic criteria:
  ADHD, 372t
  anorexia nervosa, 1599t
  Asperger disorder, 381t
  autistic disorder, 381t
  binge-eating disorder, 1601t
  bipolar disorders, 1178t
  bulimia nervosa, 1600t
  depressive disorders, 1187t
  generalized anxiety disorder, 1811t
  mental retardation, 203t
  obsessive-compulsive disorder, 1829t
  personality disorders, 1608t
    cluster A, 1612t
    cluster B, 1614t
    cluster C, 1618t
  post-traumatic stress disorder, 1844t
  schizophrenia, 236t, 236
  substance abuse vs. substance dependence, 67t
DTap, 687
Dual diagnosis, 30t, 40
Duchenne muscular dystrophy, 1076t
Ductous venosus, 1534
Ductus arteriosus, 1534
Duke University, 2335
Duloxetine, 1173
Dullness, 2004, 2004t
Dunlop traction, 1106t
Duodenal ulcers, 931
Duplex Doppler ultrasound, 1465
Duplex venous ultrasonography, 1391
Dupuytren's contracture, 1069f
Durable power of attorney, 290, 2410
Duragesic, 287t
Duration, of sound, 2005
Dutasteride (Avodart), 434, 434t
Duty, 2399
DVDs, 2375
DVT. See Deep venous thrombosis
Dwarfism, 986t

Dying. *See* Death and dying
Dysarthria, 1504
Dyscalculia, 201
Dysfunctional families:
  personality disorders and, 1609
Dysfunctional uterine bleeding (DUB):
  amenorrhea, 1748
  causes, 1748
  Client Teaching, 1751*t*
  collaborative care, 1749
  definition, 1748
  diagnostic tests, 1750
  menorrhagia, 1748
  metrorrhagia, 1748
  nursing care, 1752
  nursing diagnoses and interventions
    anxiety, 1754
    sexual dysfunction, 1754
  oligomenorrhea, 1748
  postmenopausal bleeding, 1748
  risk factors, 1749
Dysgraphia, 201
Dyslexia, 201
Dysmenorrhea:
  definition, 1693, 1748
  diagnostic tests, 1750
  etiology, 1748
  manifestations, 1749, 1749*t*
  nursing care, 1752
  pharmacologic therapies, 1750
Dyspareunia, 1694
Dysphagia, 207*t*, 1512
Dysplasia, 88
Dysplastic nevi, 184–185
Dyspnea, 582, 1221
  during pregnancy, 1575*t*
  in dying client, 618
  pneumonia and, 839
Dyspraxia, 201
Dysrhythmias:
  acute myocardial infarction and, 1368–1369
  assessment, 1316*t*
  atrioventricular (AV) conduction blocks
    characteristics, 1443–1444*t*
    pathophysiology, 1446–1448
  cardiomyopathy and, 1334, 1335*t*
  Case Study, 1461
  causes, 1438
  characteristics, 1441–1444*t*
  in children, 1439*t*
  Client Teaching, 1457*t*
  collaborative care
    cardiac mapping, 1454
    catheter ablation, 1454
    countershock, 1449
    diagnostic tests, 1448–1449
    implantable cardioverter-defibrillator, 1452
    other therapies, 1454
    pacemaker therapy, 1450–1452, 1452*t*,
      1453*t*, 1459*t*
    pharmacologic therapies, 1449
  definition, 1319, 1438
  description, 1314*t*
  developmental considerations, 1439*t*
  heart failure and, 1416
  intraventricular conduction blocks, 1448
  junctional, 1445
  manifestations, 1447*t*

  medications for, 1376, 1416
  Nursing Care Plan
    assessment, 1460*t*
Dysthymic disorder:
  definition, 1159, 1188
  diagnostic criteria, 1187*t*
  incidence, 1189
  manifestations, 1189*t*
  symptoms, 1189
  treatments, 1189*t*
Dystoninas, 243
Dysuria, 417, 417*t*
  urinary tract infections and, 874

E

e-health, 672*t*, 2251, 2383
E-mail, 2150, 2152–2153
Early pregnancy factor (EPF), 1527
Ears. *See also* Hearing
  age-related changes in, 1635, 1636*t*
  assessment, 1643–1644*t*
  diagnostic tests, 1646
  external, 1632, 1636*t*
  injuries, 1637
  inner ear, 1632s–1633, 1636*t*
  middle ear, 1632, 1636*t*
  normal presentation, 1632, 1633
  parts of, 1633*t*
Earthquake-related injuries, 2352*t*
Easter, 1781
Eating disorders:
  anorexia nervosa. *See* Anorexia nervosa
  binge-eating disorder. *See* Binge-eating disorder
  bulimia nervosa. *See* Bulimia nervosa
  Case Study, 1606
  Client Teaching, 1604*t*
  collaborative care
    clinical therapy, 1602
    diagnostic tests, 1602
    overview, 1602
  definition, 1584
  description, 1585*t*
  incidence, 1599
  manifestations, 1599–1601, 1601*t*
  nocturnal sleep-related eating disorder, 1585
  nursing diagnoses and interventions
    enhancing body image, 1604
    facilitating coping, 1604
    improving self-esteem, 1606
    managing fluids and electrolytes, 1606
  nursing process
    assessment, 1602–1603, 1602*t*
    diagnosis, 1603
    evaluation, 1606
    overview, 1602
    planning and implementation, 1603–1604, 1606
  overview, 1593
  pathophysiology and etiology, 1597–1599
  pharmacologic therapies, 1592
  Prader-Willi syndrome (PWS), 1585
  purging disorder, 1585
  risk factors, 1599
  theories on
    behavioral theory, 1598
    cognitive theory, 1598
    family factors, 1598–1599
    gender, 1599

    genetics, 1598
    intrapersonal factors, 1598
    neurobiology, 1598
    treatments, 1585*t*
EBP. *See* Evidence-based practice
ECBI (Eyberg Child Behavior Inventory), 2013*t*
Ecchymosis, 1882*t*
ECF. *See* Extracellular fluid (ECF)
Echocardiography, 1352, 1371
Echolalia, 215, 237
Echolia, 207*t*, 379
Echopraxia, 237
Eclampsia, 1468, 1470–1471
Ecologic theory, 350, 351*f*
Ecomaps, 493, 495*f*, 501, 501*f*
Economic factors, client education and, 2255
Economics, of nursing, 2215–2216, 2282
ECRI Institute, 2335
Ecstasy, 60, 68, 73
ECT. *See* Electroconvulsive therapy (ECT)
Ectoderm, 126*t*, 1528, 1529*t*
Ectopic beats, 1440
Ectopic functioning:
  laboratory indicators of, 137*t*
ED. *See* Erectile dysfunction (ED)
Edecrin, 959*t*, 963
Edema, 1880, 1883*f*, 1916. *See also* Fluid
      volume excess
  causes, 580–582, 580*t*
  definition, 529
  during pregnancy, 1574*t*
  grading pitting, 584*f*
  heart failure and, 1408
  palpating for, 584*f*
  pathophysiology and etiology, 579–581
  pulmonary, 1404–1405, 1407
  in specific conditions
    asthma, 1252–1253
Edinburgh Postnatal Depression Scale, 1202, 1203*t*
Edmonton Symptom Assessment System, 281
Education, specialized, 2280
Education for All Handicapped Children Act
      (PL 94-142), 205, 205*t*
Education levels
  of clients, 402
  of nurses, 2330, 2330*t*
Education path, 2125*t*
Education programs, 2327
Educational bias, 403
EEG. *See* Electroencephalogram (EEG), 318
Efavirenz, 713
Effective leadership, 2235, 2235*t*
Effectiveness, 2144
Effector cells, 679*f*, 681. *See also* T lymphocytes
      (T cells)
Efferent ducts, 1687
Effexor, 1173
Efficiency, 2144
Ego, 343
Ego defense mechanisms:
  compensation, 1803*t*
  denial, 1803*t*
  displacement, 1803*t*
  identification, 1803*t*
  intellectualization, 1803*t*
  introjection, 1803*t*

minimization, 1803t
projection, 1803t
rationalization, 1803t
reaction formation, 1803t
regression, 1803t
repression, 1803t
sublimation, 1803t
substitution, 1804t
undoing, 1804t
Ego differentiation, 345
Ego preoccupation, 346
Ego transcendence, 346
Ego-syntonic, 1607
Egocentricity, 2107
Egocentrism, 360t
eHealth Initiative, 2383
EHRs. *See* Electronic health records (EHRs)
Eicosapentaenoic acid (EPA), 892t
Ejaculation, 1686–1687, 1697
    rapid, 1702
    retarded, 1702
    ejection fraction, 1303
EKG. *See* Electrocardiograms
El-depryl, 217
Elasticity of the arterial wall, 1319
Elastin, 1875
Elbow replacement, 1130
Elder abuse:
    assessment, 1959
    cultural perceptions of, 1945–1946
    definition, 1945
    incidence, 1945
    institutional, 1945
    mandatory reporting of, 2413, 2414t
    manifestations, 1954t, 1956–1957
    Nursing Care Plan
        assessment, 1961t
        critical thinking, 1962t
        diagnosis, 1961t
        evaluation, 1961
        planning and implementation, 1961t
    nursing interventions, 1943
    perpetrators of, 1945
    self-neglect, 1945
    statistics on, 1936
Elderly. *See* Older adults
Elderspeak, 2158, 2158t
Elective surgery, 895
Electric shock, 2453
Electrical activity, of heart, 1312
Electrical bone stimulation, 1103
Electrical burns, 1886–1887, 1887f, 1898
Electrical hazards, 2452–2453, 2454t
Electro-oculogram (EOG), 313
Electrocardiogram (ECG):
    changes in, during angina, 1370f
    in congenital heart defects, 1352t
    definition, 1305
    description, 1327–1328t
    interpreting, 1329t
    in specific conditions
        burns, 1900
        coronary artery disease, 1371
        dysrhythmias, 1448
        heart failure, 1411
        pulmonary embolism, 1479

Electrocardiography, 1028
Electrocautery, 1901
Electroconvulsive therapy (ECT), 245, 1175,
        1189t, 1191–1192, 1191f, 1191t
Electroencephalogram (EEG), 313
Electroencephalograph (EEG) biofeedback, 45
Electrolyte-free polyethylene glycol
        (MiraLAX), 455
Electrolytes:
    in acute renal failure, 542t
    cirrhosis and, 1021
    composition, 519f
    concentrations, 520t
    definition, 517–518
    elevated, 528t
    factors affecting balance of, 526–528
    imbalances
        calcium. *See* Hypercalcemia; Hypocalcemia
        chloride. *See* Hyperchloremia; Hypochloremia
        environmental temperature and, 528
        magnesium. *See* Hypermagnesemia;
            Hypomagnesemia
        overview, 586
        phosphate. *See* Hyperphosphatemia;
            Hypophosphatemia
        potassium. *See* Hyperkalemia; Hypokalemia
        sodium. *See* Hypernatermia; Hyponatremia
    low level of, 528t
    measurement of, 518
    normal values, 532t
    regulation
        bicarbonate, 525t
        calcium, 525t
        chloride, 525t
        magnesium, 525t
        phosphate, 525t
        potassium, 524–525, 525t
        sodium, 524, 525t
    serum, 531, 532f, 540, 558
    supplements, 533t
Electromyogram (EMG), 313, 1077
Electron beam computed tomography, 1370
Electronic claims submission, 2383
Electronic communication, 2150, 2152–2153
Electronic devices, 2444
Electronic health records (EHRs), 2378–2379
    ANA position statement on, 2392t
    benefits of, 2379, 2380t
Electronic medical records (EMRs), 2378–2379,
        2390–2393, 2391f
    ANA position statement on, 2392t
    benefits of, 2390
    concerns with, 2390–2391
Electronic medication administration, 2335
Electronic patient record (EPR), 2378
Electronic prescriptions, 2383
Electronic thermometers, 1856
Electrophysiology studies, 1448–1449
Elimination, 409–410
    about, 409–423
    alterations, 410, 416–417, 418t
    assessment, 418, 418–420t
    bowel. *See* Bowel elimination
    caring interventions, 422
    definition, 409
    diagnostic tests, 420–422, 421–422t

    normal presentation, 410–413
    pharmacologic therapies, 423, 423t
    urinary. *See* Urinary elimination
ELISA. *See* Enzyme-linked immunosorbent assay
        (ELISA), 1516
Ellwood, Paul, 2428
Ellis-van Creveld syndrome, 1076t
Emancipated minors, 2404
Embolic stroke, 1500–1501
Embolus, 1476
Embryo, 5
Embryonic development, 1535, 1538–1539, 1538f
Embryonic membranes, 1528, 1529f
Emergency, defined, 2351
Emergency assessment, 2000t
Emergency contraception, 1733, 1733t, 1973
Emergency departments, 2347t
Emergency doctrine, 2404
Emergency event care, 2355t
Emergency eye wash stations, 2365
Emergency management, responsibility for, 2355
Emergency medical responders (EMRs), 2358t
Emergency medical services (EMS) system,
        2358, 2358t
Emergency Medical Services (OEMS), 2365
Emergency medical technicians (EMTs), 2358t
Emergency Medical Treatment and Labor Act
        (EMTALA), 2347t
Emergency plans, 2355
Emergency preparedness, 2351
    bioterrorism, 2357, 2357t, 2358t
    Case Study, 2359
    collaboration and, 2358
    nursing practice, 2358–2359
    overview, 2351
    site-specific disaster zones, 2356, 2356t
Emergency response, 2353–2354
    nursing competencies for, 2355, 2355t
    phases of, 2351, 2353–2355
    responsibility for, 2355
    triage, 2356, 2356f, 2356t
Emergency surgery, 895
EMG. *See* Electromyogram (EMG)
Emigration, 886
Emotional abuse:
    of children, 1946
Emotional availability, 496
Emotional contagion, 1194
Emotional factors, impacting assessment, 2007
Emotional neglect, 1947
Emotional reactions, affecting health, 645
Emotional states, 2434
Emotional stress, sleep and, 669
Emotions:
    definition, 1157
    learning and, 2251
Emotions Anonymous, 37
Empathy, 2165, 2165t, 2174
Emphysema:
    chronic obstructive pulmonary disease (COPD)
        and, 1268
    lungs depicted in, 1269f
    patient with, 1271f
Empirical data, 2327
Empirical knowledge, 2031
Employee performance, enhancement of, 2144

Empowerment, 2033
Empyema, 835, 902
EMRs. *See* Electronic medical records (EMRs)
Enabling, 2299
Enabling behavior, 30
Enamel, 656
Enbrel. *See* Etanercept
Encoding, 2149
Enculturation, 322
End-of-life care. *See also* Death and dying
    advance directives and, 289–290
    Case Study, 301
    children, 293–296
        advance care planning, 294
        ethical issues, 295–296
        evidence-based practice, 295*t*
    for children, 616–617, 617*t*
    collaborative care
        cardiopulmonary resuscitation, 297
        clinical therapies to prolong life, 296–297
        complementary and alternative medicine, 297
        feeding tubes, 297
    comfort measures, 297*t*
    compassionate, 616*f*
    competencies, 257–258, 259*t*, 288
    cultural and religious considerations in, 292–293
    definition, 257
    do-not-resuscitate orders, 290, 290*t*, 296
    ethical considerations, 2313–2315, 2313*t*
    euthanasia and, 291
    evidence-based practice, 289*t*
    hospice care, 291–292, 292*t*
    legal and ethical issues, 289–291
    manifestations, 296, 296*t*
    medications, 618*t*
    Nursing Care Plan
        assessment, 300*t*
        critical thinking, 300*t*
        diagnosis, 300*t*
        evaluation, 300*t*
        planning and implementation, 300*t*
        nursing diagnoses and interventions
        acute or chronic pain, 299
        compromised family coping, 299–300
        death anxiety, 299
    nursing process
        assessment, 298
        diagnosis, 299
        evaluation, 300
        planning and implementation, 299–300
    overview, 288
    palliative care, 291, 293–294, 294*t*
    pathophysiology and etiology, 289
End-of-life decisions, role of nurse in, 2412
End-stage renal disease (ESRD), 552. *See also*
        Chronic renal failure
Endarterectomy, 1465
Endocardial cushion defect, 1341–1342*t*
Endocrine disorders. *See also* specific disorders
    secondary hypertension and, 1424–1425
Endocrine glands, hormone release and, 980–981
Endocrine system:
    age-related changes in, 982–983, 982*t*
    alterations and treatments, 983, 983*t*
    altered function, 694*t*
    Assessment Interview, 984*t*
    benefits of exercise for, 653–654, 653*t*
    caring interventions, 987

diagnostic tests, 987
disorders of, 983*t*
fetal development, 1536*t*, 1537*t*
functions, 978*t*
metabolism and, 977–981
organs of, 978–982, 978*t*, 979*f*
pharmacologic therapies, 987, 987–988*t*
physical assessments, 984–987, 985–986*t*
pregnancy and, 1545
Endocytosis, 86*t*
Endoderm, 126*t*, 1528, 1529*t*
Endogenous insulin, 991
Endogenous pyrogens, 1860
Endogenous sources, nosocomial infections and, 787
Endometrial ablation, 1750
Endometriosis, 1753*t*
Endometrium, 1528
Endoplasmic reticulum, 86–87
Endorphins, 981
Endotoxins, 786
Enemas, 456
Energy, 2251
Enfuvirtide, 713
Engel, George L., 28
Engel's stages of grieving, 602*t*
Engrossment, 1198
Enlightenment, 330
Enmeshed families, 495
Enophthalmos, 1662
Enoxacin, urinary tract infections and, 876
Enterobacteriaceae, 770
Enterococci, 789–790
Enthusiasm, 2238
Entropion, 814, 815*f*
Enuresis, 311*t*, 414, 417, 417*t*
Environment:
    body temperature and, 1853
    communication and, 2157
    for learning, 2250
    influence on development, 342
Environmental control programs, 642
Environmental factors, impacting assessment, 2007
Environmental hazards, during pregnancy, 342
Environmental safety:
    Case Study, 2449
    client settings, 2442, 2442*t*
    heath care settings, 2443–2446, 2445*t*, 2446*t*,
        2448, 2448*t*
    overview, 2442
Environments. to support critical thinking, 2108
Enzymatic debridement, 1902
Enzyme-linked immunosorbent assay (ELISA),
        709–710, 1570
Enzymes, as tumor markers, 127
EOG. *See* Electro-oculogram (EOG)
Eosinopenia, 891*t*
Eosinophilia, 891*t*
Eosinophils, 677, 677*t*, 678*f*
EPA (Eicosapentaenoic acid), 892*t*
Ephedra, 1262
Epi-pens, 888*t*
Epidermis, 1874–1875
Epididymis, 1686*t*
Epilepsy, 968
    definition, 968
    medications, 959, 959*t*, 960*t*
    medications for, 971

in older adults, 968*t*
risk factors, 968
Epinephrine, 737, 739–740, 739*t*, 980, 1852
    for anaphylaxis, 888*t*
    arterial blood pressure and, 1423
    cellular metabolism and, 1852
Episcopalians, 1784*t*
Epispadias, 442
Epithalamus, 940
Epitope, 679
EPS (extrapyramidal side effects), 243
Equal Employment Opportunity Commission
        (EEOC), 2228
Equilibrium, 1633
Equipment-related accidents, 2445
Erectile dysfunction (ED):
    Case Study, 1716
    causes, 1713*t*
    Client Teaching, 1716*t*
    collaborative care
        diagnostic tests, 1714
        mechanical devices, 1714
        pharmacologic therapies, 1714
        surgery, 1714
    definition, 1712
    incidence, 1712
    manifestations, 1713
    nursing diagnoses and interventions
        sexual dysfunction, 1715
        situational low self-esteem, 1716
    nursing process
        assessment, 1715
        diagnosis, 1715
        evaluation, 1716
        overview, 1715
        planning and implementation, 1715–1716
    pathophysiology and etiology, 1712
    risk factors, 1713
Erection, 1686
Ergonomic devices, 2384, 2384*t*
Ergonomic keyboards, 2384*t*
Ergonomic mouse, 2384*t*
Ergonomics, 2383–2384, 2384*t*
Erickson's stages of psychosocial
        development, 1581*t*
Erikson, Erik H., 344–345
Erosion, skin, 1879*t*
Erotic stimuli, 1697
Erotomanic delusions, 240
Error prevention, 2280
Erysipelas, cellulitis and, 809, 809*f*
Erythema, 808–809, 1876
Erythema Infectiosum (Fifth Disease), 792*t*
Erythrocyte sedimentation rate (ESR), 760, 890,
        926, 1353*t*
Erythrocytes (RBCs), 678*f*, 1543
Erythropoietin, 102, 303*t*
ESBL (Extended-spectrum beta-lactamase), 789
Eschar, 1893, 1918
Escharotomy, 1901, 1901*f*
Escherichia coli:
    in large intestines, 770
    nosocomial infections and, 787
    pneumonia and, 834
    urinary tract infections and, 871
Eskalith, 1174*t*
Esophageal reflux, 43*t*

Esophageal varices, 42*t*, 1019, 1022, 1024
Esophagitis, 714*t*
ESR (erythrocyte sedimentation rate), 890
ESRD. *See* End-stage renal disease (ESRD)
Essure sterilization method, 1734
Estimated delivery date (EDD), 1538, 1561*f*
Estradiol, 129*t*, 1690
Estriol, 1519, 1534, 1690
Estrogen replacement therapy:
  coronary artery disease and, 1366
  for urinary incontinence, 443
Estrogens, 210
  during menopause, 1742
  female reproductive cycle and, 1519
  forms of, 1690
  functions, 1689–1690
  hormone replacement therapy and, 1711*t*
  menopause and, 1690
  ovarian cycle and, 1522
  plant, 1745*t*
  produced by placenta, 1534
  secondary hypertension and, 1425
  side effects, 1731*t*
Estrone, 1519, 1690
ESWL (extracorporeal shock wave lithotripsy), 469
Etanercept, 749
ETCO₂ (end-tidal carbon dioxide), 1479
Ethacrynic acid, 541*t*, 959*t*, 963
Ethambutol:
  nursing considerations and, 864*t*
  tuberculosis and, 863
Ether, 74
Ethical codes, 2227, 2281, 2333
Ethical decision making:
  models of, 2311, 2311*f*, 2311*t*
  principles of, 2308
Ethical dilemmas, 2312*t*
  academic dishonesty, 2316
  conflicting loyalties and obligations, 2313
  coping with, 2317*t*
  overview, 2312–2313
  social and technological changes and, 2312
Ethical Guidelines in the Conduct, Dissemination, and Implementation of Nursing Research (Silva), 2333
Ethical knowing, 2032
Ethical standards, 2306, 2312
Ethics:
  about, 2305–2306
  application of moral principles, 2315*t*
  bioethical issues, 2313–2315, 2313*t*, 2314–2315*t*
  bioethics, 1776
  Case Study, 2320
  codes of, 2308–2312, 2309–2310*t*
  defined, 1776, 2305
  documentation and, 2183
  morality and, 2306
  nursing, 1776, 1778
  in nursing practice, 2315–2317, 2317*t*
  in nursing research, 2332–2334, 2334*t*
  patient rights and, 2318, 2318–2319*t*, 2319*t*, 2320*t*
  strategies to assist ethical practice and decisions, 2312
  values and, 2306–2308, 2307*t*
  in working with clients and families, 2317, 2317*t*
  workplace issues, 2316, 2317*t*
Ethnic groups, 323, 622. *See also* Race/ethnicity

Etiologic agent:
  nursing interventions and, 774*t*
  role of, 771*f*, 772
Etiology:
  defined, 2065
  of nursing diagnoses, 2066, 2067*t*
Etodolac, 749*t*
Eubacterium, 770
Eupnea, 1216
Eustachian tube, 824–825, 1632, 1635
Euthanasia, 291, 2314
Euthyroid, 1041
Evaluation:
  checklist, 2100*t*
  of client responses, 2098–2101, 2099*f*
  defined, 2046, 2098
  developmental considerations, 2101*t*
  in nursing process, 2051*t*, 2098–2101, 2099*f*, 2101*t*, 2103, 2103*t*
  process
    collecting data, 2099
    comparing data with outcomes, 2099
    continuing, modifying, and terminating nursing care plan, 2100–2101
    drawing conclusions about problem status, 2100, 2101*f*
    relating nursing activities to outcomes, 2099, 2099*t*
  relationship to other nursing process phases, 2098
Evaluation phase, of policy development, 2362
Evaluation skills, 2208
Evaluation statement, 2099
Evidence-based practice, 2386
  abortion, reasons for, 2314*t*
  about, 2323–2324
  acute leukemia and lymphoma, 158*t*
  acute respiratory distress syndrome (ARDS), 1249*t*
  aging clients with MS, 1122*t*
  Alzheimer's disease, 225
  animated cartoons and knowledge of educational information, 673
  antibiotics and infection, 790
  anxiety disorders and acupuncture, 1816*t*
  assertiveness training to improve self-esteem, 1583*t*
  asthma, 1257*t*
  attitudes toward physician–nurse collaboration, 2118*t*
  back pain in pregnancy, 1576*t*
  backpack use and pain, 1081*t*
  barriers to, 2324–2325
  benefits of, 2324, 2324*t*
  bicycle helmet effectiveness, 2441*t*
  cancer and stress, 94*t*
  Case Study, 2336
  chronic obstructive pulmonary disease (COPD), 1277*t*
  clean catch, 881
  client safety and, 2444
  clinical decision making, 2044*t*
  collaborative health care for chronically ill older adults, 2117*t*
  complicated grief, 608*t*
  congenital heart defects, 1359*t*
  developing, 2334–2336
  diagnosis and treatment of African American women with breast cancer, 111*t*

  discharge teaching, 172*t*
  documentation of nursing care, 2199*t*
  effects of psychosocial stress on cardiovascular health, 1813*t*
  end-of-life care, 289*t*
  family support after death, 617*t*
  fecal incontinence, 459*t*
  fluid volume imbalances, 577*t*
  Framingham Heart Study, 1365*t*
  handwashing frequency variations, 789
  health literacy, 2259*t*
  hemodialysis, 567*t*
  hypertension, 1437
  Internet resources for, 2335*t*
  interventions to reduce prenatal illicit drug use, 61*t*
  laparoscopic cholecystectomy, 904*t*
  male catheterization, 880
  medicating for fever, 802
  natural family planning, 1726*t*
  nursing care for people with AIDS, 716*t*
  nursing delivery models and client outcomes, 2207*t*
  nursing diagnoses, 2076*t*
  nursing research, 2325–2327, 2325*t*, 2328*t*, 2329–2334
  online health information, 2252*t*
  oral rehydration therapy, 578*t*
  pain, 285*t*
  participation of clients with advanced dementia in social conversations, 2161*t*
  pediatric end-of-life care, 295*t*
  point-of-care nursing documentation, 2390*t*
  postpartum depression, 1206*t*
  promotion of, 2325
  research example, 2324*t*
  rheumatoid arthritis, 754
  self-efficacy, 348*t*
  sharing groups and the learning process, 2141*t*
  skeletal pins, 1108*t*
  smoking cessation in hospitalized patients, 56*t*
  spiritual care nursing, 1790*t*
  steps in process, 2334
    developing a question, 2334
    finding and reviewing evidence, 2335
    integrating information, 2335–2336
    sharing information, 2336
  strategies for implementing, 2331*t*
  stroke, 1510*t*
  sudden infant death syndrome (SIDS), 1289*t*
  tobacco use in adolescents, 56*t*
  treating pressure ulcers, 1922*t*
  tuberculosis screening and homeless persons, 868
  urinary incontinence, 444*t*
  VUR and prophylactic antibiotics, 877
Evidence-based Practice Centers (EPCs), 2335
Evidence-based research, 2387*t*
Evisceration, 898, 1929
Exacerbation, 638
Exaggerated grief, 606
Examining, 2000
Exanthem Sibutum, 798*t*
Excessive noise, 2452
Excisional biopsy:
  in breast cancer, 109*f*
Excitability, 1438
Excitement phase, 1697
Excoriation, 1916

Executive information systems, 2378t
Exelon, 217
Exercise, 2034–2035, 2034f
  aerobic, 652
  anaerobic, 652
  benefits of, 652–653, 653t, 654
  blood pressure and, 1309
  body temperature and, 1853
  coronary artery disease and, 1366, 1373
  definition, 652
  for depression, 1209–1210
  for diabetes management, 1007
  heart failure and, 1416
  hypertension and, 1429
  immune system and, 695
  in impaired mobility, 1077
  isokinetic, 652
  isometric, 652
  isotonic, 652
  for mood disorders, 1176
  obesity and, 1028–1029, 1031
  in osteoarthritis treatment, 1128
  preconception planning and, 1718
  range of motion, 1077
  resistive, 1077
  rheumatoid arthritis and, 751, 753
  types of, 652
Exercise ECG testing, 1370
Exercise intolerance, 1416
Exercise testing, in congenital heart defects, 1352t
Exhalation, respiratory, 1215
Exhaled carbon dioxide, in chronic obstructive
    pulmonary disease (COPD), 1272
Exocytosis, 86t
Exogenous insulin, 991
Exogenous sources:
  nosocomial infections and, 787
Exophthalmos, 1043, 1043f
Exosystem, 350
Exotoxins, 786:
Experimental study design, 2328t
Expert systems, 2385
Expressed consent, 2403
Expressive jargon, 359
Expressive speech, 357
Extended family, 485
Extended-kin network family, 485
Extended-spectrum beta-lactamase (ESBL), 789
External AV shunt, 546
External fixator device, 1101–1102, 1106t,
    1150, 1150f
Externals, 650
Extinction, 34
Extracapsular cataract extraction, 1659f
Extracapsular extraction, 1658
Extracapsular fractures, 1111
Extracellular fluid (ECF), 518, 520t, 526f
Extracorporeal shock wave lithotripsy (ESWL),
    469, 475f, 905
Extramarital sex, 1699
Extraocular structures, 1629–1630, 1630f
Extrapyramidal side effects (EPS), 243
Extreme sports, 2450f, 2450t
Extreme Unction, 1774
Exudate, 1930
  definition, 887
Exudative macular degeneration, 1676, 1677t

Eyberg Child Behavior Inventory (ECBI), 2013t
Eye color, 1635
Eye contact, 2152
Eye injuries:
  Case Study, 1667
  in children, 1665t
  client teaching
    health education, 1667t
    prevention and first aid, 1665t
  clinical therapies, 1664
  diagnostic tests, 1664
  etiology, 1661
  manifestations
    blunt trauma, 1662
    burns, 1662, 1663t
    corneal abrasion, 1661, 1663t
    detached retina, 1662, 1663t
    foreign bodies, 1663t
    penetrating injuries, 1663t
    penetrating trauma, 1662
    subconjunctival hemorrhage, 1663t
  nursing diagnoses and interventions
    impaired tissue integrity, ocular, 1665
    retinal detachment, 1666
  nursing process
    assessment, 1664
    diagnosis, 1665
    evaluation, 1667
    planning and implementation, 1665–1666
  overview, 1661
  risk factors, 1661
  surgery
    postoperative care, 1666t
    preoperative care, 1666t
  treatment
    retinal detachment, 1664
Eye movement desensitization and reprocessing
    (EMDR):
  post-traumatic stress disorder and, 1845
Eye muscles, 1630, 1630f
Eyebrows, 1629
Eyelashes, 1630
Eyelids, 1629
Eyes. See also Vision
  age-related changes in, 1635, 1636t
  assessment, 1640–1642t
  diagnostic tests, 1646
  disorders
    cataracts. See Cataracts
    glaucoma. See Glaucoma
    macular degeneration. See Macular
        degeneration
  extraocular structures, 1629, 1630, 1630f
  fetal development, 1536t, 1537t
  injuries, 1637, 1637t
  interior structure, 1631f
  intraocular structures, 1630–1631
  normal presentation, 1629, 1631
  pregnancy and, 1544
  structures, 1629f

F

F cells, 980
Facial expression, 2152, 2152f
Facial nerve, 942t
  functions, 1628t

Facilitated diffusion, 86t
Facilitated transport, 1533
Facilities management, 2388
Facility procedures, 2325t
Facility specific documentation, 2194–2195, 2195t
Factral, 1735t
Facts, 2106t
FAD (familial Alzheimer's disease), 214
FAE (fetal alcohol effects), 202
Fahrenheit:
  conversion to Celsius, 1854
Failure to observe and take appropriate action, 2401
Failure to thrive (FTT):
  case study, 394
  collaborative care, 393
  cultural factors, 393t
  definition, 392
  etiology, 392
  growth measurement, 393t
  manifestations, 392
  nursing process
    assessment, 393
    diagnosis, 393
    evaluation, 393
    planning and implementation, 393
  risk factors, 392
Faintness, during pregnancy, 1575t
Fair-mindedness, 2107
Fairbanks Center for Medical Ethics, 2306
Faith, 353, 354t, 1771
Faith-based practices:
  concerning death, 612, 2446t, 2451, 2452t
Fall prevention, 1112–1113, 1113t,
Fallopian tubes, 1525, 1688t, 1689
Falls, 2401
  fear of, 2451t
  risk factors for, 2451, 2452t
False Claims Act, 2418
False imprisonment, 2401
False pelvis, 1517, 1518f
Familial Alzheimer's disease (FAD), 214
Familiar hypercholesterolemia, 1326t
Family, 497
  about, 483–497
  advocacy for, 2300
  assessment, 492–493
  boundaries, 494–495
  of children with mental retardation, 204–205
  of client with chronic illness, 507
  competency, 497
  coping mechanisms, 497
  culture and, 485
  definition, 484
  developmental stages and tasks, 499
    couple, 499
    family with adolescents and young adults, 499
    family with infants and preschoolers, 499
    family with middle adults, 499
    family with older adults, 499
    family with school-age children, 499
  dysfunctional, 1609–1610
  effect of addictions on, 30–31
  effects of illness on, 638, 639
  emotional availability within, 496
  functions of, 484–485
  health beliefs, 493

influence on development, 342
managing conflicts with, 2130
normal presentation, 484–488
relationships within, 489–490
risk factors, 499–500, 500t
roles of, 484
sibling relationships within, 490
size, 490
support structures, 508–509
theoretical frameworks, 497–499
types of, 485–488
Family APGAR, 501, 502t
Family burden, 507–508
Family cohesion, 495–496
Family communication, 493–494
Family development, 488
Family disagreements, resolving, 38t
Family factors, impacting assessment, 2007
Family flexibility, 496
Family functioning, 488
Family health promotion, 497
  nursing process
    diagnosis, 502
    evaluation, 505
    implementation, 501–502, 505
    plan, 502, 505
  overview, 497–500
Family histories, 512, 1034, 2053t
Family life cycle, 488, 489t
Family planning:
  Case Study, 1741
  contraception. See Contraception
  genetic counseling, 1738–1739
  genetics and, 1719–1724, 1721t
  infertility counseling. See Infertility
  Nursing Care Plan
    assessment, 1740t
    critical thinking in the nursing process, 1740t
    diagnosis, 1740t
    evaluation, 1740t
    overview, 1740t
    planning and implementation, 1740t
  nursing diagnoses and interventions
    deficient knowledge, 1741
    risk for disturbed body image, 1740
    sexual dysfunction, 1741
  nursing process
    assessment, 1739
    diagnosis, 1739
    evaluation, 1741
    planning and implementation, 1739, 1741
  overview, 1717
  preconception counseling
    exercise, 1718
    nutrition, 1718
    overview, 1717
    physical examination, 1718
    preconception health measures, 1718
Family Psychosocial Screening, 2013t
Family recovery, 508–509
Family response to health alterations:
  case study, 514
  nursing process
    assessment, 512
    diagnosis, 512
    evaluation, 513–514
    implementation, 513
    plan, 512–513

overview, 506–507
pathophysiology and etiology, 507–509
Family support, 509
Family therapy, 37–38, 38t
Family values, 484
Family violence, 492, 1944–1945. See also Violence
  Assessment Interview, 1958t
Family-centered care:
  definition, 484
  elements of, 509t
  in pediatric nursing, 509–511
  promotion of, 510–511
Family-centered nursing:
  definition, 484
Farrand Training School for Nurses, 2308
Farsightedness, 1639t
FAS. See Fetal alcohol syndrome
Fascial excision, 1901
Fasciculations, 954t
Fasciectomy, 1901
Fasciotomy, 1095
FASD (fetal alcohol spectrum disorder), 59, 202
Fasting, 1773
  preoperative, 896
Fasting blood sugar, abnormal, possible causes, 129t
Fat embolism syndrome (FES), 1096
Fat-soluble vitamins, 1595, 1596t
Father–infant interactions, 1198, 1199f
Fathers. See also Parents
  adolescent pregnancy and, 1556–1557
  expectant, 1551–1552
  new, 489
  postpartum depression and, 1206
Fatigue. See also Chronic fatigue syndrome
  acute, 301
  behaviors and conditions contributing to, 302t
  Case Study, 305
  causes of, 258
  chronic, 301
  clinical therapies, 303t
  collaborative care
    complementary and alternative medicine, 304
    diagnostic tests, 302
    nonpharmacologic therapies, 303–304
    pharmacologic therapies, 303
  definition, 258, 301
  depression and, 1188
  description, 259t
  during pregnancy, 1574t
  manifestations, 302, 303t
  nursing diagnoses and interventions, 304
  nursing process
    assessment, 304
    diagnosis, 304
    evaluation, 305
    planning and implementation, 304
  pathophysiology and etiology, 301–302
  risk factors, 302
  treatment, 259t
Fats, 1593t, 1595
Faxes, 2183t
FDA. See Food and Drug Administration (FDA)
Febrile, 1854, 1859
Febrile seizures, 968, 971, 1861
Fecal assessment, 429t, 430
Fecal elimination. See Bowel elimination
Fecal impaction, 458
  digital removal of, 462

Fecal incontinence:
  definition, 458
  Evidence-Based Practice, 459t
  incidence of, 459
  manifestations, 459
  nursing diagnosis and interventions
    community-based care, 460
    risk for impaired skin integrity, 459
  nursing process
    diagnosis, 460
  in older adults, 459t
  pathophysiology, 459
  pressure ulcers and, 1916
  self-care practices for, 459t
  treatment, 459
Fecal incontinence pouch, 464
Feces, 423–424, 523
Federal agencies, 2364–2365, 2364t
Federal programs, for payment of health care
  services, 2368
Federally Qualified Health Centers, 2348
Feedback, 498, 2119, 2149, 2170, 2171t, 2249
Feedback mechanisms, 981, 981f
Feeding tubes, 297
Feet:
  care of, 1003
  complications with, diabetes mellitus and,
    999–1000
Feldene. See Piroxicam
Fellatio, 1697
Felonies, 2398
Female circumcision, 1699
Female genital mutilation (FGM), 1699, 1700t,
  1949t
Female hormones, 1519–1520
Female orgasmic disorder, 1702
Female reproductive anatomy and physiology:
  assessment, 1705–1708t
  Bartholin's glands, 1687, 1688t
  bony pelvis, 1516–1518, 1516f, 1519f
  breasts, 1691
  cervix, 1688t, 1689
  clitoris, 1688, 1688t
  external genitalia, 1687–1688
  fallopian tubes, 1688t, 1689
  internal organs, 1688–1690
  introitus, 1688
  key components, 1516–1518
  labia majora, 1687, 1688t
  labia minora, 1687, 1688t
  mammary glands, 1688t, 1691
  menstrual cycle, 1690–1691
  mons pubis, 1687, 1688t
  oogenesus and ovarian cycle, 1690, 1691f
  ovaries, 1688t, 1690
  perineum, 1688t
  pregnancy and, 1541–1545
  sex hormones
    estrogens, 1690
    progesterone, 1690
  Skene's glands, 1687, 1688t
  uterus, 1688t, 1689
  vagina, 1688, 1688t
  vestibule, 1687, 1688t
  vulva, 1687
Female reproductive cycle (FRC):
  definition, 1519
  effects of female hormones, 1519–1520

menstrual cycle, 1523
  neurohumoral basis of, 1521–1522
  ovarian cycle, 1522
Female ritual cutting (FRC), 1699
Female sexual arousal disorder, 1702
Female-to-male (FTM) transsexuals, 400, 1696
Femoral pulse, 1319f, 1320
Fenofibrate, 1374
Fenoprofen, 749t
Fentanyl, 287t
Fentanyl citrate, 287t
Ferrous sulfate, 1020
Fertility:
  female, 1718
  male, 1719
Fertility awareness-based methods:
  basal body temperature method, 1725
  calendar rhythm method, 1725
  cervical mucus method, 1725
  definition, 1725
  evidence-based practice, 1726t
  ovulation method, 1725
  symptothermal method, 1726
Fertilization, 1527f
  cellular differentiation, 1528
  definition, 1524
  moment of, 1526, 1526f
  preembryonic development and, 1527–1530
  preparation for, 1524–1525
FES. See Fat embolism syndrome (FES)
Fetal alcohol effects (FAE), 202
Fetal alcohol spectrum disorder (FASD), 59, 202
Fetal alcohol syndrome (FAS), 201, 202t, 203t, 205t
  affect on sensory perception, 1634
  characteristics of, 59
Fetal blood, 1532–1533
Fetal circulation, 1300–1302
Fetal demise, 626
Fetal development:
  assessment, 1569–1570
  circulatory system, 1534–1535, 1535f
  organ system development, 1536–1537t
  preembryonic development, 1527–1530
  stages of, 1538f, 1539–1541
  twins, 1530
Fetal heartbeat, 1548, 1569, 1570f
Fetal movement, 1546
Fetal tissue transplantation, 1137
Fetus, 1539, 1540f
Fever, 1852, 1854, 1858. See also Hyperthermia
  in children, evaluation and treatment of, 1864t
  treatment of, 1861
  types of, 1859
Fever spike, 1859
FGM (female genital mutilation), 1699,
    1700t, 1949t
Fiber, 1373
Fiberoptic bronchoscopy, 841
Fibric acid derivatives, 1374t
Fibrin, 1310, 1543, 1927
Fibrin degradation products, 1398–1399
Fibrinogen, 129t
Fibrinolytics, 1375–1376, 1479, 1506
Fibromyalgia:
  Case Study, 308
  classification of, 307t
  clinical therapies, 306t

collaborative care
  complementary and alternative medicine, 307
  diagnostic tests, 306–307
  pharmacologic therapies, 307
community-based care, 308
definition, 258
description, 259t
manifestations, 306, 306t
nursing diagnoses and interventions
  activity intolerance, 308
  fatigue, 308
nursing process
  assessment, 307
  diagnosis, 307
  evaluation, 308
  planning and implementation, 308
overview, 305
pathophysiology and etiology, 306
risk factors, 306
tender points in, 305, 306f
treatment, 259t
Fibrous joints, 1061
Fidelity, 1778
Fifth disease, 792t
Fight-or-flight response, 1423
Filtration, 521, 521f
  cellular transportation method of, 86t
Finance, 2388
Financial systems, 2378t
Finasteride (Proscar), 434
Fire extinguishers, 2451
Firearms, 1965, 2454
Fires, 2450–2451, 2458
First heart sound (S1), 1296, 1297t
First responders, 2358t
First-degree AV block, 1443t, 1447
Fissures, 1879t
Fitness. See Physical fitness
Fitzpatrick, Joyce, 2326
Fixation, 344
Flaccidity, 1505
Flagyl, 916
Flashbacks, 1842–1843
Flashover effect, 1887
Flat affect, 238
Flat warts, 1758
Flatness, 2004, 2004t
Flatulence, 427
  during pregnancy, 1575t
Flatus, 424
Fliedner, Theodore, 2287
Flight of ideas, 1179
Floccillation, 207t
Flomax, 434, 434t
Floppy drives, 2375
Flossing, 660
Flow sheets, 2187, 2189, 2191f, 2193–2194
Floxin. See Oxfloxacin
Fluid intake, 521–522, 529, 531, 542–543, 559
Fluid output, 522–523, 523t, 529, 531
Fluid replacement therapy:
  for shock, 1494–1495
Fluid restriction, 583t
Fluid volume deficit (FVD):
  assessment, 574t
  causes, 570
  in children, 570–571, 574–575, 574t

clinical therapies, 572t
collaborative care
  clinical therapies, 575–577
  diagnostic tests, 575
  intravenous fluids, 576–577
  oral rehydration, 575–576, 578t
definition, 569
description, 528t
evidence-based research, 578t
isotonic, 569
manifestations, 571–575, 572t, 575t
multisystem effects, 573f
nursing process
  assessment, 577–578
  diagnosis, 578
  evaluation, 579
  planning and implementation, 578–579
in older adults, 575, 578t
oral rehydration, 576t
pathophysiology and etiology, 569–571
risk factors, 571
risk for, 531
third spacing, 570
treatment, 528t
Fluid volume excess:
  in acute renal failure, 538t
  assessment, 574t
  causes, 581–582
  in chronic renal failure, 557t
collaborative care
  diagnostic tests, 582
  dietary management, 582–583
  fluid management, 582
  pharmacologic therapies, 582
definition, 579
interstitial, 579–581
manifestations, 581t, 582
Nursing Care Plan
  assessment, 585t
  critical thinking, 585t
  diagnoses, 585t
  evaluation, 585t
  planning and implementation, 585t
nursing process
  assessment, 583–584
  diagnosis, 584
  evaluation, 586
  planning and implementation, 586
pathophysiology and etiology, 579–582
risk factors, 531, 582
Fluids and electrolytes. See also Electrolytes
  about, 517–533
  alterations, 528–529, 528–529t
  assessment, 530t
    clinical measurements, 529, 531
    nursing history, 529
    physical assessment, 529
  Assessment Interview, 531
  body fluid composition, 518–519, 519f
  body fluid movement
    active transport, 521, 522f
    diffusion, 520–521, 521f
    filtration, 521, 521f
    osmosis, 519–520, 520f
  body fluid regulation
    antidiuretic hormone, 523, 524f
    atrial natriuretic factor, 523

fluid intake, 521–522
fluid output, 522–523
kidneys, 523
maintaining homeostasis, 523
renin-angiotensin-aldosterone system, 523
thirst mechanism, 522
caring interventions, 532
changes in older adults, 527–528
diagnostic tests
chloride excretion, 532
complete blood count, 531
osmolality, 532
serum electrolytes, 531
urine sodium, 532
urine specific gravity, 532
electrolyte regulation
normal presentation, 524–526
factors affecting balance of, 526–528
imbalances
calcium. *See* Hypercalcemia; Hypocalcemia
caring interventions, 532
Case Study, 596
in children, 570–571
chloride. *See* Hyperchloremia; Hypochloremia
cirrhosis and, 1021
conditions resulting from, 518–519
dehydration, 521
evidence-based research, 577*t*
fluid volume deficit. *See* Fluid volume deficit
fluid volume excess. *See* Fluid volume excess
isotonic, 569
magnesium. *See* Hypermagnesemia;
Hypomagnesemia
osmolar, 569
overview, 569
pharmacologic therapies, 532, 533*t*
phosphate. *See* Hyperphosphatemia;
Hypophosphatemia
potassium. *See* Hyperkalemia; Hypokalemia
sodium. *See* Hypernatremia; Hyponatremia
normal presentation, 518–528
withdrawing or withholding, 2315
Flumadine. *See* Rimantadine
Fluorescein angiogram, 1677
Fluorescein stain, 815
Fluoroimmunoassay (FIA), 1570
Fluoroquinolones:
conjunctivitis and, 816
medication administration, 807
pneumonia and, 841
Fluoxetine, 210, 1202
Flurbiprofen, 749*t*
Fluvastatin, 1374
Focal seizures, 968
Focalin, 373*t*
Focus charting, 2187, 2188*f*, 2189
Focus on Diversity and Culture. *See also*
Race/ethnicity
acceptable child behaviors, 2010*t*
African Americans and kidney disease, 562
anxiety disorders, 1811*t*
asthma, 1257*t*
autonomy, 2404*t*
chronic obstructive pulmonary disease
(COPD), 1272*t*
cirrhosis, 1016*t*
client teaching, 2267*t*
codeine use, 277*t*

complementary and alternative therapies, 751
Confucian and Buddhist religions, 1776*t*
couvade, 1552*t*
crisis, 1825*t*
culturally sensitive nursing, 2029*t*
diabetes mellitus, risk and incidence of, 1052*t*
gender-based family violence, 1944*t*
genital mutilation, 1949*t*
HIV/AIDS, 697*t*
hypertension in African Americans, 1426*t*
infectious diseases, 791
infertility treatments, 1738*t*
Jehovah's Witnesses, 564
leukemia treatment, 156*t*
mental illness, 1163*t*
mood disorders, 1180*t*
moral principles, 2315*t*
Muslim paternal attachment, 1199*t*
osteoporosis, 1034*t*
otitis media, 826
pain responses, 268*t*
personality and culture, 1587*t*
personality disorders, 1621*t*
postpartum experience, 1197*t*
post-traumatic stress disorders, 1843*t*
pregnancy, 1553*t*, 1572*t*
prostate cancer, 170*t*
religious and cultural preferences, 548
respiratory syncytial virus, (RSV)/
Bronchiolitis, 1281*t*
risk and incidence of cancer, 116*t*
risk factors for stroke, 1501*t*
seat belt use, 1988*t*
self-concept, 1588*t*
sexual health, 1700*t*
sickle cell disorder, 177*t*
sodium use, 584
sudden infant death syndrome (SIDS), 1287*t*
suicide rates, 1981*t*
tuberculosis, 860
Focused assessment by sonography in trauma
(FAST) exam, 1942
Focusing, 2177*t*
Folate, 1597*t*
Folic acid, 95, 559, 1020, 1373, 1597*t*
dietary sources, 103*t*
during pregnancy, 663*t*
Folic acid deficiency anemia, 99–100, 102*t*
Follicle-stimulating hormone (FSH), 978,
1521–1522, 1690
Follicular phase:
of ovarian cycle, 1522
Follistim, 1735*t*
Fontanels, 10 62
Food, withdrawing or withholding, 2315
Food allergy test, 736–737
Food and Drug Administration (FDA), 2364
Food and Nutrition Board (FNB), 1595
Food Guide Pyramid, 663
Food insecurity, 663*t*
Foot rest, 2384*t*
Foramen ovale, 1300, 1534
Foraminotomy, 1083
Forehead temperature, 1855
Foreign-born population, 325*f*
Forgiveness, 1772
Formal groups, 2135, 2135*t*
Formal leaders, 2233

Formal nursing care plans, 2077
Formal operation stage, 348
Formal operational thought, 364
Formulation phase, of policy development, 2362
Forseeability, 2400
Foster family, 486
Fourth heart sound (S4), 1296, 1297*t*
Fowler's position, 739, 739*f*
pneumonia and, 846
Fowler, James, 353
Fractures:
case study, 1110
classification, 1093
client teaching
fall prevention in older adults, 1104*t*
home care, 1110*t*
clinical therapies, 1098*t*
closed, 1093*f*
collaborative care
diagnostic tests, 1098
emergency care, 1098
overview, 1097
pharmacologic therapies, 1098
common, 1095*t*
complications
compartment syndrome, 1094–1095, 1096*t*, 1105
deep venous thrombosis, 1091, 1096, 1097*t*
delayed union and nonunion, 1097
fat embolism syndrome, 1096
infection, 1097, 1098*t*, 1105*t*
leg length discrepancy, 1105
malunion, 1105*t*
neurovascular injury, 1105*t*
nonunion, 1105
reflex sympathetic dystrophy, 1097
Volkmann's contracture, 1095
definition, 1065*t*, 1066, 1093
developmental considerations, 1093*t*
evidence-based practice
client with skeletal pins, 1108, 1108*t*
healing
factors affecting, 1094, 1096*t*
phases, 1093–1094
hip. *See* Hip fractures
manifestations, 1094, 1096*t*, 1098*t*
Nursing Care Plan
assessment, 1109*t*
critical thinking in the nursing process, 1109*t*
diagnoses, 1109*t*
evaluation, 1109*t*
overview, 1109*t*
planning and implementation, 1109*t*
nursing diagnoses and interventions
acute pain, 1105
clients in traction, 1101*t*
clients with a cast, 1101*t*
clients with internal fixation, 1101*t*
discharge planning and home care teaching, 1105
impaired physical mobility, 1107
maintain proper alignment, 1105
monitor neurovascular status, 1105
promote mobility, 1105
risk for disturbed sensory perception,
tactile, 1108
risk for infection, 1107
risk for peripheral neurovascular
dysfunction, 1107
nursing process

assessment, 1104
diagnosis, 1104
evaluation, 1109
overview, 1103
planning and implementation, 1104–1105,
1107–1108
open, 1093
pain management for, 1099t
pathophysiology and etiology, 1093
risk factors, 1093
stress, 1093, 1093t
treatment, 1065t
casts, 1100, 1101t, 1102, 1107
electrical bone stimulation, 1103, 1103f
external fixators, 1101, 1102f, 1106t
internal fixators, 1103f
surgery, 1101, 1101t
traction, 1099–1100, 1101t, 1105, 1106t
types, 1094, 1099f
Fragile X syndrome, 201–202, 202t, 203t, 1724
Framingham Heart Study, 1364, 1365t
Frank–Starling mechanism, 1405, 1406t
Fraternal twins, 1530, 1531f
FRC (female ritual cutting), 1699
Free clinics, 2348
Free radicals, 217
Free-floating anxiety, 1808
Freedmen's Relief Association, 2289f
Freud, Sigmund, 343–344
Friedman Family Assessment Tool (FFAM),
502–504
Friend support, 509
Friendship groups, 2135
Frontal lobe, 940
Frontier Nursing Service (FNS), 2291
Frontotemporal dementia, 206t
Frostbite, 1866–1867, 1867t
FSH. See Follicle-stimulating hormone (FSH)
FTT. See Failure to thrive
Fulguration, 143
Full consciousness, 946t
Full-thickness burns, 1889, 1889f
Fulminant colitis, 909
Functional assessments, 202
Functional decline, prevention of, 2445
Functional health patterns, 2059, 2060–2061t
Functional incontinence, 442t, 446t
Functional method, 2206
Functional nursing, 2344
Functional strength, 652
Fundal height, 1561, 1569, 1569f
Fundoscopy, 1670
Fundus, 1548f
Fungi, 771, 786t
Furadantin. See Nitrofurantoin
Furosemide, 959t, 963
in specific conditions
acute renal failure, 541t, 542
chronic renal failure, 558
Fusion and integrase inhibitors, 808
Fusobacterium, 770

G

G6PD anemia, 101
GABA. See Gamma-aminobutyric acid
Gait, 1071t, 2152
Galanin, 212
Galantamine (Reminyl), 217

Gallbladder:
disorders
cholecystitis, 902
gallstones. See Gallstones
Gallbladder disease:
overview, 902
Gallstone ileus, 902
Gallstones:
Case Study, 908–909
collaborative care
alternative therapies, 905
diagnostic tests, 903–904, 904t
nutrition, 905
pharmacologic therapies, 904–905
ultrasound, 905
common locations for, 902f
community-based care, 906t
ethnic considerations, 903t
manifestations, 902–903, 903t
Nursing Care Plan
assessment, 907t
critical thinking in the nursing process, 907t
diagnosis, 907t
evaluation, 907t
overview, 907t
planning and implementation, 907t
nursing diagnoses and interventions
imbalanced nutrition, less than body
requirements, 906–907
pain, 906
risk for infection, 907–908
nursing process
assessment, 906
diagnosis, 906
evaluation, 908
planning and implementation, 906–908
overview, 902
pathophysiology and etiology, 902–903
risk factors, 903, 903t, 906
treatment
surgery, 904t, 905
Gamblers Anonymous, 37
Gametes, 1516, 1524
Gametogenesis, 1524, 1525f
Gamma aminobutyric acid (GABA), 40, 666
Gamma-glutamyltransferase (GGT), 129t
Gamma-hydroxybutyrate (GHB), 1970
Gamma-interferon:
human immunodeficiency virus (HIV) and, 713
Gangrenous appendicitis, 893
Gangs, 2017
Ganirelix acetate, 1735t
Gardner, Howard, 2249
Gardner-Wells tongs, 1150, 1150f
Gastric analysis, 933
Gastric bypass, 1030f
Gastric lavage, 1024
Gastric outlet obstruction, 932
Gastric ulcers, 931
Gastrin, 932
Gastrinomas, 932
Gastritis, alcohol abuse and, 42t
Gastrocolic reflex, 425
Gastrointestinal system:
benefits of exercise for, 653, 653t
effects of shock on, 1487
fetal development, 1536t
pregnancy and, 1543

Gastroscopy:
in specific conditions
peptic ulcer disease, 933
Gate theory, 265
Gay and lesbian families, 487–488
GBS. See Guillain-Barré syndrome (GBS)
Gemfibrozil, 1374
Gender, 399–400
abuse and, 1951
blood pressure and, 1309
body fluid balance and, 528
communication and, 2155
conflict and, 2130–2131
influence of, on health, 644
risk factors and, 499
Gender dysphoria, 400, 1696
Gender identity, 1696–1697
Gender identity disorder, 400, 1696
Gender roles:
culture and, 1699
grief and, 604
Gender stereotypes, 1163
Gender-based family violence, 1944t
Gender-based violence, 1949–1950
Gender-bias theory:
mood disorders and, 1163–1164
personality disorders and, 1610
Gender-role behavior, 1696
General Health Questionnaire, 207t
communication and, 2155
conflict and, 2130–2131
Generalized anxiety disorder:
description and treatment, 1804t
DSM-IV-TR diagnostic criteria, 1811t
manifestations, 1811–1812
Nursing Care Plan
assessment, 1817t
critical thinking, 1817t
diagnosis, 1817t
evaluation, 1817t
planning and implementation, 1817t
Generalized seizures, 968, 971
Generalization, 2247t
Generation gap, 2238
Generation X, 2238, 2239t
Generational cohort, 2238
Generational differences, in work ethic,
2238–2241, 2239t, 2241f, 2241t
Genes, 1720
cell structure and, 87–88
phenotype, 1723
tumor suppressor, 119
Genetic counseling, 1738–1739
Genetic disorders:
chromosome structure abnormalities, 1722
emotions concerning, 1719
inheritance of. See Inheritance
monosomies, 1721
mosaicism, 1721
overview, 1720
preimplantation diagnosis, 1737–1738
sex chromosome abnormalities, 1722–1723
trisomies, 1720
Genetic testing, 1734
Genetics:
considerations in specific conditions
ADHD, 370
alcohol abuse, 41

Alzheimer's disease, 214
cardiac disorders, 1326, 1326*t*
eating disorders, 1598
macular degeneration, 1676
mood disorders, 1160, 1164*t*
musculoskeletal system, 1075, 1076*t*
personality disorders, 1608
schizophrenia, 234–235
sickle cell disorder, 177
substance abuse, 69
suicide, 1978
influence of, in health, 642
influence on development, 340–341
inheritance. *See* Inheritance
Geneva Convention, 2290
Genital herpes:
cause, 1757
collaborative care
diagnostic tests, 1758
overview, 1757
pharmacologic therapies, 1758
manifestations, 1757, 1757*f*, 1757*t*
pathophysiology, 1757
Genital intercourse, 1697
Genital warts:
collaborative care
other treatments, 1759
overview, 1758
pharmacologic therapies, 1759, 1759*t*
complications, 1758
definition, 1758
facts about, 1758*t*
incidence, 1758
manifestations, 1758, 1758*f*
pathophysiology, 1758
types, 1758
Genitourinary system:
fetal development, 1536*t*, 1537*t*
Genograms, 493, 494*f*
Genotype, 1723
Gentamicin:
urinary tract infections and, 876
Genuineness, 2175, 2175*t*
Geodon, 244*t*
Geragogy, 2245
Geriatric assessment, 2020–2024, 2020*t*, 2023*t*
Geriatric Depression Scale (GDS), 1193, 1193*t*
German measles, 342, 798–799*t*
Gestation, 1559*t*
Gestational carrier, 1738
Gestational diabetes, 989, 992, 1002
Gestures, 2152
GFR (glomerular filtration rate), 413, 923, 926
GGT. *See* Gamma-glutamyltransferase (GGT)
Gilligan, Carol, 352–353
Ginger, for morning sickness, 1576*t*
Gingiva, 656
Gingivitis, 658
common problems, 658*t*
Ginkgo biloba, 210, 972
Ginseng, 1744*t*
Glare filter, 2384*t*
Glasgow Coma Scale, 949, 949*t*, 951*t*
Glaucoma, 1637*t*, 1638, 1642*t*, 1649*t*
Case Study, 1675
in children, 1668, 1670, 1670*t*
client teaching
managing at home, 1673*t*

clinical therapies, 1669*t*
collaborative care
diagnostic tests, 1670
exercises, 1672
pharmacologic therapies, 1670, 1671*t*
surgery, 1670, 1672
definition, 1668
effects of, 1668*f*
ethnicity and, 1669*t*
manifestations, 1669, 1669*t*
medications, 1649, 1650*t*
Nursing Care Plan
assessment, 1674*t*
diagnosis, 1674*t*
evaluation, 1674*t*
overview, 1674*t*
planning and implementation, 1674*t*
nursing diagnoses and interventions
anxiety, 1673, 1675
disturbed sensory perception, visual,
1672–1673
nursing process
assessment, 1672
diagnosis, 1672
evaluation, 1675
overview, 1672
planning and implementation, 1672–1673, 1675
pathophysiology and etiology, 1668–1669
risk factors, 1669
types
angle closure, 1668–1669, 1668*f*
open angle, 1668–1669, 1668*f*
Global self, 1580
Global self-esteem, 1583
Glomerular disorders:
acute postinfectious glomerulonephritis
definition, 923
manifestations, 925
pathophysiology, 923
prognosis, 928*t*
collaborative care:
diagnosis, 926
overview, 925
pharmacologic therapies, 926–927
treatment, 927
community-based care, 928*t*
Nursing Care Plan
assessment, 929*t*
critical thinking in the nursing process, 929*t*
diagnoses, 929*t*
evaluation, 929*t*
overview, 929*t*
planning and implementation, 929*t*
nursing diagnoses and interventions
excessive fluid volume, 928
fatigue, 928
impaired skin integrity, 928
ineffective role performance, 928
risk for imbalanced nutrition, less than body
requirements, 928
risk for infection, 928
nursing process
assessment, 927
diagnosis, 927
evaluation, 929*t*
planning and implementation, 927–928
Glomerular filtrate, 410

Glomerular filtration rate (GFR), 413, 534, 923,
926, 1543
Glomerulonephritis, 889*t*. *See also* Glomerular
disorders; Nephritis
causes, 924*f*
definition, 923
Glomerulus, 410
Glossitis, 658*t*
Glossopharyngeal nerve, 942*t*, 1628*t*
Gloves, 2005*t*, 2436*t*
Glucagon, 989
Glucocorticoids, 561, 892*t*, 915*t*, 980, 1885*t*
in specific conditions
glomerular disorders, 927
multiple sclerosis, 1120
Gluconeogenesis, 989
Glucose-6-phospahte dehydrogenase (G6PD)
anemia, 101
Glucosuria, 991
Gluten-free, casein-free (GFCF) diet, 382, 383*t*
Glycogenolysis, 989
Glycosuria, 413
GnRH. *See* Gonadotropin-releasing
hormone (GnRH)
Goal statements, 2087
Goals:
components of, 2087, 2088*t*
defined, 2085
Desired outcomes, 2086
establishing client, 2085–2087, 2085*f*, 2089
guidelines for writing, 2089
long-term, 2087
purpose of, 2086
relationship to nursing diagnoses, 2087
revision of, 2101
short-term, 2087
Goiters:
definition, 985
Graves' disease and, 1041
hyperthyroidism and, 1042*t*
hypothyroidism and, 1047–1048, 1049*t*
toxic multinodular, 1043, 1043*f*
Gold compounds, 748
Gold salts, 750, 750*t*
Gold sodium, 750*t*
Goldenseal:
for gallstone, 905
Goldmark Report, 2327
Golgi apparatus, 87
GoLYTELY, 455
Gonadocorticoids, 978*t*
Gonadotropic cells, 978
Gonadotropin hormones, 978
Gonadotropin-releasing hormone (GnRH), 1521,
1690, 1735*t*
Gonads, 1516
Gonal-F, 1735*t*
Goniometer, 1071
Gonioplasty, 1672
Gonioscopy, 1670
Gonorrhea:
collaborative care
diagnostic tests, 1760
overview, 1760
complications, 1760
definition, 1760
incidence, 1760
manifestations, 1760

pathophysiology, 1760
risk factors, 1760
Good Friday, 1782
Good Samaritan, 2287
Good Samaritan laws, 2405
Goodell's sign, 1542
Goodpasture's syndrome, 693t, 729, 924
Gordon's functional health pattern framework, 2059, 2060t
Goserelin acetate, 1735t
Gould, Roger, 346
Gout, 1070
Governance, 2281
Gowns, 2436t
Graafian follicle, 1522
Grading, 125
Grady, Patricia, 2326
Graft-versus-host disease (GVHD), 155, 692, 734
Gram stain, urinary tract infections and, 875
Gram-positive organisms, 1900
Grandiosity, 240
Grandparents:
  death of, 611
  pregnancy and, 1552–1553
Granulate colony-stimulating factor (G-CSF), 93
Granulation tissue, 887, 1928
Granulocytes, 676–677, 677t, 678f
Graphesthesia, 954f
Graphic record, 2193
Graves' disease, 983t, 1041–1043, 1043f, 1046
Gravida, 1559t
Greenstick fractures, 1095t
Gretter, Lystra, 2308
Grief and loss. See also Death and dying
  about, 599–606
  alterations, 606
  Assessment Interview, 607t
  bereavement, 601
  in children, 603, 609, 610t, 613–14
    books for coping with, 612t
    death of friend, 611
    death of grandparent, 611
    death of parent, 609, 611
    other significant losses, 611
  collaborative care, 613
  complicated, 601
  definition, 601
  disenfranchised, 622t
  in early and middle adulthood, 603
  factors influencing
    age, 603–604
    cause of loss or death, 606
    culture, 604, 604t, 611
    gender, 604
    significance of loss, 604
    socioeconomic status, 605
    spiritual beliefs, 604, 605t, 612
    support system, 605
  family response
    factors influencing, 611–612
  grieving norms, 622t
  manifestations, 601
  mourning, 601
  nursing diagnoses and interventions
    facilitating grief work, 608
    providing emotional support, 608
  nursing process
    assessment, 606–607, 607t

diagnosis, 607
evaluation, 609
planning and implementation, 607–608
  in older adults, 604, 622
    factors affecting, 622
    nursing process, 624–625
  perinatal. See Perinatal loss
  of pets, 624t
  sources of
    aspect of self, 600
    external objects, 600
    familiar environment, 600
  sources of loved ones, 600
  theories of
    Engel, 601, 602t
    Kübler-Ross model, 601, 602t
    Martocchio, 601
    Rando, 601
    Sanders, 601, 603t
  types, 600
  types of grief responses, 601
  vs. depression, 1167t
Group commitment, 2136, 2137t
Group decision making, 2039–2040
Group dynamics, 2136, 2138, 2138t
Group leader, role of, 36
Group self-insurance plans, 2214
Group support sessions, 648
Group teaching, 2265
Group therapy, 35–37, 36–37t
  cognitive-behavioral, 1175
  curative factors of, 36t
  for rape victims, 1974
  for schizophrenia, 244
Groups:
  characteristics of effective, 2136, 2137t
  cohesiveness, 2138, 2139t
  decision making, 2136, 2138, 2138t
  defined, 2133
  functions, 2134, 2134t
  health care, 2140
  levels of formality, 2135
    formal, 2135, 2135t
    informal, 2135–2136, 2136t
    semiformal, 2135, 2135t
  member behaviors, 2138
  overview, 2133–2134
  power in, 2138
  problems in
    groupthink, 2139, 2140t
    monopolizing, 2139
    scapegoating, 2139
    silence and apathy, 2139
    transference and countertransference, 2139
  self-awareness/growth, 2141
  self-help, 2141, 2141t
  social support, 2141
  therapy, 2141
  types
    primary, 2134
    secondary, 2134
Groupthink, 2139, 2140t
Growth. See also Development
  definition, 339–340
  principles of, 340
  race/ethnicity and, 327
  stages of, 340, 341t
  theories of, 343–347

Growth hormone (GH), 978, 978t, 982
Growth retardation, 663t
Guided imagery, 315
Guillain-Barré syndrome (GBS):
  cause, 1679
  in children, 1681t
  definition, 1679
  incidence, 1679
  influenza vaccines and, 821
  manifestations, 1679
  pathophysiology, 1679
Guns, 1965
Gunshot wounds, 1938, 1969
Gustatory stimuli, 1628
Gut-associated lymphoid tissue (GALT), 682
GVHD. See Graft-versus-host disease (GVHD)
Gynecomastia, 1704t

H

H. pylori:
  detection of, 933
  in peptic ulcer disease, 931
H1 receptors, 888
H1-histamine receptors, 737
H1N1, 818–819, 819t. See also Influenza
H1N1 vaccine distribution, 2350, 2350f
H2 receptors, 888
HA. See Hyaluronic acid (HA)
Habit training, 445, 450
Haemophilus influenzae:
  in children, 792t
  pneumonia and, 834–835, 842t
Haemophilus influenzae type B vaccine, 687–688
Hair, 1883t
  pregnancy and, 1543–1544
Haldol, 210, 243
Halitosis, 658t
Hallucinations, 232, 238–239
Hallucinogens, 73–74, 74t
Hallux valgus, 744, 744t, 1067, 1070
Halo external fixation device, 1150, 1150f
Halo traction, 1106t
Haloperidol, 210, 243
Hamilton Depression Rating Scale, 207t
Hammertoe, 1070
Hand hygiene, 2436t
Hand restraints, 2448
Hand-off communication, 2435
Handheld devices, 2378
Handwashing, 2435
Handwritten orders, 2416
Haploid number, 1720
Haptens, 680
Haptoglobin, 129t
Hard disk drives, 2375
Hard palate, 655
Hardware, 2374–2375
Harper Model, 333f
Harrison Narcotic Act, 68
Hartmann procedure, 144
Hashimoto's thyroiditis, 693t, 729, 1048
Hassles and Uplifts Scale, 2013t
Haversian canal, 1056
Haversian system, 1056
Havighurst, Robert, 345
Hawthorn, 1417
HCG. See Human chorionic gonadotropin (HCG)
HCO₃⁻. See Bicarbonate (HCO₃⁻)

HDLs. *See* High-density lipoproteins (HDLs)
Head circumference, 2009
Head growth, infants, 2014
Head trauma, 962. *See also* Brain injury
Head-to-toe assessment, 2000, 2001*t*
Healing, 1927. *See also* Wound healing
   aging and, 1875
Health:
   about, 635–645
   concept of, 2283
   definition, 636, 637, 637*t*
   influence on development, 342
   variables affecting, 642
     age, gender, and developmental level, 644
     cognitive factors, 645
     genetic makeup, 642
     psychologic factors, 645
   vs. well-being, 635
Health agencies, audits of, 2183
Health assessment interview, 1324–1325
Health beliefs, 493, 650, 2255
Health care:
   delivery trends, 2215*t*
   factors affecting delivery of, 2120, 2341, 2343
     demand versus supply, 2213–2214
     demographics, 2342
     health literacy, 2342–2343
     separate billing for nursing services, 2214
     technology advances, 2342
   frameworks for providing
     case management, 2343–2344
     client-focused care, 2344
     managed care, 2343
   patterns of, 2053*t*
   rationing, 2213–2214
Health care access:
   barriers to
     lack of health insurance, 2346–2347, 2347*t*
     lack of usual source of care, 2347
     perceptions of need, 2347, 2347*t*
     uneven distribution of services, 2347–2348
   Case Study, 2348
   overview, 2345
   steps in, 2345
   ways to increase, 2348
Health care advance directives, 2410, 2412, 2412*t*
Health Care and Education Reconciliation Act,
     2345, 2346*t*, 2347, 2363
Health care costs, 2282, 2326, 2349
   affect of quality improvement on, 2428
   containment strategies, 2210, 2214–2215
   types of reimbursement, 2367–2369, 2368*t*
Health care decisions, developmental
     considerations and, 2042*t*
Health care disparities, 326–327
Health Care Financing Administration (HCFA),
     2194–2195, 2368
Health care home, 2347, 2348*t*
Health care information systems, 2375, 2376*f*
health care paradigm, old vs. new, 2340*t*
Health care professionals:
   changing roles of, 2114
   educating, 2299
   risk of violence and, 1965
   as source of data, 2055
   substance abuse by, 68
Health care proxy, 2410
Health care reform, 2210, 2367

Health care services:
   payment sources, 2210–2212, 2367–2368
   price controls for, 2214
   types of
     primary prevention, 2340, 2341*t*
     secondary prevention, 2340–2341, 2341*t*
     tertiary prevention, 2340–2341, 2341*t*
   uneven distribution of, 2347–2348
Health care settings:
   safety in, 2443–2446, 2445*t*, 2446*t*, 2448, 2448*t*
   types of, 2341, 2342*f*
Health care spending, 2210
Health care surrogates, 290, 2410
Health care systems, 225
   about, 2339, 2340*t*
   allocation of resources and, 2349–2351
   Case Study, 2344–2345
   emergency preparedness and, 2351
   health care access and, 2345–2348
   nursing practice, 2344
Health care teams:
   collaborative, 2117
   members of, 2116–2117*t*
Health care-associated infections (HAI). *See*
     Nosocomial infections
Health disparities:
   access to care and, 2345
   among minorities, 2342
Health education, 641, 648
Health history, 645, 656
   components of, 2053*t*
   pediatric, 2011
Health information:
   guidelines for disclosure of, 2414*t*
   on Internet, 2251–2253, 2252*t*
   protected, 2412
Health insurance:
   for children, 2346–2347
   cost of, 2213
   deductibles, 2211
   employer-sponsored, 2213
   federal programs, 2368, 2368*t*
   HMOs, 2212
   IPAs, 2212
   lack of, 2346–2347, 2347*t*
   mandatory, 2213
   Medigap policy, 2369
   PHOs, 2212
   PPAs, 2212
   PPOs, 2212
   private, 2211–2212, 2368–2369
   public, 2210–2211
   socialized, 2213
   state programs, 2368
   voluntary, 2213
Health insurance companies, rationing by, 2349
Health Insurance Portability and Accountability
     Act (HIPAA), 2001, 2153, 2317, 2333,
     2381, 2391–2392, 2412–2413, 2413*t*
Health literacy, 402–403, 671, 673, 2257–2258,
     2259*t*, 2342–2343
Health Literacy (IOM), 671
Health on the Net Foundation (HON), 2387
Health problems, risk for, 499
Health policy:
   about, 2361–2362
   accrediting bodies, 2366
   Case Study, 2370

   development of, 2362–2363, 2363*t*
   professional organizations and, 2366–2367, 2367*t*
   regulatory agencies, 2363–2365, 2364*t*
   relevance to nurses, 2362*f*
   types of reimbursement, 2367–2369, 2368*t*
Health promotion, 2254*t*, 2285, 2340
   in adolescents, 641*t*
   in children, 641*t*
   vs. disease prevention, 640, 641
   vs. health protection, 640–641
   in infants, 641*t*
   national goals and health indicators, 639–640
   national guidelines for, 2347*t*
   nurse's role in, 641–642
   nursing process
     assessment, 645–647
     diagnosis, 647
     evaluation, 648
     implementation, 648
     planning, 647, 648
   in older adults, 641*t*
Health promotion diagnosis, 2066
Health promotion interventions, 2092
Health protection, 640–641
Health Reimbursement Account (HRA), 2369
Health resources, allocation of limited, 2316
Health Resources and Services Administration
     (HRSA), 398
Health restoration, 2254*t*, 2285
Health risk appraisals, 642
Health Savings Account (HSA), 2369
Health screenings, 643*t*, 644*t*, 2341
Health services organizations, vertically integrated,
     2214–2215
Health–illness continuum, 637–638, 638*f. See also*
     Disease; Health; Illness
Health-seeking behavior, 2258–2259
Healthcare Information and Management Systems
     Society (HIMSS), 2379
HealthGrades, 2443
Healthlinks search engine, 2335
Healthy lifestyle, 645*t*, 2034–2035
Healthy People 1979, 2340
Healthy People 2010, 398, 552*t*, 639–640, 651,
     662, 686, 1127
   on interpersonal violence, 1944
   violence and injury objectives, 1936*t*
Healthy People 2020, 2340
Hearing. *See also* Ears
   assessment, 1643–1644*t*
   diagnostic tests, 1646
   in infants and children, 1635
   process of, 1632
   sensory aids, 1648*t*
   sound conduction, 1633
Hearing aids, 1653–1654, 1653*f*, 1654*f*
Hearing impairment:
   amplification for, 1653–1654
   Case Study, 1656*t*
   cochlear implants for, 1654
   collaborative care, 1653
   communication techniques for, 1655*t*
   conductive, 1651, 1653*t*
   etiology, 1651
   manifestations, 1652, 1653*t*
   nursing diagnoses and interventions
     community-based care, 1656
     disturbed sensory perception, auditory, 1655

impaired verbal communication, 1655–1656
social isolation, 1656
nursing process
assessment, 1655
diagnoses, 1655
evaluation, 1656
planning and implementation, 1655–1656
overview, 1651
presbycusis, 1652
risk factors, 1652
sensorineural, 1652, 1653t
severity levels, 1651t
surgery for, 1654
tinnitus, 1653t
Hearing loss:
effective communication and, 1648t
in older adults, 1635
safety considerations, 1649
Heart. *See also* Cardiovascular system
anatomy, physiology, and functions
action potential, 1305–1306, 1306f
cardiac cycle, 1302–1305, 1303f
cardiac output, 1303–1305
chambers and valves, 1294–1298
conduction system, 1305–1307, 1305f
coronary circulation, 1298, 1301f
heart sounds, 1295–1298, 1296f, 1297t, 1298t, 1317–1318t
internal anatomy, 1295f
layers of heart wall, 1294, 1295f
location of heart, 1294f
pericardium, 1294
pulmonary circulation, 1298, 1300f
pulse, 1307–1308
systemic circulation, 1298, 1300f
transition from fetal to pulmonary circulation, 1300–1302
chambers and valves, 1296f
definition, 1404
electrical activity of, 1312
Heart attack. *See* Acute myocardial infarction (AMI)
Heart block, 1440
Heart defects:
congenital. *See* Congenital heart defects
Heart disease. *See* Cardiovascular disease
Heart failure:
cardiomyopathy and, 1335t
Case Study, 1421
causes, 1404t
classifications
acute vs. chronic, 1407
left-sided vs. right-sided, 1407, 1407f, 1408f
low-output vs. high-output, 1407
pulmonary edema, 1407
systolic vs. diastolic, 1407
Client Teaching, 1420t
collaborative care
complementary therapies, 1417
diagnostic tests, 1411
end-of-life care, 1417
goals of, 1410
hemodynamic monitoring, 1411–1413, 1412f
nutrition and activity, 1416
pharmacologic therapies, 1413–1416
surgery, 1416–1417
compensatory mechanisms activated in, 1405–1406, 1406t
complications, 1410

etiology, 1407–1408
home activity guidelines, 1420t
incidence, 1408
manifestations
left-sided failure, 1408
other, 1408
right-sided failure, 1408
Multisystem Effects, 1409f
Nursing Care Plan
assessment, 1419t
critical thinking, 1419t
diagnoses, 1419t
evaluation, 1419t
planning and implementation, 1419t
nursing diagnoses and interventions
activity intolerance, 1418, 1420
decreased cardiac output, 1418
deficient knowledge, low-sodium diet, 1420
excess fluid volume, 1418
nursing process
assessment, 1417
diagnosis, 1418
evaluation, 1420
planning and implementation, 1418, 1420
overview, 1404–1405
physiology, 1405–1407
risk factors, 1408
stages, 1410t
Heart murmurs:
assessment, 1318t
classification, 1301–1302t
congenital heart defects and, 1349–1350
definition, 1298
distinguishing, 1299–1300t
Heart rate, 1304, 1316t, 1405
target, 652
Heart transplantation:
for cardiomyopathy, 1336
for heart failure, 1416–1417
Heart wall, 1294
Heartburn, 424
during pregnancy, 1574t
Heat balance, 1852
Heat exhaustion, 1859
Heat loss, 1852
Heat production, 1852
Heat stroke, 1859
Heel-to-shin test, 956f
Hegar's sign, 1547, 1547f
Heimlich maneuver, 2452
Helicobacter pylori:
detection of, 933
in peptic ulcer disease, 931
HELLP syndrome, 1469
Helper T cells. *See also* T lymphocytes (T cells)
human immunodeficiency virus (HIV) and, 697, 699f
immune system function and, 679, 679f, 680f, 681
Hematocrit, sepsis and, 852
Hemagglutination inhibition test, 1570
Hematochezia, 1021
Hematocrit (Hct), 129t, 531, 1308, 1490
Hematogenous spread, 857
Hematologic emergencies, 89–90
Hematoma, 1929
Hematopoiesis, 1056
Hematopoietic stem cells, 682
Hematopoietic tissues, 126t

Hematuria, 539
urinary tract infections and, 874
Hemianopia, 1502, 1503f
Hemiarthroscopy, 1112
Hemiparesis, 1505
Hemiplegia, 386t, 1147, 1505
Hemocytoblasts, 676, 678f
Hemodialysis, 416, 543–544, 543f, 559–560, 567.
See also Dialysis
Hemodynamic monitoring, 852, 1372, 1411–1413, 1412f
Hemodynamics, 1411–1413
Hemoglobin (Hgb):
abnormal, possible causes, 129t
as buffer, 4
sepsis and, 852
sickle cell disorder and, 176
Hemoglobinopathy, 176
Hemolysis, 537
Hemolytic anemia:
acquired, 100–101
causes, 100t
definition, 100
glucose-6-phospahte dehydrogenase (G6PD) anemia, 101
thalassemia, 100
Hemoptysis, 163
pneumonia and, 839
tuberculosis and, 860
Hemorrhage, 1929
in peptic ulcer disease, 932
from tumors, 122
Hemorrhagic exudate, 887
Hemorrhagic stroke, 1501
Hemorrhaging, cirrhosis and, 1021
Hemorrhoids, 424, 1574t
Hemosiderosis, 179
Hemostasis, 1927
Hemotympanum, 826
Henderson, Virginia, 2291
Heparin:
administration, 1393t
in specific conditions
deep venous thrombosis, 1392
myocardial infarction, 1376
pulmonary embolism, 1479
Hepatic encephalopathy, cirrhosis and, 1021
Hepatitis A vaccine, 688
Hepatitis B vaccine, 688–689
Hepatorenal syndrome, 1019
HepB, 688–689
Heptavalent, 690
Herbal laxatives, 457t
Herbal supplements/therapy:
for anxiety disorders, 1816
for asthma, 1262–1263
for coronary artery disease, 1383
for gallstones, 905
for heart failure, 1417
for irritable bowel syndrome, 919
for menopause, 1744t
for mood disorders, 1176
for seizure disorders, 972
for sleep disorders, 315
Herceptin, 110
Here-and-now concept, 36
Hereditary factors, 499
Heredity, cancer and, 120

Hernia, 428*t*
Herniated disk:
  client teaching
    proper body mechanics, 1084*t*
  collaborative care
    diagnostic tests, 1082
    overview, 1082
    pharmacologic therapies, 1082
  complementary and alternative therapies, 1084
  definition, 1065*t*, 1080
  diagnosis, 1080
  manifestations, 1080–1082, 1083*t*
  nursing diagnoses and interventions
    acute pain, 1085
    chronic pain, 1085
    constipation, 1085
  nursing process
    assessment, 1084
    diagnosis, 1084
    evaluation, 1085
    overview, 1084
    planning and implementation, 1084–1085
    pathophysiology and etiology, 1080–1081
    risk factors, 1081
  treatment
    conservative, 1082
    surgery, 1083–1084, 1086*t*
Herniation syndrome, 963
Heroin, 73
  effect on fetus, 58*t*
  street names, 74*t*
  use, 68
  use in pregnancy, 60
Herpes, genital. *See* Genital herpes
Herpes simplex virus (HSV), 714*t*, 814
Herpes zoster, 714*t*
Heterografts, 1903
Heterosexism, 401
Heterozygous, 1723
HHS (hyperosmolar hyperglycemic state), 996
Hib, 687–688
Hierarchy of needs, 2061, 2083, 2083*f*, 2083*t*, 2248
High holy days, 1782
High-density lipoproteins (HDLs), 1361, 1365
High-fat foods, 906*t*
High-risk cases, 2122
High-volume cases, 2122
Highly active antiretroviral therapy (HAART),
      697, 704, 710–711
Hinduism:
  dress, 1774*f*
  health-related beliefs, 1784*t*
  medical care and, 1784
Hinshaw, Ada Sue, 2332
Hip bones, 1516
Hip fractures:
  case study, 1117
  classification, 1111
  collaborative care
    diagnostic tests, 1112
    fall prevention, 1112–1113, 1113*t*
    overview, 1112
  definition, 1065*t*, 1066
  extracapsular, 1111
  home care, 1110*t*
  intracapsular fractures, 1111

  manifestations, 1112
  Nursing Care Plan
    assessment, 1116
    critical thinking in the nursing process, 1116*t*
    diagnoses, 1116*t*
    evaluation, 1116*t*
    overview, 1116*t*
    planning and implementation, 1116*t*
  nursing diagnoses and interventions
    acute pain, 1114
    impaired physical mobility, 1115
    risk for disturbed sensory perception,
        tactile, 1115
    risk for infection, 1115
    risk for peripheral neurovascular
        dysfunction, 1115
  nursing process
    assessment, 1114
    diagnosis, 1114
    evaluation, 1116
    planning and implementation, 1114–1116
  overview, 1111
  pathophysiology and etiology, 1111
  risk factors, 1111
  treatment, 1112–1113
Hip replacement, 1129
HIPAA. *See* Health Insurance Portability and
      Accountability Act (HIPAA)
HIPAA Privacy Rule, 2333
Hippocratic Oath, 2308
Hirsutism, 1883*t*
Hispanic Americans:
  autism and, 380*t*
  cancer risk and incidence, 116
  culture-specific assessment, 2010*t*
  homicide and, 1964
  hypertension in, 1425
  smoking and, 1272*t*
  stroke and, 1501*t*
  view of mental illness, 245
Histamine, 887, 887*t*, 960*t*, 964
Histamine receptors, 888
Histamine-receptor blockers:
  in specific conditions
    peptic ulcer disease, 933
Histiocytes, 678
Histoplasmosis, 706
Histrionic personality disorder:
  characteristics, 1616
    cognitive alterations, 1616
    dramatic, exhibitionistic, and egocentric
        responses, 1616
    dysfunctional interpersonal relationships, 1616
    dysphoric mood, 1616
    impaired health patterns, 1616
    impaired sexual expression, 1616
  diagnostic criteria, 1614*t*
  manifestations, 1611*t*
HIV viral load tests, 709
HIV. *See* Human immunodeficiency virus (HIV)
Hives, 1882*t*
HMOs. *See* Health maintenance
      organizations (HMOs)
Hmong, seizure beliefs of, 973*t*
Hobby group, 2135
Holism, 2006

Holistic health assessment, 2008–2009, 2010*t*,
      2011–2018, 2011*f*, 2016*t*, 2018–2020*t*,
      2020–2024, 2023*t*, 2023*t*
  adolescents, 2017
  children
    cultural considerations, 2010*t*
    special considerations, 2009, 2011–2012, 2012*t*
  growth and development, 2012, 2013*t*
  infants, 2013–2014
  life span stages and, 2012
  middle-aged adults, 2018–2019
  older adults, 2020–2023, 2020*t*
    instruments for, 2024*t*
  overview, 2008
  preschoolers, 2015
  toddlers, 2014
  young adults, 2017–2018
Holosystolic, 1342*t*
Holter monitor, 1353*t*
Holy days, 1781
Home alert systems, 2392
Home care documentation, 2195, 2195*t*
Home environment, assessment of, in older
      adults, 2020*t*
Home fires, 2451
Home hazard assessment, 2436, 2438*t*
Home Health Care Classification (HHCC), 2386
Home Observation for Measurement of the
      Environment (HOME) Inventory, 501–502
Home pregnancy tests, 1570
Home safety, 2442, 2442*t*
Home settings, computer networks in, 2392
Homeless clients, 250, 403
Homeostasis, 1793
  blood glucose, 989–990, 990*f*
  fluids and electrolytes in, 518
  maintaining, 519–520, 523
Homer's syndrome, 1145*t*
Homicide, 2457
  description, 1939*t*
  etiology, 1964
  firearm-associated, 1965
  rates, 1964
  sociocultural factors and, 1963–1964
  treatment/prevention, 1939*t*
  workplace, 1965
Homocysteine, 1366
Homografts, 1903
Homologous chromosomes, 87
Homophobia, 400
Homosexuality, incidence, 1696
Homosexuals, 400
Homozygous, 1723
Hope, 1772
Hopelessness, 222, 624
Hopkins Competency Assessment Test, 207*t*
Hormone receptors, 981
Hormone replacement therapy (HRT):
  coronary artery disease and, 1366
  for erectile dysfunction, 1714
  in menopause, 1743
  nursing considerations, 1711*t*
  warnings about, 1743
Hormones, 980–981. *See also* specific hormones
  body temperature and, 1853
  in cancer treatment, 95*t*, 172*t*

definition, 977
endocrine system, 978*t*, 980–981
female, 1519–1520
negative feedback and, 981*f*
pregnancy and, 1545
release mechanisms, 981, 982*f*
release of, 982*f*
as tumor markers, 127
Hospice care, 291–292, 292*t*
Hospital chaplains, 1790*f*
Hospital discharge, 172*t*
Hospital information system (HIS), 2375
Hospitalization:
  involuntary admission, 250
  voluntary admission, 250
Hospitals:
  magnet, 2119, 2131
  reducing environmental distractions in, 261*t*
Hot and cold theory, 1861*t*
Hot flashes, 1744
Hot zones, 2356*t*
Hot-cold belief, 650
Households, 485
hPL. *See* Human placental lactogen (hPL)
HPV. *See* Human papillomavirus (HPV)
HRSA (Health Resources and Services
    Administration), 398
HRT. *See* Hormone replacement therapy (HRT)
5-HT (5-hydroxytryptamine), 1171, 1598, 1608
Human care, theory of, 2030
Human chorionic gonadotropin (HCG), 130*t*,
    1522, 1533–1534, 1545, 1735*t*
Human dignity, 2306
Human error, 2443
Human Genome Project, 1720
Human immunodeficiency virus (HIV). *See also*
    Acquired immunodeficiency
    syndrome (AIDS)
  Case Study, 725*t*
  classification system for, 703*t*
  complementary and alternative therapies for, 715
  definition, 696–697
  description of, 693
  diagnostic tests for, 709–710, 710*t*
  etiology of, 698–701
  history of, 696–697
  incidence and prevalence of, 698–699
  investigational immune-based treatment for, 708*t*
  manifestations of, 702–708, 702*t*
  nursing care for, 708–709
  Nursing Care Plan
    assessment, 723*t*
    critical thinking, 724*t*
    diagnosis, 723*t*
    evaluation, 723*t*
    overview, 723*t*
    planning and implementation, 723*t*
  nursing diagnoses and interventions
    adherence promotion, 720
    care of infants, 719–720, 719*t*
    ineffective coping, 721
    ineffective sexuality patterns, 722
    infection prevention, 717–720
    knowledge deficit, 724
    nutrition, 722
    skin integrity, 721–722
    nursing process
      assessment, 715–716

diagnosis, 716–717
evaluation, 724
planning and implementation, 717–724
pathophysiology of, 697–698, 698*f*, 699*f*
pediatric, 710*t*, 715, 724
pharmacologic therapies
  adherence to, 711
  entry inhibitors, 713
  highly active antiretroviral therapy (HAART),
      710–711
  nonnucleoside reverse transcriptase
      inhibitors, 713
  nucleoside reverse transcriptase inhibitors
      (NRTIs), 711, 712*t*
  other, 713–715
  protease inhibitors, 713
  pregnancy and, 713–715
  prenatal care and, 697*t*
  risk factors, 701–702
  therapies for
    nonadherence to, 720
  transmission of, 698–699, 700*f*
  tuberculosis and, 857, 860
  vaccines and, 720
Human leukocyte antigen (HLA), 757, 1077*t*
Human menopausal gonadotropin (hMG), 1735*t*
Human papillomavirus (HPV), 1758
Human papillomavirus vaccine, 689
Human placental lactogen (hPL), 1533–1534, 1545
Human resource systems, 2378*t*
Human resources, 2388
Human response patterns, 2076*t*
Human Rights Guidelines for Nurses in Clinical
    and Other Research (ANA), 2333
Humanistic learning theory, 2248
Humira. *See* Adalimumab
Humor, 2150
Humoral immune response. *See* Antibody-
    mediated (humoral) immune response
Humoral immune system, in burns, 1896
Humoral immunity, 680*f*
Hunchback. *See* Kyphosis
Hurricane Katrina, 2353, 2354*f*
Hurricane-related injuries, 2352*t*
Hyaluroninc acid (HA), 1127
Hybrid devices, 2378
Hydralazine, 757
Hydralyn. *See* Hydralazine
Hydration status, assessment, 133*t*
Hydrocephalus, 2014
Hydrochloric acid, 4
Hydrocodone, 73
Hydrocolloid dressings, 1903, 1918*t*
Hydrocortisone, 914
Hydrodensitometry, 1028
Hydrogen ions, 3–4
Hydronephrosis, 433, 445, 467, 468*t*, 873
Hydrostatic pressure, 521
Hydroureter, 433
Hydroxychloroquine:
  rheumatoid arthritis and, 750*t*
  systemic lupus erythematosus (SLE) and, 761
5-hydroxytryptamine (5-HT), 1171, 1598, 1608
Hydroxyurea, 102
Hygiene, 326
Hymen, 1688
Hyperacidity, prevention in burn clients, 1901
Hyperactive behavior, 237

Hyperalgesias, 264
Hypercalcemia, 89
  clinical therapies, 593*t*
  diagnostic tests, 593*t*
  etiology, 593*t*
  manifestations, 593*t*
  medications, 593*t*
  nursing process
    assessment, 593*t*
    diagnosis, 593*t*
    interventions, 593*t*
Hypercapnia, 5, 18, 1272
Hypercarbia, 1217
Hyperchloremia:
  clinical therapies, 589*t*
  diagnostic tests, 589*t*
  etiology, 589*t*
  manifestations, 589*t*
  medications, 589*t*
  nursing process
    assessment, 589*t*
    diagnosis, 589*t*
    interventions, 589*t*
Hyperchloremic acidosis, 11
Hypercoagulability, 1884
Hypercyanotic episode, 1342
Hyperemia, 886
Hyperesthesias, 264
Hyperextension, 1144
Hyperflexion, 1144
Hyperglycemia, 990, 992, 995–996
Hyperkalemia:
  in acute renal failure, 538*t*, 548
  clinical therapies, 557*t*
  definition, 532
  diagnostic tests, 591*t*
  etiology, 591*t*
  manifestations, 556, 557*t*, 591*t*
    in children, 539*t*
  medications, 591*t*
  nursing process
    assessment, 591*t*
    diagnosis, 591*t*
    interventions, 591–592*t*
  in older adults, 416
  pharmacologic therapies, 542
Hyperlipidemia, 1361, 1365
Hypermagnesemia:
  clinical therapies, 594*t*
  diagnostic tests, 594*t*
  etiology, 594*t*
  manifestations, 594*t*
  medications, 594*t*
  nursing process
    assessment, 594*t*
    diagnosis, 594*t*
    interventions, 594–595*t*
Hypernatremia:
  clinical therapies, 587*t*, 588*t*
  definition, 532
  diagnostic tests, 587*t*
  etiology, 587*t*, 588*t*
  manifestations, 587*t*, 588*t*
  nursing process
    assessment, 587*t*
    diagnosis, 588*t*
    interventions, 588*t*

Hyperopia, 1639t
Hyperosmolar hyperglycemic state (HHS), 993t, 996
Hyperoxitest, 1353t
Hyperphosphatemia, 538
  in acute renal failure, 548
  in chronic renal failure, 556
  clinical therapies, 596t
  diagnostic tests, 596t
  etiology, 596t
  manifestations, 596t
  medications, 596t
  nursing process
    assessment, 596t
    diagnosis, 596t
    interventions, 596t
Hyperplasia, 88, 432
Hyperpyrexia, 1854, 1859
Hyperresonance, 2004, 2004t
Hypersensitivity:
  Case Study, 741
  clinical therapies, 734t
  collaborative care
    complementary and alternative therapies for, 738
    diagnostic tests, 735–737
    other therapies, 738
    pharmacologic therapies, 737–738
  community-based care, 740–741
  description of, 676, 725–726
  etiology of, 733
  manifestations of, 734–735
  nursing diagnoses and interventions
    decreased cardiac output, 739–740
    ineffective airway clearance, 739
    risk for injury, 740
  nursing process
    assessment, 738
    diagnosis, 738
    evaluation, 741
    planning and implementation, 738–741
  pathophysiology
    Type I (IgE-Mediated), 726, 726t, 727f
    Type II (Cytotoxic), 726t, 727, 728f, 729
    Type III (Immune Complex-Mediated), 726t, 729–730, 729f
    Type IV (Delayed), 726t, 730–731, 730f
  pediatric, 735t
  risk factors, 733–734
Hypersensitivity reaction, 693
Hypersomnia, 258, 309, 1188
Hypertension:
  algorithm for treating, 1428f
  Case Study, 1437
  chronic renal failure and, 556
  Client Teaching, 1435t
  collaborative care
    complementary therapies, 1433, 1433t
    diagnostic tests, 1427–1428
    goals of, 1427
    lifestyle modifications, 1428–1429, 1429t
    pharmacologic therapies, 1429–1433
    weight loss, 1429
  coronary artery disease and, 1364–1365, 1373
  definition, 1422
  description, 1314t
  diabetes mellitus and, 997
  etiology, 1425
  incidence, 1425

kidney transplants and, 562
manifestations, 1426–1427, 1427t
Nursing Care Plan
  assessment, 1436t
  critical thinking, 1437t
  diagnoses, 1436t
  evaluation, 1436t
  planning and implementation, 1436t
nursing diagnoses and interventions
  excess fluid volume, 1435
  imbalanced nutrition, more than body requirements, 1434–1435
  ineffective health maintenance, 1434
  risk for noncompliance, 1434
nursing process
  assessment, 1433
  diagnosis, 1433
  evaluation, 1435
  planning and implementation, 1433–1435
pathophysiology, 1422–1425
portal, 1017
pregnancy-induced. See Pregnancy-induced hypertension, 1293
primary, 1424
risk factors, 1425–1426, 1426t
secondary, 1424–1425
stroke and, 1501
treatment, 1314t
Hypertensive emergency, 1172, 1425, 1427t
Hypertensive encephalopathy, 1427
Hypertensive nephrosclerosis, 553t
Hyperthermia, 1852
  clinical manifestations, 1861
  collaborative care, 1861
  community-based care, 1863
  definition, 1855t, 1859
  nursing process
    assessment, 1862
    diagnosis, 1863
    evaluation, 1863
    implementation, 1863
    plan, 1863
  pathophysiology and etiology, 1859–1861
  risk factors, 1861
  treatment, 1855
Hyperthermia blanket, 1868
Hyperthyroidism. See also Hypothyroidism
  clinical therapies, 1044t
  collaborative care
    diagnostic tests, 1044, 1044t
    pharmacologic therapies, 1044
    radioactive iodine therapy (RAI), 1044–1045
    surgery, 1045
  definition, 1041
  laboratory findings in, 1044t
  manifestations, 1041–1044, 1044t
  Multisystem Effects, 1042t
  Nursing Care Plan
    assessment, 1046t
    critical thinking, 1046t
    diagnosis, 1046t
    evaluation, 1046t
    planning and implementation, 1046t
  nursing diagnoses and interventions
    disturbed body image, 1047
    disturbed sensory perception, visual, 1045, 1047

    imbalanced nutrition, less than body requirements, 1047
    risk for decreased cardiac output, 1045
  nursing process
    assessment, 1045
    diagnosis, 1045
    evaluation, 1046
    implementation, 1045–1046
    planning, 1045
  pathophysiology and etiology, 1041
  risk factors, 1041
Hypertonic dehydration, 570
Hypertonic solutions, 520
Hypertrophic scars, 1892
Hypertrophy, 652
  definition, 432
Hypertropic cardiomyopathy, 1326t, 1333–1334, 1333t
Hyperventilation, 23–25, 1253
Hyphema, 1662
Hypnotherapy, for smoking cessation, 54
Hypnotics, 217, 313–314, 314t
Hypoactive sexual desire disorder, 1702
Hypocalcemia, 538
  in chronic renal failure, 556
  diagnostic tests, 592t
  etiology, 592t
  manifestations, 592t
    in children, 539t
  medications, 592t
  nursing process
    assessment, 592t
    diagnosis, 592t
    interventions, 592t
Hypocapnia, 5
Hypochloremia:
  clinical therapies, 588–589t
  diagnostic tests, 588t
  etiology, 588t
  manifestations, 588–589t
  nursing process
    assessment, 588
    diagnosis, 589t
Hypodermis, 1875
Hypogeusia, 1635
Hypoglossal nerves, 942t, 1628t
Hypoglycemia, 993t, 996–997
Hypoglycemic agents, 1005
Hypokalemia:
  definition, 532
  diagnostic tests, 589–590t
  etiology, 589–590t
  manifestations, 589–590t
  medications, 590t
  metabolic alkalosis and, 15
  nursing process
    assessment, 589–590t
    diagnosis, 590t
    interventions, 590–591t
Hypomagnesemia:
  clinical therapies, 593–594t
  diagnostic tests, 593–594t
  etiology, 593–594t
  manifestations, 593–594t
  medications, 594t

nursing process
assessment, 593–594t
diagnosis, 593–594t
interventions, 593–594t
Hypomania:
assessment, 1182
diagnostic criteria, 1178t
manifestations, 1179, 1180t
Hyponatremia:
in acute renal failure, 548
clinical therapies, 587t
definition, 532
etiology, 587t
manifestations, 587t
in children, 539t
medications, 587t
nursing process
assessment, 587t
diagnosis, 587t
interventions, 587t
in older adults, 416
Hypophosphatemia:
clinical therapies, 595t
diagnostic tests, 595t
etiology, 595t
manifestations, 595t
medications, 595t
nursing process
assessment, 595t
diagnosis, 595t
interventions, 595–596t
Hypophysis (pituitary gland), 978
Hypoplastic left heart syndrome (HLHS),
1348–1349t
Hypoproteinemia, 1916
Hypospadia, 1735
Hypotension, 619, 1323–1324
Hypothalamus, 940
female reproductive cycle and, 1521
thermoregulation and, 1860
Hypothermia, 1852
clinical manifestations, 1862t, 1867, 1868t
collaborative care, 1867
definition, 1854–1855, 1865
induced, 1865
Nursing Care Plan, 1869
nursing process
assessment, 1868
diagnosis, 1868
evaluation, 1870
implementation, 1868, 1870
plan, 1868
pathophysiology and etiology, 1865–1867
risk factors, 1867
therapies, 1862t, 1868t
treatment, 1855
Hypothyroidism, 202. See also Hyperthyroidism
clinical therapies, 1048t
collaborative care
diagnostic tests, 1050, 1050t
pharmacologic therapies, 1050
surgery, 1050
definition, 1047
description, 983t
developmental considerations, 1052t
laboratory findings in, 1050t
manifestations, 1048, 1048t
Multisystem Effects, 1049t

Nursing Care Plan
assessment, 1051t
critical thinking, 1051t
diagnosis, 1051t
evaluation, 1051t
planning and implementation, 1051t
nursing diagnoses and interventions
constipation, 1050–1051
decreased cardiac output, 1050
risk for impaired skin integrity, 1051–1052
nursing process
assessment, 1050
diagnosis, 1050
evaluation, 1052
implementation, 1050–1052
planning, 1050
pathophysiology and etiology, 1047–1048
risk factors, 1048
skin integrity and, 1051–1052
Hypotonic dehydration, 569
Hypotonic solutions, 520
Hypovolemia, 850
definition, 535
pathophysiology, 569
pulse and, 1308
Hypovolemic shock:
in burns, 1894–1895
clinical therapies, 1491t
definition, 1488
manifestations, 1491t
stages, 1488f
Hypoxemia:
definition, 5, 1309
hypercyanotic episode and, 1342
indications
chest wall in-drawing, 1218
clubbed nail beds, 1218–1219
cyanosis, 1218
pneumonia and, 846
Hypoxia, sepsis and, 854
Hysterectomy:
abdominal, 1751
definition, 1750
postoperative care, 1751t
preoperative care, 1751t
vaginal, 1751
Hytrin, 434, 434t
critical thinking, 1460t
diagnoses, 1460t
evaluation, 1460t
planning and implementation, 1460t
nursing diagnoses and interventions
decreased cardiac output, 1458–1459
nursing process
assessment, 1457–1458
diagnosis, 1458
evaluation, 1461
planning and implementation, 1458–1459, 1461
in older adults, 1439
overview, 1438
pathophysiology, 1438, 1440
sick sinus syndrome, 1444
sinus node, 1440
supraventricular
characteristics, 1441–1442t
pathophysiology, 1440
treatment, 1314t

ventricular
characteristics, 1442–1443t
pathophysiology, 1445–1446

I

Iatrogenic, 582
Iatrogenic infections, 787
IBD. See Inflammatory bowel disease (IBD)
Ibuprofen, 275, 748, 749t, 1861t
Ibutilide, 1449
ICF. See Intracellular fluid (ICF)
ICU psychosis, 226
ICU syndrome, 226
IDEA (Individuals with Disabilities Act), 205
Ideal self, 1581
Identical twins, 1530, 1531f
Identity, development of, 1591t
Identity stressors, 1589t
Identity verification, 2443f
IDET. See Intradiscal electrothermal therapy (IDET)
Idiopathic neuropathies, 1679
IDS. See Integrated delivery systems, 2212
IEPs (individualized education plans), 205, 376
IgA, 679f, 680, 682, 692
IgD, 679f, 680–681
IgE, 679f, 680–681, 692
hypersensitivity and, 726, 726t, 727f, 733
IgG, 679f, 680, 692
IgM, 679f, 680–681, 692
IICP. See Increased intracranial pressure
Ileal pouch-anal anastomosis (IPAA), 916, 916f
Illegal activities, advocacy and, 2302
Ileostomy:
continent, 917, 917f
definition, 917
nursing care
health education for client and family, 918–919t
postoperative care, 917–918t
preoperative care, 917t
permanent, 916
temporary or loop, 916–917
Ileus, 426
Iliococcygeus, 1517t
Ilium, 1516
Illiteracy, 402–403
Illness:
about, 635–645
acute, 638
chronic. See also Chronic illness
chronic, 638
definition, 638
vs. disease, 638
effects on client and family, 638–639
impact of, on families, 506–514
Illness behaviors, 638
Illness prevention, 2254t, 2285, 2450, 2450t
Illusions, 232
Imipramine, 443
Imitation, 2247
Immigrant groups, 323
Immigrants, undocumented, 404
Immobility, 1916
Immoral activities, advocacy and, 2302
Immune complex assays, 736
Immune disorders, therapies for, 696

Immune response:
  antibody-mediated (humoral), 676
  cell-mediated (cellular), 676
  nonspecific inflammatory response, 682
  primary, 680, 680*f*
  secondary, 680
Immune surveillance, 679
Immune system:
  age and, 692–693
  altered function, 693–694
  Assessment Interview, 694
  assessment of
    health history, 694
    physical examination, 694
  benefits of exercise for, 654
  caring interventions, 695
  cells and tissues of, 682*t*
  complementary therapies, 696
  components
    antigen-presenting cells, 678
    antigens, 679–681
    granulocytes, 676–677
    leukocytes, 676
    lymphocytes, 679
    lymphoid system, 681–682
  diagnostic tests for, 695
  effects of chronic renal failure on, 556
  fetal development, 1537*t*
  function of, 676
  glucocorticoids and, 980
  pediatric differences in, 692
  pharmacologic therapies, 696
Immune-complex-dissociated p24 assay, 709–710
Immunity, 675–676
  about, 675–696
  acquired, 679
  active, 682
  alterations, 693–694
  assessment, 694, 695–696*t*
  caring interventions, 695
  complementary therapies, 696
  definition, 676
  diagnostic tests, 695
  normal presentation, 676–693
  passive, 682–683
  pharmacologic therapies, 696
Immunization guidelines, 643*t*, 644*t*
Immunizations:
  contraindications, 686
  description of, 682–683
  immune system function and, 676
  parental rights and informed consent, 686
  pediatric, 687–691
  responses to, 683
  risk of infection and, 777
  schedule, 683, 684–685*f*
Immunocompetent, 676
Immunodeficiency, 676
Immunogenicity, 680
Immunogens, 679–680
Immunoglobulins, 677*t*, 680–681
  age and, 692*f*
  pediatric levels, 692
Immunomodulators:
  in specific conditions
    multiple sclerosis, 1121*t*
Immunoradiometric assay (IRMA), 1570

Immunosuppressants:
  anemia, 102
  glomerular disorders, 926
  multiple sclerosis, 1120, 1121*t*
  rheumatoid arthritis and, 749
  transplants, 561–562
Immunotherapy, for melanomas, 190
Immunotherapy drugs:
  for hypersensitivity, 737
  systemic lupus erythematosus (SLE) and, 761*t*
Impacted fractures, 1095*t*
Impaired memory, 220
Impaired religiosity, 1785
Impairment, of coworkers, 2302
Imparting information, 2168*t*, 2169
Impedance audiometry, 828
Impetigo, 800*f*
Implanon, 1732
Implantable cardioverter-defibrillator, 1452
Implantation, 1527–1528, 1528*f*
Implementation, 2045–2046, 2046*t*
  defined, 2096
  evaluation of, 2101
  nursing interventions, 2097
  in nursing process, 2051*t*, 2096–2098, 2097*f*
  process of, 2096–2098
  relationship to other nursing process phases, 2096
  skills necessary for, 2096
Implementation phase, of policy development, 2362
Implied consent, 2403
Impotence, 1712. *See also* Erectile
    dysfunction (ED)
Impulse conduction, 1628
Impulse control, addiction and, 28
Impulsive behavior, 1588
Impulsiveness, 1610
Imuran. *See* Azathioprine
In vitro fertilization (IVF), 1736–1737
Inappropriate affect, 238
Incentive spirometry, 1227
Incest, 1947
Incident pain, 264
Incident reports, 2417
Incisions, 1880*t*
Incontinence:
  bowel. *See* Fecal incontinence
  pressure ulcers and, 1916
  urinary. *See* Urinary incontinence
Increased intracranial pressure (IICP):
  care settings, 965*t*
  Case Study, 967
  Client Teaching, 966*t*
  collaborative care, 963
    diagnostic tests, 963
    ICP monitoring, 964, 964*t*
    mechanical ventilation, 964
    pharmacologic therapy, 963, 963*t*
    physical therapy, 965
    respiratory therapy, 965
    surgery, 964
  definition, 947*t*, 948, 961
  manifestations, 962, 962*t*
  nursing interventions, 966
  nursing process
    assessment, 965
    diagnosis, 965
    evaluation, 966*t*
    planning and implementation, 965–966

  pathophysiology and etiology, 961–962
  risk factors, 962
  treatment, 947*t*, 962*t*
    medications, 959–960*t*
Incus, 1632
Independence, 2106
Independent functions, 2067
Independent interventions, 2089
Independent practice associations (IPAs), 2212
Indiana Center for Evidence-Based Nursing
    Practice, 2335
Inderal, 1815
Indicators, 2086, 2425
Indifferent parents, 491–492, 491*t*
Indinavir, 713
Indirect auscultation, 2004
Indirect Coombs' test, 736
Indirect percussion, 2003, 2004*f*
Individual conflict, 2127
Individual decision making, 2039
Individualism, 347
Individualized care plans, 2077
Individualized education plans (IEPs), 205, 376
Individualized Health Plan, 376
Individuals with Disabilities Act (IDEA), 205
Indocin. *See* Indomethacin
Indomethacin, 469, 749*t*
Inductive reasoning, 2106
Infancy, 341*t*
Infant car safety seats, 2438*t*
Infants. *See also* Newborns
  assessment of, 2013–2014
  attachment by, 2012, 2014
  body fluid balance in, 526–527, 527*f*
  body temperature of, 1858*t*
  communication by, 2155*t*
  developmental tasks in, 1581*t*
  fluid volume deficit in, 571
  grief and loss in, 610*t*
  growth and development, 354–357, 355*t*
  health promotion in, 641*t*
  neurologic assessment in, 958, 958*t*
  neurologic system in, 943
  pain perception and behavior, 269*t*
  premature, 1558*t*, 1559
  promotion of oral health in, 659
  safety measures for, 2454, 2455*t*
  sensory perception in, 1646*t*
  skin of, 1875
  sleep patterns and requirements, 668
  stress and coping in, 1802*t*
  wound care in, 1929*t*
Infected wounds, 1879
Infection control nurse, 785
Infection, 676
  about, 770–808
  acute, 771
  alterations, 785–801
  assessment, 801–804
  asymptomatic, 770
  biological threats, 790–791
  body defenses against, 773
  cancer risk and, 121
  caring interventions, 805–807
  chain of
    about, 771–772
    etiologic agent, 772
    method of transmission, 772–773

nursing interventions to break, 774–775*t*
portal of entry to susceptible host, 773
portal of exit from reservoir, 772
reservoir, 772
susceptible host, 773
children and, 775–776
chronic, 771
definition of, 770
diabetes mellitus and, 999, 1011
diagnostic tests, 804–805
health care workers and, 784–785
immune response to, 678
increased susceptibility to, 775–776
microorganisms causing, 771
normal presentation, 770–777
nosocomial, 787–789, 788*t*
older adults and, 775–776
pharmacologic therapies, 807–808*t*
precautions against
    disinfecting and sterilizing, 777–778
    isolation, 778–779, 780*t*
    protective equipment, 779–782
prevention of, 1933
    burns, 1900–1901, 1907
    sterile technique, 782, 784
sexually transmitted. *See* Sexually transmitted
    infections (STIs)
skin, 1876, 1878*t*
from tumors, 122
types of, 771
of urinary system, 418*t*
wound, 1929
Infectious disease. *See also* specific diseases
Assessment Interview, 804
complications of, 787
definition of, 770
diagnostic tests for, 804–805
mandatory reporting of, 2414, 2415*t*
    manifestations of, 804–805*t*
most common, 801*t*
nursing process
    assessment, 801–802, 804
    interventions, 805–807
    medications, 807–808
pediatric, 791, 791–799*t*
Infectious process:
in older adults, 776–777
stages of, 786–787
Inferences, 2064, 2106*t*
Inferior vena cava, 1294
Infertility:
assisted reproduction
    other techniques, 1737
    preimplantation genetic diagnosis, 1737–1738
    therapeutic insemination, 1735–1736
    in vitro fertilization, 1736–1737
causes, 1719, 1719*t*
collaborative care
    diagnostic tests, 1734
    fertility medications, 1734, 1735*t*
cultural considerations, 1738*t*
definition, 1718
incidence, 1718
medications, 1711*t*
non-Mendelian, 1723
secondary, 1718
Inflammation, 676, 682
about, 885–892

acute, 886, 888*f*
alterations, 889, 889*t*
assessment, 890
Assessment Interview, 890*t*
caring interventions, 891
cellulitis and, 808–809
chemical mediators of, 887*t*
chronic, 886
coronary artery disease and, 1366
definition, 886
diagnostic tests, 890, 891*t*
function of, 885–886
histamine receptors, 888
localized, 890
normal presentation, 886–888
nursing interventions, 891
nursing process
    assessment, 890, 890*t*
pharmacologic therapies, 891, 892*t*
signs of, 886
skin, 1876, 1878*t*
stages of, 886–887
    exudate production, 887
    reparative phase, 887
    vascular and cellular responses, 886–887
symptoms and treatment, 889*t*
treatment, 889*t*
Inflammatory bowel disease (IBD):
Case Study, 923
client teaching
    dietary instructions for children, 921*t*
collaborative care
    alternative therapies, 919
    diagnostic tests, 914
    nutrition, 916
    pharmacologic therapies, 914, 915*t*, 916
    surgery, 916–917, 917–919*t*
community-based care, 921*t*
definition, 909
incidence, 909
manifestations, 912*t*
Nursing Care Plan
    assessment, 922*t*
    critical thinking in the nursing process, 922*t*
    diagnoses, 922*t*
    evaluation, 922*t*
    overview, 922*t*
    planning and implementation, 922*t*
nursing diagnoses and interventions
    diarrhea, 920
    disturbed body image, 920
    imbalanced nutrition, less than body
        requirements, 921
nursing process
    assessment, 919
    diagnosis, 919
    evaluation, 922
    planning and implementation, 919–921, 921*t*
risk factors, 912
types
    Chrohn's disease. *See* Chrohn's disease
    ulcerative colitis. *See* Ulcerative colitis
    inflammatory breast cancer, 107
Inflammatory response:
systemic lupus erythematosus (SLE) and, 757
tuberculosis and, 856
Inflexible behavior, 1588
Infliximab, 748–749

Influence, 2235
Influenza:
avian, 818–819
care plan, 823
Case Study, 824
in children, 793*t*
definition, 818
diagnostic tests, 821
epidemics, 818
etiology, 820
H1N1, 818–819
manifestations, 820–821, 820*t*
nursing diagnoses and interventions
    disturbed sleep pattern, 823
    ineffective airway clearance, 822–823
    ineffective breathing pattern, 822
    risk of infection, 823
nursing process
    assessment, 822
    diagnosis, 822
    evaluation, 823
    planning and implementation, 822
pandemics, 819*t*
pathophysiology, 819–820
pharmacologic therapies, 821–822
pneumonia and, 835
prevention of, 820–821
risk factors, 820
treatments for, 801
vaccines, 820–821
Influenza vaccine, 689–690
Informal groups, 2135–2136, 2136*t*
Informal leaders, 2233
Informal nursing care plans, 2077
Informatics:
about, 2373–2378, 2377–2378*t*
Case Study, 2385
client safety and, 2444
clinical decision support systems, 2385–2389,
    2387*t*, 2388*t*
competencies, 2374
nursing, 2373
point-of-care devices, 2389, 2390*f*, 2390*t*
trends in, 2378–2384, 2379*f*, 2380*t*, 2381*t*,
    2382*t*, 2384*t*
Information:
acquiring, 2247*t*
Internet and, 2283
processing, 2247*t*
using, 2247*t*
Information confrontations, 2171
Information dissemination, 641
Information exchange, 2118
Information literacy skills, 2374
Information management systems, 2342
Information processing, 198
Information processing theory, 2248
Information sharing, 2336
Information sources, evaluating credibility of, 2106
Information systems:
administrative, 2375
clinical, 2375
computer, 2375
defined, 2375
hospital, 2375
nursing, 2375–2378, 2377*t*
Information technology, 2336, 2375
Informed consent, 2333–2334

children and, 2404–2405, 2405f, 2405t
client understanding and, 2403
competency for, 2404
defined, 2403
in emergency, 2404
guidelines for, 2403
protocols for, 2403
Infrared thermometer, 1857
Inguinal area:
    assessment, 428t
INH. See Isoniazid
Inhalants, 74
Inhalers, 1259, 1259t
Inheritance:
    autosomal dominant, 1723
    autosomal recessive, 1723–1724
    chromosomes, 1720
    Mendelian, 1723
    modes of, 1723
    multifactorial, 1724
    X-linked dominant, 1724
    X-linked recessive, 1724
Inhibited grief, 606
Initial (or baseline) assessment, 2000t
Initial database, 2193
Injury prevention, 2254t
    across the lifespan, 2454, 2455–2456t,
        2456–2458, 2456t
    burns and scalds, 2450t
    carbon monoxide poisoning, 2451
    Case Study, 2459
    choking, 2452
    domestic violence, 2458–2459
    electrical hazards, 2452–2453, 2454t
    excessive noise, 2452
    falls, 2451, 2452t
    firearms, 2454
    fires, 2450–2451
    overview, 2450, 2450t
    poisoning, 2451, 2453t
    radiation, 2454
    suffocation, 2452
Injuries:
    diabetes mellitus and, 1012
    immune system and, 676
    traumatic, 1937–1938
Inner ear, 1632–1633, 1636t
Innominate bones, 1516
Inotropes, 1493t
Inotropic drugs, 1493t, 1943
    sepsis and, 852–853
Input, system, 497–498
Input devices, 2374
Insensible fluid loss, 522–523
Insensible heat loss, 1853
Insensible water loss, 1853
Insomnia:
    definition, 258, 309
    depression and, 1188
    manifestations, 313t
    melatonin and, 1176
    risk factors, 311
Inspection, 2002
Inspiration, respiratory, 1215
Institute of Healthcare Improvement (IHI), 2423
Institute of Medicine (IOM):
    Crossing the Quality Chasm, 2386, 2422
    definition of quality, 2421
    To Err Is Human, 2422

on evidence-based practice, 2324
Health Literacy report, 671
on problem of underinsured, 2210t
on sleep needs, 665
Institutional abuse, 1945
Institutional review boards (IRBs), 2333
Insubordination, 2237
Insulin:
    abnormal, possible causes, 130t
    administration, 1003t
    definition, 980
    diabetes mellitus and, 1002–1005
    ectopic functioning and, 137t
    function, 989
    hypertension and, 1424
    mechanism of action, 987t
    nursing considerations, 987t
    preparations, 1002t
Insulin reaction (insulin shock), 996
Insulin resistance:
    hypertension and, 1426
Insurance. See also Health insurance
    private, 2210
    professional liability, 2402
Intake and output record, 2193
Intal. See Cromolyn sodium
Integra, 1903
Integrated delivery systems (IDSs), 2212
Integrated health care delivery system, 2343f
Integrity, 2107, 2306
    as component of professionalism, 2227, 2227t
Integumentary assessment, 1882t, 1883–1884t
Integumentary system,
Intellectual courage, 2107
Intellectual disabilities, clients with, 403
Intellectual humility, 2107
Intellectual integrity, 2107
Intellectual skills, 2096, 2248
Intellectual standards, 2109t
Intelligence, multiple, 2248–2249
Intelligence quotient (IQ), 2248
Intensity, of sound, 2005
Intentional torts, 2400–2401
Intentional trauma, 1937
Interdisciplinary teams, 2133–2141, 2135t, 2136t,
        2137t, 2138t, 2141t
    See also Groups
Interferons, 155, 713
Intergroup conflict, 2128, 2129t
Interleukin-1, 677t, 742
Interleukins, 155, 681
Intermittent claudication, 1463
Intermittent explosive disorder (IED), 1963
Intermittent fever, 1859
Internal chamber, of eye, 1631
Internal mammary artery (IMA), 1378, 1379f
Internals, 650
International Classification of Epileptic Seizures, 972
International Classification for Nursing Practice
        (ICNP®), 2386
International Council of Nurses, Code of Ethics,
        2308, 2309t
International Journal of Nursing Terminologies
        and Classifications, 2076t
International Nursing Coalition for Mass Casualty
        Education (INCMCE), 2355
International Prostate Symptom Score (IPSS),
        433t, 437t

International Red Cross, 2290
Internet, 2212, 2283
    access to, 672t, 2382–2383
    health information on, 2251–2253, 2252t
    health information on, 672t
    use by age and gender, 2252t
    use of, by older adults, 2252
Internet counseling, 648
Internet resources:
    evaluation of, 2388t
    for evidence-based research, 2335t
Interpersonal attitudes, communication and,
        2157–2158
Interpersonal conflict, 2127
Interpersonal psychotherapy (IPT), 608t, 1191
Interpersonal skills, 2096
Interpersonal violence, 1937, 1944–1945, 1953
Interpersonal violence. See also Abuse
Interpreters, 334, 2162
Interpretive confrontations, 2171
Intersex, 1696
Intersex anatomy, 400
Intersex Society of North America, 400
Interstitial fluid, 518, 519f, 580
Interstitial fluid osmotic pressure, 580
Interstitial fluid volume excess. See also Edema
Interstitial fluid volume excess, 579–581
Interstitial pneumonia, 835t
Interventional study design, 2328t
Intervertebral disks. See also Herniated disk
Intervertebral disks, 1080
Interviewing, 2000
Interviews:
    directive, 2056
    nondirective, 2056
    planning, 2057
    setting for, 2057–2058
    stages of, 2058–2059
    types of questions, 2056–2057, 2057t
    uses of, 2056
Intimacy, 1694
Intimate distance, 2156
Intimate partner abuse, 2461–2462, 2462t
Intimate partner violence (IPV), 1949–1950, 1955t
Intimidation, 2229, 2229t
Intonation, 2150
Intra-aortic balloon pump (IABP), 1382, 1382f, 1416
Intra-arterial pressure monitoring, 1411–1412
Intracapsular extraction, 1658
Intracapsular fractures, 1111, 1111f
Intracellular fluid (ICF), 518, 519f, 520t, 526f
Intracellular protein:
    as buffer, 4
Intracranial hemorrhage. See also Stroke
Intracranial hemorrhage, 1501
Intracranial hypertension. See Increased
        intracranial pressure
Intracranial pressure (ICP) monitoring, 964,
        964t, 974f
Intracranial regulation:
    about, 939–960
    alterations, 944–949, 947t
    assessment, 949, 950–58t
    caring interventions, 959
    definition, 939
    diagnostic tests, 958–59
    normal presentation, 940–944

pharmacologic therapies, 959–960, 960t
treatments, 947t
Intractable seizures, 971
Intradermal PPD test (Mantoux test), 861, 861f
Intradermal test, 736
Intradiscal electrothermal therapy (IDET), 1084
Intrafamily violence, 1942
Intragenerational family, 487
Intranets, 2379–2380
Intraocular pressure, 1668
Intraocular structures, 1630–1631
Intraoperative nursing care, 897
Intrapartum:
    definition, 1559t
Intrapartum care, 1558, 1558t
Intrapersonal communication, 2148, 2148f
Intrapersonal theory:
    mood disorders and, 1162
    personality disorders and, 1609
Intrauterine devices (IUDs), 1730–1731, 1730f
Intrauterine fetal death (IUFD), 626
Intravascular fluid, 518
Intravenous fluids:
    commonly administered, 576t, 577t
    for fluid volume deficit, 576–577
    overadministration of, 581t
Intravenous immunoglobulin (IVIg), 217
Intravenous pyelography (IVP), 469, 540, 876
Intraventricular conduction blocks, 1448
Intrinsic (intrarenal) acute renal failure. See also
        Acute renal failure
Intrinsic (intrarenal) acute renal failure, 534, 534t
Introitus, 1688
Introspection, 1580
Intuition, 2044
Intuitive decision making, 2039
Intuitive thought stage, 348
Invasion, 118
Invasion of privacy, 2401
Involuntary admission, 250
Involuntary euthanasia, 291
Iodine, recommended daily intake, 1597t
Iodine deficiency, hypothyroidism and, 1048
IOM. See Institute of Medicine
Ion trapping, 9–10
Ions, 518
Iowa Intervention Project, 2092
IPAs. See Independent practice associations, 2212
iPods, 2378
IPSS (International Prostate Symptom Score),
        433t, 437t
IPV, 691
IQ scores, 201–202
Iris, 1630, 1642t
Iron:
    anemia and, 99
    dietary sources, 103t
    hemoglobin formation and, 1310
    pregnancy and, 1543
    recommended daily intake, 1597t
    supplements, 95t, 559
Iron deficiency anemia, 97, 99, 99f, 102t. See also
        Anemia
Iron replacement therapy, 102
Iron tablets, 426
Irreversible coma, 948
Irritant contact dermatitis, 1912
Ischemia, 534, 854, 1362

Ischemic, 1304
Ischemic stroke:
    deep venous thrombosis and, 1391
    embolic, 1500–1501
    pathophysiology, 1500
    thrombotic, 1500
    transient, 1500
Ischial spines, 1516
Ischium, 1516
Islam:
    end-of-life care and, 293
    medical care and, 1783
Isobutyl nitrite, 74
Isoelectric line, 1327t
Isokinetic exercise, 652
Isolation precautions:
    overview of, 778–779
    psychosocial needs and, 782
    recommended, 780t
    types of, 779–782
Isometric exercise, 652
Isoniazid, 757
    nursing considerations and, 864t
    tuberculosis and, 862–863
Isoproterenol, 1943
Isosorbide mononitrate, 1020
Isotel. See Mannitol
Isotonic dehydration, 569
Isotonic electrolyte solutions, 576–577
Isotonic exercise, 652
Isotonic fluid volume deficit, 569
Isotonic imbalances, 569
Isotonic solutions, 520
Israel Foundation for Crohn's Disease and
        Ulcerative Colitis, 921t
IUDs. See Intrauterine devices (IUDs)
IUFD (intrauterine fetal death), 626
IVF. See In vitro fertilization (IVF)
IVIg (intravenous immunoglobulin), 217

J

Jarisch-Herxheimer reaction, 1762
Jaundice:
    cirrhosis and, 1022
JCAHO (Joint Commission on Accreditation of
        Healthcare Organizations), 670
Jehovah's Witnesses, 564, 1784, 1784t
Jewish cultures:
    infertility treatments and, 1738t
Johanna Briggs Institute, 2335
Johns Hopkins University, 2335
Johnson & Johnson, 2329
Joint arthroplasty, 1129
Joint Commission:
    as accreditation agency, 2366
    accreditation and, 2389
    mission of, 2366, 2423
    National Patient Safety Goals, 2196, 2423,
        2459, 2460t
    on client education, 2254
    on documentation, 2183
    on staff development, 2273
    patient rights and, 2318
    sentinel events and, 2423–2424
Joint Commission on Accreditation of Healthcare
        Organizations (JCAHO), 402, 670
Joint Committee of the National Council on
        Alcoholism and Drug Dependence, 40

Joint custody, 487
Joint replacement surgery, 1112
Joint(s):
    age-related changes, 1063t, 1065
    assessment, 1071, 1071t
    cartilaginous, 1061
    classification, 1061, 1061t
    definition, 1061
    disorders
        of foot, 1067, 1070f
        osteoarthritis. See Osteoarthritis (OS)
        rheumatoid arthritis. See Rheumatoid arthritis
        rotator cuff tears, 1066, 1068f
        temporomandibular joint (TMJ) syndrome, 1066
        of wrist and hand, 1066, 1068f, 1069
    fibrous, 1061
    inflammation of
        rheumatoid arthritis and, 743f
    inflammatory disease. See Rheumatoid arthritis
    range of motion, 1065, 1071–1072, 1072t
    replacement. See Total joint replacement
    synovial, 1061–1062, 1061f, 1061t
    temporomandibular, 1072f
Judaism:
    end-of-life care and, 293
    health-related beliefs, 1784t
    medical care and, 1783
Judgmental responses, 2159t
Judgments, 2106t
Junctional dysrhythmias, 1445
Junctional escape rhythm, 1442t, 1445
Jung, Carl, 347
Justice, 1778, 2308
Juvenile rheumatoid arthritis (JRA), 745, 747

K

K+. See Potassium
Kadian, 287t
Kaiserswerth School, 2287
Kaposi's sarcoma:
    acquired immunodeficiency syndrome (AIDS)
        and, 696, 705–706, 705f, 714t
Kardexes, 2193
Karyotype:
    definition, 1720
    female, 1720f
    male, 1720f
Katz Index of Independence in Activities of Daily
        Living, 2024t
Kava, 1744t, 1816
Keeping Patients Safe: Transforming the Work of
        Nurses (IOM), 2433
Kegel exercises, 445t, 450
Keloids, 1879t, 1892, 1929
Kennedy, Maureen, 2326
Kenney, Elizabeth, 2290
Keratin, 1874
Keratinization, 1874
Keratinocytes, 1874
Keratotic warts, 1758
Kernig's sign, 957t
Ketamine, 1970
Ketogenic diet, 972, 972t, 975
Ketonuria, 1001
Ketoprofen, 748, 749t
Ketosis, 990–991
Kidney biopsy, 558, 760, 926

Kidney disease:
　hypertension and, 1427
　secondary hypertension and, 1424–1425
Kidney scan, 926
Kidney stones. *See* Urinary calculi
Kidney transplant:
　immunosuppressive therapy, 561–562
　incidence, 560
　kidney allocation, 562*t*
　nursing care, 561*t*, 563*t*
　placement, 561*f*
　postoperative care, 561*t*, 563*t*
　preoperative care, 561*t*, 563*t*
　procedure, 561
　rejection of, 562
　results, 560
　source of organs, 560–561
Kidneys:
　assessment, 419*t*
　assessment techniques, 469*f*, 471*t*, 472*f*, 472*t*,
　　473*f*, 474*f*, 474*t*, 475*t*, 476*t*, 477*t*
　blood pressure and, 1424
　disorders
　　acute renal failure. *See* Acute renal failure
　　chronic renal failure. *See* Chronic renal failure
　inflammation of. *See* Nephritis
　regulation of body fluids by, 523, 527, 533
　urinary elimination by, 410–411
Kids Count Data Center, 2382
Killer T cells, 680*f*, 681
Kindling, 30*t*, 67
Kinesthesia, 1645*t*
Kinesthetic stimuli, 1628
Klebsiella pneumoniae, 834
Klinefelter syndrome, 1721*t*, 1722
Knee replacement, 1130
Knights of Saint Lazarus, 2287, 2288*f*
Knowledge:
　body of, 2280
　as component of professionalism, 2226
　developing ways of knowing, 2032
　nursing, 2006
　sources of nursing, 2327
　types of, in nursing, 2031–2032, 2031*f*
　　aesthetic, 2031
　　empirical, 2031
　　ethical, 2032
　　personal, 2032
Kock's ileostomy, 917*f*
Kohlberg, Lawrence, 351–352
Koran, 1782
Koreans and Korean Americans:
　views of older adults, 402*t*
Korotkoff's sounds, 1322, 1322*f*, 1322*t*
Korsakoff's psychosis, 30*t*, 43
Kosher food, 1773
KUB (kidneys, ureters, and bladder), 469
Kübler-Ross grief model, 601, 602*t*
Kupffer cells, 678
Kussmaul's breathing, 1221
Kussmaul's respirations, 12
Kyphosis, 1066, 1068, 1071*t*

L

Labia, 1687
Labia majora, 1687, 1688*t*
Labia minora, 1687, 1688*t*, 1707*t*
Laboratory records, as source of data, 2055

Laboratory tests. *See* Diagnostic Tests
Labyrinthitis, 824
Lacerations, 1880*t*
Lacrimal apparatus, 1630, 1636*t*
Lactic acid, 4
Lactic acidosis:
　causes, 11
　pharmacologic therapies, 12
Lactic dehydrogenase (LDH), 130*t*
Lactobacillus, 770
Lactotropic cells, 978
Lactulose, 1020
Laissez-faire leaders, 2234, 2234*t*
Lamellae, 1056
Lamictal, 1174, 1174*t*
Laminectomy:
　definition, 1083
　postoperative care, 1086*t*
　preoperative care, 1086*t*
Lamotrigine, 1174, 1174*t*
Langerhans cells, 678
Language, of interviews, 2058
Language barriers, 2251
Language deficits, 215, 2159
Language differences, 326
Language issues, 334
Laniazid. *See* Isoniazid
Laparoscopic cholecystectomy, 904*t*, 905, 908*t*
Laparotomy, 894
Lapraoscopy, 1750, 1750*f*
Large-cell carcinomas, 161*t*
Larodopa, 243
Larval therapy, 1926
Laser bronchoscopy, 165*t*
Laser iridotomy, 1672
Laser photocoagulation, 144
Laser surgery:
　prostate, 435
Laser trabeculoplasty, 1670
Lasix, 959*t*, 963. *See* Furosemide
Last Rites, 1774
Latanoprost (Xalatan), 1670, 1671*t*
Latex agglutination test, 1570
Latex allergy, 730–731, 731*t*, 731–733*t*,
　　780–781, 2438
Latter-Day Saints, 1784*t*
Lavender, 1816
Laws:
　99-457, 205
　administrative, 2398
　Americans with Disabilities Act (101–336), 205
　categories of, affecting nurses, 2399*t*
　civil, 2398
　Controlled Substance Act, 2405
　criminal, 2398
　defined, 2398
　Education for all Handicapped Children Act
　　(94–192), 205, 205*t*
　False Claims Act, 2418
　Good Samaritan, 2405
　Health Insurance Portability and Accountability
　　Act (HIPAA), 2412–2413, 2413*t*
　impacting nursing practice, 2283,
　　2402–2405, 2405*t*
　minor consent, 2405*t*
　morality and, 2306
　nursing, 2398
　Occupational Safety and Health Act, 2418

　Patient Protection and Affordable Care Act, 2418
　Patient Self-Determination Act, 250
　sources of, 2398, 2398*f*
　statutory, 2398
　tort, 2399–2401
　Whistleblower Protection Act, 2417
Laxatives, 425
　for bowel elimination, 431*t*
　for constipation, 455
　definition, 426
　herbal, 457*t*
Laënnec's cirrhosis. *See* Alcoholic cirrhosis
LDLs. *See* Low-density lipoproteins (LDLs)
Lead, 1327
Lead poisoning, 97, 2454
Leaders, 2142
　autocratic, 2233–2234, 2234*t*
　bureaucratic, 2234
　characteristics of effective, 2235*t*
　charismatic, 2234
　defined, 2233
　democratic, 2234, 2234*t*
　formal, 2233
　informal, 2233
　laissez-faire, 2234, 2234*t*
　nurses as, 2294*t*
　situational, 2234
　transactional, 2234
　transformational, 2235
Leadership:
　effective, 2235, 2235*t*
　vs. management, 2233
　overview, 2233
　shared, 2235
　theories, 2233
　　contemporary, 2234–2235
　　contingency theory, 2234
　　trait, 2233–2234
Leading questions, 2056
Lean Six Sigma, 2428
Leaning needs, assessment of, 2255
Learners, nurses and, 2244
LEARN model, 332
Learning:
　attributes of, 2244*t*
　defined, 2243, 2248
　domains, 2247
　evaluation of, 2267
　factors affecting, 2249–2251, 2250*t*, 2251*t*
　factors facilitating
　　active involvement, 2249, 2249*f*
　　environment, 2250
　　feedback, 2249
　　motivation to learn, 2249
　　nonjudgmental support, 2249
　　organization of material, 2250
　　readiness to learn, 2249
　　relevance, 2249
　　repetition, 2250
　　timing, 2250
　factors inhibiting, 2250, 2250*t*
　　cultural barriers, 2251
　　emotions, 2251
　　physiologic events, 2251
　　psychomotor ability, 2251
　observational, 2247
　older adults and, 199
　See also Teaching and learning

Learning disabilities, 200–201
Learning experience, organization of, 2262
Learning needs, 2245
　assessment interview, 2257t
　assessment of, 2254–2255, 2256t
　deficient knowledge as etiology, 2259–2260
　diagnostic labels, 2258–2259, 2259t
Learning outcomes, 2260, 2260t, 2261t
Learning styles, 2255
Learning theories, 2245
　adult learning theory, 2245, 2246t
　behaviorist theory, 2246
　categorization, 2248
　cognitive theory, 2246–2247, 2247t
　constructivism, 2248
　humanistic learning theory, 2248
　information processing theory, 2248
　mood disorders and, 1162, 1164t
　multiple intelligence, 2248–2249
　social learning theory, 2247–2248
Lea's shield, 1729
Lecithin, 219
Leflunomide, 749
Left atrium, 1294
Leg cramps:
　during pregnancy, 1575t
Legal issues, 225
　about, 2397–2406, 2400t, 2403t, 2404t,
　　2405t, 2406t
　abuse and, 1962
　additional resources for, 2406t
　advance directives, 2410, 2412, 2412t
　Case Study, 2419
　civil law, 2398
　criminal law, 2398
　documentation and, 2183
　informed consent, 2403–2405, 2405f, 2405t
　laws impacting nursing practice, 2402–2405, 2405t
　malpractice, 2398t, 2399–2400, 2400t
　mandatory reporting, 2413–2415, 2414t, 2415t
　with mental illness, 250
　minor consent laws, 2405t
　nurse practice acts, 2406–2410, 2408t, 2409t
　risk management, 2415–2417
　sexual orientation and, 401
　sources of laws, 2398, 2398f
　standard of care, 2402, 2403t
　tort law, 2399–2401
　tuberculosis, 870
　whistleblowing, 2417–2418
　See also Laws
Legionella pneumophila, 835t, 836, 842t
Legionnaires' Disease, 836, 837t
Legislation. See Laws
Legislative bodies, 2398
Legislative process, 2363t
Leininger, Madeleine, 2028
Leiomyosarcoma, 1700t
Lens, 1631, 1636t, 1642t
Lentigo maligna, 185
Lentigo maligna melanoma, 185
Leprosy, 2288f
Lesions, 1876, 1878, 1878t, 1879t, 1885t
Lethality, 1982
Let's Move program, 2364f, 2364t
Leukemia:
　Case Study, 160
　causes, 151

classification
　acute, 148
　acute lymphoblastic leukemia, 149t
　acute lymphocytic leukemia, 150t, 151f, 151t
　acute myeloid leukemia, 149, 149t, 150t
　chronic, 148
　chronic lymphocytic leukemia, 149t, 151
　chronic myeloid leukemia, 149–150, 149t
　French-American-British (FAB), 150t
　lymphocytic, 148
　myeloid, 148
clinical therapies, 153t
collaborative care
　biologic therapy, 155
　bone marrow transplant, 154–155
　chemotherapy, 153–154, 154t
　complementary therapies, 156
　diagnostic tests, 153
　radiation therapy, 154
　stem cell transplant. See Stem cell
　　transplant (SCT)
complications
　graft-versus-host disease, 155
diagnostic tests, 154t
incidence, 151
manifestations, 153, 153t
Multisystem Effects, 152
Nursing Care Plan
　assessment, 159t
　critical thinking, 159t
　diagnoses, 159t
　evaluation, 159t
　planning and implementation, 159t
nursing diagnoses and interventions
　anticipatory grieving, 159–160
　imbalanced nutrition, less than body
　　requirements, 157
　impaired oral mucous membrane, 157–158
　ineffective protection, 158–159
　risk for infection, 157
nursing process
　assessment, 156
　diagnosis, 156
　evaluation, 160
　planning and implementation, 156–160
overview, 148
pathophysiology and etiology, 148–151
risk factors, 151, 153
Leukocyte esterase test, 875
Leukocytes, 676–679, 677t, 678f, 886, 1543
Leukocytosis, 676, 886, 891t
Leukopenia, 891t
　description of, 676
　systemic lupus erythematosus (SLE) and,
　　759–760
Leukotriene modifiers, 1260t, 1262
Leukotrienes, 887t
Leuprolide acetate, 1735t
Levator ani, 1517t
Level of consciousness (LOC), 946
　altered, 944
　　fluid management, 959
　　nursing interventions, 959–960, 959t
　　nutrition and, 959
　　pharmacologic therapies, 959–960, 959t
　　surgical treatment, 959
　assessment, 949
　disorders affecting, 947–948

　in dying client, 619
　factors affecting, 946
　outcomes of altered, 948
　　brain death, 948–949
　　locked-in syndrome, 948
　　persistent vegetative state, 948
　prognosis for altered, 949
　terms used to describe, 946, 946t
Levobunolol (Betagan), 1671t
Levodopa, 243, 1138t
Levothyroxine, 1050
Lewy body dementia, 206t
LH. See Luteinizing hormone (LH)
LHRH. See Luteinizing hormone-releasing
　hormone (LHRH)
Liability, 2222–2224, 2399
Liability insurance, 2402
Libido, 343, 1712
Licensed practical nurse (LPN), 2116t
Licensed vocational nurse (LVN), 2116t
Licensure, 2407–2408
　mutual recognition model, 2408, 2408t
　revocation, 2407
　standards for, 2406
Licensure examinations, 2407
Licensure issues, 2283
Lichenification, 1876, 1879t
Lidocaine, 287t
Lidoderm, 287t
Life events:
　stressful, 1163, 1163f
Life expectancy, 368
Life Experiences Survey, 2013t
Lifestyle, 2053t
　affect on health, 645
　healthy choices, 645t
Lifestyle assessment, 645–646
Lifestyle changes:
　due to illness, 639
　health promotion and, 642
Lifestyle factors, 500
Ligaments, 1063, 1065
Ligands, agonists and antagonists, 1810f
Light palpation, 2002, 2003f
Lightning injuries, 1887
Limb restraints, 2448, 2449f
Limbic system, 1809f
Limit setting, 490, 492
Linea nigra, 1543f
Line authority, 2126
Linking, 2170
Lipid profile, 1028
Lipids, 1595
Lipoatrophy, 1005
Lipodystrophy, 1005
Lipoproteins, 1361
Lips, 655
Listening skills, 2165–2166, 2166t
Litargirio, 1896t
Literacy skills, 671, 673, 2259t
Literature, as source of data, 2055
Literature review, 2387
Lithiasis, 466
Lithium carbonate, 58t, 1173, 1174t, 1181
Lithotomy position, 2002t
Lithotripsy, 469–470, 470t
Liver, 1015–1016

Liver disease:
  Case Study, 1024
  Cirrhosis. *See* Cirrhosis
  overview, 1015–1016
Liver function tests, 863, 1411
Liver transplantation, 1020
Living wills, 289, 2410
Lobar pneumonia, 835, 835t, 837t
Lobectomy, 165t
Local agencies, 2365
Local emergency management agency
        (LEMA), 2355
Local health departments, 2365
Local infection, 771
Localized response, hypersensitivity and, 726
Locked-in syndrome, 948
Locus of control (LOC), 650
  external, 1836
  internal, 1836
Lodine. *See* Etodolac
Logical Observation Identifiers Names and Codes
        (LOINC®), 2386
Long Qt syndrome, 1326t
Long-term care, sexuality and, 1695
Long-term care documentation, 2194–2195,
        2194t, 2195t
Long-term care settings, fall prevention in, 2446t
Long-term goals, 2087
Long-term memory, 199
Loop diuretics, 959t, 963, 963t
  in specific conditions
    acute renal failure, 541t
    cirrhosis, 1020
    heart failure, 1413
Loose association, 236
Lopinavir/ritonavir, 713
Lorazepam, 959, 971, 1815
Lordosis, 1066, 1068f, 1071t
Loss, 600. *See also* Grief and loss
  sources of
    aspect of self, 600
    external objects, 600
    familiar environment, 600
    loved ones, 600
    types, 600
Lotions, 1913t
Lovastatin, 1374
Love and belonging needs, 2083t
Low back pain:
  causes, 1080
  in pregnancy, 1083t
Low-birth-weight infants, 204t
Low-density lipoproteins (LDLs), 1361, 1365, 1373
Low-literacy clients, 402–403
Low-residue diet, 918t
Low-sodium diet, 586t
Lower back pain, 264
Lower body obesity, 1026
Loyalties, conflicting, 2313
LPN. *See* Licensed practical nurse (LPN)
LSD, 58t, 74
Lubricant, 2005t
Lumbar disks, manifestations of ruptured, 1081
Lumbar injury, 1149t
Lumbar puncture, 805
Lumbar support, 2384t
Lumigan, 1671t
Lumpectomy, 110, 110f

Lund and Browder burn assessment chart, 1891f
Lung abscess, 835
Lung cancer:
  Case Study, 168–169
  cell types, 161t
  clinical therapies, 163t
  collaborative care
    complementary therapies, 165
    diagnostic tests, 164
    pharmacologic therapies, 164–165
    radiation therapy, 165
    surgery, 165, 165t
  incidence, 163
  manifestations, 163, 163t
  Multisystem Effects, 162
  Nursing Care Plan
    assessment, 167t
    critical thinking, 167t
    diagnoses, 167t
    evaluation, 167t
    planning and implementation, 167t
  nursing diagnoses and interventions
    activity intolerance, 166
    anticipatory grieving, 168
    ineffective breathing pattern, 166
    pain, 166, 168
  nursing process
    diagnosis, 166
    evaluation, 168
    lung cancer, 165–166
    planning and implementation, 166–168
  overview, 161
  pathophysiology and etiology, 161, 163
  risk factors, 163
  smoking and, 121
  TNM staging system for, 164t
Lung reduction surgery, 1273
Lung scans, 1479
Lungs:
  anatomy, physiology, and functions, 1216, 1218f,
        1224f, 1225f, 1226f
Lupus nephritis, 924. *See also* Nephritis
Lupron, 1735t
Lustral, 1201
Luteal phase:
  of ovarian cycle, 1522
Luteinizing hormone (LH), 978, 1522, 1690
Luteinizing hormone-releasing hormone
        (LHRH), 1521
Lutre-pulse, 1735t
LVN. *See* Licensed vocational nurse (LVN)
Lyme disease, 1680
Lymph, 681–682
Lymph nodes, 677t, 679f, 681–682, 681f, 695
Lymphadenopathy:
  cellulitis and, 808
  human immunodeficiency virus (HIV) and, 702
Lymphangitis, cellulitis and, 810
Lymphatic drainage, 580
Lymphedema, 108t, 110
Lymphoblasts, 678f, 679f
Lymphocytes, 676, 677t, 678f, 679–680, 679f
Lymphocytic leukemia, 148
Lymphocytopenia, 891t
Lymphocytosis, 891t
Lymphoid stem cells, 678f, 679f
Lymphoid system, 681–682, 681f
Lymphoid tissues, 677t, 681–682

Lymphomas:
  acquired immunodeficiency syndrome (AIDS)
        and, 705, 714t
Lymphopoiesis, 682
Lysosomes, 87
Lyse, 1479

M

Ma huang, 1263
MAC (mycobacterium avium complex), 704,
        706, 714t
Macrobid. *See* Nitrofurantoin
Macrodantin. *See* Nitrofurantoin
Macrolides:
  medication administration, 807
  pneumonia and, 841
Macrophages, 677t, 678, 678f, 680f, 681, 1928
Macroshock, 2453
Macrosystem, 350
Macula, 1642t, 1676
Maculae, 1633
Macular degeneration (AMD), 1637t, 1638,
        1642t, 1649t
  Case Study, 1678
  clinical therapies, 1677t
  collaborative care
    diagnostic tests, 1677
    nonpharmacologic therapies, 1677
    pharmacologic therapies, 1677
    surgery, 1677
  definition, 1676
  effects of, 1676f
  incidence, 1676
  manifestations, 1676, 1677t
  medications, 1649
  nursing process
    assessment, 1677
    diagnosis, 1677
    evaluation, 1678
    planning and implementation, 1677–1678
  pathophysiology and etiology, 1676
  risk factors, 1676
  types
    exudative, 1676, 1677t
    nonexudative, 1676, 1677t
Macules, 1878t
Magical thinking, 360t
Magnesium (Mg²⁺), 1262
  in body fluid compartments, 520t
  dysrhythmias and, 1449
  function, 525t
  imbalances. *See* Hypermagnesemia
  in intracellular fluid, 518
  recommended daily intake, 1597t
  regulation, 525–526, 525t
Magnet hospitals, 2119, 2131
Magnet Recognition Program®, 2409
Magnetic resonance imaging (MRI), 2392
  in specific conditions
    cancer, 127–128
    congenital heart defects, 1353t
    deep venous thrombosis, 1391
    multiple sclerosis, 1120
    peripheral vascular disease, 1465
    pulmonary embolism, 1228
    traumatic injury, 1942
Magnetic tape drives, 2375
Mahashivarathri, 1781

Mahoney, Mary, 2290, 2291f
Major depressive disorder (MDD):
  characteristics, 1186, 1188, 1189f
  definition, 1159
  diagnostic criteria, 1187t
  key facts, 1188t
  manifestations, 1189t
Major depressive episode, 1186, 1187t
Major histocompatibility (MHC) antigens, 1534
Maladaptive dependence, 1169
Malaise, influenza and, 818
Male circumcision, 1700
Male contraception, 1734
Male erectile disorder, 1702
Male orgasmic disorder, 1702
Male rape, 1970
Male reproductive anatomy and physiology:
  anatomy, 432f
  assessment, 1704–1705t
  breasts, 1687
  ducts and semen, 1687
  epididymis, 1686t
  male sex hormones, 1687
  penis, 1686, 1686t
  prostate gland, 1686t, 1687
  scrotum, 1686, 1686t
  seminal vesicles, 1686t, 1687
  spermatogenesis, 1687
  testes, 1686, 1686t
  urethra, 1686t
  vas deferens, 1686t
Male-to-female (MTF) transsexuals, 400, 1696
Malignant, 117
Malignant cells:
  characteristics, 117–118, 118t
Malignant hyperthermia (MH), 1860
Malignant neoplasms, 117–119, 117t
Malleus, 1632
Malnutrition, 662, 663t, 1022
Malpractice, 2399–2400, 2400t
  cases against nurses, 2398t
  strategies to prevent, 2401–2402
  suits, 2424
Mammary glands, 1688t, 1691
Mammography, 107, 109, 2211
Managed care, 2206, 2343
Management:
  conflict, 2144
  principles of, 2144–2145
  resource, 2144
  team, 2144
  time, 2144
Management functions:
  controlling, 2144
  directing, 2143
  organizing, 2143
  planning, 2143
Management theories, 2142–2145
Managers, 2142–2143, 2294t
Managing care:
  about, 2205–2207
  care coordination, 2208–2209
  Case Study, 2208
  cost-effective care, 2210–2216
  delegation, 2217–2222, 2224
  nursing practice, 2207
Mandatory health insurance, 2213
Mandatory reporting, 2413–2415, 2414t, 2415t
  of abuse, 2413, 2414t

good faith immunity and, 2413
of injuries and illnesses, 2414–2415, 2415t
of nurses in violation of NPA, 2414
other examples of, 2415
Manganese, recommended daily intake, 1597t
Mania:
  assessment, 1182
  characteristics, 1179f
  definition, 1160
  diagnostic criteria, 1178t
  manifestations, 1179, 1180t
  potential nurse reactions to clients with, 1183t
Manifestations:
  abuse, 1953, 1954–1955t, 1955–1957, 1956t
  acute myocardial infarction, 1368t
  acute renal failure, 537–539, 538t
  acute respiratory distress syndrome (ARDS),
    1235, 1238t
  acute stress disorder, 1814
  ADHD, 370–371
  adrenal tumor, 581t
  agoraphobia, 1836–1837
  alcohol abuse, 41, 42t, 43
  Alzheimer's disease, 214–216, 216t
  anemia, 97–101
  anxiety disorders, 1812t
  appendicitis, 893, 894t
  asthma, 1255–1256t
  Autism spectrum disorders, 378–380, 379t
  benign prostatic hypertrophy, 433, 433t
  bipolar disorders, 1179–1181, 1180t, 1197t, 1199t
  breast cancer, 108–109, 108t, 109t
  burns, 1892, 1894t
  cancer, 124t
  cardiomyopathy, 1334, 1335t
  cataracts, 1658
  cellulitis, 809–810, 810t
  cerebral dysfunction, 944, 945t
  cerebral palsy, 386–387, 387t
  chlamydias, 1759
  chronic obstructive pulmonary disease (COPD),
    1269–1271, 1271t
  chronic renal failure, 554–558, 557t
  cirrhosis, 1016–1017, 1017t, 1019
  colorectal cancer, 142–143, 143t
  compartment syndrome, 1096t
  confusion, 227
  congenital heart defects, 1340–1349t, 1350t
  congestive heart failure, 581t
  conjunctivitis, 814
  constipation, 455
  contact dermatitis, 1912–1913
  coronary artery disease, 1366–1369, 1369t
  crisis, 1820t, 1821t
  Crohn's disease, 912t, 914
  death, 619, 619t
  deep venous thrombosis, 1391, 1391t
  delirium, 227
  depression, 1186, 1189t
  diabetes mellitus, 991t, 992, 992t
  disseminated intravascular coagulation,
    1399, 1400t
  dysrhythmias, 1447t
  eating disorders, 1599–1601, 1600–1601t
  end-of-life care, 296, 296t
  erectile dysfunction, 1713
  eye injuries, 1661–1662, 1663t
  failure to thrive, 392
  fatigue, 302, 303t

fibromyalgia, 306, 306t
fluid volume deficit, 571–575, 572t, 575t
fluid volume excess, 581t, 582
fractures, 1094, 1096t, 1098t
gallstones, 902–903, 903t
generalized anxiety disorder, 1811–1812
genital herpes, 1757, 1757f, 1757t
genital warts, 1758, 1758f
glaucoma, 1669, 1669t
gonorrhea, 1760
gout, 1070
grief, 601
Guillian-Barré syndrome, 1679
hearing impairment, 1652, 1653t
heart failure, 1408, 1410
herniated disk, 1080f, 1081–1082, 1083t
hip fractures, 1112
HIV/AIDS, 702–707, 706–707t, 708t
hypercalcemia, 593t
hyperkalemia, 556, 591t
hypermagnesemia, 594t
hypernatremia, 587t
hyperphosphatemia, 596t
hypersensitivity, 734–735, 734t
hypertension, 1426–1427, 1427t
hyperthyroidism, 1041, 1043–1044
hypocalcemia, 592t
hypomagnesemia, 593–594t
hyponatremia, 587t
hypophosphatemia, 595t
hypothyroidism, 1048
impending death, 617t
increased intracranial pressure, 962, 962t
infections, in children, 802–803t
influenza, 820, 820t, 821t
leukemia, 153, 153t
liver cirrhosis, 581t
lung cancer, 163, 163t
macular degeneration, 1676, 1677t
menopause, 1742–1743, 1742–1743t
menstrual dysfunction, 1749, 1749t
metabolic acidosis, 12, 12t
metabolic alkalosis, 15, 15t
multiple sclerosis, 1118, 1118t
nephritis, 925, 925t
obesity, 1026, 1027t
obsessive-compulsive disorder, 1829–1831, 1830t
osteoarthritis, 1069f, 1125f, 1069f, 1126, 1126t
osteoporosis, 1035
otitis media, 826–827, 826t
pain, 266–268
panic disorder, 1813–1814
Parkinson's disease, 1135–1136, 1135f, 1135t
peptic ulcer disease, 932, 932t
perinatal loss, 627–628
peripheral neuropathy, 1680, 1680t
peripheral vascular disease, 1463, 1463t
personality disorders, 1610–1611, 1611t
phobias, 1837t
pneumonia, 839–840, 840t
post-traumatic stress disorder, 1843–1844
postpartum depression, 1201t
preeclampsia, 1469–1470
pregnancy-induced hypertension, 1470t
prenatal substance exposure, 62t
pressure ulcers, 1917
prostate cancer, 170, 170t
pulmonary edema, 1410t
pulmonary embolism, 1478, 1478t

rape-trauma syndrome, 1971–1973, 1972*t*
respiratory acidosis, 19, 19*t*
respiratory alkalosis, 23, 23*t*
respiratory syncytial virus (RSV)/Bronchiolitis, 1282, 1282*t*
schizophrenia, 235–241
scoliosis, 1068*f*, 1087
seizure disorders, 968
separation anxiety disorder, 1812–1813
sepsis, 851–852, 852*t*
shock, 1490, 1491–1492*t*
sickle cell disorder, 178–179
situational depression, 1208, 1209*t*
skin cancer, 188, 189*t*
sleep disorders, 312, 313*t*
smoking, 52, 53*t*
social phobias, 1837
specific phobias, 1838
spinal cord injury, 1146–1147, 1148*t*
stroke, 1502, 1502*t*, 1504*t*
substance abuse, 70–74
sudden cardiac death, 1455
sudden infant death syndrome (SIDS), 1287
suicide, 1981–1983, 1983*t*
syphilis, 1761, 1761*t*
systemic lupus erythematosus (SLE), 757, 759*t*, 760
tuberculosis, 860–861, 861*t*
ulcerative colitis, 912, 912*t*
urinary calculi, 467, 468*t*
urinary incontinence, 442
urinary retention, 445
urinary tract infection, 467, 874–875, 875*t*
wound healing, 1930
Manipulation, 1610
Mannitol, 541*t*, 1670
MAOIs, 1199*f*. *See* Monoamine oxidase inhibitors
MAP (mean arterial pressure), 960
Marfan's syndrome, 1076*t*, 1326*f*
Margination, 886
Marijuana, 71
effect on fetus, 58*t*
sexual functioning and, 1701*t*
street names, 74*t*
use in pregnancy, 59
Marijuana Tax Act, 68
Marital rape, 1970
Martin Chuzzlewit (Dickens), 2289
Maslow's Hierarchy of Basic Human Needs, 2061, 2083, 2083*f*, 2083*t*, 2248
basic needs, 1798, 1798*f*
meta-needs, 1798, 1798*t*
Mass casualty incidents (MCIs), 2355*t*
Massage and touch therapy:
anxiety disorders and, 1816
definition, 1084
for pain management, 280, 297
Masses, characteristics of, 2003*t*
MAST (Michigan Alcohol Screening Test), 46
Mast cells, 887
Mast cell stabilizers, 815, 816*t*, 1260*t*
Mastectomy, 107, 110
modified radical, 110, 110*f*
radical, 110
segmental, 110
Mastoid antrum, 1632
Masturbation, 1697
Materials management systems, 2378*t*
Maternal attachment behavior, 1197–1198, 1198*t*

Maternal blood, 1533
Maternal infections, 202*t*
Maternal role attainment (MRA), 1196–1197
Maternal smoking, 341
Mature minors, 2404
Maturational crises, 33
Maturity factors, 499
Mayeroff, Milton, 2028
MB-bands, 1371
McBurney's point, 893, 893*f*
McCarthy Scale of Children's Abilities, 2013*t*
McDonald's sign, 1547, 1569*f*
McMaster University, 2335
McMurray's test, 1075, 1075*t*
MCV4, 690
MDD. *See* Major depressive disorder (MDD)
MDMA (Ecstasy), 60, 73
MDR-TB (Multidrug-resistant tuberculosis), 789
MDS (Minimum Data Set), 664, 2022
Me-centered people, 1580
Mean arterial pressure (MAP), 960, 1411–1412, 1422, 1484
Measles (Rubeola), in children, 793–794*t*
Measles vaccine, 690
Meatus, urinary, 411
Mechanical debridement, 1902, 1924
Mechanical ventilation:
complications
barotrauma, 1241–1242
cardiovascular effects, 1242
gastrointestinal effects, 1242
nosocomial pneumonia, 1241
for IICP, 964
nutrition and fluids, 1243
in specific conditions
acute respiratory distress syndrome (ARDS), 1238–1243
terminal weaning, 1242–1243
types of ventilators, 1238–1239
ventilator settings, 1241, 1242*t*
weaning, 1242–1243
Meclofenamate sodium, 749*t*
Meclomen. *See* Meclofenamate sodium
Meconium, 424
Media violence, 1965
Mediastinoscopy, 165*t*
Medicaid, 2211, 2368
documentation requirements, 2195
telemedicine and, 2381
Medical abortion, 1734
Medical and Family Leave Act, 489
Medical asepsis, 771
Medical diagnoses, 2067, 2068*t*, 2072*f*
Medical errors:
deaths due to, 2443
factors increasing risk of, 2443
reducing, among children, 2416–2417
Medical home, 2347, 2348*t*
Medical records:
computerized, 2378–2379, 2380*t*, 2389–2393, 2391*f*
ANA position statement on, 2392*t*
management, 2388
paper, 2378, 2379*f*
See Client records, 2185
as source of data, 2055
Medical technology, 2214–2215
Medicare, 2210*f*, 2211, 2362, 2368
documentation requirements, 2195

Part A, 2368, 2368*t*
Part B, 2368, 2368*t*
Part C, 2368, 2368*t*
Part D, 2368, 2368*t*
Medicare Advantage, 2368
Medicare Advantage plan, 2211
Medicare payment system, 2282
Medicare reimbursement, 2211, 2214
Medication Administration, 2400*t*
adenosine, 1450*t*
adrenalcorticosteroids, 1121*t*
adrenergic agonists (mydriatics), 1671*t*
adrenergic stimulants, 1259*t*
adrenergics, 1493*t*
alpha-adrenergic blockers, 1430*t*
angiotensin II-receptor blockers, 1414*t*, 1430*t*
angiotensin-converting enzyme (ACE) inhibitors, 1414*t*, 1430*t*
anticholinergics, 1139*t*, 1259–1260*t*
anticoagulants, 1393*t*
antidysrhythmics, 1450*t*
antihypertensives, 1430–1431*t*
antiplatelet drugs, 1377*t*
antispasmodics, 1149*t*
beta-adrenergic blockers, 1430–1431*t*, 1671*t*
beta-blockers, 1450
calcium-channel blockers
for dysrhythmias, 1450
for hypertension, 1431
carbonic anhydrate inhibitors, 1671*t*
centrally acting sympatholytics, 1431*t*
children, with asthma, 1262*t*
cholesterol-lowering drugs, 1374t
colloid solutions, 1494*t*
COMT inhibitors, 1138*t*
corticosteroids, 915*t*, 1260*t*
digoxin, 1450*t*
diuretics, 1414
documentation of, 2377
dopamine agonists, 1138*t*
dopaminergics, 1138*t*
immunomodulators, 1121*t*
immunosuppressants, 1121*t*
insulin, 1003*t*
leukotriene modifiers, 1260*t*
mast cell stabilizers, 1260*t*
mesalamine, 915*t*
methylxanthines, 1259*t*
monoamine oxidase inhibitors, 1138*t*
muscle relaxants, 1121*t*
narcotics, 1907*t*
olsalazine, 915*t*
phosphodiesterase inhibitors, 1415*t*
podophyllin, 1759*t*
positive inotropic agents, 1414–1415*t*
potassium-channel blockers, 1450*t*
prostaglandin analogs, 1671*t*
sodium-channel blockers, 1450*t*
in specific conditions
ADHD, 374
asthma, 1260–1261*t*
genital warts, 1759*t*
glaucoma, 1671*t*
heart failure, 1414–1415*t*
inflammatory bowel disease, 915*t*
multiple sclerosis, 1121*t*
Parkinson's disease, 1138*t*
respiratory system alterations, 1229*t*, 1230*t*

shock, 1493*t*
  spinal cord injury, 1149*t*
sulfasalazine, 915*t*
sympathomimetic agents, 1415*t*, 1493*t*
trichloroacetic acid, 1759*t*
variances, 2417
vasodilators, 1431*t*, 1493*t*
Medication administration record, 2193
Medication dosage calculations, for children, 2416
Medication errors, 2335
  minimizing risk of, 2402
  preventing, in home, 2442*t*
  reducing, 2429
Medications. *See also* specific medications
  affect on bowel elimination, 426
  affecting urinary elimination, 415*t*
  blood pressure and, 1309
  classification of, during pregnancy, 61, 63
  disposal of unused, 2453*t*
  during pregnancy, 342, 1573, 1577, 1577*t*
  effects on skin of, 1876
  excretion of, in older adults, 416
  for acid–base imbalances, 8–10, 9*t*, 10*t*
  for acute renal failure, 540, 541*t*, 542, 542*t*
  for ADHD, 372, 373*t*
  for altered level of consciousness, 959–960, 959*t*
  for anemia, 102
  for angina, 1375
  for anxiety disorders, 1807–1808, 1807*t*,
    1814–1815
  for appendicitis, 894
  for asthma, 1258–1262
  for benign prostatic hypertrophy, 434, 434*t*
  for bipolar disorders, 1173, 1174*t*, 1181–1182
  for bowel elimination, 430, 431*t*
  for breast cancer, 110
  for burns, 1900–1901
  for cancer, 94, 95*t*, 130–131
  for cardiomyopathy, 1335–1336
  for cerebral palsy, 388
  for chlamydia, 1760
  for chronic renal failure, 558–559
  for cirrhosis, 1020
  for congenital heart defects, 1351
  for conjunctivitis, 815, 816*t*
  for constipation, 455
  for COPD, 1272–1273
  for coronary artery disease, 1373–1375
  for crisis, 1823
  for deep venous thrombosis, 1392
  for depression, 1170–1173, 1209
  for diabetes, 1002–1005
  for dysrhythmias, 1449
  for eating disorders, 1592
  for endocrine disorders, 987–988*t*
  for erectile dysfunction, 1714
  for fatigue, 303, 303*t*
  for fecal incontinence, 459
  for fibromyalgia, 307
  for fluid imbalances, 532, 533*t*
  for fluid volume excess, 582
  for fractures, 1098
  for genital herpes, 1758
  for genital warts, 1759
  for glaucoma, 1670, 1671*t*
  for glomerular disorders, 926–927
  for heart failure, 1413–1416
  for herniated disk, 1082

for hyperchloremia, 589*t*
for hyperkalemia, 591*t*
for hypernatremia, 588*t*
for hypersensitivity, 737–738
for hypertension, 1429–1433
for hyperthyroidism, 1044
for hyponatremia, 587*t*
for hypothyroidism, 1050
for IICP, 963, 963*t*
for immune system, 696
for increased intracranial pressure, 959–960*t*
for infertility, 1734, 1735*t*
for inflammation, 891, 892*t*
for influenza, 821–822
for lung cancer, 164–165
for menopause, 1743
for menstrual dysfunction, 1750
for metabolic acidosis, 12
for metabolic alkalosis, 15
for multiple sclerosis, 1120
for musculoskeletal disorders, 1079, 1079*t*
for obesity, 1028
for osteoarthritis, 1127
for osteoporosis, 1035, 1037, 1037*t*
for otitis media, 828–829
for Parkinson's disease, 1137
for peptic ulcer disease, 933–934
for perfusion, 1329, 1330–1332*t*
for peripheral vascular disease, 1465
for personality disorders, 1592
for phobias, 1838
for postpartum depression, 1201
for prostate cancer, 172–173
for pulmonary embolism, 1479–1480
for rape victims, 1973
for respiratory acidosis, 20
for respiratory alkalosis, 23
for respiratory syncytial virus
    (RSV)/bronchiolitis, 1283
for rheumatoid arthritis, 748–750
for seizure disorder, 971, 971*t*
for sepsis, 852–853
for sexual dysfunction, 1710, 1711*t*
for shock, 1490
for sleep disorders, 313–314, 314*t*
for spinal cord injury, 1149
for stroke, 1506–1507
for substance abuse, 38, 39*t*
for suicide, 1983
for syphilis, 1762
for systemic lupus erythematosus (SLE), 760
for tuberculosis, 862–863, 863–864*t*
for urinary calculi, 469
for urinary elimination, 423, 423*t*
for urinary incontinence, 443
for urinary retention, 446
for urinary tract infection, 876
for victims of violence, 1943
gallstones, 904–905
impact on sleep of, 312
inflammatory bowel disease, 914, 915*t*, 916
macular degeneration, 1677
pain, 274–278
sensory impairments, 1649, 1650*t*
sensory perception and, 1634
sexual functioning and, 1701, 1701*t*
sleep and, 669
testing of new, 399

Medigap policy, 2369
MEDLINE, 2375
Meditation, 1783, 1816
Megakaryoblasts, 678*f*
Megaloblastic anemias, 99
Meiosis, 88, 1523–1524, 1525*f*
Melanin, 184, 1874
Melanomas. *See also* Skin cancer
  classification, 185
  Client Teaching, 192
  collaborative care
    diagnostic tests, 188
    identification, 188
  definition, 184
  description, 184
  manifestations, 189*t*
  microstaging, 188–190, 190*f*
  Nursing Care Plan
    assessment, 193*t*
    critical thinking, 194*t*
    diagnoses, 193*t*
    evaluation, 193*t*
    planning and implementation, 193*t*
  precursor lesions, 184–185
  risk factors, 187, 187*t*
  treatment
    emerging treatments, 190
    immunotherapy, 190
    radiation therapy, 190
    surgery, 190
Melaocytes, 1874
Melasma gravidarum, 1543–1544
Melatonin, 219, 315, 666, 1176
Memantine (Namenda), 217
Memory, 199, 2374
  declarative, 240
  procedural, 240
Memory deficits, 240
Memory impairment, 220
Memory loss, 211
Memory T cells, 679, 679*f*, 680*f*
Mendelian (single-gene) inheritance, 1723
Meningeal irritation, 957*t*
Meninges, 940
Meningococcal Tetravalent Conjugate Vaccine, 690
Meningococcus, in children, 794*t*
Meningomyelocele, 442
Mennonites, 1784*t*
Menopause:
  affects of, 1694
  Case Study, 1746
  clinical therapies, 1742*t*
  collaborative care
    alternative therapies, 1743, 1744*t*
    diagnostic tests, 1743
    pharmacologic therapies, 1743
  coronary artery disease and, 1366
  definition, 1742
  manifestations, 1742–1743, 1742–1743*t*
  nursing diagnoses and interventions
    deficient knowledge, 1744
    disturbed body image, 1745
    ineffective sexuality pattern, 1745
    situational low self-esteem, 1745
  nursing process
    assessment, 1744
    diagnosis, 1744
    evaluation, 1746

overview, 1744
    planning and implementation, 1744–1745
osteoporosis and, 1035
overview, 1742
physiology and etiology, 1742
process of, 1690
sleep disorders and, 311
surgical, 1742
Menorrhagia, 1748
Menstrual cycle, 1690–1691
    compared with ovarian cycle, 1691f
    endometrium changes during, 1521f
    overview, 1523
    phases
        ischemic, 1523
        proliferative, 1523
        secretory, 1523
Menstrual dysfunction:
    alternative therapies, 1752
    Case Study, 1754
    collaborative care
        diagnostic tests, 1749
        overview, 1749
        pharmacologic therapies, 1750
        surgery, 1750–1751
    dysfunctional uterine bleeding, 1748
        amenorrhea, 1748
        causes, 1748
        Client Teaching, 1751t
        menorrhagia, 1748
        metrorrhagia, 1748
        oligomenorrhea, 1748
        postmenopausal bleeding, 1748
        risk factors, 1749
    dysmenorrhea, 1748–1749, 1749t
    manifestations, 1749, 1749t
    Nursing Care Plan
        assessment, 1753t
        critical thinking in the nursing process, 1753t
        diagnosis, 1753t
        evaluation, 1753t
        overview, 1753t
        planning and implementation, 1753t
    nursing process
        assessment, 1752
        diagnosis, 1752
        evaluation, 1754
        planning and implementation, 1752–1754
    overview, 1746
    pathophysiology and etiology, 1748
    premenstrual syndrome, 1746
    premenstrual syndrome. See Premenstrual syndrome (PMS)
    risk factors, 1749
Menstruation:
    definition, 1523, 1689
    during adolescence, 1693
    dysfunction, 1702t
    dysmenorrhea, 1693
Mental health issues, in older adults, 622
Mental health settings, advocacy in, 2301–2302
Mental illness, 232
    advocacy and, 250
    Asian Americans and, 1180t
    cultural considerations, 1180t
    cultural perspectives on, 245
    family burden and, 507–508
    family recovery and, 508–509

family systems and, 507
homelessness and, 250
legal issues, 250
Native Americans and, 1163t
stigma of, 250, 507
Mental retardation, 201–205, 206t
Mental status:
    assessment of, 208t
    cirrhosis and, 1021
    decreased
        and pressure ulcers, 1916
Mentoring:
    Case Study, 2271
    coaching, 2270
    overview, 2269
    precepting, 2270, 2271t
    steps in mentoring relationship, 2269–2270
Mentors, 2269, 2271t
Meperidine (Demerol), 1866
Meprobamate, 71
Mercaptopurine, 914
Mercury thermometers, 1856
Meridia, 1585
Mesalamine, 916
    administration of, 915t
Mesoderm, 126t, 1528, 1529t
Mesolimbic dopaminergic system, addiction and, 28
Mesosystem, 350
Message, in communication process, 2149
Metabolic acidosis:
    case study, 14
    causes, 6t, 7t
    collaboration, 12
    compensation, 8t
    definition, 5, 11
    laboratory values, 6t, 7t
    manifestations, 12, 12t
    nursing process, 12
        assessment, 13
        decreased cardiac output, 13
        diagnosis, 13
        evaluation, 14
        implementation, 13–14
        plan, 13
        risk for excess fluid volume, 13
        risk for injury, 13
    pathophysiology and etiology, 11
    pharmacologic therapies, 12
    risk factors, 11
    treatment, 6t
Metabolic alkalosis:
    case study, 17
    causes, 6t, 7t, 15
    collaboration, 15
    compensation, 8t
    definition, 15
    laboratory and diagnostic tests, 16
    laboratory values, 6t, 7t
    manifestations, 15, 15t
    nursing process, 16
        assessment, 16
        community care, 17
        deficient fluid volume, 17
        diagnosis, 16
        evaluation, 17
        impaired gas exchange, 16
        implementation, 16–17
        plan, 16

pathophysiology and etiology, 15
    pharmacologic therapies, 15
    risk factors, 15
    therapies, 15t
    treatment, 6t
Metabolic disorders:
    description, 983t
    medications for, 987–988
Metabolic emergencies, 89
Metabolic syndrome:
    characteristics, 1366t
    definition, 1366
    obesity and, 1027
    type 2 diabetes mellitus and, 992
Metabolic system, benefits of exercise for, 653–654, 653t
Metabolism:
    about, 977–988
    after burn injury, 1896
    alterations and treatments, 983t
    assessment, 984, 984t, 985–986t, 987
    caring interventions, 987
    definition, 977, 1597
    diabetes and. See Diabetes mellitus
    diagnostic tests, 987
    endocrine system and. See Endocrine system
    glucocorticoids and, 980
    liver disease and. See Cirrhosis
    normal presentation, 978–982
    obesity and. See Obesity
    osteoporosis and. See Osteoporosis
    pharmacologic therapies, 987, 987–988t
    pregnancy and, 1544–1545
    thyroid disease and. See Hyperthyroidism; Hypothyroidism
    thyroid hormones and, 979
Metadate, 373t
Metaphysis, osteoporosis and, 1034
Metaplasia, 88
Metaproterenol, 841
Metastasis, 106, 117–119, 119f
Metered-dose inhaler (MDI), 1259, 12 59t, 1273
Methadone, 73
    effect on fetus, 58t
    use in pregnancy, 60
Methamphetamines, 70f, 72f, 72–73
Methicillin-resistant S. aureus (MRSA), 789
Methotrexate, 749
Methylin, 373t
Methylphenidate, 372, 373t
Methylprednisolone, 561, 915t
Methylxanthines, 841, 1259, 1259t
Metipranolol (OptiPranolol), 1671t
Metronidazole, 916
Metrorrhagia, 1748
Mexican Americans:
    glaucoma in, 1669
    pain responses, 268t
Mg^{2+}. See Magnesium
MH (malignant hyperthermia), 1860
MHLC (Multidimensional Health Locus of Control) Scale, 650
Michigan Alcohol Screening Test (MAST), 46
Microalbuminuria, 998
Microdiskectomy, 1084
Microglia, 678
Microorganisms, 886
    infectious, 772t
    resident, 770t

Microstaging, 188–190, 190f
Microsytem, 350
Micturition, 412
Middle adulthood, 341t
Middle age, development in, 2012
Middle ear, 1632, 1636t
Middle ear effusion, 825
Middle Eastern culture, culture-specific
    assessment, 2010t
Middle-aged adults, 366, 368t
    assessment of, 2018–2019
    developmental tasks in, 1581t
    recommended screenings and immunizations, 644t
    stress and coping in, 1802t
Mifepristone (Mifeprex), 1734
Miliary pneumonia, 835t
Milieu therapy, 35
Millennial generation, 2238, 2239t
Milliequivalent, 518
Milrinone, 1331t
Mind Map for Critical Thinking in Nursing,
    2108, 2109f
Mind-body interactions, 645
Mindful listening, 2165–2166, 2166t
Mindfulness, 1175
Mineralocorticoids, 978t, 980
Minerals:
    overview, 1595
    recommended daily intake, 1597t
Mini Nutritional Assessment (MNA), 664
Mini-Mental Status Exam (MMSE), 207, 207t,
    219, 2013t
Minimally invasive coronary artery surgery, 1379
Minimally invasive surgery:
    for BPH, 435
Minimum Data Set (MDS), 664, 2022
Minipill, 1732
Minipress, 434t
Minnesota Evidence-Based Practice Center, 2335
Minnesota Falls Prevention Initiative, 2436
Minor consent laws, 2405t
Minor trauma, 1938
Minority groups. See Race/ethnicity
MiraLAX, 455
Mirtazapine, 1173
Miscarriage, 626
Misdemeanors, 2398
Mistaken identity, 2401
Mitigation, 2351
Mitochondria, 87
Mitosis, 88, 1523
Mitral valve, 1295
Mitt restraints, 2448, 2449f
Mittelschmerz, 1522
Mixed apnea, 310
Mixed incontinence, 442
MMR, 690
MMSE (Mini-Mental State Exam), 207, 207t
Mobility, 1056
    about, 1055–1079
    alterations, 1065–1067
    assessment, 1067, 1071, 1071–1075t, 1075, 1076t
    caring interventions, 1077–1079
    diagnostic tests, 1076–1077
    normal presentation, 1056–1065
    pharmacologic therapies, 1079, 1079t
Mobility impairments:
    abnormalities causing, 1066–1067

assistive devices
    canes, 1078–1079
    crutches, 1078
    walkers, 1078
nursing interventions
    ambulation, 1078
    exercises, 1077
    overview, 1077
    overview, 1055–1056
Modeling, 648, 2247–2248
Modified Checklist for Autism in Toddlers
    (MCHAT), 382t
Modified radical mastectomy, 110, 110f
Modified scientific method, 2044, 2044t
Molybdenum, recommended daily intake, 1597t
Mon pubis, 1688t
Mono-Gesic. See Salsalate
Monoamine oxidase (MAO), 1161, 1171
Monoamine oxidase inhibitors (MAOIs):
    client teaching, 1173
    definition, 1172
    nursing considerations, 1172
    Parkinson's disease, 1137, 1138t
    side effects, 1172
Monoblasts, 678f
Monoclonal antibodies, 806t
Monoclonal antibody infliximab, 916
Monocytes, 676–678, 677t, 678f
Monocytopenia, 891t
Monocytosis, 891t
Monogamy, 1699
Mononeuropathies, 1679
Mononucleosis, in children, 795t
Monopolizing, 2139
Monosaccharides, 1593
Monosomies, 1721
Monotheism, 1771
Monozygotic twins, 1530, 1531f
Monro-Kellie hypothesis, 961
Mons pubis, 1687
Mood and affect:
    about, 1157–1177
    assessment, 1164–1167
    bipolar disorders. See Bipolar disorders
    caring interventions
        assertive behavior, 1169
        minimizing maladaptive dependence, 1169
        preventing suicide and promoting safety,
            1168–1169, 1169t
    characteristics, 1159, 1167, 1168t
    comorbid disorders, 1158–1159
    course of
        recovery, 1158
        recurrence, 1158
        relapse, 1158
        remission, 1158
        switching, 1158
    cultural considerations, 1167, 1180t
    definition, 1157
    diabetes mellitus and, 999
    depression. See Depression
    diagnostic tests, 1170
    nonpharmacologic therapies
        alternative therapies, 1175–1177
        cognitive-behavioral therapy, 1175
        electroconvulsive therapy, 1175
        psychotherapy, 1174
    pharmacologic therapies
        antidepressants, 1170–1171

atypical depressants, 1173
developmental considerations, 1174
MAOIs, 1172–1173
mood stabilizers, 1173, 1173t, 1174t
SSRIs, 1171–1172
relapse rates, 1158
seasonal affective disorder. See Seasonal
    affective disorder (SAD)
substance-related disorders and, 1158
theories of
    biological rhythms, 1162, 1164t
    cognitive theory, 1162, 1164t
    feminist theory, 1164t
    gender bias theory, 1163–1164
    genetic, 1160, 1164t
    intrapersonal factors, 1162, 1164t
    learning theory, 1162, 1164t
    neurobiology, 1161–1162, 1164t
    overview, 1160
    sociocultural factors, 1163
    stress, 1161
    sunlight, 1162, 1164t
Mood stabilizers:
    for bipolar disorders, 1173, 1173t
    developmental considerations, 1174
    suicide and, 1983
Moore's prosthesis, 1113f
Moral behavior, 350
Moral development, 350–353, 352t, 1776
Moral issues, 2306
Moral principles, variations in applying, 2315t
Moral rules, 1777
Morality, 350 2306
    Case Study, 1781
    definition, 1776
    vs. law, 1776
    moral development, 1776
    moral principles, 1777
        accountability, 1778
        autonomy, 1777
        beneficence, 1777
        fidelity, 1778
        justice, 1778
        nonmaleficence, 1777
        responsibility, 1778
        veracity, 1778
    moral theories
        consequence-based (teleological), 1777
        principles-based (deontological), 1777
        relationship-based (caring), 1777
    Nursing Care Plan
        assessment, 1779t
        critical thinking, 1779t
        diagnosis, 1779t
        evaluation, 1779t
        planning and implementation, 1779t
    nursing practice and, 1778–1779
    nursing process
        assessment, 1779
        diagnosis, 1780
        evaluation, 1780
        overview, 1778–1779
        planning and implementation, 1780
    overview, 1776
    vs. religion, 1776
Morals, 350
Morbid obesity, 1027
Morbidity and Mortality Weekly Report
    (CDC), 2415

Mormons, 1784t
Morning sickness, 1546, 1575–1576, 1576t
Morning-after pill, 1733
Moro, 958t
Morphine, 287t
　abuse of, 73
　for dyspnea, 618t
　in end-of-life care, 618t
　in specific conditions
　　burns, 1900
　street names, 74t
Morula, 1527
Mosaicism, 1721
Mothers. See also Parents
　adolescent, 498t
　new, 489
Motivation:
　to learn, 2249, 2256–2257
　sleep and, 669
Motor coordination, 2251
Motor function, assessment, 955t
Motor nerve damage, 1680t
Motor neurons, 265
Motor vehicle crashes (MVCs), 2457–2458
　Case Study, 1993
　causes, 1988
　description, 1939t
　injury prevention, 1988–1990, 1989–1990t
　Nursing Care Plan
　　assessment, 1992t
　　critical thinking, 1992t
　　diagnosis, 1992t
　　evaluation, 1992t
　　planning and implementation, 1992t
　nursing diagnoses and interventions
　　ensure mobility, 1991
　　facilitate community-based care, 1993
　　maintain airway, 1990–1991
　　prevent infection, 1991
　　promote spiritual comfort, 1991–1992
　　provide support, 1992–1993
　nursing process
　　assessment, 1990
　　diagnosis, 1990
　　evaluation, 1993
　　planning and implementation, 1990–1993
　overview, 1988
　risk factors, 1988
　treatment/prevention, 1939t
Motrin. See Ibuprofen
Mourning, 601
Mouth, 655, 655f. See also Oral health
MP3 players, 2378
MRI. See Magnetic resonance imaging
MRSA. See Methicillin-resistant S. aureus (MRSA)
MS. See Multiple sclerosis (MS)
Mucomyst. See Acetylcysteine
Mucosa-associated lymphoid tissue, 682
Multiculturalism, 323–324, 333f
Multidimensional Health Locus of Control
　　(MHLC) Scale, 650
Multidisciplinary care plans, 2081
Multidrug-resistant tuberculosis (MDR-TB), 789
Multifocal PVCs, 1446
Multigravida, 1559t
Multiple intelligence, 2248–2249
Multiple sclerosis (MS):
　Case Study, 1124
　classification, 1118, 1118t

collaborative care
　diagnostic tests, 1120
　nutrition and fluids, 1120
　overview, 1120
　pharmacologic therapies, 1120, 1121t
　rehabilitation, 1120
　surgery, 1120
community-based care, 1124t
definition, 1065t, 1066, 1117
diagnosis, 1117
evidence-based practice
　aging clients with MS, 1122t
manifestations, 1118, 1118t
Nursing Care Plan
　assessment, 1123t
　diagnoses, 1123t
　overview, 1123t
　planning and implementation, 1123t
nursing diagnoses and interventions
　fatigue, 1122
　self-care deficit, 1123
nursing process
　diagnosis, 1122
　evaluation, 1122, 1124
　overview, 1122
　planning and implementation, 1122–1124
overview, 1117
pathophysiology and etiology, 1118
primary progressive, 1118t
progressive-relapsing, 1118t
relapsing-remitting, 1118t
risk factors, 1118
secondary progressive, 1118t
symptoms, 1066
treatment, 1065t
Multiple trauma, 1938
Multiple-puncture test (tine test), 861
Multisystem Effects:
　anemia, 98f
　cirrhosis, 1018f
　diabetes, 994f
　heart failure, 1409f
　hyperthyroidism, 1042f
　hypothyroidism, 1049f
　leukemia, 152f
　lung cancer, 162f
　rheumatoid arthritis, 746
　shock, 1486f
　stress, 1801
　systemic lupus erythematosus (SLE), 759
Mumps (Parotitis), in children, 795–796t
Mumps vaccine, 690
Mural thrombi, 1334, 1335t
Muscle relaxants:
　in specific conditions
　　multiple sclerosis, 1121t
　　musculoskeletal disorders, 1079t
Muscle(s). See also Musculoskeletal system
　age-related changes, 1063, 1063t
　anterior body, 1059f
　atrophy, 1060
　in children, 1062–1063
　fatigue, 1060
　functional properties, 1058
　movement, 1060
　muscle grading scale, 1067t
　sprain, 1063
　strength assessment, 1067t
　types, 1058, 1058t

　cardiac, 1060
　skeletal, 1058, 1058t
　smooth, 1058t
Muscle strength, 2251
Musculoskeletal system:
　age-related changes, 1062f, 1063, 1063t,
　　1064f, 1065
　alterations
　　back problems. See Back problems
　　fractures. See Fractures
　　multiple sclerosis. See Multiple sclerosis (MS)
　　osteoarthritis. See Osteoarthritis (OS)
　　Parkinson's disease. See Parkinson's disease
　　scoliosis. See Scoliosis
　　spinal cord injuries. See Spinal cord injuries
　benefits of exercise for, 653t
　McMurray's test, 1075f
　assessment
　　ballottement test, 1074f, 1074t
　　bulge test, 1074f, 1074t
　　diagnostic tests, 1076–1077, 1077t
　　gait and body posture, 1071t
　　genetic considerations, 1075, 1076t
　　health assessment interview, 1071, 1076t
　　joints, 1071t
　　McMurray's test, 1075t
　　muscle grading scale, 1067t
　　muscle strength, 1067t
　　overview, 1067
　　Phalen's test, 1074f, 1074t
　　physical assessment, 1067, 1071
　　range of motion, 1072f, 1072–1073t
　　Thomas test, 1075f, 1075t
　benefits of exercise for, 652
　composition, 1056
　fetal development, 1536t, 1537t
　functions, 1055
　inherited disorders, 1076t
　joints. See Joint(s)
　nursing interventions
　　ambulation, 1078
　　exercise, 1077
　　overview, 1077
　pregnancy and, 1544
　rehabilitative nursing, 1077
　skeleton, 1056–1058
　treatments
　　pharmacologic therapies, 1079, 1079t
Music therapy, 219, 363t, 1177
Muslims:
　health-related beliefs, 1784t
　holy days for, 1782
　paternal attachment, 1199t
　prayer, 1782f
Mutual recognition model, 2408, 2408t
Mutual pretense, 298
Myambutol. See Ethambutol
Mycobacterium avium complex (MAC), 704,
　706, 714t
Mycobacterium tuberculosis, 856
Mycophenolate mofetil, 561–562
Mycoplasma, 786t
Mycoplasma pneumoniae, pneumonia and,
　834–836, 842t
Mydriasis, 1669
Mydriatics, 1671t
Myelin sheaths, 940, 1118
Myeloblasts, 678f
Myeloid leukemia, 148

Myeloid stem cells, 678f
Myelosuppression, 93
Myocardial cells, 1306
Myocardial hypertrophy, 1312
Myocardial infarction. See Acute myocardial infarction (AMI)
Myocardial ischemia, 1362, 1362t
Myocardial perfusion imaging, 1371
Myochrysine. See Thiomalate
Myofascial pain syndrome, 264
Myofibrils, 1058
Myoglobin, 1371
Myopia, 1639t
Myotonia, 1697
Myotonic dystrophy, 1076t
Myringotomy, 827–829
Myxedema, 1045, 1047
Myxedema coma, hypothyroidism and, 1048

N

Na⁺. See Sodium
NAAL (National Assessment of Adult Literacy), 2342
Nabumetone, 749t
Nadolol, 1020
Nafarelin acetate, 1735t
Nails, 1883–1884t
Nalfon. See Fenoprofen
Naltrexone, 45
Namenda, 217
NANDA. See North American Nursing Diagnosis Association
NANDA nursing diagnoses:
  abuse, 1959
  acute renal failure, 548
  ADHD, 374
  alcohol abuse, 46, 48, 50
  Alzheimer's disease, 220, 223t
  anemia, 103
  anxiety disorders, 1817
  appendicitis, 899
  assault, 1967
  asthma, 1262
  autism spectrum disorder, 383
  benign prostatic hypertrophy, 436
  bipolar disorders, 1182
  burns, 1905
  cancer, 132
  cardiomyopathy, 1336
  cataracts, 1659
  cellulitis, 810
  cerebral palsy, 388–389
  cirrhosis, 1020–1021
  colorectal cancer, 145
  components of, 2066, 2066t
  congenital heart defects, 1355–1356
  contact dermatitis, 1914
  COPD, 1275
  coronary artery disease, 1384
  crisis, 1825
  culture, 331
  deep venous thrombosis, 1394
  defined, 2065
  depression, 1193
  diabetes mellitus, 1009
  disseminated intravascular coagulation, 1401
  dysrhythmias, 1458
  erectile dysfunction, 1715

failure to thrive, 393
family planning, 1739
fecal elimination disorders, 460
fibromyalgia, 307
fluid volume deficit, 578
fluid volume excess, 584
fractures, 1104
glaucoma, 1672
grief and loss, 607, 614, 624
heart failure, 1418
herniated disk, 1084
hip fractures, 1114
hypersensitivity, 738
hypertension, 1433
hyperthermia, 1863t
hyperthyroidism, 1045
hypothermia, 1868
hypothyroidism, 1050
increased intracranial pressure, 965
inflammatory bowel disease, 919
interrupted family processes, 513t
leukemia, 156
macular degeneration, 1677
menopause, 1744
mental retardation, 204
multiple sclerosis, 1122
nephritis, 927
NIC interventions linked to, 2093, 2094t
nutritional problems, 664
obesity, 1031
oral health, 659
osteoarthritis, 1131
otitis media, 830
pain, 284
Parkinson's disease, 1140
peptic ulcer disease, 935
perinatal loss, 629
peripheral neuropathy, 1682
peripheral vascular disease, 1466
personality disorders, 1620
phobias, 1841
pneumonia, 846
postpartum depression, 1205
pregnancy-induced hypertension, 1472
premenstrual syndrome, 1752
prenatal substance exposure, 65
pressure ulcers, 1921
prostate cancer, 173
pulmonary embolism, 1480
rape-trauma syndrome, 1975
religion, 1785
rheumatoid arthritis, 752
schizophrenia, 246
scoliosis, 1089
seizure disorders, 973–974
sexually transmitted infections, 1764
sickle cell disorder, 180–181
situational depression, 1210
skin cancer, 191
sleep disorders, 315
smoking, 54
spinal cord injury, 1151
spiritual distress, 1789
stroke, 1508
substance abuse, 79
suicide, 1983–1984
systemic lupus erythematosus (SLE), 762
tuberculosis, 865

types of, 2065–2066
urinary system disorders, 446, 446t–447t
urinary tract infections, 878
use of, in PIE documentation model, 2187
wellness diagnoses, 647
wound healing, 1931
Naprosyn. See Naproxen
Naproxen, 748, 749t
Narcissism, 1610
Narcissistic personality disorder:
  characteristics, 1616
    dysfunctional interpersonal relationships, 1617
    exhibitionism, 1617
    grandiosity, 1617
    impaired sexual expression, 1617
    labile affective response, 1617
  diagnostic criteria, 1614t
  incidence, 1616
  manifestations, 1611t
Narcolepsy:
  definition, 258, 309
  manifestations, 313t
  symptoms, 309–310
Narcotic abuse, therapies, 62t
Narcotic analgesics, 73
Narcotic Control Act, 68
Narcotics:
  administration of, 1907t
  effect on fetus, 58t
  sexual functioning and, 1701t
Narcotics Anonymous (NA), 37
Narrative charting, 2184–2185, 2185t
Nasal cannulae:
  description, 1230
  pictured, 1232f
Nasal speculum, 2005t
NasalCrom. See Cromolyn sodium
National Adult Literacy Study, 671
National Assessment of Adult Literacy (NAAL), 2342
National Association of Hispanic Nurses (NAHN), 2367t
National Association of Orthopaedic Nurses, 2367
National Black Nurses Association, 2367t
National Center for Complementary and Alternative Medicine (NCCAM), 376, 2435
National Center for Nursing Research (NCNR), 2332
National Commission for the Protection of Human Subjects of Biomedical and Behavioral Research, 2333
National Council Licensure Examination for Practical Nurses (NCLEX-PN®), 2407
National Council Licensure Examination for Registered Nurses (NCLEX-RN®), 2407
National Council of State Boards of Nursing (NCSBN), 2407–2408, 2408t
National Database of Nursing Quality Indicators™ (NDNQI), 2423
National Fire Prevention Association, 2440
National Fire Prevention's Association Life Safety Code, 2450
National Guideline Clearinghouse, 2335
National Healthcare Disparities Reports (2007), 2345
National initiatives, for quality improvement, 2423
National Institute for Nursing Research (NINR), 2326, 2329, 2332
National Institute for Occupational Safety and Health (NIOSH), 1965

National Institutes of Health (NIH), 2332, 2364
National Institutes of Health Stroke Scale, 1506t
National League for Nursing (NLN), 2367
National League for Nursing Accrediting
    Commission (NLNAC), 2366
National Organization for Associate Degree
    Nursing (N-OADN), 2280
National Patient Safety Goals (NPSGs), 2196,
    2366, 2423, 2459, 2460t
National Practitioner Data Bank (NPDB), 2398t
National Sleep Foundation, 665, 668
National Student Nurses Association (NSNA),
    2282t, 2366
National Survey on Drug Use and Health, 72
National Whistleblowers Center, 2418
Native American healing, 336
Native Americans:
    alcoholism in, 202
    culture-specific assessment, 2010t
    homicide and, 1964
    incidence of gallstones in, 903t
    mental illness and, 1163t
    otitis media in, 1634
    pain responses, 268t
    Peoplehood model of, 330
    tobacco use among, 51t
    view of mental illness, 245
    views on older adults, 402t
Natural family planning, 1725–1726, 1726t
Natural killer cells, 677t, 679, 679f, 681
Nature, 350
Nausea:
    in dying client, 618
    opioid use and, 278t
Nausea and vomiting in pregnancy (NVP), 1546,
    1546t, 1574t, 1575–1576
NCCAM (National Center for Complementary and
    Alternative Medicine), 376
Nearsightedness, 1639t
Nebulizer, 1259
Necrosis, 1915
Nedocromil, 1262
Negative feedback, 498, 2119
Negative punishment, 34
Negative reinforcement, 34
Negative symptoms, 232
Negative tilt keyboard, 2384t
Negative-pressure ventilators, 1238
Neglect, 1945–1946
Neglect syndrome, 1502–1503
Negligence, 2399
    categories of, resulting in malpractice, 2400t
    strategies to prevent incidents of professional,
        2401–2402
Nelfinavir, 713
Neomycin, 1020
Neonatal anemia, 101
Neonatal Behavioral Assessment Scale, 2013t
Neonatal stage, 341t
Neoplasms:
    benign, 117
    definition, 117
    malignant, 117–119, 117t
    metastasis, 118–119, 119f
    nomenclature, 126t
Neoplastic disease, 1876, 1878t
Nephrectomy, 560–562, 561t
Nephritis:
    Case Study, 930

classifications
    acute postinfectious glomerulonephritis, 923
    glomerulonephritis, 923
classifications
    Goodpasture's syndrome, 924
    lupus, 924
collaborative care
    diagnostic tests, 926
    overview, 925
    pharmacologic therapies, 926–927
    treatment, 927
community-based care, 928t
definition, 923
manifestations, 925, 925t
Nursing Care Plan
    assessment, 929t
    critical thinking in the nursing process, 929t
    diagnoses, 929t
    evaluation, 929t
    overview, 929t
    planning and implementation, 929t
nursing diagnoses and interventions
    excessive fluid volume, 928
    fatigue, 928
    impaired skin integrity, 928
    ineffective role performance, 928
    risk for imbalanced nutrition, less than body
        requirements, 928
    risk for infection, 928
nursing process
    assessment, 927
    diagnosis, 927
    evaluation, 929t
    planning and implementation, 927–928
pathophysiology and etiology, 923–925
risk factors, 925
treatment, 925t
Nephrolithiasis, 466
Nephrolithotomy, 470
Nephrons, 410, 410f
Nephrotic syndrome, systemic lupus
    erythematosus (SLE) and, 760
Nephrotoxins, 534–535
Nerve block, 278–279
Nervous system:
    diabetes mellitus and, 998
    fetal development, 1536t, 1537t
Nervous system. See Neurologic system, 940
Networking, 2271
Neuralgias, 264
Neurectomy, 279
Neurobiology:
    eating disorders and, 1598
    of mood disorders, 1161–1162, 1164t
    personality disorders and, 1608
Neuroendocrine route, 981
Neuroendrocine response, in heart failure,
    1405, 1406t
Neurofibrillary tangles, 212
Neurogenic bladder, 417, 873
Neurogenic shock, 1489, 1492t
Neurohypophysis (posterior pituitary), 978
Neurologic disorders, secondary hypertension
    and, 1425
Neurologic system. See also Central nervous
    system
    age-related changes
        infants and children, 943
        older adults, 943

assessment, 949
    cerebellar function, 956–957t
    children, 958t
    cranial nerves, 952–954t, 957t
    developmental considerations, 958, 958t
    diagnostic tests, 958–959
    infants, 958, 958t
    mental status, 951–952t
    motor function, 955t
    older adults, 958t
    sensory function, 954–955t
Assessment Interview, 950–951, 950–951t
cerebral dysfunction, 944
components, 940
disorders
    increased intracranial pressure. See Increased
        intracranial pressure
    seizures, 948
effects of shock on, 1487
neurons, 940
peripheral nervous system, 941, 943
Neurons, 940
    hormone release and, 981
    motor, 265
    sensory, 265
Neuropathic pain, 262
Neuropathies, classification of, 1679
Neuropeptide Y (NPY), 1598
Neurotherapy, 45
Neurotransmission, 1809f
Neurotransmission hypothesis, of mood
    disorders, 1161
Neurotransmitters. See also specific
    neurotransmitters
    dysregulation of
        eating disorders and, 1598
    impact of substance abuse on, 69
    pain and, 265
    sleep-wake cycle and, 666
Neurovascular assessment, 5 P's of, 1104
Neutral questions, 2056
Neutral thermal environment (NTE), 1854
Neutropenia, 93, 891t
Neutrophilia, 891t
Neutrophils, 677, 677t, 678f, 804f
Nevi:
    congenital, 184
    definition, 184
    dysplastic, 184–185
Nevirapine, 713
Newborns. See also Infants
    attachment formation, 1198
    body temperature of, 1854, 1858t, 1865–1866
    care of, 1558, 1558t
    father–infant interactions, 1198, 1199f
    hearing screening in, 1635
    hypothermia in, 1869–1870
    maternal attachment behavior and,
        1197–1198, 1198t
    recommended screenings and immunizations, 643t
    safety measures for, 2454, 2455t
    siblings and, 1198
    skin of, 1875
    sleep patterns and requirements, 667
    sleeping safety, 2440t
    transition from fetal to pulmonary circulation,
        1300–1302
    urinary elimination in, 413

Niacin, 1374*t*
NIC. *See* Nursing Interventions Classification
Nicotinamide, 1597*t*
Nicotine. *See also* Smoking
  addiction, 29, 247
    description, 29*t*
    treatment, 29*t*
  addictiveness of, 52
  coronary artery disease and, 1366
  definition, 51
  effect on fetus, 58*t*
  effects of, 51–52
  health problems caused by, 29
  sleep and, 669
Nicotine acetylcholine receptor agonist, 39*t*
Nicotine replacement therapy (NRT), 39*t*, 53
Nicotinic acid, 1374*t*
Nicotinic receptors, 233
Nidation, 1527–1528
Night shift workers, 669
Night sweats, 1744
Nightingale Pledge, 2308
Nightingale, Florence, 2287–2291, 2288*f*, 2308,
    2327, 2444
90-90 traction, 1106*t*
NINR. *See* National Institute for Nursing
    Research (NINR)
Nitrates:
  for angina, 1375
  for heart failure, 1415
  mechanism of action, 1331*t*
  nursing considerations, 1331*t*
Nitrite dipstick, urinary tract infections and, 875
Nitrofurantoin, 876
Nitrous oxide (laughing gas), 74
NK cells. *See* Natural killer cells
NLN. *See* National League for Nursing (NLN)
NOC. Nursing Outcomes Classification
Nociceptors, 263, 265
Nocturia, 417, 417*t*, 1408
  urinary tract infections and, 874
Nocturnal emissions, 668
Nocturnal enuresis, 414
Nocturnal frequency, 414
Nocturnal sleep-related eating disorder, 1585
Nodular melanoma, 185
Nodules, 1878*t*
Noise, excessive, 2452
Nolo contendere, 2407
Nolvadex, 110
Nominal group technique (NGT), 2136, 2138*t*
Non-English speakers, 2162–2163
Non-Mendelian (multifactorial) inheritance, 1723
Non-small-cell carcinomas, 161
Nonbreather masks:
  description, 1231
  pictured, 1233*f*
Noncompliance, 2259, 2259*t*
Nondirective interviews, 2056
Nonexudative macular degeneration, 1676, 1677*t*
Noninvasive ventilation (NIV), 1239
Nonjudgmental support, 2249
Nonmaleficence, 1777, 2308, 2315*t*, 2334
Nonnucleoside reverse transcriptase inhibitors
    (NNRTIs), 713, 808
Nonopioids, 275
  ceiling effect, 275
  misconceptions, 276*t*

narrow therapeutic index, 275
  for pain management, 275
Nonphenothiazine antipsychotics, 243
Nonprogrammed decisions, 2040
Nonshivering thermogenesis (NST), 1866
Nonspecific inflammatory response, 682
Nonspecific responses, immune system and, 676
Nonsteroidal anti-inflammatory drugs (NSAIDs):
  ceiling effect, 275
  for inflammation, 891, 892*t*
  narrow therapeutic index, 275
  for pain management, 274–275
  in specific conditions
    musculoskeletal disorders, 1079*t*
    osteoarthritis, 1127
    peptic ulcer disease, 931
    rheumatoid arthritis, 748, 749*t*
Nonunion, 1097, 1105
Nonverbal communication, 326, 2149, 2151–2152,
    2151*f*, 2157*t*
Nonverbal cues, for emotional states, 1158
Nonvolatile acids, 4
Noradrenaline, 666, 980
Norepinephrine (NE), 980, 1598, 1608, 1852
  arterial blood pressure and, 1423
  cellular metabolism and, 1852
  heart rate and, 1405
Norepinephrine uptake inhibitors (SSNIs):
  for fibromyalgia, 307
Normal sinus rhythm, 1440, 1441*t*
Normative commitment, 2231
Norms, 2068, 2069*t*
Norplant, 1732–1733
North American Nursing Diagnosis Association
    (NANDA), 2065, 2214, 2376
Norton's Pressure Area Risk Assessment Form
    Scale, 1921
Nosocomial infections:
  causes, 788*t*
  description of, 787–788
  pneumonia, 834
  prevention of, 788–789
  urinary tract infections and, 872
Novarel, 1735*t*
Novartis Microlipid, 972*t*
NPSGs (National Patient Safety Goals), 2196
NREM (non-rapid-eye-movement) sleep, 666–667
NRT (nicotine replacement therapy), 53
NSAIDs. *See* Nonsteroidal anti-inflammatory drugs
NST (nonshivering thermogenesis), 1866
NTE (neutral thermal environment), 1854
Nuclear detonation, 2353*t*
Nuclear family, 485
Nuclear imaging, in cancer, 128
Nucleation, 466
Nuclectomy, 1083
Nucleic acids, 679
Nucleolus, 86
Nucleoside reverse transcriptase inhibitors
    (NRTIs), 710–711, 712*t*, 713, 808
Nucleus, 86, 87*t*
Null cells. *See* Natural killer cells
Nulligravida, definition, 1559*t*
Nuremberg Code, 2333
Nuremberg Trials, 2333
Nurse administrator, 2295
Nurse anesthetist, 2294
Nurse educators, 2295

Nurse entrepreneurs, 2295
Nurse informaticist, 2391
Nurse Licensure Compact, 2408, 2408*t*
Nurse managers, 2142
Nurse practice acts (NPAs), 2292, 2398, 2402
  components of, 2407*t*
  credentialing and, 2409
  licensure and, 2407–2408
  mandatory reporting of nurses in violation of, 2414
  overview, 2406–2407
  relationship between administrative rules,
    position/advisory statements and, 2407*f*
  student nurses and, 2409
Nurse practitioners, 2293
Nurse researchers, 2295
Nurse Spiritual Therapeutics Scale, 1790*t*
Nurse staffing, 2428
Nurse-midwife, 2294
Nurses:
  as advocates, 2306, 2331–2332
  as collaborators, 2114–2115, 2115*t*
  as learners, 2244
  as member of health care team, 2116*t*
  as teachers, 2244
  changing role of, 2114
  educational levels of, 2327, 2330, 2330*t*
  guidelines for legal protection, 2417*t*
  impact of laws and standards on, 2409*f*
  laws affecting, 2399*t*
  malpractice cases against, 2398*t*
  malpractice suits against, 2424
  need for assistance by, 2097
  racial diversity among, 404*t*
  resource allocation and, 2350
  role of, in research, 2330–2332
  role of, with families, 507
  roles and functions of, 2293–2295, 2294*t*
  self-care for, 2034–2035
  supervision of delegated care by, 2098
  types of, and client outcomes, 2207*t*
Nurses' Health Study, 2332
Nurses' Health Study II, 2332
Nurse–client relationship, 2399, 2401
Nurse–physician relationship, 2131
Nursing:
  as caring, 2030
  commitment to profession of, 2230–2232
  concept of, 2283
  critical values of, 2281
  culturally sensitive, 2029*t*
  definitions of, 2291–2292
  functional, 2344
  historical perspectives on, 2287–2290
  primary, 2207, 2344
  recipients of, 2292
  settings for, 2292
  socialization to, 2281–2282
  team, 2206–2207, 2344
  theoretical definitions of, 2291
  types of knowledge in, 2031, 2031*f*
    aesthetic, 2031
    developing ways of knowing, 2032
    empirical, 2031
    ethical, 2032
    personal, 2032
Nursing activities:
  documentation of, 2098
  relating to outcomes, 2099, 2099*t*

Nursing administration, computers in, 2388–2389
Nursing assessment, 2193
Nursing care:
  cost effectiveness of, 2326
  providing competent, 2416
Nursing care coordination. See Care coordination
Nursing care delivery systems, 2344
Nursing Care Plans:
  acute myocardial infarction, 1387–1388t
  acute renal failure, 549t
  acute respiratory distress syndrome (ARDS), 1250t
  ADHD, 375t
  alcohol withdrawal, 49t
  alcoholic cirrhosis, 1023t
  Alzheimer's disease, 223t, 223–224t
  anemia, 105t
  anxiety disorders, 1817t
  appendicitis, 900t
  asthma, 1265t
  benign prostatic hypertrophy, 438t
  bipolar disorders, 1184t
  borderline personality disorder, 1623t
  bowel elimination disorders, 463t
  breast cancer, 114t
  bulimia nervosa, 1605t
  burns, 1910t
  cancer, 139–140t
  cataracts, 1674t
  cellulitis, 811t
  cerebral palsy, 390t, 391t
  chronic obstructive pulmonary disease (COPD),
    1278t, 1279t
  chronic pain, 286t
  colorectal cancer, 147t
  continuing, modifying, and terminating,
    2100–2101
  crisis, 1826t
  deep venous thrombosis, 1396t
  delirium, 229t
  depression, 1194t
  developing, 2077–2079, 2081–2083
  developmental considerations, 2095t
  disseminated intravascular coagulation, 1402t
  diversity in planning health care, 405–406t
  documents included in, 2078f
  dysrhythmias, 1460t
  elder abuse, 1961–1962t
  end-of-life care, 300t
  endometriosis, 1753t
  end-stage renal disease, 566t
  family planning, 1740t
  fluid volume excess, 585t
  formal, 2077
  formats for, 2081
  fractures, 1109t
  gallstones, 907t
  glaucoma, 1674t
  Graves' disease, 1046t
  guidelines for writing, 2081–2083
  heart failure, 1419t
  hip fractures, 1116t
  HIV infection, 723–724t
  hypertension, 1436–1437t
  hypothermia, 1869
  hypothyroidism, 1051t
  impaired urinary elimination, 452t
  individualized, 2077
  informal, 2077
  leukemia, 159t
  lung cancer, 167t
  melanoma, 193–194t
  morality issues, 1779t
  motor vehicle crashes, 1992t
  multiple sclerosis, 1123t
  nephritis, 929t
  obesity, 1032t
  obsessive-compulsive disorder, 1833t
  osteoarthritis, 1132–1133t
  osteoporosis, 1039t
  otitis media, 831t
  Parkinson's disease, 1141t
  peptic ulcer disease, 936t
  perinatal loss, 631t
  phobias, 1840–1841t
  pneumonia, 847t
  postpartum depression, 1205t
  post-traumatic stress disorder, 1847t
  pregnancy-induced hypertension, 1474t
  prenatal substance exposure, 64t
  pressure ulcers, 1925t
  prostate cancer, 174t
  pulmonary embolism, 1481t
  rape, 1976t
  religion, 1786t
  respiratory acidosis, 21t
  respiratory syncytial virus (RSV)/
    Bronchiolitis, 1284t
  rheumatoid arthritis, 755t
  risk for impaired parenting, 505
  schizophrenia, 249
  scoliosis, 1090–1091t
  seizure disorders, 973t
  septic shock, 854t, 1497–1498t
  sexually transmitted infections, 1763t
  sickle cell anemia, 182t
  situational depression, 1210t
  sleep disorders, 317t
  smoking, 55t
  spinal cord injury, 1154t
  spiritual distress, 1791t
  standardized, 2077–2081, 2080f
  stroke, 1511–1512t
  substance abuse, 79t
  suicidal client, 1985t
  syphilis, 1764t
  tuberculosis, 869t
  type 1 diabetes mellitus, 1013–1014t
  types, 2193
  ulcerative colitis, 922t
  urinary calculi, 479t
  urinary tract infections, 879t
  ventricular septal defect, 1358t
Nursing codes of ethics, 1776, 1778, 2308–2311,
    2309–2310t
Nursing competencies, for promoting client
    safety, 2444
Nursing diagnoses, 2065–2076, 2065f, 2076t
  assigning priorities to, 2084t
  collaborative problems compared with, 2067,
    2068t, 2072f
  communication, 2161
  components of, 2066, 2066t
  defined, 2065
  deriving desired outcomes from, 2085t
  formulating, 2069–2071t
  identification of, 2090–2091t, 2102–2103t
  medical diagnoses compared with, 2067,
    2068t, 2072f
  ongoing development of, 2074, 2076
  relationship of desired goals/outcomes to, 2087
  types of, 2065–2066
  See also NANDA nursing diagnoses
  Nursing Diagnosis: The International Journal of
    Nursing Language and Classification, 2076
Nursing discharge/referral summaries, 2194
Nursing economics, 2215–2216
Nursing education, 2327
Nursing education program accreditation, 2366
Nursing expertise, 2286t
Nursing health history,
  assessment of learning needs during,
    2254–2255, 2256t
  components of, 2053t
Nursing history, 2193
Nursing Home Reform Act, 1962
Nursing informatics, 2373. See also Informatics
Nursing information systems, 2375–2378, 2377t
Nursing interventions:
  consideration of consequences of, 2090
  criteria for choosing, 2090
  defined, 2077
  delegation of, 2092
  identification of, 2090–2091t, 2102–2103t
  implementation of, 2097
  redesign of, 2101
  relationship to problem status, 2092
  selection of, 2089–2090
  taxonomy, 2092–2093, 2093–2094t, 2094t
  types of, 2089–2090
  writing individualized, 2090, 2092
Nursing Interventions Classification (NIC),
    2092–2093, 2093–2094t, 2214, 2376, 2386
Nursing knowledge, 2006, 2327
Nursing languages, 2376, 2386
Nursing laws, 2398
Nursing leaders, 2290–2291
Nursing Management Minimum Data Set
    (NMMDS), 2386
Nursing Minimum Data Set (NMDS), 2191, 2386
Nursing Outcome Classifications (NOCs), 1868,
    2085–2086, 2086t, 2214, 2376, 2386
Nursing practice, 509
  accountability and, 2284, 2326
  applying critical thinking to, 2110–2111, 2110t
  contemporary, 2291–2293, 2293t
  cost-conscious, 2216
  decision making and, 2046
  ethical issues in, 2315–2317, 2317t
  factors influencing
    consumer demands, 2282–2283
    demography, 2283–2284
    economics, 2282
  in family-centered care, 509t
  health promotion and, 641–642
    information and telecommunications, 2283
    legislation, 2283
    science and technology, 2283
  HIPAA compliance and, 2413t
  laws impacting, 2402–2405, 2405t
  new nurses perceptions of, 2281t
  standards of, 2293, 2293t
Nursing presence, 2032–2033
Nursing process:
  abuse, 1957–1962

health promotion and illness prevention in, 641t,646t
hearing loss in, 1651
hypothermia in, 1870
injury prevention in, 2458
Internet use by, 672t
interventions for general population, 2023t
interventions for high-risk populations, 2023t
leading causes of death, 2023t
learning needs, 2256t
mental health issues, 622
minorities, 622
neurologic assessment in, 958t
neurologic system in, 943
nursing care plans for, 2095t
nutrition and, 1595t
pain in, 273, 273t
pain perception and behavior, 269t
physical changes in, 367–368, 369t
poisoning in, 2453t
postoperative care, 898, 898t
prevention of functional decline in, 2445
promotion of oral health in, 659–660
recommended screenings and immunizations, 644t
safety issues and, 2434
safety measures, 2456t
sensory perception in, 1635
sexuality in, 1694–1695
sleep disorders and, 311–312
sleep patterns and requirements, 669
sleep promotion in, 318t
spirituality in, 1772t
stress and coping in, 1802t
substance abuse in, 78t
tooth and gum problems in, 656
urinary elimination in, 414
use of Internet by, 2252
wound care in, 1929t
wound healing in, 1930t
Olecranon bursitis, 1068
Olfactory cells, 1633
Olfactory nerves, 942t, 1628t
Olfactory sense. See Smell
Olfactory stimuli, 1628
Oligomenorrhea, 1748
Oligospermia, 1735
Oliguria, 416, 417t, 1469–1470
Olsalazine, administration of, 915t
Omaha System, 2386
Omalizumab, 737–738
Omega-3 fatty acids, 218, 245, 1176
Omnibus Budget Reconciliation Act (OBRA), 2022, 2194
On-the-job instruction, 2274
Oncogenes, 119
Oncologic emergencies, 89–90
Oncologic imaging, 127–128
Oncology, 116
Oncotic pressure, 520, 580
Online health information, 672t, 2251–2253, 2252t
Oocytes, 1524, 1690
Oogenesis, 1524, 1690
OPCD. See Obsessive-compulsive personality disorder
Open awareness, 298
Open fractures, 1093, 1095t
Open reduction and internal fixation (ORIF), 1101
Open-angle glaucoma, 1668–1669, 1669t.
    See also Glaucoma

Open-ended questions, 2056, 2057t, 2167t, 2170
Opening stage, of interview, 2058
Operant conditioning, 347
Ophthalmics, 1670
Opiates, 73, 74t
Opioid antagonists, 39t
Opioids:
    endogenous, 1598
    for pain management, 274
    side effects, 277, 278t
    in specific conditions
        burns, 1900
        traumatic injury, 1943
    strong, 277
    types
        full agonists, 276
        mixed agonists-antagonists, 276
        partial agonists, 276
    weak or mixed, 276
Opportunistic infections:
    definition of, 771
    human immunodeficiency virus (HIV) and, 676
    treatments for, 714t
Ophthalmoscope, 2005t
Opinions, 2106t
Optic disc, 1642t
Optic nerve, 942t, 1628t
Optimism, 2238
OPTN (Organ Procurement and Transplantation Network), 2349–2350
Oral approach, 1655
Oral cavity, 655, 655f
Oral contraceptives, 1711t
    benefits, 1732
    combined estrogen-progestin, 1731
    contraindications, 1731
    coronary artery disease and, 1366
    secondary hypertension and, 1425
    side effects, 1731t
Oral hairy leukoplakia, 706
Oral health, 658
    developmental considerations, 656
    nursing process
        assessment, 656, 658
        diagnosis, 659
        evaluation, 661
        implementation, 659–661
        in older adults, 660t
        planning, 659
    overview, 655–656
    promotion of, 659
Oral rehydration, 575–576, 576t, 578t
Oral suction tube, 1245f
Oral temperature, 1855–1856
Oral thermometers, 1856
Oral-genital sex, 1697
Orbital blowout fracture, 1662
Orchiectomy, 172–173
Order of Deaconesses, 2287
Oregon Evidence-Based Practice Center, 2335
Oregon Health Plan, 2349
Orem's self-care model, 2059, 2060t
Organ of Corti, 1632, 1652
Organ Procurement and Transplantation Network (OPTN), 2349–2350
Organ transplantation, bioethics of, 2313
Organic solvents, 74
Organization-level plans, 2143
Organizational chart, 2126, 2126f

Organizational commitment, 2230
Organizational conflict, 2128
Organizing, 2143
Orgasmic disorders, 1702, 1702t
Orgasmic phase, 1697
Orientation, 2272
ORIF. See Open reduction and internal fixation (ORIF)
Ornish diet, 1383
Oropharynx, 655
Ortho Evra, 1732
Orthopaedic procedures, deep venous thrombosis and, 1391
Orthopnea, 582, 1221, 1408
Orthostatic hypotension, 1323
Orthotic devices, rheumatoid arthritis and, 751
Orudis. See Ketoprofen
Oseltamivir, 821
OSHA. See Occupational Safety and Health Administration (OSHA)
OSHA regulations, 2364f
Osmitrol. See Mannitol
Osmolality, 520, 532, 852
Osmolar imbalances, 569
Osmosis, 86t, 519–520, 520f
Osmotic diuretics, 541t, 959t, 963, 963t, 1670
Osmotic pressure, 520
Osseous tissue, 1056
Ossicles, 1633
Ossification, 1058
Osteoarthritis (OA):
    Case Study, 1133
    classification, 1125
    collaborative care
        conservative treatment, 1128
        diagnostic tests, 1127
        exercise, 1128
        nonpharmacologic treatment, 1127
        overview, 1127
        pharmacologic therapies, 1127
        rest to control symptoms, 1128
        surgery, 1129–1130
        viscosupplementation, 1129
        weight loss, 1128
    community-based care, 1131t
    complementary and alternative therapies, 1130
    complications, 1126–1127
    definition, 1065t, 1066
    incidence, 1125
    manifestations, 1069, 1125–1126, 1126t
    Nursing Care Plan, 1133t
        assessment, 1132t
        diagnoses, 1132t
        evaluation, 1132t
        overview, 1132t
        planning and implementation, 1132t
    nursing diagnoses and interventions
        chronic pain, 1131
        impaired physical mobility, 1133
        self-care deficit, 1133
    nursing process
        assessment, 1131
        diagnosis, 1131
        evaluation, 1133
        overview, 1131
        planning and implementation, 1131, 1133
    overview, 1125
    pathophysiology and etiology, 1125–1126
    race/ethnicity and, 1125t

rheumatoid arthritis (RA) and, 742–743, 743*t*
risk factors, 1126
treatment, 1065*t*
Osteoblasts, 652, 1056
Osteoclasts, 652, 1056
Osteocytes, 1056
Osteodystrophy, 540, 556
Osteon, 1056
Osteophytes, 1126
Osteoporosis:
  Case Study, 1040
  collaborative care
    diagnostic tests, 1036
    dietary management, 1036
    medications, 1037, 1037*t*
    physical therapy, 1036
  definition, 1033
  description, 983*t*
  manifestations, 1035, 1036*t*
  Nursing Care Plan, 1039*t*
    assessment, 1039*t*
    critical thinking, 1039*t*
    diagnosis, 1039*t*
    evaluation, 1039*t*
    planning and implementation, 1039*t*
  nursing diagnoses and interventions
    acute pain, 1038
    exercise, 1040
    healthy behavior, 1040
    imbalanced nutrition, less than body
      requirements, 1038
    risk for injury, 1038
  nursing process
    assessment, 1038
    diagnosis, 1038
    evaluation, 1040
    implementation, 1038
    planning, 1038
  overview, 1033
  pathophysiology and etiology, 1034
  risk factors, 1034–1035
  spinal changes from, 1036*f*
Osteotomy, 1129
Ostomy, 144*f*, 916–917, 917–919*t*
Other-centered people, 1580
Otitis externa, 824
Otitis interna, 824
Otitis Media, 1634*t*
  acute, 825–827, 827*f*
  Case Study, 832–833
  chronic, 825
  collaborative care
    alternative therapies, 829
    diagnostic tests, 828
    overview, 828
    pharmacologic therapies, 828–829
    surgery, 829
  cultural factors for, 826
  definition, 824
  with effusion, 825–827, 827 *f*
  etiology, 825
  immunizations and, 829
  manifestations, 826–827, 827*f*, 828*f*
  Nursing Care Plan
    assessment, 831*t*
    critical thinking, 831*t*
    diagnoses, 831*t*
    evaluation, 831*t*

planning and implementation, 831*t*
nursing diagnoses and interventions
  acute pain, 830
  disturbed sensory perception, auditory, 832
  fatigue, 832
  knowledge deficit, 832
  risk for caregiver role strain, 830, 832
  risk for delayed growth and development, 832
nursing process
  assessment, 829–830, 830*f*
  diagnosis, 830
  evaluation, 832
  planning and implementation, 830, 832
  pathophysiology, 824–825
risk factors, 825
serous, 825–827
treatments for, 801
Otoscope, 826, 2005*t*
Outcome standards, 2425
Outcomes management, 2425–2426
Outlet dystocia, 1518
Outpatient care, 2282
Output, 498
Output devices, 2375
Ovarian cycle, 1521*f*, 1522, 1690, 1691*f*
Ovarian follicles, 1522, 1522*f*, 1690
Ovarian hormones, 1519–1520, 1521*f*
Ovaries, 1519, 1688*t*, 1690
  pregnancy and, 1542
Overactive bladder, 442
Overdelegation, 2222
Overdose, 44, 75
Overeaters Anonymous, 37
Overflow incontinence, 442*t*
Overnutrition, 662, 2009, 2113
Overreactive affect, 238
Overt conflict, 2128
Overweight:
  in children, 2009
  nutritional status and, 662
  prevalence, 663*t*
Ovulation, 1690
  definition, 1522
  progesterone and, 1519–1520
Ovum, 1524–1525, 1526*f*, 1527*f*
Oxaprozin, 749*t*
Oxazepam, 1815, 1020
Oxybutynin, 423*t*, 443
Oxycodone (OxyContin), 73, 73*f*, 287*t*
Oxygen delivery systems, 1233*t*
Oxygen therapy, 1493
Oxygenation. *See also* Respiration;
    Respiratory system
  about, 1215–1233
  alterations in, 1218–1221, 1220*t*
  assessment, 1222–1223, 1223*t*, 1224–1225*t*, 1225
  clinical therapies, 1230–1233
  definition, 1215
  diagnostic tests, 1226–1229, 1228*t*
  normal presentation, 1216–1218
  pediatric differences, 1309
  pharmacologic therapies, 1229–1230
Oxymizer:
  description, 1230
  pictured, 1232*f*
Oxytocin, 413, 978

P

Pace, of speech, 2150
Pacemakers, 1450–1452, 1451*f*, 1452*t*, 1453*t*, 1459*t*
PaCO₂:
  defintion, 5
  in metabolic acidosis, 6*t*
  in metabolic alkalosis, 6*t*
  normal value, 5
  in respiratory acidosis, 5, 6*t*, 7*t*
  in respiratory alkalosis, 5, 6*t*, 7*t*
PACU (postanesthesia care unit), 897
PACU nurse, 897
Paget's disease, 107
Pain:
  acute
    characteristics, 262–263
    vs. chronic pain, 257*t*
    definition, 257
    description, 259*t*
    treatment, 259*t*
  alternative therapies, 266, 266*t*
  Assessment Interview, 281*t*
  breakthrough, 264
  cancer, 123–124, 257, 264
  Case Study, 287
  central, 264
  children and, 270–273
    behavioral consequences, 271
    developmental aspects, 272–273
    misconceptions, 272*t*
    neonatal, 270–271
    physiological consequences, 271
  chronic
    vs. acute pain, 257*t*
    characteristics, 263
    definition, 257
    description, 259*t*
    treatment, 259*t*
  collaborative care
    complementary and alternative medicine, 280
    diagnostic tests, 273
    nonpharmacological invasive therapies,
      278–279
    nonpharmacological pain management,
      279–280, 280*t*
    WHO three-step analgesic approach, 274–275
  community-based care, 286–287
  definition, 256, 262
  descriptors of, 256–257
  duration, 257
  in dying, 618
  etiology, 262
  factors affecting responses to
    developmental stage, 268–269, 269*t*
    environment and support people, 269–270
    ethnic and cultural values, 268
    meaning of pain, 270
    past pain experiences, 270
  history, 280–281
  incident, 264
  intensity, 262, 281–282
  location, 262
  management, 256
    barriers to, 266
    evidence-based practice, 285*t*
    standards, 272*t*
  manifestations, 266–268, 303*t*

medications
  analgesics, 274t, 287t
  coanalgesics, 274, 274t, 277–278
  drug abuse history and, 279t
  nonopioids, 274–275, 274t
  NSAIDs, 274–275
  opioids, 274, 276–277
  placebos, 278
  WHO three-step analgesic approach,
    274–275, 274f
of musculoskeletal system
  assessment, 1067
myths and misconceptions about, 270
neuropathic, 262
Nursing Care Plan
  assessment, 286t
  critical thinking, 286t
  diagnosis, 286t
  evaluation, 286t
  overview, 286t
  planning and implementation, 286t
nursing process
  assessment, 280–282
  diagnosis, 284
  evaluation, 287
  planning and implementation, 284–286
older adults and, 273, 273t
pathophysiology and etiology, 265–266
phantom, 264
postoperative, 264, 266
proprioceptive reflex to, 267f
psychogenic, 264
rating scales, 281–282, 282f
referred, 262
risk factors, 266
sensitization, 271
sleep disorders and, 312
stimuli, 265t
theories
  gate theory, 265
  pattern theory, 265
  specific theory, 265
types, 262, 264
Pain management flow sheet, 283f
Pain threshold, 271
Pain tolerance, 271
Palate, 655
Palliation, 131
Palliative care. See also End-of-life care
  complementary and alternative medicine in, 297
  definition, 291
  pediatric, 293–294, 294t
Palliative procedure, 1351
Pallidotomy, 1137
Palmar grasp, 958t
Palpation, 1222, 2002–2003, 2003f
Pancreas:
  definition, 980
  pregnancy and, 1545
Pandemic, 2351
Panic disorder:
  description and treatment, 1804t
  levels of severity, 1813t
  manifestations, 1813–1814
Pannus, 742–743, 743f
Pantothenic acid, 1597t
PaO₂:
  definition, 5
  normal value, 5

Papaverine, 1714
Paper medical records, 2378, 2379f
Papillary layer, 1875
Papilledema, 18
Papular warts, 1758
Papules, 1878t
Paracentesis, cirrhosis and, 1022
Paradoxical sleep. See REM sleep
Paraldehyde, 71
Parallel communication, 2118
Parallel functioning, 2118
Parallel play, 358, 358f
Paralysis
  assessment of communication and, 2160
  types, 1147f
Paramedical technologists, 2116t
Paramedics, 2358t
Paraneoplastic syndrome, 123, 124t
Paranoia, 232
Paranoid personality disorder:
  characteristics, 1611
    exclusion, 1612
    projection, 1612
    suspiciousness and mistrust, 1612
  diagnostic criteria, 1612t
  manifestations, 1611t
Paraphasia, 207t, 215
Paraphrasing, 2169, 2175, 2178t
Paraplegia, 1147
Parasites, 771, 786t
Parasomnias:
  bruxism, 311t
  definition, 258, 310
  enuresis, 311t
  periodic limb movements disorder, 311t
  sleeptalking, 311t
  somnambulism, 311t
Parasympathetic nervous system (PNS),
    1423–1424
Parasympathomimetics, 423t
Parathyroid glands, 978t, 979–980
Parathyroid hormone (PTH), 978t, 979
  abnormal, possible causes, 130t
  bone remodeling and, 1058
  ectopic functioning and, 137t
  effects of, 556
Parental control, 490, 491t
Parental roles, 484
Parental warmth, 490, 491t
Parenteral nutrition:
  in specific conditions
    acute renal failure, 543
Parenthood, transition to, 488
Parenting:
  definition, 490
  influence on development, 342
  styles, 490–492
Parents:
  anticipatory guidance for, 2439–2440
  authoritarian, 490, 491t
  authoritative, 490–491
  communication with, 335t
  death of, 609, 611
  emotional availability of, 496
  guidelines for collaboration with, 511t
  indifferent, 491–492, 491t
  influences of, on child, 489–490
  limit setting by, 490
  permissive, 491, 491t

presence of, during procedures, 484
of sick children, 2011
single, 486
teen, 486
who are addicts, 30–31
Paresis, in compartment syndrome, 1096t
Paresthesias, 24t, 556, 1096t, 1679
Parietal lobe, 940
Parkinsonian gait, 956t
Parkinsonism, 1066
Parkinson's disease (PD):
  Case Study, 1142
  Client Teaching, 1140t
  collaborative care
    deep brain stimulation, 1137
    diagnostic tests, 1137
    pharmacologic therapies, 1137
    rehabilitation, 1139
    surgery, 1137
  community-based care, 1142t
  complications, 1137
  definition, 1065t, 1066, 1134
  incidence, 1066
  manifestations, 1135, 1135t
    abnormal posture, 1135
    autonomic and neuroendocrine effects, 1136
    bradykinesia, 1136t
    constipation, 1136t
    dementia, 1136t
    interrelated effects, 1137
    loss of normal reflexes, 1136t
    mood and cognition, 1136
    rigidity and bradykinesia, 1135
    sleep disturbances, 1137
    tremor, 1135
  Medication Administration, 1138t
  Nursing Care Plan
    assessment, 1141t
    critical thinking in the nursing process, 1141t
    diagnosis, 1141t
    evaluation, 1141t
    overview, 1141t
    planning and implementation, 1141t
  nursing diagnoses and interventions
    disturbed sleep pattern, 1142
    imbalanced nutrition, less than body
      requirements, 1140
    impaired physical mobility, 1140
    impaired verbal communication, 1140
  nursing process
    assessment, 1139
    diagnosis, 1140
    evaluation, 1142
    overview, 1139
    planning and implementation, 1140, 1142
  overview, 1134
  pathophysiology and etiology, 1134
  risk factors, 1134
  stages of, 1134t
  symptoms, 1066
  treatment, 1065t
Parlodel, 1735t
Parotitis, 658t, 795–796t
Paroxetine, 1201
Paroxysmal atrial tachycardia, 1444
Paroxysmal nocturnal dyspnea, 1408
Paroxysmal supraventicular tachycardia (PSVT),
    1442t, 1444–1445
Partial agonists, 276

Partial seizures, 968
Partial-thickness burns, 1889, 1889f, 1894t
Participative decision making, 2039
Passive behavior, 1169
Passive communicators, 2179, 2179t
Passive immunity, 682–683
Passover, 1781
Patch test, 736
Patch testing, 1913
Patches, skin, 1878t
Patent airway, 1218
Patent ductus arteriosus (PDA), 1339, 1340t
Patent ductus arteriosus (PDA) closure, 1354t
Paternal attachment, 1198, 1199t
Pathogenesis, 636
Pathogenicity:
    definition of, 770
Pathogens, 786t
    definition of, 770–771
    infection control and, 785–786
Pathologic fractures, 1093
Pathological grief, 606
Patient advocates, nurses as, 2331–2332
Patient Care Data Set (PCDS), 2386
Patient Protection and Affordable Care Act, 2418
Patient responsibilities, 2320t
Patient rights:
    overview, 2318
    protection of, 2318, 2318–2319t, 2319t, 2320t
Patient Safety and Quality: An Evidence-Based
        Handbook for Nurses (AHRQ), 2423, 2433
Patient Self-Determination Act, 250, 290, 294t,
        2283, 2301, 2318, 2410
Patient-controlled analgesia (PCA), 1086t, 1900
Patient-centered care, 2444
Patient/family education path, 2125t
Patients, 2292
Patient's Bill of Rights (AMA), 670, 2254
Pattern theory, 265
Patterns of health care, 2053t
Pauciarticular juvenile rheumatoid arthritis
        (JRA), 745
Paxil, 1201
Payment structures, 2214
Payroll systems, 2378t
PCA. See Patient-controlled analgesia (PCA)
PCP (phencyclidine), 58t, 60, 73
PCPs. See Primary care providers (PCPs)
PCV7, 690
PD. See Parkinson's disease
PDAs (personal digital assistants), 2378
PDD. See pervasive developmental
        disorders (PDD)
PDs. See Personality disorders
Peak expiratory flow rate (PEFR), 1227–1228
Peck, Robert, 345–346
Pedagogy, 2245
Pedia pulse, 1320
Pediatric cardiology, 1313
Pediatric health care home, 2348t
Pediatric nursing, family-centered care in,
        509–511
Pediatric research studies, 2334, 2334t
Pediatric Symptom Checklist, 2013t
Pedigree, 1723
Pedophiles, 1947
Peer coaching, 2275
Peer review, 2425
Pelvic cavity, 1517

Pelvic diaphragm, 1517
Pelvic examinations:
    urinary tract infections and, 876
Pelvic floor, 411-412, 1517, 1517t, 1518f
Pelvic floor muscle exercises, 445t, 450
Pelvic inlet, 1517
Pelvic outlet, 1518
Pelvis, female, 1516–1519, 1516f, 1519f, 1520f
Penetrating injury, of eye, 1662, 1663t, 1664
Penetrating trauma, 1938
Penetrex. See Enoxacin
D-penicillamine, 748, 750t
Penicillin-resistant Streptococcus pneumoniae
        (PRSP), 789
Penicillins:
    medication administration, 807
    pneumonia and, 841
Penile implants, 1714, 1715f
Penis:
    anatomy, physiology, functions, 1686, 1686t
    assessment, 1704t
Penumbra, 1500
Peoplehood model, 330
Peplau, Hildegard, 35, 1796–1797
Peppermint tea, 919
Peptic ulcer disease (PUD):
    Case Study, 937
    collaborative care
        diagnostic tests, 933
        nutrition, 934
        pharmacologic therapies, 933–934
        surgery, 934
    common sites affected by, 931f
    community-care settings, 937t
    complications, 932, 933t, 934
    definition, 930
    incidence, 930
    manifestations, 932, 932t
    Nursing Care Plan
        assessment, 936t
        critical thinking in the nursing care process, 936t
        diagnoses, 936t
        evaluation, 936t
        overview, 936t
        planning and implementation, 936t
    nursing diagnoses and interventions
        deficient fluid volume, 936–937
        disturbed sleep pattern, 935
        imbalanced nutrition, less than body
            requirements, 935
        pain, 935, 935t
    nursing process
        assessment, 934
        diagnosis, 935
        evaluation, 937
        overview, 934
        planning and implementation, 935–937
    pathophysiology and etiology, 931
    risk factors, 931, 932t
    superficial, 931f
    treatment, 932t
        for complications, 934
    Zollinger-Ellison syndrome, 932
Peptic ulcers, 930
Peptide hormones, 981
Perceived loss, 600
Perception, 199
    checking, 2170
    validating, 2178t

definition, 1629
Perceptions, 2156
Percussion, 2003–2004, 2004f, 2004t
    chronic obstructive pulmonary disease (COPD)
        and, 1273
    definition, 1222
    pneumonia and, 843, 843f
Percussion (reflex) hammer, 2005t
Percutaneous cholecystostomy, 905
Percutaneous coronary revascularization (PCR),
        1372f, 1376–1378, 1378t
Percutaneous ultrasonic lithotripsy, 476f
Perforated appendix, 893
Perforating injury, of eye, 1662, 1663t, 1664
Perforation, 893–894, 932
Performance assessment, 2425
    audits, 2426
    outcomes management, 2425–2426
    peer review, 2425
    utilization reviews, 2426
Perfusion:
    about, 1294–1332
    assessment, 1316–1318t
    caring interventions, 1326, 1329
    diagnostic tests, 1326
    pharmacologic therapies, 1329, 1330–1332t
Perianal assessment, 429t
Pericarditis, 1369
    rheumatoid arthritis and, 747
    systemic lupus erythematosus (SLE) and, 759–760
Pericardium, 1294
Peripheral vascular disease, 998
Perimenopausal period:
    definition, 1742
    manifestations, 1743t
Perinatal loss:
    Case Study, 633
    definition, 626
    fetal testing, 627t
    factors associated with
        fetal factors, 626t
        maternal factors, 626t
        placental and other factors, 626t
    grieving, 628
    manifestations, 627–628
    maternal testing, 627t
    Nursing Care Plan
        assessment, 631t
        critical thinking in the nursing process, 631t
        diagnosis, 631t
        evaluation, 631t
        overview, 631t
        planning and implementation, 631t
    nursing diagnoses and interventions
        caring or couple with previous loss in
            pregnancy, 632
        facilitating familys grief work, 630, 632
        preparing family birth, 629
        providing discharge care, 630
        referring family to community services, 632
        supporting family in viewing stillborn infant, 630
    nursing process
        assessment, 628
        diagnosis, 629
        evaluation, 632
        planning and implementation, 629–632
    overview, 626
    pathology and etiology, 626

pathophysiology and etiology, 626–627
risk factors, 627
Perinatal mortality rate (PMR), 626
Perineal prostatectomy, 171, 440
Perineum, 1517, 1688t, 1708t
Periodic limb movements disorder (PLMD), 311t
Periodontal disease, 656, 658, 658t
diabetes mellitus and, 999
Perioperative nursing care:
definition, 894
diagnosis, 895t
PeriOperative Nursing Data Set (PNDS), 2386
Periosteum, 1056
Peripartum cardiomyopathy, 1334
Peripheral atherosclerosis, 1463t, 1464t
Peripheral nerves, 1679
Peripheral nervous system (PNS):
components, 940
cranial nerves, 941
diabetes mellitus and, 998
functions, 1679
neurons, 265
spinal nerves, 943
Peripheral neuropathy, 707
Case Study, 1683
Charcot-Marie-Tooth syndrome, 1680
clinical therapies, 1680t
collaborative care
alternative therapies, 1681
diagnostic tests, 1681
definition, 1679
diabetes mellitus and, 998–999
Guillain-Barré syndrome, 1679
manifestations, 1680, 1680t
nursing diagnoses and interventions
disturbed sensory perception, 1682
pain, 1682
nursing process
assessment, 1681–1682
diagnosis, 1682
evaluation, 1682
planning and implementation, 1682
pathophysiology and etiology, 1679–1680
prognosis, 1680
risk factors, 1680
treatment, 1681
types, 1679
Peripheral obesity, 1026
Peripheral pulse, 1307
Peripheral vascular disease (PVD):
Case study, 1468
Client Teaching, 1466t
collaborative care
clinical therapies, 1465
complementary therapies, 1465
diagnostic tests, 1464–1465
overview, 1463–1464
pharmacologic therapies, 1465
surgery, 1465
definition, 1462
etiology, 1462
manifestations, 1463
nursing diagnoses and interventions
activity intolerance, 1467
impaired skin integrity, 1467
ineffective tissue perfusion, peripheral,
1466–1467
pain, 1467

nursing process
assessment, 1466
diagnosis, 1466
evaluation, 1467
overview, 1465–1466
planning and implementation, 1466–1467
pathophysiology, 1462
risk factors, 1462–1463
Peripheral vascular resistance, 1308, 1422–1423
Peristalsis, 773
Peritoneal dialysis, 416, 543, 546, 547t, 559–560.
See also Dialysis
Peritonitis, 893, 894t, 932
Permanent teeth, 657
Permissive parents, 491, 491t
Pernicious anemia, 99
Perseverance, 2107
Persistent vegetative state, 948
Personal appearance, 2152
Personal competence, 1591t
Personal digital assistants (PDAs), 2378
Personal distance, 2156
Personal health information (PHI), 2391
Personal identity, 1582, 1589
Personal knowing, 2032
Personal payment, for health care services,
2212, 2369
Personal Protective Equipment (PPE), 2365, 2435
Personal space, 326, 2058t, 2156–2157, 2156f
Personality, 343, 350
in adolescence, 364
culture and, 1587t
definition, 1607
identifying areas of strength, 1590t
infancy, 357
parameters of, 349t
preschool age, 361
in school-age years, 363
toddlers, 358
Personality disorders (PDs):
Case Study, 1624
characteristics, 1587, 1610, 1621t
in children, 1587t
clinical features
behavior, 1588
emotions, 1588
impaired sense of self, 1588
thinking patterns, 1588
cluster A (odd-eccentric)
characteristics, 1611
diagnostic criteria, 1612t
paranoid personality disorder, 1611–1613,
1611–1612t
schizoid personality disorder, 1611–1612t, 1613
schizotypal personality disorder,
1611–1612t, 1613
cluster B (dramatic-emotional)
antisocial personality disorder,
1611t, 1614t, 1617
borderline personality disorder, 1611t,
1614–1616, 1614t
characteristics, 1613
diagnostic criteria, 1614t
histrionic personality disorder, 1611t,
1614t, 1616
narcissistic personality disorder, 1611t, 1614t,
1616–1617

cluster C (anxious-fearful)
avoidant personality disorder, 1611t, 1618, 1618t
characteristics, 1617
dependent personality disorder, 1611t,
1618t, 1619
diagnostic criteria, 1618t
obsessive-compulsive personality disorder,
1611t, 1618t, 1619
collaborative care
alternative therapies, 1619, 1620t
cognitive-behavioral therapy, 1619
dialectical behavior therapy, 1619
overview, 1619
pharmacologic therapies, 1619
cultural considerations in, 1621t
definition, 1587, 1607
description, 1585t
diagnostic criteria, 1608t
ego-syntonic, 1607
family education, 1624t
manifestations, 1610–1611, 1611t
nursing diagnoses and interventions
improving family communication, 1624
maintaining boundaries, 1622
modifying cognitive distortions, 1622,
1623t, 1624
teaching, 1622
nursing process
assessment, 1620
diagnosis, 1620
evaluation, 1624
overview, 1620
planning and implementation, 1621–1622,
1623t, 1624
overview, 1607
pathophysiology and etiology, 1607–1608
pharmacologic therapies, 1592
risk factors, 1610
theories on
family theory, 1609
gender-bias theory, 1610
genetics, 1608
intrapersonal factors, 1609
neurobiology, 1608
sociocultural factors, 1609
treatments, 1585t
types of, 1587
Personality traits, 1607
Perspiration, 1853
Pertussis vaccine, 687
Pertussis (Whooping Cough), 796t
Pervasive developmental disorder not otherwise
specified (PDD-NOS), 378, 379t
Pervasive developmental disorders (PDDs), 378.
See also Autistic spectrum disorders
PES format, 2072, 2073t
Pessimists, 2238
PET. See Positron emission tomography (PET)
Pew Internet and American Life Project,
672t, 2382
Peyer's patches, 681f, 682
PGD. See Preimplantation genetic
diagnosis (PGD)
PGs. See Prostaglandins (PGs)
pH, 3
arterial blood
in metabolic acidosis, 6t, 7t

in metabolic alkalosis, 6*t*, 7*t*
in respiratory acidosis, 6*t*, 7*t*
in respiratory alkalosis, 6*t*
serum levels
in respiratory alkalosis, 7*t*
Phagocytic cells, 677–678
Phagocytosis, 86*t*, 677*t*, 681, 1928
Phalen's test, 1074, 1074*t*
Phantom pain, 264
Pharmacists, 218*t*, 2116*t*
Pharmacologic therapies:
cognitive disorders, 210
Phase of mutual recognition, 1198
Phencyclidine (PCP):
use in pregnancy, 60
Phenobarbital, 58*t*, 971
Phenothiazine chlorpromazine (Thorazine), 242
Phenothiazines, 242
Phenotype, 1723
Phenylketonuria, 202
Phenytoin, 959, 971
PHI. *See* Protected health information
Philadelphia chromosomes, 149–150, 150*f*
Phimosis, 1704*t*
PHOs. *See* Physician/hospital organizations
Phobias:
Assessment Interview, 1839*t*
Case Study, 1842
collaborative care
cognitive-behavioral therapy, 1839, 1839*t*
journal writing, 1839
pharmacologic care, 1838
description and treatment, 1804*t*
developmental considerations, 1837*t*
manifestations, 1837*t*
agoraphobia, 1836–1837
social phobias, 1837
specific phobias, 1838
Nursing Care Plan
assessment, 1840*t*
critical thinking, 1841*t*
diagnosis, 1840*t*
evaluation, 1840*t*
planning and implementation, 1840*t*
nursing process
assessment, 1839
assessment interview, 1839*t*
diagnosis, 1841
evaluation, 1841
planning and implementation, 1841
overview, 1835
pathophysiology and etiology, 1835–1836
risk factors, 1836
Phocomelia, 1723
Phosphate (PO$_4$–):
as buffer, 4
function, 525*t*
imbalances. *See* Hyperphosphatemia
in intracellular fluid, 518
regulation, 525*t*, 526
regulation. *See* Hypophosphatemia
Phosphatidyl serine, 218
Phosphodiesterase inhibitors, 1415*t*
mechanism of action, 1331*t*
nursing considerations, 1331*t*
Phosphoric acid, 4

Phosphorus (P):
in musculoskeletal system assessment, 1077*t*
recommended daily intake, 1597*t*
Photodynamic therapy, 1649, 1677
Photophobia, 1669*t*
conjunctivitis and, 814
Physical abuse, 1945, 1946*f*
Physical activity, 652. *See also* Exercise
Physical agents, 886
Physical attending, 2166, 2166*t*
Physical dependence, 30*t*
Physical examination, 645, 2000–2005, 2059
addressing client situations, 2001*t*
assessment of learning needs and, 2255
client preparation, 2001
environment preparation, 2001
equipment, 2005, 2005*t*
head-to-toe assessment, 2000, 2001*t*
methods, 2002–2005
auscultation, 2004–2005
inspection, 2002
palpation, 2002–2003, 2003*f*
percussion, 2003–2004, 2004*f*, 2004*t*
normal and abnormal findings, 2000
positioning, 2001, 2002*t*
purposes, 2000–2001
types, 2000
Physical fitness, 651–652
Physical fitness assessment, 645
Physical neglect, 1946
Physical restraints, 2445. *See also* Restraints
Physical therapists, 2116*t*
Physical therapy, for stroke, 1507
Physician assistants (PAs), 2117*t*
Physician management systems, 2378*t*
Physician–nurse collaboration, 2118*t*
Physician–nurse relationship, 2131
Physician/hospital organizations (PHOs), 2212
Physicians, 2116*t*
Physician's orders, implementing, 2416
Physiologic anemia of infancy, 101
Physiologic anemia of pregnancy, 1310, 1543
Physiologic events, learning and, 2251
Physiologic needs, 2083*t*
Physiological pain, 262
Piaget, Jean, 198, 347, 348*t*, 360*t*
Pica, 97
PIE documentation model, 2187
Pinocytosis, 86*t*, 1533
Pinpointing, 2170
Piroxicam, 749*t*
Pitch, 2004
Pituitary gland:
definition, 978
pregnancy and, 1545
Pityrosporum oxale (yeast), 770
Placebo effect, 278
Placebos, 278, 2328*t*
Placenta:
definition, 1530
development of, 1528, 1530–1531
exchange of substances across, 1531
fetal side, 1532*f*
functions, 1533–1534
endocrine, 1533–1534
immunologic, 1534

metabolic, 1533
transport, 1533
maternal side, 1532*f*
placental circulation, 1532–1533
vascular arrangement of, 1532*f*
Placenta previa, 60
Plague, 2357*t*
Plan:
developing nursing care plans, 2077–2079,
2081–2083
in nursing process, 2051*t*, 2077–2093, 2077*f*, 2091*t*
standardized approach, 2078–2081
types of planning, 2077
Plan B, 1733
Plan of care, of POMR, 2187
Plan-Do-Study-Act cycle (PDSA), 2427, 2427*t*
Planned Parenthood, 2291
Planning, 2038–2039, 2143
contingency, 2143
strategic, 2143
Planning process:
delegating implementation, 2092
establishing client goals, 2085–2087, 2085*f*, 2089
overview, 2083
selecting nursing interventions and activties,
2089–2090
setting priorities, 2083–2085, 2084*t*
writing individualized nursing interventions,
2090, 2092
Plant estrogens, 1745*t*
Plaque, 656
formation, 1361–1362, 1462
Plaquenil. *See* Hydroxychloroquine
Plaques, 1118, 1878*t*
Plasma:
in extracellular fluid, 518, 519*f*
pregnancy and, 1543
Plasma cells, 678*f*, 679, 679*f*, 680*f*, 681–682
Plasma d-dimer levels, 1479
Plasma exchange therapy, 927
Plasma protein, as buffer, 4
Plasmapheresis, 738, 750–751, 927
Platelet (thrombocyte) count, 130*t*, 153
Play:
associative, 360
cooperative, 363
dramatic, 361
in infancy, 356
parallel, 358, 358*f*
preschoolers, 360–361
school-age children, 362–363
solitary, 356
in toddlerhood, 358
Play therapist, 1282
Play therapy, for burn victims, 1908*t*
Pleasure model, of addiction, 28
Plethysmography, 1391
Pleura, 1216
Pleural effusion, 747, 835
Pleuritis, 835
Pleximeter, 2004
Plexor, 2004
PLISSIT model, 1694
Plumbism, 2454
PMR (perinatal mortality rate), 626
PMS. *See* Premenstrual syndrome (PMS)

Pneumatic retinopexy, 1664
Pneumococcal Conjugate Vaccine, 690
Pneumococcal infection, in children, 797t
Pneumocystis carinii, 834, 836, 842t
Pneumocystis carinii pneumonia (PCP), 696, 703–704, 714t
Pneumomediastinum, 1242
Pneumonectomy, 165t
Pneumonia, 714t
  acute bacterial, 834–836
  aspiration, 837
  Case Study, 849
  collaborative care
    chest physiotherapy, 843–844
    clinical treatments, 842
    complementary therapies, 844
    diagnostic tests, 841
    immunizations, 841, 845
    overview, 840–841
    oxygen therapy, 842–843
    pharmacologic therapies, 841–842
  definition, 833
  inflammatory response and, 834f
  influenza vaccines and, 845
  Legionnaires' disease, 836
  manifestations, 839–840, 840t
  manifestations of infectious, 837t
  multisystem effects, 840
  nosocomial infections and, 787–788
  Nursing Care Plan
    assessment, 847t
    critical thinking, 847t
    diagnoses, 847t
    evaluation, 847t
    interventions, 847t
    planning and implementation, 847t
  nursing diagnoses and interventions
    activity intolerance, 848
    home care, 848
    ineffective airway clearance, 846
    ineffective breathing pattern, 848
  nursing process
    assessment, 845–846
    diagnosis, 846
    evaluation, 848
    pediatric assessment, 845t
    pediatric differences and, 846t
    planning and implementation, 846
  in older adults, 834
  pathogenesis of, 836f
  pathophysiology, 833–834
  patterns of lung involvement in, 835t
  pediatric differences and, 837, 838f, 839–841, 839f
  Pneumocystis carinii, 836, 837t
  prevention of, 840
  primary atypical, 836, 837t
  risk factors, 837, 839
  therapies for
    antibiotics, 842t
    chest physiotherapy, 843
    clinical treatments, 842
    complementary and alternative, 844
    medications, 841–842
    oxygen therapy, 842–843, 842f, 843f
  viral, 836, 837t
Pneumopericardium, 1242

Pneumothorax:
  definition, 1221
  result of barotrauma, 1242
  tuberculosis and, 861
PNS. See Peripheral nervous system
PO₄−. See Phosphate
Podophyllin, 1759t
Point of maximal impulse (PMI), 1307
Point of service (POS), 2369
Point-of-care devices, 2389, 2390f, 2390t
Poisoning, lead, 2454
Poisoning prevention, 2451, 2453t
Polar body, 1522
Policies, 2079
Policy making, phases of, 2362
Poliomyelitis, in children, 797t
Poliovirus vaccine, 691
Polyarticular juvenile rheumatoid arthritis (JRA), 745
Polycystic kidney disease, 553t
Polycythemia, 1309
Polydipsia, 246, 416, 991
Polyethylene glycol electrolyte solution (GoLYTELY), 455
Polygamy, 1699
Polymerase chain reaction, 862
Polymorphonuclear leukocytes, 729f
Polyneuropathies, 1679
Polypeptides, 679
Polyphagia, 991
Polyps, 141
Polysaccharides, 679–680, 1593
Polysomnography (PSG), 313
Polysubstance abuse, 30t, 45, 67
Polytheism, 1771
Polyuria, 416, 417t, 582, 991
POMR. See Problem-oriented medical records
Popliteal pulse, 1320
Populations, 2327
POR. See Problem-oriented records
Portal hypertension, 1017
Portal systemic encephalopathy, 1019
Positive attitude, as component of professionalism, 2228
Positive end-expiratory pressure (PEEP), 1240t, 1241
Positive feedback, 498, 2119
Positive inotropic agents, 1414–1415t
Positive punishment, 34
Positive reinforcement, 34, 648, 2246
Positive symptoms, 232
Positive-pressure ventilators:
  description, 1238–1239
  modes of ventilation, 1239–1241, 1240t
  pictured, 1239f
Positron emission tomography (PET), 1120, 2392
Post-traumatic stress disorder (PTSD):
  Assessment Interview, 1846t
  Case Study, 1848
  collaborative care
    acupuncture, 1845
    eye movement desensitization and reprocessing (EMDR), 1845
    pharmacologic therapies, 1845
  description and treatment, 1804t
  DSM-IV-TR diagnostic criteria, 1844t

  health care, 1848
  heart surgery and, 1359t
  manifestations, 1843–1844
  Nursing Care Plan
    assessment, 1847t
    critical thinking, 1847t
    diagnosis, 1847t
    evaluation, 1847t
    planning and implementation, 1847t
  nursing process
    assessment, 1846
    assessment interview, 1846t
    diagnosis, 1846
    evaluation, 1848
    planning and implementation, 1846–1847
  overview, 1842
  pathophysiology and etiology, 1842–1843
  rape and, 1972–1973
  risk factors, 1843
Postanesthesia care unit (PACU), 897
Postcoital contraception, 1733
Postconception age periods, 1538
Postconventional stage, 352t
Postdoctoral study, 2330
Posterior cavity, of eye, 1631
Posterior pituitary (neurohypophysis), 978
Posterior syndrome, 1145t
Posterior tibial pulse, 1320
Posthepatic cirrhosis, 1016
Postherpetic neuralgia, 264
Postictal period, 970
Postmenopausal bleeding, 1748
Postnecrotic cirrhosis, 1016
Postoperative complications:
  cardiovascular, 897
  elimination, 897
  respiratory, 897
Postoperative nursing care:
  complications, 897
  head-to-toe assessment, 897
  immediate, 897
  older adults, 898, 898t
  pain management, 897
  surgical wounds, 897–898
  when client is stable, 897
Postoperative pain, 264, 266
Postpartum, 1559t
Postpartum blues, 1159, 1200
Postpartum care, 1558, 1558t
Postpartum depression:
  about, 1159
  Case Study, 1207
  clinical therapies, 1201t
  collaborative care
    other therapies, 1202
    overview, 1201
    pharmacologic therapies, 1201
    support groups, 1202
  community-based care, 1206
  definition, 1159, 1160t, 1201
  fathers and, 1206
  manifestations, 1201t
  Nursing Care Plan
    assessment, 1205t
    critical thinking, 1205t

diagnosis, 1205t
evaluation, 1205t
planning and implementation, 1205t
nursing process, 1202–1207t
overview, 1196
prevention strategies, 1207t
prevention, identification, and intervention for, 1206t
recurrence, 1174
risk factors, 1201
suicide risk and, 1201
treatments, 1160t
Postpartum Depression Predictors Inventory Revised (PDPI-R), 1202, 1203–1204t
Postpartum major mood disorder, 1201. See also Postpartum depression
Postpartum period:
bowel elimination in, 424
characteristics, 1196
cultural considerations, 1197t, 1199
development of family attachment in, 1197
maternal attachment behavior, 1197–1198, 1198t
siblings in, 1198
social support during, 1200
urinary elimination in, 413
Postpartum psychiatric disorders:
classification, 1200
postpartum depression. See Postpartum depression
postpartum psychosis. See Postpartum psychosis
Postpartum psychosis:
clinical therapies, 1201t
definition, 1159
incidence, 1200
manifestations, 1201t
symptoms, 1200
Postrenal acute renal failure, 534, 534t. See also Acute renal failure
Postsynaptic neurons, 265f
Postterm labor:
definition, 1559t
Postural drainage:
chronic obstructive pulmonary disease (COPD) and, 1273–1274
pneumonia and, 843–844, 844f
Posture, 1071t, 2152
Potassium (K+), 1593t
abnormal, possible causes, 130t
in body fluid compartments, 520t
diabetic ketoacidosis and, 996
function, 525t
imbalances. See Hyperkalemia; Hypokalemia
in intracellular fluid, 518
regulation, 524–525, 525t
Potassium chloride, 10
Potassium-channel blockers, 1450t
Potential Complication (PC), 2073
Power, groups, 2138
Poverty:
nutritional status and, 663t
as risk factor, 499–500
violence and, 1964
PPAs. See Preferred provider arrangements
PPI (proton-pump inhibitor), 933
PPOs. See Preferred provider organizations

Prader-Willi syndrome (PWS), 1585
Pravastatin, 1374
Prayer, 1782–1783, 1786–1787, 1787t
Prazosin (Minipress), 434t, 1432
Precepting, 2270, 2271t
Preceptors, 2270, 2271t, 2272
Precipitating factors, 1937
Preconception counseling:
exercise, 1718
genetic counseling, 1738–1739
nutrition, 1718
overview, 1717
physical examination, 1718
preconception health measures, 1718
Preconceptual phase, 348t
Preconventional stage, 352t
Prediabetes, 1000
Predisposing factors, 1937
Prednisolone, 915t
Prednisone, 561, 915t, 926
Preeclampsia:
collaborative care
antepartal management, 1470–1471
intrapartal management, 1471
postpartal management, 1471–1472
definition, 1468
etiology, 1469
HELLP syndrome and, 1469
manifestations, 1469–1470
mild, 1469
pathophysiology, 1469
severe, 1469–1471
Preembryonic development, 1527–1530
amniotic fluid, 1528–1530
anatomy and physiology of reproductive system, 1541–1542
cellular differentiation, 1528
cellular multiplication, 1527
implantation, 1527–1528
yolk sac, 1530
Preferred provider arrangements (PPAs), 2212
Preferred provider organizations (PPOs), 2212, 2369
Prefrontal cortex, 940, 1161
Pregnancy:
abuse during, 1950
adolescent
factors contributing to, 1553–1554
family and social network reactions to, 1557
partners of adolescent mothers, 1556–1557
reaction to, 1555t, 1557t
risks to child, 1556
risks to mother, 1554–1556
anatomy and physiology of, 1541–1545
breasts, 1542
cardiovascular system, 1542–1543
central nervous system, 1544
endocrine system, 1545
eyes, 1544
gastrointestinal system, 1543
metabolism, 1544–1545
musculoskeletal system, 1544
respiratory system, 1542
skin and hair, 1543–1544
urinary tract, 1543
antepartum care, 1558

assessment
client history, 1559–1561
fetal development, 1569–1570
initial, 1562–1569t
pelvic adequacy, 1570
physical examination, 1561, 1569–1570
uterine, 1561, 1569
asthma and, 1258
back problems in, 1082t, 1083t
bowel elimination in, 424
Braxton Hicks contractions in, 1533, 1542
cardiovascular changes in, 1309–1310
caring interventions
pharmacologic therapies, 1577, 1577t
prenatal education, 1571–1573
relief of common discomforts, 1573, 1574–1575t, 1575–1577
cocaine use in, 71
constipation in, 454
cultural values and, 1553, 1572
developmental tasks of expectant couple, 1548–1549
diagnostic tests, 1570, 1571t
eclampsia in, 1468, 1470–1471
embryonic development, 1535, 1538–1539
first trimester, 57
fluid volume deficit in, 571
grandparents and, 1552–1553
health care during, 204
human immunodeficiency virus (HIV) and, 701, 710–711, 713–715
hypertension and, 1425
illness during, 342
intrapartum care, 1558
length of, 1535, 1538
medications during, classification of, 61, 63
nutrition during, 341, 663t
parental reactions to, 1548–1552, 1549t
periodontal disease during, 656
postpartum care, 1558
postural changes during, 1544f
preeclampsia in. See Preeclampsia
proper lifting in, 1082f
psychologic responses to, 1548–1553
psychotropic medication use during, 1174
risk factors, 1561
siblings and, 1552
signs of, 1545–1549
diagnostic (positive), 1548
objective (probable), 1546–1548, 1547t
subjective (presumptive), 1546, 1546t
smoking during, 52, 60
substance abuse, 57
substances commonly abused in, 58–60
systemic lupus erythematosus (SLE) and, 760
urinary elimination in, 412–413
urinary tract infections and, 874
weight gain during, 1544–1545
Pregnancy tests, 1548, 1570, 1942
Pregnancy-induced hypertension, 1315, 1425
Case Study, 1475
collaborative care
antepartal management, 1470–1471
intrapartal management, 1471
postpartal management, 1471–1472
etiology, 1469

manifestations, 1469–1470, 1470t
Nursing Care Plan
  assessment, 1474t
  critical thinking, 1474t
  diagnoses, 1474t
  evaluation, 1474t
  planning and implementation, 1474t
nursing diagnoses and interventions
  community-based nursing care, 1473
  hospital-based nursing care, 1473
  nursing management during labor and birth,
    1473, 1475
  nursing management during postpartal
    period, 1475
nursing process
  assessment, 1472
  diagnosis, 1472
  evaluation, 1475
  planning and implementation, 1472–1473, 1475
overview, 1468
pathophysiology, 1468–1469
risk factors, 1469
Pregnyl, 1735t
Preimplantation genetic diagnosis (PGD),
  1737–1738
Prejudice, 398
Preload, 1304, 1343t
Premarital sex, 1699
Premature atrial contractions (PAC), 1441t, 1444
Premature infants, 1558t, 1559
  birth of, 626
  cognitive disorders and, 204t
  risk for IICP in, 962
Premature junctional contractions, 1445
Premature ventricular contractions (PVC), 1442t,
  1445–1446
Premenstrual dysphoric disorder (PMDD), 1746
Premenstrual syndrome (PMS):
  alternative therapies, 1752
  collaborative care, 1749
  definition, 1746
  manifestations, 1749
  nursing diagnoses and interventions
    acute pain, 1752
    anxiety, 1754
    ineffective coping, 1753
    sexual dysfunction, 1754
  nursing process
    assessment, 1752
    diagnosis, 1752
    evaluation, 1754
    overview, 1752
    planning and implementation, 1752, 1754
  pathophysiology and etiology, 1748
  pharmacologic therapies, 1750
  physiology and etiology, 1748
  risk factors, 1749
Prenatal care, 57
Prenatal development:
  embryonic development, 1535, 1538–1539
  fetal development, 1539–1541
  placenta
    development of, 1530–1531
    functions, 1533–1534
    placental circulation, 1532–1533
  preembryonic development, 1527–1530
Prenatal education, 1571–1573

Prenatal influences, on development, 341
Prenatal screening, 1561
Prenatal substance exposure:
  alcohol, 59, 62t
  caffeine, 59
  Case Study, 65–66
  cocaine, 62t
  cocaine and crack, 59
  collaborative care, 63
  fetal effects
    barbiturates, 58t
    depressants, 58t
    narcotics, 58t
    T's and Blues, 58t
  heroin, 60
  incidence, 61
  manifestations, 62t
  marijuana, 59
  MDMA (ecstasy), 60
  methadone, 60
  narcotics, 62t
  nicotine, 62t
  Nursing Care Plan
    assessment, 64t
    complementary therapies, 63
    critical thinking, 64t
    diagnosis, 64t
    evaluation, 64t
    planning and implementation, 64t
  nursing process
    assessment, 63
    diagnosis, 65
    evaluation, 65
    planning and implementation, 65
  overview, 57
  pathophysiology and etiology, 58–61
  phencyclidine (PCP), 60
  risk factors, 61, 62t
  tobacco, 60
Prentiff Cavity Rim, 1729
Preoperative nursing care, 895
  client and family teaching, 896
  client preparation, 896
  fasting, 896
Preorgasmic women, 1702
Preparedness, 2351
Prenal acute renal failure, 534, 534t. See also
  Acute renal failure
Presbycusis, 1636t
Presbyopia, 1639t
Preschool children:
  assessment of, 2015
  communication with, 2155t
  grief and loss in, 610t
  growth and development, 359–361
  pain perception and behavior, 269t
  promotion of oral health in, 659
  recommended screenings and immunizations, 643t
  safety measures, 2456, 2455t, 2457f
  sleep patterns and requirements, 668
Preschool stage, 341t
Prescription drugs:
  addiction to, 73
  illicit use of, 68
  Medicare coverage of, 2211, 2368, 2368t
Presencing, 1789, 2032–2033

Presidential Advisory Commission on Consumer
  Protection and Quality in the Health Care
  Industry, 2422
Pressure trauma, 2353t
Pressure ulcers:
  Braden Scale for Predicting Pressure Sore
    Risk, 1920f
  case study, 1926t
  collaborative care, 1918
  definition, 1915
  imbalanced nutrition and, 1922
  manifestations, 1917
  Nursing Care Plan
    assessment, 1925t
    critical thinking and the nursing process, 1925t
    diagnosis, 1925t
    evaluation, 1925t
    expected outcomes, 1925t
    planning and implementation, 1925t
  nursing process, 1918–1926
  pathophysiology and etiology, 1915
  prevention of, 1923–1924, 1924t, 1931t,
    2092, 2444
  risk factors, 1916–1917
  risk for compromised human dignity/situational
    low self-esteem, 1923
  risk for impaired skin integrity/impaired skin
    integrity, 1921–1922
  risk for infection and, 1922
  staging of, 1917t
  treatment of, 1918t, 1922t, 1924, 1926, 1926t
Pressure-support ventilation (PSV), 1240t, 1241
Presynaptic neurons, 265f
Preterm labor:
  definition, 1559t
Pretibial myxedema, 1043
Preven, 1733
Prevention interventions, 2092
Priapism, 177–178, 1702t
Price controls, for health care services, 2214
Prick (epicutaneous or puncture) test, 736
Primary care, delivery of, 2341
Primary care providers (PCPs), 2369
Primary germ layers, 1528, 1528f
Primary groups, 2134
Primary hypertension, 1424
Primary immune response, 680, 680f
Primary intention healing, 1927
Primary nursing, 2207, 2344
Primary prevention, 2340, 2341t
Primary sources, 2054
Primigravida, 1559t
Primipara, 1559t
Primordial germ cells, 1525f
Principal investigators, nurses as, in research
  study, 2330
Principles-based theories, 1777
Prinzmetal's angina, 1362
Priority decisions, 2038
Priority setting, 2083–2085, 2084t
Pritikin diet, 1383t
Privacy, 2309, 2317, 2413
  invasion of, 2401
Privacy Rule, 2412
Private health insurance, 2368–2369
Private insurance, 2210–2212
Probing questions, 2159t

Problem list, of POMR, 2186, 2186f
Problem solving:
  approaches to, 2043–2045
    intuition, 2044
    research method, 2044, 2044t
    trial and error, 2043
  compared with critical thinking and decision making, 2041t
Problem statement, 2066
Problem status, drawing conclusions about, 2100, 2101f
Problem-focused assessment, 2000t
Problem-oriented medical records (POMRs), 2185–2187
Problem-oriented records (PORs), 2185–2187
Problem-solving process, 2038
Problems, 2039
  clarification of, 2040, 2041t
  determining, 2071
Procainamide, 757
Procalcitonin (CTpr), 804
Procan-SR. See Procainamide
Procedural memory, 240
Procedure-related accidents, 2445
Procedures, 2079
Process addictions, 28, 29t
Process standards, 2425
Processing, 2172, 2172t
Productivity, 2144
Proerythroblasts, 678f
Profession:
  criteria of, 2280–2281
  defined, 2280
Professional behaviors:
  about, 2225–2226
  associated with ethical nursing, 2307t
  Case Study, 2229–2230
  components of professionalism, 2226–2228, 2228f
    appearance, 2226–2227, 2227f
    compassion, 2228, 2228f
    competence, 2226
    integrity, 2227, 2227t
    knowledge, 2226
    positive attitude, 2228
    teamwork, 2227, 2227t
  unprofessional behaviors, 2228–2229, 2229t
  work ethic and, 2236–2238, 2239t, 2240–2242
Professional commitment, 2230–2232
  factors of, 2230–2231
  stages of development, 2231–2232
  stress management and, 2232
  types of, 2231
Professional development:
  historical perspectives, 2287–2290
  overview, 2287
Professional journals, 2324
Professional liability insurance, 2402
Professional misconduct, charges of, 2407
Professional negligence, 2399–2400, 2400t
  strategies to prevent, 2401–2402
Professional nursing associations, 2291
Professional nursing organizations, 2141
Professional organizations, 2281, 2300, 2366–2367, 2367t
Professional standards review organizations, 2210
Professional status, of nursing profession, 2325
Professional support, 509

Professional values, 2306
Professionalism, 2280
Professionalization, 2280
Progesterone, 1690
  during pregnancy, 1545
  female reproductive cycle and, 1519–1520
  for infertility, 1735t
  in pregnancy, 424
  produced by placenta, 1534
Progestin:
  contraceptives, 1732–1733
  side effects, 1731t
Programmed decisions, 2040
Progress notes, 2194
  of POMR, 2187, 2188f
Prohibition, 68
Prolactin, 978
Prometrium, 1735t
Prompted voiding, 450
Prone position, 2002t
Pronestyl. See Procainamide
Prophylaxis, in tuberculosis, 862
Propionibacterium acnes, 770
Propoxyphene, 276
Propranolol, 1815
Proprioception, 1502
Proprioceptive reflex, 267f
Proptosis, 1043
Proscar, 434, 434t
Prospective payment system (PPS), 2211
Prostaglandin analogs, 934, 1671t
  for glaucoma, 1670
Prostaglandin E, 1714
Prostaglandins (PGs), 887t, 1520, 1525, 1545, 1650t
Prostate:
  hyperplasia, 432
  hypertrophy, 415, 432. See also Benign prostatic hypertrophy
  palpation of, 435f
  surgery, 435
  transurethral resection of, 436f
Prostate cancer:
  Case Study, 175
  Client Teaching, 175
  collaborative care
    diagnostic tests, 170
    hormone therapy, 172t
    pharmacologic therapies, 172–173
    radiation therapy, 171t, 172
    surgery, 170–171, 172t
  manifestations, 170, 170t
  Nursing Care Plan
    assessment, 174t
    critical thinking, 174t
    diagnoses, 174t
    evaluation, 174t
    overview, 174t
    planning and implementation, 174t
  nursing diagnoses and interventions
    pain, 175
    sexual dysfunction, 174–175
    urinary incontinence, 173
  nursing process
    assessment, 173
    diagnosis, 173
    evaluation, 175
    overview, 173
    planning and implementation, 173–175

overview, 169
pathophysiology and etiology, 169
risk factors, 169
screening guidelines, 132t
staging, 171t
treatment, 171t, 172t
Prostate examinations, 876
Prostate gland, 1686t, 1687, 1705t
Prostate-specific antigen (PSA), 125, 127, 130t, 434, 436
Prostatectomy, 170–171, 171f, 435, 436f, 444
  Client Teaching, 440t
  discharge instructions following, 439t, 440
  postoperative care, 437–440
  preoperative care, 436–437
Prostatic hypertrophy, 418t
Prostatitis, 872
  definition, 432
Prostatodynia:
  definition, 432
Protease inhibitors, 713
  medication administration, 808
Protected health information (PHI), 2153, 2183, 2412
Protective factors, 350, 1937
Protective services, 1949, 1962
Protein, 1595
  as tumor markers, 127
  complete and incomplete sources, 927, 927t
Protein hormones, 981
Protein-calorie malnutrition, 662
Proteinuria, 540, 558, 1469
  systemic lupus erythematosus (SLE) and, 759–760
Protestant Christianity:
  medical care and, 1784
Proteus, 770
Protocols, defined, 2079
Proton-pump inhibitor (PPI), 933, 1149
Proventil. See Albuterol sulfate
Provider–client relationship, 2399
Proxemics, 2156–2157, 2156f
Proximodistal growth, 340, 340f
Prozac, 210, 1202
PRSP (Penicillin-resistant Steptococcus pneumoniae), 789
Pruritis, 1914t
Pruritus, 278t, 1876
PRV, 691
PSA. See Prostate-specific antigen (PSA)
Pseudoaddiction, 28
Pseudomonas aeruginosa, 834
Psychedelics, 73–74
Psychiatric rehabilitation, 244
Psychogenic pain, 264
Psychogeriatric Dependency Rating Scale, 207t
Psychologic dependence, 30t
Psychological battering, 1949
Psychological data, 2053t
Psychological factors:
  impacting assessment, 2007
  influencing health, 645
Psychomotor ability, learning and, 2251
Psychomotor domain, 2247
Psychomotor retardation, 1188
Psychoneurologic system:
  benefits of exercise for, 653t, 654
Psychosis, 232

Psychosocial development:
  in adolescence, 364, 366
  infancy, 356–357, 356t
  preschool years, 360–361, 361t
  school-age years, 362–363, 363t
  stages of, 1581t
  toddlerhood, 358, 359t
Psychosocial skills, 34
Psychosocial theories, 343–347
Psychostimulants, 71–73
Psychotherapy:
  for depression, 1190
  interpersonal, 1191
  for mood disorders, 1174
Psychotropics, effect on fetus, 58t
PTH. See Parathyroid hormone (PTH)
Ptosis, 1641f, 1641t
PTSD. See Post-traumatic stress disorder (PTSD)
Ptyalism, 1574t
Puberty, 364, 2012
Pubic arch, 1518
Pubis, 1516
Public distance, 2157
Public insurance, 2210–2211
Public laws. See Laws
Pubococcygeus, 1517t
Puborectalis, 1517t
Pubovaginalis, 1517t
PUD. See Peptic ulcer disease
Puerperium, 1196
Puerto Ricans, pain responses, 268t
Pulmonary angiogram, 1228
Pulmonary angiography, 1479
Pulmonary artery (PA) catheter, 1412–1413, 1413f
Pulmonary artery pressure monitoring, 1412–1413, 1413f
Pulmonary atresia, 1344t
Pulmonary blood flow:
  defects decreasing, 1339, 1342, 1350–1351
  defects increasing, 1339, 1350
  pulmonary embolism and, 1476–1477
Pulmonary circulation, 1298, 1300f
Pulmonary edema, 1404–1405, 1407
  complications, 1410
  manifestations, 1410t
Pulmonary embolism:
  Case Study, 1483
  Client Teaching, 1480t
  collaborative care
    diagnostic tests, 1479
    pharmacologic therapies, 1479–1480
    surgery, 1480
  definition, 1476
  etiology, 1477
  manifestations, 1478, 1478t
  Nursing Care Plan
    assessment, 1481t
    critical thinking, 1481t
    diagnoses, 1481t
    evaluation, 1481t
    planning and implementation, 1481t
  nursing diagnoses and interventions
    anxiety, 1482t
    decreased cardiac output, 1481–1482
    impaired gas exchange, 1480–1481
    ineffective protection, 1482

nursing process
    assessment, 1480
    diagnosis, 1480
    evaluation, 1482
    planning and implementation, 1480–1482
  physiology, 1476–1477
  risk factors, 1477
Pulmonary function tests (PFTs), 19, 164
  in chronic obstructive pulmonary disease (COPD), 1272
  purpose and description, 1227, 1228t
Pulmonary system:
  aging and, 1312
Pulmonary vascular resistance, 1300–1301
Pulmonic stenosis (PS), 1343t
Pulp cavity, 656
Pulse:
  apical, 1307, 1316t, 1320
  assessment, 1318–1320
  definition, 1307
  developmental considerations, 1321t
  factors affecting, 1307–1308
  peripheral, 1307
  sites, 1319–1320, 1319f, 1320t
  variations in, 1308t
Pulse deficit, 1316t, 1320
Pulse oximetry, 841
  purpose and description, 1227
  in specific conditions
    burns, 1900
    chronic obstructive pulmonary disease (COPD), 1272
Pulse pressure, 1308, 1422, 1484
Pulse rhythm, 1319
Pulse volume, 1319
Pulses Profile, 2024t
Punctuality, 2236–2237, 2237f
Punctures, 1880t
Punishment, 34–35, 492
Pupil, 1630–1631, 1636t
Pupillary assessment, 1640t
Pupillary light reflex, 1631
Pure (basic) research, 2329
Purging, 1584, 1600
Purging disorder, 1585
Purified protein derivative (PPD) of tuberculin, 861
Pursed-lip breathing, emphysema and, 1270
Purulent exudate, 887, 1930
Pus, 1930
Pustules, 1878t
PVC. See Premature ventricular contractions (PVC)
PVD. See Peripheral vascular disease (PVD)
Pyelography, 540
Pyelolithotomy, 470
Pyelonephritis:
  manifestations of, 875
  urinary tract infections and, 872
Pyogenic bacteria, 1930
Pyorrhea, 658
Pyrazinamide:
  nursing considerations and, 864t
  tuberculosis and, 863
Pyrexia, 1854. See also Hyperthermia
Pyridoxine, recommended daily intake, 1596t

Psychosocial development:
  in adolescence, 365, 365t
Pyuria, 874

Q

Quadriplegia, 386t, 1147
Quadrivalent, 689
Qualifiers, 2066
Qualitative research, 2328t
Quality:
  defined, 2421
  of sound, 2005
Quality and Safety Education Project for Nurses, 2444
Quality assurance, 2388–2389
Quality assurance systems, 2378t
Quality First: Better Health Care for all Americans (President's Advisory Commission), 2422
Quality improvement, 2422, 2444
  about, 2421–2422
  affect on costs, 2428
  Case Study, 2430
  continuous, 2427–2428
  creating blame-free environments, 2429–2430
  identification of key processes for, 2427, 2427t
  implementing, 2423
    breach of care, 2424, 2424t
    root cause analysis, 2424
    sentinel events, 2423–2424
  improving quality of care, 2428–2429
  measurement of, 2426–2428
  national initiatives, 2423
  need for, 2422–2423
  nurse staffing and, 2428
  nursing practice, 2430
Quality management, 2422
Quality management plans, 2425
Quality management programs, 2424–2426
Quantitative research, 2328t
Questioning, 2170
Questions:
  closed, 2056, 2057t
  leading, 2056
  neutral, 2056
  open-ended, 2056, 2057t
  Socratic, 2105, 2106t, 2108
Questran, 905
Quetiapine fumarate, 244t
Quickening, 1546, 1546t, 1569

R

RA. See Rheumatoid arthritis (RA)
RACE acronym, 2451
Race/ethnicity:
  biological variations due to, 327–328
  blindness and, 1658t
  blood pressure and, 1309, 1424
  definition, 323, 404
  end-of-life care and, 292–293
  family-centered care and, 511t
  glaucoma and, 1669t
  health care disparities and, 326–327
  human immunodeficiency virus (HIV) and, 699

hypertension and, 1426
methamphetamine use by, 70f
mood disorder considerations and, 1167
osteoporosis and, 1034
postpartum period and, 1199–1200
risk factors and, 499
U.S. population by, 324f, 325f
vision impairment and, 1649t
Radial pulse, 1319, 1319f
Radiation, 1852, 2454, 2458
Radiation burns, 1887, 1898
Radiation cataracts, 1657
Radiation exposure injury, 2353t
Radiation therapy:
in cancer, 131
intraoperative, 112
in specific conditions
breast cancer, 111–112
colorectal cancer, 144
leukemia, 154
lung cancer, 165
melanoma, 190
prostate cancer, 171t, 172
Radiological dispersion bomb (dirty bomb)
blast, 2353t
Radical mastectomy, 110
Radical prostatectomy, 170–171, 171t
Radioactive iodine therapy (RAI), 1044–1045
Radioallergosorbent test (RAST), 735
Radiographic studies:
in specific conditions
acute renal failure, 540
Radiologic examination, 805, 1076
Radionuclide imaging, 1372
Radon, 163
RAI (radioactive iodine therapy), 1044–1045
RAI (Resident Assessment Instrument), 2022
Ramadan, 1781–1782
Random access memory (RAM), 2374
Range of motion (ROM):
assessment, 1071–1072, 1071f, 1072–1073t
exercises, 753, 1077
of joints, 1065, 1071, 1072t
Rape:
acquaintance, 1970
Case Study, 1977
date, 1950, 1970–1971, 2462
definition, 1970
etiology, 1971
factors in
gender-bias factors, 1971
interpersonal factors, 1971
intrapersonal factors, 1970
sociocultural factors, 1971
male, 1970
marital, 1970
Nursing Care Plan
assessment, 1976t
critical thinking, 1976t
diagnosis, 1976t
evaluation, 1976t
planning and implementation, 1976t
physical injuries from, 1972, 1975
responses to, 1971–1973

risk factors, 1971
victim assessment, 1974t
Rape drugs, 1970
Rape-trauma syndrome:
collaborative care
diagnostic tests, 1973
group therapy, 1974
pharmacologic therapies, 1973
description, 1939t
manifestations, 1971–1973, 1972t
nursing diagnoses and interventions
encouraging calming techniques, 1977
identifying and prioritizing concerns,
1975–1976
provide community resources, 1977
supporting coping behaviors, 1976–1977
nursing process
assessment, 1974–1975
diagnosis, 1975
evaluation, 1977
planning and implementation, 1975–1977
overview, 1970
pathophysiology and etiology, 1970–1971
treatment/prevention, 1939t
Rapid cycling, 1160
Rapidly progressive glomerulonephritis
(RPGN), 924
Rapists, 1970–1971
Rapport, 2056, 2058
establishing with children, 2176t
RAPs (Resident Assessment Protocols), 2022
RAS (reticular activating system), 666, 944, 1629f
Rashkind-Balloon atrial septostomy, 1354t
Rational pharmacy, 274
Rationale, 2081
Rationing, 2349
Ray, Marilyn Anne, 2028–2029
Raynaud's phenomenon:
systemic lupus erythematosus (SLE) and, 760
RBCs. See Red blood cells (RBCs)
Read-only memory (ROM), 2374
Readiness for enhanced religiosity, 1785
Readiness to learn, 2249, 2256
Reading skills, 2258
Reality female condom, 1728, 1728f
Reasonable professional nurse standard, 2399
Reasoning:
deductive, 2106
inductive, 2106
Recent memory, 199
Receptive speech, 357
Receptor, 1628
Receiver, in communication process, 2149
Reciprocity, 1198
Recombinant follicle-stimulating hormone
(rFSH), 1735t
Recording, 2182
Records, 2182. See also Client records
Recovery, 32
Recovery phase, of emergency response,
2354–2355
Rectal temperature, 1855–1856
Recurrent stroke, 1502
Red blood cells (RBCs):
abnormal, possible causes, 130t

in anemia, 96–97, 99f, 100
transfusion, in sickle cell disorder, 179–180
Red clover, 1744t
Red reflex, 1642t
Reentry phenomenon, 1440
Referral, 2118
Referral summaries, 2194
Referred pain, 262
Reflecting, 2168–2169, 2168t, 2175
Reflection, 2108–2109, 2177t
Reflex incontinence, 446t
Reflex sympathetic dystrophy, 1097
Reflexes, 941, 941f
Reflux, 424, 872f
Refraction, 1631–1632
Refractoriness, 1438
Refractory hypoxemia, 1234
Refractory period, 1306
Regeneration, 1927
tissue, 887
Regional enteritis. See Crohn's disease
Registered nurses (RNs), 2206
Regulator cells, 681
Regulatory agencies, 2363–2365, 2364t
Regurgitation, 1369
Rehabilitation:
after joint replacement, 1130
in multiple sclerosis, 1120
in Parkinson's disease, 1139
Reimbursement, 2183
Reimbursement types, 2367–2369, 2368t
Reinforcement, 34–35
Relafen. See Nabumetone
Relapsing fever, 1859
Relationship-based theories, 1777
Relationships, communication and, 2157
Relaxation response, 1209
Relaxation therapy, 390t
Relaxation training, 1175
Relaxin, 1545
Relenza. See Zanamivir
Relevance, of communication, 2150
Relevance, of learning, 2249
Reliability, 2237
Religion, 325. See also specific religions
alterations, 1784–1785
Buddhism, 1784
Case Study, 1788
characteristics of, 1781
Confucianism, 1776t
definition, 1771
denominations, 1783
end-of-life care and, 293
grief and, 612
health-related information on specific
religions, 1784t
Hinduism, 1784
holy days, 1781–1782
Islam, 1783
Jehovah's Witnesses, 1784
Judaism, 1783
medical care and, 1783
monotheism, 1771
vs. morality, 1776

Nursing Care Plan
  assessment, 1786t
  critical thinking, 1786t
  diagnosis, 1786t
  evaluation, 1786t
  nursing diagnoses and interventions
    assisting clients with prayer, 1786–1787
    supporting religious practices, 1785, 1787t
  nursing process
    assessment, 1785
    diagnosis, 1785
    evaluation, 1787
    planning and implementation, 1785–1787
  nursing profession and, 2287–2288
  overview, 1781
  polytheism, 1771
  prayer and meditation, 1782–1783, 1786, 1787t
  Protestant Christianity, 1784
  Roman Catholicism, 1784
  sacred symbols, 1782
  sacred writings, 1782
  sexuality and, 1700
  similarities among, 1781
  spirituality and, 1771
Religious beliefs:
  health effects of, 645
  on birth, 1774
  on death, 1774
  on diet and nutrition, 1773
  on dress, 1774
  on healing, 1773
Religious delusions, 240
Religious rituals, grief and, 612f
REM (rapid-eye-movement) sleep, 666–667
Remeron, 1173
Remicade, 916
Reminyl, 217
Remission, 153, 638
Remittent fever, 1859
Renal and bladder ultrasound, 876
Renal arteries, 471f
Renal biopsy, 540
Renal failure, 415, 418t. See also Acute renal
    failure; Chronic renal failure
  characteristics, 534
  definition, 534
  in older adults, 554t
  systemic lupus erythematosus (SLE) and, 760
Renal function:
  age-related changes in, 415
  in specific conditions
    burns, 1900
Renal function studies, 1428
Renal insufficiency, 537
Renal osteodystrophy, 556
Renal replacement therapy, 543–546, 559–562.
    See also Dialysis
Renal rickets, 556
Renal system:
  acid–base balance and, 5
  aging and, 1312
  effects of shock on, 1487
Renal ultrasonography, 469, 540, 558
Renin, 980
Renin-angiotensin-aldosterone system, 523, 980,
    1423–1424
Repetitive motion disorders, 2383
Repetitive stress injuries (RSIs), 2383

Repetitive transcranial magnetic stimulation
    (rTMS), 1175
Replication studies, 2332
Repolarization, 1306
Reporting, 2200–2202, 2201t
Reports, 2182
  change-of-shift, 2200, 2200f, 2201t
  telephone, 2201
Reproduction, 1516. See also Conception;
    Pregnancy
  about, 1516–1557
  assessment, 1559–1561, 1562–1569t, 1569–1570
  caring interventions, 1570–1573, 1574–1575t,
    1575–1577
  conception and fetal development, 1523–1541
  diagnostic tests, 1570
  female reproductive system, 1516–1523
  pharmacologic therapies, 1577, 1577t
Repronex, 1735t
Res ipsa loquitur, 2400
Research:
  computers in, 2386–2387, 2387t
  data collection and analysis, 2387
  dissemination, 2387
  evidence-based, 2386, 2387t
  literature review, 2387
  nursing, 2280
  on Web, 2387–2388, 2388t
  problem identification, 2386
  study design, 2387
  utilization of, 2386
Research consumer, nurse as, 2294t
Research findings:
  evaluation of, 2331
  users of, 2331
Research guidelines, 2333–2334
Research journals, nursing, 2325t
Research problems, identification of, 2330
Research process, 2044, 2044t
Research questions, 2334
Research studies, 2327, 2329t
  pediatric, 2334, 2334t
Research team members, nurses as, in research
    study, 2330
Research utilization, 2331
Reservoirs:
  nursing interventions and, 774t
  portal of exit from, 772, 772t
    nursing interventions and, 774t
  role of, 771f, 772, 772t
Residency programs, 2272
Resident Assessment Instrument (RAI), 2022
Resident Assessment Protocols (RAPs), 2022
Resident Utilization Guidelines (RUGs), 2022
Residual urine, 413
Resilience, 350, 1208, 1609
Resiliency, 497
Resiliency theory, 350
Resistive behaviors, 2173
Resistive exercises, 1077
Resolution phase, 1699
Resonance, 2004, 2004t
Resource allocation:
  Case Study, 2351
  examples of, 2349–2350
  nurses and, 2350
  overview, 2349
Respect, 2119, 2158, 2174

Respiration:
  alterations in rate
    apnea, 1221
    bradypnea, 1221
    tachypnea, 1221
  definition, 1215
  difficulties in
    Biot's respirations, 1221
    Cheyne-Stokes respirations, 1221
    dyspnea, 1221
    Kussmaul's breathing, 1221
    orthopnea, 1221
  factors affecting
    alveolar surface tension, 1217
    oxygen and carbon dioxide levels, 1217
    ventilation-perfusion (V-Q) ratio, 1218
  hypoxemia, 1218–1219
  normal presentation
    breath sounds, 1216–1217
    hypercarbia, 1217
  sickle cell anemia and, 1219, 1221
  variations in, 1308t
Respiratory acidosis:
  acute, 18–19, 19t, 21t
  case study, 22
  causes, 6t, 7t, 18
  chronic, 18–19, 19t
  collaborative care, 19
  compensation, 8t
  definition, 5
  diagnostic tests, 19
  laboratory values, 6t, 7t
  manifestations, 19, 19t
  Nursing Care Plan
    assessment, 21t
    critical thinking in the nursing process, 21t
    diagnosis, 21t
    evaluation, 21t
    planning and implementation, 21t
  nursing process, 20
    anxiety, 20–21
    assessment, 20
    community care, 21–22
    diagnosis, 20
    evaluation, 22
    impaired gas exchange, 20
    implementation, 20–22
    ineffective airway clearance, 20
    plan, 20
    risk for injury, 21
  pathophysiology and etiology, 18
  pharmacologic therapies, 20
  respiratory support in, 20
  risk factors, 18
  therapies, 19t
  treatment, 6t
Respiratory alkalosis:
  case study, 25
  causes, 6t, 7t, 23
  collaborative care, 23
  definition, 5, 23
  development considerations, 24
  laboratory values, 6t, 7t
  manifestations, 23, 23t
  nursing process, 24
    assessment, 24
    diagnosis, 24
    evaluation, 25

implementation, 24–25
plan, 24
pathophysiology and etiology, 23
pharmacologic therapies, 23
respiratory therapies, 23–24
risk factors, 23
therapies, 23t
treatment, 6t
Respiratory depression, opioid use and, 277, 278t
Respiratory health:
directives for maintaining
air quality management, 1219
smoking cessation, 1219
vaccination, 1219
factors affecting
air quality, 1219
illnesses and disorders, 1219
lifestyle behaviors, 1219
medications, 1219
Respiratory inspiration, 1230f
Respiratory rate:
alterations
bradypnea, 1221
tachypnea, 1221
value ranges by age, 1217t
Respiratory syncytial virus (RSV)/Bronchiolitis:
Case Study, 1286
collaborative care
clinical therapies, 1283
diagnostic tests, 1282, 1283t
pharmacologic therapies, 1283
manifestations, 1282, 1282t
Nursing Care Plan
assessment, 1284t
critical thinking, 1284t
diagnoses, 1284t
evaluation, 1284t
planning and implementation, 1284t
nursing diagnoses and interventions
activity intolerance, 1285
fluid volume deficit, 1285
impaired gas exchange, 1285
impaired nutrition, 1285
ineffective airway clearance, 1284–1285
ineffective breathing pattern, 1285
nursing process
assessment, 1283
diagnosis, 1283
evaluation, 1285
planning and implementation, 1283–1284
overview, 1281
pathophysiology and etiology, 1281
risk factors, 1281–1282
treatment, 1220t
Respiratory system:
acid–base balance and, 4–5
alterations and treatments
acute respiratory distress syndrome (ARDS), 1220t
asthma, 1220t
causes, 1221
chronic obstructive pulmonary disease (COPD), 1220t
respiratory syncytial virus (RSV), 1220t
sudden infant death syndrome (SIDS), 1220t
anatomy of, 1217f
anatomy, physiology, and functions
lower respiratory system, 1217
bronchi and alveoli, 1216–1217

defense systems, 1216
lungs, 1216, 1224f, 1225f
pleura, 1216
trachea, 1216
upper respiratory system, 1216
defense systems, 1216
mouth, 1216
nose, 1216
assessment
assessment interview, 1224t
benefits of exercise for, 653, 653t
collaborative care
assisting with activities of daily living, 1234
laboratory and diagnostic testing, 1229
medication administration, 1229
monitoring activity tolerance, 1234
nutrition, 1234
oxygen administration, 1230–1231
pharmacologic therapies, 1229
secretion clearance, 1229
smoking cessation, 1230
thoracic catheter, 1231
diagnostic tests, 1226–1229
effects of shock on, 1487
factors affecting respiration and ventilation
alveolar surface tension, 1216
oxygen and carbon dioxide levels, 1217
ventilation-perfusion (V-Q) ratio, 1218
fetal development, 1537t
physical assessment
breath sounds, 1222–1223, 1222t
musculature, 1223t
nose, 1223t
overview, 1222–1223
skin, 1223t
thorax, 1223t
pregnancy and, 1542
treatments for, 947
Respiratory therapists, 2117t
Respiratory therapy, 965
Respondeat superior, 2400
Response, in communication process, 2149
Responsibility, 1778, 2126, 2144, 2279–2280
of nursing students, 2409
Rest pain, 1463
Restraints:
alternatives to, 2448t
chemical, 2446
injuries from, 2446
legal implications of, 2446
monitoring and intervention flow sheet, 2447f
physical, 2445
selection of, 2446
types of, 2448
use of, 2445–2446
Restrictive cardiomyopathy, 1333–1334, 1333t
Restrictive procedures, 1030
Restrictive/malabsorptive procedures, 1029–1030
Retarded ejaculation, 1702
Rete testis, 1687
Retention. See Urinary retention
Reticular activating system (RAS), 666, 944, 1629f
Reticular layer, 1875
Retina, 1631, 1636t, 1642t
Retinal detachment, 1662, 1664, 1666
Retractions:
in pediatric asthma, 1254
pneumonia and, 839, 839f
sites in pediatric asthma, 1255f

Retrograde conduction, 1445
Retrograde ejaculation, 1735
Retrograde pyelography, 540
Retropubic prostatectomy, 171, 439
Retrospective audit, 2426
Rett's disorder, 378
Revascularization procedures:
coronary artery bypass grafting, 1378–1379, 1379t, 1380–1382t
percutaneous coronary revascularization, 1376–1378, 1378t
for peripheral vascular disease, 1465
transmyocardial laser revascularization, 1382
Reverse delegation, 2222
Reverse triage, 2356
ReVia, 45
Revised Behavior Problem Checklist, 371t
Reward deficiency syndrome, 28
Reye's syndrome, 820–821, 1861
Rhabdomyolysis, 535
Rheumatoid arthritis (RA):
Case Study, 756
collaborative care
complementary therapies, 751
diagnostic tests, 748
overview, 747–748
pharmacologic therapies, 748–750
physical and occupational therapy, 751
rest and exercise, 751
surgery, 750–751
deformities of chronic advanced, 744f, 744t
description of, 693, 742
etiology of, 742–743
evidence-based practice, 754
manifestations, 743–747
extra-articular manifestations, 745
increased risk of coronary heart disease, 745, 747t
joint manifestations, 744–745
joints, 1069, 1069f, 1070f
juvenile rheumatoid arthritis, 745, 747
pericarditis, 747t
pleural effusion, 747t
uveitis, 747t
vasculitis, 747t
medications for, 748–750, 749t, 750t
multisystem effects of, 746
Nursing Care Plan
assessment, 755t
critical thinking, 755t
diagnosis, 755t
evaluation, 755t
expected outcomes, 755t
overview, 755t
planning and implementation, 755t
nursing diagnoses and interventions
chronic pain, 752–753
disturbed body image, 753–754
fatigue, 753
impaired mobility, 754
ineffective role performance, 753
psychosocial effects and, 751
nursing process
assessment, 752
diagnosis, 752
evaluation, 754
nursing care plan, 755
planning and implementation, 752–754

osteoarthritis and, 743t
pathophysiology of, 742
risk factors, 743
self-management of, 752t
therapies for, 748–749
Rheumatoid factor (RF), 1077t
Rheumatoid nodules, 745, 745f
Rhinorrhea, 819, 1282
Rhizotomy, 279
Rhonchi, 1222t
Ribavirin, 821, 1283
Riboflavin, recommended daily intake, 1596t
Ribonucleic acid (RNA), 86
Ribosomes, 86
Ribs, 1307
Richards, Linda, 2290
Rickettsia, 786t
Ridaura capsules. See Auranofin
Rifadin. See Rifampin
Rifampin:
    nursing considerations and, 864t
    tuberculosis and, 863
Right atrium, 1294
Right ventricle, 1294
Rimactane. See Rifampin
Rimantadine, 821
Ringer's solution, 576–577, 576t, 1899
Rinne test, 1643f, 1643t, 1646
Risk assessment, 2436, 2438t, 2450
Risk factors, 645, 1937
    defined, 2065
    resiliency theory and, 350
Risk for impaired religiosity, 1785
Risk for injury, 2437–2438
Risk management, 2429, 2429t
    implementing physician's orders and, 2416
    incident reports, 2417
    overview, 2415
    strategies for, 2415–2417
Risk management systems, 2378t
Risk nursing diagnosis, 2065
Risks, determining, 2071
Risperdal, 210, 244t, 1181
Risperidone, 243, 1181
Risperidone fumarate, 244t
Ritalin, 372, 373t
Ritonavir, 713
Rituals, challenging of, 2107
Rivastigmine (Exelon), 217
RNs. See Registered nurses
RNA (ribonucleic acid), 86
Roach, M. Simone, 2029
Robert Wood Johnson foundation, 2330
Rofecoxib, 275
Rohypnol, 1970
Role, 1582
Role ambiguity, 1583
Role conflicts, 1583, 2127
Role development, 1582
Role mastery, 1582
Role models, positive, 2235
Role performance, 1582–1583, 1590
Role strain, 1583
Role stressors, 1589t
Roles, communication and, 2157
Roman Catholicism:
    health-related beliefs, 1784t
    medical care and, 1784

Romberg test, 956t, 958t
Root, tooth, 656
Root cause analysis, 2424
Rooting, 958t
Rosenbaum chart, 1639t
Roseola (Exanthem Subitum, Sixth Disease):
    in children, 798t
Rosh Hashanah, 1782
Ross Carbohydrate Free formula, 972t
Ross Polycose, 972t
Rotator cuff tears, 1066, 1068
Rotavirus, in children, 798t
Rotavirus vaccine, 691
Roux-en-Y gastric bypass surgery, 1029–1030
Rowasa, 916
Roy's adaptation model, 2059, 2060t
RPGN (rapidly progressive glomerulonephritis), 924
RTI International–University of North Carolina at
    Chapel Hill, 2335
rTMS (repetitive transcranial magnetic
    stimulation), 1175
RU 486, 1734
Rubella (German Measles), 342
    in children, 798–799t
Rubella vaccine, 690
Rubeola, 793t, 794t
RUGs (Resident Utilization Guidelines), 2022
Rules, family, 496
Ruptured disk. See Herniated disk
Rural Health Clinics Act, 2210
Russell traction, 1106t

S

Sabbath, 1781
Sacred symbols, 1782, 1783f
Sacroiliac joints, 1516–1517
Sacrum, 1517
SAD. See Seasonal affective disorder (SAD)
SAFE KIDS coalitions, 2440
Safer sex, 2461, 2462t
Safety:
    about, 2433–2434
    anticipatory guidance and, 2439–2440, 2440t,
        2441t
    assessment, 2436, 2438t
    automobile, 2440f, 2440t
    Case Study, 2439
    environmental, 2442–2446, 2442t, 2446t,
        2448–2449, 2448t
    factors affecting
        ability to communicate, 2434
        age and development, 2434, 2434t
        cognitive awareness, 2434
        complementary and alternative medicine, 2435
        culture, 2435
        emotional state, 2434
        lifestyle, 2434
        mobility and health status, 2434
        sensory-perceptual alterations, 2434
    fall prevention, 2446t
    home, 2442, 2442t
    for hospitalized children, 2445t
    injury and illness prevention, 2450–2454, 2450t,
        2452–2453t, 2454t, 2455–2456t,
        2456–2459, 2456t
    National Patient Safety Goals, 2459, 2460t
    nursing practice, 2439

nursing process, 2436–2439, 2438t
promoting, across the lifespan, 2454,
    2455–2456t, 2456–2458, 2456t
promotion of client, 2444–2446, 2445t, 2446t,
    2448, 2448t
responsible sexual behavior, 2461–2462, 2462t
standard precautions, 2435, 2436t
workplace, 2442, 2443f
Safety and security needs, 2083t
Safety awareness, 2435
Safety strap restraints, 2448
Salflex. See Salsalate
Salicylic acid, 11
Saline, 520
Saliva, 655
Salmeterol, 1273
Salsalate, 748
SAMe (S-adenosylmethionine), 219, 1176
Same-sex couples, 487–488
Samples, 2329
Sanders, phases of bereavement, 603t
Sandimmune. See Cyclosporine
Sandwich Generation, 488
Sanger, Margaret, 2291
Sanguineous (hemorrhagic) exudate, 1930
Saquinavir, 713
Sarafem, 1202
Sarcopenia, 1063
Satiety, 1025, 1598
Scalds, 2450t
Scales, 1879t
Scanning speech, 215
Scapegoating, 2139
Scar tissue, 887
Scars, 1879t, 1929
    hypertrophic, 1892
    keloids, 1892
SCD. See Sudden cardiac death (SCD)
SCDDs (state councils on developmental
    disabilities), 205
Scheduled toileting, 445
Scheduling decisions, 2038
Schemas, 1175
Schistocytes, 1399
Schizoaffective disorder, 235
Schizoid personality disorder:
    characteristics, 1613
    diagnostic criteria, 1612t
    genetic factors in, 1608
    manifestations, 1611t
Schizophrenia:
    age-specific characteristics, 241–242
    alternative therapies, 245
    assertive community treatment, 245
    case study, 252
    catatonic type, 236t
    central nervous system abnormalities, 233t
    collaborative care, 242
    comorbid disorders, 236–237
    cultural factors, 234
    definition, 232
    disorganized type, 236t
    DSM-IV-TR diagnostic criteria, 236t
    electroconvulsive therapy, 245
    group therapy, 244
    homelessness and, 250
    impaired sensory filtering in, 233f
    incidence, 234, 235f

interventions
  family education, 247–248
  nicotine addiction, 247
  positive reinforcement, 247
manifestations, 235–241
  affect, 238
  catatonic, 237–238
  cognitive function, 239–241
  effects on interpersonal relationships, 241
  perceptions, 238–239
Nursing Care Plan, 249
  assessment, 249
  critical thinking in the nursing process, 249
  diagnosis, 249
  evaluation, 249
  implementation, 249
  planning, 249
nursing process
  assessment, 245–246
  diagnosis, 246
  evaluation, 248, 250
  implementation, 246–248
  plan, 246
overview, 232
paranoid type, 236t
pathophysiology and etiology, 232–234
pharmacologic therapies, 242–244
psychiatric rehabilitation, 244
residual type, 236t
risk factors, 234–235
safety issues, 250
symptoms, 232, 234–236, 237t
therapies, 237–238
undifferentiated type, 236t
Schizophreniform disorder, 235
Schizotypal personality disorder:
  characteristics, 1613
  diagnostic criteria, 1612t
  genetic factors in, 1608
  manifestations, 1611t
School age stage, 341t
School-age children:
  assessment of, 2015–2017
  communication with, 2155t
  grief and loss in, 610t
  growth and development, 362–364
  pain perception and behavior, 269t
  promotion of oral health in, 659
  recommended screenings and immunizations, 643t
  safety measures, 2455t, 2456
  sleep patterns and requirements, 668
Schools:
  violence in, 1965
SCI. See Spinal cord injury (SCI)
Sciatica:
  definition, 1081
Scientific advances, 2283
Scientific method, 2044, 2044t, 2327
Scientific research, 2327, 2328t, 2329, 2329t
Scleral buckling, 1664
Scleroderma, 693t
Sclerosing cholangitis, 912
Scoliosis:
  assessment, 1071t
  causes, 1087
  client teaching
    home care after spinal surgery, 1091t

collaborative care
  clinical therapy, 1087–1088
  diagnostic tests, 1087
  surgery, 1087f, 1088
definition, 1065t, 1066, 1087
diagnosis, 1080, 1087f, 1089f
evidence-based practice
  adolescent self-image and braces, 1088t
functional, 1071t
manifestations, 1068, 1083t, 1087
Nursing Care Plan
  assessment, 1090t
  critical thinking in the nursing process, 1091t
  diagnosis, 1090t
  evaluation, 1091t
  overview, 1090t
  planning and implementation, 1090t
nursing process
  assessment, 1088–1089
  diagnosis, 1089
  evaluation, 1091
  planning and implementation, 1089, 1091
pathophysiology and etiology, 1087
risk factors, 1087
treatment, 1065t
Scope and Standards of Practice (ANA), 1776
Screening, 2341
Screening Tool for Autism in Two-Year-Olds, 382t
Scriptures, 1782
Scrotum, 1686, 1686t, 1705t
SCT. See Stem cell transplant (SCT)
Seasonal affective disorder (SAD), 1162, 1189, 1189t
Seat belt use, 1988
Second heart sound (S2), 1296, 1297t
Second malignant neoplasm (SMN), 90
Second-degree AV block, 1443t, 1447
Secondary cancers, 90
Secondary care, delivery of, 2341
Secondary cataracts, 1657
Secondary groups, 2134
Secondary hypertension, 1424–1425
Secondary immune response, 680
Secondary infertility, 1718
Secondary intention healing, 1927
Secondary prevention, 2340–2341, 2341t
Secondary sex characteristics, 1519
Secondary sources, 2054
Secondary storage, 2375
Secondhand smoke, 51–52, 53t, 60, 1718
Security Rule of HIPAA, 2183
Sedation, opioid use and, 277, 278t
Sedation scale, 277t
Sedatives, for sleep disorders, 313–314, 314t
Sedentary lifestyle, osteoporosis and, 1035
Segmental mastectomy, 110
Segmental pressure measurements, 1464
Segmental resection, 165t
Seizure disorders. See also Epilepsy
  Case Study, 975
  collaborative care
    clinical therapies for children, 965f, 971–972
    diagnostic tests, 970
    pharmacologic therapy, 971, 971t
    surgery, 972
  complementary therapies, 972
  definition, 947t, 968

developmental considerations
  adolescents, 974t, 975
  adults, 974t, 975
  children, 974t
manifestations, 968
Nursing Care Plan
  assessment, 973t
  critical thinking in the nursing process, 973t
  diagnosis, 973t
  evaluation, 973t
  overview, 973t
  planning and implementation, 973t
nursing interventions, 974–975
nursing process
  assessment, 972–973, 972t
  diagnosis, 973–974
  planning and implementation, 974–975
pathophysiology and etiology, 968
risk factors, 968
treatment, 947t
  medications, 959, 959t, 960t
Seizures:
  clonic phase, 970
  cultural influences and, 973t
  definition, 948
  febrile, 968, 971, 1861
  focal, 968
  generalized, 968, 971
  intractable, 971
  postictal period, 970
  tonic phase, 968
Selective estrogen-receptor modulators (SERMs), 988t
Selective perception, 239
Selective serotonin, 307
Selective serotonin reuptake inhibitors (SSRIs):
  client teaching, 1172
  definition, 1171
  for depression, 1189t
  developmental considerations, 1174
  effects of, 1171
  for fatigue, 303t
  for fibromyalgia, 307
  nursing considerations, 1171
  for PMS, 1749
  in specific conditions
    anxiety disorders, 1815
    eating disorders, 1602
    personality disorders, 1592
    phobias, 1838
Selegiline (El-depryl), 217
Selenium, recommended daily intake, 1597t
Self, 645
  about, 1579–1592
  alterations, 1584, 1585t
    eating disorders. See Eating disorders
    personality disorders. See Personality disorders
  assessment, 1588–1590, 1588t
  caring interventions, 1590, 1591–1592t
  components of
    body image, 1582, 1582f, 1589
    personal identity, 1582, 1589
    role performance, 1582–1583, 1590
    self-esteem, 1583, 1590
  definition, 1579
  dimensions of, 1580

factors affecting
  family and culture, 1584, 1584f
  history of success and failure, 1584
  illness, 1584
  resources, 1584
  stage of development, 1583
  stressors, 1584, 1589, 1589t
formation of, 1580–1581, 1581t
normal presentation, 1580–1584
nursing interventions
  enhancing self-esteem, 1590, 1591–1592t
  identifying areas of strength, 1590
  pharmacologic therapies, 1592
Self-actualization, 2083t
Self-assessment, 2108
Self-awareness, 1580
Self-awareness/growth groups, 2141
Self-care, 2034–2035
Self-care deficit, urinary incontinence and, 443t
Self-care model, 2059, 2060t
Self-destructive behaviors, 1981
Self-determination, 2248, 2308
Self-disclosure, 2169, 2169t
Self-employment-based health insurance, 2369
Self-efficacy, 348, 348t
Self-esteem:
  assertiveness training to improve, 1583t
  assessment, 1590
  Assessment Interview, 1589t
  definition, 1583
  enhancement of, 1590, 1591–1592t
  global, 1583
  obesity and, 1031–1032
  specific, 1583
Self-esteem needs, 2083t
Self-esteem Questionnaire, 2035t
Self-esteem stressors, 1589t
Self-help groups, 2141, 2141t
Self-mutilation, 1620f
Self-neglect, 1945, 1961–1962t
Self-perceptions, 645
Self-protective groups, 2135
Self-talk, 2148, 2148f
Semen, 1525, 1687
Semicomatose, 946t
Semiformal groups, 2135, 2135t
Seminal vesicles, 1686t, 1687
Sender, in communication process, 2149
Senile purpura, 1875
Sensation, diminished and pressure ulcers, 1916
Senses, 207. See also specific senses
Sensitization, 271
Sensorimotor phase, 348t
Sensory acuity, 2251
Sensory aids, 1647, 1648t
Sensory deficits, 2160
Sensory deprivation, 1647
Sensory function, assessment, 954–955t
Sensory impairment, 1649
Sensory memory, 199
Sensory nerve damage, 1680t
Sensory neurons, 265
Sensory neuropathies, 1680
Sensory overload, 239, 1647
Sensory perception:
  about, 1627–1650
  age-related changes in, 1635, 1636t, 1637
  alterations, 1637–1638

assessment
  client environment, 1639
  mental status and cognition, 1638
  nursing history, 1638
  physical, 1642–1643
  social support network, 1639, 1642
  taste and smell, 1643, 1645
Assessment Interview, 1638t
caring interventions, 1646–1649
definition, 1628
developmental considerations, 1646t
diagnostic tests, 1645
factors affecting
  congenital and hereditary conditions, 1634
  culture, 1634
  isolation, 1634
  lifestyle and personality, 1635
  medication and illness, 1634
  stress, 1634
hearing. See Hearing
hyperthyroidism and, 1045–1047
injuries, 1637, 1637t
normal presentation
  ears, 1632–1633
  eyes, 1629–1631
pharmacologic therapies, 1649, 1650t
smell, 1634–1635
taste, 1633, 1635
therapeutic interventions
  adjusting environmental stimuli, 1647
  communicating effectively, 1648, 1648t
  managing acute sensory deficits, 1647
  overview, 1646
  preventing sensory deprivation, 1647
  preventing sensory overload, 1647
  promoting health sensory function, 1647
  promoting use of other senses, 1647
  safety considerations, 1648
  sensory aids, 1647, 1648t
touch, 1634
vision. See Vision
Sensory-perceptual alterations, 2434
Sentinel events, 2366, 2423–2424, 2446
Sentinel node biopsy, 110
Separation anxiety disorder, 1812–1813
Sepsis:
  Case Study, 855
  collaborative care
    diagnostic tests, 852
    fluid replacement, 853
    oxygen therapy, 853
    pharmacologic therapies, 852–853
  definition, 771, 850
  etiology of, 850–851
  manifestations, 851–852, 852t
  nursing process
    assessment, 853
    diagnosis, 853
    evaluation, 855
    older adults and, 853
    planning and implementation, 854–855
  pathophysiology, 850
  portals of entry for, 850–851
  risk factors, 851
  severe, 850
  treatments for, 801
Septal defect, 1339

Septic shock, 89, 1489, 1492t, 1497t
  definition, 850
  development of, 851f
  infectious diseases and, 787
  Nursing Care Plan
    assessment, 854t
    critical thinking, 854t
    diagnoses, 854t
    evaluation, 854t
    interventions, 854t
    planning and implementation, 854t
  refractor, 850
Septicemia, 1489
  cellulitis and, 809–810
  definition of, 771
  infectious diseases and, 787
  pneumonia and, 840
  septic shock and, 850
  urinary tract infections and, 787
Serax, 1815
Seroconversion, 697
Serologic testing, 805, 841, 933
Serophene, 1735t
Seroquel, 244t
Serosanguineous exudate, 1930
Serotonin, 1171
  aggression and, 1963
  eating disorders and, 1598
  personality disorders and, 1608
Serous exudate, 887, 1930
Seroxat, 1201
Sertraline, 210, 1201
Serum bilirubin, 903, 904t
Serum bicarbonate, 5
Serum cardiac enzymes, 1490
Serum cholesterol, 1028, 1365t, 1370
Serum complement levels, systemic lupus erythematosus (SLE) and, 760
Serum creatine, 926, 1411
Serum creatinine:
  renal function and, 540, 553f
  in specific conditions
    chronic renal failure, 558
    sepsis and, 852
    systemic lupus erythematosus (SLE) and, 760
Serum digoxin level, 1353t
Serum electrolytes, 19, 532f, 1411, 1490
  electrolyte imbalances and, 531
  renal function and, 540
  sepsis and, 852
  in specific conditions
    burns, 1900
    chronic renal failure, 558
    fluid volume deficit, 575
    nephritis, 926
Serum enzymes, sepsis and, 852
Serum glucose, 1028
Serum lipid panel, 1353t
Serum osmolality, 130t, 532
Serum potassium, 1428
Serum protein analysis, 1884
Serum sickness, 729, 734, 1272
Service orientation, 2280
Seven Habits of Highly Effective People (Covey), 2235, 2235t
Seventh-Day Adventists, 1784t
Sex Addicts Anonymous, 37

Sex chromosomes, 87–88, 340
Sex hormones:
  female, 1690
  male, 1687, 1712
Sex offenders, 1970–1971
Sexual abuse:
  child, 1947–1949
  eating disorders and, 1598
  manifestations, 1955t, 1956t
  personality disorders and, 1609
Sexual activity:
  anal stimulation, 1697
  genital intercourse, 1697
  guidelines for safe practices, 718
  oral-genital sex, 1697
  responsible, 2461–2462, 2462t
Sexual assault, 1936. See also Rape-trauma
    syndrome
Sexual assault nurse examiner (SANE), 1975t
Sexual aversion disorder, 1702
Sexual dysfunction:
  caring interventions, 1710
  diabetes mellitus and, 1012, 1694
  dissatisfaction problems, 1703
  erectile dysfunction. See Erectile dysfunction
  factors influencing
    cognitive factors, 1701
    health factors, 1701
    medications, 1701, 1701t
    psychological factors, 1700
    relationship factors, 1701
    sociocultural factors, 1700
  menstrual dysfunction, 1702t
  orgasmic disorders, 1702t
    female, 1702
    male, 1702
  pharmacologic therapies, 1710, 1711t
  prostate cancer and, 174–175
  risk factors, 1703
  sexual arousal disorders, 1702t
    female, 1702
    male erectile disorder, 1702
  sexual desire disorders
    hypoactive sexual desire disorder, 1702
    sexual aversion disorder, 1702
  sexual pain disorders
    causes, 1703
    priapism, 1702t
    vaginismus, 1703
    vestibulitis, 1703
    vulvodynia, 1703
  in women
    dyspareunia, 1694
Sexual harassment, 2228–2229
Sexual health:
  characteristics of, 1695t
  components of
    body image, 1695
    gender identity, 1696
    gender-role behavior, 1696
    sexual self-concept, 1695
  cultural influences on, 1700t
  definition, 1695
Sexual orientation, 400–401, 1696
Sexual pain disorders, 1702t, 1703
Sexual response cycle:
  desire phase, 1697

excitement phase, 1697
orgasmic phase, 1697
physiological changes, 1697, 1698t
resolution phase, 1699
Sexual self-concept, 1695
Sexuality:
  about, 1685–1712
  in adolescence, 365–366
  age-related changes, 1712
  alterations, 1700–1703
  assessment, 1703
    female reproductive system, 1705–1708t
    male reproductive system, 1704–1705t
  Assessment Interview
    men, 1709t
    women, 1709
  caring interventions, 1710
  development and, 1691
    adolescence, 1692t, 1693
    childhood, 1692t, 1693
    older adults, 1693t, 1694–1695
    young and middle adulthood, 1692t, 1694
  diagnostic tests, 1710
  factors influencing
    culture, 1699–1700
    family, 1699
    personal expectations and ethics, 1700
    religion, 1700
  female anatomy and physiology, 1687–1691, 1688t
  inappropriate sexual behavior, 1710, 1710t
  long-term care and, 1695
  pharmacologic therapies, 1710, 1711t
  reproductive anatomy and physiology
    male, 1686–1687
  in school-age children, 363–364
  varieties of
    erotic preferences, 1697
    gender identity, 1696–1697
    sexual orientation, 1696
Sexually transmitted infections (STIs), 2461
  in adolescents, 1693, 1755
  Case Study, 1766
  characteristics, 1756
  chlamydias. See Chlamydias
  complications, 1756
  definition, 1755
  facts about, 1755t
  genital herpes. See Genital herpes
  genital warts. See Genital warts
  gonorrhea. See Gonorrhea
  HIV/AIDS and, 1756
  incidence and prevalence, 1755–1756, 1755t
  manifestations, 1702t
  Nursing Care Plan
    assessment, 1763t
    critical thinking in the nursing process, 1763t
    diagnosis, 1763t
    evaluation, 1763t
    overview, 1763t
    planning and implementation, 1763t
  nursing diagnoses and interventions
    acute pain, 1765
    deficient knowledge, 1765
    sexual dysfunction, 1765
  nursing process
    assessment, 1762
    diagnosis, 1764

evaluation, 1765
overview, 1762
planning and implementation, 1764–1765
overview, 1755
prevention and control, 1756
resources for clients with, 1757t
syphilis. See Syphilis
Shaken baby syndrome, 1951
Shared Electronic Health Record (SEHR), 2378
Shared governance, 2206, 2235
Shared leadership, 2235
Shared psychotic disorder, 235
Sharp debridement, 1924
Shearing forces, 1916
Shigella, 770
Shock:
  anaphylactic, 1489–1490, 1492t
  cardiogenic, 1488–1489, 1491t
  Case Study, 1498–1499
  clinical therapies, 1491–1492t
  collaborative care
    diagnostic tests, 1490
    fluid replacement therapy, 1494–1495
    oxygen therapy, 1493
    pharmacologic therapies, 1490
  definition, 1483
  description, 1314t
  distributive, 1489, 1492t
  effects of, on body systems
    cardiovascular system, 1485
    gastrointestinal system, 1487
    neurologic system, 1487
    renal system, 1487
    respiratory system, 1487
    skin, temperature, thirst, 1487
  etiology, 1487–1490
  hypovolemic, 1488, 1491, 1894–1895
  manifestations, 1490, 1491–1492t
  medical treatment for, 1943
  Multisystem Effects, 1486t
  neurogenic, 1489, 1492t
  Nursing Care Plan
    assessment, 1497t
    critical thinking, 1498t
    diagnoses, 1497t
    evaluation, 1497t
    planning and implementation, 1497
  nursing diagnoses and interventions
    anxiety, 1496, 1498
    decreased cardiac output, 1495–1496
    ineffective tissue perfusion, 1496
  nursing process
    assessment, 1495
    diagnosis, 1495
    evaluation, 1498
    planning and implementation, 1495–1496, 1498
  obstructive, 1489, 1492t
  overview, 1483–1484
  pathophysiology, 1484
  risk factors, 1490
  septic, 1489, 1492t, 1497t
  stages
    early, reversible, and compensatory,
      1484–1485
    intermediate or progressive, 1485
    refractory of irreversible, 1485
  treatment, 1314t

Shock-wave lithotripsy, 475*f*, 905
Short Portable Mental Status Questionnaire
  (SPMSQ), 207*t*
Short staffing, 2316, 2317*t*
Short-term goals, 2087
Short-term memory, 199
Shoulder replacement, 1130
Shunt, 1349
Sibling relationships, 490
Sibutramine, 1585
Sick sinus syndrome (SSS), 1444
Sickle cell anemia, 102*t*. *See also* Sickle
  cell disorder
  and respiration, 1219, 1221
  definition, 176
  description, 176*t*
  Nursing Care Plan
    assessment, 182*t*
    critical thinking, 182*t*
    diagnoses, 182*t*
    evaluation, 182*t*
    planning and implementation, 182*t*
  pain and, 180*t*
Sickle cell crisis:
  definition, 177
  precipitating factors, 178
  types, 178*t*
Sickle cell disorder:
  Case Study, 183
  children with, 180*t*, 181*t*
  Client Teaching, 181
  collaborative care
    diagnostic tests, 179
    hydration, 179
    other therapies, 180
    oxygenation, 179
    pain control, 179
    prevention and treatment of infection, 179
    red blood cell transfusion, 179–180
    complications, 176–177
  definition, 176
  manifestations, 178–179
  nursing diagnoses and interventions
    acute pain, 181
    caregiver role strain, 183
    delayed growth and development, 181, 183
    risk for impaired tissue perfusion, 181
    risk for infection, 181
  nursing process
    assessment, 180
    diagnosis, 180–181
    evaluation, 183
    planning and implementation, 181, 183
  pathophysiology and etiology, 176–177
  risk factors, 177
  stroke and, 1502
  types
    combination, 176*t*
    sickle cell anemia, 176*t*
    sickle cell syndrome, 176*t*
    sickle cell trait, 176*t*
Sickle cell syndrome, 176*t*
Sickle cell trait, 176*t*, 177
Sickling, 176, 178
Sickness funds, 2213
Side rails, 2444

SIDS. *See* Sudden infant death syndrome
Sigma Theta Tau International Honor Society of
  Nursing, 2324, 2329, 2335, 2367
Sigmoid colostomy, 143–144
Sign language, 1655*t*
Signs, 2054
Simple appendicitis, 893
Simple face masks:
  description, 1232–1233
  pictured, 1232*f*
Simple fractures, 1093
Simple mastectomy, 110
Simple Triage and Rapid Transport (START)
  System, 2356*t*
Simplicity, of speech, 2150
Sims position, 2002*t*
Simvastatin, 1374
Single adults, 488
Single parents, 486, 1163
Single-causation theory, of disease, 638
Sinoatrial (SA) node, 1305
Sinus arrhythmia, 1316, 1440, 1441*t*
Sinus bradycardia, 1440, 1441*t*
Sinus node dysrhythmias, 1440
Sinus rhythms, 1440
Sinus tachycardia, 1440, 1441*t*
Site-specific disaster zones, 2356, 2356*t*
Sitting position, 2002*t*
Situational crises, 33
Situational depression:
  Case Study, 1211
  clinical therapies, 1209*t*
  collaborative care
    exercise, 1209–1210
    pharmacologic therapies, 1209
  definition, 1159, 1160*t*
  manifestations, 1208, 1209*t*
  Nursing Care Plan
    assessment, 1210*t*
    diagnosis, 1210*t*
    evaluation, 1210*t*
    planning and implementation, 1210*t*
  nursing diagnoses and interventions
    depression, 1210
    disrupted family processes, 1211
    helplessness, 1211
  nursing process
    assessment, 1210
    diagnosis, 1211
    planning and implementation, 1211
  overview, 1208
  resilience factors, 1208
  risk factors, 1208
  treatments, 1160*t*
Situational leaders, 2234
Situational losses, 600
Six Sigma, 2428
Sixth Disease, 798*t*
Sjögren's syndrome, 693*t*
Skeletal frame, 328
Skeletal pins, 1108*t*
Skeletal traction, 1100, 1100*f*, 1106*t*
Skeleton. *See also* Musculoskeletal system
  appendicular, 1056
  axial, 1056
  bones. *See* Bone(s)

pediatric differences in, 1062
Skene's glands, 1687, 1688*t*, 1707*t*
Skin:
  age-related changes, 1875, 1876*t*, 1877*t*
  diagnostic tests, 1884
  dry, 1914*t*
  edema, 1880
  fetal development, 1537*t*
  functions of, 1874
  integumentary assessment, 1882*t*, 1882–1884*t*
  layers, 1874*f*
    dermis, 1875
    epidermis, 1874–1875
    subcutaneous tissue, 1875
  pregnancy and, 1543–1544, 1548
  sensory receptors in, 1853
  wounds. *See* Wounds, 1878
Skin assessment record, 2194
Skin biopsy, 1884
Skin cancer, 1878*t*
  ABCD rule, 189*t*
  Case Study, 194
  collaborative care
    melanoma, 188–190
    nonmelanoma, 188
  manifestations, 188, 189*t*
  nursing diagnoses and interventions
    anxiety, 192, 194
    hopelessness, 192
    impaired skin integrity, 191–192
  nursing process
    assessment, 191, 191*t*
    diagnosis, 191
    evaluation, 194
    planning and implementation, 191–194
  overview, 184
  pathophysiology and etiology, 184–187
  risk factors, 187–188, 187*t*
  types
    basal cell, 185–186, 186*f*, 186*t*
    melanoma. *See* Melanomas
    nonmelanoma, 185–187
    squamous cell, 186–187, 187*f*
Skin color, 328
Skin disorders:
  classification of, 1876, 1878*t*
  medications for, 1913*t*
  signs and symptoms, 1876
Skin grafts, 1901*f*, 1902*f*
Skin integrity:
  cirrhosis and, 1022
  diabetes mellitus and, 1010–1011
  hypothyroidism and, 1051
Skin integrity. *See* Tissue integrity
Skin lesions, 1876, 1878, 1878*t*, 1879*t*, 1885*t*
Skin pigmentation, skin cancer and, 188
Skin Prep Granulex, 1918*t*
Skin tests, in hypersensitivity reactions, 736, 736*f*
Skin traction, 1099–1100, 1106*t*
Skinner, B.F., 347
SLE. *See* Systemic lupus erythematosus (SLE)
Sleep:
  circadian rhythms, 666
  factors affecting, 669
  functions of, 667
  NREM, 666–667

overview, 665
physiology of, 666–667
REM, 667
requirements, 258
    adolescents, 668
    adults, 668
    infants, 668
    newborns, 667
    older adults, 669
    preschoolers, 668
    school-age children, 668
    toddlers, 668
smoking and, 52
types of, 666–667
Sleep apnea:
    characteristics, 258, 310
    clinical therapies, 314–315
    community-based care, 318
    manifestations, 313t
    risk factors, 311
    stroke and, 1501
    treatments, 310
    types
        central, 310
        mixed, 310
        obstructive, 310
Sleep architecture, 666
Sleep cycles, 667
Sleep deprivation, 665, 667t
    consequences of, 258, 310
    manifestations, 313t
Sleep disorders, 665
    about, 258
    Assessment Interview, 316t
    Case Study, 318
    collaborative care
        complementary and alternative medicine, 315
        diagnostic studies, 313
        overview, 312
        pharmacologic therapies, 313–314, 314t
    depression and, 1188
    description, 259t
    hypersomnia, 258, 309
    incidence, 258, 311
    insomnia. See Insomnia
    insufficient sleep, 310
    manifestations, 312, 313t
    mood disorders and, 1170
    narcolepsy, 258, 310, 313t
    Nursing Care Plan
        assessment, 317t
        critical thinking, 317t
        diagnosis, 317t
        evaluation, 317t
        planning and implementation, 317t
    nursing diagnoses and interventions, 317
    nursing process
        assessment, 315
        diagnosis, 315
        evaluation, 318
        planning and implementation, 316–318
    older adults and, 311–312, 318
    overview, 309
    parasomnias, 258, 310
    risk factors, 311
    sleep apnea. See Sleep apnea

treatment, 259t
Sleep hygiene, 260
Sleep in America poll, 669
Sleep patterns:
    adolescents, 668
    adults, 668
    infants, 668
    newborns, 667
    older adults, 669
    preschoolers, 668
    regular, 667
    school-age children, 668
    toddlers, 668
Sleep quality, 669
Sleep-wake cycle, mood disorders and, 1162
Sleeptalking, 311t
Sleeve resection, 165t
Small-cell carcinomas, 161, 161t
Smallpox, 2357t
Smart phones, 2378
Smell, 1634–1635, 1643, 1645, 1645t, 1649
Smoke poisoning, 1895
Smoking:
    by adolescents, 56t
    and respiratory health, 1219
    cancer risk and, 52, 53t, 121
    Case Study, 57
    cessation
        complementary therapies, 53
        difficulty of, 52
        evidence-based practice, 56t
        interventions for, 1231t
        nicotine replacement therapy, 53
        in pregnancy, 62t
        programs, 53
        withdrawal symptoms, 52
    chemicals found in tobacco and, 52t
    chronic bronchitis and, 1268
    chronic obstructive pulmonary disease (COPD)
        and, 1269, 1274
    collaborative care, 53
    coronary artery disease and, 1365–1366, 1372
    cultural views of, 51t
    deaths from, 51–52
    during pregnancy, 52
    effect on fetus, 58t
    heart disease and, 52
    Hispanics and, 1272t
    hypertension and, 1429
    lung cancer and, 163
    manifestations, 52, 53t
    Nursing Care Plan, 55t
        assessment, 55t
        critical thinking in the nursing process, 55t
        diagnosis, 55t
        evaluation, 55t
        planning and implementation, 55t
    nursing process
        assessment, 54, 54t
        diagnosis, 54
        evaluation, 56
        overview, 54
        planning and implementation, 54–55
    overview, 51
    pathophysiology and etiology, 51–52

preconception planning and, 1718
pregnancy and, 1573
in pregnancy, 60
risk factors, 52
sleep and, 669
sleep disturbances and, 52
stroke and, 1501
Snellen chart, 1639t
Snowstorm-related injuries, 2352t
SOAP format, 2187, 2188f
SOAPIE format, 2187
SOAPIER format, 2187, 2188f
Social anxiety disorders. See Social phobias
Social behaviors, 326
Social cognitive theory, 2248
Social data, 2053t
Social distance, 2156
Social justice, 2307
Social learning theory, 347–348, 1950–1951,
    2247–2248
Social microcosm, 35
Social phobias, 1837
Social support groups, 2141
Social support systems:
    assessment of, in older adults, 2022
    cultural aspects of, 646t
    facilitation of, 648
    review of, 646
Social workers, 2117t
Socialization, 2226
    defined, 2281
    to nursing, 2281–2282
Socialized insurance, 2213
Socialized medicine, 2213
Societal attitudes, toward nursing, 2289–2290
Sociocultural factors:
    mood disorders and, 1163
    personality disorders and, 1609
Sociocultural characteristics, communication
    and, 2156
Socioeconomic influences:
    on nutritional health, 663t
Sociologic factors, 499–500
Socratic questioning, 2105, 2106t, 2108
Sodium (Na$^+$), 518, 1593t
    abnormal, possible causes, 130t
    in body fluid compartments, 520t
    in diet, 584t, 586t
    foods high in, 583t
    function, 525t
    hypertension and, 1426
    imbalances. See Hypernatremia
    imbalances. See Hyponatremia
    regulation, 524, 525t
    retention, 582–583
    urine excretion, 532
Sodium bicarbonate:
    in specific conditions
        acidosis, 8–9, 9t, 10t
        acute renal failure, 542t
        chronic renal failure, 558
        metabolic acidosis, 12
Sodium chloride, 10, 518
Sodium nitroprusside, 1415
Sodium oxybate, 309

Sodium polystyrene sulfonate, 542, 542*t*, 559
Sodium-channel blockers, 1449, 1450*t*
Soft palate, 655
Software, 2374
Solganal. *See* Aurothioglucose
Solitary play, 356
Solutes, 518, 520
Solvents, 519–520
Somatic cells, 88, 1720
Somatic delusions, 240
Somatic neuropathies, 998–999, 1679
Somatic pain, 263
Somatization, 1167
Somatosensory evoked potential (SSEP), 1077
Somatostatin, 989
Somatotropic cells, 978
Somatotropin, 978
Somnambulism, 311*t*
Somnology, 665
Somogyi phenomenon, 995
Sordes, 658*t*
Sound conduction, 1633
Source-oriented records, 2184–2185, 2185*t*
Southern California Evidence-Based Practice
    Center–RAND Corporation, 2335
Spastic hemiparesis, 956*t*
Spasticity, 1505
Special gradient acoustic reflectometry, 828
Special Interest Professional Organizations, 2367*t*
Specialized education, 2280
Specialty practice organizations, 2367
Specific gravity, 532
Specific phobias:
    manifestation, 1838
    table of specific phobias, 1838*t*
Specific reactivity, 680
Specific response. *See* Immune response
Specific self-esteem, 1583
Specific theory, of pain, 265
Speech audiometry, 1646
Speech therapy, for stroke, 1507
Speizer, Frank, 2332
Sperm, 1525, 1526*f*
Spermatogenesis, 1524, 1687
Spermicides, 1727
Sphincter muscles, 411, 412*f*
Sphygmomanometer, 1030, 1321, 1321*f*
SPICES, 2024*t*
Spinal cord, 941
Spinal cord injury (SCI):
    assessment findings in acute, 1149*t*
    Case Study, 1155
    causes, 1145, 1146*f*
    classification, 1144
    collaborative care
        diagnostic tests, 1148
        emergency care, 1148
        pharmacologic therapies, 1149
    community-based care, 1153*t*
    complete, 1144, 1146
    complications
        autonomic dysreflexia, 1147
        by body system, 1148*t*
        paraplegia and quadriplegia, 1147

upper and lower motor neuron deficits, 1147
    forces resulting in, 1144
    incomplete, 1144, 1145*t*, 1146
    manifestations, 1146–1147, 1148*t*
    Medication Administration, 1149*t*
    Nursing Care Plan
        assessment, 1154*t*
        critical thinking in the nursing process, 1154*t*
        diagnoses, 1154*t*
        evaluation, 1154*t*
        planning and implementation, 1154*t*
    nursing diagnoses and interventions
        alteration in perfusion, 1152
        impaired gas exchange, 1151
        impaired physical mobility, 1151
        impaired urinary elimination and
            constipation, 1152
        ineffective breathing patterns, 1152
        low self-esteem, 1153
        sexual dysfunction, 1153
    nursing process
        assessment, 1151
        diagnosis, 1151
        evaluation, 1155*t*
        overview, 1151
        planning and implementation, 1151–1153, 1155
    overview, 1143
    pathophysiology and etiology, 1143–1145
    risk factors, 1066, 1145
    sites of pathology, 1144
    treatment
        stabilization and immobilization, 1150
        surgery, 1150
Spinal cord stimulation (SCS), 279
Spinal fusion, 1083, 1088
Spinal nerves, 943, 943*f*
Spinal shock, 1146, 1149*t*
Spine abnormalities:
    assessment, 1071*t*
    curvature, 1062
    kyphosis, 1066, 1071*t*
    lordosis, 1066, 1071*t*
    scoliosis. *See* Scoliosis
Spiral fractures, 1094, 1095*t*
Spirit titer, 1770*f*
Spiritual beliefs:
    grief and, 604, 605*t*
    health effects of, 645
    of nurse, 1790*t*
Spiritual counseling, 1790
Spiritual development, 353, 353*t*, 354*t*
    developmental considerations
        children, 1772*t*
        older adults, 1772*t*
    stages of, 1773*t*
Spiritual distress, 1771
    Case Study, 1791
    characteristics of, 1788
    as etiology, 1788
    Nursing Care Plan
        assessment, 1791*t*
        critical thinking, 1791*t*
        diagnosis, 1791*t*
        evaluation, 1791*t*
        planning and implementation, 1791*t*

nursing diagnoses and interventions
    providing presence, 1789
    referring clients for spiritual counseling, 1790
nursing process
    assessment, 1789
    diagnosis, 1789
    evaluation, 1790
    planning and implementation, 1789–1790
    overview, 1788
Spiritual health, 1771*t*
    assessment of, 646
    benefits of exercise for, 654
    definition, 1770
    indicators of, 1771*t*
Spiritual skills, 34
Spiritual support, 509
Spiritual well-being, 1770
Spirituality. *See also* Religion
    about, 1769–1775
    assessment
        clinical assessment, 1775
        nursing history, 1775
    Assessment Interview, 1775*t*
    components of
        religion, 1771
        spiritual distress, 1771
        spiritual health and well-being,
            1770–1771, 1771*t*
        spiritual needs, 1770, 1770*t*
    core aspects
        faith, 1771
        forgiveness, 1772
        hope, 1772
        transcendence, 1772
    end-of-life care and, 293
    grief and, 612
    morality. *See* Morality
    overview, 1769–1770
    practices affecting nursing care
        birth beliefs, 1774
        death, 1774
        diet and nutrition, 1773
        dress, 1774
        guidelines, 1772
        healing beliefs, 1773
    spiritual development, 1772, 1772–1773*t*
    spiritual distress. *See* Spiritual distress
Spleen, 677*t*, 679*f*, 681–682, 681*f*
Splenic sequestration, 178*t*
splenomegaly, 1017
Splints, 1108*t*
Splitting, 1615
SPMSQ (Short Portable Mental Status
    Questionnaire), 207*t*
Spontaneous abortion, 626
Spontaneous bacterial peritonitis, 1019
Sprains, 1063
Sputum grain stain, 841
Sputum smear, 862
Sputum specimen, in lung cancer, 164
Squamous cell cancer, 186–187, 187*f*, 189*t*.
    See also Skin cancer
Squamous cell carcinomas, 161*t*
SSRIs. *See* Selective serotonin reuptake
    inhibitors (SSRIs)

St. John's Wort, 1176
Stab wounds, 1938
Stable angina, 1362, 1367t
Staff authority, 2126
Staff development, 2272–2273, 2273t
Staff education:
　Case Study, 2275
　evaluation of, 2274–2275
　on-the-job instruction, 2274
　orientation, 2272
　other educational techniques, 2274
　overview, 2272
　staff development process, 2273
Staffing shortages, 2316, 2317t
Staghorn stones, 466
Staging, of cancer, 107, 125
Standard of care, 2402, 2403t
Standard precautions, 2435, 2436t
Standardized nursing care plans, 2077–2081, 2080f
Standardized nursing languages (SNLs), 2376, 2386
Standards, 2068, 2069t, 2425
Standards of care, 2078, 2079f, 2280
Standards of Clinical Nursing Practice (ANA),
　　2402, 2403t, 2410
Standards of practice, 2280, 2293, 2293t, 2410
Standards of Professional Performance, 2293, 2293t
Standards of Professional Performance (ANA),
　　2244, 2244t, 2327, 2328t
Standing orders, 2080
Stanford-Binet Intelligence Scale: Fourth
　　Edition, 2013t
Stapedectomy, 1654
Stapes, 1632
Staphylococcus, 1900
Staphylococcus aureus, 770, 787, 789, 834, 842t
Staphylococcus epidermidis, 770
Staphylococcus saprophyticus, 871
Staples, removal, 898
Starling's law of the heart, 1304
State agencies, 2365
State board of nursing (BONs), 2406–2407
State boards of nursing, 2398
State Child Health Insurance Program (SCHIP), 2368
State Children's Health Insurance Program, 2362
State Children's Health Insurance Program
　　(SCHIP), 2211
State councils on developmental disabilities
　　(SCDDs), 205
State divisions of health and human services, 2365
State licensing, 2283
Statements, differentiating types of, 2106t
Statins:
　mechanism of action, 1330t
　Medication Administration, 1374t
　nursing considerations, 1330t
　in specific conditions
　　COPD, 1273
　　hyperlipidemia, 1373
Status asthmaticus, 1253
Status epilepticus, 947t, 959
　definition, 971
　management of, 971t
Status quo, challenging of, 2107
Statute of limitations, 2400
Statutory laws, 2398

Steatorrhea, 933
Stem cell transplant (SCT), 155
Stem cells, 676, 678f
Step-down therapy, 1433
Stepfamily, 486–487
Steppage gait, 956t
Stepping, 958t
Stereognosis, 1628
Stereotaxic thalamotomy, 1137
Stereotypes, 2159t
Stereotyping, 323, 398
Stereotypy, 379
Steri-Strips, 898
Sterile field, 782
Sterile technique:
　definition of, 771
　general care and, 782, 784
Sterility, 1718
Sterilization, 778
　definition, 1733
　tubal ligation, 1733
　vasectomy, 1733
Sternum, 1307
Steroid hormones, 981
Stethoscope, 2004
Stigma, 250, 376t, 507
Stillbirth, 626
Stillborn. See also Perinatal loss
Stimulants:
　for fatigue, 303t
　sleep and, 669
Stimulus, 1628
STIs. See Sexually transmitted infections (STIs)
Stoma, 916, 917f
Stomatitis, 157, 658t
Stool, 423–424
Stool softeners, 455
Stool toileting refusal (STR), 457t
STR (stool toileting refusal), 457t
Straight traction, 1099–1100
Strategic National Stockpile, 2358
Strategic planning, 2143
Strattera, 373t
Stratum basale, 1874
Stratum corneum, 1875
Stratum granulosum, 1874
Stratum lucidum, 1875
Stratum spinosum, 1874
Strengths, determining, 2071
Streptococcal exoenzymes, 926
Streptococcus, 770, 1900
Streptococcus A, in children, 799–800t
Streptococcus mutans, 770
Streptococcus pneumoniae:
　in oropharynx, 770
　penicillin-resistant, 790
　pneumonia and, 834–835, 842t
Streptokinase, 1376
Streptomycin, 864t
Stress and coping, 646. See also Stressors
　about, 1793–1808
　alterations from normal coping
　　generalized anxiety disorder, 1804t
　　obsessive-compulsive disorder (OCD), 1804t
　　panic disorder, 1804t

　　phobias, 1804t
　　post-traumatic stress disorder (PTSD), 1804t
　　treatments for, 1804t
　assessment
　　checklist, 1806t
　　nursing history and assessment interview,
　　　1805, 1805t
　　physical examination and observation,
　　　1805–1806
　　successful nursing interactions with anxious
　　　clients, 1805t
　Assessment Interview, 1805t
　blood pressure and, 1309
　body temperature and, 1853
　cancer and, 94t, 121
　caring interventions
　　cognitive-behavioral therapy (CBT),
　　　1806–1807
　　psychotherapy, 1806–1807
　definition, 1793
　developmental concerns, 1802t
　ego defense mechanisms, 1802–1804
　factor affecting stress response, 1798t
　glucocorticoids and, 980
　hypertension and, 1426, 1429
　indicators of
　　cognitive, 1801–1802
　　physiological, 1800, 1800t
　　psychoemotional, 1800–1801
　　spiritual, 1802
　life events causing, 1163, 1163f
　management, 2232
　mood disorders and, 1161, 1163
　Multisystem Effects, 1801
　pharmacologic therapies, 1807–1808
　pulse and, 1308
　response-based models
　　general adaptation syndrome (GAS), 1794
　　local adaptation syndrome (LAS), 1794
　　stages, 1794–1795, 1795f
　　　alarm reaction, 1795
　　　exhaustion stage, 1795, 1795f, 1796t
　　　resistance stage, 1794–1795, 1795f
　sensory perception and, 1634
　sleep and, 669
　stimulus-based models, 1794
　stress management for nurses, 1807
　transactional model
　　cognitive appraisal, 1795–1797
　　Hildegard Peplau, 1796–1797
　　nursing transactional model, 1796, 1796f
Stress electrocardiography, 1371
Stress fractures, 1093, 1093t
Stress incontinence, 442, 442t, 446t, 450t
Stress response. See coping
Stress testing, 1464
Stress ulcers, 1896
Stressors:
　classification
　　acute and time limited, 1797, 1797t
　　chronic intermittent, 1797, 1797t
　　chronic permanent, 1797, 1797t
　　sequential events following initial stressor,
　　　1797, 1797t

definition, 1794
types of stressors
  developmental stressors, 1797t
  environmental stressors, 1797–1798, 1797t
  hassles, 1797, 1797t
  internal stressors, 1797, 1797t
Stretch marks, 1544
Striae, 428t, 1544
Strictureplasty, 916
Stridor, 1222t
Stroke:
  Case Study, 1513
  clinical therapies, 1504t
  collaborative care
    diagnostic tests, 1505
    pharmacologic therapies, 1506–1507
    rehabilitation, 1507
    surgery, 1507
  complications
    cognitive and behavioral changes, 1503
    communication disorders, 1503–1504
    elimination disorders, 1505
    gastrointestinal, 1503t
    genitourinary, 1503t
    integument, 1503t
    motor deficits, 1504–1505
    musculoskeletal, 1503t
    neurologic, 1503t
    respiratory, 1503t
    sensory-perceptual deficits, 1502–1503
  definition, 1499
  description, 1315t
  diabetes mellitus and, 997
  evidence-based practice, 1510t
  hemorrhagic, 1501
  hypertension and, 1427t
  ischemic
    embolic, 1500–1501
    pathophysiology, 1500
    thrombotic, 1500
    transient, 1500
  manifestations, 1502, 1502t, 1504t
  National Institutes of Health Stroke Scale, 1506t
  Nursing Care Plan
    assessment, 1511t
    critical thinking, 1512t
    diagnosis, 1511t
    evaluation, 1511t
    planning and implementation, 1511t
  nursing diagnoses and interventions
    impaired physical mobility, 1509
    impaired swallowing, 1512
    impaired urinary elimination and risk for
      constipation, 1509, 1512
    impaired verbal communication, 1509
    ineffective tissue perfusion, cerebral,
      1508–1509
    self-care deficit, 1509
  nursing process
    assessment, 1508
    diagnosis, 1508
    evaluation, 1512
    overview, 1507–1508
    planning and implementation, 1508–1510, 1512
  overview, 1499
  pathophysiology and etiology, 1499–1501
  risk factors, 1501–1502

sickle cell anemia and, 177
treatment, 1315t
treatment stages, 1505
Stroke volume (SV), 1303, 1405, 1483
Structural deficits, affecting communication, 2160
Structural-functional theory, 498–499
Structure standards, 2425
Structuring, 2170
Struvite stones, 466, 467t
Student care plans, 2081
Student nurses, 2281
Stupor, 946t
Subclinical infection, 770
Subconjunctival hemorrhage, 1662
Subculture groups, 323
Subcultures, 326f
Subcutaneous tissue, 1875
Subdermal implants, 1732–1733
Subfertility, 1718
Subjective data, 2054, 2054t
Subjective family burden, 508
Subjective Global Assessment (SGA), 664
Subluxation, 744
Substance abuse:
  addictive substances, 69f
    amphetamines, 68, 72–73
    caffeine, 71
    central nervous system depressants, 71
    cocaine, 68, 71–72
    hallucinogens, 73–74
    heroin, 68, 73
    inhalants, 74
    marijuana, 71
    methadone, 73
    methamphetamine, 72–73
    nicotine, 51
    opiates, 73
    prescription drugs, 68
    psychostimulants, 71–73
    street names, 74t
  assessment, 31–32, 32t
    history of past substance abuse, 78
    medical and psychiatric history, 78
    open-ended questions for, 77, 77t
    psychosocial issues, 78
    screening tools, 78
  Case Study, 82
  causes, 28
  client teaching, 81t
  co-occuring disorders, 67
  codependency, 30–31
  collaborative care, 75
  costs of, 68
  criminalization of, 68
  deaths related to, 68
  definition, 66
  description, 29t
  diagnostic tests, 32, 75
  DSM-IV-TR diagnostic criteria, 67t
  during pregnancy, 342
  effect on children, 31
  effects on families, 29–31
  impaired nurses, 68–69, 69t
  incidence, 66, 68
  interpersonal violence and, 1953
  interventions, 32
  kindling effect and, 67

manifestations, 70–74
nicotine, 51
Nursing Care Plan
  assessment, 79t
  critical thinking, 79t
  diagnosis, 79t
  evaluation, 79t
  planning and implementation, 79t
nursing diagnosis and interventions, 80
  chronic low or situational low self-esteem, 80
  deficient knowledge, 81
  disturbed sensory perceptions, 81
  disturbed thought processes, 81
  imbalanced nutrition, less than body
    requirements, 80
  ineffective coping, 80
  ineffective denial, 80
  risk for injury and risk for violence, 80
nursing interventions
  behavioral therapy, 34–35
  communication, 33
  crisis intervention, 33–34
  family intervention, 33
  family therapy, 37–38, 38t
  group therapy, 35–37, 36–37t
  milieu therapy, 35
nursing process
  assessment, 77–78, 77t
  diagnosis, 79
  evaluation, 81
  overview, 77
  planning and implementation, 79–81
in older adults, 78t
osteoporosis and, 1035
overdose
  emergency care, 75
  signs and treatment, 76–77t
overview, 66–67
pain management and, 279t
pathophysiology and etiology, 67–68
pharmacologic therapies, 38, 39t
polysubstance, 45, 67
in pregnancy, 57
relapse, 81t
risk factors, 61, 62t, 69
  biologic, 69
  genetic, 69
  psychologic, 69
  sociocultural factors, 70, 70t
  in teenagers, 70t
schizophrenia and, 236
statistics, 29
stroke risk and, 1502
vs. substance dependence, 28
terminology, 29, 30t
treatment, 29t
  group therapy, 36t
  withdrawal, 75, 75t
treatment programs, 77
warning signs, 63t
withdrawal, 75, 75t
withdrawal symptoms, 66
Substance Abuse and Mental Health Services
  Administration, 2335
Substance dependence:
  definition, 66
  DSM-IV-TR diagnostic criteria, 67t

Substance-related disorders, 1158
Substances, action at brain receptor sites, 69f
Subsystems, 497
Sucking, 958t
Sucralfate, 934
Suction catheters, 1245, 1245f
Suctioning:
  developmental considerations, 1246t
  in specific conditions
    acute respiratory distress syndrome (ARDS), 1245–1246
Sudden cardiac death (SCD):
  causes, 1454t
  Client Teaching, 1458t
  collaborative care
    advanced life support, 1455
    basic life support, 1455
    care for family, 1456–1457, 1457t
    postresuscitation care, 1455–1456
  definition, 1454
  etiology, 1454
  manifestations, 1455
  risk factors, 1454–1455
Sudden infant death syndrome (SIDS):
  Case Study, 1290
  Client Teaching, 1289
  collaborative care
    modeling protective behaviors, 1288
    psychosocial needs of the family, 1288
  health care, 1289–1290
  manifestations, 1287
  nursing diagnoses and interventions
    knowledge deficit related to risk factors, 1289
  nursing process
    assessment, 1288
    diagnosis, 1288
    evaluation, 1289
    planning and implementation, 1288–1289
  overview, 1286
  pathophysiology and etiology, 1286–1287
  risk factors, 1287, 1287t
  treatment, 1220t
Suffocation, 2452
Suicidal behavior, 1978, 1981–1982
Suicide, 236, 2457–2458
  antidepressants and, 1170–1171, 1190
  assessment, 1192
  assisted, 2314
  Case Study, 1986
  collaborative care, 1983
  definition, 1978
  description, 1939t
  developmental considerations, 1980t
  etiology, 1979
  facts about, 1980t
  incidence, 1978, 1980f
  manifestations, 1983t
    affect, 1982
    behavior, 1981–1982
    cognition, 1982
    interpersonal relationships, 1982–1983
    self-destructive behaviors, 1981
  Nursing Care Plan
    assessment, 1985t
    critical thinking, 1985t
    diagnosis, 1985t

evaluation, 1985t
    planning and implementation, 1985t
  nursing diagnoses and interventions
    maintain safety, 1984
    prevent future suicidal behavior, 1984
    promote problem solving, 1984
    support families of victims, 1984–1985
  nursing process
    assessment, 1983
    diagnosis, 1983–1984
    evaluation, 1985–1986
    planning and implementation, 1984–1985
  overview, 1978
  pathophysiology
    behavioral theory, 1979
    comorbid disorders, 1979
    genetics, 1978
    interpersonal factors, 1979
    neurobiology, 1978–1979
    social factors, 1979
  pharmacologic therapies, 1983
  postpartum depression and, 1201
  prevention, 1168–1169, 1169t
  protective factors, 1983
  risk factors, 1979–1981, 1980t
  statistics on, 1936
  treatment/prevention, 1939t
Suicide rates, 1981t
Sulfasalazine, 748, 750t, 914, 915t
Sulfate, in intracellular fluid, 518
Sulfonamides, 807
Sulfuric acid, 4
Sulindac, 749t
Summarizing, 2172, 2178t
Sun exposure, 187–188, 2458
Sunburn, 1896
Sundown syndrome, 226
Sundowning, 215
Sunlight, mood disorders and, 1162, 1164t
Superego, 343
Superficial burns, 1888, 1894t
Superficial spreading melanoma, 185
Supine (horizontal recumbent) position, 2002t
Supine hypotensive syndrome, 1310, 1310f, 1542–1543
Supplemental Nutrition Assistance Program, 663t
Supplemental Security Income (SSI), 2211, 2368
Support braces/gloves, 2384t
Support groups, for addiction, 36–37
Support people, as source of data, 2054
Support structures, 508–509
Suppressor T cells, 679f, 681. See also
  T lymphocytes (T cells)
Suppuration, 1930
Suprapubic prostatectomy, 171, 439
Suprasystems, 497
Supraventricular aortic stenosis, 1326t
Supraventricular dysrhythmias, 1444–1445
Supraventricular rhythms, 1440
  characteristics, 1441–1442t
  normal sinus rhythm, 1440
  sick sinus syndrome, 1444
  sinus node dysrhythmias, 1440
  supraventricular dysrhythmias, 1444–1445
Supraventricular tachycardia, 1460t

Surface temperature, 1851, 1852
Surfactant, in respiration, 1217
Surge capacity, 2351
Surgery:
  bowel elimination following, 426
  burns
    autografting, 1901–1902
    escharotomy, 1901, 1901f
    surgical debridement, 1901
  classification of, 895
  elective, 895
  emergency, 895
  intraoperative nursing care, 897
  laser, 435
  minimally invasive, 435
  nursing care
    bladder neck suspension, 443t
    procedures, 908t
    prostatectomy, 436–440, 439–440t
  postoperative nursing care
    complications, 897
    head-to-toe assessment, 897
    immediate, 897
    older adults, 898, 898t
    pain management, 897
    surgical wounds, 897–898
    when client is stable, 897
  preoperative nursing care, 895
    client and family teaching, 896
    client preparation, 896
    fasting, 896
    prostatectomy, 436–437
  procedures
    adenoidectomy, 315
    adenotonsillectomy, 314t
    appendectomy, 893f, 894
    arthroplasty, 1112
    arthroscopy, 1076, 1129
    bariatric, 1029–1030
    breast reconstruction, 110–111
    cardiac transplantation, 1336, 1416–1417
    cardiomyoplasty, 1417
    carotic angioplasty, 1507
    carotid endarterectomy, 1507
    cerebral hemispherectomy, 972
    cerebral palsy, 388
    colectomy, 916
    colostomy, 144
    cordotomy, 279
    coronary artery bypass grafting, 1378–1379, 1380–1382t
    dilation and curettage, 1734
    diskectomy, 1083
    endarterectomy, 1465
    endometrial ablation, 1750
    fasciotomy, 1095
    foraminotomy, 1083
    gonioplasty, 1672
    hysterectomy, 1750–1751, 1751t
    intracranial, 964
    intradiscal electrothermal therapy (IDET), 1084
    joint arthroplasty, 1129
    laminectomy, 1083, 1086t
    laparoscopic cholecystectomy S, 908t
    laparoscopic cholecystectomy, 904t, 905

laser iridotomy, 1672
laser photocoagulation, 144
laser trabeculoplasty, 1670
liver transplantation, 1020
lumpectomy, 110
lung reduction surgery, 1273
mastectomy, 110
microdiskectomy, 1084
minimally invasive coronary artery surgery, 1379
myringotomy, 829
nephrectomy, 560–562, 561t
neurectomy, 279
nuclectomy, 1083
open reduction and internal fixation, 1101
osteotomy, 1129
ostomy, 916–917, 917–919t
pallidotomy, 1137
prostatectomy, 170–171, 171f, , 435–440, 436f,
    439–440t
rhizotomy, 279
spinal fusion, 1083, 1088
stapedectomy, 1654
stereotaxic thalamotomy, 1137
strictureplasty, 916
therapeutic D&C, 1750
thyroidectomy, 1045
tonsillectomy, 315
trabeculectomy, 1670
tympanocentesis, 829
tympanoplasty, 1654
ureteroplasty, 876–877
uvulopalatopharyngoplasty, 315
venous thrombectomy, 1392
ventricular reduction, 1417
in specific conditions
breast cancer, 110–111
cancer, 130
cardiomyopathy, 1336
cataract, 1658–1659, 1660t
cirrhosis, 1020
colorectal cancer, 143–144
congenital heart defects, 1354–1355t
COPD, 1273
coronary artery disease, 1378–1382
deep venous thrombosis, 1392
diabetes mellitus, 1007–1008
erectile dysfunction, 1714
eye, 1666t
fractures, 1101
glaucoma, 1670, 1672
hearing impairment, 1654
heart failure, 1416–1417
herniated disk, 1083, 1085, 1086t
hip fractures, 1112
hyperthyroidism, 1045
hypothyroidism, 1050
inflammatory bowel disease, 916–917,
    917–919t
lung cancer, 165, 165t
macular degeneration, 1677
melanomas, 190
menstrual dysfunction, 1750–1751
multiple sclerosis, 1120
obesity, 1029–1030
osteoarthritis, 1129–1130
otitis media, 829
Parkinson's disease, 1137
peptic ulcer disease, 934

peripheral vascular disease, 1465
prostate cancer, 170–171, 172t
prostate, 170–171, 171f, , 435–440, 436f,
    439–440t
pulmonary embolism, 1480
rheumatoid arthritis, 750–751
scoliosis, 1088
spinal cord injury, 1150
stroke, 1507
urinary incontinence, 443
urinary tract infections and, 876
transurethral, 435
urinary system
    bladder neck suspension, 443t
    lithotripsy, 469–470, 470t
    prostatectomy, 444
    for urinary retention, 446
Surgical asepsis, principles and practices of,
    783–784t
Surgical debridement, 1901
Surgical menopause, 1742
Surgical wounds, postoperative care, 897–898
Susceptible host:
    defenses for, 777
    definition of, 773
    nursing interventions and, 775t
    portal of entry to, 773, 773f
        nursing interventions and, 774–775t
    role of, 773f
Suspension traction, 1100
Sutures, removal, 898
Swan-Ganz catheter, 1412–1413, 1413f
Swan-neck deformity, 744, 744t
Swanson, Nolan and Pelham Questionnaire II
    Teacher and Parent Rating Scale
    (SNAP-IV), 371t
Symmetrel. See Amantadine
Symmetry, 1222
Sympathetic nervous system (SNS):
    arterial blood pressure and, 1423–1424
    sympathetic tone and, 1484
Sympathetic tone, 1484
Sympathomimetic agents, 1415t, 1449, 1493t
Sympathy, 2165
Symptoms, 2054
Symptothermal method, 1726
Synarel, 1735t
Synchronized cardioversion, 1449
Synchronized intermittent mandatory ventilation
    (SIMV), 1240t, 1241
Syncope, 1334, 1335t, 1350
Syndrome diagnosis, 2066
Synovectomy, 750
Synovial joints, 1061–1062, 1061t
Synovitis, 1070f, 1073t
Synovium, rheumatoid arthritis and, 743f
Syphilis:
    collaborative care
        diagnostic tests, 1762
        overview, 1762
        pharmacologic therapies, 1762
    definition, 1760
    incidence, 1761
    latent and tertiary, 1762
    manifestations, 1761, 1761t
    Nursing Care Plan
        assessment, 1764t
        critical thinking in the nursing process, 1764t

        diagnosis, 1764t
        evaluation, 1764t
        overview, 1764t
        planning and implementation, 1764t
    pathophysiology, 1761
    primary, 1761
    secondary, 1761
    transmission, 1760
Syrup of Ipecac, 1602
Systematic decision making, 2039
Systematic Nomenclature of Medicine Clinical
    Terms (SNOMED CT®), 2386
Systematized delusions, 239
Systemic blood flow, 1342, 1351
Systemic circulation, 1298, 1300f
Systemic infection, 771
Systemic inflammatory response syndrome
    (SIRS), 850
Systemic juvenile rheumatoid arthritis (JRA), 745
Systemic lupus erythematosus (SLE), 924
    Case Study, 765
    in children, 762
    chronic renal failure and, 553t
    Client Teaching, 764
    collaborative care
        complementary therapies, 761
        diagnostic tests, 760
        other treatments, 761
        pharmacologic therapies, 761
    description of, 693, 756
    etiology of, 757
    manifestations of, 757–760, 757f, 760t
    Multisystem Effects, 759
    nursing diagnoses and interventions
        avoidance of triggers for disease flares, 763
        impaired health maintenance, 764–765
        ineffective protection, 763–764
        maintain fluid balance, 763
        manage side effects of medications, 763
        prevent infection, 763
        promote rest and comfort, 763
        promote skin integrity, 762–763
        provide emotional support, 763
    nursing process
        assessment, 762
        diagnosis, 762
        evaluation, 765
        planning and implementation, 762–765
    pathophysiology of, 756–757
    risk factors, 757
    self-care for, 764
    therapies for, 761
    treatments for, 762
Systemic response, hypersensitivity and, 726
Systemic vascular resistance, 1301–1302
Systems, 497
Systems theory, 497–498
Systole, 1296, 1302
Systolic blood pressure, 1422
Systolic pressure, 1308

T

T cells. See T lymphocytes (T cells)
T lymphocytes (T cells):
    immune system function and, 677t, 678–679,
        679f, 680f, 681
    systemic lupus erythematosus (SLE) and, 756

T-cell (cell-mediated) function, 692f
T-tubes:
nursing care of client with, 905t
placement, 905f
T₄. See Thyroxine
Taboo, 1572t
Tachyarrhythmias, 1439t
Tachycardia, 1319
Tachydysrhythmia, 1440
Tachypnea, 1221
influenza and, 822
pneumonia and, 840
Tactile sense, 1634, 1649
Tactile stimuli, 1628
Talk test, 652
Talmud, 1782
Talwin, 58t
Tamiflu. See Oseltamivir
Tamoxifen citrate, 110
Tamsulosin (Flomax), 434, 434t
Tangential excision, 1901
Tapestry of life, 1592t
Tardive dyskinesia, 243
Tartar, 656, 658
Task forces, 2140
Taste, 1633, 1635, 1643, 1645
Tax Equity and Fiscal Responsibility Act
(TEFRA), 2214
Taxonomy II, 2075, 2075f
TCAs. See Tricyclic antidepressants
Tdap, 687
Teacher–learner relationship, 2244
Teachers, nurses as, 2244, 2294t
Teaching aids, developing written, 2258t
Teaching and learning, 670–671, 673
about, 2243–2244, 2244t
art of teaching, 2244–2245
Case Study, 2253
characteristics of effective teaching, 2245t
client education, 2254–2269, 2254t, 2256–2257t,
2258t, 2259t, 2259t, 2261t, 2263t, 2264t,
2267t, 2268t
compliance and, 2245
defined, 2243
developmental considerations, 2256t
domains of learning, 2247
evaluation of teaching, 2268
factors affecting learning, 2249–2251, 2250t, 2251t
factors facilitating learning
active involvement, 2249, 2249f
environment, 2250
feedback, 2249
motivation to learn, 2249
nonjudgmental support, 2249
organization of material, 2250
readiness to learn, 2249
relevance, 2249
repetition, 2250
timing, 2250
factors inhibiting learning, 2250, 2250t
cultural barriers, 2251
emotions, 2251
physiologic events, 2251
psychomotor ability, 2251
guidelines for teaching, 2262–2264, 2264f
learning needs, 2245
learning theories, 2245–2249, 2246–2247t

mentoring, 2269–2271, 2271t
nurses and, 2244
nursing process compared with teaching
process, 2255t
online health information and, 2251–2253, 2252t
staff education, 2272–2275
teaching tools for children, 2264t
terminology, 2245
Teaching groups, 2140
Teaching plan:
development of, 2260–2262, 2261t, 2262t
guides for, 2261
implementation, 2262, 2264–2267
sample, 2261t
Teaching priorities, 2260
Teaching process, documentation of, 2268
Teaching strategies:
behavior modification, 2265–2266
client contracting, 2265
computer-assisted instruction, 2265
discovery/problem-solving technique, 2265
group teaching, 2265
selecting, 2261, 2262f
transcultural teaching, 2266–2267
types of, 2263t
Teaching–learning process, 2243
Team dynamics, 2020
Team nursing, 2206–2207, 2344
Teams, 2140, 2144
Teamwork, 2227, 2227t, 2444
Tebrazid. See Pyrazinamide
Technical skills, 2096
Technological advances, 2283
Technology:
advances in, and health care delivery, 2342
ethical dilemmas and, 2312
Teenage mothers, 498t
Teenage parents, 486
Teenage pregnancy. See Adolescent pregnancy
Teenagers. See Adolescents
Teeth, 656–657
Tegretol, 217, 1174, 1174t
Telecommunications, 2283
Telehealth, 2283, 2380–2381
applications, 2381, 2382t
barriers to client participation in, 2382–2383
barriers to implementation of, 2381–2382
benefits, 2381t
global, 2381t
Telenursing, 2283
Teleological theories, 1777
Telephone counseling, 648
Telephone orders, 2201
Telephone reports, 2201
Temperament, 340
in adolescence, 364
infancy, 357
preschool age, 361
in school-age years, 363
toddlers, 358
Temperament theory, 349–350, 349t
Temperature, blood pressure and, 1424
Temperature conversion, 1854
Temperature-sensitive tape, 1857
Temporal artery, 1856
Temporal artery thermometer, 1857
Temporal lobe, 940

Temporal pulse, 1319, 1319f
Temporomandibular joint (TMJ) syndrome, 1066
Temporomandibular joints, 1072
Ten Commandments, 2333
Tender points, 258, 305, 306f
Tendonitis, 1073t
Tendons, 1063, 1065
Teratogenesis, 58
Teratogens, 57, 1538, 1572–1573
Teratospermia, 1735
Terazosin (Hytrin), 434, 434t, 1432
Term, 1559t
Terminology, for documentation, 2196,
2196–2198t
Territoriality, 2157
Tertiary care, delivery of, 2341
Tertiary intention healing, 1927
Tertiary prevention, 2340–2341, 2341t
Testes, 1686, 1686t, 1712
Testosterone, 1687, 1712, 1714
produced by placenta, 1534
Tetanus:
in children, 800t
Tetanus immunization, 1943
Tetanus toxoid, 687
Tetanus vaccine:
in burn clients, 1901
Tetanus-diphtheria (Td) booster, 1664t
Tetanus-diphtheria-pertussis (Tdap) booster, 1664t
Tetany, 548, 986t
Tetracyclines:
medication administration, 807
Tetralogy of Fallot, 1343–1344t
Tetraplegia, 1147
TH. See Thyroid hormone
Thalamic pain, 264
Thalamus, 940
Thalassemia, 100, 102t
THC (delta-9-tetrahydrocannabinol), 71
Theophylline, 841, 1259, 1262
Therapeutic communication:
addiction and, 33
barriers to, 2172
Case Study, 2178
overview, 2164–2165
techniques, 2167–2168t
accepting, 2177t
acknowledging, 2168t
active listening, 2177t
attentive listening, 2165–2166, 2166t
avoiding self-disclosure, 2169, 2169t
clarifying, 2167–2168t, 2169, 2169t, 2177t
collaborating, 2177t
common mistakes, 2172
confronting, 2171–2172
empathizing, 2165, 2165t
exploring, 2177t
focusing, 2168t, 2177t
giving feedback, 2170, 2171t
imparting information, 2168t, 2169
linking, 2170
offering self, 2167t
open-ended questions, 2167t
paraphrasing, 2169, 2178t
perception checking, 2167t, 2170
physical attending, 2166, 2166t
pinpointing, 2170

presenting reality, 2168*t*
processing, 2172, 2172*t*
questioning, 2170
reflecting, 2168–2169, 2168*t*
reflection, 2177*t*
restatement, 2178*t*
restating or paraphrasing, 2167*t*
structuring, 2170
summarizing, 2172, 2178*t*
summarizing and planning, 2168*t*
using silence, 2166, 2167*t*, 2168
using touch, 2167*t*
validating perceptions, 2178*t*
with children and families, 2176, 2177–2178*t*
Therapeutic insemination:
definition, 1735
therapeutic donor insemination (TDI), 1735–1736
therapeutic husband insemination (THI), 1735
Therapeutic relationships:
characteristics of, 2173*t*
developing, 2175–2176
introductory phase, 2173, 2173*t*
overview, 2172–2173
phases of, 2173
introductory phase, 2174*t*
preinteraction phase, 2173, 2174*t*
termination phase, 2174*t*, 2175, 2175*t*
working phase, 2174*t*, 2174–2175, 2175*t*
Therapy groups, 2141
Thermal burns, 1886, 1886*f*, 1898
Thermometers, 1855, 1857
Thermoregulation. *See also* Hyperthermia;
Hypothermia
about, 1851–1858
definition, 1852
diagnostic tests, 1858
interventions, 1858
in newborns, 1854
normal presentation, 1852–1853
physical assessment, 1854–1855, 1857
process of, 1853
Thiamin, recommended daily intake, 1596*t*
Thiamine depletion, 43
Thiazide diuretics, 469, 1429
Thiomalate, 750*t*
Third heart sound (S3), 1296, 1297*t*
Third National Congress on the State of the
Science in Nursing Research, 2326
Third-party reimbursement, 2212
Third spacing, 570, 572*t*
Third-degree AV block, 1444*t*, 1447
Thirst mechanism, 522
Thomas test, 1075, 1075*t*
Thompson and Thompson model of ethical
decision making, 2311*t*
Thoracentesis, 835, 1229
Thoracic cage, 1307
Thoracic catheter, 1233–1234
Thoracic computed tomography (CT), 1228
Thoracic injury, 1149*t*
Thoracotomy, 165*t*
Thorax, 1218*t*
Thorazine, 242
Thought broadcasting, 240
Thought insertion, 240

Thought withdrawal, 240
Threshold potential, 1306
Thrombocytes (platelets), 678*f*
Thrombocytopenia, 89, 759–760
Thromboemboli, 1476, 1477*f*
Thrombolytics:
mechanism of action, 1332*t*
nursing considerations, 1332*t*
Thrombophlebitis. *See* Deep venous thrombosis
Thrombotic crisis, 178
Thrombotic stroke, 1500
Throughput, 498
Thunderstorm-related injuries, 2352*t*
Thymosin, 682
Thymus gland:
age and, 692
human immunodeficiency virus (HIV) and, 708*t*
immune system function and, 677*t*, 679, 679*f*, 681–682, 681*f*
risk of infection and, 777
Thyroglobin, 979
Thyroid agents, 988*t*
Thyroid crisis, 1043–1044
Thyroid disease:
hyperthyroidism. *See* Hyperthyroidism
hypothyroidism. *See* Hypothyroidism
overview, 1041
Thyroid function tests, 1411
Thyroid gland, 978*t*, 980*f*
definition, 979
palpating, 985*f*
pregnancy and, 1545
Thyroid hormone (TH):
control of, 981
decreased levels, 1048
definition, 1041
description, 978*t*
elevated levels of, 1043–1044
function, 979
Graves' disease and, 1041, 1043, 1043*f*
hyperthyroidism and, 1041
toxic multinodular goiter and, 1043, 1043*f*
Thyroid hormone levels, mood disorders and, 1161
Thyroid profile, 1028
Thyroid storm, 1043–1044
Thyroid-stimulating hormone (TSH), 978, 1043
Thyroidectomy, 1045
Thyroiditis, 1043
Thyrotoxicosis, 1041
Thyrotropic cells, 978
Thyroxine, 979, 1852
Thyroxine (T4), 137, 978*t*
TIA. *See* Transient ischemic attack (TIA)
Tibetan Book of the Dead, 1774
TICS (Telephone Interview for Cognitive Status), 207*t*
Time, 326, 2109
Time management, 2144
Time management decisions, 2038
Timed Up and Go (TUG) test, 2451
Timing, of communication, 2150
Timolol (Timoptic), 1671*t*
Tinea pedis, cellulitis and, 809
Tinnitus, 1652
Tissue:
granulation, 887

osseous, 1056
regeneration of, 887
Tissue integrity:
about, 1873–1885
alterations, 1875–1876, 1878–1880, 1879*t*
assessment, 1880
Assessment Interview, 1880–1881*t*
caring interventions, 1884
diagnostic tests, 1884
integumentary assessment, 1882–1883*t*, 1884*t*
normal presentation, 1874–1875
risk for impaired
pressure ulcers and, 1921–1922
therapeutic interventions for alterations in, 1884
pharmacologic therapies, 1884, 1885*t*
wounds, 1878. *See* Wounds
Tissue plasminogen activator (tPA), 1510
TMS (transcranial magnetic stimulation), 245
TNF (tumor necrosis factor), 916
TNM staging system, 125, 126*t*
for colorectal cancer, 142–143
for lung cancer, 164*t*
To Err Is Human (IOM), 2324, 2422, 2433, 2443
Tobacco, 51, 52*t*. *See also* Smoking
use in pregnancy, 60
Tobacco cessation. *See* Smoking cessation
Tobacco smoking. *See* Smoking
Today vaginal sponge, 1730
Toddlerhood, 341*t*
Toddlers:
assessment of, 2014
developmental tasks in, 1581*t*
grief and loss in, 610*t*
growth and development, 357–359
pain perception and behavior, 269*t*
promotion of oral health in, 659
recommended screenings and immunizations, 643*t*
safety measures, 2454, 2455*t*
sleep patterns and requirements, 668
Tofranil, 443
Toileting:
assistance, 451
facilitation of, 462*t*
scheduled, 445
Token economies, 35
Tolectin. *See* Tolmetin
Tolerance, 28, 30*t*
Tolmetin, 749*t*
Tolterodine, 443
Tone, 1483
Tongue, 655
Tongue blades (depressors), 2005*t*
Tonic neck, 958*t*
Tonic phase, 968
Tonicity, 520
Tonometry, 1646, 1670
Tonsillectomy, 315
Tonsils, 677*t*, 681–682, 681*f*
Tooth decay, prevention of, 660*t*
Top-down sampling, 1161*f*
Topamax, 1585
Topiramate, 1585
Torah, 1782
Tornado-related injuries, 2352*t*
Torsades de pointes, 1446, 1446*f*
Torsemide, 541*t*

Tort law, 2399–2401
  intentional torts, 2400–2401
  strategies to prevent incidents of professional
      negligence, 2401–2402
  unintentional torts
    negligence, 2399
    professional negligence, 2399–2400, 2400t
Torts, 2398
Total anomalous pulmonary venous return, 1346t
Total care, 2206
Total communication, 1655t
Total incontinence, 442, 446t
Total joint replacement, 1112
  cemented vs. uncemented, 1129
  complications, 1130
  definition, 1129
  elbow, 1130
  hip, 1129, 1129f
  knee, 1130, 1130f
  Nursing Care Plan
    assessment, 1132t
    critical thinking in the nursing process, 1133t
    diagnoses, 1132t
    evaluation, 1132t
    overview, 1132t
    planning and implementation, 1132t
  physical therapy and rehabilitation, 1130
  shoulder, 1130
Total lymphoid irradiation, 751
Total parenteral nutrition (TPN), 916, 921t
Total protein, 130t
Total quality management (TQM), 2426–2427, 2427t
Touch, 1634, 1645t, 1649
Touch therapy, 219
Toxic megacolon, 912
Toxic multinodular goiter, 1043, 1043f
Toxic shock syndrome, 850
Toxoplasmosis, 704, 714t
Trabeculectomy, 1670
Trachea:
  anatomy, physiology, and functions, 1216
  pediatric differences in, 837, 838f
Trachoma, 814
Traction:
  definition, 1099
  examples of, 1150
  types, 1100, 1101t, 1106t, 1150
Traditional beliefs, 330
Traditional family, 485–486
Traditional nursing process approach, 2376
Trait theories of leadership, 2233–2234
Tranquilizers, effect on fetus, 58t
Trans fatty acids, 1372
Transactional leaders, 2234
Transactional model of stress and coping:
  appraisal, 1798
  coping, 1798–1799
    types of coping, 1799, 1799t
  reappraisal and adaptation, 1799
Transcatheter closure, 1354t
Transcellular fluid, 518
Transcendence, 1772
Transcendental meditation, 1433t
Transcranial blood flow, monitoring of, 964
Transcranial magnetic stimulation (TMS), 245, 1175

Transcultural nursing, 2028
Transcultural teaching, 2266–2267
Transcutaneous oximetry, 1465
TransCyte, 1903
Transductive reasoning, 360t
Transference, 2139
Transformational leaders, 2235
Transfusion reaction, hypersensitivity and,
      725–726, 727
Transgenderism, 1696
Transient ischemic attack (TIA), 1500
Transjugular intrahepatic portosystemic shunt
      (TIPS), 1024
Translators, 2058, 2058t
Translocation, 1722
Transmission of infection:
  methods of
    airborne, 773
    direct, 772–773
    indirect, 773
  nursing interventions and, 774t
  precautions against, 778–779, 780t, 788–789
Transmyocardial laser revascularization, 1382
Transparent dressing, 1918t
Transplacental immunity, 683
Transposition of the great arteries (TGA), 1345t
Transsexuals, 400, 1696
Transurethral microwave thermotherapy, 435
Transurethral needle ablation (TUNA), 435
Transurethral resection of the prostate (TURP),
      435, 438
Transurethral surgery, 435
Transverse diameter, 1517
Transverse loop colostomy, 144
Trastuzumab, 110
Trauma:
  assessment, 1940–1941
  caring interventions, 1943
  common mechanisms of injury, 1937–1938, 1938t
  components of, 1937–1938
  definition, 1937
  diagnostic tests, 1941–1942
  effects on family, 1941
  personality disorders and, 1609
  prevention, 1938–1940
  rape-trauma syndrome. See Rape-trauma syndrome
  types
    blunt, 1938
    minor, 1938
    multiple, 1938
    penetrating, 1938
Trauma prevention, 1103, 1104t
Traumatic cataracts, 1657
Travatan, 1671t
Travoprost (Travatan), 1671t
Trazodone (Desyrel), 217
Treated wounds, 1880
Treatment providers, educating, 2299
Treatments, 2092
Treaty of Geneva, 2290
Tremor, in Parkinson's disease, 1135
Tremors, 955t
Triage, 1943, 2356, 2356f, 2356t
Tricosal. See Choline magnesium trisalicylate
Tri-Council for Nursing, 2290
Tricuspid atresia, 1344t

Tricuspid valve, 1295
Tricyclic antidepressants (TCAs):
  anxiety disorders, 1815
  client teaching, 1171
  definition, 1170
  depression, 1189t
  fatigue, 303t
  fibromyalgia, 307
  developmental considerations, 1174
  drug interactions with, 1171
  nursing considerations, 1171
  side effects, 1170–1171
  uses of, 1170
Trigeminal nerve, 942t, 1628t
Triglycerides, 1025, 1361, 1365, 1365t
Triiodothyronine, 979
Trilisate. See Choline magnesium trisalicylate
Trimethoprim (TMP), 876
Trimethoprim-sulfamethoxazole (TMP-SMZ):
  in specific conditions
    otitis media, 828
    urinary tract infections and, 876
Tripitakas, 1782
Triplet, 1446
Tripod position, emphysema and, 1270
Trisomies, 1720–1721, 1721t. See also Down
      syndrome
Trochlear nerve, 942t, 1628t
Trophoblast, 1527
Troponins, 1371
Trousseau's sign, 592t, 986t
True pelvis, 1517, 1518f
Truncus arteriosus, 1345–1346t
Trusopt, 1670, 1671t
Trust, 2119, 2173, 2176, 2444
Truth, Sojourner, 2288, 2289f
L-tryptophan, 669
TSH (thyroid-stimulating hormone), 978, 1043
Tsunami-related injuries, 2352t
Tubal ligation, 1733
Tubercle, 856
Tuberculin tests, 164
Tuberculosis:
  acquired immunodeficiency syndrome (AIDS)
      and, 704
  Case Study, 870–871
  collaborative care
    diagnostic tests, 862
    pharmacologic therapies, 862–863
    screening, 861–862, 861t, 866
  cultural factors for, 860
  definition, 856
  etiology, 857
  extensively drug resistant (XDR) strains, 860
  extrapulmonary, 857
  interpreting test results, 861t
  latent infection, 865t
  manifestations, 860–861, 860t
  miliary, 857
  multidrug-resistant (MDR) strains, 857, 860
  Nursing Care Plan
    assessment, 869t
    critical thinking, 869t
    diagnoses, 869t
    evaluation, 869t
    planning and implementation, 869t

nursing diagnoses and interventions
assessing for home care, 866
deficient knowledge, 865–867
ineffective therapeutic regimen management, 867
older adults and, 866
risk for infection, 867–868
nursing process
assessment, 865
diagnosis, 865
evaluation, 870
planning and implementation, 865–868, 870
pathogenesis of, 858–859f
pathophysiology, 856–857
primary, 856
pulmonary, 856–857
reactivation, 856–857
risk factors, 857, 860
therapies for
nursing considerations and, 863t, 864–865t
pharmacologic therapies, 863–864t
prophylaxis, 862
treatments for, 801
Tuberculosis (TB), 706, 714t
Tuberculosis empyema, 860
Tubman, Harriet, 2288, 2288f
Tufts New England Medical Center, 2335
Tularemia, 2358t
Tumor lysis syndrome, 89
Tumor markers, 126–127
Tumor necrosis factor (TNF), 916
Tumor necrosis factor alpha (TNF-a), 708t, 742
Tumor suppressor genes, 119
Tumor-associated antigen (TAA), 119
Tumors. See also Cancer
benign, 117
classification, 125–126
growth of, 117
invasion, 118
malignant, 117–119
metastasis, 118–119, 119f
nomenclature, 126t
ontologic imaging, 127–128
skin, 1878t
space-occupying lesions, 90
staging, 125, 126t
TUNA (Transurethral needle ablation), 435
Tuning fork, 2005t
Turner syndrome, 1721t, 1722, 1722f
TURP (transurethral resection of the prostate),
435, 438
TURP syndrome, 439
Tuskegee Study, 2332
Twelve-step programs, 37, 37t
Twins:
development of, 1530
fraternal, 1530, 1531f
identical, 1530, 1531f
Two-career family, 486
Two-point discrimination, 955f
Tylenol, 275
Tympanic membrane, 824, 827f, 828, 1632, 1644f,
1644t, 1855–1856
Tympanocentesis, 828–829
Tympanogram, 828
Tympanometry, 1646
Tympanoplasty, 1654

Tympanostomy tubes, 829
Tympany, 2004, 2004t
Type 1 diabetes mellitus. See also Diabetes
mellitus
clinical manifestations, 990–991, 991t
clinical therapies, 991t
Nursing Care Plan, 1013–1014t
pathophysiology and etiology, 990
risk factors, 990
Type 1 DM. See Type 1 diabetes mellitus
Type 2 diabetes mellitus. See also Diabetes
mellitus
clinical manifestations, 992, 992t
clinical therapies, 992t
hypoglycemic agents and, 1005
pathophysiology and etiology, 991
risk factors, 991–992
Type 2 DM. See Type 2 diabetes mellitus
Type and crossmatch, 735
Tyramine, 1172, 1172t
Tyrosine, 1176

U

UAPs. See Unlicensed assistive personnel
Ulcerative colitis, 693t. See also Inflammatory
bowel disease
characteristics, 910t
complications, 909, 912
definition, 889t, 909
incidence, 909
manifestations, 909, 912, 912t
Nursing Care Plan
assessment, 922t
critical thinking in the nursing process, 922t
diagnoses, 922t
evaluation, 922t
overview, 922t
planning and implementation, 922t
pathophysiology and etiology, 909–910, 912
treatment, 889t
Ulcers:
arterial, 1464t
Curling's, 1896, 1901
definition, 930
duodenal, 931
gastric, 931
peptic. See Peptic ulcer disease
pressure. See Pressure ulcers
skin, 1879t
venous, 1464t
Ulnar deformity, 744t
Ulnar deviation, 1069f
Ultrafiltration, 544
Ultrasonic examination, 805
Ultrasonic lithotripsy, 476f
Ultrasound:
during pregnancy, 1548, 1570
in cancer, 128
in specific conditions
appendicitis, 894
Ultraviolet radiation:
skin cancer and, 187–188
Umbilical cord, 1530
Unconscious mind, 343
Underdelegation, 2222

Underground Railroad, 2288, 2288f, 2289f
Underinsured, 2210t, 2345
Undernutrition, 662, 663t, 2010, 2013
Underwater weighing, 1028
Undocumented immigrants, 404
Unethical activities, advocacy and, 2302
Unifocal PVCs, 1446
Uniform Anatomical Gift Act, 2313
Uniform languages, 2386
Unilateral decision making, 2039
Unilateral lobar pneumonia, 834
Uninsured, 2345–2347, 2347t
Unintentional torts:
negligence, 2399
professional negligence, 2399–2400, 2400t
Unintentional trauma, 1937. See also Motor
vehicle crashes
Unipolar disorder, 1159–1160. See also Major
depressive disorder (MDD)
Unit-based discussions, 2306
United Ostomy Associations of America, Inc, 921t
United States:
health care values of, vs. other countries, 2213t
payment for health care in, 2210–2212
Universal precautions, 778
University of Alberta, 2335
University of Connecticut, 2335
University of Ottawa, 2335
University of Texas Academic Center for
Evidence-Based Practice (ACE), 2335
University of Texas Health Science Center, 2335
Unlicensed assistive personnel (UAPs), 2116t,
2206–2207
delegation to, 2217–2218, 2218t
functional nursing and, 2344
Unprofessional behaviors, 2228–2229, 2229t
Unresolved grief, 606
Unstable angina, 1362
Untreated wounds, 1880
Upper body obesity, 1026
Upper gastrointestinal (GI) series, 933
Urea, 541t
Urea breath test, 933
Ureaphil. See Urea
Uremia:
clinical therapies, 557t
definition, 554
manifestations, 557t
multisystem effects, 555f
neurologic effects, 556
Ureteral stent, 876, 877f
Ureteral stones, 468t
Ureterolithotomy, 470
Ureteroplasty, 876
Ureters, 411
Urethra, 1686t
age-related changes in, 416
female, 412f
function of, 411
male, 412f
Urethritis, 872
Urge incontinence, 442, 442t, 446t
Urgency:
urinary, 417, 417t
urinary tract infections and, 874

Uric acid, 130t, 1077t
Uric acid stones, 466, 467t
Urinalysis:
  infection, 805
  normal and abnormal findings, 421–422t
  in specific conditions
    acute renal failure, 540
    burns, 1900
    chronic renal failure, 558
    heart failure, 1411
    hypertension, 1428
    nephritis, 926
    systemic lupus erythematosus (SLE), 760
    urinary calculi, 468
    urinary tract infections and, 875
Urinary bladder:
  female, 412f
  function of, 411
  male, 412f
Urinary calculi:
  Case Study, 480
  Client Teaching, 478t
  collaborative care
    diagnostic tests, 468–469
    pharmacologic therapy, 469
    surgery, 469–470, 470t
  complications
    hydronephrosis, 467
    infection, 468
    obstruction, 467
  composition of, 466
  definition, 466
  kidney stones, 468t
    definition, 418t
    treatment, 418t
  manifestations, 467, 468t
  Nursing Care Plan
    assessment, 479t
    critical thinking in the nursing process, 480t
    diagnoses, 479t
    evaluation, 479t
    overview, 479t
    planning and implementation, 479t
  nursing diagnoses and interventions
    acute pain, 477
    deficient knowledge, 478
    health promotion, 478
    impaired urinary elimination, 477–478
    preparing for client discharge, 478
  nursing process
    assessment, 470
    diagnosis, 470
    evaluation, 480
    planning and implementation, 470, 477–478
  pathophysiology and etiology, 466
  risk factors, 467, 467t
  treatment, 467t, 468t
  types, 466
Urinary elimination:
  alterations, 418t
  altered, 416–417, 417t
  Assessment Interview, 421t
  care settings, 448t
  Client Teaching, 449t

factors affecting
  developmental factors, 413, 414
  fluid and food intake, 414
  medications, 414, 415t
  muscle tone, 414
  pathologic conditions, 414–415
  psychosocial factors, 414
  surgical and diagnostic procedures, 415
habits, 410
home care, 449t
infants, 414
kidneys role in, 410
in newborns, 413
nocturnal frequency, 414
normal presentation, 410–412
Nursing Care Plan
  assessment, 452t
  critical thinking in the nursing process, 452t
  diagnosis, 452t
  planning and implementation, 452t
nursing interventions, 422
in older adults, 414
pharmacologic therapies, 423, 423t
in pregnancy, 412–413
preschoolers, 414
role of kidneys in, 411
school-age children, 414
Urinary frequency, 417t
  definition, 417
  during pregnancy, 1546t, 1574t, 1576
Urinary hesitancy, 417
Urinary incontinence, 417t
  acute, 442
  causes, 442
  chronic, 442
  community-based care, 451
  definition, 418t, 441
  etiology and pathophysiology, 441–442
  evidence-based practice, 444t
  home care, 450
  incidence and prevalence, 441
  manifestations, 442
  nursing care
    evaluation, 452
    implementation, 449–451
    planning, 448
  nursing diagnosis and interventions
    assisting with toileting, 451
    coping with social isolation, 451
    maintaining normal voiding habits, 450, 451t
    maintaining skin integrity, 450
    nursing interventions and diagnoses, 447t
  nursing process
    assessment, 446
  in older adults, 443t
  pressure ulcers and, 1916
  prostate cancer and, 173
  risk factors, 442
  treatment, 418t
    client teaching, 444
    complementary therapies, 444
    health promotion, 444
    medications, 443
    surgery, 443–444
  types, 442t

Urinary output, 423
Urinary retention, 417t, 418t
  benign prostatic hypertrophy and, 433
  causes, 445
  definition, 445
  etiology and pathophysiology, 445
  manifestations, 445
  nursing care
    evaluation, 452
    implementation, 449–451
    planning, 448
  nursing diagnosis and interventions, 447t
    promoting urination, 450
  nursing process
    assessment, 446
    diagnosis, 446
  opioid use and, 278t
  risk factors, 445
  treatment, 446
  voluntary, 445
Urinary stasis:
  urinary tract infections and, 873
Urinary system:
  age-related changes in, 415–416
  assessment, 418, 418–419t
  benefits of exercise for, 653t, 654
  diagnostic tests, 420, 421–422t
  disorders
    overview, 441
    retention. See Urinary retention
    urinary incontinence. See Urinary incontinence
    urinary retention. See Urinary retention
  infection of, 418t
Urinary tract:
  anatomic structures, 410f
  pregnancy and, 1543
Urinary tract infection (UTI):
  asymptomatic, 874–875
  Case Study, 882
  collaborative care
    complementary therapies, 877–878
    diagnostic tests, 875–876
    pharmacologic therapies, 876
    surgery, 876
  community-based care for prevention of, 880
  definition, 871
  etiology, 872–873
  from urinary calculi, 468
  manifestations, 467, 874–875
  nosocomial infections and, 787
  nursing diagnoses and interventions
    impaired urinary elimination, 880–881
    ineffective health maintenance, 881
    pain, 878–880
  nursing process
    assessment, 878
    diagnosis, 878
    evaluation, 881–882
    planning and implementation, 878–881
  pathophysiology, 872
  risk factors, 873–874, 873t
  treatments for, 801
Urination, 412
Urine, 522
  characteristics of normal and abnormal, 420t
  residual, 413

Urine creatine, 926
Urine culture, 558
Urine drug screen, 1942
Urine osmolality, 130t, 532
Urine output, by age, 413t
Urine production, altered, 416
Urine specific gravity, 532, 575, 852
Uroflowmetry, 436
Urogenital system, 411
Urolithiasis. *See* Urinary calculi
Uroxatral, 434
Ursodiol, 904
Urticaria, 1882t
U.S. Advisory Commission on Consumer
    Protection and Quality in the Health Care
    Industry, 2319t
U.S. Department of Health and Human Services:
    See Department of Health and Human Services
    (DHHS), 2364
U.S. Department of Health and Human Services
    (DHHS), 2340
U.S. Department of Health, Education and Welfare
    (HEW), 2333
U.S. Drug Enforcement Agency, 2405
U.S. drug schedules, 2406t
USB flash drives, 2375
USB ports, 2375
Usual source of care, 2347, 2348t
Uterine cancer:
    leiomyosarcoma, 1700t
    screening guidelines, 132t
Uterine relaxants, 1577t
Uterine stimulants, 1577t
Uterus, 1688t, 1689
    implantation of fertilized ovum in, 1527–1528
    pregnancy and, 1541–1542, 1547
    UTI. *See* Urinary tract infection (UTI)
Utilitarianism, 1777
Utility, 1777
Utilization reviews, 2388–2389, 2426
Uvea, 1631
Uveitis, 747, 912
Uvula, 655
Uvulopalatopharyngoplasty (UPPP), 315

V

Vaccines. *See also* Immunizations; specific vaccines
    client education about, 673
    description of, 682–683
    human immunodeficiency virus (HIV) and,
        713, 720
Vacuum constriction device (VCD), 1714
Vacuum-assisted closure, 1918t
Vacuum-assisted closure (VAC) device:
    for burns, 1904
Vagal nerve stimulator, 972
Vagina, 1542, 1688, 1688t, 1708t
Vaginal discharge, during pregnancy, 1574t
Vaginal hysterectomy, 1751
Vaginal speculum, 2005t
Vaginal sponge, 1730, 1730f
Vaginismus, 1703
Vaginitis, 714t

Vagus nerve, 942t
    functions, 1628t
Vagus nerve stimulation (VNS), 1176
Valdecoxib, 275
Valerian, 315
Validation, 2064–2065, 2064t
Valium, 971, 1815
Valproate (Depakote), 217
Valproic acid, 1174t
Valsalva maneuver, 1454
Value decisions, 2038
Values, 2156
    clarifying client, 2307–2308
    defined, 2306
    essential to professional nursing, 2306–2307, 2307t
    professional, 2306
Values clarification, 2306
Valve disease:
    description, 1314t
    treatment, 1314t
Vancomycin-intermediate or -resistant *S. aureus*
    (VISA/nlor VRSA), 789
Vancomycin-resistant *Enterococcus* (VRE), 789
Vanderbilt Parent and Teacher Scales, 371t
Vanderbilt University, 2335
Vaporization, 1853
Vapotherms:
    description, 1230
    pictured, 1232f
Variance, 2192, 2192f, 2417
Varicella virus vaccine, 691
Varicose veins, during pregnancy, 1574t
Vas deferens, 1686t
Vascular dementia, 206t
Vascular system, aging and, 1312
Vasculitis:
    rheumatoid arthritis and, 747
    systemic lupus erythematosus (SLE) and, 760
Vasectomy, 1733
Vasoactive drugs, sepsis and, 852–853
Vasocongestion, 1697
Vasoconstrictors, 1493t
Vasodilators:
    administration, 1431t, 1493t
    mechanism of action, 1330t
    nursing considerations, 1330t
    in specific conditions
        heart failure, 1413, 1415
        hypertension, 1431t, 1432
        shock, 1493
Vasoocclusive crisis, 178, 178t
Vasopressin, 978, 1423
Vasopressors, 1149, 1943
Vedas, 1782
Vena caval syndrome, 1310, 1310f
Venal caval filters, 1392, 1392f
Venal caval syndrome, 1542–1543, 1542f
Venereal diseases. *See* Sexually transmitted
    infections (STIs)
Venlafaxine, 1173
Venous pressure monitoring, 1412
Venous stasis, 1462
Venous thrombectomy, 1392

Venous ulcers, 1464t
Ventilation, 18
Ventilation-perfusion (V-Q) relationships,
    1218, 1222f
Ventilation-perfusion scans (V-Q scans):
    in chronic obstructive pulmonary disease
        (COPD), 1272
    purpose and description, 1228–1229
Ventilation. *See* Respiration
Ventricles, 1294–1295
Ventricular aneurysm, 1369
Ventricular assist devices (VADs), 1382
Ventricular bigeminy, 1446
Ventricular dysrhythmias, 1445–1446
Ventricular fibrillation (VF), 1443t, 1446
Ventricular gallop, 1296
Ventricular hypertrophy, 1406t
Ventricular reduction surgery, 1417
Ventricular rhythms, 1440, 1442–1443t
Ventricular septal defect (VSD), 1341t, 1358t
Ventricular tachycardia (VT), 1443t, 1446
Ventricular trigeminy, 1446
Venturi masks:
    description, 1231
    pictured, 1233f
Veracity, 1778, 2308, 2315t
Verbal abuse, 2131–2132
Verbal communication, 2149–2151, 2161, 2161t
Verbal cues, for emotional states, 1157
Verbal orders, 2201, 2416
Vernix caseosa, 1541
Verteporfin, 1677
Vertical transmission, 697
Vertically integrated health services organizations,
    2214–2215
Vertigo, 1638t
Very-low-birth-weight (VLBW) infants, 1869
Very-low-density lipoproteins (VLDLs), 1361
Vesicles, 1878t
Vesicoureteral junction, 446f
Vesicoureteral reflux, 872–873, 877
Vest restraints, 2448
Vestibule, 1687, 1688t
Vestibulitis, 1703
Vestibulocochlear nerve, 942t
Veterans, 2239t
Vibration:
    chronic obstructive pulmonary disease (COPD)
        and, 1273
    pneumonia and, 843, 843f
    Vicodin (hydrocodone), 73
Videoconferencing, 2381
Vietnam War, 2289
Vietnam Women's Memorial, 2290f
Violence. *See also* Abuse; Assault; Trauma
    about, 1935–1943
    alterations, 1937–1940
    assessment, 1940–1941
    caring interventions, 1942–1943
    cycle of, 1937, 1937t
    dating, 1950, 2461–2462, 2462t
    diagnostic tests, 1941–1942
    domestic, 2458–2459

factors leading to, 1937
family, 492
forms of
abuse, 1937
trauma, 1937–1938
gender-based, 1949–1950
gender-based family violence, 1944t
interpersonal, 1937, 1944–1945
intimate partner, 1949–1950
intrafamily, 1942
media, 1965
normal presentation, 1937
pharmacologic therapies, 1943
prevention, 1938–1940, 1939t
problem of, 1935–1936
sociocultural factors and, 1963–1964
statistics on, 1935–1936
Violence prevention programs, 1966
Vioxx, 275
Viral hemorrhagic fevers (VHF), 2357t
Viral pneumonia, 801
Virazole. See Ribavirin
Virchow's triad, 1390
Virions, 697
Virulence, variations in, 770
Viruses, 786t
cancer development and, 120, 120t
definition of, 771
VISA (Vancomycin-intermediate or -resistant
S. aureus), 789
Visceral, 1628
Visceral neuropathies:
diabetes mellitus and, 999
Visceral pain, 263
Viscosupplementation, 1129
Viscous, 1308
Vision, 2235. See also Eyes
age-related changes in, 1635, 1636t
alterations
cataracts, 1637t, 1638
glaucoma, 1637t, 1638, 1649, 1650t
macular degeneration, 1637t, 1638, 1649, 1649t
assessment, 1639t, 1641–1642t
diagnostic tests, 1646
hyperthyroidism and, 1045–1047
impairment
effective communication, 1648t
in older adults, 1649t
safety considerations, 1648, 1649
in neonates, 1635
refraction, 1631–1632
sensory aids, 1648t
Vision assessment, 862, 1639t
Visual cortex, 940
Visual field testing, 1670
Visual hallucinations, 239
Visual impairment, 1635
Visual stimuli, 1628
Vital signs, assessment of, 529
Vitamin A, recommended daily intake, 1596t
Vitamin B:
for mood disorders, 1176
recommended daily intake, 1596t, 1597t
Vitamin B12, 95, 99, 1373
dietary sources, 103t

parenteral, 102
Vitamin B12 deficiency anemia, 99, 102t
Vitamin B6, 1373
Vitamin C, recommended daily intake, 1596t
Vitamin D, 559, 1595, 1596t
Vitamin E, recommended daily intake, 1596t
Vitamin K, 1020, 1596t
Vitamins:
definition, 1595
fat-soluble, 1595, 1596t
recommended daily intake, 1595, 1596t
water-soluble, 1595, 1596–1597t
Vitiligo, 1882t
VLBW. See Very-low-birth-weight (VLBW) infants
VNS (vagus nerve stimulation), 1176
Voiding, 412
Voiding cystourethrography, 876
Volatile acids, 4
Volatile nitrites, 74
Volkmann's contracture, 1095
Voltaren. See Diclofenac
Voluntary admission, 250
Voluntary insurance, 2213
Vomiting:
dehydration from, 571
opioid use and, 278t
VRE (Vancomycin-resistant Enterococcus), 789
VRSA (Vancomycin-intermediate or -resistant
S. aureus), 789
Vulnerability, 1808
Vulnerability factors, 1937
Vulnerable populations, 403–404, 2300–2302
Vulnerable Populations Model for Research and
Practice, 403
Vulva, 1687
Vulvodynia, 1703
Vygotsky, Lev, 198, 345

W

Waist circumference, 1028
Wald, Lillian, 2290
Walkers, 1078
Walking, 1078
Wandering, by older adults, 2458
War, nursing profession and, 2288–2289
Warfarin, 2442t
administration, 1393t
in specific conditions
deep venous thrombosis, 1392
pulmonary embolism, 1479
Warm zones, 2356t
Warts, genital. See Genital warts
Wasting syndrome:
acquired immunodeficiency syndrome (AIDS)
and, 704f
human immunodeficiency virus (HIV) and, 722
Water. See also Body fluids
in body fluids, 518
functions, 518
Water metabolism, during pregnancy, 1545
Water-soluble vitamins, 1595, 1596–1597t
Weapons, 1964–1965
Web-based client education, 2393
Web-based research, 2387–2388, 2388t

Weber test, 1643f, 1643t, 1646
Wechsler Preschool and Primary Scale of
Intelligence—Revised (WPPSI-R), 2013t
Wedge resection, 165t
Weight gain, during pregnancy, 1544–1545
Weight loss, hypertension and, 1429
Weight measurement, to assess fluid status, 529
Weight-bearing activity, 652–653
Weight-loss programs:
obesity and, 1031
Well-being, 635, 637
Wellbutrin, 1173, 1190
Wellness, 637, 637f
about, 635–645
wellness assessment programs, 642
wellness diagnoses, 647
Wellness diagnosis, 2066
Wellness models, 2060
Wellness promotion, 2285
Wernicke-Korsakoff syndrome, 43
Wernicke's encephalopathy, 42t, 43
Westerhoff, John, 353
Western blot antibody testing, 709
Wet-to-dry gauze dressing, 1918t
Wharton's jelly, 1530
Wheals, 1878t
Wheezing, 1222t
Whistleblower Protection Act, 2417
Whistleblower Protection Program, 2418
Whistleblowers, 2418
Whistleblowing, 2417–2418
White blood cell (WBC) count, 804–805
sepsis and, 852
for inflammation, 890, 891t
in specific conditions
hypersensitivity, 735
shock, 1490
White blood cell (WBC) differential, 804–805
pneumonia and, 841
sepsis and, 852
urinary tract infections and, 875
White blood cells (WBCs):
abnormal, possible causes, 130t
cellulitis and, 808
in leukemia, 148, 151
White blood cells (WBCs). See Leukocytes
Whitman, Walt, 2288
Whooping cough, 796t
Williams syndrome, 1326t
Withdrawal symptoms, 67
Withdrawal syndrome, 30t
Withdrawing or withholding life-sustaining
therapy (WWLST), 2314, 2315t
Wocial, Lucia, 2306
Wolff's law, 1058
Women, Infants and Children (WIC) program,
663t
Women's roles, 2287
Wong-Baker FACES Rating Scale, 282, 282f
Work-role preoccupation, 345
World Health Organization (WHO):
definition of health, 636
three-step pain management approach,
274–275, 274f

World view, 329
Work ethic:
    attendance and punctuality, 2236–2237
    attitude and enthusiasm, 2238
    generational differences in, 2238, 2239t,
        2240–2241, 2241f, 2241t
    overview, 2236
    reliability and accountability, 2237
Work groups, 2135
Workplace, managing conflict in, 2130
Workplace bullying, 2131–2132
Workplace ergonomics, 2383–2384, 2384t
Workplace issues, ethical considerations, 2316, 2317t
Workplace safety, 2442, 2443f
World War I, 2288
World War II, 2288
Wound care:
    developmental considerations, 1929t
    home care assessment, 1931t
    prevention of pressure ulcers and, 1931t
Wound cultures, 1884
Wound healing:
    burns, 1890, 1892
    case study, 1933
    collaborative care, 1930
    complications of, 1929
    developmental considerations in, 1930
    factors affecting, 1929–1930
    factors inhibiting, 1930t
    infection prevention, 1933
    manifestations, 1930
    moist, 1931
    nursing process
        assessment, 1930–1931
        diagnosis, 1931
        evaluation, 1933
        planning and implementation, 1931
    in older adults, 1930t
    overview, 1927

    phases of, 1928f
        inflammatory phase, 1927–1928
        maturation phase, 1928–1929
        proliferative phase, 1928
    positioning and, 1933
    types of, 1927
Wound vacuum, 1904f
Wounds:
    burn, 1902
    debridement of, 1924
    dehiscence, 898
    depth of, 1880
    evisceration, 898
    gunshot, 1938, 1969
    stab, 1938
    surgical
        postoperative care, 897–898
    treated, 1880
    types of, 1878, 1880, 1880t
    untreated, 1880
Wrist rests, 2384t
Written communication, 2153–2154
Written teaching aids, 2258t

X

X chromosomes, 1722
X-linked dominant inheritance, 1724
X-linked recessive inheritance, 1724
X-ray imaging:
    of tumors, 127
    burns, 1900
Xalatan, 1670, 1671t
Xanax, 1814–1815
Xenografts, 1903
Xenophobia, 398
Xerostomia, 138t
Xolair. See Omalizumab
XXY chromosome, 1721t
Xyrem, 309–310

Y

Yankauer suction tube, 1245f
Yoga, 45
    anxiety disorders and, 1816
    for mood disorders, 1176
    obsessive-compulsive disorder and, 1831
    prenatal substance exposure and, 63
Yolk sac, 1530
Yom Kippur, 1781–1782
Young adulthood, 341t
Young adults, 366, 366t
    assessment of, 2017–2018
    development in, 2012
    developmental tasks in, 1581t
    recommended screenings and immunizations, 643t
    safety measures, 2457

Z

Zanamivir, 821
Zidovudine, 710–711, 712t, 713
    human immunodeficiency virus (HIV) and, 697
Zinc, 1262, 1677
    recommended daily intake, 1597t
Zip drive disks, 2375
Ziprasidone, 244t
Zoladex, 1735t
Zollinger-Ellison syndrome, 932
Zoloft, 210, 1201
Zolpidem, 313
Zona pellucida, 1527
Zygote, 88, 1524, 1527
Zyprexa, 210, 244t, 1181